a LANGE me

CURRENT
Diagnosis & Treatment
Nephrology & Hypertension

SECOND EDITION

Edited by

Edgar V. Lerma, MD, FACP, FASN, FPSN (Hon)

Clinical Professor of Medicine
Section of Nephrology
Department of Internal Medicine
University of Illinois at Chicago College
 of Medicine/Advocate Christ Medical Center
Oak Lawn, Illinois
Associates in Nephrology
Chicago, Illinois

Mitchell H. Rosner, MD, MACP

Henry B. Mulholland Professor of Medicine
 Chair, Department of Medicine
University of Virginia Health System
Charlottesville, Virginia

Mark A. Perazella, MD, FACP

Professor of Medicine
Director, Acute Dialysis Services
Medical Director, Yale Physician Associate Program
Section of Nephrology
Department of Internal Medicine
Yale University School of Medicine
New Haven, Connecticut

New York   Chicago   San Francisco   Athens   London   Madrid   Mexico City
New Delhi   Milan   Singapore   Sydney   Toronto

Current Diagnosis & Treatment: Nephrology & Hypertension, Second Edition

1 2 3 4 5 6 7 8 9 LCR 22 21 20 19 18 17

ISBN 978-1-259-86105-5
MHID 1-259-86105-8
ISSN 1943-832X

Notice

Medicine is an ever-changing science. As new research and clinical experience broaden our knowledge, changes in treatment and drug therapy are required. The author and the publisher of this work have checked with sources believed to be reliable in their efforts to provide information that is complete and generally in accord with the standards accepted at the time of publication. However, in view of the possibility of human error or changes in medical sciences, neither the author nor the publisher nor any other party who has been involved in the preparation or publication of this work warrants that the information contained herein is in every respect accurate or complete, and they disclaim all responsibility for any errors or omissions or for the results obtained from use of the information contained in this work. Readers are encouraged to confirm the information contained herein with other sources. For example and in particular, readers are advised to check the product information sheet included in the package of each drug they plan to administer to be certain that the information contained in this work is accurate and that changes have not been made in the recommended dose or in the contraindications for administration. This recommendation is of particular importance in connection with new or infrequently used drugs.

This book was set in Minion Pro by Cenveo® Publisher Services.
The editors were Amanda Fielding and Kim J. Davis.
The production supervisor was Catherine Saggese.
Project management was provided by Harleen Chopra of Cenveo Publisher Services.

Contents

Section IX. Kidney Disease in Special Populations

Section X. Special Topics in Nephrology

Authors

Emaad Abdel-Rahman, MD, PhD
Department of Medicine, University of Virginia,
  Charlottesville, Virginia
Chapter 55

Blaise Abramovitz, DO
Nephrology Fellow, Renal Electrolyte and Hypertension
  Division, The Hospital of the University of Pennsylvania,
  Philadelphia, Pennsylvania
Chapter 12

Anjali Acharya, MBBS
Associate Professor Albert Einstein College of Medicine, Bronx,
  New York
Chapter 42

Talal A. Alfaadhel, MBBS, FRCP(C)
Assistant Professor, Department of Medicine, King Saud
  University, Riyadh, Saudi Arabia
Chapter 27

Kisra Anis, MBBS
Assistant Professor Albert Einstein College of Medicine, Bronx,
  New York
Chapter 42

William S. Asch, MD, PhD
Yale University School of Medicine, Yale New Haven Hospital
  Transplantation Center, New Haven, Connecticut
Chapter 52

Stephen R. Ash, MD, FACP
HemoCleanse Technologies, LLC and Ash Access Technology,
  Inc., Lafayette, Indiana
Chapter 56

George L. Bakris, MD
ASH Comprehensive Hypertension Center, Section of
  Endocrinology, Diabetes and Metabolism, The University of
  Chicago Medicine, Chicago, Illinois
Chapter 40

Seki A. Balogun, MBBS
Department of Medicine, University of Virginia, Charlottesville,
  Virginia
Chapter 55

James E. Balow, MD
Clinical Director, NIDDK, National Institutes of Health,
  Bethesda, Maryland
Chapter 33

William M. Bennett, MD
Medical Director of Transplantation, and Director of Renal
  Research, at Legacy Health Systems in Portland, Oregon
Chapter 14

Ursula C. Brewster, MD
Associate Professor of Medicine, Section of Nephrology,
  Yale School of Medicine, New Haven, Connecticut
Chapter 54

Daniel C. Cattran, MD, FRCP(C)
Senior Scientist, Toronto General Research Institute; Professor
  of Medicine, University of Toronto, Toronto, Ontario,
  Canada
Chapter 27

Elliot Charen, MD
Assistant Professor of Medicine at Icahn School of Medicine at
  Mount Sinai, Division of Nephrology and Hypertension at
  Mount Sinai Beth Israel, New York, New York
Chapter 57

Debbie L. Cohen, MD
University of Pennsylvania, Renal, Electrolyte and
  Hypertension Division, Philadelphia, Pennsylvania
Chapter 41

Neera K. Dahl, MD, PhD
Section of Nephrology, Yale University School of Medicine,
  New Haven, Connecticut
Chapter 39

Robert J. Desnick, PhD, MD
Dean for Genetic and Genomic Medicine; Professor and
  Chairman Emeritus, Department of Genetic and Genomic
  Sciences, Icahn School of Medicine at Mount Sinai,
  New York, New York
Chapter 47

Dominique Dorsainvil, MD
Yale University School of Medicine, Department of Internal
  Medicine, Section of Nephrology, New Haven, Connecticut
Chapter 38

Thomas D. DuBose, Jr, MD, MACP, FASN
Emeritus Professor of Medicine, Department of Internal
  Medicine, Wake Forest School of Medicine and University
  of Virginia School of Medicine, Winston-Salem,
  North Carolina
Chapter 5

James Dylewski, DO
Department of Medicine, Division of Renal and Hypertension, University of Colorado, Aurora, Colorado
Chapter 24

William J. Elliott, MD, PhD
Professor of Preventive Medicine, Internal Medicine and Pharmacology; Chair, Department of Biomedical Sciences; Chief, Division of Pharmacology, Pacific Northwest University of Health Sciences, Yakima, Washington
Chapter 44

Michael Emmett, MD, MACP
Department of Internal Medicine, Baylor University Medical Center, Dallas, Texas, Baylor-Scott & White Healthcare; Professor of Medicine, Texas A&M School of Medicine and Clinical Professor of Medicine, University of Texas Southwestern, Dallas, Texas
Chapter 4

Fernando C. Fervenza, MD, PhD
Professor of Medicine, Division of Nephrology and Hypertension, Mayo Clinic College of Medicine, Rochester, Minnesota
Chapter 27

Ashley Frazer-Abel, PhD
Assistant Research Professor, Department of Medicine, Division of Rheumatology, University of Colorado, Aurora, Colorado
Chapter 35

Samantha L. Gelfand, MD
Instructor in Internal Medicine, Department in Internal Medicine, Yale University School of Medicine, New Haven, Connecticut
Chapter 54

David Geller, MD, PhD
Section of Nephrology, Yale University School of Medicine, New Haven, Connecticut; Section of Nephrology, West Haven VA Hospital, West Haven, Connecticut
Chapter 39

Muriel Ghosn, MD
University of Pennsylvania, Renal, Electrolyte and Hypertension Division, Philadelphia, Pennsylvania
Chapter 41

Debbie S. Gipson, MD, MSPH
Professor of Pediatrics, University of Michigan School of Medicine, Ann Arbor, Michigan
Chapter 26

Edward R. Gould, MD
Vanderbilt University School of Medicine, Nashville, Tennessee
Chapter 23

Nikolas B. Harbord, MD
Division of Nephrology and Hypertension, Mount Sinai Beth Israel, Icahn School of Medicine at Mount Sinai, New York, New York
Chapter 57

Raymond C. Harris, MD
Division of Nephrology, Vanderbilt University School of Medicine and Nashville Veterans Affairs Hospital, Nashville, Tennessee
Chapter 53

Brenda B. Hoffman, MD
Associate Professor of Clinical Medicine, Perelman School of Medicine, University of Pennsylvania, Philadelphia, Pennsylvania
Chapter 50

Vicki J. Hwang, PhD
Division of Nephrology, Department of Internal Medicine, University of California, Davis, California
Chapter 28

Maria V. Irazabal, MD
Division of Nephrology and Hypertension, Mayo Clinic, Rochester, Minnesota
Chapter 45

Anushya Jeyabalan, MD
Fellow, Department of Renal, Electrolyte and Hypertension, Hospital of the University of Pennsylvania, Philadelphia, Pennsylvania
Chapter 12

Kenar D. Jhaveri, MD
Professor of Medicine, Hofstra Northwell School of Medicine, Division of Nephrology, North Shore University Hospital and Long Island Jewish Medical Center, Great Neck, New York
Chapter 17

Belinda Jim, MD
Associate Professor Albert Einstein College of Medicine, Bronx, New York
Chapter 42

Kamyar Kalantar-Zadeh, MD, PhD, MPH
Division of Nephrology and Hypertension, University of California Irvine School of Medicine; and Division of Nephrology and Hypertension, Los Angeles Biomedical Research Institute at Harbor-UCLA Medical Center; and David Geffen School of Medicine at UCLA; Orange, California
Chapter 22

Elaine S. Kamil, MD
Pediatric Nephrology, Cedars-Sinai Medical Center; Clinical
Heath Sciences Professor of Pediatrics, David Geffen School
of Medicine at UCLA, Los Angeles, California
Chapter 25

Clifford E. Kashtan, MD, FASN
Department of Pediatrics, University of Minnesota Medical
School, Minneapolis, Minnesota
Chapter 46

Sana F. Khan, MD
University of Virginia Health System, Charlottesville, Virginia
Chapter 11

Sidney Kobrin, MD
Associate Professor, Renal Division, Hospital of the University
of Pennsylvania, Philadelphia, Pennsylvania
Chapter 8

Holly M. Koncicki, MD, MS
Assistant Professor, Department of Internal Medicine, Division
of Nephrology, Brookdale Department of Geriatrics and
Palliative Medicine, Icahn School of Medicine at Mount
Sinai, New York, New York
Chapter 58

Laura Kooienga, MD
Renal Fellow, University of Colorado School of Medicine,
Denver, Colorado
Chapter 24

Joel D. Kopple, MD
Division of Nephrology and Hypertension and Department
of Medicine; Los Angeles Biomedical Research Institute
at Harbor-UCLA Medical Center; David Geffen School of
Medicine at UCLA and UCLA Fielding School of Public
Health, Torrance, California
Chapter 22

Kar Neng Lai, MD, DSc
Emeritus Chair Professor, Department of Medicine, University
of Hong Kong, Hong Kong, China
Chapter 36

Edgar V. Lerma, MD, FACP, FASN, FPSN (Hon)
Clinical Professor of Medicine, Section of Nephrology,
Department of Internal Medicine, University of Illinois
at Chicago College of Medicine/Advocate Christ Medical
Center, Oak Lawn, Illinois; Associates in Nephrology,
Chicago, Illinois
Chapter 1

Nelson Leung, MD
Division of Nephrology and Hypertension, Division of
Hematology, Mayo Clinic, Rochester, Minnesota
Chapter 34

Jeremy S. Leventhal, MD
Assistant Professor of Medicine, Division of Nephrology, Icahn
School of Medicine at Mount Sinai, New York, New York
Chapter 36

Julia Lewis, MD
Vanderbilt University School of Medicine, Nashville, Tennessee
Chapter 23

Gregg Y. Lipschik, MD
Clinical Associate Professor, Department of Medicine
Perelman School of Medicine, University of Pennsylvania,
Philadelphia, Pennsylvania
Chapter 5

Joseph B. Lockridge, MD
Assistant Professor of Medicine and Medical Director,
Portland VA Medical Center, Transplantation Kidney,
Portland, Oregon
Chapter 14

Randy L. Luciano, MD, PhD
Department of Internal Medicine, Section of Nephrology,
Yale University School of Medicine, New Haven, Connecticut
Chapter 38

Jeanne P. Macrae, MD
Associate Professor of Clinical Medicine, SUNY Downstate
College of Medicine, Brooklyn, New York
Chapter 5

Niti Madan, MD
Division of Nephrology, Department of Internal Medicine,
University of California, Davis, California
Chapter 28

Hector M. Madariaga, MD
Department of Medicine, Good Samaritan Medical Center,
Brockton, Massachusetts
Chapter 1

David Martins, MD
Assistant Professor of Medicine, Charles Drew University,
Los Angeles, California
Chapter 42

Piyush Mathur, MBBS, DNB
Senior Consultant Nephrologist, Department of Nephrology,
Santokba Dulabhji Memorial Hospital, Jaipur, India
Chapter 51

Ravindra L. Mehta MD, FACP, FRCP
Professor Emeritus of Medicine, Department of Medicine,
University of California San Diego, La Jolla, California
Chapter 51

Beckie Michael, DO, FASN
Marlton Nephrology and Hypertension Clinical Associate
Professor of Medicine, Rowan School of Osteopathic
Medicine, Marlton, New Jersey
Chapter 16

Sharon M. Moe, MD, FASN
Stuart A. Kleit Professor of Medicine; Director, Division
of Nephrology, Indiana University School of Medicine;
Section Chief Nephrology, Roudebush Veterans
Administration Medical Center, Indianapolis, Indiana
Chapter 21

Dennis G. Moledina, MD
Research Fellow in Nephrology, Yale School of Medicine,
Program of Applied Translational Research, New Haven,
Connecticut
Chapter 37

Bruce A. Molitoris, MD
Distinguished Professor of Medicine, Indiana University School
of Medicine; Roudebush VA Medical Center, Indianapolis,
Indiana
Chapter 9

Shahriar Moossavi, MD, PhD
Associate Professor of Internal Medicine/Nephrology, Division
of Nephrology, Wake Forest University Health Sciences,
Winston-Salem, North Carolina
Chapter 49

Georges N. Nakhoul, MD
Department of Nephrology and Hypertension, Glickman
Urological and Kidney Institute, Cleveland Clinic; Cleveland
Clinic Lerner College of Medicine (CCLM) of Case Western
Reserve University (CWRU), Cleveland, Ohio
Chapter 20

Joseph V. Nally, MD
Department of Nephrology and Hypertension, Glickman
Urological and Kidney Institute, Cleveland Clinic; Cleveland
Clinic Lerner College of Medicine (CCLM) of Case Western
Reserve University (CWRU), Cleveland, Ohio
Chapter 20

Samih H. Nasr, MD
Professor of Laboratory Medicine and Pathology, Mayo Clinic,
Rochester, Minnesota
Chapters 31, 34

Saed Nemr, MD, FACP
Yale University School of Medicine, Yale New Haven Hospital
Transplantation Center, New Haven, Connecticut
Chapter 52

Thomas D. Nolin, PharmD, PhD
Associate Professor, Center for Clinical Pharmaceutical
Sciences, Department of Pharmacy and Therapeutics,
School of Pharmacy, Department of Medicine Renal-
Electrolyte Division, School of Medicine, University of
Pittsburgh, Pittsburgh, Pennsylvania
Chapter 59

Keith C. Norris, MD, PhD
Professor of Medicine, David Geffen School of Medicine at
UCLA, Los Angeles, California
Chapter 42

Gregorio T. Obrador Vera, MD, MPH
Dean and Professor of Medicine, Universidad Panamericana
School of Medicine, Mexico City, Mexico; Adjunct Assistant
Professor of Medicine, Tufts University School of Medicine,
Boston, Massachusetts
Chapter 18

Ali J. Olyaei, PharmD
Professor of Medicine and Pharmacotherapy, Pharmacy
Practice/ Nephrology and Hypertension, Oregon State
University/Oregon Health and Sciences University,
Portland, Oregon
Chapter 14

Nishita Parikh, MD
Instructor of Medicine, Hofstra Northwell School of Medicine;
Division of Nephrology, North Shore University Hospital
and Long Island Jewish Medical Center, Great Neck,
New York
Chapter 17

Mark A. Perazella, MD, FACP
Professor of Medicine; Director, Acute Dialysis Services;
Medical Director, Yale Physician Associate Program,
Section of Nephrology, Department of Internal Medicine,
Yale University School of Medicine, New Haven,
Connecticut
Chapter 15

Phuong-Mai T. Pham, MD
Associate Clinical Professor of Medicine, Department of
Medicine, Nephrology Division, VA Greater Los Angeles
Healthcare System, North Hills, California
Chapter 48

Phuong-Thu T. Pham, MD, FASN
Clinical Professor of Medicine, Department of Medicine,
Nephrology Division, David Geffen School of Medicine at
UCLA, Los Angeles, California
Chapter 48

Robert Provenzano, MD, FACP, FASN
Vice President Medical Affairs, Office of Chief Medical Officer, DaVita Healthcare Partners, Denver, Colorado
Chapter 19

Shaker S. Qaqish, MD
Nephrology Fellow, Department of Medicine, Nephrology Division, UCLA-Olive View Medical Center, Sylmar, California
Chapter 48

Jai Radhakrishnan, MD, MS
Professor of Medicine at Columbia University Medical Center; Clinical Chief, Nephrology, New York Presbyterian Hospital, Columbia Campus, New York, New York
Chapter 32

Mandana Rastegar, MD, EdM
Section of Nephrology, Greater Los Angeles VA Healthcare System and the David Geffen School of Medicine at UCLA, Los Angeles, California
Chapter 13

Andrew J. Rees, MB, FRCP, FRSB, FMedSci
Professor Emeritus, Clinical Institute of Pathology, Medical University of Vienna, Vienna, Austria
Chapter 30

Renu Regunathan-Shenk, MD
Assistant Professor of Medicine, Division of Renal Diseases and Hypertension, George Washington University School of Medicine, Washington, District of Columbia
Chapter 32

Robert F. Reilly, MD
Associate Chief of Staff for Education, Central Alabama Veterans Affairs Health Care System, Montgomery, Alabama
Chapter 7

Michael V. Rocco, MD, MSCE
Vardaman M. Buckalew Jr. Professor of Internal Medicine, Section on Nephrology, Wake Forest School of Medicine, Winston-Salem, North Carolina
Chapter 49

Michael J. Ross, MD
Chief, Division of Nephrology; Professor of Medicine; Professor of Developmental and Molecular Biology, Albert Einstein College of Medicine/Montefiore Medical Center, Bronx, New York
Chapter 36

Michael R. Rudnick, MD, FACP, FASN
Associate Professor of Medicine, Perelman School of Medicine of the University of Pennsylvania, Philadelphia, Pennsylvania
Chapter 12

Luis M. Ruilope, MD
Director Cardiorenal Investigation, Institute of Investigation, Hospital 12 Octubre, Madrid
Chapter 43

Theodore F. Saad, MD
Nephrology Associates, P.A., Newark, Delaware
Chapter 56

Samar M. Said, MD
Assistant Professor, Department of Laboratory Medicine and Pathology, Mayo Clinic, Rochester, Minnesota
Chapter 31

Alan Segal, MD
Associate Professor and Program Director, Nephrology Fellowship, University of Vermont Medical Center, Burlington, Vermont
Chapter 2

Julian Segura, MD, PhD
Head of Hypertension Unit, Department of Nephrology, Hospital 12 de Octubre, Madrid, Spain
Chapter 43

Anushree Shirali, MD
Section of Nephrology, Yale University School of Medicine, New Haven, Connecticut
Chapter 13

Stuart M. Sprague, DO
Chief, Division of Nephrology and Hypertension, NorthShore University HealthSystem; Clinical Professor of Medicine, University of Chicago Pritzker School of Medicine, Evanston, Illinois
Chapter 6

Hillel Sternlicht, MD
Assistant Professor of Medicine, Division of Nephrology and Hypertension, Lenox Hill Hospital-Northwell Health, New York, New York
Chapter 42

Richard H. Sterns, MD
Professor of Medicine, Emeritus University of Rochester School of Medicine and Dentistry, Rochester General Hospital, Rochester, New York
Chapter 3

Jonathan Suarez, MD
University of Pennsylvania, Renal, Electrolyte and Hypertension Division, Philadelphia, Pennsylvania
Chapter 41

Sydney C. W. Tang, MD, PhD
Chair of Renal Medicine and Yu Professor in Nephrology ,
    Department of Medicine, The University of Hong Kong,
    Hong Kong, China
Chapter 36

Isaac Teitelbaum, MD
Professor of Medicine, University of Colorado, Aurora,
    Colorado
Chapter 24

Joshua M. Thurman, MD
Professor of Medicine, University of Colorado School of
    Medicine, Division of Renal Diseases and Hypertension,
    Aurora, Colorado
Chapter 35

Vicente E. Torres, MD, PhD
Division of Nephrology and Hypertension, Mayo Clinic,
    Rochester, Minnesota
Chapter 45

Raymond R. Townsend, MD
Renal, Electrolyte and Hypertension Division, University of
    Pennsylvania, Philadelphia, Pennsylvania
Chapter 41

Howard Trachtman, MD
Professor of Pediatrics, NYU School of Medicine, New York,
    New York
Chapters 26, 29

Faruk H. Turgut, MD
Department of Medicine, Mustafa Kemal University, Hatay,
    Turkey
Chapter 55

Rimda Wanchoo, MD
Associate Professor of Medicine, Hofstra Northwell School of
    Medicine; Division of Nephrology, North Shore University
    Hospital and Long Island Jewish Medical Center,
    Great Neck, New York
Chapter 17

Robert H. Weiss, MD
Division of Nephrology, Department of Internal Medicine and
    Comprehensive Cancer Center, University of California,
    Davis, California; Medical Service, Sacramento VA Medical
    Center, Sacramento, California
Chapter 28

Michael R. Wiederkehr, MD
Professor, Division of Nephrology, Baylor University Medical
    Center-Baylor Scott & White Healthcare, Texas A&M
    College of Medicine, Dallas, Texas
Chapter 4

James F. Winchester, MD, FRCP (Glas)
Adjunct Professor of Medicine, Icahn School of Medicine at
    Mount Sinai, New York, New York
Chapter 57

Florence Wong, MD, FRACP, FRCP(C)
Division of Gastroenterology, Department of Medicine,
    Toronto General Hospital, University of Toronto, Ontario,
    Canada
Chapter 10

Hala Yamout, MD
Department of Medicine, Division of Nephrology, St. Louis
    University Medical Center, Veterans Affairs St. Louis Health
    Care System, St. Louis, Missouri
Chapter 40

Muhammad Sohail Yaqub, MD
Associate Professor of Clinical Medicine, Indiana University
    School of Medicine, Indianapolis, Indiana
Chapter 9

Jane Y. Yeun, MD
Division of Nephrology, Department of Internal Medicine and
    University of California, Davis, California; Medical Service,
    Sacramento VA Medical Center, Sacramento, California
Chapter 28

Preface

The second edition of *Current Diagnosis & Treatment: Nephrology & Hypertension* features practical, up-to-date, referenced information on the care of patients with diseases involving the kidneys and hypertension. It also covers dialysis, transplantation, critical care nephrology, interventional nephrology, palliative care nephrology, and clinical renal pharmacology as well as a new area of specialization—onco-nephrology. This book emphasizes the clinical aspects of kidney care while also presenting important underlying principles. *Current Diagnosis & Treatment: Nephrology & Hypertension* provides a practical guide to diagnosis, understanding, and treatment of the medical problems of all adult patients in an easy-to-use and readable format. The current edition also includes clinically based questions and answers to build on the material in the chapters.

INTENDED AUDIENCE

In the tradition of all Lange medical books, this second edition of *Current Diagnosis & Treatment: Nephrology & Hypertension* is a concise yet comprehensive source of up-to-date information. For medical students, it can serve as an authoritative introduction to the specialty of nephrology and an excellent resource for reference and review. Residents in internal medicine (and other specialties) and most especially, nephrology fellows in training, will appreciate the detailed descriptions of diseases and diagnostic and therapeutic procedures. General internists, family practitioners, hospitalists, nurses and nurse practitioners, physician assistants, and other allied health-care providers who work with patients with kidney diseases will find this a very useful reference on management aspects of renal medicine. Moreover, patients and their family members who seek information about the nature of specific diseases and their diagnosis and treatment may also find this book to be a valuable resource.

COVERAGE

Fifty-nine chapters cover a wide range of topics, including fluid, electrolyte, and acid-base disorders, acute and chronic kidney failure, glomerular and tubulointerstitial diseases, hypertension, systemic diseases with renal manifestations, renal replacement therapies, renal transplantation, geriatric nephrology, interventional nephrology, palliative care nephrology, clinical renal pharmacology, and onco-nephrology.

These and many other diseases are covered in a crisp and concise manner. Striking just the right balance between comprehensiveness and convenience, *Current Diagnosis & Treatment: Nephrology & Hypertension* emphasizes the practical features of clinical diagnosis and patient management while providing a comprehensive discussion of pathophysiology and relevant basic and clinical science. With its consistent formatting chapter by chapter, this text makes it simple to locate the practical information you need on diagnosis, testing, disease processes, and up-to-date treatment and management strategies.

The book has been designed to meet the clinician's need for an immediate refresher in the clinic as well as to serve as an accessible text for thorough review of the specialty for the boards. The concise presentation is ideally suited for rapid acquisition of information by the busy practitioner.

ACKNOWLEDGMENTS

We wish to thank our contributing authors for devoting their precious time and offering their wealth of knowledge in the process of completing this important book. These authors have contributed countless hours of work in regularly reading and reviewing the literature in this specialty, and we have all benefited from their clinical wisdom and commitment.

We would like to thank Kim Davis, the managing editor of this textbook, for her expert assistance in managing the flow of manuscripts and materials among the chapter authors, editors, and publisher. Her attention to detail was enormously helpful. This book would not have been completed without the help of Amanda Fielding, Catherine Saggese, Anju Joshi, and of course, the unwavering support of James Shanahan.

Edgar V. Lerma, MD, FACP, FASN, FPSN (Hon)
Mitchell H. Rosner, MD, MACP
Mark A. Perazella, MD, FACP

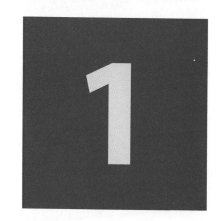

Approach to the Patient with Renal Disease

Hector M. Madariaga, MD

Edgar V. Lerma, MD, FACP, FASN, FPSN (Hon)

General Considerations

Any patient with renal disease can present either as an outpatient or inpatient consultation. Some patients may be referred because of abnormal urinary findings, such as hematuria or proteinuria, or abnormal laboratory work such as an elevated serum creatinine, which may have been incidentally discovered during routine clinical evaluation or as part of initial employment requirements. Depending on the stage of renal disease, patients can present with mild edema, generalized pruritus, or more advanced signs and symptoms of uremia, such as decreased appetite, weight loss, dysgeusia, pruritus, and change in mental status. In general, the symptoms and signs of patients presenting with renal disease are nonspecific (Table 1–1) and some patients may present only with an elevation in serum creatinine.

To narrow the differential diagnosis, it is important to determine whether the disease is acute, subacute, or chronic on presentation. There is usually an overlap in these stages, and at times, it may not be evident as to how long the disease process may have been existing. Certainly, a patient, who presents with an elevated serum creatinine that was documented to be normal a few days previously, has an acute presentation, whereas a patient, who presents with a previously elevated serum creatinine that has been rising steadily over the past several months to years, has a chronic disease. Often, acute exacerbations of chronic renal disease are common presentations.

The next step is to determine which segment or component of the renal anatomy is involved. This is subdivided into prerenal, renal (Table 1–2), or postrenal.

Prerenal disease refers to any process that decreases renal perfusion, such as intravascular volume depletion, hypotension, massive blood loss, or third spacing of fluids. It is also due to congestive heart failure or advanced liver cirrhosis, whereby decreased effective circulating volume decreases blood flow toward the kidneys (see Chapter 9).

Postrenal disease refers to any obstruction that impedes urinary flow through the urinary tract. Examples include benign prostatic hypertrophy, bladder issues, nephrolithiasis, pelvis masses, or gynecological malignancy (see Chapter 16).

Renal involvement is further subdivided into vascular, glomerular (see Chapters 24–36), or tubulointerstitial disease (see Chapters 37 and 38), depending on which segment is involved.

Assessment of Glomerular Filtration Rate

Glomerular filtration rate (GFR) cannot be directly measured; however, the gold standard to measure GFR is inulin clearance. This test is not commonly performed in clinical practice due to its cumbersome characteristics as it requires a continuous intravenous infusion, several blood samples, bladder catheterization, and is expensive. Inulin is freely filtered at the glomerulus and is neither secreted nor reabsorbed in the tubules. Other methods to measure GFR are filtration markers such as nonradioactive iothalamate, iohexol, diethylenetriaminepentaacetic acid (DTPA), or ethylenediaminetetraacetic acid (EDTA); just like inulin, these filtration markers are not used commonly in clinical practice (see https://www.ncbi.nlm.nih.gov/pubmed/19833901).

The most common method of assessing renal function is by estimation of the glomerular filtration rate (eGFR). The eGFR gives an approximation of the degree of renal function. Daily eGFR in normal subjects ranges between 150 and 250 L/24 h or 100 and 120 mL/min/1.73 m² of body surface area. eGFR is decreased in those with renal dysfunction and is used to monitor renal function in those with chronic kidney disease. Knowing renal function is critical in allowing proper dosing of medications that are cleared from the body by the kidney.

There are several methods by which eGFR can be estimated. Twenty-four hour creatinine clearance and equations such as

Table 1–1. Symptoms and signs at presentation of patients with renal disease.

Easy fatigability
Decreased appetite
Nausea and vomiting
Generalized pruritus
Shortness of breath
Sleep disturbances
Urinary hesitancy, urgency, or frequency
Microscopic or gross hematuria
Proteinuria
Frothy appearance of urine
Flank pain, mostly unilateral (may be bilateral)
Mental status changes, eg, confusion
Pallor
Weight loss or gain
Lower extremity "pitting" edema
Ascites
Pulmonary edema or congestion
Pleural or pericardial effusion
Pericarditis
Uncontrolled hypertension

Table 1–2. Causes of acute renal failure.

Prerenal
Intravascular volume depletion
    Blood loss
    Gastrointestinal losses, eg, vomiting, diarrhea
    Third spacing or redistribution of fluids, eg, burns, pancreatitis
Hypotension
    Myocardial infarction
    Sepsis
Decreased renal perfusion
    Congestive heart failure
    Renal artery stenosis
    Medications, eg, nonsteroidal anti-inflammatory drugs, ACE inhibitors,
        angiotensin receptor blockers and diuretics in the setting
        of volume depletion

Renal
Glomerular
    Rapidly progressive glomerulonephritis, thrombotic thrombocytopenic
        purpura
Tubular
    Acute tubular necrosis
        Ischemic
        Nephrotoxic
        Endogenous: Rhabdomyolysis
        Exogenous: Radiocontrast nephropathy, aminoglycosides, cisplatin
Interstitial
    Acute tubulointerstitial nephritis, eg, drugs (antibiotics), infections
Vascular
    Vasculitides, eg, ANCA-mediated diseases, renal artery/vein thromboses

Postrenal
Obstructive uropathy
    Intrinsic: Nephrolithiasis, papillary necrosis, prostate/bladder diseases
    Extrinsic: Retroperitoneal fibrosis, cervical carcinoma

ACE, angiotensin-converting enzyme; ANCA, antineutrophilic cytoplasmic antibody.

the Cockroft–Gault formula, chronic kidney disease epidemiology collaboration (CKD-EPI) equation, and the Modification of Diet in Renal Disease (MDRD) Study formula. Such options have been validated against measured methods of determining GFR (Table 1–3).

It is important to realize that using the serum creatinine alone to estimate GFR is inaccurate for several reasons. First, a small amount of creatinine is normally secreted by the proximal tubule (10–40% of urinary creatinine is derived from tubular secretion), and this amount tends to increase as progressive renal decline occurs, thereby overestimating the true GFR value. Similarly, there are factors that increase serum creatinine without truly affecting renal function, such as dietary meat (protein) intake, muscle mass volume, and certain medications that interfere with tubular secretion of creatinine such as cimetidine, famotidine, trimethoprim, probenecid, ranolazine, and dronedarone. Elderly patients, those with cachexia, amputees, as well as patients with spinal cord injury or disease, tend to have less muscle mass, hence, lower serum creatinine values, but this may not translate into higher GFR values (Table 1–4).

The 24-hour urine collection is used to determine creatinine clearance. Urine collection can be cumbersome, particularly in the elderly and in those with either fecal or urinary incontinence; some of the other limitations include an incomplete or prolonged urine collection (see further how to correct this) and states in which there is a variation of creatinine secretion such as liver cirrhosis, sickle cell disease, nephrotic syndrome, and medications.

To determine if a 24-hour urine collection is complete, the following reference is used:

For males, Urine creatinine × Urine volume = 20–25 mg/kg/24 h

For females, Urine creatinine × Urine volume = 15–20 mg/kg/24 h

A common method to estimate creatinine clearance is by the following equation:
Cockroft–Gault formula:

$$\text{Creatinine clearance} = \frac{(140 - \text{Age in years}) \times \text{Weight (kg)}}{\text{Plasma creatinine} \times 72}$$

Due to less muscle mass in females, a factor of 0.85 is multiplied by the creatinine clearance to arrive at the estimated creatinine clearance.

Table 1–3. Methods to estimate renal function.

Serum creatinine
Inaccurate with early or advanced stages of kidney disease
Affected by age, gender, muscle mass, and some medications

24-hour urine creatinine clearance
Cumbersome
Can overestimate the true GFR

Estimation equations
Cockroft–Gault formula
    Highly dependent on serum creatinine (see above) MDRD study formula
    Not tested in different populations, eg, the elderly and obese,
        or ethnicities

Radioisotopic clearance
Best measure of GFR
Invasive
Uses radioisotopes
Available only in certain academic institutions

GFR, glomerular filtration rate; MDRD, Modification of Diet in Renal Disease.

The equation was first reported in 1976, an era where obesity rates were low. This equation has certain limitations; for instance, it tends to overestimate kidney function in patients who are morbidly obese and/or have significant edema. This equation does not adjust for body surface area; hence, caution is advised when interpreting results as it may overestimate creatinine clearance by 10–40%. MDRD formula:

$$GFR = 175 \times \text{Serum creatinine}^{-1.154} \times \text{Age}^{-0.203}$$
$$\times [0.742 \text{ if female}] \times [1.21 \text{ if black}]$$

This equation was published in 1999, and the trial included white patients and nondiabetics with a mean GFR

Table 1–4. Factors that can affect levels of BUN and creatinine, independent of renal function.[a]

Increase BUN
High protein intake, eg, high-meat diet, hyperalimentation
Gastrointestinal bleeding
Corticosteroids
Tetracycline
High catabolic state

Increase creatinine
High protein intake, eg, creatine supplements
Trimethoprim
Cimetidine (blocks tubular secretion of creatinine)
Ketones (interfere with the Jaffe reaction, used in some laboratories
    to measure creatinine)

BUN, blood urea nitrogen.
[a]Low BUN and creatinine is usually observed in those with decreased muscle mass, eg, muscle wasting diseases and amputees.

of 40 mL/min/1.73 m². It is reasonably accurate in patients with stable CKD, nonhospitalized, and is less accurate in obese patients, nonwhite ethnicities, and kidney transplant recipients.

Both equations tend to be inaccurate in patients with normal or close to normal GFR.

CKD-EPI equation:

$$GFR = 141 \times \min (S_{cr}/\kappa, 1)^{\alpha} \times \max(S_{cr}/\kappa, 1)^{-1.209} \times 0.993^{\text{Age}}$$
$$\times 1.018 \text{ [if female]} \times 1.159 \text{ [if black]}$$

The equation was published in 2009 and was developed for a better assessment of kidney function in patients with a GFR of greater than 60 mL/min/1.73 m². It included patients with and without kidney disease, and it performs better in individuals with higher GFR, in the elderly, patients with higher body mass index (BMI), and in certain subgroups defined by age, sex, race, diabetes, and prior solid organ transplantation (see https://www.ncbi.nlm.nih.gov/pubmed/20557989).

Clinical Findings

A. Symptoms and Signs

The majority of patients with renal disease, especially when mild, are asymptomatic. For those with symptomatic renal disease, most of the symptoms are nonspecific (see Table 1–1) and can be referred to almost any body organ. Examples include constitutional symptoms such as generalized weakness, malaise, decreased appetite, shortness of breath, sleep disturbances, and symptoms and signs of fluid overload. Edema develops when eGFR is less than 10 mL/min/1.73 m² and can be treated with diuretics. Some patients may present with gross hematuria or flank discomfort. Abnormal urination such as increased urgency or frequency may commonly indicate underlying urologic pathology; however, they are also seen in infections or inflammatory diseases involving any part of the urinary tract. In certain connective tissue disorders such as scleroderma, the kidneys are commonly affected. For instance, it can manifest as scleroderma renal crisis and may present as acute kidney injury (AKI), hypertensive crisis, and proteinuria (see https://www.ncbi.nlm.nih.gov/pubmed/22087012). In addition, renal involvement is quite common in systemic lupus erythematosus presenting as AKI and hematuria, cellular casts, and proteinuria (nephritis) prompting a native kidney biopsy for further evaluation.

B. Laboratory Findings

1. Urinalysis—The most important diagnostic test used in a patient with renal disease is the urinalysis. The urine specimen is obtained by doing a midstream catch for males, while in females, the labia majora should be cleaned and then separated to avoid contamination. Urine specimen should be examined within 60 minutes of voiding.

Initially, a dipstick examination is performed, and this includes assessment of the urine specific gravity, pH, leukocytes, nitrites, urobilinogen, protein, blood, ketones, bilirubin, and glucose (Table 1–5).

Microscopic examination of the urine sediment corroborates the findings on the initial dipstick analysis. The presence of various crystals, cells, casts, bacteria, and fungal elements is then reported (see Table 1–5). To perform, at least 10 mL of urine is collected in a tube and centrifuged at 3000 rpm (revolutions per minute) for 5 minutes. Then, the supernatant is poured, and the pellet is resuspended by shaking the tube. The next step is to get a pipette to place approximately 50 μL (small drop) on a glass slide and a coverslip. Then slide is placed under a brightfield or phase-contrast microscope and then analyzed to look for abnormal findings.

Certain patterns of findings on urinalysis are indicative of certain specific diagnoses. For instance, in the patient presenting with AKI, muddy brown and granular casts may indicate acute tubular necrosis (ATN), whereas the presence of red blood cell casts and dysmorphic red blood cells is indicative of glomerulonephritis. High-grade proteinuria is suggestive of glomerular disorders.

2. Urinary indices—Measurement of urine sodium (urine Na) in a random urine specimen is helpful in the differential diagnosis of AKI of prerenal causes and ATN. Urine Na less than 20 mEq/L points to prerenal causes of AKI, for instance, intravascular volume depletion due to fluid losses or sequestration, hypotension, sepsis, etc. On the other hand, urine Na greater than 40 mEq/L suggests ATN. To adjust for the influence of urine concentration, the following equation is recommended:

$$\text{Fractional excretion of Na}\,(FE_{Na}\%)$$
$$= \frac{\text{Urine Na} \times \text{plasma creatinine} \times 100}{\text{Plasma Na} \times \text{urine creatinine}}$$

An FE_{Na} less than 1% points to prerenal disease, while an FE_{Na} greater than 2% suggests ATN. There are certain clinical scenarios where there is a low FeNa such cardiorenal or hepatorenal disease, indicating decreased perfusion as patients appeared to be sodium-avid (see https://www.ncbi.nlm.nih.gov/pubmed/7073153). Limitations to the use of urinary indices include prior infusion with normal saline or administration of diuretics.

An FEUrea is another tool that can be used in the assessment of AKI. It is usually less than 35% if the cause is prerenal and more than 50–65% in ATN. Evidence suggests that the formula is more accurate in patients on diuretics. This is discussed in further detail in Chapter 9.

3. Urinary biomarkers—Several urinary biomarkers are currently being developed to distinguish prerenal AKI and

Table 1–5. Interpretation of urinalysis findings.

Dipstick testing
Specific gravity
   Reflects the ability to concentrate urine in states of volume depletion
pH
   Normal range: 4.5–8
   <5.3: Renal tubular acidosis
   >7.0: Infection with urease-producing organisms, such as *Proteus*
Blood
   1–2 red blood cells per high-power field
   Seen in glomerulonephritides, nephrolithiasis
Glucose
   Seen in poorly controlled diabetes, Fanconi syndrome (type 2 proximal renal tubular acidosis)
   Not reliable for the diagnosis of diabetes
Protein
   Detects only albumin, hence insensitive in detecting microalbuminuria
Nitrite
   Indicates the presence of microorganisms that convert urinary nitrate to nitrite
Leukocyte exterase
   Pyuria

Microscopy
Casts
   Hyaline
      Nonspecific
   Granular
      Nonspecific
      Acute tubular necrosis: Pathognomonic "muddy-brown" granular casts
   Waxy and broad
      Nonspecific
      Advanced renal disease
   Fatty
      Nephrotic syndrome: Oval fat bodies that appear as "Maltese crosses" on polarized micoscopy
   Red blood cells
      Sine qua non of glomerulonephritis
   White blood cells
      Urinary tract infections, eg, pyelonephritis, cystitis
      Tubulointerstitial nephritis
      Renal tuberculosis
Crystals
   Uric acid
      Requires an acidic urine pH
   Calcium phosphate and calcium oxalate
      Require an alkaline urine pH
   Magnesium ammonium phosphate (struvite)
      Seen in urinary tract infections caused by urease-producing organisms, eg, *Proteus* and *Klebsiella*
   Cystine
      Diagnostic of autosomal recessive cystinuria
Epithelial cells
   If >15–20, may be indicative of poorly catched urine specimen
Myoglobin
   Rhabdomyolysis

ATN, but mostly to detect tubular injury earlier. These include neutrophil gelatinase-associated lipocalin (NGAL), kidney injury molecule (1-KIM), liver-fatty-binding protein (L-FABP), urinary interleukin-18 (IL-8), tissue inhibitor of metalloproteinases-2 (TIMP-2), and urinary insulin-like growth factor-binding protein 7 (IGFB7). The last two biomarkers were approved by the Food and Drug Administration (FDA) in 2014 (see https://www.ncbi.nlm.nih.gov/pubmed/25535301).

C. Imaging Studies

In the evaluation of the patient with renal disease, various radiographic studies are available. Usually, they are performed either alone or in combination, to diagnose the different pathologies affecting the genitourinary tract (Table 1–6).

The most common imaging modality used is renal ultrasonography, because it is safe, noninvasive, easy to perform, and avoids the use of radiation or contrast media. Important detailed information that can be obtained through ultrasonography includes the size and shape of the kidneys, the presence of calculi, echogenicity, and identification of a mass or cyst. Asymmetry of the kidneys usually indicates a unilateral disease process. The presence of hydronephrosis is an indication of obstruction along the ipsilateral ureter (if unilateral) or at the level of the bladder or lower (if bilateral).

Increased echogenicity is a common finding that indicates chronic kidney disease.

The plain film of the abdomen may give information about the kidney size and shape, as well as radiopaque (calcium containing) calcifications. Common limitations

include its inability to detect radiolucent stones (uric acid) and inability to image the renal parenchyma.

Computed tomography (CT) scanning provides more detailed information about the structure of the kidneys, as it can also differentiate simple from complex cysts. Noncontrast-enhanced spiral CT scan is the imaging modality of choice for the diagnosis of nephrolithiasis. CT angiography is used in staging of renal cell carcinoma, as well as in demonstrating renal vein thrombosis. Its main disadvantages are the use of contrast media as well as radiation.

Magnetic resonance imaging (MRI) also provides detailed structural information about the kidneys. In the past, magnetic resonance angiography (MRA) with gadolinium contrast has been used extensively in the evaluation of the renovascular disease, diabetic nephropathy, renal transplants, renal masses, and pediatric anomalies. Evidence published in 2006, revealed a link between gadolinium and nephrogenic systemic fibrosis in patients with CKD and thus, there has been a significant decline in its use in patients with renal disease. In fact, some experts recommend not using gadolinium in those with an estimated GFR of less than or equal to 30 mL/min, including those who are dependent on renal replacement therapy or dialysis.

Renal angiography is commonly used in the diagnosis of renal artery stenosis. Because iodinated contrast media is used, caution is advised, especially in patients with baseline renal dysfunction due to increased risk of contrast-associated nephropathy. Prophylactic measures such as volume expansion with normal saline are recommended prior to contrast administration.

The main indications for radionuclide studies (radioisotope scanning with ^{99m}Tc dimercaptosuccinic acid [DMSA]) include early detection of urinary obstruction and urine leaks postsurgery or trauma, as well as vesicoureteric reflux (voiding cystourethrogram).

Retrograde and antegrade pyelography are used primarily during placement of ureteral stents or nephrostomy tubes. Because they utilize radiation, other noninvasive imaging modalities such as ultrasonography and CT scanning have been used more commonly in the diagnosis of urinary tract obstruction, including identification of the site of obstruction.

D. Special Tests

Renal biopsy—Percutaneous renal biopsy is used in situations in which evaluation of the patient's history, physical examination, as well as noninvasive testing (including serum and urine tests and imaging studies) do not provide a diagnosis. In some cases, biopsy may also provide important prognostic information.

The indications for performing a renal biopsy include (1) unexplained persistent hematuria or proteinuria, especially if associated with progression of renal dysfunction,

Table 1–6. Imaging studies and various renal indications.

Renal ultrasonography
Renal failure Microscopic and/or gross hematuria
Proteinuria/nephritic syndrome
Obstructive uropathy/hydronephrosis
Nonobstructing stones in the renal collecting system or proximal ureter
Renal allograft rejection
Percutaneous renal biopsy

CT scan with contrast enhancement
Renal vein thrombosis
Renal infarction

CT scan without contrast
Renal parenchyma infection, eg, abscess, pyelonephritis
Nephrocalcinosis
Renal artery stenosis
Retroperitoneal fibrosis
Percutaneous renal biopsy

Intravenous pyelography
Obstructive uropathy/hydronephrosis, eg, stones, papillary necrosis

CT, computed tomography.

(2) nephrotic syndrome, (3) acute nephritis, and (4) unexplained acute or rapidly progressive renal decline.

The most common complication arising from a percutaneous renal biopsy is bleeding. The patient's ability to coagulate normally should be ascertained by verifying coagulation tests prior to the procedure (partial thromboplastin time, prothrombin time, international normalized ratio and platelet count). Patients should also be advised to hold acetylsalicylic acid and/or nonsteroidal anti-inflammatory drugs at least 1 week prior to the planned renal biopsy. Patients requiring maintenance chronic anticoagulation with the vitamin K antagonist, warfarin, should stop it 4–7 days prior to procedure and should be placed on heparin. However, holding anticoagulation should be based on their risk of thromboembolism and if this is low, warfarin can be stopped without bridging with heparin. In the other hand, patients taking one of the novel oral anticoagulants, such as apixaban, should discontinue the medication for at least 48 hours prior to procedure and resume once hemostasis has been established; typically the following day after the procedure.

Postbiopsy, many patients may develop transient microscopic hematuria, while transient gross hematuria has been described in 3–10% of cases. Arteriovenous fistulas arising as complications of renal biopsies as demonstrated by color Doppler studies have been described in the literature as well.

The major contraindications to percutaneous renal biopsy can be divided into (1) those involving the kidneys and (2) those involving the patient. Examples of contraindications affecting the kidneys are the presence of multiple cysts either unilaterally or bilaterally, the presence of a renal mass, a solitary functioning kidney, the presence of active renal or perirenal infection, and unilateral or bilateral hydronephrosis. Patient-related contraindications include an uncooperative patient, uncontrolled severe hypertension, intractable bleeding disorder, and morbid obesity. It must be noted, however, that with the exception of intractable bleeding disorder, most of the contraindications are relative rather than absolute. Therefore, the actual clinical situation often dictates whether a contraindication can be overridden. Recently, it has been shown that percutaneous renal biopsy may be performed in those with solitary kidneys. Several published reports have demonstrated that even for those with solitary functioning kidneys, the risk of general anesthesia (during open renal biopsy) far outweighs the risk of requiring surgery and subsequent nephrectomy. Therefore, in selected cases, percutaneous renal biopsy may be performed in the presence of a solitary functioning kidney.

Hematuria

Hematuria is the presence of red blood cells in the urine, and it can be either gross or microscopic. In the initial evaluation of a patient with gross hematuria, it must be determined whether the urine discoloration is truly secondary to pathologic bleeding within the urinary tract. Patients who are menstruating or postpartum should not be evaluated for hematuria. In the absence of true hematuria, the urine may appear grossly red following the intake of certain medications, such as rifampin, phenothiazine, or phenazopyridine (analgesic), or the intake of beets in certain predisposed individuals. It is also important to differentiate hematuria from other causes of red urine such as hemoglobinuria and myoglobinuria. The latter is usually seen in those with acute rhabdomyolysis. Microscopic examination of the urine should always be performed to confirm true hematuria (Figure 1–1).

Microscopic hematuria is defined as the presence of more than two red blood cells (RBCs) per high-power field (hpf). It is usually detected incidentally by urine dipstick examination.

Careful history taking is of paramount importance in the evaluation of patients with hematuria. Important historical information usually provides diagnostic clues. For instance, the occurrence of concomitant flank pain with radiation to the ipsilateral testicle or labia suggests underlying nephrolithiasis; burning on urination or dysuria may point to possible urinary tract infection, and a recent upper respiratory tract infection may suggest either postinfectious glomerulonephritis or even IgA nephropathy. A family history of hematuria is also vital, as certain diseases tend to run in families, such as polycystic kidney disease or even sickle cell nephropathy. Likewise, thin basement membrane disease and benign familial hematuria tend to occur in families, and notably have a benign course. Exercise-induced hematuria is seen in adolescents who exercise vigorously.

In elderly individuals, or those above 50 years of age, the finding of gross or microscopic (even transient) hematuria should trigger an extensive evaluation to rule out malignancy involving the genitourinary tract. The incidence of bladder cancer and other malignancies involving the kidneys and the ureters is significantly elevated, particularly in those with a prolonged history of tobacco smoking and analgesic use. The occurrence of symptoms of increased urgency and frequency with hematuria in this population should suggest urinary tract obstruction secondary to either benign prostatic hypertrophy (BPH) or prostatic malignancy.

Using urine microscopy, the presence of dysmorphic RBCs or RBC casts should suggest glomerular disorders as the primary etiology of hematuria. This is one of the indications for performing a percutaneous renal biopsy.

Proteinuria

Normal urine protein excretion is 150 mg/day. Anything above this value is considered overt proteinuria. Proteinuria usually implies that there is a defect in glomerular permeability. In general, proteinuria can be classified into three types: (1) glomerular, (2) tubular, or (3) overflow.

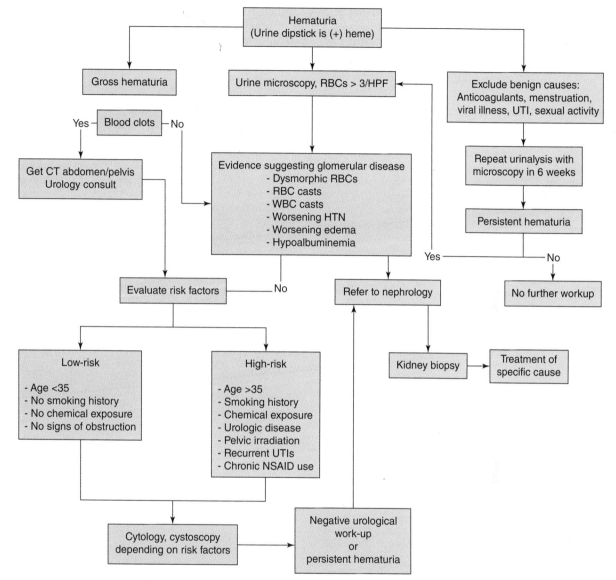

▲ **Figure 1–1.** Evaluation of hematuria in adults. (Adapted from *Comprehensive Clinical Nephrology*, 5th ed.)

Glomerular proteinuria includes diabetic nephropathy and other common glomerular disorders (see Chapters 37–39). It is usually caused by increased filtration of albumin and other proteins across the glomerular capillary wall. There are also causes of glomerular proteinuria that have a rather benign course, such as orthostatic and exercise-induced proteinuria. These latter causes are characterized by significantly lower degrees of proteinuria, less than 2 g/day.

Tubular proteinuria is usually seen in those with underlying tubulointerstitial diseases, typically less than 2 g/day and

the urine dipstick may be negative. They often have defective re-absorptive capacities in the proximal tubules, such that the proteins, instead of being normally reabsorbed, are excreted in the urine. In contrast to glomerular proteinuria, whereby macromolecules such as albumin are leaked out, in tubular proteinuria, it is mostly low-molecular-weight proteins (<25,000 Da), such as β_2-microglobulin, retinol-binding protein, polypeptides, and immunoglobulin light chains.

Last, overflow proteinuria is exemplified by multiple myeloma, where there is an overabundance of immunoglobulin light chains secondary to overproduction. In other words, proteinuria occurs because the amount of protein produced exceeds the maximum threshold for reabsorption in the tubules. Other clinical scenarios occur in rhabdomyolysis (myoglobulin) and acute myelomonocytic leukemia (lysozyme) and in rate cases, polymyositis.

Whereas both glomerular and tubular proteinuria are secondary to abnormalities involving the glomerular capillary and tubular walls, respectively, in overflow proteinuria, the problem is the overproduction of certain proteins.

When performing a urinalysis, the dipstick examination can detect only albumin, and not the low-molecular-weight proteins. In fact, it can detect it only when proteinuria is greater than 300–500 mg/day. Hence, one of its most important limitations is its inability to detect microalbuminuria, which corresponds to the earliest phase of diabetic nephropathy. However, the sulfosalicylic acid test (SSA) can detect all types of proteins in the urine, including low-molecular-weight proteins, but this is rarely performed in routine practice.

Quantification of the degree of proteinuria is accomplished by performing a 24-hour urine collection, which can be cumbersome, especially in elderly individuals or those with concomitant fecal or urinary incontinence.

The urine protein-to-creatinine (using a random urine specimen) ratio has been shown to have a good correlation with 24-hour urine protein determination.

Orthostatic or postural proteinuria, by definition, is characterized by increased urine protein excretion in the upright position and normal urine protein excretion in the supine position. It is a benign condition, seen mostly among adolescents, the mechanism of which is not clearly understood. The diagnosis is established by performing a split urine collection, as follows: (1) The first morning void is discarded, (2) a 16-hour upright collection is obtained between 7 AM and 11 PM, with the patient performing normal activities and finishing the collection by voiding just before 11 PM (the times can be adjusted according to the normal times at which the patient awakens and goes to sleep), (3) the patient should assume a recumbent position 2 hours before the upright collection is finished to avoid contamination of the supine collection with urine formed when in the upright position, and (4) a separate overnight 8-hour collection is obtained between 11 PM and 7 AM.

Patients with orthostatic proteinuria do not progress to end-stage renal disease; in fact, proteinuria resolves spontaneously in the majority of affected patients.

KEY READINGS

Garcia DA, Crowther MA. Reversal of warfarin: case-based practice recommendations. Circulation 2012;125:2944.

Marckmann P, et al. Nephrogenic systemic fibrosis: suspected causative role of gadodiamide used for contrast-enhanced magnetic resonance imaging. J Am Soc Nephrol 2006;17:2359.

Tschuppert Y, et al. Effect of dronedarone on renal function in healthy subjects. Br J Clin Pharmacol 2007;64:785.

Wilhelm-Leen E, et al. Estimating the risk of radiocontrast-associated nephropathy. J Am Soc Nephrol 2017;28:653.

Zhang JL, et al. New magnetic resonance imaging methods in nephrology. Kidney Int 2014;85:768.

■ CHAPTER REVIEW QUESTIONS

1. A 67-year-old male patient is evaluated in the emergency department with a 3-day history of fever, chills, and malaise. He denies having any urinary symptoms, for example frequency, dysuria, and urgency. He states that 2 days ago he noticed watery stools, approximately 6–8 times a day accompanied by nausea and non-bilious vomiting. His medical history is remarkable for hypertension and osteoarthritis. His medications include lisinopril, metformin, furosemide, naproxen, and multivitamins.

   On physical examination, his vital signs are stable: blood pressure is 132/88 mm Hg, heart rate is 92 beats/min, respiratory rate is 17 breaths/min, and he is afebrile. The rest of the physical examination is unremarkable.

   Chest X-ray and electrocardiogram (ECG) are within normal limits.

   Laboratory data:
   Blood urea nitrogen (BUN) 70 mg/dL
   Serum creatinine 2.8 mg/dL
   Serum potassium 4.5 mEq/dL
   Serum sodium 146 mEq/dL
   Fractional excretion of sodium: 1.7%
   Fractional excretion of urea: 7.5%

   What is the most likely diagnosis?
   A. Prerenal acute kidney injury
   B. Interstitial nephritis
   C. Obstructive nephropathy
   D. Acute tubular necrosis

2. A 27-year-old female is being evaluated in the inpatient psychiatry unit due to elevated creatinine. The patient is currently hospitalized because of new-onset severe depression and suicidal ideation after she had a fight with her boyfriend. She does not have a remarkable past medical history, except for chronic tobacco smoking. Her current medications include citalopram, folic acid, and trimethoprim-sulfamethoxazole which she recently started 4 days ago for a presumptive urinary tract infection. For the last 3 days, she has had nausea, but not vomiting with some episodes of loose stools, which she attributes to the hospital food.

Physical examination: blood pressure is 112/77 mm Hg, pulse rate is 62 beats/min, and respiratory rate of 17 breaths/min. The rest of the physical examination is normal.

Laboratory data:
Serum sodium: 133 mEq/dL
Serum potassium: 5.6 mEq/dL
Serum creatinine: 1.9 mg/dL

Rest of the serum electrolytes are normal.

What is the cause of the elevated creatinine?
A. Laboratory error
B. Prerenal acute kidney injury
C. Interstitial nephritis
D. Urinary tract infection
E. The antibiotic

3. A 19-year-old man is evaluated at his primary care physician's office due to intermittent microscopic hematuria found on routine urinalysis. He is a lacrosse player. He denies any dysuria, urgency, or increase in urinary frequency and he takes no medications. He recalls that his grandfather and his father may have had the same issues, but never developed any complications related to their kidneys nor require dialysis or transplantation. Physical examination is unremarkable.

Laboratory data reveal a normal basal metabolic panel with a normal creatinine and normal liver function tests. Urine protein creatinine ratio is 0.1 mg/g.

What is the most appropriate next step in the management of this patient?
A. Kidney biopsy
B. Abdomen and pelvis tomography
C. Reassurance
D. Drug screening

4. A 28-year-old female is being evaluated for intermittent proteinuria. As part of her work as a school bus driver, she had a routine urinalysis that revealed 3+ protein. Her primary care provider obtained a urine protein-to-creatinine ratio of 1.2 mg/g. She occasionally runs 1–2 miles, three times a week. She denies any recent strenuous exercise, fever, seizures, or gastrointestinal symptoms. As her primary care physician wanted to confirm the results, he performed a 24-hour urine collection, which revealed 140 mg/day of protein. Once a nephrologist evaluated her, a 24-hour urine collection was performed again, revealing 600 mg of protein.

On her physical examination, blood pressure is 130/84 mm Hg, heart rate is 75 beats/min, and respiratory rate is 14 breaths/min. She is afebrile. Cardiopulmonary examination is unremarkable. Abdomen is benign and there is no costovertebral tenderness. Lower extremity exam reveals no pitting edema.

What is the best next step in the management of this patient?
A. Perform a 24-hour urine collection
B. Perform a urine-to-protein creatinine ratio
C. Perform a split 24-hour urine collection
D. Kidney biopsy

5. A 19-year-old male patient underwent an annual screening for his job and was discovered to have proteinuria. A 24-hour urine collection revealed 2.9 g of proteinuria per day. He is asymptomatic. He takes diclofenac 100 mg at least two or three times per week for occasional lumbar back pain. He denies any previous exposure to herbal supplements. His last HIV screening test was negative.

Physical examination revealed a blood pressure of 123/78 mm Hg, heart rate of 98 beats/min, respiratory rate of 15 breaths/min. BMI is 42 kg/m². Cardiopulmonary examination is unremarkable. Abdomen is soft and nontender. Lower extremities with 2+ edema.

He undergoes a percutaneous kidney biopsy that reveals FSGS.

Of the following risk factors, which is the most likely cause of FSGS on this patient?
A. NSAIDs
B. Obesity
C. Age
D. HIV
E. All of the above

Disorders of Extracellular Volume: Hypovolemia and Hypervolemia

Alan Segal, MD

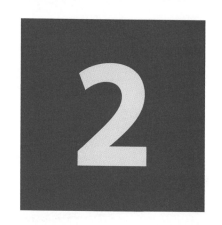

EVALUATION OF THE EXTRACELLULAR VOLUME

General Considerations

Life most likely began in or very near an ocean where the predominant cation was sodium (Na^+). That is, life is *supported* by a solution high in Na^+. Life itself *developed* from single cells where potassium (K^+) would become the predominant cation of the cytoplasm. From that ancient time to present day animal cells, the intracellular fluid (ie, the ICF, the first space of *life*) remains high in K^+ while the extracellular fluid (ie, the ECF, the second space of *life support*) remains high in Na^+.

Initially, the cyclical ebb and flow of the ocean provided nutrients via diffusion, but as organisms became larger and more complex, another system was needed to deliver nutrients and excrete wastes. Ultimately, this became the cardiovascular system consisting of the heart—a pump to provide the driving force (ie, blood pressure) for transport—and the blood vessels (permeabilities) through which the nutrients flow. This system also features circulation into an excretory system (ie, kidney), where key regulation of ECF volume (ie, sodium balance) occurs.

Life on land results in a constant loss of water and salt. Therefore, the fundamental challenge terrestrial animals (including humans) face is the ability to ingest and conserve adequate water and salt to maintain body tonicity and ECF volume, respectively. Disorders of body tonicity—discussed in Chapter 3 are disturbances in *water balance* that relate to sodium *concentration*. That is, hypernatremia usually occurs in states of net free water loss (ie, dehydration) and hyponatremia occurs in states of relative free water excess.

In contradistinction, disorders of ECF volume—the subject of this chapter—are disorders of *sodium balance* and relate to total body sodium *content*. A person is said to be *euvolemic* when the volume of isotonic fluid in their ECF, as judged from the history and physical examination, is optimal. That is, the ECF is large enough to ensure adequate arterial perfusion of the tissues but without evidence of interstitial fluid volume expansion (edema) or depletion. Hypovolemia exists when a net loss of sodium (eg, via skin, gut, or kidney) leads to ECF volume depletion. On the other hand, hypervolemia exists when a net gain of sodium leads to ECF volume overload. Hypervolemia is usually a result of organ dysfunction (eg, congestive heart failure, liver cirrhosis, kidney failure) but may also occur with aggressive volume resuscitation as seen during the treatment of early sepsis.

The distribution of body fluid volumes in health are given in Table 2–1. With reference to the ECF volume, a steady state will exist whenever the Na^+ excretion rate (output) equals the Na^+ ingestion rate (input). In normal individuals, this steady state occurs when their ECF volume is judged to be euvolemic.

The control of ECF volume is inextricably linked to the regulation of sodium balance by the kidney. Clinical euvolemia refers to that range of ECF volumes such that steady state Na^+ balance occurs without evidence of hypoperfusion (eg, hypotension) or expansion of the interstitial component of the ECF (ie, edema). For example, it is important to note that a patient with edema due to compensated congestive heart failure is in steady state with respect to Na^+ balance, but that steady state is achieved at the *cost* of ECF (interstitial) expansion because of organ dysfunction.

Disorders of ECF volume have long presented a challenge in the understanding of body fluid volume regulation because the elements of ECF volume being "sensed" by the afferent limb of the control system are not firmly established, and indeed, may change dynamically, as follows. For a euvolemic person with normal organ function, the interstitium may behave as low compliance system so that small increases in interstitial volume lead to steep increases in interstitial pressure, which in turn generates a robust natriuretic signal to the kidney across a wide range of sodium intake. For example, there is evidence that increases in renal interstitial pressure

Table 2–1. Body fluid distribution.

Compartment Volume in 70-kg Person	Amount	Volume (L)
Total body fluid	60% of body weight	42
Intracellular fluid (ICF)	40% of body weight	28
Extracellular fluid (ECF)	20% of body weight	14
Interstitial fluid	Two-thirds of ECF	9.4
Plasma fluid	One-third of ECF	4.6
Venous fluid	85% of plasma fluid	3.9
Arterial fluid	15% of plasma fluid	0.7

lead to a decrease in apical Na^+ transporters in the proximal tubule, producing a natriuresis. Such a mechanism is consistent with the model of *pressure-natriuresis* established by Guyton and colleagues in the 1960s.

In contrast, the interstitium may behave as a higher compliance system in a patient with congestive heart failure and edema such that additional increases in interstitial volume cause only small changes in interstitial pressure. This would effectively decrease the slope of the pressure-natriuresis curve, allowing more interstitial expansion before an adequate natriuresis is achieved to come into another (more edematous) steady state.

The relation between cardiac outflow and peripheral arterial resistance has been called the "effective arterial blood volume" (EABV). The EABV refers to a conceptual component of ECF volume that "senses" the fullness of the arterial system (or the effectiveness at which perfusion of organs is occurring), which provides the feedback signal that regulates Na^+ handling by the kidney. Under normal circumstances, the EABV might equal the actual arterial blood volume, which allows a person with normal organ function to maintain euvolemia across a wide range of sodium intake. This system may become dysregulated in the presence of organ dysfunction.

HYPOVOLEMIA

ESSENTIALS OF DIAGNOSIS

- ▶ History of blood loss, gastrointestinal (GI) losses, or excessive sweating.
- ▶ History of diuretic use.
- ▶ Tachycardia and postural hypotension.
- ▶ The jugular venous pulse is not visible.

▶ General Considerations

Over the millennia, the kidney has developed a remarkable ability to conserve sodium. Indeed, every segment of the nephron possesses a different transport element designed to reabsorb Na^+ from the urine. The *renin–angiotensin–aldosterone system* (RAAS) is the major hormone system that acts on the kidney to promote salt reabsorption in states of ECF volume depletion (hypovolemia). The neurohormonal response to hypovolemia also includes activation of the sympathetic nervous system (SNS) and, to some extent, release of arginine vasopressin (AVP, also known as antidiuretic hormone, ADH). The key clinical corollary is to always give volume (ie, isotonic saline) to ECF volume-depleted patients.

Hypovolemia reflects a decrease in ECF volume, and sodium depletion implies ECF volume depletion (and vice versa). The ECF volume decreases when losses (NaCl losses or losses of ECF) exceed input. Simply reducing dietary NaCl intake leads to a modest decline in ECF volume. Typical western diets include about 4–6 g/day (~170–260 mmol) of Na^+. For example, if a person with a serum [Na] of 140 mmol/L reduced their daily dietary Na^+ intake by 2 g (87 mmol), their ECF volume would decrease by $(87/140) = 0.62$ L. Although reduced NaCl intake can lead to mild ECF volume depletion, the effects are usually not clinically significant because normal kidneys can reduce urinary NaCl excretion to very low levels.

ECF losses frequently occur via one of four routes: gastrointestinal, renal, integumentary, or into a "third space" (eg, pleural effusion, ascites).

Gastrointestinal losses can be external (eg, vomiting, diarrhea, external fistulas) or internal (eg, third spacing as in pancreatitis). A history of vomiting or diarrhea often precipitates ECF volume depletion, especially because gastrointestinal disorders are frequently associated with reduced intake. Cholera is one of the best examples of severe loss of essentially isotonic saline due to the profound secretory diarrhea caused by the cholera enterotoxin.

Losses via the skin can also be external (eg, sweating), and severe burns can cause excessive losses, both external and internal.

When sodium depletion is a result of skin or gastrointestinal tract losses, the urine [Na] and fractional excretion of sodium (FENa) will be low if the kidney is functioning normally. In these so-called 'prerenal' states of renal hypoperfusion, the urine [Na] will often be less than 15 mmol/L with a FENa less than 1%. Excessive renal losses—usually accompanied by a urine [Na] greater than 20 mmol/L and an increased FENa—can be secondary to salt-wasting disorders of the kidney, to the administration of salt-wasting diuretic drugs, or to osmotic losses via the urine, such as occur during poorly controlled diabetes. The major causes of salt-wasting disorders are listed in Table 2–2.

Table 2–2. Salt-wasting disorders.

I. Intrinsic Renal
   A. Chronic kidney disease
   B. Postacute kidney injury
   C. Postobstructive nephropathy
   D. Renal tubule acidosis
   E. Bartter syndrome
   F. Gitelman syndrome
II. Extrinsic Renal
   A. Mineralocorticoid deficiency
      1. Addison disease
      2. Isolated hypoaldosteronism
   B. Natriuretic peptide-mediated
      1. Cerebral (renal) salt wasting
      2. SIADH
III. Drug-Induced
   A. Solute diuresis
      1. Mannitol
      2. Urea
      3. Glucose
      4. Bicarbonate
   B. Diuretics
      1. Proximal, eg, acetazolamide
      2. Loop, eg, furosemide, torsemide, bumetanide
      3. DCT, eg, hydrochlorothiazide, chlorthalidone, indapamide
      4. CCT, eg, spironolactone, eplerenone, amiloride, triamterene

CCT, cortical collecting tubule; DCT, distal convoluted tubule; SIADH, syndrome of inappropriate secretion of antidiuretic hormone.

► Clinical Findings

A. Symptoms and Signs

The evaluation of the patient with hypovolemia should include an appropriate history, careful physical examination, and key laboratory data. The history should focus on any potential loss of sodium or fluids that could have occurred via the gut (vomiting, diarrhea), skin (sweating), or kidney (polyuria, diuretic use). A history of previous renal disease, familial salt wasting, or diuretic use points to salt wasting (see Table 2–2). Symptoms of polyuria, polydipsia, and polyphagia suggest diabetes. Generic symptoms of ECF volume depletion include thirst and salt craving. Patients with Addison disease frequently manifest symptoms of lassitude. Individuals with inherited salt wasting frequently describe the desire to drink pickle (salt brine) juice or ingest large amounts of salty foods. When ECF volume depletion is more severe (approaching 7–10% of body weight), the symptoms result from reduced plasma volume; these include weakness, dizziness/lightheadedness, syncope, and eventually loss of consciousness.

A complete physical examination should always be performed looking for both specific signs of ECF volume depletion (detailed below) and potential causes (eg, acute abdomen, bowel obstruction, etc).

1. Skin and mucous membranes—If the skin on the thigh, calf, or forearm is pinched in normal subjects, it will immediately return to its normally flat state when the pinch is released. The speed at which the skin returns to its normal flat state after being pinched is often called "skin turgor." A diminished turgor has frequently been suggested to indicate depletion of the ECF volume, but a systematic review found this sign to have no diagnostic value in adult patients. In contrast, dry axillae may suggest ECF volume depletion, whereas moist axillae argue against it. Dryness of the mucous membranes of the mouth and nose and longitudinal furrows on the tongue have also been shown to indicate ECF volume depletion. Other signs may include a delay in capillary refill, decreased peripheral pulses, cool extremities, and oliguria. It is important to remember that all of these findings are not diagnostic in themselves and need to be evaluated with caution and in the context of the clinical presentation.

2. Pulse and arterial blood pressure—Changes in pulse rate and arterial pressure may indicate ECF volume depletion. When the ECF volume depletion is mild, only postural changes may be evident. Clinicians measuring postural changes should wait at least 2 minutes before measuring the supine vital signs and 1 minute after standing before measuring the upright vital signs. Counting the pulse for 30 seconds and doubling the result is more accurate than 15 seconds of observation. In normovolemic individuals, a postural pulse increment of more than 30 beats/min is uncommon, affecting only about 2–4% of individuals. The most helpful physical findings in the setting of blood loss are severe postural dizziness (preventing measurement of upright vital signs) or a postural pulse increment of 30 beats/min or more. Postural changes on sitting are much less reliable. After excluding those unable to stand, postural hypotension has no incremental diagnostic value.

3. Jugular venous pressure—The reduction in the vascular volume observed with hypovolemia occurs primarily in the venous circulation (which normally contains 70% of the blood volume), thereby leading to a decrease in venous pressure. As a result, estimation of the jugular venous pressure can be useful to confirm the diagnosis of hypovolemia and to assess the adequacy of volume replacement. Details concerning examination of the jugular venous pressure are presented below (ECF volume expansion). It is important to remember that a low jugular pressure (wherein the jugular pulse cannot be observed) may be normal and is consistent with, but never diagnostic of, hypovolemia.

B. Laboratory Findings

Most information concerning the state of ECF volume is obtained from the history and physical examination. In some situations, laboratory tests can provide additional suggestive information. For example, for extrarenal losses, corroborative results would include (1) a low urine [Na], (2) a FENa less than 1%, and (3) a BUN:Cr ratio greater than 20. The basis of the latter is that under conditions of renal hypoperfusion, urea is avidly reabsorbed whereas creatinine is not reabsorbed and a small percentage is secreted into the tubule.

It is worth reemphasizing that abnormalities of serum sodium concentration should not be used to imply a disorder of ECF volume. This is because abnormalities in serum sodium concentration reflect defects in water balance. A hyponatremic patient may be hypovolemic, euvolemic, or hypervolemic, depending on clinical circumstances. Nevertheless, abnormal values for serum Na concentration suggest consideration of volume disorders. Further, abnormalities of serum K, Cl, or HCO_3 also suggest disorders of ECF volume. As an example, hypokalemic metabolic alkalosis is commonly associated with chloride depletion (eg, vomiting, loop and thiazide diuretics), often with concomitant ECF depletion. More rarely, hypokalemic alkalosis may also be associated with hypervolemia (eg, primary aldosteronism, apparent mineralocorticoid excess); thus constellations of electrolyte abnormalities should not generally be used to diagnose disorders of ECF volume.

Some laboratory findings do provide useful indices that correlate or can be used to corroborate the impression of ECF volume depletion as assessed from the history and physical examination. As mentioned, the ratio of blood urea nitrogen to creatinine (when both expressed in the same units) frequently exceeds 20:1 when azotemia results from depletion of the ECF volume. Hemoconcentration (a rise in the hematocrit and hemoglobin concentration) and increases in serum uric acid concentration may also be observed. In the setting of acute kidney injury, a FENa less than 1% suggests prerenal azotemia, which may be the result of true ECF volume depletion. Yet prerenal azotemia (ie, hypoperfusion of the kidney) also occurs in the setting of congestive heart failure and cirrhosis, where the ECF volume is expanded, but EABV is reduced. Thus, urine chemistry may help to determine the state of the "effective" arterial volume, but is less useful for determining ECF volume itself. As mentioned, hypokalemic metabolic alkalosis may be associated with an ECF volume depleted or expanded state. In that setting, a urine Cl concentration of less than 10–15 mM is often taken as evidence that the alkalosis is related to chloride/ECF volume depletion, which should be chloride responsive.

A measured central venous pressure provides definitive evidence of the filling pressure of the venous circulation. Placement of a pulmonary artery catheter can provide information about the left-sided filling pressure, but this technique has become less commonly employed because controlled studies suggest that it does not improve outcome.

A. Imaging Studies

Depletion or expansion of the ECF volume may be estimated by ultrasound or echocardiography. This approach is often restricted to patients in the intensive care unit but appears to be reliable. Ultrasound is used to detect the respiratory variation in the diameter of the inferior vena cava (IVC) using M-mode in a spontaneously breathing patient. The percent difference between the maximal and minimal IVC diameter is called the collapsibility index. When the IVC is underfilled, the compliance and collapsibility index are increased, so large respiratory variations in vena cava dimensions suggest reduced intravenous volume and predict fluid responsiveness. On the other hand, an IVC with a small collapsibility index makes volume depletion less likely.

B. Special Tests

Determination of the clinical volume status is sometimes particularly challenging due to multiple factors including patient's body habitus, inaccurate weights, and/or absence of clinical symptoms and signs of ECF depletion or overload. Several novel noninvasive techniques have emerged that hold promise for improving the clinician's ability to assess volume status and guide therapy; namely, measurements of bioimpedance and photoplethysmography.

Bioimpedance measurements exploit the differing conductivity of body fat (a nonconductor) and fat-free mass (conductor). Once quantified from five body regions (trunk, upper limbs, and lower limbs), the volume of fat-free mass can be derived, from which the volume of the ICF and ECF can be estimated.

Photoplethysmography is a noninvasive optical technique similar to pulse oximetry whereby signal waveforms related to cardiac output and respiration can be processed to yield hemodynamic information that can be related to changes in blood volume. Photoplethysmographic methods and devices are now becoming available for use in the critical care unit and dialysis unit, where determining clinical volume status can be particularly challenging.

▶ Differential Diagnosis

The differential diagnosis of true ECF volume depletion is often made from the history and physical examination as discussed, with the support of certain laboratory information.

Determining that the sodium loss occurred via the skin (sweating, burns, etc), gastrointestinal tract (vomiting, diarrhea, GI bleed, etc), or kidney (diuretics, osmotic diuresis, etc) is usually clear, but in some cases the specific etiology may be less obvious. For example, individuals with eating disorders may go to great lengths to conceal surreptitious vomiting (bulimia) or diuretic/laxative abuse.

The presence of hypokalemia with metabolic acidosis suggests GI loss of potassium bicarbonate via laxatives, and low values for the urine [Na] and urine [K] would be expected. In the setting of lower GI losses, the urine [Cl] is often elevated due to the excretion of ammonium chloride (NH_4Cl) as the kidney responds to the hypokalemia and metabolic acidosis by stimulation of ammoniagenesis.

Vomiting and loop/thiazide ingestion will both result in metabolic alkalosis, so the differential diagnosis can be difficult. If not clear from the history, the urine electrolytes can be helpful as follows: shortly after vomiting, the urine [Na] is often elevated (due to bicarbonaturia), but the urine [Cl] may be low. With loop/thiazide diuretic (ab)use, the urine [Cl] may be increased. If suspected, a urine diuretic screen can be helpful.

A number of rare inherited or acquired diseases of kidney ion transport feature renal salt wasting. Depending on their severity and the clinical setting, salt-wasting disorders may present as unrelenting polyuria with life-threatening depletion of the ECF volume or as mild but troubling syndromes in which depletion of the ECF volume is nearly undetectable. Several clinical features, however, are typical of most salt-wasting disorders. These features include malaise, lassitude, fatigability, and salt craving. When mild, these symptoms can be subtle enough to lead to diagnostic difficulty. A classification of salt-wasting disorders is shown in Table 2–2.

A careful family history is crucial if a rare autosomal recessive "salt-wasting nephropathy" is suspected. Genetic mutations of transport proteins in the loop of Henle (ie, Bartter syndrome) or the thiazide-sensitive cotransporter in the early distal convoluted tubule (ie, Gitelman syndrome) both lead to hypokalemic metabolic alkalosis with ECF volume depletion. Bartter syndrome tends to present prior to adolescence and volume depletion is more prominent. Those with Gitelman syndrome tend to present during adolescence and symptoms of muscle weakness predominate. Urine electrolytes will show hypercalciuria in Bartter syndrome, but hypocalciuria in Gitelman syndrome. Hypomagnesemia is also characteristic of the latter.

Complications

Recall that the intracellular fluid (ICF) is the "first space" because it is the space of life (eg, nucleus, DNA, organelles, cytoplasm, cytoskeleton, cell membrane, etc) while the ECF volume is the "second space" and serves in the role of life support. As such, ECF volume depletion presents risks to adequate tissue perfusion and normal organ (eg, brain, heart, liver, gut, kidney) function. Therefore, progressive and/or severe hypovolemia causes organ dysfunction, including prerenal azotemia. The kidney is especially sensitive to hypoperfusion due to depletion of the ECF volume or the EABV, and responds by increasing retention of NaCl and water. These effects tend to restore ECF volume, but if untreated, prerenal azotemia can progress to ischemic acute tubule necrosis and uremia. When even more severe, ECF volume depletion can lead to a state of hypovolemic shock in which the perfusion of vital organs is inadequate to meet physiological needs. In this setting, frank hypotension is present, the patient is cool and often dusky, and the mentation is impaired. In hypovolemic shock states such as these, lactate levels often rise and can be a helpful laboratory measure.

Treatment

The essential factors in treating hypovolemic patients are to stop ongoing losses and replace the ECF volume deficit. Clearly, the treatment team should address ongoing blood, urinary, gastrointestinal, or sweat losses appropriately, and diuretics should be discontinued.

The route and choice of repletion method depends on the severity of symptoms, the nature and magnitude of the losses, and the presence of superimposed disorders of osmolality (Table 2–3). Mild ECF volume depletion frequently responds to provision of dietary NaCl and water. One of the most common causes of ECF volume depletion worldwide is infectious diarrhea, especially in children. Oral rehydration solutions (ORS) have become the repletion standard by which all but the most serious cases are treated (Table 2–4). These have had a dramatic impact on mortality.

When the ECF volume depletion is more severe, resuscitation with intravenous fluids is indicated. Intravenous saline or Ringer lactate have been shown to restore ECF volume and hemodynamic stability effectively. If one has an idea of the fluid weight the patient has lost, the amount of volume to replete can be estimated to a target weight. The rate of repletion often depends on the urgency of the situation, with mentation and urine output serving as surrogates of tissue perfusion while postural measurements of blood pressure and pulse are monitored. The hemodynamic response to a rapid infusion (bolus) of normal saline and/or measurements of central pressure may also be useful.

Blood products such as fresh-frozen plasma and packed red blood cells are the most effective volume expanders because they are confined to the intravascular space, but come at an increased cost and there is a very small risk of infection. Isotonic (normal) saline is an effective ECF volume expander, but one must remember 75% will end up in the interstitial space. Isotonic saline is usually preferred in patients with upper GI losses (eg, vomiting). In those with diarrhea or underlying kidney disease, Ringer lactate has the advantage of avoiding hyperchloremic acidosis, which some studies have suggested increases the risk of acute kidney injury in large-volume resuscitations. Ringer lactate should be avoided in patients with ongoing lactic acidosis, in whom the administered lactate will not be metabolized. Use of albumin or starch-containing solutions does not appear to improve effectiveness and starch solutions have been associated with a risk of acute kidney injury. A solution of 5% dextrose in water (d5W) is not an effective volume expander because it will distribute to all of body water, so 67% will end up in the ICF. It should never be used for ECF volume repletion.

The rate of crystalloid administration cannot be derived from empirical formulas. In general, crystalloid may be administered at a rate 50–100 mL/h greater than ongoing losses, unless the patient is profoundly volume depleted. For

Table 2–3. Treatment of ECF volume depletion in children.

	No Signs of Dehydration	Some Dehydration	Severe Dehydration
Mental state	Well, alert	Restless, irritable	Lethargic
Appearance of eyes	Normal	Sunken	Sunken
Thirst	Not thirsty	Thirsty, drinks eagerly	Drinks poorly
Skin pinch	Normal	Returns slowly	Returns very slowly
Estimated degree of dehydration	<5% or <50 mL/kg	5–10% or 50–100 mL/kg	>10% or >100 mL/kg
Suggested treatment	Treat at home Give more fluids than normal Give zinc supplements Continue to feed child Reassess if worsening	Rehydration at health center; give ORS-based on weight; assess response; give zinc, food on discharge	Intravenous rehydration in hospital where possible; if not available, nasogastric ORS is suggested

ECF, extracellular fluids; ORS, oral rehydration solutions.
Source: Reproduced with permission from Cheng AC: Infectious diarrhea in developed and developing countries. *J Clin Gastroenterol* 2005;39:757.

patients who are severely hypotensive or in septic shock, a goal-directed approach that combines early central venous pressure (CVP) monitoring with crystalloid administration to maintain the CVP at 8–12 mm Hg has been shown to improve outcomes. Repeated 500-mL boluses of crystalloid can be given every 30 minutes to achieve a CVP of 8–12 mm Hg. One exception to this rule is for patients who are bleeding. In this situation, blood products rather than crystalloids are recommended, with the goal of increasing the hematocrit up to a maximum of 35%. Values above this are associated with potential complications.

When ECF volume depletion is persistent due to ongoing renal losses, maneuvers to supplement intake or reduce those losses are useful. Ingestion of a high salt diet or the use of the synthetic mineralocorticoid, fludrocortisone, may be useful to treat patients with inherited or acquired salt-wasting disorders.

▶ **Prognosis**

The prognosis of hypovolemia in the absence of septic shock is usually excellent, as long as corrective maneuvers are instituted promptly. Most authorities attribute substantial reductions in childhood mortality to the use of oral rehydration solutions to treat infectious diarrhea in developing countries.

Table 2–4. Composition of oral rehydration solutions (ORS).

	Recommended Rehydration Therapy			Not Recommended	
	"Standard" ORS (WHO, 1975)	Reduced-Osmolarity ORS (WHO, 2002)	Rice-Based ORS (eg, Ceralyte)	Gatorade	Coke
Glucose (g/L)	111	75	—	—	—
Carbohydrate (g/L)	—	—	40	60	110
Sodium (mEq/L)	90	75	50–90	20	6
Potassium (mEq/L)	20	20	20	3	
Chloride (mEq/L)	80	65	40	14	26
Citrate (mEq/L)	10	10	30	3	
Osmolarity (mOsm/L)	311	245	225–275	350	650

Source: Reproduced with permission from Cheng AC: Infectious diarrhea in developed and developing countries. *J Clin Gastroenterol* 2005;39:757.

KEY READINGS

Bentzer P et al: Will this hemodynamically unstable patient respond to a bolus of intravenous fluids? JAMA 2016;316:1298.

Moritz ML, Ayus JC: Maintenance intravenous fluids in acutely ill patients. N Engl J Med 2015;373:1350.

Myburgh JA, Mythen MG: Resuscitation fluids. N Engl J Med 2013;369:1243.

EXTRACELLULAR FLUID VOLUME EXPANSION (EDEMATOUS DISORDERS)

▶ General Considerations

Hypervolemia reflects an increase in ECF volume, and generalized ECF volume overload implies total body sodium overload (and vice versa). A person is said to be *clinically hypervolemic* when the volume of isotonic fluid in their ECF is increased compared to euvolemia, and this surfeit can be inferred from the history and assessed on physical examination (eg, generalized edema). The presence of peripheral and/or pulmonary edema (expansion of the "second space") is usually due to underlying organ dysfunction such as congestive heart failure, cirrhosis, or kidney disease (eg, nephrotic syndrome). The term anasarca is applied when edema fluid also transfers into "third spaces" (eg, pleural effusion, ascites) and is widespread.

As discussed at the outset of this chapter, the effective arterial blood volume (EABV) is a concept that relates the cardiac output and the peripheral arterial resistance. In a normal individual, the actual EABV likely correlates well with the conceptual EABV, so that the total size of the ECF required for maintaining steady state sodium balance is a normal "euvolemic" size. In congestive heart failure (CHF), the decrease in cardiac performance leads to changes in the ECF volume and the EABV, and modifies the relation between them. The patient with compensated CHF can also maintain sodium balance in the steady state, but at a cost of a larger ECF volume. That is, the price of decreased cardiac function is hypervolemia. Therefore, a decrease in sodium intake (ie, a low-salt diet) is a cornerstone of care for these patients because the workload of the heart is directly related to the size of the ECF, and a decrease in sodium intake allows steady state to be achieved at a smaller ECF volume.

For example, consider a patient with CHF with an expanded ECF volume (as manifested by peripheral pitting leg edema) who has a plasma [Na] of 136 mmol/L and eats 6 g (261 mmol) of Na^+ per day. A reduction to a 2-g Na^+ (87 mmol) diet would result in a 1.3-L decrease in ECF volume because (261 − 87) mmol ÷ 136 mmol/L = 1.3 L. Steady state requires that one "excrete what you eat" and the reduction in dietary Na^+ allows steady state to be achieved at a lower ECF volume.

What about hypoalbuminemia as a cause of edema? Whereas total body sodium overload is necessary and sufficient to produce hypervolemia and/or edema in the steady state, hypoalbuminemia is neither necessary nor sufficient to produce edema in the steady state. Some examples follow: (1) A patient with edema from CHF may have a normal serum albumin, (2) albumin infusions do not reverse edema and ascites in a cirrhotic patient in the steady state, (3) individuals born without albumin do not have edema, and (4) severely hypoalbuminemic patients with nephrotic syndrome due to minimal change disease who respond to treatment begin to lose their edema before any significant increase in serum albumin has occurred. Most patients with generalized edema—except those with capillary leak syndromes associated with hypersensitivity, inflammation, and angioneurotic edema—are total body sodium overloaded. Another important exception may be the patient with flash pulmonary edema. The issue for patients with hypoalbuminemia is that often a fall in oncotic pressure leads to a fall in EABV and secondary sodium retention by the kidney leads to the development of edema.

Although total body sodium overload leads to generalized edema (ie, an increase in total body interstitial fluid), it should be noted that generalized edema may have a predilection for specific areas of the body. For example, cirrhotic physiology features the aggravating factors of portal hypertension and hypoalbuminemia, which leads to the formation of ascites (third spacing) when lymphatic drainage is overwhelmed. The effects of gravity will also influence the distribution of interstitial edema. During the usual hours of upright posture, accumulation of the edema fluid in the dependent parts of the body should be expected, whereas excessive hours at bed rest in the supine position will predispose to edema accumulation in the sacral and periorbital areas.

In discussing causes of ECF volume expansion below, emphasis will be placed on diagnosis and treatment of the ECF volume expansion itself. Other chapters (for nephrotic syndrome) or other volumes in this series (for congestive heart failure and cirrhotic ascites) should be consulted for additional details about specific diagnostic and treatment approaches.

CONGESTIVE HEART FAILURE

ESSENTIALS OF DIAGNOSIS

- ▶ History of dyspnea on exertion, orthopnea, and edema.
- ▶ Rales, an S3, and edema.
- ▶ The jugular pressure exceeds 3 cm above the sternal angle.
- ▶ Pulmonary vascular congestion is present on chest X-ray.
- ▶ Determination of B-type natriuretic peptide concentration is useful, when the cause of dyspnea is in doubt.

► Clinical Findings

A. Symptoms and Signs

Heart failure is the leading cause of morbidity among older adults in the country. Of the more than 1 million hospitalized per year, half will be readmitted within 6 months and up to one-third will die within 1 year. Early clinical symptoms of congestive heart failure occur before overt physical findings of pedal edema and pulmonary congestion. These symptoms relate to the gain in intravascular and interstitial volume resulting from compensatory renal sodium and water retention that accompanies arterial underfilling. Patients may experience dyspnea well before signs of pulmonary edema develop because of left ventricular dysfunction and an increased work of breathing. The latter is caused by fluid expansion into the pulmonary interstitium, which increases the weight of the lungs and increases lung stiffness. Exertion exacerbates the sensation of dyspnea.

The patient may present with a history of weight gain, weakness, dyspnea on exertion, decreased exercise tolerance, paroxysmal nocturnal dyspnea, and orthopnea. Nocturia may occur because in the supine position, peripheral edema can be reabsorbed back into the vascular space, which increases venous return, cardiac output (Starling law), and renal perfusion. Sympathetic tone and the activity of the RAAS are also decreased in the supine position, which helps explain why patients with congestive heart failure may lose considerable weight during the first few days of hospitalization (bed rest) without the administration of diuretics. Although overt edema is not detectable early in the course of congestive heart failure, the patient may complain of swollen eyes on awakening and tight rings and shoes, particularly at the end of the day. As much as 3–4 L of fluid can be retained before overt edema occurs.

1. Jugular venous pressure—As discussed above, the jugular venous pressure provides evidence of the state of the venous circulation on the right side of the heart and is very useful in evaluating patients with dyspnea. Many clinicians recommend estimating the CVP by assessing the internal jugular vein, but most formal analyses indicate that estimates of venous pressure can also be made from the external jugular vein, which runs across the sternocleidomastoid muscle. The patient should initially be recumbent, with the trunk elevated at 15–45° and the head turned slightly away from the side to be examined. The right-sided veins are preferred for assessment of venous pressure.

The external jugular vein is identified by placing the forefinger above the clavicle and pressing lightly. This will occlude the vein, which will then distend as blood continues to enter from the cerebral circulation. The external jugular vein can usually be seen more easily by shining a beam of light obliquely across the neck. At this point, the occlusion should be released and the vein occluded superiorly

to prevent distention by continued blood flow. The venous pressure can now be measured, since it will be approximately equal to the vertical distance between the upper level of the fluid column within the vein and the level of the right atrium (estimated as being 5–6 cm below the sternal angle). The normal venous pressure is 1–8 cm H_2O or 1–6 mm Hg (1.36 cm H_2O is equal to 1.0 mm Hg).

Alternatively, the internal jugular vein can be examined. In this case, the venous pulsations are best distinguished from arterial pulsations by their diffuse, multiphasic negative deflections (representing three troughs, the x, x_1, and y descents, respectively). In most situations, moreover, the venous pressure declines during inspiration, whereas the arterial pressure does not.

Although precise estimates of jugular venous pressure may be attempted, these techniques have had limited accuracy in controlled studies. Comparisons of measured and estimated jugular venous pressures suggest that clinicians tend to underestimate the venous pressure. Based on reviews of empirical trials, it has been suggested that the clinicians should attempt to determine only whether the jugular pressure is more than 3 cm H_2O above the sternal angle. If so, the venous pressure is elevated. More precise estimates of the jugular venous pressure do not generally add diagnostic information.

Measurement of the CVP is useful because it is often related directly to the left ventricular end diastolic pressure (LVEDP). There are clinical settings, however, in which the CVP does not provide a reliable estimate of the LVEDP and should not be used to guide therapy. First, some patients with pure left-sided heart failure exhibit normal CVP when the LVEDP is elevated. Conversely, the CVP overestimates the LVEDP in patients with pure right-sided heart failure or cor pulmonale. These patients may have high central venous pressures even in the presence of inadequate left-sided filling pressures.

2. Cardiac and pulmonary examinations—Cardiac failure is often associated with enlargement of the heart, either from left ventricular hypertrophy or dilated cardiomyopathy. A laterally displaced point of maximal impact has a high sensitivity and specificity for heart failure. Third heart sounds (an S3 gallop) also have both diagnostic and prognostic value in this situation. Evidence of pulmonary congestion (wet pulmonary crackles) and pleural effusions (third spacing, especially on the right side) are also consistent with an expanded ECF volume due to heart failure.

3. Extremities—As shown in Table 2–1, two-thirds of body fluid resides inside cells (ie, the ICF), and one-third resides outside cells (the ECF). The patient with generalized edema has an excess of ECF. The ECF resides in the vascular compartment (plasma fluid) and between the cells (interstitial fluid). In the vascular compartment, approximately 85% of the fluid resides on the venous side of the circulation and 15% on the arterial side. An excess of interstitial fluid constitutes edema. With digital pressure the interstitial fluid can generally be moved from the area of pressure and thus has been described as "pitting." If digital pressure does not cause pitting, either interstitial fluid cannot move freely or edema is absent. Pitting is more frequently demonstrated by using gentle pressure for longer periods of time rather than stronger pressure for shorter periods. In severe cases, pitting edema due to an expanded interstitium may extend from the feet to above the knees and even into the hips and abdominal wall. Presacral edema may be present as dependent edema while supine. Nonpitting edema can occur with lymphatic obstruction (ie, lymphedema) or regional fibrosis of subcutaneous tissue, which may occur with chronic venous stasis.

4. Other physical findings—Additional signs suggestive of the presence of heart failure that may be present include an abnormal hepatojugular reflux, a narrow pulse pressure, irregularly irregular pulse (atrial fibrillation due to dilated atria), and pulsus alternans.

B. Laboratory Findings

For dyspneic patients, the serum concentration of B-type natriuretic peptide (BNP) and N-terminal pro-BNP (NT-proBNP) may provide useful information above that provided by the history and physical examination. Although the test has only marginal value for classifying patients whose dyspnea is easily determined to be either cardiac or pulmonary, based on clinical parameters, it is very useful when the diagnosis is less than clear. Thus, determination of B-type natriuretic peptide concentration should be reserved for dyspneic patients in whom a diagnosis is in doubt.

BNP and NT-proBNP levels are increased in patients with LV dysfunction and heart failure (HF). A BNP less than 100 pg/mL has a high negative predictive value for HF, but will exceed 400 pg/mL in most patients with dyspnea due to HF, although it will not exclude the presence of a second cause of dyspnea (eg, a patient with HF and pneumonia). An NT-proBNP level under 300 pg/mL has a high negative predictive value for HF, but HF as the cause of dyspnea should be considered if the NT-proBNP exceeds 450 pg/mL (age under 50), 900 pg/mL (age 50–75), or 1800 pg/mL (age over 75).

Occult hypothyroidism or hyperthyroidism may present as congestive heart failure that is treatable; these conditions may be diagnosed with appropriate laboratory testing.

C. Imaging Studies

1. Chest X-ray—For dyspneic patients in whom ECF volume expansion is suspected, a posteroanterior (PA) and lateral chest radiograph is important, since the presence of cardiomegaly, pulmonary venous congestion (eg, cephalization of the pulmonary vessels), interstitial edema, Kerley-B lines, or pleural effusion is helpful in confirming the presence of volume overload and heart failure.

2. Echocardiogram—The echocardiogram provides invaluable information concerning the state of left ventricular contractility. The anatomy and movement of the chambers can be visualized and functional information relating to cardiac hemodynamics can be extracted. Categorization of heart failure into "systolic" dysfunction versus "diastolic" dysfunction provides both prognostic and therapeutic information. Some information about LVEDP can also be obtained.

▶ Differential Diagnosis

Patients with heart failure typically present with either edema or dyspnea. Edema may also result from nephrotic syndrome, cirrhosis of the liver, or local factors. Nephrotic-range proteinuria (>3.5 g/day) in the setting of hypoproteinemia suggests an important component of nephrosis. Typical stigmata of hepatic cirrhosis (eg, hepatomegaly, spider angiomata, caput medusa, and ascites) and laboratory abnormalities suggesting the same are often diagnostic of liver disease. Perhaps the most common diagnostic difficulty, however, is to determine whether dyspnea is the result of pulmonary or cardiac disease. As discussed above, the constellation of typical historical and physical findings of heart failure may point strongly to it as etiology, precluding the need for additional tests. When doubt is present, determination of the B-type natriuretic peptide level and echocardiography may prove invaluable.

▶ Treatment

Treatment of systolic dysfunction involves the use of angiotensin-converting enzyme (ACE) inhibitors, angiotensin receptor blockers (ARBs), β-adrenergic blocking drugs, digitalis glycosides, and aldosterone blocking drugs. Details of specific treatments can be found in the companion volume, *Current Diagnosis and Treatment in Cardiology*. The current discussion will focus on treatment of ECF volume overload itself.

A. Dietary Salt Restriction

The daily sodium intake in the United States is typically 4–6 g (1 g of sodium contains 43 mmol; 1 g of sodium chloride contains 17 mmol of sodium). By not using added salt at meals, the daily sodium intake can be reduced to 4 g (172 mmol), whereas a typical "low-salt" diet contains 2 g (86 mmol). Diets lower in sodium chloride content can be prescribed, but many individuals find them unpalatable. If salt substitutes are used, it is important to remember that these often contain potassium chloride; therefore potassium-sparing diuretics (eg, spironolactone, eplerenone, triamterene, amiloride) should not be used with potassium-containing salt substitutes.

Other drugs that increase serum potassium concentration must also be used with caution in the presence of salt substitute intake, including angiotensin converting enzyme inhibitors (ACEIs), ARBs, β-blockers, and nonsteroidal anti-inflammatory drugs (NSAIDs). When prescribing dietary therapy for an edematous patient, it is important to emphasize that sodium chloride restriction is required, even if diuretic drugs are employed. The therapeutic potency of diuretic drugs varies inversely with the dietary salt intake.

B. Diuretic Drugs

All commonly used diuretic drugs act by increasing urinary sodium excretion, that is, by acting as natriuretics. They can be divided into five classes, based on their predominant site of action along the nephron (Table 2–5). Osmotic diuretics (eg, mannitol) and proximal diuretics (eg, acetazolamide) are not employed as primary agents to treat edematous disorders. Loop diuretics (eg, furosemide) block the Na^+-K^+-$2Cl^-$ triple cotransporter, distal convoluted tubule diuretics (eg, hydrochlorothiazide) block the Na^+-Cl^- cotransporter, and collecting duct diuretics (eg, amiloride, spironolactone) block the epithelial Na^+ channel (ENaC) and mineralocorticoid receptor, respectively. All play important, but distinct, roles in treating edematous patients.

The goal of diuretic treatment of heart failure is to reduce ECF volume and to maintain the ECF volume at the reduced level in the steady state. This requires an initial natriuresis,

Table 2–5. Physiological classification of diuretic drugs.

Osmotic diuretics
Proximal diuretics
Carbonic anhydrase inhibitors
Acetazolamide
Loop diuretics (maximal FE_{Na} = 30%)
Na-K-2Cl inhibitors
Furosemide
Bumetanide
Torsemide
Ethacrynic acid
DCT diuretics (maximal FE_{Na} = 9%)
Na-Cl inhibitors
Chlorothiazide
Hydrochlorothiazide
Metolazone
Chlorthalidone
Indapamide[a]
Many others
Collecting duct diuretics (maximal FE_{Na} = 3%)
Na channel blockers
Amiloride
Triamterene
Aldosterone antagonists
Spironolactone
Eplerenone

CD, collecting duct; DCT, distal convoluted tubule.
[a]Indapamide may have other actions as well.

but at steady-state urinary sodium chloride excretion returns close to baseline despite continued diuretic administration. Importantly, an increase in sodium and water excretion does not prove therapeutic efficacy if ECF volume does not decline. Conversely, a return to "basal" levels of urinary sodium chloride excretion does not indicate diuretic resistance. The continued efficacy of a diuretic is documented by a rapid return to ECF volume expansion that occurs if the diuretic is discontinued.

It is important to establish a therapeutic goal—usually a target weight—when initiating loop diuretic treatment for edema. If a low initial dose does not lead to natriuresis, it can be doubled repeatedly until the maximum recommended dose is reached (Table 2–6). When a diuretic drug is administered by mouth, the magnitude of the natriuretic response is determined by the intrinsic potency of the drug, the dose, the bioavailability, the amount delivered to the kidney, the amount that enters the tubule fluid (most diuretics act from the luminal side), and the physiologic state of the individual. Except for diuretics that act in the proximal tubule, the maximal natriuretic potency of a diuretic can be predicted from its site of action. Table 2–5 shows that loop diuretics can increase fractional Na excretion to 30%, distal convoluted tubule (DCT) diuretics can increase it to 9%, and Na channel blockers can increase it to 3% of the filtered load.

More than 90% of patients admitted for heart failure are treated with loop diuretics, but up to 30% exhibit diuretic resistance (see below). The intrinsic diuretic potency of a diuretic is defined by its dose–response curve, which is generally sigmoid. Loop diuretics often described as "threshold drugs" because they are ineffective until a certain concentration appears in the urine. When starting loop diuretic treatment, it is important to ensure that the dose reaches the steep part of the dose–response curve before adjusting the dose frequency. In normal individuals, the relative potency of the loop diuretics is 40 mg furosemide equals 20 mg torsemide equals 1 mg bumetanide.

Because loop diuretics act rapidly, many patients will note an increase in urine output within several hours of taking the drug; this can be helpful in establishing that an adequate dose has been reached. Loop diuretics are short acting, so any increase in urine output more than 6 hours after a dose is unrelated to drug effects. This is the reason that most loop diuretic drugs should be administered at least twice daily, when given by mouth.

The bioavailability of diuretic drugs varies widely, between classes of drugs, between different drugs of the same class, and even within drugs. The bioavailability of loop diuretics ranges from 10% to 100% (mean of 50% for furosemide, 80–100% for bumetanide and torsemide). Limited bioavailability (eg, due to bowel edema) can usually be overcome by appropriate dosing, but some drugs, such as furosemide, are variably absorbed by the same patient on different days making precise titration difficult. It is customary to double the furosemide dose when changing from intravenous to oral therapy, but the relation between intravenous and oral dose may vary. For example, the

Table 2–6. Ceiling doses of loop diuretics.[a]

	Furosemide (mg)		Bumetanide (mg)		Torsemide (mg)	
	IV	PO	IV	PO	IV	PO
Renal insufficiency	80	80–160	2–3	2–3	50	50
GFR 20–50 mL/min						
GFR = 20 mL/min	200	240	8–10	8–10	100	100
Severe acute renal failure	500	NA	12	NA		
Nephrotic syndrome	120	240	3	3	50	50
Cirrhosis	40–80	80–160				1
	1–2	10–20				10–20
Congestive heart failure	40–80	160–240	2–3	2–3	20–50	50

GFR, glomerular filtration rate.

[a]Ceiling dose indicates the dose that produces the maximal increase in fractional sodium excretion. Larger doses may increase net daily natriuresis by increasing the duration of natriuresis without increasing the maximal rate.

Source: Reproduced with permission from Brady HR, Wilcox CS, eds: *Therapy in Nephrology & Hypertension*, WB Saunders, 1999.

amount of sodium excreted during 24 hours is similar when furosemide is administered to a normal individual by mouth or by vein despite its 50% oral bioavailability. This paradox results from the fact that oral furosemide absorption is slower than its clearance, leading to "absorption-limited" kinetics. For example, the peak natriuretic effect occurs 75 minutes after oral furosemide, but only 30 minutes after intravenous furosemide. Thus, effective serum furosemide concentrations persist longer when the drug is given by mouth because a reservoir in the gastrointestinal tract continues to supply furosemide to the body. This relation holds for a normal individual. Thus, it is difficult to predict the precise relation between oral and intravenous doses.

Patients with kidney disease will generally require higher doses of diuretics than individuals with normal kidney function, in part because of the lower filtered load of Na$^+$ that occurs when the glomerular filtration rate (GFR) is reduced. For example, the ceiling dose of oral furosemide in those without kidney disease is 40 mg, whereas up to 240 mg may be required in the setting of CHF and a GFR below 20 mL/min. Bumetanide and torsemide are generally more effective than furosemide in the setting of heart failure; torsemide has the longest half-life. The ceiling doses for the loop diuretics under various conditions are shown in Table 2–6.

Complications of diuretic therapy are shown in Table 2–7. Although hyponatremia may be a complication of diuretic treatment, furosemide can help to ameliorate hyponatremia in some patients with congestive heart failure when combined with ACE inhibitors, probably by improving cardiac output. Hypokalemia and hypomagnesemia are frequent complications of diuretic treatment in patients with heart failure because of secondary hyperaldosteronism.

This increases sodium delivery to the distal sites at which aldosterone stimulates potassium secretion. Severe renal magnesium wasting may also occur in the setting of secondary hyperaldosteronism and loop diuretic administration. Since both magnesium and potassium depletion cause similar deleterious effects on the heart, and potassium repletion is very difficult in the presence of magnesium depletion, supplemental replacement of both of these cations is frequently necessary in patients with cardiac failure. These complications have become less common with the advent of mineralocorticoid receptor antagonist treatment. It should be noted that furosemide, torsemide, and bumetanide all contain sulfonamide groups, so patients with severe allergy

Table 2–7. Complications of diuretics.

Contraction of the vascular volume
Orthostatic hypotension (from volume depletion)
Hypokalemia (from loop and DCT diuretics)
Hyperkalemia (from spironolactone, eplerenone, triamterene, and amiloride)
Gynecomastia (spironolactone)
Hyperuricemia
Hypercalcemia (thiazides)
Hypercholesterolemia
Hyponatremia (especially with DCT diuretics)
Metabolic alkalosis
Gastrointestinal upset
Hyperglycemia
Pancreatitis (DCT diuretics)
Allergic interstitial nephritis

DCT, distal convoluted tubule.

should be treated with ethacrynic acid, although it has been associated with severe ototoxicity.

Although thiazides are the cornerstone therapy for hypertension, they are used in the treatment of ECF volume overload in combination with loop diuretics, especially in patients who develop diuretic resistance (discussed later). Metolazone is a thiazide-like diuretic taken orally to promote volume removal, especially in patients with CHF or the cardiorenal syndrome. It is well absorbed, used at doses from 2.5 mg daily to 10 mg twice daily, and maintains efficacy even in those with kidney disease. To avoid excessive diuresis and relative volume contraction, patients taking metolazone and a loop diuretic should weigh themselves daily and be aware of a target weight.

Treatment of CHF and cirrhotic ascites with aldosterone antagonists (spironolactone and eplerenone) may be complicated by hyperkalemia. It is currently recommended that serum potassium be monitored 1 week after initiating therapy with an aldosterone blocker, after 1 month, and every 3 months thereafter. Patients should be counseled regarding a low-potassium diet and a serum potassium above 5.5 mmol/L should prompt an evaluation for medications such as potassium supplements or NSAIDs that might be contributing to the hyperkalemia. If such factors are not detected, the dose of aldosterone blocker should be reduced to 25 mg every other day. It is prudent to avoid use of aldosterone blockers in patients with a creatinine clearance less than 30 mL/min and to be cautious in those with a creatinine clearance between 30 and 50 mL/min. Those patients should be followed up even more closely than recommended above. The emerging availability of a new generation of potassium lowering drugs (patiromer and sodium zirconium cyclosilicate) may play a major role in helping patients tolerate mineralocorticoid receptor antagonist therapy.

KEY READING

Qavi AH, Kamal R, Schrier RW: Clinical use of diuretics in heart failure, cirrhosis, and nephrotic syndrome. Int J Nephrol Volume 2015, Article ID 975934, 9 pages.

DIURETIC RESISTANCE

ESSENTIALS OF DIAGNOSIS

▸ Inadequate diuresis despite maximal doses of loop diuretics.

▸ Exclude occult nephrotic syndrome.

▸ Exclude complicating drug use, such as NSAIDs.

▸ Exclude excessive dietary NaCl intake (24-hour Na excretion measurement).

▶ General Considerations

The major goal of diuretic therapy is to achieve a net natriuresis in order to decongest ECF volume overloaded patients with peripheral edema, pulmonary edema, ascites, and/or congestive nephropathy. A patient can be considered to be diuretic resistant when appropriate and near maximal doses of loop diuretics along with dietary sodium restriction fail to produce an adequate decrease in ECF volume in the setting of CHF (with or without cardiorenal syndrome), cirrhotic physiology, or nephrotic syndrome. When faced with apparent diuretic resistance, a number of assessments should be made, as follows:

• Is there optimal adherence to the diuretic regimen? For example, are adverse side effects leading to nonadherence?

• Is the patient adequately salt restricted? This may be assessed by measuring the daily urinary Na^+ excretion to ensure adherence with a low-salt diet.

• Has therapy for the underlying primary disorder or syndrome been optimized? For example, is a RAAS blocker being used to reduce the afterload (in a patient with heart failure) or proteinuria (in a patient with nephrotic syndrome)?

• Are factors that alter the pharmacokinetics of the diuretic present? For example, bowel edema can reduce drug absorption and bioavailability, and kidney disease reduces the concentration of the drug reaching the site of action in the tubule lumen.

• Are factors that alter the pharmacodynamics of drug action present? Effective natriuresis requires an adequate GFR without extreme Na^+ avidity of the nephron. For example, the SNS and RAAS may be profoundly activated in patients with severe CHF or cirrhosis, which reduces GFR and renders the proximal and distal parts of the nephron to be highly Na^+ avid. At the same time, the action of loop diuretics increases Na^+ delivery to the early DCT, which stimulates compensatory hypertrophy and increased activity of the DCT cells, which significantly limits natriuresis.

• Is hypoalbuminemia and/or hyperalbuminuria present? Both occur in nephrotic syndrome. Hypoalbuminemia will increase the volume of distribution because both loop and thiazide diuretics are highly protein bound. To make matters worse, albumin leaking across the glomerulus into the tubule will bind diuretics and blunt their natriuretic effect (although there is evidence that refutes this mechanism).

• Finally, are there other medications present that could interfere with diuretic action? Prostaglandins are required for the full diuretic effect of loop diuretics, so NSAIDs and COX-2 inhibitors will blunt diuresis. Medications such as cimetidine, trimethoprim, and probenecid—which compete with the secretion of diuretics into the proximal tubule—must be avoided.

▶ Clinical Findings

A. Symptoms and Signs

The major symptoms and signs of diuretic resistance are those that indicate ECF volume expansion, as described above. The most troublesome cause of diuretic resistance is progression of the underlying disease, because this situation may be difficult to address. Yet, it is always important to seek evidence of reversible or unexpected causes, so that appropriate and effective treatment can be designed. Perhaps the most common cause of diuretic resistance is impaired diuretic delivery to the active site. Most diuretics, including the loop diuretics, DCT diuretics, and amiloride, act from the luminal surface. Although diuretics are small molecules, most circulate tightly bound to protein and reach the tubule fluid primarily by secretion, and diuretic resistance occurs when drugs do not reach the tubule fluid at sufficient levels. Uremic anions, NSAIDs, probenecid, and penicillins all inhibit loop and DCT diuretic secretion into the tubule fluid. Thus, a history of renal failure or use of one of the above-mentioned drugs should always be sought. Chronic kidney disease shifts the loop diuretic dose–response curve to the right, requiring a higher dose to achieve maximal effect. Patients with chronic kidney disease are often given doses below those that are required to achieve therapeutic efficacy.

B. Laboratory Findings

One common cause of apparent diuretic resistance is excessive dietary sodium chloride intake. When sodium chloride intake is high, renal sodium chloride retention can occur between natriuretic periods, maintaining the ECF volume expansion. A careful history of dietary salt intake is always essential, but measuring the sodium excreted during 24 hours can be useful in diagnosing excessive intake. If the patient is at steady state (the weight is stable), then the urinary sodium excreted during 24 hours is equal to the dietary sodium chloride intake. If sodium excretion exceeds 100–120 mmol/day (approximately 2–3 g sodium/day), then dietary sodium chloride consumption is too high and dietary counseling should be undertaken. If the sodium excretion exceeds 100–120 mmol/day this also indicates that the patient is not diuretic resistant; this rate of sodium excretion should be sufficient to induce negative salt balance.

As noted above, diuretic resistance is common in chronic kidney disease. Further, diuretic treatment itself, especially in the setting of ACE inhibitors, may predispose to acute kidney injury. Both acute and chronic renal disease lead to diuretic resistance, and measurement of blood urea nitrogen and serum creatinine is always important.

▶ Treatment

Several strategies are available to achieve effective control of ECF volume in patients who do not respond to full doses of effective loop diuretics.

A. Combination Diuretic Therapy

A diuretic of another class may be added to a regimen that includes a loop diuretic to achieve sequential tubular segment blockade of sodium absorption (Table 2–8). This strategy produces true synergy; the combination of agents is more effective than the sum of the responses to each agent alone. DCT diuretics are the class of drug most commonly combined with loop diuretics. They inhibit adaptive changes (ie, hypertrophy) in the distal nephron that increase the reabsorptive capacity of the tubule and limit the potency of loop diuretics. Further, DCT diuretics have longer half-lives than loop diuretics. These drugs therefore prevent or attenuate NaCl retention during the periods between doses of loop diuretics (which should not exceed 8 hours), thereby increasing their net effect. When two diuretics are combined, the DCT diuretic is generally administered some time before the loop diuretic (1 hour is reasonable) in order to ensure that NaCl transport in the distal nephron is blocked when it is flooded with solute. When intravenous therapy is indicated, chlorothiazide (500–1000 mg) may be employed. In addition to the ability to block the Na^+-Cl^- cotransporter in the DCT, it also inhibits carbonic anhydrase in more proximal segments, further promoting a natriuresis. Metolazone is the oral DCT diuretic most frequently combined with loop diuretics because its half-life is relatively long and because it has been reported to be effective even when renal failure is present. Acetazolamide can be used for patients with a marked metabolic alkalosis.

Table 2–8. Combination diuretic therapy (to add to a ceiling dose of a loop diuretic).

Distal convoluted tubule diuretics
Metolazone 2.5–10 mg PO daily[a]
Hydrochlorothiazide (or equivalent) 25–100 mg orally daily
Chlorothiazide 500–1000 mg intravenously
Proximal tubule diuretics
Acetazolamide 250–375 mg daily or up to 500 mg intravenously
Collecting duct diuretics
Spironolactone 100–200 mg daily
Amiloride 5–10 mg daily

[a]Metolazone is generally best given for a limited period of time (3–5 days) or should be reduced in frequency to three times per week once extracellular fluid volume has declined to the target level. Only in patients who remain volume expanded should full doses be continued indefinitely, based on the target weight.

Source: Reproduced with permission from Brady HR, Wilcox CS, eds: *Therapy in Nephrology & Hypertension*, WB Saunders, 1999.

The dramatic effectiveness of combination diuretic therapy is accompanied by complications in a significant number of patients. Massive fluid and electrolyte losses have led to circulatory collapse during combination therapy and patients must be followed carefully and weigh themselves every day. The lowest effective dose of DCT diuretic should be added to the loop diuretic regimen; patients can frequently be treated with combination therapy for only a few days and then placed back on a single drug regimen; when continuous combination therapy is needed low doses of DCT diuretic (eg, 2.5 mg metolazone) administered only two or three times per week may be sufficient. Patients must also be closely monitored for electrolyte disturbances such as hypokalemia.

B. Continuous Diuretic Infusion

For hospitalized patients who are resistant to diuretic therapy, a different approach is to infuse loop diuretics continuously (Table 2–9). Continuous diuretic infusions have several advantages over bolus diuretic administration. First, because they avoid peaks and troughs of diuretic concentration, continuous infusions prevent periods of positive NaCl balance (postdiuretic NaCl retention) from occurring. Second, continuous infusions are more efficient than bolus therapy (ie, the amount of NaCl excreted per mg of drug administered is greater). Third, some patients who are resistant to large doses of diuretics given by bolus have responded to continuous infusion. Fourth, diuretic response can be titrated; in the intensive care unit where obligate fluid administration must be balanced by fluid excretion, excellent control of NaCl and water excretion can be obtained. Finally, complications associated with high doses of loop diuretics, such as ototoxicity, appear to be less common when doses are administered as continuous infusion. Total daily furosemide doses exceeding 1 g have been tolerated well when administered continuously over 24 hours. One approach is to administer a loading dose of 20 mg furosemide followed by a continuous infusion at 4–60 mg/h. In patients with preserved renal function, therapy at the lower dosage range should be sufficient. When renal failure is present, higher doses may be used, but patients should be monitored carefully for side effects such as ECF volume depletion and ototoxicity.

C. Bolus Versus Continuous Diuretic Infusion

In the Diuretic Optimization Strategies Evaluation (DOSE) trial, 308 patients with acute decompensated heart failure (ADHF) were prospectively randomized in a double-blind multicenter study to either low or high dose furosemide bolus every 12 hours or a continuous infusion of low or high dose furosemide. Patients were eligible if they presented within the previous 24 hours with ADHF, defined as having at least one symptom (dyspnea, orthopnea, edema) and one sign (pulmonary rales, peripheral edema, ascites, or pulmonary vascular congestion on chest radiograph). Patients also had to have a history of chronic heart failure and have been maintained on an oral dose of the equivalent of 80–240 mg furosemide for at least 1 month. Patients were excluded if systolic blood pressure was less than 90, they required intravenous vasodilators or inotropes, or had a serum creatinine greater than 3 mg/dL.

Patients were randomized into four groups in a 2-by-2 design, where the two variables were low- versus high-dose intravenous (IV) furosemide via bolus every 12 hours versus continuous infusion. Patients in the low-dose group received IV furosemide at the same level as their oral home dose, while the high-dose group received IV furosemide at 2.5 times the level of their oral home dose. Patients randomized to the furosemide bolus group also received a continuous infusion of placebo saline, and patient randomized to the furosemide continuous infusion group also received boluses of placebo saline (ie, the double blind/double dummy design). The home furosemide dose was ~130 mg/day for each of the four groups, and the average [Na] and creatinine for each group was 138 mmol/L and 1.5 mg/dL, respectively. Over the 72-hour study, patients in the low-dose group received a median of 358 mg IV furosemide while those in the high-dose group received a median of 773 mg IV furosemide. At 48 hours into the study, the treating physician had the option of either increasing the IV furosemide dose by 50% or switching to open label oral diuretics. Patients in the low-dose group were more likely to need the 50% increase while patients in the high-dose group were more likely to be switched to oral diuretics.

The major result of the DOSE trial was that there was *no difference* between bolus versus continuous infusion for the two primary endpoints, which were the patient's global assessment of symptoms and the mean change in serum creatinine. This result differed from smaller studies that suggested continuous infusion was superior to bolus therapy. There was, however, a significant improvement in patient reported dyspnea, net fluid loss, and freedom from congestion (jugular venous pressure less than 8 cm H_2O, no

Table 2–9. Continuous infusion of loop diuretics.

Diuretic	Starting Bolus (mg)	Infusion Rate (mg/h)		
		GFR <25 mL/min	GFR 25–75 mL/min	GFR >75 mL/min
Furosemide	40	20 then 40	10 then 20	10
Bumetanide	1	1 then 2	0.5 then 1	0.5
Torsemide	20	10 then 20	5 then 10	5

GFR, glomerular filtration rate.

orthopnea, zero to trace edema) at 72 hours in those receiving the continuous infusion.

KEY READING

Felker GM et al: Diuretic strategies in patients with acute decompensated heart failure. N Engl J Med 2011;364:797.

D. Ultrafiltration

Acute decompensated heart failure (ADHF) is one of the top causes of hospitalization in older adults and has the highest rate of readmission. Many of these patients have cardiorenal syndrome, and a number of recent studies have attempted to address whether extracorporeal venovenous ultrafiltration (UF) therapy is a superior alternative to pharmacological therapy with diuretics. In 2007, the Ultrafiltration Versus Intravenous Diuretics for Patients Hospitalized for ADHF (UNLOAD) trial showed promising results for UF.

In 2012, however, the Cardiorenal Rescue Study in ADHF (CARRESS-HF) trial failed to show any benefit of UF. In this trial, patients had to have 2+ peripheral edema, jugular venous pressure greater than 10 cm of H_2O, and pulmonary edema or pleural effusion on chest radiograph. Patients on IV vasodilators, inotropes, or creatinine greater than 3.5 mg/dL were excluded. UF was performed at a rate of 200 mL/h for a median of 40 hours. For stepped diuretics, IV furosemide was used as needed to achieve a daily urine volume of 3–5 L/day, with the median dose being 120 mg/day. Nearly half of the patients also received metolazone. Kidney function deteriorated more in the UF group, which also had more serious adverse effects. The authors stated that given "the high cost and complexity of ultrafiltration, the use of this technique … does not seem justified for patients hospitalized for ADHF, worsened renal function, and persistent congestion." It is important to realize that the patients undergoing UF in this trial were not diuretic resistant and this may be the subgroup where UF may be of benefit when no other pharmacological therapies are effective.

In 2015, the Aquapheresis Versus Intravenous Diuretics and Hospitalization for Heart Failure (AVOID-HF) trial was stopped early due to poor recruitment. Although it too showed no significant difference, the design was to individualize UF therapy for each patient. Therefore, it appears that optimized diuretic protocols will be used for management of ADHF at least until an appropriately powered study can be completed comparing adjustable UF with stepped pharmacological therapy.

KEY READING

Bart BA et al: Ultrafiltration in decompensated heart failure with cardiorenal syndrome. N Engl J Med 2012;367:2296.

HEPATIC CIRRHOSIS

ESSENTIALS OF DIAGNOSIS

- ▶ History of alcoholism or viral hepatitis.
- ▶ Stigmata of chronic liver disease including jaundice and spider angiomata.
- ▶ Signs of portal hypertension including ascites.
- ▶ Laboratory abnormalities include elevated bilirubin and reduced albumin.

▶ General Considerations

As discussed at the outset, disorders of ECF volume relate to changes in EABV, which in turn is the relation between cardiac output and peripheral arterial resistance. In CHF, the primary abnormality is a decrease in cardiac output, which results in activation of the SNS, RAAS, and other neurohormonal effector mechanisms that bring about a secondary increase in peripheral arterial resistance to maintain blood pressure. In cirrhosis of the liver, the primary abnormality appears to be a decrease in peripheral arterial resistance with a secondary increase in cardiac output. As cirrhosis with worsening portal hypertension progresses, splanchnic arterial vasodilation occurs, most likely due to increased production and/or decreased degradation of nitric oxide. Splanchnic vasodilation and decreased systemic vascular resistance—hallmarks of advanced cirrhosis—result in arterial underfilling. That is, although blood and plasma volume are increased, EABV is decreased, which activates the same neurohormonal effector mechanisms (SNS, RAAS, and ADH) that leads to salt and water retention, with development of peripheral edema and hyponatremia. The simultaneous presence of the cirrhotic physiology with portal hypertension predisposes to the formation of ascites (third spacing).

Diuretic resistance is common in cirrhosis with ascites because of the extreme Na^+ avidity of the proximal tubule, which limits distal Na^+ delivery to sites where loop, DCT, and CCD diuretics work. Further mechanisms of diuretic resistance include bowel edema (decreases drug absorption) and an increased volume of distribution due to hypoalbuminemia. Of course, any complications that may develop (eg, hypotension, bleeding varices, spontaneous bacterial peritonitis) will exacerbate the situation and increase the probability of diuretic resistance.

▶ Treatment

Options for treating cirrhotic ascites and edema include dietary NaCl restriction, diuretic drugs, large-volume paracentesis, peritoneovenous shunting, portosystemic shunting (usually transjugular intrahepatic portosystemic shunting or TIPS), and liver transplantation. Each of these approaches has a role in the treatment of cirrhotic ascites, but most patients (until end stage) can be treated successfully with dietary Na$^+$ restriction, diuretics, and, when necessary, large-volume paracentesis. A 2 g Na$^+$ limit is mandatory when ascites is present, and oral fluid restriction is necessary when serum [Na] falls below 125 mmol/L. The latter requires fluid intake be less than urine volume, which is not always possible.

Keeping mean arterial blood pressure above 82 mm Hg appears to be important for survival, and midodrine may improve systemic and splanchnic hemodynamics. ADH receptor antagonists (vaptans) have been used in the treatment of hyponatremia and ascites, and although serum [Na] improved, a large study showed mortality was higher in those using vaptan for recurrent ascites. Hepatotoxicity has been reported with vaptans, albeit at significantly higher doses than those typically used to treat hyponatremia.

A. Diuretics

The initial therapy of cirrhotic ascites is supportive, including dietary sodium restriction (<2000 mg sodium). When these maneuvers prove inadequate, diuretic treatment should begin with spironolactone. Spironolactone has several advantages over loop diuretics in this situation. First, spironolactone is more effective than furosemide as a single agent in reducing cirrhotic ascites. Second, spironolactone is a long-acting diuretic (half-life ~20 hours) that can be given once per day in doses ranging from 25 to 400 mg/day. Third, unlike most other diuretics, hypokalemia does not occur when spironolactone is administered. Hypokalemia increases renal ammoniagenesis and can precipitate encephalopathy.

The most common side effects of spironolactone are painful gynecomastia and hyperkalemia. Gynecomastia is less common with the more selective antagonist, eplerenone (half-life 4–6 hours), which may be substituted, but less information concerning its effectiveness in treating cirrhotic ascites is available. Amiloride, another K$^+$-sparing diuretic, can be used as an alternative, although spironolactone tends to be more effective.

For patients who do not respond to a low dose of spironolactone, spironolactone can be combined with furosemide, starting at 100 mg spironolactone/40 mg furosemide (to a maximum of 400 mg spironolactone/160 mg furosemide). This regimen has the advantages of once per day dosing and minimal hypokalemia. Torsemide may be more effective than furosemide. Patients who do not respond to this therapy are considered to have refractory ascites. Some authorities recommend a thiazide be added to spironolactone therapy rather than a loop diuretic. If the thiazide is not effective after 3 days, it should be replaced with a loop diuretic.

The appropriate rate of diuresis depends on the presence or absence of peripheral edema. Because mobilizing ascitic fluid into the vascular compartment is slow (approximately 500 mL/day), the rate of daily diuresis should be limited to 0.5 L/day if peripheral edema is absent. In the presence of edema, most patients can tolerate up to 1.0 L/day of fluid removal. Since ascites in the decompensated cirrhotic patient is associated with substantial complications including (1) spontaneous bacterial peritonitis (50–80% mortality), which does not occur in the absence of ascites; (2) impaired ambulation, decreased appetite, and back and abdominal pain; (3) elevated diaphragm with decreased ventilation predisposing to hypoventilation, atelectasis, and pulmonary infections; and (4) negative cosmetic and psychological effects, the treatment of the ascites with diuretics and sodium restriction is appropriate. The approach outlined above is successful in approximately 90% of patients and complications are rare. In earlier studies in which there were complications of diuretic therapy, more aggressive diuretic regimens were often used.

B. Large-Volume Paracentesis

Total paracentesis in increments over 3 days or, more commonly, at one episode has been shown to have few complications; in some studies paracentesis appears to have a lower incidence of complications than does diuretic treatment. Paracentesis (abdominal decompression) can be limited to 5 L if the ascites is responding to diuretics; otherwise the goal is to maximize fluid removal. Albumin replacement is necessary in the latter case, and especially important when ascites is present without peripheral edema.

When peripheral edema is absent, albumin (6–8 g for each liter of ascitic fluid removed) should always be infused to reduce hemodynamic compromise. The use of albumin remains controversial in patients with concomitant edema. Patients often favor paracentesis over diuretic treatment because symptoms improve more rapidly, but diuretics and salt restriction continue to be primary approaches and are required between paracentesis, even in those patients who cannot be maintained on diuretics alone.

C. Portosystemic Shunting

Portosystemic shunting is now usually performed via transjugular intrahepatic portosystemic shunt (TIPS). Uncontrolled trials suggested that TIPS increases urine output, reduces ascites, and reduces diuretic usage. In a meta-analysis TIPS was found to be effective in reducing ascites, but was also shown to carry a substantial complication rate, including inducing encephalopathy. Therefore it remains reserved for truly refractory patients who will not receive a liver transplant. Similar considerations apply to peritoneovenous (LeVeen) shunting. In controlled trials, peritoneovenous shunting was shown to reduce ascites more effectively than paracentesis or diuretics, but this was associated with a high rate of complications, and there was no survival advantage of the shunt.

D. Liver Transplantation

The development of ascites in a previously compensated cirrhotic patient is an indication for liver transplantation. In view of the morbidity and mortality associated with decompensated cirrhosis, liver transplantation is an important treatment for the ECF volume expansion that accompanies cirrhotic ascites. Worsening of ascites in a previously stable individual is most often caused by progressive liver disease but should also compel the search for hepatocellular carcinoma and portal vein thrombosis.

KEY READING

Ge PS, Runyon BA: Treatment of patients with cirrhosis. N Engl J Med 2016;375:767.

NEPHROTIC SYNDROME

ESSENTIALS OF DIAGNOSIS

- ▸ Signs of ECF volume expansion, including edema.
- ▸ Proteinuria greater than 3.5 g/day.
- ▸ Hypoalbuminemia.
- ▸ Hyperlipidemia may or may not be present.
- ▸ Kidney function may be normal or impaired.

▸ General Considerations

Another major cause of edema is the nephrotic syndrome, the clinical hallmarks of which include proteinuria (>3.5 g/day), hypoalbuminemia, hypercholesterolemia, and edema. Nephrotic edema may be mistaken for congestive heart failure if evidence for proteinuria or hypoalbuminemia is not sought. The lower the plasma albumin concentration, the more likely the occurrence of anasarca; the degree of sodium intake is, however, also a determinant of the degree of edema. The nephrotic syndrome has many causes (see Chapter 24). This discussion will focus on treatment of ECF volume expansion in nephrosis.

▸ Pathogenesis

Although edema formation in nephrotic syndrome (NS) also involves activation of the SNS, RAAS, and increased AVP levels, the pathogenesis of ECF volume expansion in nephrotic syndrome is more variable than the pathogenesis in congestive heart failure or cirrhotic ascites. Traditionally, ECF volume expansion in nephrotic syndrome was believed to depend on underfilling of the arterial circulation (ie, a decreased EABV). Several observations have raised questions about the "underfill" hypothesis; rather a role for primary renal sodium chloride

retention in the pathogenesis of nephrotic edema has been suggested (the "overfill" hypothesis). While "primary" renal NaCl retention may contribute to nephrotic edema in many patients, it is not often the only mechanism, and it appears therefore that nephrotic syndrome reflects a combination of primary renal sodium chloride retention and relative underfilling. In one study of over 200 patients, plasma volume was reduced in a third, increased in a quarter, and normal in the rest. The major consequence of the presence of a component of primary renal sodium retention is that nephrotic patients often tolerate relatively aggressive diuretic regimens without undue consequences. On the other hand, diuretics may worsen kidney function in those who may be underfilled.

▸ Treatment

The initial focus of therapy must be aimed at treatable underlying causes of nephrotic syndrome such as minimal change disease, membranous nephropathy, systemic lupus erythematosus or drugs (eg, phenytoin, NSAIDs) (see chapters on specific disease processes for additional details).

A. Diuretics

The treatment of the edema in nephrotic patients involves dietary sodium restriction and diuretics, as in other volume expansion disorders. As mentioned, because nephrotic patients may not be as underfilled as patients with cirrhosis or congestive heart failure, diuretics are often well tolerated.

Loop diuretics are always used as initial therapy. For several reasons, however, nephrotic patients are often quite resistant to these drugs. Although low serum albumin concentrations may increase the volume of diuretic distribution and albumin in the tubule lumen may bind to diuretics, these factors are not considered to be predominant causes of resistance. Rather, diuretic resistance likely reflects a combination of reduced glomerular filtration rate (from the ongoing glomerular disease) and intense renal sodium chloride retention (reflecting both primary renal sodium retention and a redistribution of fluid from the vascular compartment to the interstitium). For example, there is evidence that primary sodium retention in nephrotic syndrome can result from stimulation of the Na^+/H^+ exchanger in the proximal tubule, while certain proteases contained in the filtered protein can activate the epithelial sodium channel (ENaC) along the collecting duct.

B. Albumin

Administration of albumin to patients with the nephrotic syndrome can be costly and cause pulmonary edema. Mixing albumin with a loop diuretic (6.25 g albumin per 40 mg furosemide) may induce a diuresis in severely hypoalbuminemic patients. Co-administration of furosemide and albumin may be more effective than either albumin or furosemide alone, but only marginally so. In general, albumin should be reserved for the most refractory patients who are severely hypoalbuminemic.

KEY READING

Qavi AH, Kamal R, Schrier RW: Clinical use of diuretics in heart failure, cirrhosis, and nephrotic syndrome. Int J Nephrol 2015; 2015:975934.

▶ Acknowledgment

The author would like to acknowledge the contributions of David H. Ellison, who wrote the previous version of this chapter.

■ CHAPTER REVIEW QUESTIONS

Diagnosis/Treatment of Moderate and Severe Diarrhea due to Cholera

1. A localized outbreak of cholera occurs after severe flooding in the Gulf States. Patients are suffering a spectrum of gastrointestinal losses, but the fluid ("rice-water" stools) has a [Na] of 135–140 mM, a [Cl] of 100 mM, and a [HCO_3] of 25 mM. There are many patients, but, fortunately, most have mild-moderate losses and can be treated with standard oral rehydration solutions (ORS). A smaller number of patients suffering more severe losses (based on physical examination) will require intravenous fluid (IVF) therapy.

   Which behavior/physical examination findings would most support the use of IVF therapy?
   A. Restless/irritable
   B. Thirsty and drinks eagerly
   C. Poor skin turgor
   D. Urinary fractional excretion of Na (FENa) less than 1%
   E. Lethargic/obtunded

2. Which of the following is the best choice of IV solution to administer?
   A. 5% dextrose in water
   B. 0.45% (half-isotonic) saline
   C. 0.9% (isotonic) saline
   D. 0.45% saline with 75 mM bicarbonate added
   E. 3% (hypertonic) saline

Diagnosis/Treatment of Acute Decompensated Heart Failure and Diuretic Resistance

3. A 72-year-old man with a history of congestive heart failure is admitted 2 days after Thanksgiving for worsening dyspnea even at rest. Symptoms first became noticeable about 30 hours ago, and he has also noted swelling of his feet, ankles, and legs below the knee. Home medications include aspirin 81 mg daily, cimetidine 300 mg twice daily, furosemide 40 mg daily, and lisinopril 20 mg daily. For the past 4 days he has also been taking ibuprofen 400–600 mg 2–3 times daily for lower back pain. Vital signs show blood pressure is 136/85 with a heart rate of 92 beats/min and respirations at 28 breaths/min. He is afebrile; oxygen saturation is 90% on room air. Physical examination shows a chronically ill-appearing man in mild-moderate respiratory distress. Cardiovascular examination shows an elevated jugular venous pressure at 14 cm water, an S3 gallop, and 2+ pitting leg edema. Lungs show pulmonary crackles half way up bilaterally. Ascites is not present. The remainder of the examination is unremarkable, but his weight is 6 kg higher than that measured in cardiology clinic 1 month ago. Labs reveal plasma [Na] 134 mM (nl 136-144), [K] 3.7 mM (nl 3.5–5), [tCO_2] 26 mM (nl 22–28), BUN 42 mg/dL, Cr 1.8 mg/dL (baseline 1.2). The fractional excretion of sodium (FENa) is 0.6%. Chest X-ray shows bilateral pulmonary edema with Kerley B-lines and a small to moderate right pleural effusion.

   In addition to being placed on a low-Na diet, supplemental oxygen by nasal cannula, and discontinuation of ibuprofen, which of the following is the most reasonable initial approach to diuretic management?
   A. Furosemide 80 mg orally twice daily
   B. Furosemide 160 mg orally twice daily
   C. Furosemide 40 mg IV bolus (over 10 minutes)
   D. Furosemide 100 mg IV bolus (over 20 minutes)
   E. Furosemide 160 mg IV bolus (over 40 minutes)

4. The patient now becomes resistant to the maximal dose of furosemide (200 mg). In addition to discontinuing the cimetidine, which of the following is the most appropriate next step?
   A. Add oral metolazone at 10 mg prior to the first IV furosemide bolus of the day.
   B. Add oral hydrochlorothiazide at 50 mg prior to first IV furosemide bolus of the day.
   C. Add IV chlorothiazide at 500 mg prior to the first IV furosemide bolus of the day.
   D. Add oral spironolactone at 50 mg twice daily.
   E. Add oral amiloride at 10 mg twice daily.

Treatment of Cirrhosis

5. A 67-year-old man with a long history of nonalcoholic fatty liver disease has now developed stigmata of cirrhosis due to nonalcoholic steatohepatitis (NASH). He now presents complaining of abdominal distention developing over the past several weeks. He denies pain or jaundice, hematemesis, or melena. He does relate that he experiences some increased shortness of breath while recumbent. There have been no fevers or chills. Medications only include a high protein nutritional supplement (two 474 mL cans nightly) and a multivitamin. Vital signs show a blood pressure of 118/75 (MAP 89.3 mm Hg), heart rate of 80 beats/min, respiratory rate of 20 breaths/min, temperature 37.2°C, and oxygen saturation of 98% on room air. Physical examination shows spider angiomata, but normal cardiac and pulmonary findings. The abdomen is distended with a fluid wave and shifting dullness consistent with ascites. There is no peripheral edema. Labs reveal normal electrolytes with a plasma [Na] of 136 (nl 136–144) and creatinine of 0.8 mg/dL. Serum albumin is 3.2 g/dL. Sampling of the ascitic fluid revealed a serum-ascites albumin gradient (SAAG) consistent with portal hypertension. His weight is noted to be 7 kg heavier than 6 months previous.

In addition to a salt-restricted diet (< 2000 mg sodium per day), which of the following initial treatment plans is most appropriate?

A. Furosemide orally 40 mg daily
B. Spironolactone orally 100 mg daily
C. Large-volume paracentesis
D. Spironolactone 100 mg orally daily and furosemide orally 40 mg daily
E. Spironolactone 100 mg daily and hydrochlorothiazide 50 mg daily

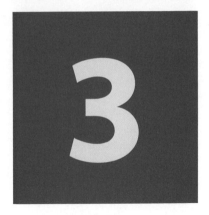

3

Disorders of Water Balance: Hyponatremia and Hypernatremia

Richard H. Sterns, MD

HYPONATREMIA

ESSENTIALS OF DIAGNOSIS

- ▶ Hyponatremia develops when water intake exceeds water losses.
- ▶ Most cases of hyponatremia are caused by impaired water excretion due to excess antidiuretic hormone (ADH).
- ▶ The reason for excess ADH can be determined by a clinical assessment of extracellular volume status and measurement of urine chemistries.

▶ General Considerations

Hyponatremia frequently occurs in hospitalized patients because acute illnesses often promote antidiuretic hormone (ADH) secretion. Outside the hospital, hyponatremia can be a side effect of medications, most notably thiazide diuretics and antidepressants, and it is a common problem among alcoholics, particularly heavy beer drinkers. Identifying the cause of persistent hyponatremia is important, because it can be an indication of serious, unsuspected underlying illnesses, such as adrenal insufficiency and small cell lung cancer. Hyponatremia can also develop in patients with heart failure and hepatic cirrhosis, and its appearance portends a bad prognosis. Chronic hyponatremia, even when mild, causes impaired cognition, gait disturbances, osteoporosis, falls and fractures. Very low serum sodium concentrations can result in serious neurological complications, either from hyponatremia itself, or from overzealous efforts to correct it.

▶ Pathogenesis

Excretion of dilute urine is the normal defense against hyponatremia (Figure 3–1). On a typical Western diet with normal kidneys, adults can match 18 L of daily water intake with 18 L (750 mL/h) of maximally dilute urine (urine osmolality 50 mOsm/kg). Psychotic patients can develop acute water intoxication within several hours, despite a normal ability to excrete water, if they drink more than 1 L/h. More often, patients with hyponatremia have impaired water excretion and become hyponatremic on more modest water intakes; in most cases, the reason is too much antidiuretic hormone (ADH), a hormone released from the posterior pituitary that promotes water reabsorption by the kidney. The presence of ADH is reflected by urine that is not maximally dilute (urine osmolality >100 mOsm/kg) and is, rather, sometimes very concentrated (up to a maximum urine osmolality of 1200 mOsm/kg).

ADH levels should normally be low when the serum sodium concentration falls, but an inadequate circulating volume (due to volume depletion, heart failure, or hepatic cirrhosis), can stimulate ADH secretion despite low serum sodium levels; in such cases, the kidney avidly reabsorbs sodium. ADH-mediated hyponatremia with a normal circulation is considered "inappropriate." Because sodium excretion is controlled by effective intravascular volume, and not the serum sodium concentration or ADH, the syndrome of inappropriate ADH secretion (SIADH) is characterized by sodium excretion that equals or exceeds sodium intake.

In some cases, impaired water excretion is persistent, so that patients are always at risk of hyponatremia, unless their water intake is restricted or the effect of ADH is thwarted. In other cases, impaired water excretion is reversible, so that hyponatremia may correct itself through excretion of excess water in a dilute urine.

The plasma sodium concentration usually determines the tonicity of extracellular fluid. Hypotonicity makes cells swell, which is most important in the brain. Given enough time (about 48 hours), brain cells adapt to hyponatremia by extruding intracellular solutes called organic osmolytes. Because it takes more time for the brain to reaccumulate organic osmolytes than to lose them, too much correction of hyponatremia

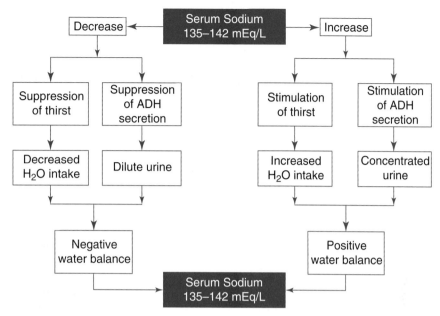

▲ **Figure 3–1.** Normal osmoregulation.

in too short a time (>8 mEq/L/day) in susceptible patients can damage astrocytes, resulting in the osmotic demyelination syndrome. Overcorrection of hyponatremia is often caused by recovery of the ability to excrete dilute urine, which can raise the serum sodium concentration by greater than 2 mEq/L/h.

▶ **Prevention**

Hyponatremia can be avoided in the hospital by limiting the prescription of hypotonic intravenous fluids (eg, 5% dextrose in water, 0.45% saline) to patients whose serum sodium concentrations are high, and by checking serum sodium levels daily when patients are treated with intravenous fluids or diuretics. Because the stress of surgery almost always results in ADH secretion, hypotonic fluids should almost never be given during the first two postoperative days, and, because patients with high ADH levels can extract water from saline, large volumes of isotonic fluids (eg, 0.9% saline, lactated Ringers) should be avoided in postoperative patients and in other patients with SIADH.

Thiazide diuretics are one of the most common causes of hyponatremia; they should not be prescribed to heavy beer drinkers or patients with psychotic polydipsia and they should be temporarily withheld when patients are acutely ill or undergo surgical procedures.

▶ **Clinical Findings**

A. Symptoms and Signs

The symptoms and signs of hyponatremia result from cerebral edema if the condition develops rapidly (<24 hours) and

from an adaptive reduction in cell solute that helps minimize brain swelling if the condition develops more gradually. Although no consistent correlation between the degree of hyponatremia and neurological manifestations exists, patients with seizures and altered sensorium generally have serum sodium concentrations less than 120 mEq/L.

Acute hyponatremia developing over less than 48 hours is more likely to present with severe symptoms due to the lack of complete cerebral adaptation. In acute hyponatremia, symptoms of headache, nausea and vomiting, delirium or lethargy reflect increased intracranial pressure that may rapidly progress to seizures, coma, respiratory arrest, or fatal herniation. In contrast, "chronic" hyponatremia, developing over more than 48 hours, even when severe, does not cause severe brain swelling due to the brain's adaptations to hypotonicity. Symptoms of nausea, vomiting, confusion, lethargy, gait disturbances, and, occasionally, seizures, in chronic hyponatremia reflect altered brain chemistry caused by the adaptive loss of cellular osmolytes. Sometimes, chronically hyponatremic patients may appear to be asymptomatic despite extremely low serum sodium concentrations, but formal testing will reveal abnormalities in cognition and gait. Adaptations that protect against lethal brain swelling in chronic hyponatremia make the brain vulnerable to permanent injury if hyponatremia is corrected too rapidly.

B. Laboratory Findings

Laboratory findings depend on the cause of hyponatremia, and they are helpful in the differential diagnosis. Because

Table 3–1. Hyponatremia with a urine osmolality (Uosm) <100 mOsm/kg.

Condition	Mechanism
Psychosis with polydipsia	Water intake episodically >1 L/h exceeding maximum capacity to excrete water
Beer potomania Tea and toast diet	Low-protein diet reduces urine urea excretion and results in low rate of solute excretion and limited urine volume despite maximally dilute urine: Urine volume = Rate of solute excretion/Uosm
Reversible cause of hyponatremia	Urine becomes maximally dilute once cause of hyponatremia resolves • After saline therapy in hypovolemic hyponatremia • After discontinuation of thiazide diuretic • After discontinuation of medication causing SIADH • After steroid therapy in adrenal insufficiency

Table 3–2. Clues to a diagnosis of hypovolemic hyponatremia.

- Urine sodium concentration <20 mEq/L
- Urine osmolality <100 mOsm/kg after administration of 0.9% saline
- Abnormal serum bicarbonate
  - High: vomiting or gastric drainage, diuretics
  - Low: diarrhea
- Abnormal serum potassium
  - High: Addison disease
  - Low: vomiting, diarrhea, or diuretics

direct laboratory measurement of ADH (vasopressin) is technically difficult, yielding unreliable results, urine osmolality is used as a "bioassay" for the hormone, and actual measurement of vasopressin is unnecessary. The urine osmolality is usually high (or, at least not low), reflecting persistent secretion of ADH, but there are exceptions (Table 3–1).

Urine sodium concentrations vary, depending on the condition responsible for persistent secretion of ADH. If the cause is hypovolemia, heart failure, or hepatic cirrhosis, the kidney responds with increased reabsorption of filtered sodium and urine sodium concentrations are less than 20 mEq/L; if the cause is Addison disease (primary adrenal insufficiency) the kidney wastes sodium, and urine sodium concentrations are greater than 20 mEq/L despite hypovolemia; if the cause is SIADH, urine sodium excretion matches or exceeds sodium intake and urine sodium concentrations are usually greater than 30 mEq/L; if the cause is a thiazide diuretic, the urine sodium may also be greater than 30 mEq/L, mimicking SIADH.

If hypovolemia is due to vomiting, urinary sodium levels may not be low because high serum bicarbonate levels increase urine bicarbonate excretion (an anion), which obligates excretion of sodium and potassium; in this situation, hypovolemia can be confirmed by measuring the urinary chloride concentration, which is typically less than 10 mEq/L.

Several laboratory clues can help distinguish between SIADH and hypovolemic hyponatremia (Table 3–2). The serum potassium and serum bicarbonate concentrations are normal in patients with SIADH. Hyperkalemia suggests the possibility of hyponatremia due to Addison disease; hypokalemia or high serum bicarbonate suggests hypovolemic hyponatremia due to vomiting or diuretics; low serum

bicarbonate suggests hypovolemic hyponatremia due to diarrhea.

Blood urea nitrogen (BUN), creatinine, and uric acid also vary depending on the cause of hyponatremia. Oliguric renal failure limits the ability to excrete water regardless of ADH levels and both the BUN and creatinine are elevated. In SIADH, BUN and uric acid levels are low and serum creatinine is normal. In hyponatremia caused by hypovolemia or decreased effective vascular volume, BUN and uric acid levels are elevated.

C. Imaging Studies

Computed tomography (CT) scans may reveal cerebral edema in severe acute hyponatremia; evidence of brain swelling resolves after treatment. When rapid correction of chronic hyponatremia leads to the osmotic demyelination syndrome, Magnetic resonance imaging (MRI) is initially normal, but repeat scans after 2 weeks reveal lesions in the pons, basal ganglia, and subcortical white matter. In patients with persistent SIADH of unknown cause, CT scans of the head and chest are indicated to exclude neuroendocrine tumors of the sinuses, pituitary disease, brain tumors, or lung cancer.

▶ Differential Diagnosis

Hyponatremia should be approached systematically (Figure 3–2):

Step 1: Measure urine osmolality—Urine osmolality helps distinguish between hyponatremia caused by an inability to appropriately dilute the urine (to a urine osmolarity <100 mOsm/kg) and hyponatremia that develops despite a normal ability to dilute the urine (see Table 3–1). If urine osmolality is less than 100 mOsm/kg, hyponatremia may have been caused by excessive fluid ingestion or inadequate solute intake. However, if the measurement was *after* infusion of isotonic saline, dilute urine may represent recovery from hypovolemic hyponatremia. In either case, excretion of maximally dilute urine will rapidly correct hyponatremia spontaneously.

Step 2: Exclude non-hypotonic hyponatremia—Usually, a low plasma sodium concentration means that body

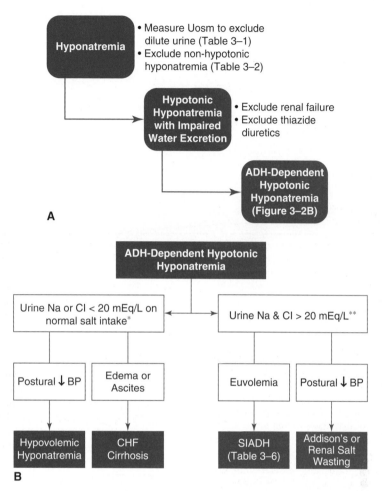

▲ **Figure 3–2 A.** Diagnostic approach to hyponatremia. **B.** Diagnostic approach to ADH-dependent hypotonic hyponatremia.

fluids are too dilute (hypotonicity) and that corrective measures are needed, but there are important exceptions (Table 3–3). The most common is hyperglycemia, a *hypertonic* condition that lowers plasma sodium by causing a shift of water out of cells. If hyperglycemia is present, add 2 mEq/L to the reported sodium concentration for every 100 mg/dL increase in plasma glucose.

If a condition associated with non-hypotonic hyponatremia is present (see Table 3–3), the serum sodium concentration should be remeasured using the laboratory's autoanalyzer. The repeat serum sodium concentration is compared to the plasma sodium concentration measured with a sodium-sensing electrode (available on blood-gas machines) in undiluted blood or plasma; in addition, the plasma osmolality is measured with an osmometer and the value is compared to the plasma osmolality calculated

from the repeat serum sodium, blood glucose, and BUN (see Table 3–3).

Measurement of plasma osmolality is unnecessary, and occasionally confusing, in the absence of conditions that cause non-hypotonic hyponatremia. For example, hyponatremic patients who have been drinking alcohol have hypotonicity, but osmolality may be normal because ethanol is measured by the osmometer. Because urea is also detected by the osmometer, plasma osmolality may also be normal in hypotonic hyponatremia caused by renal failure.

Step 3: Exclude oliguric renal failure and thiazide diuretics—Patients with severe renal failure are unable to excrete excess water and become hyponatremic despite suppression of ADH secretion. Urine osmolality is typically close to plasma osmolality regardless of the plasma

Table 3–3. Causes of non-hypotonic hyponatremia.

Condition	Plasma Osmolality	Osmolar Gap[a]	Direct Na-Sensing Electrode[b]
Hyperglycemia	High	No gap	Plasma Na low
IV Mannitol	High	Gap present	Plasma Na low
Absorption of glycine and other irrigants during prostate or intrauterine surgery	Normal or slightly low	Gap present	Plasma Na low
Hyperlipidemia (pseudohyponatremia)	Normal	Gap present	Plasma Na normal
Hypercholesterolemia with jaundice—lipoprotein X (pseudohyponatremia)	Normal	Gap present	Plasma Na normal
Hyperproteinemia—plasma cell dyscrasias (pseudohyponatremia)	Normal	Gap present	Plasma Na normal

[a]An osmolar gap is present if the plasma osmolality (Posm) measured by an osmometer is >10 mOsm/kg higher than Posm calculated from the serum sodium concentration (in mmol/L), blood glucose (in mg/dL), and BUN (in mg/dL):

$$\text{Calculated Posm} = 2\,[Na^+] + Gluc/18 + BUN/2.8$$

[b]In pseudohyponatremia, the aqueous portion of a serum sample is reduced by protein or lipid. Autoanalyzers employing a dilution step sample an abnormally low amount of plasma water, artifactually lowering the measured sodium concentration. Measurement with a sodium sensing electrode in undiluted plasma is free of this artifact.

sodium concentration. The patient may also be edematous due to impaired sodium excretion.

Thiazide diuretics impair the ability to dilute the urine while preserving the ability to excrete concentrated urine. Patients taking thiazides may present with clinical features identical to those found in SIADH. The thiazide should be discontinued and the patient's ability to excrete water should be reassessed after 2–3 weeks off the drug.

Step 4: Assess volume status and measure the urine sodium and chloride—At this stage in the differential diagnosis, it has been established that the patient has hypotonic hyponatremia, does not have oliguric renal failure, is not taking thiazides, and is excreting urine that is not maximally dilute. Therefore, hyponatremia can be attributed to the continued presence of ADH (or, very rarely, an inherited abnormality of the ADH receptor). By assessing volume status clinically and measuring the urine sodium and chloride, hypovolemic hyponatremia, and hyponatremia caused by congestive heart failure (CHF) or hepatic cirrhosis can be distinguished from SIADH (see Figure 3–2).

1. Hypovolemic hyponatremia—In hypovolemic hyponatremia, nonosmotic release of ADH occurs in response to hypovolemia. Despite serum hypoosmolality, circulating ADH causes urinary concentration, water retention, and hyponatremia. A patient with hypovolemia has a deficit of total body sodium resulting from either extrarenal or renal sodium losses. The sodium deficit may result in postural hypotension and prerenal azotemia; however, secondary retention of water partially corrects hypovolemia, masking these clinical findings. Extrarenal sodium loss can occur from the gastrointestinal tract in the form of vomiting or diarrhea, from sweat, or through third-space fluid sequestration. These conditions are usually evident from the history. Renal sodium loss is common after diuretic administration or during osmotic diuresis. More rarely, renal sodium loss can be caused by salt-losing nephropathy (eg, after cis-platinum chemotherapy), or mineralocorticoid deficiency. Hypovolemia caused by vomiting results in a urine chloride less than 20 mEq/L while other causes of extrarenal sodium loss result in a urine sodium less than 20 mEq/L. If patients with hypovolemic hyponatremia are given isotonic saline, the stimulus for ADH secretion is abolished, the urine becomes dilute, and the plasma sodium concentration will return to normal.

2. Edematous hyponatremia—In patients with hyponatremia caused by heart failure or cirrhosis, both total body sodium and total body water are increased, but total body water is increased to a greater amount. These disease states all have a low effective circulating arterial volume that results in excessive thirst and ADH release. The degree of hyponatremia often correlates with the severity of the disorder and is an important prognostic factor. In the absence of diuretics, the urinary sodium concentration is typically less than 10 mEq/L. Administration of isotonic saline worsens edema and fails to decrease urine osmolality or correct hyponatremia.

3. Euvolemic hyponatremia—Hyponatremic patients who are unable to dilute their urine appropriately, who do not have renal failure and are not taking thiazide diuretics, and are neither hypovolemic, nor edematous can be classified as having SIADH (Table 3–4). In SIADH, however, ADH is inappropriately released and the urine, consequently, is concentrated. Despite abnormal water handling, sodium regulatory mechanisms remain intact and patients do not become edematous; urine sodium excretion matches sodium intake. Hypouricemia is commonly seen in SIADH due to both dilution and increased uric acid elimination. If patients with SIADH are given isotonic saline, the urine remains concentrated, and the excess sodium is excreted in the urine, potentially exacerbating hyponatremia.

Step 5. If the patient has SIADH, determine its cause— A diagnosis of SIADH is like a diagnosis of "fever"; it is essential to determine its cause. Particularly in smokers, small cell lung cancer and head and neck tumors should be excluded, and, if no other cause is found, it is important to rule out hypopituitarism. SIADH is most commonly associated with medication administration (Table 3–4). With widespread use, selective serotonin reuptake inhibitor (SSRI) antidepressants are frequent causative agents, particularly among the elderly. Pulmonary or central nervous system (CNS) disease, infection, and trauma are responsible for the remainder of cases. SIADH is also been frequently described in association with human immuno-deficiency virus (HIV) infection.

Table 3–4. Causes of the syndrome of inappropriate ADH secretion (SIADH).

Tumors	Small cell carcinoma of the lung (most common) Head and neck tumors • Squamous carcinoma • Esthesioneuroblastoma of the sinuses
Pulmonary disorders	Infectious (bacterial, viral, and fungal pneumonia and tuberculosis) Functional (asthma, acute respiratory failure, and mechanical ventilation)
Neurologic disorders	Head trauma and brain surgery Neoplasms (primary and metastatic) Vascular (hemorrhage, infarction, and vasculitis) Infection (meningitis, brain abscess, and encephalitis) Miscellaneous (Guillain–Barré syndrome, multiple sclerosis, hydrocephalus, Shy–Drager syndrome)
Endocrine disorders[a]	Glucocorticoid deficiency (hypopituitarism) Severe hypothyroidism (controversial)
Drugs	Antidiuretic hormones (vasopressin, desmopressin, and oxytocin) Antiarrhythmics (amiodarone, lorcainide, propafenone) Antibiotics (ciprofloxacin, rifabutin, vidarabine) Anticonvulsant drugs (carbamazepine, oxcarbazepine, sodium valproate, levetiracetam) Antineoplastic agents (cyclophosphamide, vincristine, and vinblastine) Diabetic agents (chlorpropamide and tolbutamide) "Ecstasy" (3,4-methylenedioxymethamphetamine) Nonsteroidal anti-inflammatory drugs Psychotropic agents (tricyclic antidepressants, serotonin and norepinephrine reuptake inhibitors, monoamine oxidase inhibitors) Proton pump inhibitors
Other causes	Nausea Surgical procedures and anesthesia Alcohol withdrawal AIDS

[a]Many authors do not include endocrine disorders in the differential diagnosis of SIADH. We include because unrecognized glucocorticoid deficiency caused by pituitary disease often presents with clinical features typical of SIADH. When hypothyroidism causes hyponatremia, it is usually severe enough as to present with myxedema coma.

Complications

Untreated hyponatremia is associated with an increased incidence of falls and fractures. If the serum sodium falls below 120 mEq/L in less than 24 hours, it results in cerebral edema and, rarely, death from herniation. Rapid correction of chronic hyponatremia can cause permanent brain damage due to demyelinating brain lesions (osmotic demyelination syndrome).

Treatment

A. Severe Hyponatremia in the Hospital

When hyponatremia develops in the hospital, or when patients are admitted to the hospital because of hyponatremia, there is a serious risk of major morbidity and mortality, particularly if the serum sodium is less than 120 mEq/L. There are three important goals in this setting:

- Ensure that the serum sodium concentration falls no further.

- Raise the serum sodium concentration enough to relieve hyponatremic symptoms and prevent neurological complications from the untreated electrolyte disturbance.

- Avoid neurological injury due to overcorrection.

Thiazide diuretics and medications known to cause hyponatremia should be discontinued if possible and fluid intake should be restricted. In most cases, restricting fluid intake to less than 1 L/24 hours will be sufficient to avoid worsening of hyponatremia. Treatment with isotonic saline is only indicated when the patient is clearly hypovolemic. In patients who are not hypovolemic, no more than 1 L of 0.9% saline should be given in 24 hours, because in SIADH, isotonic saline may cause the serum sodium to fall further and may precipitate or aggravate neurologic symptoms. In patients with acute postoperative hyponatremia who have already been given large volumes of isotonic or hypotonic saline, the plasma sodium concentration may fall spontaneously if the electrolyte concentration in the urine is higher than the plasma sodium concentration; in such cases, a small volume of hypertonic saline may be needed, regardless of symptoms, just to keep the serum sodium from falling.

1. Emergency therapy—Patients at high risk of herniation or complications from seizures (Table 3–5) require emergency treatment with hypertonic saline to rapidly increase the serum sodium by 4–6 mEq/L. This is best achieved with 100 mL bolus infusions of 3% saline, repeated as needed every 10–15 minutes to a maximum dose of 4 mL/kg body weight.

A more gradual onset of hyponatremia (over 48 hours or more) carries virtually no risk of herniation, even when the serum sodium is less than 100 mEq/L. In the past, it was believed that the serum sodium must be rapidly raised to a "safe level" above 120 mEq/L or even above 130 mEq/L. There is no evidence to support this practice and it places patients with extremely low serum sodium concentrations at risk of developing neurological complications from overcorrection. When the duration of hyponatremia is unknown, it should be presumed to be chronic with a risk of osmotic demyelination syndrome (ODS). While some clinicians may choose to begin therapy with 3% saline in patients with serum sodium concentrations <115 mEq/L to reduce the risk of seizures, correction should not exceed 8 mEq/L/24 h (see below).

2. Avoiding overcorrection and ODS—Chronically hyponatremic patients with serum sodium concentrations less than 120 mEq/L may develop ODS if hyponatremia is corrected by too much in too short a time. Because this complication of therapy reflects apoptosis of astrocytes, clinical findings are delayed, emerging 1 to several days after treatment of hyponatremia. In severe cases of the syndrome, patients may be left with permanent, severe, and sometimes fatal brain damage. Conditions that increase the risk of developing ODS are listed in Table 3–6. Susceptibility to ODS may be reduced by giving thiamine to patients suspected of malnutrition and by correcting hypokalemia and hypophosphatemia.

ODS can be avoided by limiting correction of hyponatremia to no more than 8 mEq/L/day. An increase of 8 mEq/L

Table 3–5. Indications for emergency treatment of hyponatremia.

- Acute self-induced water intoxication associated with
  - Psychosis with polydipsia
  - Competitive exercise (marathon runners)
  - Use of "ecstasy"
- Symptomatic acute (<24 hours) postoperative hyponatremia
- Symptomatic hyponatremia with intracranial pathology
- Hyponatremia with seizures or coma

Table 3–6. High risk of osmotic demyelination after correction of chronic hyponatremia.[a]

- Serum Na <105 mEq/L
- Hypokalemia
- Alcoholism
- Malnutrition
- Liver disease

[a]Chronic hyponatremia is defined as a known duration of >48 hours. Hyponatremia is presumed to be chronic when the duration of hyponatremia is unknown.

represents the *limit*, not to be exceeded, and not the *goal* of therapy. To avoid overshooting the mark, correction efforts should target a *daily* increase of 4–6 mEq/L/day. This does not preclude prompt, rapid correction in the first few *hours* of therapy because an increase of 4–6 mEq/L is sufficient to relieve the most serious complications of untreated hyponatremia. This strategy can be described by an easy to remember rule of sixes (where the abbreviation "sx's" stands for symptoms):

"Six a day for safety so six in 6 hours for severe sx's and *stop*."

The rule means that correction efforts can be front-loaded in the first few hours for severely symptomatic patients, and once the goal is achieved, further correction is postponed for subsequent days.

Avoiding overcorrection can be challenging, because many patients have reversible defects in water excretion (see Table 3–1). Once the cause of hyponatremia is eliminated (eg, after repair of hypovolemia with intravenous saline), the urine becomes appropriately dilute, and excretion of electrolyte-free water will spontaneously and rapidly correct hyponatremia. For this reason, predictive formulas are unreliable guides and it is essential to monitor urine output and to measure the serum sodium values frequently (at least every 4–6 hours) until the serum sodium has been increased above 125 mEq/L. If a water diuresis emerges during therapy, urinary water losses should either be matched with intravenous D5W or stopped with desmopressin (a synthetic ADH). Alternatively, in patients with reversible causes of hyponatremia (see Table 3–1), desmopressin can be administered proactively at the beginning of therapy, with repeat doses every 8 hours, so that when endogenous ADH secretion ceases, the urine remains concentrated; the serum sodium is then increased gradually with a concurrent slow infusion of 3% saline. Desmopressin is discontinued once the serum sodium has been raised above 125 mEq/L.

Hypokalemic patients often have reversibly impaired water excretion caused by diuretics or vomiting. Overcorrection is particularly common in hypokalemic patients because replacement of potassium increases the serum sodium concentration; sodium, which had moved intracellularly to replace cellular potassium, returns to the extracellular fluid when potassium is repleted.

B. Mild to Moderate Hyponatremia

Because even mild hyponatremia can increase the risk of falls, restoring normonatremia is an appropriate goal. Hypovolemic patients are primarily seen in the hospital and hyponatremia corrects readily after treatment with isotonic saline. Hospitalized patients with hyponatremia caused by heart failure, cirrhosis, or SIADH will require fluid restriction; its effectiveness can be predicted by measuring the summed concentrations of sodium and potassium in the urine. If the urine ($Na^+ + K^+$) concentration is less than half the serum sodium concentration, fluid restriction should result in gradual correction of hyponatremia; if the urine cation concentration is higher than the serum sodium concentration, fluid restriction will be ineffective and other measures will be required.

3. Loop diuretics and salt—For most ambulatory patients and for many persistently hyponatremic patients in the hospital, fluid restriction is not a satisfactory treatment. Some patients respond to loop diuretics, like furosemide, which limit the ability of ADH to concentrate the urine by impairing formation of the concentration gradient in the renal medulla. Furosemide given two or three times daily with less dietary sodium restriction can be effective in patients with heart failure and cirrhosis. Salt tablets (2 g three times daily) combined with furosemide can be effective in some patients with SIADH.

4. ADH (vasopressin) antagonists—The vasopressin antagonist conivaptan, which is given intravenously, is an option in the hospital, and tolvaptan, an oral antagonist are options for both hospitalized and ambulatory patients with heart failure and SIADH. These agents, knows as "vaptans" block the ADH receptor in the collecting duct, resulting in a dilute urine and increased urinary water losses. Conivaptan is more expensive and less predictable than 3% saline and it causes phlebitis, but it can be useful in patients with heart disease who do not tolerate a sodium load. Tolvaptan can also be given in the hospital, and it has been proven in controlled trials to be effective in restoring normonatremia in outpatients. However, the FDA recommends that tolvaptan be started in the hospital and that patients be given drug holidays because of concerns about hepatotoxicity. These barriers, lack of evidence of improved outcomes, and cost limit their use.

5. Urea—Oral urea is another option for the management of outpatient hyponatremia; in uncontrolled studies control of hyponatremia is comparable to that achieved with tolvaptan. Urea increases water excretion by inducing an osmotic diuresis. Urea is available as a medical food (www.ure-na.com) in flavored packets.

Hyponatremia associated with heart failure or hepatic cirrhosis is generally chronic and relatively mild. Treatment involves sodium and water restriction, the use of loop diuretics, and management of the underlying disorder. V_2-receptor antagonists like tolvaptan have been shown to promote excretion of electrolyte-free water thereby making them another option for treatment of hypervolemic hyponatremia. Treatment may improve clinical signs and symptoms, but no long-term benefits have been proven.

▶ Prognosis

Hyponatremia is associated with an increased mortality rate, but it is not known if this is due to the low serum sodium concentration or to the underlying disorders that cause hyponatremia. The short-term prognosis for patients with symptomatic hyponatremia is excellent and a full recovery of neurological symptoms can be anticipated if correction limits are adhered to. The prognosis for patients who develop osmotic demyelination syndrome is guarded, but even those with severe manifestations, requiring ventilator support, can recover fully; for this reason, withdrawal of care should not be considered for several months.

▶ When to Refer/When to Admit

Because of the potential for serious neurological morbidity, patients with serum sodium concentrations less than 120 mEq/L and hyponatremic patients with neurologic symptoms should be admitted to the hospital. Referral to a specialist is recommended for hyponatremic patients with seizures or coma, for all patients with serum sodium concentrations less than 110 mEq/L, and for patients with sodium concentrations less than 120 mEq/L who have conditions that put them at high risk of developing osmotic demyelination (see Table 3–6). Endocrine consultation is useful in the evaluation of suspected hypopituitarism or Addison disease.

KEY READINGS

Sterns RH: Disorders of plasma sodium—causes, consequences, and correction. N Engl J Med 2015;372:55.
Verbalis JG et al: Diagnosis, evaluation, and treatment of hyponatremia: expert panel recommendations. Am J Med 2013;126:S1.

HYPERNATREMIA

ESSENTIALS OF DIAGNOSIS

▸ Hypernatremia develops when water losses exceed water intake and patients are unable to seek water themselves.

▸ Urine osmolality can help distinguish between renal and extrarenal water losses.

▶ General Considerations

Hypernatremia frequently occurs in hospitalized patients because acute illnesses often limit the ability to seek water.

Outside the hospital, hypernatremia can develop in debilitated nursing home patients with deficient thirst caused by multiple cerebrovascular accidents. More rarely, hypothalamic disease causing both adipsia and diabetes insipidus can present with severe chronic hypernatremia.

Pathogenesis

Hypernatremia (a serum sodium concentration >145 mEq/L) is usually caused by the failure to replace fluid losses. Sweat and urinary losses caused by diabetes insipidus are nearly "pure" electrolyte-free water, almost devoid of electrolytes. Other fluid losses are "hypotonic," containing a good deal of electrolyte, but at a lower concentration than normal plasma; these losses can be thought of as a mixture of isotonic saline and electrolyte-free water. Less commonly, hypernatremia is caused by a large intake of concentrated salt, a disorder known as acute salt poisoning. The renal concentrating mechanism normally minimizes electrolyte-free water losses as the plasma sodium concentration rises, but thirst prevents hypernatremia regardless of how much water is lost (see Figure 3–1). Thirst is such an effective defense that hypernatremia typically does not develop, even in the setting of severe diabetes insipidus, unless the thirst mechanism is impaired or access to water is restricted.

The serum sodium concentration reveals nothing of the patient's extracellular volume status, which is a function of the *amount* of sodium in the body, not the sodium *concentration*. Patients with hypernatremia can be salt overloaded or sodium depleted. However, all patients with hypernatremia have cellular dehydration and need water replacement to restore normal cell volume.

Prevention

Hypernatremia can be prevented by providing patients with enough electrolyte-free water to match their water losses. If the serum sodium concentration is rising, it means that water intake is insufficient and should be increased. Electrolyte-free water can be provided by encouraging oral water intake, by adding water to tube feedings, or by infusing 5% dextrose in water intravenously. In patients with neurogenic diabetes insipidus, excessive water losses can be prevented with daily administration of desmopressin.

Clinical Findings

A. Symptoms and Signs

Hypernatremia is always reflective of a hyperosmolar state. In response to hyperosmolality, water shifts from the relatively hypotonic intracellular space to the extracellular compartment resulting in decreased cellular volume. Such water shifts are most important in the brain. Depending on the acuity and severity of hypernatremia, changes in brain cell volume are associated with a spectrum of neurologic symptoms. Irritability, lethargy, muscle spasticity, seizures, coma, and death may all occur. If hypernatremia develops over more than 24 hours, the brain adapts by accumulating intracellular osmolytes that act to restore cellular tonicity and volume. Chronic hypernatremia may, therefore, be less symptomatic at the same degree of hypernatremia than if it had occurred acutely. Due to the accumulation of osmolytes, chronic hypernatremia carries the attendant risk of cerebral edema if rapidly corrected.

B. Laboratory Findings

The plasma osmolality is always high in hypernatremia and there is no need to measure it. Urine osmolality and urine specific gravity will be maximally concentrated (>600 mOsm/kg and as high as 1200 mOsm/kg; urine specific (sp) gravity 1.015–1.030) if hypernatremia is caused by extrarenal water losses and the kidneys are normal. By contrast, the urine may be dilute (urine osmolality <300 mOsm/kg and as low as 50 mOsm/kg; urine sp gravity <1.010 and as low as 1.001) if hypernatremia is caused by diabetes insipidus (see below). Measurement of urine sodium, potassium, glucose, urea nitrogen, and creatinine helps further define the cause and magnitude of urinary losses. When hypotonic fluid losses containing substantial amounts of sodium are the cause of hypernatremia, there may be laboratory findings of hypovolemia: a high BUN/creatinine ratio; a low or high serum bicarbonate concentration, hypokalemia; and, an increase in serum hematocrit (Hct) over baseline. Such findings are absent when hypernatremia is caused by pure electrolyte-free water losses unless the serum sodium concentration is extremely high.

C. Imaging Studies

Imaging studies are only helpful in patients suspected of having neurogenic diabetes insipidus. Magnetic resonance imaging of the hypothalamic—pituitary region may reveal the etiology. Normally the posterior pituitary produces a bright spot on T1-weighted images that may be characteristically absent in neurogenic diabetes insipidus.

Differential Diagnosis

Unlike hyponatremia, which requires a methodical, diagnostic approach, the differential diagnosis of hypernatremia is relatively straightforward. The goals are to identify the reason why water was not replaced, to identify the source and magnitude of excess electrolyte-free water losses, and to determine if there were also isotonic fluid losses that require replacement. These are primarily therapeutic issues and are discussed in the therapy section that follows.

The biggest challenge in differential diagnosis is in the small subset of hypernatremic patients who are polyuric. The same approach is used in the evaluation of polyuria in patients who are able to replace their water losses and have normal serum sodium concentrations.

In all patients with hypernatremia, urine osmolality should be measured. A value greater than 700 mOsm/kg excludes a urinary source for the lost water, while a value less than 400 mOsm/kg indicates that renal water conservation is severely compromised. Patients with intermediate values should be reevaluated after partial rehydration has reduced the serum sodium concentration to less than 150 mEq/L.

A. Evaluation of Polyuria

The evaluation of polyuria should be approached systematically (Figure 3–3):

Step 1: Exclude osmotic diuresis—In an osmotic diuresis, excretion of solute (urine osmolality × daily urine volume) is greater than 900 mOsm/day. If urine volume is not known, it can be estimated from the urine creatinine concentration; assuming that daily urine creatinine excretion is 1 g/day, the urine volume in liters equals 100 divided by the urine creatinine concentration in mg/dL. An osmotic diuresis caused by saline or mannitol should be obvious by reviewing what has been administered intravenously, while polyuria caused by glycosuria should be apparent by measuring blood and urine glucose. Osmotic diuresis due to urea can occur in catabolic patients and in patients who have received high dose steroids; the urine osmolality may be considerably higher than 300 mOsm/kg, but electrolyte-free water excretion is high because the urine electrolyte concentration is low.

Step 2: Assess the response to desmopressin—Hypernatremic patients who excrete dilute urine (urine osmolality <300 mOsm/kg) have diabetes insipidus (DI). Polyuric patients with normal serum sodium concentrations need to be water deprived until the serum sodium concentration is greater than 145 mEq/L in order to make that diagnosis, but the water deprivation test is unnecessary and potentially dangerous in patients who are already hypernatremic. Neurogenic DI, caused by ADH deficiency, responds to subcutaneous desmopressin (2–4 mcg) or aqueous vasopressin (5 units) with an increase in urine osmolality while in nephrogenic DI the urine remains dilute.

Step 3: Determine the cause of DI

1. Neurogenic DI—Since vasopressin is produced in the hypothalamus and released from the posterior pituitary gland, any disease process involving the hypothalamic–pituitary axis may lead to vasopressin deficiency and neurogenic DI (Table 3–7). Common causes include head trauma, pituitary surgery, infection, primary or metastatic malignancy, thrombosis, and granulomatous disease. Congenital forms have been described but are rare. An unusual form of diabetes insipidus resistant to vasopressin has been described in pregnancy. Rather than renal insensitivity to the hormone, placentally derived circulating vasopressinase neutralizes circulating vasopressin. Desmopressin (DDAVP) is not affected by vasopressinase and is effective in treating the disease.

2. Nephrogenic DI—Nephrogenic diabetes insipidus may be acquired or congenital (see Table 3–7). The acquired form is much more common. Any advanced form of chronic renal failure may impair urinary concentrating ability,

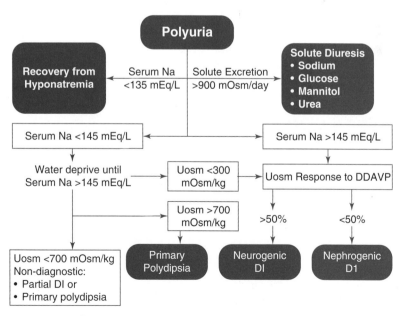

▲ **Figure 3–3.** Diagnostic approach to polyuria.

Table 3–7. Causes of diabetes insipidus.

Neurogenic (central) diabetes insipidus
- Congenital
  - Autosomal dominant (late onset)
  - Wolfram syndrome
- Acquired
  - Tumors, neurosurgery, traumatic brain injury, interruption of pituitary vascular supply, infiltrative diseases, IgG4 disease, and autoimmune disease

Nephrogenic diabetes insipidus
- Congenital
  - X-linked (V_2 vasopressin receptor)
  - Recessive (aquaporin defects)
- Acquired
  - Electrolyte abnormalities: hypokalemia, hypercalcemia
  - Drugs: lithium, demeclocycline, methoxyflurane
  - Pregnancy (vasopressinase)

but polyuria is unusual. Various pharmacologic agents, particularly lithium and demeclocycline frequently cause nephrogenic DI. If nephrogenic DI develops after long-term lithium treatment it is often irreversible; patients may become severely hypernatremic after surgical procedures, if their water losses are not replaced.

Complications

The complications of hypernatremia depend on how rapidly it developed. Severe hypernatremia can ensue within minutes after acute salt poisoning, an uncommon disorder, that occurs after intrauterine administration of hypertonic saline for therapeutic abortion, suicidal ingestion of salty fluids (eg, soy sauce) or table salt, or child abuse; the disorder presents with dramatic, and often fatal neurological findings associated with brain hemorrhages. A less abrupt, but still acute onset of hypernatremia over 24 hours, due to diabetes insipidus, can result in osmotic demyelination, with brain lesions similar to those that develop after rapid correction of hypernatremia. When hypernatremia develops over several days, brain cells adapt to the disturbance by accumulating extra organic osmolytes that persist as hypernatremia is corrected. If infants with chronic hypernatremia are rapidly rehydrated, they develop cerebral edema and seizures. For this reason, limited correction is advised for all patients with severe, chronic hypernatremia.

Treatment

Patients with hypernatremia need water. The water prescription should replace both the water deficit and ongoing water losses. The net loss of 3 mL of water per kg body weight will increase the serum sodium concentration by about 1 mEq/L. This relationship can be used to plan fluid therapy. For example, consider a 69-kg man on tube feeding whose serum sodium concentration is now 150 mEq/L and whose serum sodium had been increasing by an average 1 mEq/L/day for the past 10 days. Because 200 mL of water were required to raise the serum sodium concentration by 1 mEq/L, the amount of water needed to correct the deficit and return the serum sodium to 140 mEq/L is approximately 2 L. In addition to replacing the deficit with 2 L of water, given orally or as 5% dextrose in water intravenously, the patient needs an extra 200 mL of water added to his feedings each day to keep up with ongoing losses. In patients with chronic hypernatremia, it is reasonable to avoid correction rates greater than 10 mEq/L/day, because more rapid rates have resulted in cerebral edema in hypernatremic infants. If hypernatremia is known to be acute, it should be corrected as rapidly as it developed.

Patients who have become hypernatremic because of gastric fluid losses, glycosuria, or osmotic or loop diuretics, are sodium depleted and volume depleted despite their high serum sodium concentration. Patients with hypovolemic hyponatremia can be corrected with hypotonic saline (0.45% NaCl in 5% dextrose in water); because this solution is ½ electrolyte-free water and ½ isotonic saline, the needed volume is twice the calculated water deficit.

Particularly in the ICU, hypernatremia may be associated with sodium overload. This occurs in patients who had been treated with large volumes of isotonic saline for septic or cardiogenic shock and whose ongoing electrolyte-free water losses were not replaced. Hypernatremic patients who are edematous can be treated by administering loop diuretics, which promote excretion of urine that is ½ electrolyte free water and ½ isotonic saline, and replacing urine output with 5% dextrose in water.

Prognosis

Hypernatremia is associated with a high mortality rate, but it is likely that this reflects the underlying conditions responsible for it. The short-term neurologic prognosis for chronic hypernatremia is excellent, but severe acute hypernatremia can result in permanent brain damage.

When to Refer/Admit

Patients with serum sodium concentrations above 154 mEq/L should be admitted to the hospital for intravenous hydration. Subspecialty referral is recommended for the evaluation and treatment of patients with suspected diabetes insipidus.

KEY READINGS

Lindner G, Funk GC: Hypernatremia in critically ill patients. J Crit Care 2013;28:216.e11.

Robertson GL: Diabetes insipidus: differential diagnosis and management. Best Pract Res Clin Endocrinol Metab 2016;30:205.

Sterns RH: Disorders of plasma sodium—causes, consequences, and correction. N Engl J Med 2015;372:55.

■ CHAPTER REVIEW QUESTIONS

1. A 30-year-old woman competing in her first marathon is brought to the hospital after collapsing at the end of the race. She is confused and delirious and complains of a headache. Vital signs show blood pressure (BP) is 150/90 mm Hg, heart rate (HR) is 60 beats/min, and temperature is 37.4°C. Physical examination reveals no jugular venous distention, crackles at the lung bases, normal heart sounds, no organomegaly, a trace of pre-tibial edema, and no focal neurological findings.

   Laboratory Data:
   Serum Na 119, K 3.5, Cl 90, CO_2 22 mmol/L
   BUN 4, creatinine 0.5 mg/dL, glucose 80 mg/dL

   Which ONE of the following is the BEST next step
   A. Give 2 L of 0.9% saline by IV bolus.
   B. Order urine osmolality and urine chemistries.
   C. Give desmopressin.
   D. Give intravenous furosemide.
   E. Give 100 mL of 3% saline as a bolus.

2. A 40-year-old man with a history of heavy beer drinking and hypertension treated with hydrochlorothiazide, is brought to the hospital after being found on the floor of his apartment. He is confused and delirious, fighting with caregivers. Vital signs show blood pressure is 95/60 mm Hg, heart rate is 100 beats/min, and temperature is 37.5°C. Physical examination reveals no jugular venous distention, scleral icterus, clear lungs, normal heart sounds, hepatomegaly, no edema, and no focal neurological signs.

   Laboratory Data:
   Serum Na 104, K 2.5, Cl 75, CO_2 35 mmol/L
   BUN 20, creatinine 1, glucose 70 mg/dL

   He is given 2 L of 0.9% saline, 100 mg thiamine, and 40 mEq of KCl in the end of the day (ED). Four hours later his BP has increased to 120/80 mm Hg but his neurologic condition is unchanged. Repeated laboratory data show:
   Serum Na 110, K 2.4, Cl 80, CO_2 30 mmol/L

   Which ONE of the following is the BEST next treatment?
   A. Conivaptan
   B. 100 mL of 3% saline as a bolus
   C. 0.9% saline at 100 mL/h
   D. 3% saline at 30 mL/h
   E. Desmopressin

3. A 60-year-old man with a long history of bipolar disease undergoes elective coronary artery bypass surgery. The next morning, vital signs are normal, but he is found to be lethargic with no localizing neurological signs.

   Laboratory Data:
   Serum Na 158, K 4, Cl 100, CO_2 24 mmol/L
   BUN 30, creatinine 1.4, glucose 100 mg/dL
   Urine osmolality 160 mOsm/kg, urine creatinine 20 mg/dL

   Which ONE of the following is the BEST next step?
   A. Conduct a water deprivation test.
   B. Give 1 L bolus of 0.9% saline.
   C. Give 0.45% saline at 100 mL/h.
   D. Give intravenous furosemide.
   E. Give 5% dextrose at 300 mL/h.

4. A 70-year-old woman with lung cancer presents with a seizure. A CT scan of the head reveals metastatic lesions and she is treated with high dose steroids. Two days later her urine output is found to be 4.5 L in 24 hours.

   Laboratory Data:
   Serum Na 147, K 4, Cl 114, CO_2 25 mmol/L
   BUN 30, creatinine 0.8, glucose 180 mg/dL
   Urine osmolality 500 mOsm/kg, Na 30 mmol/L, creatinine 22 mg/dL

   Which ONE of the following is the MOST likely cause of the large urine output?
   A. Syndrome of inappropriate antidiuretic hormone secretion (SIADH)
   B. Cerebral salt wasting
   C. Neurogenic diabetes insipidus
   D. Osmotic diuresis
   E. Kidney metastases

5. A 50-year-old woman complains of progressive lethargy and frequent falls. She is alert and oriented but slow to answer questions. Vital signs show blood pressure is 140/80 mm Hg, heart rate is 80 beats/min, respiratory rate is 16 breaths/min, and temperature is 37°C. There is no jugular venous distention. Chest shows rhonchi and wheezes, heart sounds are normal, no organomegaly, no edema.

   Laboratory Data:
   Serum Na 120, K 4, Cl 90, CO_2 25 mmol/L
   BUN 4, creatinine 0.6, glucose 100 mg/dL
   Urine osmolality 790 mOsm/kg, urine Na 100, K 50 mmol/L

   Which ONE of the following is LEAST likely to be effective in increasing her serum sodium concentration?
   A. 0.9% saline
   B. Conivaptan
   C. Tolvaptan
   D. Water restriction
   E. Urea

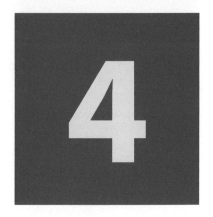

Disorders of Potassium Balance: Hypo- and Hyperkalemia

Michael Emmett, MD, MACP

Michael R. Wiederkehr, MD

▶ General Considerations

Potassium is the principal cation of the intracellular fluid (ICF) where its concentration is between 120 and 150 mEq/L. The extracellular fluid (ECF) and plasma potassium concentration [K] is much lower—in the 3.5- to 5-mEq/L range. This very large transcellular gradient is maintained by active K transport via the Na/K ATPase pumps present in all cell membranes and the ionic permeability characteristics of these membranes. The resulting 30–40 fold transmembrane [K] gradient is the principal determinant of the transcellular resting potential gradient, which is about 90 mV, with the cell interior negative (Figure 4–1). Normal cell function requires maintenance of the ECF [K] within a relatively narrow range. This is particularly important for excitable cells such as myocytes, conducting tissues, and neurons. The pathophysiologic effects of hypokalemia and hyperkalemia on these cells result in most of the clinical manifestations.

Individual potassium intakes vary widely—a typical western diet provides between 50 and 100 mEq K/day and about 90% of the ingested K is absorbed by the gastrointestinal (GI) tract. Under steady-state conditions, an equal amount is lost from the body. Most is excreted in urine and a small amount in stool and sweat. Homeostatic mechanisms maintain plasma [K] between 3.5 and 5.0 mEq/L. A large ingested meal may contain more potassium than is present in the entire ECF. Yet the serum K concentration generally varies by less than 10%. This homeostasis is achieved by the integrated action of multiple regulatory systems. The normal postprandial rise in insulin concentration drives both K and glucose into the intracellular compartment. Although postprandial insulin release is primarily stimulated by increased plasma glucose concentrations, potassium also directly stimulates pancreatic β-cells to release insulin. Insulin deficiency and/or resistance can increase plasma [K]. In addition a postprandial "feed-forward" system, which is not yet fully understood, increases urine K excretion in response to oral K loads independent of changes in

serum K or known K regulating hormones. Urine K excretion also has a circadian rhythm component. Epinephrine and norepinephrine also rapidly regulate transcellular K balance and become especially important during and following vigorous exercise. Hyperadrenergic states such as alcohol withdrawal and hyperthyroidism, β-sympathomimetics such as the tocolytic terbutaline, and theophylline poisoning can generate hypokalemia due to translocation of K from the ECF into cells.

Hyperchloremic acidosis (and other inorganic or mineral acidoses) shifts K out of cells. However, the much more common organic metabolic acidoses (lactic and ketoacidosis) do not directly generate much K shift. Both respiratory acidosis and respiratory alkalosis generate some K shift from cells to the ECF. It had been assumed that the alkalemia produced by respiratory alkalosis would drive K into cells, but studies found that the opposite occurred. The small *increase* in plasma [K] with respiratory alkalosis is probably due to concomitant α-adrenergic stimulation. The hypertonicity generated by hyperglycemia will shift both water and K from the intracellular space to the ECF. Hypokalemia per se will also cause K to shift from the intra- to the extracellular space.

The movement of K from the ECF into cells is generated by insulin, β-adrenergic activity, and, to a lesser degree, metabolic alkalosis.

KEY READINGS

Adrogué HJ, Madias NE: Changes in plasma potassium concentration during acute acid-base disturbances. Am J Med 1981;71:456.

Aronson PS, Giebisch G: Effects of pH on potassium: new explanations for old observations. J Am Soc Nephrol 2011;22:198.

Gumz ML, Rabinowitz L, Wingo CS: An integrated view of potassium homeostasis. N Engl J Med 2015;373:60.

Perez GO, Oster JR, Vaamonde CA: Serum potassium concentration in acidemic states. Nephron 1981;27:233.

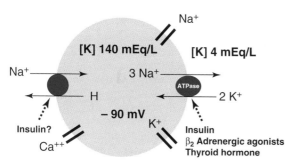

▲ **Figure 4–1.** Transcellular ion movement. Most cells contain these pumps, antiporters, and channels. The effects of insulin, catecholamines, and thyroid hormones on K transport are shown.

▶ Pathogenesis

Potassium absorption in the small intestine is not thought to be regulated, but potassium secretion by colonic and rectal epithelial cells is regulated. Colon and rectal K secretion increases in response to chronic hyperkalemia and increased aldosterone levels (eg, in patients with chronic kidney disease [CKD]). However, the net effect on K balance is usually very small because despite potential large variation in the K concentration of stool water the volume of water in formed stool is very small. Consequently, the absolute amount of K lost in stool is a minor contributor to overall K balance despite potentially large changes in stool K concentration. Major stool K loss can only occur if patients have high-volume, electrolyte-rich, watery diarrhea.

The main regulator of body K balance is the kidney. Plasma potassium is freely filtered (600–800 mEq/day) and then largely reabsorbed in the proximal tubule and thick ascending loop of Henle. Therefore, the amount of K delivered to the more distal nephron segments is only about 10–15% of filtered K, and the K concentration of fluid leaving the loop of Henle is relatively low. The distal tubule, the connecting tubule (CNT), and the cortical collecting duct (CCD) are the sites at which major regulation of K excretion occurs. Sodium (Na) reabsorption is indirectly linked to K and H secretion in these tubule segments and is affected by the luminal fluid flow rate, the amount of Na delivered to these segments, how readily the anions associated with the Na in the tubule fluid are absorbed, and the activity of the mineralocorticoids, especially aldosterone. In the CNT and CCD, Na is absorbed through epithelial Na channels (ENaC) present on the luminal surface of the predominant (principal) cells in these segments. Tubule absorption of large amounts of Na, especially when delivered with a poorly absorbed anions (Cl, HCO_3, and others), generates a negative electrical charge within the lumen. This intraluminal negative "potential difference" (PD) enhances the secretion of K and H (Figure 4–2).

Aldosterone regulates the rate of Na absorption through these ENaC channels at multiple levels. It enhances energy (ATP) generation, increases Na-K ATPase pump density and activity, and increases the density of "open" ENaC channels.

In normal individuals, high renin and aldosterone activity is usually associated with low CNT/CCD Na delivery. For example, high salt intake expands the ECF volume, reduces renin and aldosterone levels, and increases distal delivery and

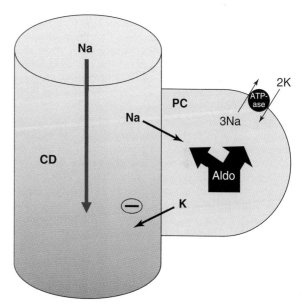

▲ **Figure 4–2.** K handling by the cortical collecting duct (CCD). Aldosterone has multiple effects on electrolyte transport in the connecting tubule (CNT) and CCD. Sodium (Na) absorption increases as a result of stimulation of basolateral Na/K ATPase activity and an increased number and "open state" status of luminal Na channels (ENaC). The influx of Na, which is generally more rapid than its associated anions, causes a negative charge to develop within the lumen. The negative luminal charge stimulates the transit of positive charges (K and H) into the lumen.

Volume-contracted states lead to avid Na reabsorption in proximal tubule segments and relatively reduced Na delivery to the CCD. Volume contraction also markedly stimulates renin activity and aldosterone levels increase. Although aldosterone levels are high, the reduced delivery of Na to the distal nephron sites prevents a major increase in K and H secretion.

Volume-expanded states reduce proximal tubule Na reabsorption and increase distal nephron Na delivery. Volume expansion also decreases renin activity and aldosterone levels fall. Despite low aldosterone levels, appropriate secretion of K and H is maintained as a result of generous Na delivery to distal tubule segments.

excretion of Na. The high distal Na and fluid delivery counterbalances low aldosterone activity in regard to distal tubule K and H secretion. The net effect is a "normal" rate of renal K and H secretion and excretion despite low aldosterone levels. Conversely, when low salt intake contracts the ECF, this activates renin activity and aldosterone levels increase. Simultaneously, distal Na delivery is reduced. Under these conditions, low CNT/CCD Na delivery is associated with high aldosterone activity. Again, a relatively "normal" rate of K and H secretion and excretion are maintained. This reciprocal interplay between aldosterone (and renin) activity and distal Na delivery is very important for the maintenance of normal Na, K, and acid-base balance when physiologic changes in salt and fluid intake occur. It is critical for simultaneous maintenance of both volume and electrolyte homeostasis. Multiple other regulatory systems (such as the WNK kinases) fine-tune these physiologic interactions.

A number of pathologic conditions can disrupt the systems described in the previous paragraph. For example, the simultaneous existence of generous Na delivery to the CNT/CCD and high aldosterone activity are generally a pathologic state. When this occurs, CNT/CCD K and H secretion will be pathologically driven and result in inappropriate excretion of K and acid into the urine. Hypokalemia and metabolic alkalosis will develop. The classic cause of high distal Na delivery and high aldosterone activity is primary hyperaldosteronism. Volume expansion, hypertension hypokalemia, and metabolic alkaloses will develop. Another state of simultaneous high aldosterone activity and generous delivery of Na to the CNT/CCD is the use of thiazide and/or loop diuretics. They contract ECF volume and stimulate the renin/aldosterone system but simultaneously inhibit Na reabsorption in the loop of Henle and distal tubule Na. Thus high aldosterone activity occurs together with generous distal Na delivery. Hypokalemia and metabolic alkalosis ensue.

Conversely, the simultaneous existence of reduced delivery of Na to the CNT/CCD Na and low aldosterone activity will markedly decrease the excretion of K and protons into the urine leading to hyperkalemia and metabolic acidosis. For example, this may develop in patients with hypoaldosteronism who become volume contracted.

KEY READINGS

Agarwal R, Afzalpurkar R, Fordtran JS: Pathophysiology of potassium absorption and secretion by the human intestine. Gastroenterology 1994;107:548.

Giebisch GH, Wang WH: Potassium transport—an update. J Nephrol 2010;23:S97.

Sterns RH, Spital A: Disorders of internal potassium balance. Semin Nephrol 1987;7:399.

Youn JH, McDonough AA: Recent advances in understanding integrative control of potassium homeostasis. Annu Rev Physiol 2009;71:381.

▶ Clinical Manifestation

Nerve cells, cardiac conduction tissue, and muscle cells are especially sensitive to changes in transcellular voltage, and therefore are most affected by hypo- or hyperkalemia. Figure 4–3 shows how either condition can cause muscle weakness.

Hypokalemia generally causes the resting potential across cell membranes to become more negative—or hyperpolarized. The pathophysiologic and clinical result of cellular hyperpolarization varies depending on the type of cell. Muscle cells become resistant to depolarization and excitation. Severe hypokalemia can result in a *hyper*polarization block and flaccid paralysis. It may also cause rhabdomyolysis and paralytic ileus. In contrast, cardiac conducting tissue becomes *more readily* depolarized and excitable. Ventricular myocyte repolarization is slowed by hypokalemia. Also, the classic electrocardiographic (ECG) findings of hypokalemia include atrial and ventricular arrhythmias, a prolonged QT interval, depression of the ST segment, low-amplitude T waves, and the development of U waves.

Hypokalemia also affects the kidney; renal manifestations include metabolic alkalosis, nephrogenic diabetes insipidus,

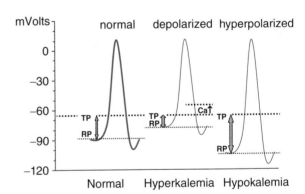

▲ **Figure 4–3.** Muscle and cardiac cell depolarization and hyperpolarization are affected by extracellular potassium. Muscle contraction requires cells to depolarize from the resting potential (RP) to the threshold potential (TP). Hyperkalemia moves the RP closer to the TP and can result in depolarization muscle paralysis. In cardiac conduction tissue, hyperkalemia blocks the sodium channel and this slows conduction. Hypokalemia hyperpolarizes cells and this also impairs depolarization. Cardiac conducting tissue becomes more readily depolarized and excitable. The flaccid paralysis caused by either hypokalemia or hyperkalemia can be clinically similar. Calcium infusions raise the TP (among other effects), ameliorating the effects of hyperkalemia, while hypocalcemia has the opposite effect.

and formation of renal cysts. Chronic hypokalemia has also been implicated in the development of hypertension.

Hyperkalemia causes the resting potential across cell membranes to become less negative—or hypopolarized. Muscle cells become less excitable and cannot normally repolarize. Clinical manifestations include fatigue, myalgia, and muscle weakness (legs > arms), hyporeflexia, paresthesias, and muscle cramps. Severe hyperkalemia causes flaccid paralysis due to a *depolarization block*. Muscle weakness may progress to ascending paralysis, hypoventilation, and respiratory failure. In the heart, the depolarized state generated by hyperkalemia generates a complex pathophysiologic cascade. The earliest manifestation is usually accelerated repolarization which generates T-wave peaking and a shortened QT interval. Hyperkalemia also inactivates Na channels in cardiac conduction tissue and myocytes, and this slows initial phase of the action potential and reduces its magnitude. The P-wave amplitude falls, and the PR interval and QRS complex are widened. Overall, cardiac cells become much less excitable. Figure 4–4 shows typical ECG changes.

The clinical manifestations of an abnormal plasma [K] vary greatly and depend on (a) the magnitude of the abnormality, (b) acuity of onset, (c) the relative contributions of cellular K shifts versus changes in total body K, and (d) coexisting abnormalities which either potentiate or blunt the [K] effects, including underlying heart disease, drugs (digoxin, antiarrhythmic agents), hypo- or hypercalcemia or hypermagnesemia, cardiac pacing devices, and others.

The resting membrane potential of all cells is largely determined by the ratio of intracellular and extracellular [K] (K_i/K_e). Acute K shifts into or out of the intracellular space has a small impact on intracellular [K] because this space contains 98% (~3000 mEq) of total body K at a relatively high concentration. However, the effect on the extracellular concentration can be dramatic, because the total quantity of K in this compartment is relatively small (~60 mEq) and its concentration is relatively low. Therefore, acute K shifts will markedly affect the K_i/K_e ratio and can cause rapid and profound hyperpolarization—or depolarization—with muscular, neurological, and cardiac effects (Figure 4–5). In contrast,

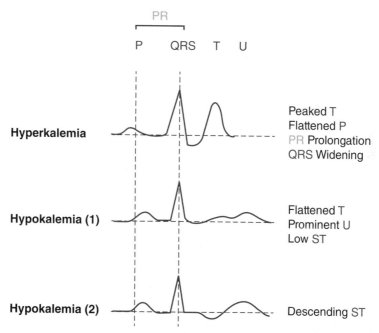

▲ **Figure 4–4.** Electrocardiographic tracings with hypokalemia and hyperkalemia. Hyperkalemia initially causes peaking ("tenting") of T waves and a shortened QT interval (accelerated repolarization) and then progresses to widening of the QRS and PR intervals (slowed depolarization), sinus bradycardia and arrest, atrioventricular-block, fusion of QRS with T (sine-wave appearance), idioventricular rhythm, and finally ventricular tachycardia and fibrillation, and asystole.

Hypokalemia causes ST depression, flattening of the T waves, and prominent U waves (slowed repolarization). This progresses to fusion of the T and U waves into a single wave, and the ST segment becomes negative and descending. The QT interval lengthens, especially if hypocalcemia or hypomagnesemia is present. Increased excitability generates atrial and ventricular arrhythmias.

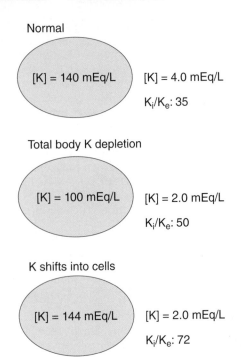

Normal

$[K] = 140$ mEq/L $[K] = 4.0$ mEq/L

K_i/K_e: 35

Total body K depletion

$[K] = 100$ mEq/L $[K] = 2.0$ mEq/L

K_i/K_e: 50

K shifts into cells

$[K] = 144$ mEq/L $[K] = 2.0$ mEq/L

K_i/K_e: 72

▲ **Figure 4–5.** K distribution with intracellular K shift versus K depletion. The resting membrane potential is primarily generated by the ratio of intracellular to extracellular potassium (K_i/K_e).

Total body K depletion reduces both intracellular and extracellular [K]. The K_i/K_e ratio increases and the cell becomes hyperpolarized.

A transcellular shift of K into cells slightly increases intracellular [K] and markedly reduces extracellular [K]. Therefore, the K_i/K_e ratio increases more markedly, cellular hyperpolarization can be very severe and produce clinical symptoms. Hypokalemic periodic paralysis may be an exception in regards to hyperpolarization versus depolarization. A defect in K exit from cells may simultaneously increase intracellular K, reduce extracellular K, and generate a *depolarized* state.

states of chronic K depletion reduce both intra- and extracellular K levels, and thereby have a smaller effect on K_i/K_e ratio with less severe clinical manifestations. Furthermore, K shifts produce much more rapid changes in plasma [K], and thus the clinical effects are often more dramatic than with states of total body K depletion.

Comorbid illness such as coronary heart disease will amplify the clinical importance of both hypo- and hyperkalemia by increasing the risk of serious arrhythmia. Hyperkalemic effects on cardiac conduction are well documented and are the principal reason it constitutes a medical emergency (see Figure 4–4). The cardiac risks of hypokalemia are less well established. Although increased risk of ectopy is established for patients with acute myocardial infarction and those treated with digoxin and a number of antiarrhythmics agents, the adverse impact of moderate hypokalemia for most patients remains unclear.

Calcium also plays an important role in myocyte depolarization. Hypocalcemia reduces the depolarization threshold potential and renders the cardiac myocyte more excitable. Conversely, hypercalcemia reduces membrane excitability by increasing the depolarization threshold (see Figure 4–3). This calcium-related shift of depolarization threshold is one aspect of the mechanisms by which calcium infusions reverse cardiac toxicity of hyperkalemia.

KEY READINGS

Adrogue HJ, Madias NE: Changes in plasma potassium concentration during acute acid-base disturbances. Am J Med 1981; 71:456.

Agarwal R, Afzalpurkar R, Fordtran JS: Pathophysiology of potassium absorption and secretion by the human intestine. Gastroenterology 1994;107:548.

Bia MJ, DeFronzo RA: Extrarenal potassium homeostasis. Am J Physiol 1981;240:F257.

Gennari FJ: Disorders of potassium homeostasis. Hypokalemia and hyperkalemia. Crit Care Clin 2002;18:273.

Macdonald JE, Struthers AD: What is the optimal serum potassium level in cardiovascular patients? J Am Coll Cardiol 2004; 43:155.

Rossignol P et al: Emergency management of severe hyperkalemia: guideline for best practice and opportunities for the future. Pharmacol Res 2016 Nov;113:585.

▶ Hypokalemia

A serum [K] below 3.5 mEq/L defines hypokalemia. Table 4–1 lists the more common causes and clinical conditions associated with this disorder. They include diuretics, vomiting/nasogastric (NG) suction, and large-volume watery diarrhea (or laxatives). These etiologies are usually readily apparent unless the patient is using drugs covertly or secretly vomiting. More detailed evaluation is necessary when the frequent causes of hypokalemia have been excluded.

Hypokalemia due to transcellular K shifts often generates impressive clinical presentations. Examples include several forms of hypokalemic periodic paralysis, the administration of β_2-agonists, theophylline poisoning, and conditions that enhance β-agonist activity such as hyperthyroidism and hypothermia. Insulin drives K into cells and can promote hypokalemia. Barium poisoning and chloroquine overdose block cellular K channels, and thereby cause pathologic K accumulation within the ICF and profound hypokalemia. Potassium accumulation within cells also occurs with a rapid expansion of cell mass. This may occur with refeeding after a prolonged period of starvation, with rapidly growing

Table 4–1. Hypokalemia.

Renal Losses
  Diuretics
  Vomiting, NG suction, congenital chloride wasting diarrhea
  Osmotic diuresis (uncontrolled diabetes and others)
  Drugs
    Excretion of nonreabsorbable anions
    Fludrocortisone and others
    Licorice (see text)
    Tubular toxicity (aminoglycosides, cisplatin, and others)
  Primary hyperaldosteronism
  Liddle syndrome
  Cushing disease
  Renal tubular acidosis types I and II (when treated with $NaHCO_3$)
  Bartter and Gitelman syndrome
  Magnesium deficiency
Extrarenal Losses
  Diarrhea, laxatives
  Ileostomy/short bowel
  Ureteral diversion into colon
  Ogilvie syndrome (colonic pseudo-obstruction)
  Villous adenoma
Transcellular Shift
  Insulin
  β_2-Adrenergic agonists
  Thyrotoxicosis
  Periodic paralysis
  Theophylline
Barium, chloroquine, cesium
Rapid expansion of cell mass
Anabolic states
Treatment phase of pernicious anemia
Rapidly growing malignancy

malignant tumors, and when patients with severe pernicious anemia are treated with vitamin B_{12}.

Patients with hypokalemic periodic paralysis often have a dramatic clinical presentation. At least two distinct subtypes of this syndrome have been characterized: a rare familial form (usually due to an autosomal dominant mutation affecting a calcium channel) and a much more common acquired type associated with hyperthyroidism. Hyperthyroid periodic paralysis is especially prevalent among young men (20–40 years old) of Asian ancestry (Native American Indians and Hispanic men are also at higher risk of developing this disorder if they become hyperthyroid). These patients typically present with profound acute muscle paralysis affecting mainly proximal limb muscle groups (legs > arms) with sparing of ocular and respiratory muscles. Deep tendon reflexes are generally absent. Paralysis often develops after a period of exercise, which increases β-agonist activity or following ingestion of carbohydrates, which increases insulin levels. Each of these hormones drives K into cells. The clinical features of thyrotoxicosis may be subtle. A prior history of recurrent episodes of weaknesses is common. Plasma [K] usually falls below 2 mEq/L, and hypophosphatemia and mild hypomagnesemia may also occur. Although acute treatment with small amounts of exogenous K salts is generally appropriate, rebound hyperkalemia often develops since total body stores are normal. Therefore K replacement must be implemented very cautiously. Treatment with nonselective β-blockers such as propranolol is helpful, and correction of the hyperthyroid state is usually curative. The pathophysiology of this disorder is thought to include the action of thyroid hormone on the Na/K ATPase, an exaggerated response to insulin, and the hyperadrenergic state of hyperthyroidism. The genetic and racial predisposition is probably due to inherited mutations of muscle ion transporters and channels which remain subclinical until magnified by the hyperthyroid state. There may be a blockage of specific K channels which prevent K from exiting muscle cells.

When hypokalemia is associated with reduced total body K stores, this may be the result of excessive gastrointestinal or renal losses, or a combination of both. Quantitating the 24-hour urine potassium excretion can help define the etiology. The kidney responds to K deficits by reducing K excretion to less than 20–30 mEq/day. Therefore, reduction of renal K excretion to this range in a patient with hypokalemia usually indicates that the hypokalemia is due to a transcellular shift or that gastrointestinal K losses may be responsible. Higher K excretion in hypokalemic patients indicates "inappropriate" renal K wasting. However, it must be recognized the renal K losses can occur intermittently, with intervening periods of appropriate K conservation. For example, diuretics cause excess renal K losses, but urine K excretion falls to an appropriately low range when the diuretic effect wears off. Similarly, vomiting or NG suction will generate excess renal K loss during the active phase of vomiting or suction (when the kidney is excreting a relatively large amount of Na and K bicarbonate salts into the urine, but K excretion will fall into the "appropriate" low range when the patient enters the "equilibrium phase" and the urine bicarbonate and electrolyte excretion fall sharply.

If a 24-hour urine collection cannot be accomplished, alternative useful measurements are the transtubular [K] gradient (TTKG) and the urine [K]/Cr ratio. The TTKG is a calculation which attempts to predict the plasma to urine [K] ratio in the tubule fluid exiting the CCD before water reabsorption occurs downstream where medullary water reabsorption increases the tubule fluid/urine [K]. The TTKG is calculated as:

$$TTKG = \frac{U[K] \times P[Osm]}{P[K] \times U[Osm]}$$

The P[Osm] is generally assumed to be about 300 mOsm/L for purposes of this calculation.

A TTKG below 3 indicates appropriate renal K conservation in a patient with hypokalemia. However, the TTKG becomes uninterpretable if urine osmolality is less than 300, or when distal nephron sodium delivery is very low; that is, urine sodium falls below 20 mEq/L.

The urine [K]/Cr ratio is another method of "correcting" the urine [K] for the urine concentration. This ratio is generally less than 13 mEq K/g Cr when the kidney is appropriately conserving K in the face of hypokalemia.

Assessment of volume status and blood pressure provides additional diagnostic clues. Patients with hypokalemia, volume expansion, and hypertension may have primary or exogenous hypermineralocorticoidism. An increased plasma aldosterone level (normal 5–20 ng/dL) *and* a simultaneous suppressed plasma renin activity (PRA—normal 1–3 ng/mL/h) indicate autonomous aldosterone secretion. An aldosterone/PRA ratio greater than 30 together with an elevated aldosterone level (>20 ng/dL) is consistent with primary hyperaldosteronism. Autonomous hyperaldosteronism may be due to a unilateral aldosterone secreting adenoma (Conn syndrome), various forms of bilateral adrenal hyperplasia (including glucocorticoid-remediable aldosteronism), or very rarely, adrenal cancer. Although radiological evaluation often points to a specific syndrome, bilateral adrenal vein sampling is often required if surgical intervention is considered.

Pseudohyperaldosteronism is characterized by many of the biochemical and clinical features of an autonomous mineralocorticoid excess state but with suppressed aldosterone levels. It may be due to secretion of a nonaldosterone mineralocorticoid. Examples include adrenal tumors secreting the mineralocorticoid deoxycorticosterone (DOC), some forms of congenital adrenal hyperplasia (17- and 11-hydroxylase deficiency), and conditions, which cause glucocorticoids to develop potent mineralocorticoid properties. The reason glucocorticoids do not normally activate the mineralocorticoid receptor is presence of the enzyme 11β-hydroxysteroid dehydrogenase type 2, near mineralocorticoid receptors. This enzyme inactivates glucocorticoids (but not mineralocorticoids). If this enzyme is absent or inhibited, physiologic levels of glucocorticoids will produce a mineralocorticoid excess state. The enzyme is congenitally absent or defective in patients with the "apparent mineralocorticoid excess" (AME) syndrome. They develop a hyperaldosteronism like disorder with hypokalemia, metabolic alkalosis, volume expansion, and hypertension. An acquired form of this disorder is generated by glycyrrhetinic acid, which is present in true licorice, in several decongestants available in Europe, and in some brands of chewing tobacco (eg, RedMan). Excessive use/ingestion of these products can result in the same clinical and biochemical presentation. Also, 11β-hydroxysteroid dehydrogenase type 2 may be overwhelmed by the markedly elevated cortisol levels in some patients with Cushing syndrome, in particular the form due to ectopic adrenocorticotropic hormone secretion.

Liddle syndrome is a disorder with the biochemical and clinical features of a classic mineralocorticoid excess state except all known mineralocorticoids are present in very low concentrations. The disorder is due to an autosomal dominant mutation, which causes excess numbers of epithelial Na channels (ENaC) in the CT and CCD to remain in a persistently open state despite the absence of mineralocorticoid stimulation. Clinical and biochemical findings mimic a nonaldosterone mineralocorticoid excess state—volume expansion, hypertension, hypokalemia, metabolic alkalosis, and suppressed levels of renin and aldosterone.

Secondary hyperaldosteronism exists when high aldosterone levels are generated by high renin levels (and angiotensin II levels). The high renin may be due to ECF volume contraction. This may occur with diarrhea, diuretic therapy, or genetic renal salt-wasting syndromes such as Bartter or Gitelman syndrome. Secondary hyperaldosteronism also occurs in patients with renal artery stenosis and in some patients with severe hypertension whose major renal arteries are anatomically open—probably as a result of reduced blood flow in smaller vessels. Another very rare cause of secondary hyperaldosteronism are tumors, which secrete renin and thereby generate a state of hyperaldosteronism, hypertension, and hypokalemia.

When secondary hyperaldosteronism is due to thiazide or loop diuretic use or due to genetic renal salt wasting (Bartter/Gitelman syndrome), distal renal tubule NaCl delivery is relatively high. Whenever this occurs together with hyperaldosteronism, distal tubule K and H secretion is activated. Hypokalemia and metabolic alkalosis result.

As mentioned above, Bartter and Gitelman syndromes mimic the effects of loop or thiazide diuretics. Gitelman syndrome is due to a defect of the thiazide sensitive NaCl transporter in the early distal renal tubule (or other mutations which indirectly reduce the activity of this ion transporter). Bartter syndrome is caused by generic mutations that impair the function of the Na-K-2Cl transporter in the thick ascending limb of Henle that is inhibited by loop diuretics (or other mutations which indirectly blunt the activity of this ion transporter). These disorders are characterized by similar clinical and biochemical abnormalities: volume contraction, hypotension, hypokalemia with renal K and NaCl wasting, metabolic alkalosis, high renin and aldosterone levels, and, sometimes, very high levels of urinary prostaglandins. Several characteristics distinguish Bartter from Gitelman syndrome. Bartter syndrome generates hypercalciuria and moderate hypomagnesemia while Gitelman syndrome reduces urine calcium excretion and generates severe hypomagnesemia. Several subtypes of Bartter syndrome are very severe and typically present in infancy or childhood while Gitelman syndrome is usually a relatively milder disorder and may not be recognized until adulthood. It may be difficult to discern the patients with these genetic disorders from patients who are surreptitiously using diuretics. The clinical features can be identical and blood and urine electrolytes very similar. Urine assay for diuretics and the identification of specific genetic mutations may be required for definitive diagnosis. Also, the urine chloride concentration can be helpful. It will generally be persistently elevated (>20 mEq/L) with Bartter or Gitelman syndrome but will often "cycle" from low to high with diuretic use (high when the diuretic activity is present and low when the diuretic effect has waned).

Osmotic diuresis can generate hypokalemia and hypernatremia and is relatively common in the intensive care unit (ICU). The two most common causes of osmotic diuresis are glucose-induced osmotic diuresis generated by poorly controlled blood glucose levels and urea-induced osmotic diuresis due to catabolic states, acute illness, high-dose steroids, parenteral nutrition or tube feeding, and during recovery from acute kidney injury. Osmotic diuresis causes the delivery of relatively large amounts of sodium salts to the CNT/collecting tubule (CCT), where K and H secretion are stimulated. Several nephrotoxic drugs, including aminoglycoside antibiotics, amphotericin B, cisplatin, and foscarnet, can also increase distal tubule Na delivery in the face of relative ECF volume contraction and thereby generate K wasting. Some of these drugs also cause renal magnesium wasting and hypomagnesemia. Hypomagnesemia also promotes kaliuresis. Patients with acute myeloid or lymphoblastic leukemia may develop proximal and/or distal tubule dysfunction which can cause hypokalemia. Metabolic acidosis, hyponatremia, hypocalcemia, hypophosphatemia, and hypomagnesemia may also develop in these patients.

When Na is delivered to the distal nephron with poorly reabsorbed anions, K and H secretion are increased. This effect is magnified when ECF contraction elevates renin and aldosterone (see Figure 4–2). This pathologic sequence can develop in patients treated with high-dose Na-penicillin, during the development and treatment of diabetic ketoacidosis (Na-β-hydroxybutyrate), and with inhalation of toluene/glue (Na-hippurate and benzoate). It also occurs with vomiting or NG suction when NaHCO$_3$ is delivered to the distal tubule. Similar mechanisms generate hypokalemia when patients with proximal renal tubular acidosis (RTA type 2) are treated with exogenous bicarbonate salts. Although patients with classic distal tubular acidosis (RTA type 1) have accelerated distal tubule Na-K exchange and develop hypokalemia, renal K excretion and hypokalemia *improve* with NaHCO$_3$ therapy in these patients—in part because ECF volume expands and aldosterone levels fall.

The colon can secrete K and also normally absorbs chloride in exchange for HCO$_3$. Consequently, watery diarrhea can generate metabolic acidosis and hypokalemia. This is particularly pronounced with cholera and cholera-like syndromes. If urine enters the colon, or a segment of ileum (ileal loop bladder), urinary chloride is exchanged for HCO$_3$. In addition, K is secreted. This results in hypokalemia and a hyperchloremic metabolic acidosis. This occurs when ureters are anastomosed into the sigmoid colon, colon segments are interposed between the kidney and bladder, and when ileal loop bladders become partially obstructed and thereby result in prolonged urinary contact time in the intestinal segment. Several other GI disorders can generate severe K wasting and hypokalemia. Colonic pseudo-obstruction (Ogilvie syndrome) is sometimes associated with the loss of large volumes of diarrheal fluid with a very high K concentration. A very small fraction of villous adenomas secrete large amounts of mucous with high K concentrations. A rare genetically inherited condition called congenital chloride-wasting diarrhea results in metabolic alkalosis with hypokalemia. In this disorder, much of the K loss is via the kidney in addition to the stool (HCO$_3$ is intermittently excreted into the urine with Na and K). In many ways, this disorder is analogous to the acid-base and K pathology generated by vomiting or NG suction.

KEY READINGS

Choi MJ, Ziyadeh FN: The utility of the transtubular potassium gradient in the evaluation of hyperkalemia. J Am Soc Nephrol 2008;19:424.

Ethier JH et al: The transtubular potassium concentration in patients with hypokalemia and hyperkalemia. Am J Kidney Dis 1990;15:309.

Scheinman SJ et al: Genetic disorders of renal electrolyte transport. N Engl J Med 1999;340:1177.

▶ Treatment of Hypokalemia

When conditions which are likely to generate hypokalemia exist, it is important to initiate measures which will prevent or ameliorate the development of hypokalemia. Combination of loop and thiazide diuretic therapy is a particularly kaliuretic regimen. Adding an aldosterone antagonist (spironolactone or eplerenone) or a distal tubule Na channel blocker (amiloride or triamterene) to the diuretic regimen will reduce K losses. Angiotensin-converting enzyme inhibitors (ACE-I) and angiotensin receptor blockers (ARBs) can also reduce renal K losses generated by diuretics—in part by reducing aldosterone levels.

Potassium replacement is necessary when K losses reduce body K. As discussed above, exogenous K salts are sometimes used to treat the acute clinical manifestations generated by large K shifts into cells. However, it is imperative that such replacement be undertaken very cautiously since total body K stores under these conditions are normal and rebound hyperkalemia will often occur as the condition reverses.

Oral K salts are the safest method for replacement and should be utilized whenever possible. Although potassium-rich foods (dried fruit, nuts, bananas, oranges, tomatoes, spinach, potatoes, and meat) are generally recommended, they are often inadequate because their K content is relatively low compared to total calories and because the K in food is mainly in the form of organic K salts (see below). Therefore therapeutic K salts are often required to replenish major deficits. Although the relationship is not very tight, a plasma [K] between 3 and 3.5 mEq/L represents a K deficit of 200–400 mEq, while plasma [K] between 2 and 3 mEq/L requires 400–800 mEq.

Potassium replacement salts are divided into two broad classes: potassium chloride (KCl) and potassium bicarbonate ($KHCO_3$) or bicarbonate precursors. Many organic K salts can be metabolized, and when this occurs, HCO_3 is generated mole for mole. KCl is the most appropriate and effective replacement for K deficits associated with metabolic alkalosis. Conversely, alkalinizing K salts ($KHCO_3$, K-citrate, K-acetate, K-gluconate) are best for hypokalemia conditions associated with metabolic acidosis, such as RTA, or chronic diarrhea. Alkalizing K salts are more palatable and better tolerated than oral KCl. However, organic K salts should not be used to treat hypokalemia associated with metabolic alkalosis. In those conditions, alkalinizing K salts are poorly retained and less effectively correct the K deficit and metabolic alkalosis. Table 4–2 lists the various forms of oral potassium salts.

When the oral route cannot be used, or total K deficits are severe, intravenous (IV) replacement becomes necessary. A parenteral fluid KCl concentration of 20–40 mEq/L is generally well tolerated. IV fluid KCl concentrations of 60 mEq/L and greater are painful and may cause peripheral vein necrosis. When the IV administration of a large volume of fluid is contraindicated in a patient with a major K deficit, IV K concentrations of up to 200 mEq/L (20 mEq in 100 mL of isotonic saline) may be given into a central vein, but the administration rate should not exceed 10–20 mEq/h. Central venous administration of very concentrated K solutions requires a rate-controlling pump. The IV solution to which the KCl is added should also be considered, because dextrose infusion will increase insulin and shift K into cells. This could temporarily worsen hypokalemia.

KEY READINGS

Coca SG, Perazella MA, Buller GK: The cardiovascular implications of hypokalemia. Am J Kidney Dis 2005;45:233.

Gennari FJ: Hypokalemia. N Engl J Med 1998;339:451.

Manoukian MA, Foote JA, Crapo LM: Clinical and metabolic features of thyrotoxic periodic paralysis in 24 episodes. Arch Intern Med 1999;159:601.

Norris KC, Levine B, Ganesan K: Thyrotoxic periodic paralysis associated with hypokalemia and hypophosphatemia. Am J Kidney Dis 1996;28:270.

Stewart PM: Mineralocorticoid hypertension. Lancet 1999; 353:1341.

Unwin RJ, Luft FC, Shirley DG: Pathophysiology and management of hypokalemia: a clinical perspective. Nat Rev Nephrol 2011;7:75.

Warnock DG: Hereditary disorders of potassium homeostasis. Best Pract Res Clin Endocrinol Metab 2003;17:505.

Weiner ID, Wingo CS: Hypokalemia—consequences, causes, and correction. J Am Soc Nephrol 1997;8:1179.

West ML et al: New clinical approach to evaluate disorders of potassium excretion. Miner Electrolyte Metab 1986;12:234.

▶ Hyperkalemia

The causes of hyperkalemia, defined as a serum [K] above 5.0 mEq/L, are listed in Table 4–3. Acute or chronic renal failure is by far the most common cause or major contributor to hyperkalemia. When the kidney and the renin-angiotensin-aldosterone system (RAAS) function normally, the plasma [K] is maintained in the normal range despite

Table 4–2. Oral potassium salts.

KCL	KCl elixir	15 mEq/20 mL	
	KCl extended release tablets	8 or 10 mEq/tablet	Micro-K, K-Lor, Slow-K, K-Dur, Kaon-Cl, Klor-Con, Klotrix
	KCl powder	20 or 25 mEq/pack	Kay Ciel, Klor-Con
	KCl solution	20 mEq/15 mL	Kchlor, Kay Ciel, Kaon-Cl
$KHCO_3$ and metabolizable K-organic salts	$KHCO_3$ effervescent tablets	25 mEq/tablet	K-Lyte effervescent tablets, Klor-Con/EF
	K Citrate liquid	2 mEq/mL	Polycitra-K
	K Citrate tablets	5, 10, or 15 mEq/tablet	Urocit-K
	K gluconate liquid/tablets	6.7 mEq/5 mL	Kaon Elixir, Glu-K
		2 and 2.5 mEq/tablet	
	K HCO_3/organic anion mixtures	15 mEq/5 mL	Tri-K, K-Lyte DS
		50 mEq/tablet	

The brand names are those that are more commonly used; other brands are also available.

Table 4–3. Hyperkalemia.

Renal Retention
    Acute renal failure
    Chronic renal failure (especially interstitial renal disease)
    Drugs (see text)
    Addison disease
    Renal tubular acidosis type IV
    Pseudohypoaldosteronism
Tissue Release and Transcellular Shifts of K
    Tissue breakdown (hemolysis, rhabdomyolysis, ischemia, tumor lysis)
    Insulin deficiency
    Hyperosmolarity
    Hyperchloremic metabolic acidosis
    Drugs (succinylcholine, digoxin toxicity)

wide extremes in intake. Therefore, persistent hyperkalemia almost always indicates impaired renal excretion, either due to intrinsic kidney pathology or inadequate/inappropriate endocrine signaling. Rapid K shifts from the intracellular fluid space to the ECF can generate acute hyperkalemia, despite normal renal and endocrine function. Hyperkalemia due to these shifts is exacerbated by coexistent renal dysfunction and/or hormonal derangements.

Before initiating treatment of hyperkalemia or evaluating its etiology, the possibility of artifactual or pseudohyperkalemia must be considered. It can be related to the collection and/or preparation of the blood specimen or an artifact of the K measurement procedure itself. Potential causes include repeated fist clenching during phlebotomy, prolonged tourniquet application, hemolysis due to traumatic venipuncture particularly with small gauge needles, delayed processing of the specimen (especially when placed on ice), and K release from white blood cells when severe leukocytosis (usually >$100 \times 10^3/\mu L$) exists or from platelets when extreme thrombocytosis (usually >$1000 \times 10^3/\mu L$) exists. Some patients have a propensity to leak K from red blood cells (RBCs) ex vivo due to an inherited RBC membrane defects.

Hyperkalemia is associated with an increased risk of death. However, the strongest association is in patients with hyperkalemia and normal renal function. The risk declines as CKD stage progresses, with CKD stage 5 having the lowest risk in one study, and ESRD apparently having a protective effect in another study.

A transcellular shift of K from the intra- to the extracellular space may be caused by direct damage or destruction of cell membranes. This occurs with tumor lysis related to chemotherapy, acute intravascular hemolysis due to infection, transfusion reactions, severe hemolytic anemia, hemolysis occurring within a large hematoma, extensive burns, rhabdomyolysis, and with intestinal ischemia/necrosis.

Excessive K efflux may also occur when the cell membranes are intact. Certain drugs, metabolic disorders, and

inherited diseases can generate this class of hyperkalemia. The muscle relaxant succinylcholine consistently promotes cellular K efflux and can generate profound hyperkalemia, especially in patients with an underlying neuromuscular or renal disorder. Drugs that block β-agonist activity also favor K efflux from cells. Therapeutic digitalis levels inhibit Na/K ATPase in cardiac myocytes, and this is primarily responsible for the drug's positive inotropic effect. However, toxic levels of digitalis also inhibit Na/K ATPase pumps in muscle cells throughout the body and thereby generates extreme hyperkalemia. Potassium translocation from cells to the ECF also occurs with insulin deficiency or resistance, certain hyperosmolar conditions such as hyperglycemia, and some forms of inorganic (usually hyperchloremic) metabolic acidoses. It was previously assumed that all forms of acidemia, especially those due to metabolic acidosis, caused protons to move into cells with reciprocal K efflux. However, organic metabolic acidoses, such as keto- and lactic acidosis, do not generate significant K shifts. When hyperkalemia develops in these patients, it is usually the result of other pathophysiological processes and not the academia per se. For example, hyperkalemia occurs frequently with lactic acidosis but is principally due to tissue ischemia/necrosis and concomitant renal insufficiency. Hyperkalemia is also a common finding in diabetic ketoacidosis and is due to the combination of insulin deficiency, hyperosmolarity (hyperglycemia), and decreased renal perfusion, rather than the academia per se. The infusion of some inorganic acids, such as HCl, will generate a direct K shift out of cells. Genetic defects of cell membrane ion transporters, usually epithelial Na-channels, cause the syndrome of *hyper*kalemic periodic paralysis.

Nonphysiologic states of hypoaldosteronism (ie, not secondary to ECF expansion) can generate chronic hyperkalemia because of reduced distal tubule (CNT/CCD) K secretion. This is exacerbated by concomitant renal insufficiency or markedly reduced distal tubule Na delivery. Pathologic hypoaldosteronism may be the consequence of a direct block of adrenal aldosterone synthesis (due to congenital or acquired enzyme defect or adrenal damage) or secondary to dysregulation of the signals mediating aldosterone synthesis and release. The most important physiologic regulator of systemic aldosterone is angiotensin II activity, and the most common form of pathologic hypoaldosteronism is due to reduced renin activity and hence angiotensin II levels. This state of "hyporeninemic hypoaldosteronism" often develops in patients with long-standing diabetes mellitus as a result of interstitial renal disease with atrophy and/or destruction of the renin-secreting cells in the juxtaglomerular apparatus. Other interstitial renal diseases, such as those associated with sickle cell disease, analgesic nephropathy, and chronic urinary outlet obstruction (especially in elderly men), may produce a state of hyporeninemic hypoaldosteronism as well. Elderly patients may develop hyporeninemic hypoaldosteronism in the setting of reduced renal function which is often underappreciated because of their low muscle mass.

Hypoaldosteronism directly slows the rate of distal tubule proton secretion. In addition, hyperkalemia inhibits renal ammonia synthesis and reduces NH_4Cl excretion. These defects combine to generate a syndrome of hyperkalemic, hyperchloremic metabolic acidosis called renal tubular acidosis type 4. Correction of the hyperkalemia increases urine ammonia excretion and often reverses the metabolic acidosis.

Inhibition or blockade of the RAAS—i.e. Renin → angiotensin I → angiotensin II → aldosterone → activation of distal tubule Na reabsorption and K (and H) secretion at any step will promote the development of hyperkalemia. Clinically important causes include

1. Suppressed renin secretion: β-blockers, nonsteroid anti-inflammatory drugs (NSAIDs), cyclosporine, and tacrolimus

2. Blockade of renin action on angiotensinogen: aliskiren

3. Impaired angiotensin II generation: angiotensin converting enzyme inhibitors (ACE-I)

4. Blockade of type I angiotensin II receptor: angiotensin receptor blockers (ARB)

5. Inhibition of aldosterone synthetic pathway: heparin, ketoconazole

6. Destruction of the adrenal gland: autoimmune disease, infection

7. Competitive antagonism of mineralocorticoid receptors: spironolactone, eplerenone

8. Blockade of the CNT/CCT epithelial sodium channels: triamterene, amiloride, trimethoprim, and pentamidine

9. Blunted renal epithelial response to aldosterone: inherited disorders (the congenital pseudohypoaldosteronism syndromes)

The development of hyperkalemia in patients with diabetes mellitus is due to a number of potential pathologies including autonomic sympathetic neuropathy which reduces renin levels and blunts β-adrenergic activity, and multiple often prescribed medications such as ACE-I, ARB, aldosterone antagonists, and NSAID (see below). Renal function is often reduced and these patients may also ingest excess K in the form of salt substitute. With suboptimal diabetic control, the combined effects of insulin deficiency and hyperglycemia may generate marked acute hyperkalemia.

The contribution of reduced renal K excretion to the development of hyperkalemia is usually readily apparent. If it is not obvious a quantitative urine collection to measure daily K excretion is helpful. Chronic hyperkalemia should stimulate renal K excretion and the 24-hour urine should contain more than 80 mEq. If a quantitative urine collection cannot be obtained, the TTKG (described in the

hypokalemia section) should be greater than 10, provided urine osmolality is above 300 mOsm/L and urinary Na excretion above 20 mEq/L.

KEY READINGS

Adrogue HJ et al: Determinants of plasma potassium levels in diabetic ketoacidosis. Medicine 1986;65:163.

Allon M: Hyperkalemia in end-stage renal disease: mechanisms and management. J Am Soc Nephrol 1995;6:1134.

Einhorn LM et al: The frequency of hyperkalemia and its significance in chronic kidney disease. Arch Intern Med 2009;169:1156.

Greenberg A: Hyperkalemia: treatment options. Semin Nephrol 1998;18:46.

Hughes-Austin JM et al: The relation of serum potassium concentration with cardiovascular events and mortality in community-living individuals. Clin J Am Soc Nephrol 2017;12:245.

Juurlink DN et al: Rates of hyperkalemia after publication of the Randomized Aldactone Evaluation Study. N Engl J Med 2004; 351:543.

Montford JR, Linas S: How Dangerous is hyperkalemia? J Am Soc Nephrol 2007;28.

Perazella MA: Drug-induced hyperkalemia: old culprits and new offenders. Am J Med 2000;109:307.

Wiederkehr MR, Moe OW: Factitious hyperkalemia. Am J Kidney Dis 2000;36:1049.

▶ Treatment of Hyperkalemia

Before addressing the treatment of hyperkalemia, it is important to emphasize the importance of initiating measures to prevent its occurrence in patients who are susceptible to its development. These patients should restrict their dietary potassium intake. Lists of potassium-rich food sources (potatoes, tomatoes, oranges, and other fruit) should be given to these patients, and they benefit from counseling by a dietitian. Potassium-rich sources to be avoided also include many salt substitutes, herbal medicines, and a variety of dietary supplements.

A number of commonly used medications which inhibit or antagonize the renin-angiotensin-aldosterone axis contribute to the development of hyperkalemia. They include ACE-I, angiotensin 2 receptor blockers, calcineurin inhibitors, β-blockers, digoxin, nonsteroidal anti-inflammatory drugs, and potassium sparing diuretics. The aldosterone antagonists spironolactone and eplerenone are commonly used for management of systolic congestive heart failure, proteinuric renal disease, and resistant hypertension.

There is no consensus about the exact level of hyperkalemia which requires urgent intervention, and the terminology of "mild," "moderate," and "severe" hyperkalemia is inconsistent. We suggest adjustments in medications and/or diet whenever the potassium level exceeds the upper limit of normal. Generally, urgent intervention is indicated when the potassium level exceeds 6.0–6.5 mEq/L.

Emergency intervention for hyperkalemia can be divided into a three-phased approach:

1. Direct reversal of cardiotoxic effects—membrane stabilization
   a. Intravenous calcium
2. Translocating K into cells
   a. Insulin infusion with glucose (insulin alone if hyperglycemia exists)
   b. Adrenergic agonists such as albuterol
   c. NaHCO$_3$ infusion
3. Increasing K excretion
   a. Via the kidney by ECF volume expansion and kaliuretic diuretics
   b. Via the gastrointestinal tract by K-binding agents and induction of diarrhea
   c. Via dialysis for patients with severe acute or chronic renal failure

Hyperkalemia decreases the resting potential of the myocyte membrane and produces a spectrum of ECG abnormalities, including peaked T waves, a prolonged PR segment, progressive widening of QRS, bundle branch block, and bradycardia (Figure 4–3). However, these ECG changes are unreliable and inconsistent, and a normal ECG should not delay immediate action in the setting of severe hyperkalemia (if pseudohypokalemia is unlikely or has been ruled out). Life-threatening cardiac arrhythmias can develop without warning. Calcium infusion stabilizes the myocardium by opposing the depolarizing effects of hyperkalemia (Figure 4–4). Increasing ECF calcium raises the threshold potential and also speeds cardiac impulse propagation. The calcium may act by reversing hyperkalemia-induced inactivation of voltage gated sodium channels. Calcium infusions are generally safe in the absence of overt hypercalcemia, marked hyperphosphatemia, or digitalis toxicity. One ampule (10 mL) of 10% calcium gluconate contains 93 mg or 4.65 mEq of elemental calcium. It is administered as a slow IV push via a peripheral IV over 2–5 minutes. An alternative formulation is calcium chloride; 1 ampule (10 mL) of calcium chloride 10% contains about three times as much elemental calcium (273 mg or 13.6 mEq) as 1 ampule of calcium gluconate. However, it is generally recommended that calcium chloride be administered via a central line because extravasation of calcium chloride can cause tissue necrosis. The beneficial effect of IV calcium on the ECG is seen almost immediately. The dose of calcium may be repeated if ECG abnormalities persist or recur. It is important to understand that calcium infusions do not directly affect the plasma [K]. Therefore, other treatments that reduce plasma [K] must be initiated together with, or immediately after, the calcium infusion. Also, although IV calcium infusions work rapidly—within 1–3 minutes—the myocardial electrical stabilizing effect of calcium only continues for about ½–1 hour.

Insulin, β_2-agonists, and NaHCO$_3$ all drive extracellular potassium into cells. Insulin stimulates Na-K ATPase and probably the Na-H exchanger (Figure 4–1). It reliably reduces plasma [K] by 0.5–1 mEq/L within 10–20 minutes. The maximum K-lowering effect of insulin requires supraphysiologic insulin levels. The usual dose is 10 units of regular insulin via IV push. Subcutaneous, intramuscular, and "low-dose" IV infusions should not be utilized because adequate plasma insulin levels will not be achieved. Of course, glucose must also be administered with the insulin to avoid hypoglycemia unless the patient is hyperglycemic (glucose >250 mg/100 mL). A reasonable approach is to administer 1 ampule (50 mL) of 50% glucose, followed by an intravenous infusion of 10% glucose at about 75 mL/h. Hyperglycemia should be avoided because it increases tonicity which will shift fluid and K (by "solvent drag") from intracellular fluid to the extracellular space. The glucose infusion is required to avoid late hypoglycemia because the glucose-lowering effect of the bolus of insulin peaks at about 1 hour, may last up to 2 hours, and persists even longer in patients with CKD. Therefore, the glucose and K levels should be carefully monitored. Although the infusion of glucose alone will stimulate endogenous insulin secretion (in nondiabetic patients), it is not recommended because the resulting insulin levels are inadequate. Although short-acting insulins such as insulin lispro (Humalog) and insulin aspart (NovoLog) may be safer alternatives, they have not yet been well studied for this indication.

The β_2-agonist albuterol stimulates Na-K ATPase and transfers K into cells. This effect is additive to that of IV insulin and occurs within 30–60 minutes. Because parenteral albuterol is not available in the United States, the drug can only be administered via the respiratory tract by nebulization. The dose of albuterol for this purpose is relatively high: 10–20 mg in 4 mL of saline (4–8 fold the bronchodilation dose). Albuterol is relatively contraindicated when acute cardiac ischemia or severe myocardial disease exists. It is important to emphasize that some patients do not respond to albuterol. Therefore, it should always be combined with an insulin infusion.

Hypertonic NaHCO$_3$ has several mechanisms of action in reversing the effects of hyperkalemia. It increases intracellular Na by stimulating Na-H exchangers and NaHCO$_3$ cotransporters. The resulting higher intracellular Na concentration activates cellular Na-K ATPase which moves K into cells. The NaHCO$_3$ solution in ampules is very hypertonic: 44 mEq NaHCO$_3$ in 50 mL translates to 892 mOsm/L. This osmotic salt load causes a rapid influx of fluid into the ECF space and expansion lowers [K] by dilution. However, this effect can also precipitate acute pulmonary edema and/ or cardiac decompensation in susceptible persons. If kidney function is not markedly impaired, NaHCO$_3$ will generate a diuresis which decreases K. Although several studies have shown NaHCO$_3$ to be relatively ineffective in reducing

K concentrations, it has not been studied in patients with significant metabolic acidosis. Last, the increase in ECF Na concentration could be beneficial in partially reversing the inhibition of voltage sensitive sodium channels generated by hyperkalemia.

Stabilization of the myocardial membrane with calcium and translocation of potassium into the intracellular space are rapid and effective interventions for hyperkalemia. Ultimately, however, an important goal is to remove excess K from the body by renal, gastrointestinal, and/or extracorporeal means. If kidney function is adequate, loop and thiazide diuretics (and especially in combination) are effective kaliuretic agents. Thiazide diuretics are particularly helpful for patients with hyporeninemic hypoaldosteronism. This class of agents is generally less useful in advanced CKD (with the exception of metolazone), where loop diuretics are more commonly utilized. For acute management, high-dose IV push furosemide (or other loop diuretics) generally works rapidly and effectively. These drugs may be used in combination with saline or $NaHCO_3$ in volume contracted patients ("forced diuresis"). Monitoring hourly urine output is a useful way to follow the response. IV or oral loop diuretics remain effective even as kidney function approaches "end stage." In diabetics with hypoaldosteronism due to hyporeninemia (RTA type 4), or medication-induced hypoaldosteronism (calcineurin inhibitors cyclosporine or tacrolimus), the addition of the mineralocorticoid agent fludrocortisone, increases renal potassium excretion. Mineralocorticoids are generally indicated if the patient's volume status is contracted. They may also be useful when combined with a diuretic that increases delivery of Na to the distal renal tubule principal cell where luminal Na is exchanged for potassium in the presence of a mineralocorticoid hormone.

Stool potassium excretion is increased by administration of laxatives to generate electrolyte-rich diarrhea and by binding gastrointestinal luminal K to a nonabsorbable polymers, resins, and other substances.

Sodium polystyrene sulfonate (SPS, Kayexalate) is an Na-charged resin which has been used since the 1950s. It releases Na and in exchange for K but also Mg, Ca, NH_4, and protons. The conditions in the distal colon and rectum are most optimal for K binding to this resin. Kayexalate has a sand-like/gritty constituency which is unpalatable. It swells within the GI tract and is often associated with GI side effects. SPS is usually premixed with sorbitol, which speeds its transit through the gut and acts to avoid constipation but sometimes lead to diarrhea. SPS-sorbitol suspensions have been associated with intestinal necrosis. Although very uncommon, this complication is often fatal. Intestinal necrosis was initially attributed to very hypertonic (70%) sorbitol mixtures, but subsequent reports also implicated reduced sorbitol concentrations (33%) and even sorbitol-free SPS. Furthermore, multiple studies have demonstrated that potassium binding to SPS is relatively inefficient. SPS has a delayed effect of several hours and should not be used for acute K lowering.

Two new potassium binders, patiromer calcium and sodium zirconium silicate (ZS-9) have recently been developed. Patiromer is a nonabsorbed, synthetic, nonswelling polymer which is formed into smooth spherical 100-μm-diameter beads. Patiromer's active exchange groups are initially charged with Ca. After ingestion, the active sites exchange the Ca for K, but Mg, NH_4, and protons also compete for binding on the polymer. Conditions in the colon are most favorable for K exchange. Depending on the dose of patiromer, the daily fecal potassium excretion is about 15–20 mmol. The potassium lowering effect of patiromer is typically delayed by about 7 hours. Therefore, the drug is not approved for the treatment of acute hyperkalemia. Side effects are mainly gastrointestinal (flatulence, diarrhea, and nausea). Some of the released Ca is absorbed, and some is excreted in the stool (bound to phosphate and other anions). Hypomagnesemia may occur. Because patiromer can potentially bind to co-administered drugs, it should be administered at least 3 hours before or 3 hours after other oral medications.

Sodium zirconium cyclosilicate (ZS-9) is a selective cation-exchanging crystal that releases Na and binds K (and NH_4). It is taken as a tasteless, odorless, insoluble powder that is mixed with water and given with food. The exchange process occurs throughout the entire GI tract and is largely independent of the ambient pH. It has a more than 25-fold selectivity for K over Ca and Mg. Zirconium cyclosilicate binds K at least nine times more effectively than SPS. The release and systemic absorption of Na can cause weight gain and edema. It does not swell in the GI tract, and the incidence of adverse events has thus far been very low. Complaints of diarrhea are similar to placebo. Zirconium cyclosilicate apparently does not bind other oral medications. Because it works throughout the entire GI tract, it has a rapid onset of action and thus could be useful for the treatment of both acute and chronic hyperkalemia. Ingestion of 10 g of zirconium silicate lowered serum potassium levels by 0.4 mEq/L at 1 hour and 0.7 mEq/L at 4 hours. However, sodium zirconium cyclosilicate has not yet been approved by the FDA. While the long-term safety of these new agents is yet to be established, it is likely that they will play important roles in the treatment of the hyperkalemic patient and will probably replace SPS as a gastrointestinal K binding agent.

Hemodialysis is a highly effective, but invasive, modality to reduce the potassium concentration. Hemodialysis rapidly removes 25–50 mEq/h of potassium from the extracellular space. Although serum level is promptly reduced, significant postdialysis rebound occurs because extracellular potassium equilibrates with intracellular stores. It is commonly employed in hyperkalemic patients with end stage renal disease (ESRD) and also in critically ill patients who can develop sudden hyperkalemia as a result of tissue necrosis (in particular rhabdomyolysis) and/or hemolysis.

KEY READINGS

Packham DK et al: Sodium zirconium cyclosilicate in hyperkalemia. N Engl J Med 2015;372:222.

Palmer BF: Managing hyperkalemia caused by inhibitors of the renin-angiotensin-aldosterone system. N Engl J Med 2004;351:585.

Rossignol P et al: Emergency management of severe hyperkalemia: guideline for best practice and opportunities for the future. Pharmacol Res 2016;113:585.

Sterns RH, Grieff M, Bernstein PL: Treatment of hyperkalemia: something old, something new. Kidney Int 2016;89:546.

Weir MR et al: Patiromer in patients with kidney disease and hyperkalemia receiving RAAS inhibitors. N Engl J Med 2015;372:211.

■ CHAPTER REVIEW QUESTIONS

1. A 40-year-old man with HIV/AIDS admitted to the hospital with weakness. He had a recently diagnosed mycobacterial infection which is being treated. Current medications include tenofovir-emtricitabine plus raltegravir, isoniazid, rifampin, pyridoxine, and trimethoprim-sulfamethoxazole.

   Laboratory studies include blood urea nitrogen (BUN) 15, creatinine 1.6, glucose 110, sodium 137, potassium 6.3, chloride 104, and bicarbonate 26. Discontinuation of which of the following medications is most likely to reduce his serum potassium concentration?
   A. Rifampin
   B. Trimethoprim-sulfamethoxazole
   C. Pyridoxine
   D. Tenofovir-emtricitabine

2. A 50-year-old man is admitted for evaluation of weakness and palpitations. Two weeks ago pernicious anemia was diagnosed and he was begun on vitamin B_{12} injections 6 days ago. Now he has developed worsening diffuse weakness and palpitations. Examination shows him to be pale and anxious. Pulse is irregular. Bowel sounds are diminished. Deep tendon reflexes are markedly decreased.

   His hematocrit has increased from 18 to 28 g%. Platelet count increased from 70,000 to 90,000. BUN was 15 mg% and creatinine was 1.1 mg%, which were both stable. Electrolytes 2 weeks ago: sodium 140, potassium 3.9, chloride 105, and bicarbonate 22. Electrolytes now: sodium 139, potassium 2.5, chloride 104, and bicarbonate 23. A urine potassium-to-creatinine ratio is 15 mEq/g. ECG shows frequent ventricular extrasystole and prominent U waves. Kidney, ureter, and bladder (KUB) X-ray shows dilated loops of the small intestine. Blood gas: pH 7.48, PCO_2 32, PO_2 is 100. Which of the following is the most likely cause of his acute hypokalemia?

   A. Renal potassium wasting
   B. Sequestration of potassium in small bowel fluid
   C. Respiratory alkalosis
   D. B_{12} administration

3. A 76-year-old woman is admitted to the hospital after falling and fracturing her right hip. Following admission she undergoes a right hip replacement. She is receiving pain medication and has now developed abdominal discomfort. Over the next 24 hours her abdomen swells, and X-rays show a diffusely enlarged colon containing a great deal of fluid. She has also developed watery diarrhea. Her electrolytes on admission were normal. Now she has developed hypokalemia with potassium of 2.5 mEq/L. Which of the following is the most likely etiology for her hypokalemia?
   A. Very high stool potassium output due to active K secretion
   B. Increased urinary potassium losses
   C. Potassium shift into cells
   D. Electrolyte artifact
   E. Poor K intake

4. A 25-year-old man was involved in a motor vehicle accident resulting in marked blunt trauma to the abdomen. He required extensive abdominal surgery which included revascularization of his small bowel and resection of a segment of small bowel. He is now in the intensive care unit receiving nasogastric suction which is removing a large amount of gastric fluid. He has developed severe metabolic alkalosis with hypokalemia (HCO_3 = 42; K = 2.8 mEq/L). Which of the following mechanisms is the most likely cause of the hypokalemia in this patient?
   A. Potassium loss in the aspirated NG fluid
   B. Potassium loss into the urine
   C. Potassium shift into cells
   D. Potassium loss in stool

5. A 40-year-old man is seen by his physician for a routine examination and is found to have asymptomatic hypertension. Electrolytes show he is hypokalemic (3.0 mEq/L) and has bicarbonate of 32 mEq/L. A renin-aldosterone ratio shows that both renin and aldosterone levels are markedly reduced. Which of the following diagnostic possibilities should be considered in this patient?
   A. Primary hyperaldosteronism due to a unilateral adenoma (Conn syndrome)
   B. Licorice ingestion
   C. Bartter syndrome
   D. Hypokalemic periodic paralysis

6. For many years Kayexalate was the only available GI potassium-binding medication. Now a new and more potent binding agent called patiromer has been approved by the FDA. When Kayexalate binds potassium, it releases sodium. Which counter ion is released from patiromer?
   A. Magnesium
   B. Calcium
   C. Sodium
   D. Lanthanum

Acid–Base Disorders

Thomas D. DuBose, Jr, MD, MACP, FASN

Gregg Y. Lipschik, MD

Jeanne P. Macrae, MD

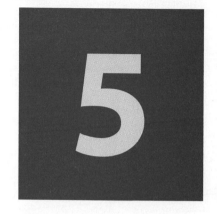

▼ METABOLIC ACIDOSIS

Thomas D. DuBose, Jr, MD

▶ General Considerations

A. Introduction

Metabolic acidosis is one of four cardinal acid–base disorders and is characterized by a decrease in the serum [HCO_3^-] or [tCO_2] below the value of 22 mEq/L. Because respiratory alkalosis can also cause a decline in plasma [HCO_3^-] below normal, it is necessary to measure blood pH to distinguish between the two disorders. With metabolic acidosis, the pH is typically below the normal range of 7.35–7.45, while in respiratory alkalosis the pH is customarily above the normal range. Chronic respiratory alkalosis is the only acid base disorder for which the compensatory response can return the blood pH to normal (fully compensated). Therefore, an arterial blood gas is needed to make the precise acid base diagnosis. In addition, the clinical setting in which the disorder occurs is also helpful and is discussed below. Finally, other clinical tools (such as the serum anion gap [AG]) and simple calculations (comparison of the change in [HCO_3^-] with the change in the AG from their respective normal values) can aid in making the appropriate acid–base diagnosis. Metabolic acidosis may occur because of an increase in endogenous organic acid production (such as lactate and ketoacids), a loss of bicarbonate (as with diarrhea), or an accumulation of endogenous acids because of inappropriately low excretion of net acid by the kidney (as in chronic kidney disease).

B. Neurorespiratory Response to Acidemia

The neurorespiratory control of ventilation is a critically important response to an acid load, and primary metabolic acidosis elicits predictable compensatory respiratory responses (secondary changes in $Paco_2$). In general, a fall in systemic arterial pH is sensed by the chemoreceptors that stimulate ventilation and, therefore, reduce $Paco_2$. The fall in blood pH that would otherwise occur in uncompensated metabolic acidosis is blunted, therefore, but is not returned to the normal value, when metabolic acidosis is part of a simple (or single) acid base disturbance. Typically, the $Paco_2$ declines by an average of 1.25 mm Hg for each 1.0 mEq/L drop in HCO_3^- concentration. The appropriate value for the $Paco_2$ with physiologic compensation in steady-state metabolic acidosis can be estimated from the patient's serum HCO_3^- concentration by application of the classical Winter equation:

$$Paco_2 = 1.5 (HCO_3^-) + 8 \pm 2 \text{ (mm Hg)}$$

An easier but less accurate approach requires one to simply add the number 15 to the patient's [HCO_3^-] to quickly estimate the predicted (or compensatory) value for $Paco_2$ (valid in the pH range of 7.2–7.5). Approximately 12–24 hours is required to achieve full respiratory compensation for metabolic acidosis. However, since the decline in $Paco_2$ is limited by the accompanying hypoxia and cannot fall below about 10–12 mm Hg, the blood pH is less well defended by respiration when the plasma HCO_3^- concentration is less than 10 mEq/L.

When metabolic acidosis occurs and the $Paco_2$ falls within the range of the predicted compensatory response (as derived from the Winter equation), those values denote a **simple** metabolic acidosis. For example, consider a patient presenting with diarrhea of 3 days and the following laboratory values: Na = 140, Cl = 115, K = 3.0, and HCO_3 = 15; arterial pH = 7.32, and a $Paco_2$ = 30. Clearly this patient has metabolic acidosis, and since the predicted $Paco_2$ (from the Winter equation) is equal to 30 mm Hg (or exactly the same value as the measured $Paco_2$), the findings together, corroborate that the acid–base disorder is a **simple** metabolic acidosis. In contrast, measured values for $Paco_2$ that are outside the predicted range by ±3 mm Hg (ie, <27 or >33), indicate a mixed disturbance, metabolic acidosis plus respiratory alkalosis, and metabolic acidosis plus respiratory acidosis, respectively. Therefore, if a patient with a similar history, but different laboratory values: Na = 140, Cl = 100, HCO_3 = 15; arterial pH = 7.38, and $Paco_2$ = 26, then these laboratory values indicate the presence of a **mixed** acid base disturbance, specifically, in this example: mixed metabolic acidosis and respiratory alkalosis. Note that the presence of a metabolic acidosis is supported additionally, in this example by the existence of a high anion gap (AG = 25 mEq/L). The use of the AG in acid–base analysis is expanded in the following section.

C. Calculation and Application of the Anion Gap (AG)

There are two major categories of metabolic acidosis in the clinical setting: high-AG and non-AG acidosis. Therefore, the accurate diagnosis of clinical acid–base disorders requires attention to the AG. The AG is calculated as: AG = $Na^+ - (Cl^- + HCO_3^-)$. The value for plasma $[K^+]$ is typically omitted from the calculation of the AG, by laboratories in the United States. The "normal" value for the AG reported by clinical laboratories has been declined with improved methodology for measuring plasma electrolytes, and ranges from 6 to 12 mmol/L, with an average of approximately 10 mmol/L. Those unmeasured anions normally present in plasma include anionic proteins (eg, albumin), phosphate, sulfate, and organic anions. When organic acid anions, such as acetoacetate, betahydroxyacetate, or lactate, accumulate in extracellular fluid (ECF), the AG increases, causing a **high-AG acidosis**. An increase in the AG is most often due to an increase in unmeasured anions, but less commonly, may be due to a decrease in unmeasured cations (calcium, magnesium, potassium), or, conversely, the AG may increase because of an increase in anionic albumin. A decrease in the AG can be due to (1) an increase in unmeasured cations; (2) the addition to the blood of abnormal cations, such as lithium (lithium intoxication) or cationic immunoglobulins (plasma cell dyscrasias); (3) a reduction in the plasma anion albumin concentration (nephrotic syndrome, liver disease, or malabsorption); or (4) hyperviscosity and severe hyperlipidemia, which can lead to an underestimation of sodium and chloride concentrations.

The AG should always be corrected for the prevailing albumin concentration (for each g/dL decrease in albumin below the normal value of 4 g/dL, add 2.5 mEq/L to the traditionally calculated AG to obtain the "corrected" AG. The normal AG in patients with a normal serum albumin concentration and otherwise normal metabolic status is approximately 10 mEq/L. Corrected AG values above 10 mEq/L represent a high AG metabolic acidosis.

A high AG acidosis typically denotes the accumulation of organic acids to the ECF. This may occur if the anion does not undergo glomerular filtration (eg, uremic acid anions), or if, because of alteration in metabolic pathways (ketoacidosis, L-lactic acidosis), the anion cannot be utilized immediately. Theoretically, with a pure AG acidosis, the increment in the AG above the normal value of 10 ± 3 mEq/L (ΔAG) should equal the decrease in bicarbonate concentration below the normal value of 25 mEq/L (ΔHCO_3^-). When this relationship is considered, circumstances in which the increment in the AG exceeds the decrement in bicarbonate (ΔAG > ΔHCO_3^-) suggest a **mixed acid base disorder**, and in this example, the coexistence of a metabolic alkalosis. Circumstances in which the increment in the AG is less than the decrement in bicarbonate (ΔAG < ΔHCO_3^-) suggest the coexistence of a non-AG metabolic acidosis.

The high AG is significant clinically even if the $[HCO_3^-]$ or pH is normal. A high AG is usually due to accumulation of non–chloride-containing acids that contain inorganic (phosphate, sulfate), organic (ketoacids, lactate, uremic organic anions), exogenous (salicylate or ingested toxins with organic acid production), or unidentified anions. A detailed list of causes of high AG acidosis is displayed in Table 5–1. Common causes of a high gap acidosis (HAG acidosis) include (1) lactic acidosis, (2) ketoacidosis, (3) toxin- or poison-induced acidosis, and (4) uremic acidosis. The presence of metabolic acidosis, a normal AG, and hyperchloremia denotes the presence of a normal or non-AG metabolic acidosis (NAG acidosis) and will be discussed following a review of the causes of the high AG acidoses.

KEY READING

Vichot AA, Rastegar A: Use of anion gap in the evaluation of a patient with metabolic acidosis. Am J Kidney Dis. 2014;64:653.

▶ Clinical Examples of High AG Acidosis (Table 5–1)

A. Lactic Acidosis

Lactic acid can exist in two forms: L (levorotatory)-lactic acid and D (dextrorotatory)-lactic acid. In mammals, only the levorotatory form is a product of mammalian metabolism. D-Lactate can accumulate in humans only as a by-product of metabolism of carbohydrate by bacteria which abnormally accumulate and overgrow in the gastrointestinal tract as might occur with a "blind loop" in bowel, with jejunal bypass, or short bowel syndrome. L-Lactic acidosis is one of the most common forms of a high AG acidosis. Hospital chemistry laboratories routinely measure L-lactic acid levels, not D-lactic acid levels. Consequently, the clinician who suspects D-lactic acidosis must ask the clinical laboratory to specifically measure D-lactic acid.

Table 5–1. Causes of high anion gap metabolic acidosis.

Conditions associated with type A lactic acidosis
    Hypovolemic shock
    Cholera
    Septic shock
    Cardiogenic shock (low-output or high-output heart failure)
    Regional hypoperfusion
    Severe hypoxia
        Severe asthma
        Carbon monoxide poisoning
        Severe anemia
Conditions associated with type B lactic acidosis
    Liver disease
    Diabetes mellitus
    Catecholamine excess
    Thiamine deficiency
    Intracellular inorganic phosphate depletion
        Intravenous fructose
        Intravenous xylose
        Intravenous sorbitol
    Alcohols and other ingested compounds metabolized by alcohol
        dehydrogenase
        Ethanol, Methanol, Ethylene glycol, Propylene glycol
    Mitochondrial toxins
    Salicylates
    Cyanide
    2,4-dinitrophenol
    Nonnucleoside antireverse transcriptase drugs
    Other drugs
    Metastatic tumors (large tumors with regional hypoxemia or
        liver metastasis)
    Major motor seizure-prolonged
    Inborn errors of metabolism
D-Lactic acidosis
    Short bowel syndrome
    Ischemic bowel
    Small-bowel obstruction
Ketoacidosis
    Diabetic
    Alcoholic
    Starvation
Other toxins
    Salicylates
    Paraldehyde
    Pyroglutamic acid
Uremia (late renal failure)

Lactic acid metabolism, although similar to that of pyruvate, is in a metabolic cul-de-sac with pyruvate as its only outlet. In most cells, the major metabolic pathway for pyruvate is oxidation in the mitochondria to acetyl-coenzyme A by the enzyme pyruvate dehydrogenase within the mitochondria.

According to the historical classification of the L-lactic acidoses, type A L-lactic acidosis is due to tissue hypoperfusion or acute hypoxia, whereas type B L-lactic acidosis is associated with common diseases, drugs or toxins, and hereditary and miscellaneous disorders. Lactate concentrations are mildly increased in various nonpathologic states (eg, exercise), but the magnitude of the elevation is generally small. A lactate concentration greater than 4 mmol/L (normal is 0.67–1.8 mmol/L) is taken as evidence that the metabolic acidosis is the result of lactic acid acidosis.

Tissue underperfusion and acute underoxygenation at the tissue level (tissue hypoxia) are the most common causes of type A lactic acidosis. Inadequate cardiac output, of either the low-output or the high-output variety, is the most frequent cause, but severe arterial hypoxemia can also generate L-lactic acidosis. The prognosis is related to the increment in plasma L-lactate and the severity of the acidemia.

A number of medical disorders (without tissue hypoxia) may cause type B L-lactic acidosis. Hepatic failure reduces hepatic lactate metabolism, and leukemia increases lactate production. Severe anemia, especially as a result of iron deficiency or methemoglobinemia, may cause lactic acidosis. Among patients in the critical care unit the most common cause of L-lactic acidosis is bowel ischemia and infarction. Malignant cells produce more lactate than normal cells even under aerobic conditions. This phenomenon is magnified if the tumor expands rapidly and outstrips its blood supply. Therefore, exceptionally large tumors may be associated with severe L-lactic acidosis. Seizures, extreme exertion, heat stroke, and tumor lysis syndrome may all cause L-lactic acidosis.

Several drugs and toxins predispose to L-lactic acidosis. Of these, metformin is the most widely reported to have this effect, but is relatively uncommon. Nevertheless, metformin-induced lactic acidosis is at higher risk in patients with chronic kidney disease (and is contraindicated when the serum creatinine exceeds 1.4 mg/dL), or whenever there is hypoperfusion or hypotension, including severe volume depletion (especially in the elderly), shock, septicemia, congestive heart failure (CHF), or a recent myocardial infarction.

In patients with HIV infection, nucleoside analogs predispose to toxic effects on mitochondria by inhibiting DNA polymerase-γ. Therefore, hyperlactatemia is common with anti-HIV therapy, but the serum L-lactate level is usually only mildly elevated. However, with severe concurrent illness pronounced lactic acidosis may occur in association with hepatic steatosis and a high mortality.

B. Treatment of L-Lactic Acid Acidosis

The overall mortality of patients with L-lactic acidosis is approximately 60%, but approaches 100% in those with coexisting multiorgan dysfunction. The most important and effective therapy for L-lactic acidosis is to correct the underlying condition initiating the disruption in normal lactate metabolism. In general this requires attention to cessation of acid production by improvement of tissue oxygenation, restoration of the circulating fluid volume, improvement or augmentation of cardiac function, surgical resection of ischemic tissue (eg, infarcted bowel), and antibiotics may all be necessary for type A L-lactic acidosis.

Limited administration of intravenous $NaHCO_3$ is advocated for acute, severe acidemia (pH of <7.0) to improve myocardial inotropy and lactate utilization. Nevertheless, $NaHCO_3$ therapy in large amounts can depress cardiac performance and exacerbate academia, because, paradoxically, bicarbonate therapy activates phosphofructokinase, which is regulated by intracellular pH, thereby increasing lactate production. For all of these reasons, $NaHCO_3$ should be used very cautiously with the goal of increasing the plasma $[HCO_3^-]$ to a value of no more than 5–8 mmol/L.

If the underlying cause of the L-lactic acidosis can be remedied, blood lactate will be reconverted to HCO_3^-. The bicarbonate derived metabolically from lactate conversion is additive to any new HCO_3^- generated by kidney mechanisms during acidosis and from exogenous alkali therapy might lead to an "overshoot" alkalosis.

KEY READINGS

Kim HJ, Son YK, An WS: Effect of sodium bicarbonate administration on mortality in patients with lactic acidosis: a retrospective analysis. PLoS One 2013;8:e65283.

Mirrakhimov AE et al: Propofol infusion syndrome in adults: a clinical update. Crit Care Res Pract 2015;2015:260385.

C. D-Lactic Acidosis

The typical clinical features of D-lactate acidosis are episodic encephalopathy and high AG acidosis in association with short bowel syndrome. D-Lactic acidosis has been described in patients with bowel obstruction, jejunal bypass, short bowel, or ischemic bowel disease. Ileus or stasis is associated with overgrowth of flora in the gastrointestinal tract, which is exacerbated by a high-carbohydrate diet. D-Lactate acidosis occurs when fermentation by colonic bacteria in the intestine causes D-lactate to accumulate so that it can be absorbed into the circulation. Serum D-lactate levels of greater than 3 mmol/L confirm the diagnosis. Treatment with a low-carbohydrate diet and antibiotics (neomycin, vancomycin, or metronidazole) is often effective.

D. Ketoacidosis

1. Diabetic ketoacidosis—Diabetic ketoacidosis (DKA) is due to increased fatty acid metabolism and accumulation of ketoacids (acetoacetate and β-hydroxybutyrate) as a result of insulin deficiency or resistance and elevated glucagon levels. DKA is usually seen in insulin-dependent diabetes mellitus upon cessation of insulin therapy or during an illness, such as an infection, gastroenteritis, pancreatitis, or myocardial

infarction, which increases insulin requirements acutely. The accumulation of ketoacids accounts for the increment in the AG, which is accompanied, most often, by hyperglycemia (glucose level of >300 mg/dL).

2. Alcoholic ketoacidosis—Chronic alcoholics, particularly binge drinkers, who discontinue food intake while continuing alcohol consumption, may develop the "alcoholic" ketoacidosis. Often the onset of vomiting and abdominal pain with volume depletion leads to cessation of alcohol consumption. The metabolic acidosis may be severe but is accompanied by only modestly deranged glucose levels, which are usually low but may be slightly elevated. The net result of the deranged metabolic state is ketosis. The acidosis is primarily due to elevated levels of ketones, which exist predominantly in the form of β-hydroxybutyrate because of the altered redox state induced by the metabolism of alcohol. Compared with patients with DKA, patients with AKA have lower plasma glucose concentrations and higher β-hydroxybutyrate/acetoacetate and lactate/pyruvate ratios. Because the standard clinical tests for ketone bodies do not accurately detect the reduced ketoacid β-hydroxybutyrate, AKA patients with severe ketoacidosis comprised mostly of β-hydroxybutyrate may go undetected in the setting of a negative test for ketones if the clinician does not have a high index of suspicion. The typical high AG acidosis is often mixed with metabolic alkalosis (vomiting), respiratory alkalosis (alcoholic liver disease), lactic acidosis (hypoperfusion), and/or non-gap metabolic acidosis (kidney excretion of ketoacids). Finally, elevation in the osmolar gap is usually accounted for by an increased blood alcohol level, but the differential diagnosis should always include ethylene glycol and/or methanol intoxication.

E. Drug- and Toxin-Induced High AG Acidosis

1. The osmolar gap and toxin-induced metabolic acidosis—Under most physiologic conditions, Na^+, urea, and glucose generate the osmotic pressure of blood. Serum osmolality may be calculated according to the following expression:

$$\text{Osmolality} = 2[Na^+] + \frac{[BUN]}{2.8} + \frac{[Glucose\,(mg/dL)]}{18}$$

The calculated and determined osmolality should agree within 10 mOsm/kg. When the measured osmolality exceeds the calculated osmolality by more than 10 mOsm/kg, one of two circumstances prevails. First, the serum Na^+ may be spuriously low, as occurs with hyperlipidemia or hyperproteinemia (pseudohyponatremia). Second, osmolytes other than sodium salts, glucose, or urea may have accumulated in plasma. Examples include infused mannitol, radiocontrast media, or other solutes, such as the alcohols, ethylene glycol, and acetone. For these examples, the difference between the osmolality calculated from the above equation and the measured osmolality is proportional to the concentration of the unmeasured solute. This difference is known as the *osmolal (or osmolar) gap,* and becomes a very reliable and helpful screening tool in assessing for toxin-associated high AG acidosis.

F. Ethylene Glycol

Accidental or intentional ingestion of ethylene glycol (EG), used in antifreeze, leads to a high AG metabolic acidosis and a significantly elevated osmolar gap. The consequences are due to the metabolic products of EG metabolism by alcohol dehydrogenase and include severe central nervous system, cardiopulmonary, and kidney damage. Disparity between the measured and calculated blood osmolality (high osmolar gap) is typically noted, especially in the first few hours after ingestion. However, over time, as the EG is metabolized, the osmolar gap begins to fall and the AG begins to rise so that in advanced EG intoxication, the AG will be very high but the osmolar gap will narrow. The high AG is attributable to the ethylene glycol metabolites oxalic acid, glycolic acid, and other incompletely identified organic acids. L-Lactic acid production also increases as a result of a toxic depression in the reaction rates of the citric acid cycle and altered intracellular redox state.

G. Methanol

Methanol has wide application in commercially available solvents and is used for industrial and automotive purposes. Sources include windshield wiper fluid, paint remover or thinner, deicing fluid, canned heating sources, varnish, and shellac. Ingestion of methanol (wood alcohol) causes metabolic acidosis in addition to severe optic nerve and central nervous system manifestations resulting from its metabolism to formic acid from formaldehyde. Lactic acids and ketoacids as well as other unidentified organic acids may contribute to the acidosis. Because of the low molecular mass of methanol (32 Da), an osmolar gap is usually present early in the course but declines as the AG increases, the latter reflecting the metabolism of methanol. Therapy is generally similar to that for ethylene glycol intoxication, including general supportive measures, fomepizole administration, and hemodialysis.

H. Propylene Glycol

Propylene glycol is used as a vehicle for intravenous medications and some cosmetics and, as all of the toxic alcohols, is metabolized to lactic acid by hepatic alcohol dehydrogenase. Numerous intravenous preparations contain propylene glycol as the vehicle (lorazepam, diazepam, pentobarbital, phenytoin, nitroglycerin, and TMP-SMX), and may accumulate and cause a high AG plus high osmolar gap acidosis

in patients receiving continuous infusion or higher dosages of these agents, especially in the presence of chronic kidney disease, chronic liver disease, alcohol abuse, or pregnancy. The acidosis is the result of accumulation of L-lactic acid, D-lactic acid, and L-acetaldehyde, but typically abates with cessation of the offending agent.

I. Pyroglutamic Acid

Pyroglutamic acid, or 5-oxoproline, is an intermediate in the γ-glutamyl cycle for the synthesis of glutathione. Acetaminophen ingestion may deplete glutathione, causing an increase in the formation of γ-glutamyl cysteine, which is metabolized to pyroglutamic acid. Accumulation of this intermediate has been reported in critically ill patients taking acetaminophen who are often critically ill, usually with sepsis. Such patients have severe high AG acidosis and alterations in mental status.

J. Uremia

Advanced chronic kidney disease eventually converts the non-gap metabolic acidosis of stage 3–4 chronic kidney disease (CKD) to the typical high AG acidosis, or "uremic acidosis" of stage 5 CKD. Poor filtration plus continued reabsorption of poorly identified uremic organic anions contributes to the pathogenesis of this metabolic disturbance.

K. Salicylate

Intoxication with salicylate is more common in children than in adults, and may result in the development of a high AG metabolic acidosis. However, adult patients with salicylate intoxication usually present with pure respiratory alkalosis or mixed respiratory alkalosis–metabolic acidosis. A portion of the increase in the AG is due to the increase in plasma salicylate concentration, and the remainder is due to high ketone concentrations, as well as increased L-lactic acid production, due to a direct drug effect and the result of the salicylate-induced decrease in P_{CO_2}.

KEY READINGS

Boutin CA, Laskine M: Ketoacidosis in a non-diabetic adult with chronic EtOH consumption. J Clin Med Res 2016;8:919.

Kraut JA, Xing SX: Approach to the evaluation of a patient with an increased serum osmolal gap and high-anion-gap metabolic acidosis. Am J Kidney Dis 2011;58:480.

► Non-Gap Metabolic Acidosis

A. General Concepts

Metabolic acidosis with a normal AG (hyperchloremic or non-AG acidosis) indicates that HCO_3^- in the plasma has been effectively replaced by Cl^-, so that the AG does not change. The majority of disorders in this category are caused by (1) loss of bicarbonate from the gastrointestinal tract (diarrhea) or from the kidney (proximal renal tubular acidosis [RTA]), or (2) inappropriately low renal acid excretion (classical distal RTA [cDRTA], generalized distal RTA [type 4 RTA], or the non-AG acidosis of acute and chronic kidney disease). The major challenge in distinguishing these causes is to be able to determine if the response by the kidney is appropriate for the prevailing acidosis. With non-gap acidosis of extrarenal etiology, the kidney will respond appropriately by increasing net acid excretion (as with a non-gap acidosis from a gastrointestinal origin). In contrast, when the kidney responds inappropriately, as manifest by low, rather than augmented urine acid excretion, the non-gap acidosis can be ascribed to a kidney tubule disorder. The differential diagnosis of the non-gap acidoses is outlined in Table 5–2.

Diarrhea results in the loss of large quantities of HCO_3^- decomposed by reaction with organic acids. Since diarrheal stools contain a higher concentration of HCO_3^- and decomposed HCO_3^- than plasma, volume depletion and metabolic acidosis develop. Hypokalemia occurs because large quantities of K^+ are lost from stool and because volume depletion causes secondary hyperaldosteronism, which enhances K^+ secretion by the collecting duct. Instead of an acid urine pH as might be anticipated with chronic diarrhea, a pH of 6.0 or more is often noted, especially with diarrhea of several days duration. A urine pH that appears to be evaluated for the clinical acidosis occurs because chronic metabolic acidosis and hypokalemia each increase kidney ammonia (NH_3) production. The increased amount of renal ammonia then combines with protons (H^+) to form ammonium (NH_4^+) for urine excretion. The resulting increase in urine NH_3/NH_4^+ buffer will increase urine pH. Because urinary NH_4^+ excretion is typically low in patients with RTA and high in patients with diarrhea, urinary NH_4^+ excretion should be estimated or measured. Since most clinical laboratories do not typically measure urine NH_4^+, in the presence of non-gap metabolic acidosis one can estimate urine NH_4^+ by calculating the urine anion gap (UAG), using the following equation:

$$UAG = [Na^+ + K^+]_U - [Cl^-]_U$$

where U denotes the urine concentration of these electrolytes. The calculated UAG is often used as a surrogate for an actual measurement of urine NH_4^+. By convention, the UAG should become progressively negative as the rate of ammonium excretion increases in response to acidosis or to acid loading in non-gap acidosis of extrarenal origin such as diarrhea. A negative UAG (> –20 mEq/L) implies, therefore, that sufficient NH_4^+ is present in the urine. Conversely, when the UAG is positive (the urine concentration of $Na^+ + K^+$ is greater than that of Cl^-), the urine can be assumed to contain little or no NH_4^+. A positive UAG suggests the presence of a renal tubular mechanism for the hyperchloremic acidosis, such as cDRTA, or DRTA type 2 (with hypokalemia) or hypoaldosteronism with hyperkalemia (type 4 RTA).

Nevertheless, it should be noted that if a patient has ketonuria, drug anions (penicillins or aspirin), or toluene metabolites in the urine, the UAG is not reliable and should not be used. In such circumstances the urinary ammonium concentration ($U_{NH_4^+}$) may be estimated more reliably from the urine osmolal gap, which is the difference in the measured urine osmolality (U_{osm}), and the urine osmolality calculated from the urine [$Na^+ + K^+$] and the urine urea and glucose (all expressed in mmol/L):

$$U_{NH_4^+} = 0.5(U_{osm} - [2(Na^+ + K^+) + Urea + Glucose]_U$$

Calculated urinary ammonium concentrations of 75 mEq/L or more would be anticipated if kidney tubular function is intact and the kidney is responding to the prevailing metabolic acidosis by appropriately increasing ammonium

Table 5–2. Causes of non-anion gap acidosis.

Extra-Renal Causes
Diarrhea
Other GI losses of bicarbonate and bicarbonate precursors
　(eg, tube drainage)
Post-treatment of ketoacidosis (dilutional)

Renal Causes Not Due to Renal Tubular Acidosis
Ureteral diversion (eg, ileal loop, ureterosigmoidostomy)
Progressive chronic kidney disease (stages 3–4)
Toluene ingestion (excretion of hippurate)
Drugs
　With associated hypokalemia
　　Carbonic anhydrase inhibitors (acetazolamide and topiramate)
　　Amphotericin B
　With associated hyperkalemia
　　Amiloride,
　　Triamterene,
　　Spironolactone,
　　Trimethoprim
　With normal potassium
　　$CaCl_2$, $MgSO_4$ ingestion
　　Cholestyramine
Exogenous acid loads (NH_4Cl, acidic amino acids in total parenteral
　nutrition [TPN], sulfur)
Post-hypocapnic state

Renal Tubular Acidosis
With hypokalemia
　Type 1 (classical distal) RTA
　Type 2 (proximal) RTA
　Type 3 (mixed proximal and distal) RTA (carbonic anhydrase II
　　deficiency)
With hyperkalemia
　Type 4 (generalized distal RTA)
　　Hypoaldosteronism (hyporeninemic and isolated)
　　Aldosterone resistance
　　Voltage defect in collecting duct

production and excretion. Values below 25 mEq/L denote inappropriately low urinary ammonium concentrations, and favor the diagnosis of RTA.

Severe non-AG or hyperchloremic metabolic acidosis with hypokalemia may also occur in patients with ureteral diversion procedures. The pathogenesis of the NAG acidosis is based on the fact that the ileum and the colon are both endowed with Cl^-/HCO_3^- exchangers. Therefore, when Cl^- from the urine enters the gut or pouch, the HCO_3^- concentration in the pouch increases as a result of the exchange of HCO_3^- for Cl^-, so that ultimately, HCO_3^- is excreted. Moreover, K^+ secretion is stimulated, which, together with HCO_3^- loss, can result in a non-AG metabolic acidosis with hypokalemia. Therefore, the history and physical examination must establish whether a ureteral diversion has been performed.

Loss of functioning kidney parenchyma in progressive kidney disease is associated with metabolic acidosis. Typically, the acidosis is a non-AG acidosis when the glomerular filtration rate (GFR) is between 20 and 50 mL/min but may convert to the typical high AG acidosis of uremia with more advanced chronic kidney disease, when the GFR is typically less than 15–20 mL/min. The principal defect in urinary acidification of stages 3–4 CKD is that ammoniagenesis is reduced in proportion to the loss of functional kidney mass. Medullary NH_4^+ accumulation and trapping in the outer medullary collecting tubule may also be impaired. Because of adaptive increases in K^+ secretion by the collecting duct and colon, the acidosis of chronic kidney disease is typically normokalemic. Non-AG metabolic acidosis accompanied by hyperkalemia is almost always associated with a generalized dysfunction of the distal nephron. However, K^+-sparing diuretics (amiloride, triamterene), as well as calcineurin inhibitors, nonsteroidal anti-inflammatory drugs (NSAIDs), angiotensin converting enzyme (ACE) inhibitors, angiotensin II receptor blockers (ARBs), β-blockers, pentamidine, and heparin may all impair K^+ and H^+ secretion by the collecting duct and cause hyperkalemia with a non-gap metabolic acidosis. Because hyperkalemia augments the development of acidosis by suppressing urinary net acid excretion, discontinuing these agents while reducing the serum K^+ allows ammonium production and excretion to increase, and aids in repair of the acidosis.

KEY READING

Rastegar M, Nagami GT: Non-anion gap metabolic acidosis: a clinical approach to evaluation. Am J Kidney Dis 2016;16: 30515.

B. Proximal Renal Tubular Acidosis

The initial step in urinary acidification involves reabsorption of filtered HCO_3^- in the proximal tubule, a process that returns 80% of the filtered HCO_3^- to the blood. If reabsorption by the proximal tubule is impaired, more of the filtered HCO_3^- will be delivered to more distal segments. This increase in HCO_3^- delivery overwhelms the limited capacity for bicarbonate reabsorption by the distal nephron, and bicarbonaturia occurs, net acid excretion ceases, and metabolic acidosis follows. Enhanced Cl^- reabsorption, stimulated by ECF volume contraction causes hyperchloremic (non-AG) chronic metabolic acidosis. With progressive metabolic acidosis and decreased serum HCO_3^- levels, the filtered HCO_3^- load declines progressively. As plasma HCO_3^- concentration decreases progressively, the defective HCO_3^- reabsorptive capacity will reach a point where the distal tubule can reabsorb the lower filtered load of HCO_3^-. As less bicarbonate is excreted, the urine pH will decline. As a consequence, the serum HCO_3^- concentration usually reaches a nadir of 15–18 mEq/L, and the systemic acidosis no longer progresses. Therefore, in untreated patients with proximal RTA who are in a steady state, the serum HCO_3^- is typically 15–18 mEq/L and the urine pH is acid (<5.5). As is typical in proximal RTA, administration of bicarbonate causes a progressive amount of bicarbonate to be excreted in the urine so that the fractional excretion of bicarbonate ($FeHCO_3^-$) will eventually exceed 15% or more, and the urine pH becomes alkaline.

The causes of proximal RTA are summarized in Table 5–3. Proximal RTA can present in one of three ways: (1) acidification is the only defective function, (2) there is a more generalized proximal tubule dysfunction with multi-transporter abnormalities (most common), and (3) as a part of a mixed proximal and distal RTA (type 3). Inheritance patterns for isolated proximal RTA include autosomal recessive and autosomal dominant. Isolated pure bicarbonate wasting is typical of autosomal recessive proximal RTA with accompanying ocular abnormalities and occurs because of mis-sense mutations of the gene SLCA4 that encodes for the basolateral transporter, NBCe1. A rare variant, inherited as an autosomal dominant trait, has been described and appears to be a mutation of the gene that encodes the apical Na^+/H^+ exchanger, NHE-3, and is associated with short stature. Familial disorders associated with acquired proximal RTA include cystinosis, tyrosinemia, hereditary fructose intolerance, galactosemia, glycogen storage disease type 1, Wilson disease, and Lowe syndrome.

Additionally, features of both proximal RTA (bicarbonate wasting), and distal acidification abnormalities are evident in patients with autosomal recessive RTA (mixed proximal and distal, or type 3 RTA). The inherited form of type 3 RTA has been attributed to a defect in the CA2 gene that encodes for carbonic anhydrase II (CAII), an intracellular form of the enzyme distributed to the cytoplasm of the proximal tubule and distal tubule. In addition to metabolic acidosis, the phenotype includes osteopetrosis, and ocular abnormalities.

Table 5–3. Clinical disorders associated with proximal RTA (type 2 RTA).

1. Primary disorders
   Inherited—isolated pure bicarbonate wasting
      Autosomal recessive: mutations of NBCe1/*SLC4A4*
        (several examples associated with ocular abnormalities)
      Autosomal dominant: mutation of NHE-3 with short
        stature (defect not determined)
   Familial disorders associated with PRTA
      Cystinosis
      Tyrosinemia
      Hereditary fructose intolerance
      Galactosemia
      Glycogen storage disease (type 1)
      Wilson disease
      Lowe syndrome

2. Acquired disorders
   Multiple myeloma, amyloidosis, light chain nephropathy
   Chemotherapeutic agents
      Ifosfamide
   Carbonic anhydrase inhibitors
      Topiramate
      Acetazolamide
      Sulfamylon
   Heavy metals
      Lead, copper, cadmium, mercury
   Renal transplantation
   Paroxysmal nocturnal hemoglobinuria

3. Mixed proximal and distal RTA (type 3 RTA)
   Carbonic anhydrase II deficiency-osteopetrosis and ocular
      abnormalities
      (Guibaud-Vainsel syndrome)

The majority of cases of proximal RTA fit into the category of generalized proximal tubule dysfunction with multi-transport abnormalities manifest as glycosuria, aminoaciduria, hypercitraturia, and phosphaturia, and referred to as *Fanconi syndrome.*

Although proximal RTA is more common in children, the most common causes of acquired proximal RTA in adults include either multiple myeloma and light chain nephropathy, in which increased excretion of immunoglobulin light chains injures the proximal tubule epithelium, or chemotherapeutic drug injury of the proximal tubule (eg, ifosfamide). RTA due to ifosfamide toxicity, lead intoxication, and cystinosis is more common in children. Carbonic anhydrase inhibitors cause pure bicarbonate wasting but not Fanconi syndrome. Topiramate, widely used in the prevention of migraine headaches, or for treatment of a seizure disorder is a potent carbonic anhydrase inhibitor, and is an important cause of non-AG metabolic acidosis (approximately 15–25% of patients on this agent). The acidosis typically subsides when topiramate is discontinued.

C. Classical Distal Renal Tubule Acidosis

The mechanisms involved in the pathogenesis of cDRTA (type 1 RTA) with hypokalemia, have been better appreciated with the discovery of the genetic and molecular bases of the inherited forms of this disease. Most studies suggest that the inherited forms of cDRTA are due to defects in either the basolateral HCO_3^-/Cl^- exchanger (SLC4A1), or subunits of the H^+-ATPase (*ATP6V1B1* and *ATP6V0A4*) in the type A intercalated cell of the collecting duct.

While the classical finding is an inability to acidify the urine maximally in the face of systemic acidosis (to a urine pH of <5.5), attention to urine ammonium excretion rather than urine pH alone is essential in the diagnosis of this disorder. Patients with impaired collecting duct H^+ secretion and cDRTA exhibit uniformly low excretion rates of NH_4^+ when the degree of systemic acidosis is taken into consideration. Low NH_4^+ excretion equates with inappropriately low regeneration of HCO_3^- by the kidney, and demonstrates that the kidney is responsible for causing or perpetuating the chronic metabolic acidosis. Low NH_4^+ excretion in classical distal RTA occurs because of the failure to trap NH_4^+ in the medullary collecting duct as a result of higher than normal tubule fluid pH in this segment. The clinical features of cDRTA are summarized in Table 5–4.

Medullary interstitial disease, which commonly occurs in conjunction with distal RTA, may impair NH_4^+ excretion by interrupting the medullary countercurrent system for NH_4^+. The complete form of classical distal RTA is manifest by a non-AG acidosis and hypokalemia in patients not receiving alkali therapy. The clinical spectrum of complete cDRTA may include stunted growth, hypercalciuria, hypocitraturia, osteopenia, nephrolithiasis, and nephrocalcinosis. The disturbances in bone and calcium metabolism, as well as hypocitraturia are a direct consequence of chronic metabolic acidosis. The dissolution of bone is due to calcium resorption and mobilization from bone in response to the acidosis and through activation of the pH sensitive G protein-coupled receptor, OGR1, which resides in bone. Other common electrolyte abnormalities, not due to acidosis include

Table 5–4. Clinical features of acquired classical distal RTA.

Urine AG positive with induced or spontaneous metabolic acidosis
Abnormally low NH_4^+ excretion
Urine pH >5.5
Modest bicarbonaturia (FeHCO$_3^-$ >5%, <10%)
Hypokalemia
Absence of Fanconi syndrome
Abnormal calcium metabolism (hypercalciuria, nephrocalcinosis, nephrolithiasis, bone disease)
Low urine citrate
Hyperglobulinemia

hypokalemia, hypernatremia and salt wasting, and polyuria due to nephrogenic diabetes insipidus. The hypokalemia may be due to a signaling pathway involving activation and release of PGE2 by β-intercalated cells that directly communicate to enhance sodium absorption and potassium secretion by activation of the epithelial sodium channel (ENaC) and big potassium (BK) channels in collecting duct principal cells. Because chronic metabolic acidosis also decreases the production of citrate, the resulting hypocitraturia in combination with hypercalciuria together dramatically increase urinary stone formation and set the stage for the development of nephrocalcinosis. Distal RTA occurs frequently in patients with Sjögren syndrome and is due to the inability to traffic and insert the H$^+$-ATPase into the apical membrane properly because of autoantibodies and infiltration of lymphocytes. The numerous causes of both inherited and acquired defects resulting in classical distal RTA are summarized in Table 5–5 and sources of alkali therapy used commonly to treat cDRTA is listed in Table 5–6.

D. Generalized Distal Renal Tubular Acidosis

The coexistence of hyperkalemia and a non-gap metabolic acidosis indicates a generalized dysfunction in the cortical and medullary collecting tubules. Hyperkalemia is an important mediator of the kidney response to acid–base balance, because it independently reduces ammonium production and excretion. Chronic hyperkalemia decreases ammonium production in the proximal tubule and other nephron segments, inhibits absorption of NH$_4^+$ in the mTAL, reduces medullary interstitial concentrations of NH$_4^+$ and NH$_3$, and decreases entry of NH$_4^+$ and NH$_3$ into the medullary collecting duct, all leading to a marked reduction in urinary ammonium excretion. The potential for development of a hyperchloremic metabolic acidosis is greatly augmented when a reduction in functional kidney mass (GFR of <60 mL/min) coexists with hyperkalemia or when aldosterone deficiency or resistance is present. The numerous causes of generalized distal RTA are summarized in Table 5–7.

1. Drug-induced renal tubular secretory defects in type 4 RTA—Drugs may impair renin or aldosterone elaboration or cause mineralocorticoid resistance in patients with CKD, and produce effects that mimic the clinical manifestations of the acidification defect seen in the generalized form of distal RTA with hyperkalemia. Examples include NSAIDs or COX-2 inhibitors, spironolactone and eplerenone, β-adrenergic antagonists, heparin, and ACE inhibitors and ARBs.

2. Voltage defect of collecting duct—Autosomal recessive PHA-1, is a prototypical voltage defect, and is the result of a loss-of-function mutation of the gene that encodes one of the α-, β-, or γ-subunits of the epithelial sodium channel in the collecting, or ENaC. The typical phenotype of children with PHA-1 includes vomiting, hyponatremia, failure to thrive, and respiratory distress. They usually respond well to

Table 5–5. Disorders associated with classical hypokalemic distal RTA.

Inherited
1. Autosomal dominant
   a. Abnormality of the basolateral HCO$_3^-$/Cl$^-$ exchanger (AE-1) due to SLC4A1 mutation
2. Autosomal recessive
   a. Deficiency or abnormality of the H$^+$-ATPase
      Autosomal recessive ATP6V1B1 mutation with deafness
      Autosomal recessive ATP6V0A4 mutation with or without deafness
   b. Carbonic anhydrase II deficiency—mixed PRTA-DRTA

Acquired Defect of the H$^+$-ATPase
Sjögren syndrome
Secondary to Systemic Disorders

Autoimmune diseases	
Hyperglobulinemic purpura	Fibrosing alveolitis
Cryoglobulinemia	Chronic active hepatitis
Sjögren syndrome	Primary biliary cirrhosis
Thyroiditis	Polyarteritis nodosa
HIV nephropathy	
Hypercalciuria and Nephrocalcinosis	
Primary hyperparathyroidism	Vitamin D intoxication
Hyperthyroidism	Idiopathic hypercalciuria
Medullary sponge kidney	Wilson disease
Fabry disease	Hereditary fructose intolerance
X-linked hypophosphatemia	Hereditary sensorineural deafness
Drug- and Toxin-Induced Disease	
Amphotericin B	
Mercury	
Vanadate	Lithium
Hepatic cirrhosis	Classic analgesic nephropathy
Ifosfamide	Foscarnet
Topiramate	Acetazolamide
Tubulointerstitial Diseases	
Balkan nephropathy	Renal transplantation
Chronic pyelonephritis	Leprosy
Obstructive uropathy	Jejunal bypass with hyperoxaluria
Vesicoureteral reflux	
Associated with Genetically Transmitted Diseases	
Ehlers–Danlos syndrome	Hereditary elliptocytosis
Sickle cell anemia	Marfan syndrome
Medullary cystic disease	
Hereditary sensorineural deafness	Carnitine palmitoyltransferase I
Osteopetrosis with carbonic II deficiency	

high-salt intake that concomitantly corrects the electrolyte and acid–base manifestations.

Amiloride and triamterene may be associated with hyperkalemia, because these potassium-sparing diuretics occupy and block the apical Na$^+$-selective channel (ENaC) in the

Table 5–6. Sources of alkali for therapy of RTA.

$NaHCO_3$ tablets
 325 mg [3.8 mEq]
 650 mg [7.6 mEq]
Shohl solution (Na^+ citrate and citric acid)
 Sodium citrate solution (500 mg and citric acid 334 mg per 5 mL)
  HCO_3^- equivalent 1 mEq/mL and Na^+ 1 mEq/mL
Baking soda (60 mEq/tsp)
K-Lyte (25 or 50 mEq/tablet)
Polycitra (K^+ Shohl)
Granules, effervescent (Brioschi)

collecting duct principal cell. Occupation of ENaC inhibits Na^+ absorption and reduces the negative transepithelial voltage, which alters the driving force for K^+ secretion.

The calcineurin inhibitors cyclosporine A and tacrolimus may be associated with hyperkalemia in the transplant recipient as a result of inhibition of the basolateral Na^+-K^+-ATPase and the consequent decrease in intracellular [K^+] and the transepithelial potential, which together reduce the driving force for K^+ secretion. Calcineurin inhibitors may also inhibit K^+ secretion by directly interfering with function of the K channel, renal outer medullary potassium (ROMK). An additional explanation for the association of hyperkalemia, volume expansion, and hypertension, a syndrome that resembles the phenotype of familial hyperkalemic hypertension or PHA-2, is enhanced activity of Na-Cl cotransporter (NCC) in the distal convoluted tubule (DCT).

E. The Acidosis of Progressive Kidney Failure

The metabolic acidosis of CKD associated with a chronic reduction in GFR is typically a non-gap metabolic acidosis for a GFR in the range of 20–30 mL/min, but typically converts to the high AG variety as kidney insufficiency progresses and GFR falls below 15 mL/min. Unlike patients with classical distal RTA, patients with primary kidney disease have a normal ability to lower the urine pH during acidosis. Therefore, this disorder is not considered as one of the renal tubular acidoses. The net distal H^+ secretory capacity is qualitatively normal and can be increased by buffer availability in the form of PO_4^{3-} or by non-reabsorbable anions. The principal defect is an inability to produce or to excrete NH_4^+ sufficient to match net endogenous acid production. Consequently, the kidneys cannot quantitatively excrete all of the metabolic acids produced daily, especially if the patient is ingesting a typical Western diet, and net positive acid balance supervenes.

There have been important advances recently in elucidating the serious consequences of chronic metabolic acidosis in patients with CKD. It has been demonstrated that metabolic acidosis is uniquely deleterious and accelerates CKD progression, augments dissolution of bone and impaires hydroxylation of 25-hydroxycholecalciferol, that

Table 5–7. Generalized abnormality of distal nephron with hyperkalemia.

Mineralocorticoid Deficiency
Primary Mineralocorticoid Deficiency
 Combined deficiency of aldosterone, desoxycorticosterone, and cortisol
  Addison disease
  Bilateral adrenalectomy
  Bilateral adrenal destruction
   Hemorrhage or carcinoma
 Congenital enzymatic defects
  21-Hydroxylase deficiency
  3β-Hydroxydehydrogenase deficiency
  Desmolase deficiency
 Isolated (selective) aldosterone deficiency
  Chronic idiopathic hypoaldosteronism
  Heparin (unfractionated or low molecular weight [LMW]) in critically ill patient
  Familial hypoaldosteronism
   Corticosterone methyloxidase deficiency, types 1 and 2
  Primary zona glomerulosa defect
  Transient hypoaldosteronism of infancy
  Persistent hypotension and/or hypoxemia in critically ill patient
 Angiotensin II–converting enzyme inhibition
  Endogenous
  ACE Inhibitors and AT_1 receptor antagonists (ARBs)
Secondary Mineralocorticoid Deficiency
 Hyporeninemic hypoaldosteronism
  Diabetic nephropathy
  Tubulointerstitial nephropathies
   Nephrosclerosis
   Nonsteroidal anti-inflammatory agents
   Acquired immunodeficiency syndrome
   IgM monoclonal gammopathy

Mineralocorticoid Resistance
 Pseudohypoaldosteronism type 1 (PHAI)—autosomal dominant

Renal Tubular Dysfunction (Voltage Defect)
 Pseudohypoaldosteronism type 1 (PHAI)—autosomal recessive
 Pseudohypoaldosteronism type 2 (PHAII)—autosomal recessive
 Drugs that impair Na^+ channel function in collecting duct
  Amiloride
  Triamterene
  Trimethoprim
  Pentamidine
 Calcineurin inhibitors (interfere with Na^+, K^+-ATPase in CCT)
  Cyclosporin A
  Tacrolimus
 Drugs that inhibit aldosterone in collecting duct
  Spironolactone
  Eplerenone
 Disorders causing tubulointerstitial nephritis
  Lupus nephritis
  Methicillin nephrotoxicity
  Obstructive nephropathy
  Kidney transplant rejection
  Sickle-cell disease

together lead to renal osteodystrophy. In addition chronic acidosis also causes sarcopenia from enhanced skeletal muscle protein degradation with subsequent loss of functional muscle strength, and activity, such as gait speed. Therefore, for all of these reasons, more attention is being devoted currently to securing recommendations that would lead to a wider view of the importance of correcting the metabolic acidosis with alkali therapy. Moreover, beyond overt metabolic acidosis (as defined by a serum $[HCO_3^-]$ of <24 mEq/L), evidence is accumulating revealing that there may be significant consequences in patients with very early CKD (eg, stage 2). For example, patients with early CKD progress more rapidly when they ingest a higher dietary acid load, as is typical of the Western diet. The subsequent high endogenous net acid production, and may cause more rapid progression of CKD even before the serum $[HCO_3^-]$ falls into the range of the typical clinical recognition of acidosis ($[HCO_3^-]$ in the normal range). Several smaller trials clearly indicate that the typical finding in patients with CKD that progress in this group is a higher than normal net endogenous acid load and an elevated net acid excretion. Additional large randomized clinical trials are badly needed in this area so that the apparent benefit of either alkali therapy or consumption of diets that emphasize fruits and vegetables, can be offered to the large segment of the early CKD population that appear to fall into this category. Moreover, additional studies are needed to establish the pathophysiological basis of this adverse response to dietary acid loads in patients with CKD.

KEY READINGS

Banerjee T et al: High dietary acid load predicts ESRD among adults with CKD. J Am Soc Nephrol 2015;26:1693.

Goraya N, Simoni J, Jo C, Wesson DE: Dietary acid reduction with fruits and vegetables or bicarbonate attenuates kidney injury in patients with a moderately reduced glomerular filtration rate due to hypertensive nephropathy. Kidney Int 2012;81:86.

Kraut JA, Madias NE: Metabolic acidosis of CKD: an update. Am J Kidney Dis 2016;67:307.

Raphael KL et al: Bicarbonate concentration, acid-base status, and mortality in the Health, Aging, and Body Composition Study. Clin J Am Soc Nephrol 2016;11:308.

Wesson DE, Pruszynski J, Cai W, Simoni J: Acid retention with reduced glomerular filtration rate increases urine biomarkers of kidney and bone injury. Kidney Int 2017;91:914.

▼ METABOLIC ALKALOSIS

Thomas D. DuBose, Jr, MD

▶ Introduction

The primary defect in metabolic alkalosis is an inability of the kidney to excrete an excessive amount of bicarbonate present in extracellular fluid. This disorder occurs because of primary factors that generate the net gain of bicarbonate and the cumulative impact of secondary factors that maintain the alkalosis. Disorders that generate metabolic alkalosis include vomiting, diuretics, chloride and volume depletion, hypokalemia, and primary or secondary hyperaldosteronism. Differentiation of these many causes requires attention to the patient's ECF volume status, blood pressure, and potassium stores. Although uncommon, excessive exogenous alkali loads may also cause metabolic alkalosis under certain circumstances. This chapter summarizes the pathophysiologic basis of each disorder and develops, within this framework, an approach to the therapy and ultimate correction of this acid–base disorder.

▶ Pathogenesis

The pathogenesis of metabolic alkalosis involves two linked components: (1) *generation* and (2) *maintenance. Generation* occurs by net gain of bicarbonate ions (HCO_3^-) or, more commonly, net loss of nonvolatile acid (usually HCl by vomiting) from the extracellular fluid. Although the kidneys have an impressive capacity to excrete HCO_3^- under normal circumstances, that ability is impaired significantly in the maintenance stage of metabolic alkalosis so that the kidneys fail to excrete HCO_3^-. Bicarbonate may be retained in the ECF because of volume contraction, a low glomerular filtration rate (GFR), as well as depletion of body stores of chloride (Cl^-) or potassium (K^+). Retention, rather than excretion, of excess alkali by the kidney is promoted when: (1) volume depletion, Cl^-, and K^+ deficiency exist in combination with a reduced GFR, or (2) hypokalemia prevails because of autonomous hyperaldosteronism. In the first example, alkalosis is typically corrected by administration of NaCl and KCl, whereas, in the latter example, it is necessary to address the alkalosis by pharmacologic or surgical intervention rather than saline administration.

▶ Differential Diagnosis

To establish the cause of metabolic alkalosis, it is necessary to assess the extracellular fluid volume (ECV) status, the recumbent and upright blood pressure, and the serum potassium and chloride concentrations. In hypertensive patients with chronic hypokalemia, it is also helpful to evaluate the renin-angiotensin system. For example, the presence of chronic hypertension and chronic hypokalemia in an alkalemic patient suggests either mineralocorticoid excess or a hypertensive patient receiving diuretics. Low plasma renin activity and urine $[Na^+]$ and $[Cl^-]$ values greater than 20 mEq/L in a hypertensive patient not taking diuretics are consistent with primary mineralocorticoid excess.

The combination of hypokalemia and alkalosis in a nonedematous patient with a low or normal BP may be caused by, vomiting, exogenous alkali, Bartter or Gitelman syndrome, magnesium deficiency or diuretic ingestion. Determination of urine electrolytes (especially [Cl⁻]) and screening of the urine for diuretics may be helpful. When the urine chloride concentration is measured (Table 5–8), it should be considered in context with assessment of the ECV status of the patient. A low urine $[Cl^-]$ (ie, <10 mEq/L) indicates avid Cl^- retention by the kidney and denotes ECV depletion even if the urine Na^+ is high (ie, >20 mEq/L), whereas a high urine $[Cl^-]$ in the absence of concurrent diuretic use suggests inappropriate chloride loss resulting from a renal tubular defect or mineralocorticoid excess. If the urine is alkaline with an elevated urine $[Na^+]$ and $[K^+]$ but urine $[Cl^-]$ is lower than 10 mEq/L, the diagnosis is usually either vomiting (overt or surreptitious) or alkali ingestion. If the urine is relatively acidic and has low concentrations of Na^+, K^+, and Cl^-, the most likely possibilities are previous vomiting, the posthypercapnic state, or previous diuretic ingestion. If, on the other hand, neither the urine $[Na^+]$, $[K^+]$, nor $[Cl^-]$ is depressed, magnesium deficiency, Bartter or Gitelman syndrome, or active diuretic use should be considered.

▶ Clinical Causes of Metabolic Alkalosis

A. Metabolic Alkalosis due to Exogenous Bicarbonate Loads

1. Alkali administration—Administration of base to individuals with normal kidney function rarely causes alkalosis since the normal kidney has a high capacity for HCO_3^- excretion. Nevertheless, in patients with coexistent hemodynamic disturbances, alkalosis may develop because the normal capacity to excrete HCO_3^- has been exceeded. Examples include patients receiving oral or intravenous HCO_3^-, acetate loads (parenteral hyperalimentation solutions), citrate loads (transfusions, continuous renal replacement therapy,

---

Table 5–8. Causes of metabolic alkalosis.

Exogenous HCO₃⁻ Loads
  Acute alkali administration
  Milk-alkali syndrome
  Use of NaOH in "freebasing" of crack cocaine
  Street cocaine "cut" with baking soda
  Baking soda pica in pregnancy
  Bicarbonate precursors (citrate, acetate) in chronic or acute
     kidney disease
  Alkali NG tube feedings, particularly in settings of low GFR
	Bartter syndrome
	Gitelman syndrome
	Carbohydrate refeeding after starvation
	Pendred syndrome (during thiazide diuretic use or intercurrent illness)
	
	ECV Expansion, Hypertension, K⁺ Deficiency, and Hypermineralocorticoidism
	- Associated with high renin
	  Renal artery stenosis

Effective ECV Contraction, Normotension, K⁺ Deficiency, and Secondary
  Hyperreninemic Hyperaldosteronism
- Gastrointestinal origin
  Vomiting
  Gastric aspiration
  Congenital chloridorrhea
  Villous adenoma
  Combined administration of sodium polystyrene sulfonate (Kayexalate)
    and aluminum hydroxide
  Cystic fibrosis and volume depletion
  Gastrocystoplasty
  Chronic laxative abuse
  Cl⁻ deficient infant formula
	Accelerated hypertension
	  Renin-secreting tumor
	  Estrogen therapy
	
	- Associated with low renin
	  Primary aldosteronism
	    Adenoma
	    Hyperplasia
	    Carcinoma
	    Glucocorticoid suppressible
	  Adrenal enzymatic defects
	    11β-Hydroxylase deficiency
	    17α-Hydroxylase deficiency

- Kidney origin
  Diuretics (remote use of thiazides or loop diuretics)
  Edematous states
  Posthypercapnic state
  Hypercalcemia–hypoparathyroidism
  Recovery from lactic acidosis or ketoacidosis
  Nonreabsorbable anions (eg, intravenous penicillin derivatives such
    as carbenicillin or ticarcillin)
  Mg²⁺ deficiency
  K⁺ depletion
	Cushing syndrome or disease
	    Ectopic corticotropin
	    Adrenal carcinoma
	    Adrenal adenoma
	    Primary pituitary
	  Other
	    Licorice
	    Carbenoxolone
	    Chewing tobacco (containing glycyrrhizinic acid)
	
	Gain-of-Function Mutation of ENaC with ECV Expansion, Hypertension,
	  K⁺ Deficiency, and Hyporeninemic Hypoaldosteronism
	  Liddle syndrome

ECV, extracellular fluid volume; ENaC, epithelial sodium channel; GFR, glomerular filtration rate.

or infant formula), or antacids in conjunction with cation-exchange resins (aluminum hydroxide and sodium polystyrene sulfonate). Moreover, metabolic alkalosis may develop when there is a coexisting problem that results in enhanced reabsorption of HCO_3^-, such as volume depletion, a reduction in GFR, potassium depletion, or hypercapnia.

In patients with acute kidney injury or advanced chronic kidney disease, overt alkalosis can develop after alkali administration because the capacity to excrete HCO_3^- is exceeded or coexistent hemodynamic disturbances have caused enhanced HCO_3^- reabsorption. Baking soda ingestion should be considered in CKD patients, especially when baking soda is used as a home remedy for dyspepsia. The use of tube feedings in elderly patients in long-term care facilities has been associated with metabolic alkalosis as tube feeding preparations in the elderly are a common and underappreciated source of alkali loads. Plasma electrolytes should be monitored more frequently in these patients. Other examples of acute metabolic alkalosis resulting from alkali ingestion include the association of pica for baking soda in pregnancy.

2. Milk-alkali syndrome—A long-standing history of excessive ingestion of milk and antacids, termed milk-alkali syndrome, is a historically important cause of metabolic alkalosis, but there has been a resurgence since the 1990s following increased use of calcium carbonate and vitamin D for osteoporosis. The majority of contemporary patients with this form of milk-alkali syndrome are asymptomatic women with incidental hypercalcemia, previously unappreciated CKD, and hypophosphatemia. Older women on diuretics and ACE inhibitors appear to be at higher risk. Both hypercalcemia and vitamin D excess increase renal tubular HCO_3^- reabsorption. A critical component of this syndrome is reduced GFR. Patients with this disorder are prone to developing nephrocalcinosis, progressive CKD, and metabolic alkalosis. Discontinuation of alkali ingestion is usually sufficient to correct the alkalosis, but the kidney disease may be irreversible if nephrocalcinosis is advanced.

3. Citrate administration—If citrate is used for regional anticoagulation (eg, in CRRT), metabolic alkalosis can occur, depending on the amount of citrate delivered to the patient. The metabolism of citrate by the liver and skeletal muscle causes a net gain of HCO_3^-. Strategies have been advanced to reduce the complications of regional trisodium citrate anticoagulation by using anticoagulant citrate dextrose formula A, and the incidence of metabolic alkalosis has declined in this circumstance.

B. Metabolic Alkalosis Associated With Effective Intravascular Volume Contraction and Secondary Hyperreninemic Hyperaldosteronism

1. Gastrointestinal origin—Gastrointestinal loss of H^+, Cl^-, Na^+, and K^+ from vomitus or gastric aspiration during active vomiting, causes continued addition of HCO_3^- to plasma across the basolateral membrane of the gastric parietal cell in exchange for Cl^-. This causes the elevated plasma $[HCO_3^-]$ to exceed the reabsorptive capacity of the proximal tubule, and to increase renal HCO_3^- excretion. The accompanying loss of fluid and electrolytes results in contraction of the ECV and stimulation of the renin-angiotensin system and reduced GFR, thereby increasing the capacity of the renal tubule to reabsorb HCO_3^-. Excess angiotensin II stimulates Na^+/H^+ exchange by the proximal tubule. Aldosterone and endothelin also stimulate the proton-transporting adenosine triphosphatase (H^+-ATPase) in the distal nephron, resulting in enhanced capacity for distal nephron HCO_3^- absorption and, paradoxically, aciduria. When the excess $NaHCO_3$ reaches the distal tubule, potassium secretion is enhanced by aldosterone and the delivery of the poorly reabsorbed anion, HCO_3^-. Thus the predominant cause of hypokalemia is urinary loss of K^+, and not gastrointestinal potassium wasting.

Hypokalemia has selective effects on renal tubular bicarbonate absorption and ammonium production that are counterproductive to metabolic alkalosis. Hypokalemia dramatically increases the activity of the proton pump (H^+/K^+-ATPase) in the cortical and medullary collecting tubule for reabsorbing K^+, but this occurs at the expense of both enhanced net acid excretion and HCO_3^- absorption. Hypokalemia also increases ammonium production independently of acid–base status, which, in the face of enhanced H^+ secretion, results in increased ammonium production and excretion; this in turn adds new bicarbonate to the systemic circulation (increase in net acid excretion). Therefore, hypokalemia plays an important role in the seemingly maladaptive response of the kidney to maintain the alkalosis. Because of contraction of the ECV and hypochloremia, there is avid conservation of Cl^- by the kidney, and is evident clinically as a low urinary chloride concentration (see Table 5–9). Therapy should include correction of the contracted ECV with isotonic NaCl and repletion of the K^+ deficit as KCl. Such therapy corrects the acid–base disorder because it restores the ability of the kidney to excrete excess bicarbonate.

A. GASTROCYSTOPLASTY—Augmentation of the bladder by gastrocystoplasty, although uncommon, has been used as an alternative to enterocystoplasty. Implantation of a segment of vascularized stomach into the bladder in children with reduced bladder capacity has been associated with hypokalemia, hypochloremia, and metabolic alkalosis. Gastrointestinal complications have also been reported. Oral potassium chloride should be administered chronically.

B. CONGENITAL CHLORIDORRHEA—Congenital chloridorrhea is a rare autosomal-recessive disorder, that causes metabolic alkalosis by an extrarenal mechanism of severe diarrhea, fecal acid loss, and HCO_3^- retention. The disease is the result of mutations in the *SLC26A3* gene that disrupt the ileal and colonic HCO_3/Cl^- anion exchange mechanism so that Cl^- cannot be reabsorbed in the GI tract, but the parallel Na^+/H^+ ion exchanger remains functional, allowing Na^+ to be reabsorbed and H^+ to be secreted into the lumen. Therefore, the stool has high concentrations of H^+ and Cl^-, causing Na^+ and HCO_3^- retention in the extracellular fluid. The alkalosis is sustained by concomitant ECV contraction, hyperaldosteronism, and K^+ deficiency. Delivery of Cl^- to the distal nephron is low because of volume contraction. As in cystic fibrosis, this low delivery of Cl^- results in impaired HCO_3^- secretion by the β-intercalated cell. Therapy consists of oral supplementation of sodium and potassium chloride. Administration of proton pump inhibitors may reduce chloride secretion by the parietal cells and improve the diarrhea. The long-term outcome is good with daily supplementation of NaCl and KCl.

C. VILLOUS ADENOMA—Metabolic alkalosis has been described in cases of villous adenoma. K^+ depletion probably induces the alkalosis since colonic secretion is alkaline.

2. Renal origin—The generation of metabolic alkalosis through renal mechanisms involves three processes for increasing distal nephron H^+ secretion and enhancing net acid excretion (ammonium) excretion: (1) high delivery of Na^+ salts to the distal nephron, (2) excessive elaboration of mineralocorticoids, and (3) K^+ deficiency.

A. DIURETICS—Drugs that induce distal delivery of sodium salts, such as thiazide and loop diuretics, diminish ECV without altering total body bicarbonate content. Consequently, the serum $[HCO_3^-]$ increases. The chronic administration of diuretics generates a metabolic alkalosis by increasing distal salt delivery, thereby enhancing K^+ and H^+ secretion by the collecting tubule. The alkalosis is maintained by persistent contraction of the ECV, secondary hyperaldosteronism, K^+ deficiency, and activation of the H^+/K^+-ATPase, as long as diuretic administration continues. Hypokalemia also enhances ammonium production and excretion. Repair of the alkalosis is achieved by withholding the diuretic, providing isotonic saline to correct the ECV deficit, and repleting potassium.

B. BARTTER SYNDROME—Both classic Bartter syndrome and the antenatal variety are inherited as autosomal-recessive disorders that impair salt absorption in the thick ascending limb (TAL) of the loop of Henle. The phenotype of this disorder is therefore, copious salt wasting, volume depletion, and activation of the renin-angiotensin system. These manifestations are the result of loss-of-function mutations of one of the genes that encode transporters involved in NaCl absorption in the TAL. The most prevalent disorder is a mutation of the gene *NKCC2*, which encodes the $Na^+/K^+/2Cl^-$-cotransporter on the apical membrane. A second mutation has been discovered in

the gene *KCNJ1*, which encodes the ATP-sensitive apical K^+ conductance channel (ROMK) that operates in parallel with the $Na^+/K^+/2Cl^-$-cotransporter to recycle K^+. Both defects can be associated with antenatal Bartter syndrome or with classic Bartter syndrome. A mutation of the *CLCNKb* gene encoding the voltage-gated basolateral chloride channel (ClC-Kb) is associated with a quantitatively milder defect, and is rarely associated with nephrocalcinosis. All of the described defects have the same manifestations: loss of Cl^- transport in the TAL, causing enhanced delivery of NaCl that stimulates K^+ and H^+ secretion by the collecting tubule, causing hypokalemia and metabolic alkalosis.

Antenatal Bartter syndrome has been observed in consanguineous families in association with sensorineural deafness, a syndrome linked to chromosome 1p31. The responsible gene, *BSND*, encodes a subunit, barttin that colocalizes with the ClC-Kb channel in the TAL and K^+-secreting epithelial cells in the inner ear. Barttin appears to be necessary for the function of the voltage-gated chloride channel. Expression of ClC-Kb is lost when coexpressed with mutant barttins. Therefore, mutations in *BSND* define an additional category of patients with Bartter syndrome.

Because of the ECV contraction and secondary hyperreninemic hyperaldosteronism, plus increased delivery of Na^{Cl} to the distal nephron, patients manifest metabolic alkalosis, urinary K^+ wasting, and hypokalemia. Secondary overproduction of prostaglandins, juxtaglomerular apparatus hypertrophy, and vascular pressor unresponsiveness ensue. Most patients have hypercalciuria and normal serum magnesium levels, distinguishing this disorder from Gitelman syndrome.

Bartter syndrome may be inherited as an autosomal-recessive defect. Most patients are homozygotes or compound heterozygotes for different mutations in one of these four genes, whereas a few patients with the clinical syndrome have no discernible mutation in any of these genes. Additionally, activating mutations in the calcium-sensing receptor, CaSR, on the basolateral cell surface of the TAL inhibit the function of ROMK recapitulating the phenotype of inherited Bartter syndrome. Such CaSR defects may be inherited as an autosomal dominant disorder, or may be acquired, as has been reported in patients receiving aminoglycoside antibiotics.

For diagnosis, Bartter syndrome must be distinguished from surreptitious vomiting, diuretic administration, and laxative abuse. The finding of a low urinary Cl^- concentration is helpful in identifying the vomiting patient (Table 5–9). The urinary Cl^- concentration in a patient with Bartter syndrome would be expected to be normal or increased, rather than depressed.

The therapy for Bartter syndrome focuses on repair of the hypokalemia through inhibition of the renin-angiotensin-aldosterone system or the prostaglandin-kinin system, using propranolol, amiloride, spironolactone, prostaglandin inhibitors, and angiotensin-converting enzyme inhibitors,

Table 5–9. Categorization of metabolic alkalosis using urinary electrolytes.

Low Urinary [Cl⁻] (<10 mEq/L)	High or Normal Urinary [Cl⁻] (>15–20 mEq/L)
Normotension Vomiting, nasogastric Aspiration Diuretics Posthypercapnia Bicarbonate treatment of organic acidosis K⁺ deficiency	**Hypertension** Primary aldosteronism Cushing syndrome Renal artery stenosis Renal failure plus alkali therapy
Hypertension Liddle syndrome	**Normotension or Hypotension** Mg²⁺ deficiency Severe K⁺ deficiency Bartter syndrome Gitelman syndrome Diuretics

as well as direct repletion of the deficits of potassium and magnesium.

C. **Gitelman syndrome**—Patients with Gitelman syndrome resemble the Bartter syndrome phenotype in that an autosomal-recessive metabolic alkalosis is associated with hypokalemia, normal-to-low blood pressure, volume depletion with secondary hyperreninemic hyperaldosteronism, and juxtaglomerular hyperplasia. However, the consistent presence of hypocalciuria and the frequent presence of hypomagnesemia are useful in distinguishing Gitelman syndrome from Bartter syndrome on clinical grounds. These unique features mimic the effects of chronic thiazide diuretic administration. Missense mutations of the gene *SLC12A3*, which encodes the thiazide-sensitive sodium chloride cotransporter in the distal convoluted tubule (NCC), account for the clinical features, including the classic finding of hypocalciuria. However, it is not clear why these patients have pronounced hypomagnesemia.

Compared to Bartter syndrome, Gitelman syndrome becomes symptomatic later in life and is associated with milder salt wasting. A large study of adults with proven Gitelman syndrome and NCC mutations showed that salt craving, nocturia, cramps, and fatigue were more common than in sex-matched and age-matched controls. Women experience exacerbation of symptoms during menses, and they may experience complicated pregnancies.

Treatment for Gitelman syndrome consists of a diet high in potassium and potassium salts, typically with the addition of magnesium supplementation. Amiloride is often more helpful than spironolactone or eplerenone, with dose escalation to as much as 10 mg twice daily. Amiloride may be used in combination with spironolactone or eplerenone. Importantly, almost all patients with Gitelman syndrome exhibit some degree of substantial salt craving. In such

cases the offending high salt foods should be identified and avoided. Dietary salt loading increases distal delivery of NaCl and greatly amplifies K⁺ secretion by the cortical collecting tubule. Angiotensin-converting enzyme inhibitors or angiotensin receptor blockers have been suggested in selected patients for which frank hypotension is not a complication.

D. **Nonreabsorbable anions and magnesium deficiency**—Administration of large quantities of non-reabsorbable anions, such as with penicillin derivatives like carbenicillin, can enhance distal acidification and K⁺ secretion by increasing the negative transepithelial potential difference. Mg²⁺ deficiency frequently accompanies hypokalemia, and both electrolyte abnormalities must be corrected to ameliorate the metabolic alkalosis.

E. **Post-lactic acidosis or ketoacidosis**—When an underlying stimulus for the endogenous generation of lactic acid or keto acid is removed rapidly, as with the repair of circulatory insufficiency or administration of insulin therapy, the lactate or ketones are metabolized to yield an equivalent amount of HCO_3^-. Other sources of new HCO_3^- are additive to the original alkali generated by organic anion metabolism to create a surfeit of HCO_3^-. Such sources include new HCO_3^- added to the blood by the kidneys as a result of enhanced acid excretion during the preexisting period of acidosis, and exogenous alkali administered during the treatment phase of the acidosis. Acidosis-induced contraction of the ECV acts to sustain the alkalosis.

F. **Posthypercapnia**—Prolonged CO_2 retention with chronic respiratory acidosis enhances tubular HCO_3^- absorption and the generation of new HCO_3^- (increased net acid excretion). If the partial pressure of carbon dioxide in arterial blood (Pa_{CO_2}) is returned to normal by mechanical ventilation or other means, metabolic alkalosis results from the persistently elevated $[HCO_3^-]$. Associated ECV contraction does not allow complete repair of the alkalosis by correction of the Pa_{CO_2} alone, and alkalosis persists until isotonic saline is infused.

3. Metabolic alkalosis associated with hyperaldosteronism and hypertension

A. **Associated with high renin**—Hyperreninemia promotes conversion of angiotensin I to angiotensin II, causing severe vasoconstriction and aldosterone release. The clinical features of functional renal artery stenosis are related primarily to activation of the renin-angiotensin-aldosterone system causing renovascular hypertension (contralateral kidney) and ischemic nephropathy (affected kidney). Patients typically present with resistant hypertension that may be unresponsive to high doses of multiple antihypertensive agents. In addition, approximately 20% of adult patients also exhibit hypokalemia and metabolic alkalosis. Additional examples of metabolic alkalosis, hypokalemia, and hypertension can also occur with renin-secreting tumors of the kidney, accelerated hypertension, and estrogen therapy.

B. ASSOCIATED WITH LOW RENIN

4. Primary hyperaldosteronism—Increased aldosterone levels may result from autonomous adrenal overproduction or secondary aldosterone release caused by the overproduction of renin by the kidneys. In both situations, the normal feedback of ECV on aldosterone production is disrupted, and hypertension is the result of ECF volume expansion. Excessive production of aldosterone also increases net acid excretion and may result in metabolic alkalosis, which is worsened by associated K^+ deficiency. ECV expansion from salt retention causes hypertension and antagonizes the reduction in GFR. Tubule acidification is enhanced by aldosterone and by K^+ deficiency, through an increase in the activity of the H^+-ATPase and H^+, K^+-ATPase, respectively. The kaliuresis worsens K^+ depletion, resulting in a urinary concentrating defect, polyuria, and polydipsia.

5. Liddle syndrome—Liddle syndrome is a monogenetic disorder causing an inherited form of hypertension presenting in childhood, accompanied by hypokalemia and metabolic alkalosis. These features resemble those of primary hyperaldosteronism, but renin and aldosterone levels are suppressed (pseudohyperaldosteronism). The defect is attributed to an abnormality in the gene that encodes the β or the γ subunit of the renal epithelial Na^+ channel (ENaC) on the apical membrane of principal cells in the cortical collecting duct. This defect leads to constitutive activation of the renal sodium channel. Either mutation results in deletion of the cytoplasmic tail (C-terminus) of the affected subunit. The C-termini contain a PY amino acid motif that is highly conserved, and essentially all mutations in Liddle syndrome patients involve disruption or deletion of this motif. This causes an increase in the surface localization of the ENaC complex by failing to internalize the channels from the cell surface. Ultimately, persistent Na^+ absorption results in volume expansion, hypertension, hypokalemia, and metabolic alkalosis.

6. Glucocorticoid-remediable hyperaldosteronism—Glucocorticoid-remediable hyperaldosteronism is an autosomal-dominant form of hypertension, the features of which resemble primary aldosteronism (hypokalemic metabolic alkalosis and volume-dependent hypertension). However, in this disorder glucocorticoid administration corrects the hypertension as well as the excessive excretion of 18-hydroxysteroid in the urine. This disorder occurs from an unequal crossover between two genes located in close proximity on chromosome 8, resulting in the glucocorticoid-responsive promoter region of the gene encoding the 11-β-hydroxylase (*CYP11B1*) attaching to the structural portion of the *CYP11B2* gene encoding aldosterone synthase.

The chimeric gene produces excess amounts of aldosterone synthase unresponsive to serum potassium or renin levels; however, production can be suppressed by glucocorticoid administration. Although a rare cause of primary aldosteronism, it is important to diagnose since the treatment is unique and the syndrome can be associated with severe hypertension and stroke, especially during pregnancy.

7. Cushing syndrome—Abnormally high glucocorticoid production as a result of adrenal adenoma, carcinoma, or ectopic corticotropin production causes metabolic alkalosis. The alkalosis may be ascribed to coexisting mineralocorticoid (deoxycorticosterone and corticosterone) hypersecretion. Alternatively, glucocorticoids may have the capability of enhancing net acid secretion and NH_4^+ production through cross-reactivity with mineralocorticoid receptors.

8. Miscellaneous conditions—Ingestion of licorice or licorice-containing chewing tobacco can cause a typical pattern of mineralocorticoid excess. Glycyrrhizinic acid contained in authentic licorice inhibits 11β-hydroxysteroid dehydrogenase. This enzyme is responsible for converting cortisol to cortisone, an essential step in protecting the mineralocorticoid receptor from cortisol. When the enzyme is inactivated, cortisol can occupy type I mineralocorticoid receptors, mimicking aldosterone. Genetic apparent mineralocorticoid excess (AME) resembles excessive ingestion of licorice, with volume expansion, low renin and aldosterone levels, and a salt-sensitive form of hypertension that may include metabolic alkalosis and hypokalemia. In genetic AME, 11β-hydroxysteroid dehydrogenase is defective, and monogenic hypertension develops. Hypertension responds to thiazides and spironolactone, but without abnormal steroid products in the urine.

Symptoms of Metabolic Alkalosis

Patients with metabolic alkalosis experience changes in central and peripheral nervous system function similar to those of hypocalcemia. This results from binding of free calcium to anionic protein sites exposed in alkalemia, lowering the ionized calcium concentration. Symptoms may include confusion, obtundation, and a predisposition to seizures, paresthesia, muscular cramping, tetany, aggravation of arrhythmias, and hypoxemia in chronic obstructive pulmonary disease. Related electrolyte abnormalities include hypokalemia and hypophosphatemia.

Treatment of Metabolic Alkalosis

The maintenance phase of metabolic alkalosis represents a failure of the kidney to excrete bicarbonate efficiently because of chloride or potassium deficiency, continuous mineralocorticoid elaboration, or both. Treatment depends on the cause of the metabolic alkalosis, and it is primarily directed at correcting the underlying stimulus for HCO_3^- generation and restoring the ability of the kidney to excrete the excess HCO_3^-.

A history of vomiting, diuretic use, or alkali therapy, and assessment of the urine chloride concentration, arterial blood pressure, and volume status (particularly the presence or absence of orthostasis), help to guide diagnosis and treatment.

A high urine chloride level and hypertension suggest that primary mineralocorticoid excess is present. If primary aldosteronism is diagnosed, correction of the underlying cause (adenoma, bilateral hyperplasia, Cushing syndrome) will reverse the alkalosis. Patients with bilateral adrenal hyperplasia may respond to spironolactone. Normotensive patients with a high urine chloride level may have Bartter or Gitelman syndrome if diuretic use or vomiting can be excluded. A low-urine chloride level and relative hypotension suggest a chloride-responsive metabolic alkalosis such as vomiting or nasogastric suction. Loss of $[H^+]$ by the stomach or kidneys can be mitigated by the use of proton pump inhibitors or the discontinuation of diuretics. The second aspect of treatment is to remove the factors that sustain HCO_3^- reabsorption, such as ECV contraction or K^+ deficiency. Although K^+ deficits should be repleted, NaCl therapy is usually sufficient to reverse the alkalosis if ECV contraction is present, as indicated by low urine $[Cl^-]$.

Patients with congestive heart failure or unexplained volume expansion represent special challenges in the critical care setting. Patients with a low-urine chloride concentration, usually indicative of a "chloride-responsive" form of metabolic alkalosis, may not tolerate normal saline infusion. Renal HCO_3^- loss can be accelerated by administration of the carbonic anhydrase inhibitor acetazolamide (250 mg intravenously) if associated conditions preclude infusion of saline (ie, clinical evidence of congestive heart failure). Acetazolamide is usually effective in patients with adequate kidney function, but can exacerbate urinary K^+ losses causing hypokalemia. Dilute hydrochloric acid (0.1 N HCl) infused into a central vein is rarely recommended and should be avoided. Several potentially serious complications, such as hemolysis, venous sclerosis, and imprecise dosing, result in a very high risk-to-benefit ratio.

KEY READINGS

Feldman M et al: Respiratory compensation to a primary metabolic alkalosis in humans. Clin Nephrol 2012;78:365.

Gennari FJ: Pathophysiology of metabolic alkalosis: a new classification based on the centrality of stimulated collecting duct ion transport. Am J Kidney Dis 2011:626.

Huber L, Gennari FJ: Severe metabolic alkalosis in a hemodialysis patient. Am J Kidney Dis 2011;58:144.

Kandasamy N et al: Life-threatening metabolic alkalosis in Pendred syndrome. Eur J Endocrinol 2011;165:167.

Mæhle K et al: Metabolic alkalosis is the most common acid-base disorder in ICU patients. Crit Care 2014;28:420.

Peixoto AJ, Alpern RJ: Treatment of severe metabolic alkalosis in a patient with congestive heart failure. Am J Kidney Dis 2013;61:822.

Pucci G et al: Acute renal failure and metabolic alkalosis in a patient with colorectal villous adenoma (McKittrick-Wheelock syndrome). Surgery 2013;154:643.

Yi JH et al: Metabolic alkalosis from unsuspected ingestion: use of urine pH and anion gap. Am J Kidney Dis 2012;59: 577.

▼ RESPIRATORY ACID–BASE DISORDERS

Gregg Y. Lipschik, MD & Jeanne P. Macrae, MD

The respiratory acid–base disorders, respiratory alkalosis and respiratory acidosis, are commonly seen in intensive care units and emergency rooms, as well as in general practice. Both are caused by changes in alveolar ventilation that lead to a rise or fall in the partial pressure of CO_2 in arterial blood (Pco_2). The clinical importance of these disorders, however, is very different. While respiratory alkalosis rarely requires specific treatment, respiratory acidosis accompanies some of the most dramatic presentations of illness a physician will see.

CO_2 is produced by metabolism and eliminated by ventilation. Alveolar CO_2 concentration is conveniently measured as Pco_2. Pco_2 is inversely proportional to alveolar ventilation (V_A), so that anything that increases V_A (an increase in respiratory rate or tidal volume or improved ventilation-perfusion [V/Q] matching) causes a decrease in Pco_2, and anything that decreases V_A (a decrease in respiratory rate or tidal volume, or severe V/Q mismatch, leading to increased physiologic dead space) causes an increase in Pco_2.

Understanding the diagnosis and treatment of the respiratory acid–base disorders requires knowledge of the buffer systems that serve to protect against alterations in hydrogen ion concentration and pH. As CO_2 enters the blood, it combines with H_2O to form carbonic acid (H_2CO_3), which dissociates into bicarbonate (HCO_3^-) and hydrogen ions:

$$CO_2 + H_2O \leftrightarrow H_2CO_3 \leftrightarrow HCO_3^- + H^+$$

Most of the H^+ ions produced by this addition of CO_2 to the blood combine with intracellular buffers including hemoglobin, and this tissue buffering minimizes the elevation in hydrogen ion concentration and the corresponding fall in pH.

In respiratory acid–base disturbances, a primary rise or fall in Pco_2 (respiratory acidosis or alkalosis, respectively) will result in a change in pH unless a proportional change in HCO_3^- occurs to compensate. The initial response to a primary change in Pco_2 is tissue buffering of the change with movement of intracellular HCO_3^- to or from the extracellular fluid. Subsequently, renal HCO_3^- excretion is adjusted, and serum HCO_3^- changes further to defend against pH changes.

RESPIRATORY ALKALOSIS

ESSENTIALS OF DIAGNOSIS

▶ Low PCO_2 and high pH.

▶ Acute respiratory alkalosis: HCO_3^- falls 2 mEq/L for each 10 mm Hg fall in PCO_2 (in minutes).

▶ Chronic respiratory alkalosis: HCO_3^- falls 5 mEq/L for each 10 mm Hg fall in PCO_2 (over days). pH may return to normal!

▶ If calculated compensation is too little or too much, another acid–base abnormality (a mixed disorder) must be present.

▶ General Considerations

Respiratory alkalosis is the result of hyperventilation produced by a variety of influences. It rarely requires specific treatment other than for the underlying condition. In fact, overly aggressive efforts to treat respiratory alkalosis itself are often fruitless or dangerous and occasionally cause respiratory acidosis.

▶ Pathogenesis

With hyperventilation, CO_2 is eliminated out of proportion to its production, the bicarbonate equilibrium described above shifts to the left (see below), hydrogen ions are utilized, and pH rises. This decrease in PCO_2 (hypocapnia) and rise in pH constitute **respiratory alkalosis**.

$$CO_2 + H_2O \leftarrow H_2CO_3 \leftarrow HCO_3^- + H^+$$

Acute reduction in PCO_2 releases H^+ from tissue buffers, titrating HCO_3^- and decreasing its concentration. Eventually, decreased PCO_2 also inhibits renal tubular reabsorption and generation of HCO_3^-, the serum level falls further, and pH returns toward normal.

▶ Prevention

The only common cause of respiratory alkalosis that can be prevented occurs in a mechanically ventilated patient when the chosen ventilator settings produce too high a rate of minute ventilation. This may be difficult to distinguish from the situation in which a ventilated patient develops a respiratory alkalosis because of dyspnea, pain, anxiety, or the underlying disease (see **Treatment** below).

▶ Clinical Findings

A. Symptoms and Signs

Chronic respiratory alkalosis is generally asymptomatic, as the blood pH is near normal (Table 5–10). In acute respiratory alkalosis, patients may experience dyspnea, dizziness, anxiety,

Table 5–10. Clinical manifestations of respiratory alkalosis.[1]

Neuromuscular
Related to cerebral vasospasm and decreased perfusion
Lightheadedness
Confusion
Syncope
Related to decreased to ionized calcium or decreased availability of calcium
Seizures (or decreased seizure threshold)
Paresthesias
Muscular cramps, tetany
Cardiovascular
Tachycardia
Ventricular arrhythmias
Gastrointestinal
Nausea and vomiting
Other
Dyspnea
Anxiety
Decreased ionized calcium

[1]Most signs and symptoms are seen with acute respiratory alkalosis.

and acral or circumoral paresthesias. Symptoms are related to both decreased ionized calcium and reduced cerebral blood flow (see below).

B. Laboratory Findings

Respiratory alkalosis is diagnosed by arterial blood gas analysis showing a high pH, decreased PCO_2, and variably decreased serum HCO_3^-. It must be distinguished from metabolic acidosis in which the PCO_2 and HCO_3^- are also decreased but pH is low. Accurate diagnosis requires knowledge of the magnitude of the expected compensation (fall in HCO_3^-) and the duration of the abnormality. An initial decrease in HCO_3^- occurs in minutes in response to respiratory alkalosis, but full renal compensation for chronic respiratory alkalosis takes days to develop. The data describing appropriate compensation for acute and chronic respiratory alkalosis come from studies of hyperventilation in normal volunteers.

1. Acute respiratory alkalosis: HCO_3^- falls 2 mEq/L for each 10 mm Hg fall in PCO_2 (in minutes).

2. Chronic respiratory alkalosis: HCO_3^- falls 5 mEq/L for each 10 mm Hg fall in PCO_2 (over days). *pH may return to normal!*

3. If calculated compensation is too little or too much, another acid–base abnormality (a mixed disorder) must be present.

C. Imaging Studies and Special Tests

Imaging studies and specialized testing are generally not helpful in the diagnosis and management of respiratory alkalosis, although such testing may be appropriate in the management of the underlying disorder.

Differential Diagnosis

Most conditions causing hyperventilation and respiratory alkalosis (with the exception of mechanical ventilation) do so via central respiratory stimulation, increasing the minute ventilation and alveolar ventilation and therefore lowering the P_{CO_2}. Table 5–11 lists the common causes.

Table 5–11. Causes of respiratory alkalosis.

Supratentorial
Anxiety
Pain
Fever

Pulmonary
Hypoxia from all causes
　　Hypoxic pulmonary or cardiac disease
　　High altitude
Pulmonary disorders causing respiratory alkalosis with or without hypoxia
　　Conditions causing decreased compliance
　　　　Pneumothorax
　　　　Pneumonia
　　　　Pulmonary edema
　　　　Interstitial lung disease
　　　　Less severe chest wall disorders
　　Pulmonary embolism
　　Bronchospasm
　　Auto-PEEP in mechanically ventilated patients

Central nervous system
Meningitis, encephalitis
Intracranial tumors
Cerebrovascular accident
Head trauma

Drugs
Aspirin and other salicylates
Progesterone
Theophylline
Catecholamines
Thyroxine

Miscellaneous conditions
Excessive mechanical ventilation
Pregnancy
Sepsis (particularly gram-negative)
Liver disease
Exercise
Acute reversal of metabolic acidosis
Thyrotoxicosis
Alcohol withdrawal
Beri-beri

PEEP, positive end-expiratory pressure.

Anxiety and pain are common causes of hyperventilation and respiratory alkalosis; the act of obtaining a blood gas sample is likely to produce sufficient hyperventilation to demonstrate an acute respiratory alkalosis. Hypoxia in patients with respiratory disease is also very common and often overlooked as a cause of respiratory alkalosis.

The cause of respiratory alkalosis in both liver failure and pregnancy is believed to be elevated levels of both progesterone and estradiol. Progesterone increases ventilation by acting on central nervous system progesterone receptors, while estradiol is thought to increase the number of these receptors. Increased levels of progesterone and estradiol are part of the normal physiologic milieu of pregnancy, while in liver failure they are caused by the inability of the diseased liver to metabolize free hormones.

Aspirin, although its effect in causing hyperventilation is well known, commonly causes a mixed acid–base pattern: respiratory alkalosis and metabolic acidosis. The same pattern is seen in gram-negative sepsis. The hyperventilation seen with gram-negative sepsis, or even with fever alone, is caused by the effects of inflammatory mediators, most prominently tumor necrosis factor and the interleukins.

Complications

Alkalosis directly enhances neuromuscular excitability and modestly decreases serum ionized calcium. As mentioned above, these changes in ionized calcium levels cause paresthesias, numbness, and muscle twitching. With severe alkalosis, tetany may result. Severe alkalosis and hypocapnia can cause dizziness, confusion, and loss of consciousness due to cerebral vasospasm with decreased cerebral blood flow. In fact, intentional production of respiratory alkalosis (using mechanical ventilation) and subsequent cerebral vasospasm is a commonly used short-term treatment for increased intracranial pressure.

Respiratory alkalosis, like metabolic alkalosis, may cause hypokalemia through an intracellular shift of potassium ions. The resultant hypokalemia is generally mild with few clinical features and does not require treatment.

Treatment

Respiratory alkalosis itself is rarely a clinically important problem. Sedation, analgesia, and antipyretics (for anxiety, pain, and fever, respectively) are often sufficient therapy.

In other cases, treating the underlying problem (oxygen for hypoxia, hemodialysis for severe aspirin overdose, treating infections for a patient with sepsis) is necessary. In patients with respiratory alkalosis complicating mechanical ventilation, simply adjusting ventilator settings or changing the mode of ventilation should not be considered an adequate "treatment." These maneuvers can produce an apparent improvement in arterial blood gases but at the cost of a fatigued or dyspneic patient whose reason for hyperventilation remains undiagnosed and untreated. While settings should be checked for appropriateness, a more effective approach to treating alkalosis in this setting is to search for underlying causes of hyperventilation and treat them. Typically, pain, anxiety, or dyspnea due to a concurrent or new condition (pneumonia, pulmonary edema, bronchospasm, pulmonary embolism, retained secretions) is the cause of a new respiratory alkalosis in a previously stable mechanically ventilated patient.

▶ Prognosis

Prognosis in respiratory alkalosis is entirely dependent on the underlying cause; patients may recover from an episode of anxiety-related hyperventilation in minutes or remain chronically subject to increased ventilatory drive from severe lung diseases such as interstitial fibrosis.

▶ When to Refer/When to Admit

As for **Prognosis** (earlier), decisions about triage for patients with acute or chronic respiratory alkalosis depend on the underlying cause; respiratory alkalosis itself is rarely a reason to admit or refer a patient.

RESPIRATORY ACIDOSIS

ESSENTIALS OF DIAGNOSIS

- ▸ High P_{CO_2} and low pH.
- ▸ Acute respiratory acidosis: HCO_3^- rises 1 mEq/L for each 10 mm Hg rise in P_{CO_2} (in minutes).
- ▸ Chronic respiratory acidosis: HCO_3^- rises 3.5 mEq/L for each 10 mm Hg rise in P_{CO_2} (over days).
- ▸ If calculated compensation is too little or too much, another acid–base abnormality (a mixed disorder) must be present.

▶ General Considerations

Unlike respiratory alkalosis, respiratory acidosis, particularly acute respiratory acidosis caused by severe pulmonary disease or sedative overdose, may produce dangerous hypercapnia and acidosis and often requires urgent treatment.

▶ Pathophysiology

With hypoventilation, elimination of CO_2 is unable to keep pace with its metabolic production, CO_2 is retained, and the equilibrium above shifts to the right. Excess hydrogen ions are produced, and pH falls. This rise in P_{CO_2} (hypercapnia) and fall in pH constitute **respiratory acidosis**.

$$CO_2 + H_2O \rightarrow H_2CO_3 \rightarrow HCO_3^- + H^+$$

Decreased ventilation quickly results in increased P_{CO_2} because metabolic production of CO_2 is so rapid. Acutely, tissue buffering slightly raises HCO_3^-, limiting the pH drop. Eventually, renal acid excretion increases, HCO_3^- reabsorption is stimulated, serum HCO_3^- rises, and pH returns toward normal.

Two pathophysiologic mechanisms produce hypercapnia and respiratory acidosis: Severe V/Q mismatch of the dead space (high V/Q) type and alveolar hypoventilation. Again, since P_{CO_2} is inversely proportional to V_A, any process that decreases V_A (alveolar hypoventilation or severe V/Q mismatch) causes a rise in P_{CO_2}.

In patients with chronic respiratory disease and hypercapnia, excess supplemental oxygen can cause hypoventilation (via blunted hypoxic drive) and V/Q mismatch (via the release of hypoxic vasoconstriction), causing worse hypercapnia and respiratory acidosis (see **Prevention** and **Differential Diagnosis**, below). In this situation, the Haldane effect, release of hemoglobin-bound CO_2, also contributes slightly to the resulting hypercapnia.

▶ Prevention

Few of the causes of respiratory acidosis can be prevented. One exception (see **Pathogenesis**, above and **Differential Diagnosis**, below) is the iatrogenic acute respiratory acidosis that can result from overzealous oxygen administration in patients with severe, chronic respiratory disease who are adapted to hypercapnia and dependent on hypoxia to stimulate ventilation. In these patients, oxygen should be administered by low flow (nasal cannula) or controlled dose (Venturi mask) methods to deliver the minimal F_{IO_2} necessary to correct hypoxemia.

In addition, extreme care should be used in administering sedative drugs to patients with underlying hypercapnic lung disease.

▶ Clinical Findings

A. Symptoms and Signs

The symptoms and signs of respiratory acidosis (Table 5–12) depend on how quickly the acidosis develops (because a rapid rise in brain P_{CO_2} is not quickly compensated for by a rise in brain HCO_3^-) and are related to its effect on brain pH. Hypercapnia lowers brain pH and produces cerebral vasodilation, increased cerebral blood flow, and increased intracranial pressure with symptoms and signs similar to the effects of narcotic agents. Early symptoms may include blurred vision, headache, restlessness, tremors, and delirium. These may progress to drowsiness, lethargy, and coma as P_{CO_2} rises and pH falls.

B. Laboratory Findings

Respiratory acidosis is diagnosed by arterial blood gas analysis showing a low pH, elevated P_{CO_2}, and variably elevated serum HCO_3^-. Respiratory alkalosis must be distinguished from metabolic alkalosis in which the P_{CO_2} and

Table 5–12. Clinical manifestations of respiratory acidosis.[1]

Neuromuscular (presumably related to cerebral vasodilation and increased cerebral blood flow)
Headache
Drowsiness, restlessness, lethargy, coma
Delirium
Headache
Papilledema (rare)
Myoclonus

Cardiovascular
Tachycardia
Ventricular arrythmias

Other
Dyspnea
Hypoxia and related symptoms (as CO_2 replaces O_2 in the alveolus)

[1]Signs and symptoms are worse with acute or rapidly developing respiratory acidosis.

HCO_3^- are also elevated, but pH is high. When a blood gas is not immediately available, or when questioning the duration of respiratory acidosis, the measured serum HCO_3^- may also be helpful. In an appropriate clinical setting, a significantly elevated serum HCO_3^- from a previous arterial blood gas (at least a few days prior) is indirect evidence of a chronic respiratory acidosis. As mentioned, however, an elevated serum HCO_3^- may also represent metabolic alkalosis.

As for respiratory alkalosis, accurate diagnosis requires knowledge of the magnitude of the expected compensation (rise in HCO_3^-) and the duration of the abnormality. An initial increase in HCO_3^- from tissue buffering occurs in minutes in response to respiratory acidosis, but maximal renal compensation for chronic respiratory acidosis takes days to develop. The data describing appropriate compensation for acute and chronic respiratory acidosis come from several studies of dogs, normal humans, and patients with severe underlying pulmonary disease.

1. Acute respiratory acidosis: HCO_3^- rises 1 mEq/L for each 10 mm Hg rise in Pco_2 (in minutes).

2. Chronic respiratory acidosis: HCO_3^- rises 3.5 mEq/L for each 10 mm Hg rise in Pco_2 (over days).

3. If calculated compensation is too much or too little, another process (a mixed disorder) must be present.

C. Imaging Studies and Special Tests

Imaging studies and specialized testing are generally not helpful in the diagnosis and management of respiratory acidosis, although such testing may be appropriate in the management of the underlying disorder.

▶ Differential Diagnosis

Common causes of respiratory acidosis are listed in Table 5–13.

A. Acute Respiratory Acidosis

Acute respiratory acidosis most frequently results from iatrogenic or intentional overdose of a sedative drug (opiates, benzodiazepines). These drugs suppress central respiratory drive causing alveolar hypoventilation, hypercapnia, and respiratory acidosis. Severe, acute exacerbations of any respiratory disease (eg, asthma) can also cause acute respiratory acidosis. These conditions produce severe V/Q mismatch and a high work-of-breathing with respiratory muscle fatigue, both leading to hypercapnia and respiratory acidosis.

Table 5–13. Causes of acute and chronic respiratory acidosis.

Acute
Pulmonary
  Airway problems
    Status asthmaticus
    Laryngospasm
  Parenchymal problems
    Severe pneumonia
    Severe pulmonary edema
    Any acute, severe pulmonary disease
  Other
    Excess supplemental oxygen in patients with chronic hypercapnia
    Disconnection or failure of mechanical ventilation
Nonpulmonary
  Drugs
    Anesthetics
    Sedative drugs (opiates, methadone, benzodiazepines)
    Neuromuscular blockers
    Aminoglycosides
  Flail chest
    Spinal cord injury
    Cardiopulmonary arrest

Chronic (may also cause acute acidosis)
Pulmonary
  Severe chronic obstructive pulmonary disease
  Other severe chronic lung diseases (interstitial fibrosis)
Nonpulmonary
  Obstructive sleep apnea
  Obesity hypoventilation syndrome
  Myxedema
  Neuromuscular and chest wall disease
    Brainstem infarct
    Guillain–Barré syndrome
    Myasthenia gravis
    Muscular dystrophy
    Poliomyelitis
    Kyphoscoliosis
    Diaphragmatic paralysis
    Amyotrophic lateral sclerosis

One important, preventable cause of acute respiratory acidosis is the administration of supplemental oxygen to patients with chronic respiratory disease and hypercapnia (see **Pathophysiology** and **Prevention**, above).

B. Chronic Respiratory Acidosis

The most important and most common cause of chronic respiratory acidosis is severe emphysema (chronic obstructive pulmonary disease [COPD]). In this condition, severe V/Q mismatch and respiratory muscle weakness/dysfunction produce hypoventilation, hypercapnia, and respiratory acidosis. Obesity-hypoventilation syndrome is another common cause of chronic respiratory acidosis. Other severe respiratory (eg, pulmonary fibrosis), neuromuscular (Guillain–Barré syndrome, muscular dystrophy), and chest wall (kyphoscoliosis) diseases are less common causes of chronic respiratory acidosis. These conditions are characterized by severe V/Q mismatch, respiratory muscle dysfunction, and/or hypoventilation, leading to hypercapnia.

Chronic use or abuse of opiate drugs (eg, for control of chronic pain or in methadone maintenance programs) is another cause of chronic respiratory acidosis; treatment is generally not necessary but caution is warranted as these patients are at high risk for further decompensation, particularly if concurrent respiratory disease ensues.

C. "Acute-on-Chronic" Respiratory Acidosis

Patients with severe but compensated respiratory diseases and chronic respiratory acidosis may develop an acute respiratory acidosis when an acute insult (pneumonia, pulmonary embolus, flare of the underlying disease) occurs. The pathophysiologic mechanisms at work here are usually severe V/Q mismatch due to the underlying disease and hypoventilation due to respiratory muscle fatigue and an increased work of breathing.

▶ Complications

Unlike respiratory alkalosis, respiratory acidosis is often clinically important. Severe respiratory acidosis and hypercapnia simulate the effects of opiates. They can cause hypotension, confusion and obtundation, and ultimately coma (see Table 5–14 and **Symptoms and Signs,** above). Hypercapnia causes cerebral vasodilation, which may result in increased intracranial pressure and papilledema.

Since hyperventilation is the primary defense against metabolic acidosis, patients with chronic respiratory disease who develop metabolic acidosis are at greater risk and may need early mechanical ventilation.

▶ Treatment

Treatment is focused on improving ventilation. When chronic respiratory acidosis results from respiratory disease, optimally treating the underlying condition (eg, COPD) will simultaneously treat the acidosis.

When acute (or acute-on-chronic) respiratory acidosis is caused by acute exacerbations of chronic respiratory disease or drug overdose, mechanical ventilation may be necessary as well as specific antidotes for the drug ingested.

Although CO_2 production is one of the determinants of alveolar and arterial Pco_2, it is rare for increased CO_2 production to play a significant role in the development of respiratory acidosis. Still, it is occasionally possible to improve hypercapnia in cases of end-stage pulmonary disease by decreasing CO_2 production with a low carbohydrate diet and by avoiding overeating or overfeeding. These measures are rarely necessary or useful in other clinical settings.

▶ Prognosis

Prognosis in respiratory acidosis depends on and is determined by the underlying etiology of the disorder. Patients

Table 5–14. Recognition, causes, and therapy of respiratory acid–base disorders.

Acid–Base Disorder	Primary pH Change	Pco₂ Change	Expected Compensation	Common Causes	Therapy
Acute respiratory acidosis	↓	Pco_2 ↑	HCO_3^- ↑1/↑ 10 in Pco_2	Narcotics, acute or acute-on-chronic lung disease	Therapy of lung disease, mechanical ventilation, specific antidotes
Chronic respiratory acidosis	↓	Pco_2 ↑	HCO_3^- ↑3.5/↑10 in Pco_2	Chronic lung disease	Therapy of lung disease
Acute respiratory alkalosis	↑	Pco_2 ↓	HCO_3^- ↓2/↓10 in Pco_2	Fever, pain, anxiety, mechanical ventilation	Sedation, analgesia, antipyretics
Chronic respiratory alkalosis	↑	Pco_2 ↓	HCO_3^- ↓5/↓10 in Pco_2	Chronic liver disease, pregnancy, aspirin overdose, and sepsis (with metabolic acidosis)	Therapy of underlying disease

may recover fully from acute acidosis associated with drug overdose or exacerbation of asthma. Patients with severe, hypercapnic obstructive lung disease generally follow an inexorably downhill course.

When to Refer/When to Admit

As for **Prognosis** (above), triage decisions for patients with acute and chronic respiratory acidosis depend on the underlying cause, chronicity, and severity of the acidosis. Patients with chronic respiratory acidosis caused by (for example) stable chronic obstructive lung disease, obesity-hypoventilation syndrome or methadone maintenance are generally safely followed as outpatients. Those with acute respiratory acidosis from opiate overdose or with acute, severe respiratory disease (eg, asthma or COPD exacerbations) are best managed in intensive care units, often with mechanical ventilation.

■ CHAPTER REVIEW QUESTIONS

1. A 22-year-old woman is referred for evaluation of progressive weakness of 5 months duration. The patient denies vomiting or ingestion of diuretics, but notes "salt craving" as manifest by eating highly salty food snacks several times daily. On physical examination the BP is 100/60 and declines to 80/42 with standing. There is no jugular vein distention (JVD) or peripheral edema and the examination of the heart reveals normal heart sounds and no murmurs, rubs or gallops.

Laboratory Data:
Metabolic profile: Na 140, K 2.8, Cl 90, tCO_2 38, BUN 28, Cr 1.1, Serum Osm 297
Urine: Na 46, K 42, Cl 56, pH 5.0, Osm 450
Arterial blood gas: pH 7.48, PCO_2 50, HCO_3^- 36

Which ONE response from the list below best describes the acid–base disorder in this patient?
A. Mixed metabolic acidosis—metabolic alkalosis
B. Metabolic alkalosis—respiratory acidosis
C. Metabolic alkalosis
D. Respiratory acidosis

2. A 44-year-old woman was referred from a local hospital after presenting with flaccid paralysis. Severe hypokalemia was documented (2.0 mEq/L) and an infusion containing KCl was initiated, prior to transfer to your hospital. The laboratory data on arrival to St. Nephron Hospital follow:

Laboratory Data:	Units
Sodium	140 mEq/L
Potassium	2.3 mEq/L
Chloride	115 mEq/L
Bicarbonate	15 mEq/L
Anion gap	10 mEq/L
BUN	22 mg/dL
Creatinine	1.4 mg/dL

Arterial Blood Gases:
pH	7.32 U
$Paco_2$	30 mm Hg
HCO_3	15 mEq/L

Urinalysis

pH = 6.0, normal sediment without white or red blood cell casts and no bacteria. The urine protein to creatinine ratio was 0.150 g/g. Urinary electrolyte values: Na^+ 35, K^+ 40, Cl^- 18 mEq/L.

From the list below choose the one BEST description of the acid–base disorder.
A. Chronic respiratory alkalosis
B. High AG metabolic acidosis
C. Non-AG metabolic acidosis
D. Mixed metabolic acidosis—respiratory alkalosis

3. A 58-year-old woman with CKD secondary to chronic glomerulonephritis (CGN) who is managed conservatively and has an established baseline S_{Cr} of 1.8, and BUN of 28, is admitted with protracted vomiting of several days duration. Significant orthostatic hypotension is noted on PE and the patient appears to be volume depleted clinically.

The following laboratory data were obtained on admission:
Na = 145, K = 4, Cl = 100, HCO_3 = 25 mEq/L
BUN = 75, Cr = 5, Alb = 3.8
pH = 7.4, PCO_2 = 40, HCO_3 = 25

From the following list select the ONE correct statement that most accurately characterizes the diagnosis of the acid–base disturbance in this patient.
A. Metabolic alkalosis
B. High AG metabolic acidosis
C. Mixed metabolic acidosis—metabolic alkalosis
D. Mixed metabolic acidosis—metabolic alkalosis and respiratory acidosis
E. None of the above

4. A 67-year-old woman is admitted to the surgical service with acute cholecystitis that is treated by nasogastric suction and replacement of fluid losses with hypotonic saline containing 10 mEq KCl/L. The ECG is normal. The Nephrology Consultation Service is asked to evaluate the patient. The following laboratory data are obtained:

Na = 138, K = 2.8, Cl = 85, and $HCO_3^- = 42$ mEq/L
pH = 7.54, $Pco_2 = 51$, $Po_2 = 92$ mm Hg
Urine Na = 42, Urine K = 45, and Urine Cl = 6 mEq/L
Urine pH = 6.9

Which ONE of the following best describes the acid–base disorder in this patient?
A. Mixed respiratory acidosis and metabolic alkalosis
B. Mixed respiratory alkalosis and metabolic alkalosis
C. Metabolic acidosis
D. Metabolic alkalosis

5. A 22-year-old man was admitted with a history of depression and suicidal ideation. His friends indicated that the patient had experienced recent emotional problems stemming from a failed relationship. The patient was obtunded on admission to the emergency department (ED), but there were no focal neurological deficits. The remainder of the physical examination was unremarkable.

Initial Laboratory Data:

	Units
Na^+	140 mEq/L
K^+	5 mEq/L
Cl^-	105 mEq/L
HCO_3^-	10 mEq/L
Glucose	115 mg/dL
BUN	15 mg/dL
Creatinine	0.9 mg/dL
Ionized calcium	4.0 mg/dL
Plasma osmolality	325 mOsm kg/H_2O
Anion gap	25 mEq/L
Plasma ketones trace	
L-Lactate	1.16 mmol/L

Arterial blood gas (room air): pH = 7.26, $Paco_2 = 23$ mm Hg, $Pao_2 = 100$ mm Hg, $[HCO_3^-] = 10$

Urinalysis revealed crystalluria, with a mixture of "envelope" and "needle"-shaped crystals.

Choose the one BEST description of the patient's acid–base disturbance from the list below.
A. Compensated metabolic acidosis
B. High AG metabolic acidosis
C. Mixed high AG acidosis plus respiratory alkalosis
D. Mixed metabolic acidosis and metabolic alkalosis

6. A 44-year-old woman with a history of short bowel syndrome is admitted with a history of diarrhea of 4 days duration and weakness. Significant orthostatic hypotension is noted on admission to the ED.

Laboratory Data:
Na = 140, K = 2.0, Cl = 115, $HCO_3 = 15$,
pH = 7.32, $Paco_2 = 30$, $Pao_2 = 94$, $HCO_3 = 15$
Urine pH = 6.0, glucose = negative, ketones = slightly positive, protein = negative, Sp. Gr. = 1.031
Urine electrolytes: Na = 15, K = 10, Cl = 45

Which ONE of the following represent the MOST correct description(s) of the acid–base disturbance in this case?
A. Non-AG metabolic acidosis
B. High AG metabolic acidosis
C. Respiratory alkalosis and metabolic alkalosis
D. Mixed non-AG acidosis and respiratory alkalosis

7. A 70-year-old man has been mechanically ventilated in the intensive care unit after a stroke with stable laboratory values for 5 days. On day 6, he seems agitated and his routine morning arterial blood gas shows the following result:

pH 7.49 Pco_2 30 mm Hg HCO_3^- 22 mmol/L

What is the MOST appropriate response to this change?
A. Change the ventilator mode to synchronized intermittent mechanical ventilation (SIMV).
B. Look for a cause of pain or dyspnea.
C. Decrease ventilator tidal volume or rate.
D. Check patient's liver function tests.

8. You are consulted post-op about a 65-year-old diabetic man with complications of diabetic neuropathy and renal insufficiency, admitted for elective coronary artery bypass graft surgery. His admission chest X-ray showed an elevated right hemi-diaphragm. The surgeon reported that he might have nicked a nerve in the left mediastinum. Now, almost 3 days post-op, his respiratory rate is 30. An arterial blood gas done on 2 L/min of nasal oxygen shows: pH 7.32, Pco_2 50 mm Hg, Po_2 85 mm Hg, HCO_3 25 mmol/L.

Which of the following is MOST likely?
A. His renal disease is the cause of his acidosis.
B. Neuropathy paralyzed the right hemi-diaphragm, then the surgeon nicked the left phrenic nerve, causing a paralyzed left hemi-diaphragm and respiratory acidosis.
C. Whatever the cause of his acidosis, he probably did not have it before the surgery.
D. Supplemental oxygen suppressed his hypoxic drive, causing hypercapnia.

Disorders of Calcium Metabolism: Hypocalcemia and Hypercalcemia

Stuart M. Sprague, DO

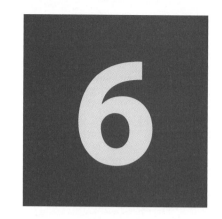

CALCIUM BALANCE

Serum calcium concentrations are normally tightly controlled within a narrow range, usually 8.5–10.5 mg/dL. However, the serum calcium concentration comprises less than 1% of the total body calcium content and is a poor reflection of overall total body calcium. The remainder of total body calcium is stored in bone. Serum calcium concentration comprises ionized calcium (approximately 40%), which is physiologically active, while the remainder of the calcium is bound predominantly to albumin (approximately 45%) and to a much lesser extent to anions (approximately 15%) such as citrate, bicarbonate, and phosphate. In the presence of acidosis, there is a relative increase in the ionized calcium component of the total serum calcium. Serum levels of ionized calcium are maintained in the normal range by the secretion of parathyroid hormone.

In normal individuals, the net calcium balance (intake–output) varies with age. Children and young adults are usually in a slightly positive net calcium balance to enhance linear growth; beyond age 25–35, when bones stop growing, the calcium balance tends to be neutral. Normal individuals have protection against calcium overload by virtue of their ability to increase renal excretion of calcium and reduce intestinal absorption of calcium by actions of parathyroid hormone and the activated form of vitamin D (calcitriol). However, in chronic kidney disease, the ability to maintain normal calcium homeostasis, including a normal serum ionized calcium level and appropriate calcium balance for age is lost.

Calcium absorption across the intestine occurs via a vitamin D dependent, saturable (transcellular) and independent, nonsaturable (paracellular) pathway. In states of adequate dietary calcium, the paracellular mechanism prevails, but the vitamin D dependent pathways are critical in calcium deficient states. In general, 15–25% of ingested calcium is absorbed. Normal ionized serum calcium is maintained by the secretion of parathyroid hormone which will increase bone resorption to release calcium into the circulation as well as to enhance calcium reabsorption by the kidneys. Parathyroid hormone also has an indirect effect by increasing the production of calcitriol by the kidney, which will act to increase the transcellular gastrointestinal absorption of calcium.

HYPOCALCEMIA

ESSENTIALS OF DIAGNOSIS

- ▶ Decreased ionized serum calcium concentration or a decreased albumin corrected serum calcium concentration.
- ▶ Defect or deficiency in the parathyroid hormone and/or vitamin D axis, resulting in decreased GI absorption or inability to mobilize calcium from bone.
- ▶ Excessive tissue deposition such as occurs with massive tissue death or trauma, such as in rhabdomyolysis, tumor lysis, or acute pancreatitis.
- ▶ Hyperphosphatemia results in complexation with high phosphate load, which may occur with excessive oral phosphate ingestion, phosphate enemas, or chronic kidney disease.
- ▶ Excessive deposition of calcium in bone in patients with osteoblastic metastasis, such as prostate cancer.
- ▶ May occur transiently in patients with severe sepsis or other serious illnesses.

▶ General Considerations

The incidence of hypocalcemia is difficult to quantify as there have been very few studies. Among intensive care patients, hypocalcemia was reported to range between 15% and 88%. Transient hypocalcemia is common after both thyroid and parathyroid surgery, with up to 2% having permanent hypocalcemia. Hypocalcemia commonly occurs in the following conditions; chronic and acute renal failure, vitamin D deficiency, hypomagnesemia, acute pancreatitis, hypoparathyroidism, and infusion of phosphate, citrate, or calcium-free albumin. Death from hypocalcemia is rare but has been reported. Severe hypocalcemia may result in paresthesias, seizures, cardiovascular collapse, hypotension unresponsive to fluids and vasopressors, and dysrhythmias. The age distribution of hypocalcemia is contingent on the underling disorder. In children, nutritional deficiencies are more frequent; in adults, kidney disease predominates.

▶ Prevention

The key to prevention is to identify potential clinical scenarios in which hypocalcemia may develop. In particular, patients who are undergoing extensive thyroid or parathyroid surgery need to be closely monitored postoperatively. The use of vitamin D and oral calcium supplements should be considered following surgery with monitoring of serum calcium concentrations. If vitamin D deficiency is identified it should be corrected, if possible, prior to surgery.

▶ Clinical Findings

A. Signs and Symptoms

The clinical manifestations of acute hypocalcemia are rather specific and relate to the neuromuscular actions of hypocalcemia. Early symptoms include perioral and digital paresthesias. Signs of acute hypocalcemia include intermittent muscle spasms (tetany), which result from increased neuromuscular irritability after stimulation. Specifically, the development of carpopedal spasm (adduction of thumb, flexion of wrists and metacarpals, and extension of fingers). The manifestations of hypocalcemia can be elicited by testing for the Trousseau sign (inflating a sphygmomanometer cuff above systolic pressure for 3 minutes and finding carpopedal spasm of the affected limb) or the Chvostek sign (twitching of facial muscles after tapping on the facial nerve anterior to the ear). These signs of neuromuscular irritability may progress to seizures, laryngospasm, and bronchospasm and therefore represent a medical emergency when seen. In addition to the neuromuscular irritability, cardiac abnormalities including prolonged QT interval, arrhythmias, particularly in patients on digitalis, heart failure, and hypotension may develop as well, particularly in the critical care setting. These abnormalities are typically seen when patients have a serum calcium level that is greater than 30% below the normal range.

Chronic hypocalcemia is associated with neuropsychiatric manifestations including dementia or mental retardation in children and other psychiatric syndromes, including depression and anxiety. In addition, idiopathic hypoparathyroidism, an important cause of chronic hypocalcemia, may be associated paradoxically with intracerebral calcifications, particularly in the basal ganglia, and a Parkinsonian syndrome may result from basal ganglia damage. Other manifestations of chronic hypocalcemia may include subcapsular cataracts, dry skin, osteopenia/osteoporosis, and abnormal dentition.

B. Laboratory Findings

The first step in the evaluation of a patient with hypocalcemia is to verify with repeat measurement (total serum calcium corrected for albumin or ionized calcium) that there is a true decrease in the serum calcium concentration. If there is hypoalbuminemia, since serum calcium is approximately 40% bound to albumin, then the calcium should be corrected. For each 1 g/dL reduction in the serum albumin concentration the total calcium concentration should be increased by approximately 0.8 mg/dL. If the diagnosis of hypocalcemia is in doubt, either because the patient's symptoms are atypical or the patient's serum calcium concentration is only slightly low, serum ionized calcium should be measured. It should be ascertained that the laboratory is known to measure ionized calcium reliably.

Other measurements that may be helpful include serum magnesium, creatinine, phosphate, the vitamin D metabolites calcidiol (25-hydroxyvitamin D) and calcitriol (active vitamin D hormone, 1,25-dihydroxyvitamin D), alkaline phosphatase, and amylase. In addition, urinary measurements of calcium, creatinine, and magnesium. Finally, an electrocardiogram should be performed in patients with moderate to severe hypocalcemia to evaluate for QT prolongation.

▶ Differential Diagnosis

The various disorders that result in hypocalcemia are listed in Table 6–1. The predominant hormonal regulator of serum calcium concentrations are parathyroid hormone and vitamin D. Thus, it is useful to characterize hypocalcemia broadly as whether it is associated with low or high parathyroid hormone concentration. Hypocalcemia associated with hypoparathyroidism occurs when there is destruction of the parathyroid glands (autoimmune, postsurgical, radiation), abnormal parathyroid gland development, or altered regulation of parathyroid hormone production and secretion. The most common cause of hypoparathyroidism is surgical.

Surgical hypoparathyroidism may occur following thyroid, parathyroid, or radical neck surgery for head and neck cancer. In the absence of a total parathyroidectomy, it is usually transient, with recovery in days, weeks, or months. However, it may also be permanent or intermittent. Transient hypoparathyroidism is generally due to compromise of the blood supply to or removal of one or more

Table 6–1. Major causes of hypocalcemia.

Low Parathyroid Hormone	High Parathyroid Hormone	Medications	Disorders of Magnesium
Genetic disorders • Abnormal gland development • Abnormal secretion • Activating mutation of calcium sensing receptor	**Vitamin D deficiency**	**Antiresorptive** • Calcitonin • Bisphosphonates • Denosumab	**Hypomagnesemia**
Postsurgical • Thyroidectomy • Parathyroidectomy • Neck dissection	**Parathyroid hormone resistance** • Missense mutation • Pseudohypoparathyroidism	**Calcimimetics** • Cinacalcet • Etelcalcetide	**Severe hypermagnesemia**
Autoimmune • Autoimmune polyglandular syndrome	**Renal disease**	**Calcium chelators** • EDTA • Citrate • Phosphate	
Radiation	**Sequestration of calcium from circulation** • Hyperphosphatemia • Tumor lysis syndrome • Acute pancreatitis • Osteoblastic metastasis • Acute respiratory alkalosis	**Foscarnet**	
Hungry bone syndrome • Post-parathyroidectomy		**Phenytoin**	

parathyroid glands during surgery. Transient hypoparathyroidism occurs in up to 20% of patients after surgery for thyroid cancer and permanent hypoparathyroidism occurs in 0.8–3.0% of patients after total thyroidectomy. Partial parathyroidectomy may also cause transient hypoparathyroidism, resulting from suppression of the remaining parathyroid tissue by prior hypercalcemia. Patients who have severe and long standing hyperparathyroidism may develop the hungry bone syndrome. This is associated with severe and prolonged hypocalcemia as well as hypophosphatemia. The bones recovering from their persistent resorptive state, from prolonged and severe, undergo aggressive bone mineralization extracting both calcium and phosphorus from the circulation. Hypocalcemia due to hungry bone syndrome may persist despite recovery of PTH secretion from the remaining normal glands. Thus, serum PTH concentrations may be low, normal, or even elevated.

Acquired hypoparathyroidism not related to surgery is frequently the result of an autoimmune disease. Permanent hypoparathyroidism can result from immune-mediated destruction of the parathyroid glands. Alternatively, hypoparathyroidism may result from activating antibodies to the calcium-sensing receptor that decrease PTH secretion. Autoimmune hypoparathyroidism may also occur as a feature of polyglandular autoimmune syndrome type I (Whitaker syndrome), which is a familial disorder associated with chronic mucocutaneous candidiasis and adrenal insufficiency.

Other rare causes of hypoparathyroidism include irradiation and storage or infiltrative diseases of the parathyroid glands (hemochromatosis, Wilson disease, granulomas, or metastatic cancer). Genetic defects may result in X-linked or in autosomal recessive hypoparathyroidism due to abnormal parathyroid gland development or production of abnormal parathyroid hormone peptides. Finally, there can be activating mutations of the calcium sensing receptor such that parathyroid hormone is not released at serum calcium concentrations that normally trigger parathyroid hormone release. In contrast to other causes of hypocalcemia, urinary calcium excretion is normal or high, presumably due to increased activation of the calcium sensing receptor in the kidney.

Hypocalcemia associated with hyperparathyroidism is generally the result of appropriately increased parathyroid hormone production as a result of the hypocalcemia in an attempt to mobilize calcium from bone and to increase renal calcium reabsorption and calcitriol production. Hypocalcemia results when these compensatory mechanisms are inadequate to restore the serum calcium to normal.

Vitamin D deficiency or tissue resistance to the action of vitamin D may cause hypocalcemia with a high PTH. Causes of vitamin D deficiency include poor intake or malabsorption coupled with reduced exposure to ultraviolet light, decreased 25-hydroxylation of vitamin D in the liver to form calcidiol, increased 24-hydroxylation of vitamin D to inactive metabolites, decreased 1-hydroxylation of calcidiol to calcitriol in the kidney, and decreased calcitriol action.

The most common cause of an acquired decrease in renal production of calcitriol is chronic kidney disease (CKD). In addition to the calcitriol deficiency associated with CKD, the retention of phosphate and development of hyperphosphatemia further decreases the ionized calcium concentration. Hypocalcemia is typically relatively mild and does not occur until stage 4 CKD.

Acidosis may result in decreased ionized calcium may occur in the presence of normal albumin and in the absence of total serum hypocalcemia. Changes in blood pH can alter the equilibrium constant of the calcium binding to albumin, with acidosis reducing the binding and alkalosis enhancing it. Thus, in critically ill or postsurgical patients, correcting total calcium for albumin is not necessarily accurate because of changes in pH and affinity of calcium binding. Consequently, when there is clinical suspicion of hypocalcemia and there are major shifts in blood pH, it is most prudent to directly measure the ionized calcium level in order to determine the presence of hypocalcemia.

Pseudohypoparathyroidism is a rare group of heterogeneous disorders that present in childhood and are characterized by unresponsiveness to parathyroid hormone in bone and kidney, due to an alteration in the postreceptor parathyroid hormone signaling pathway. In type 1, binding of the PTH receptor fails to elicit the generation of cyclic AMP as there is inactivation mutation of the gene for the G protein mutation. In type 2, the receptor is normal but the cellular response to cyclic AMP is deficient. Clinical presentation is hypocalcemia, hyperphosphatemia, and hyperparathyroidism.

In addition to both acute and chronic renal disease that results in hyperphosphatemia-associated hypocalcemia, hyperphosphatemia from the excessive intake of phosphate (either oral or via phosphate enemas) or excess tissue breakdown (rhabdomyolysis, tumor lysis) can cause acute hypocalcemia. Hypocalcemia results from calcium-phosphate deposition into bone as well as into extraskeletal tissue.

Malignancies that develop osteoblastic metastases, predominantly prostate or breast cancer, may develop hypocalcemia. The presumed cause is deposition of calcium in the newly formed bone around the tumor. The hypocalcemia results in secondary hyperparathyroidism.

Hypocalcemia is also a frequent finding in patients with acute pancreatitis, where it is associated with precipitation of calcium soaps in the abdominal cavity. The actual mechanism remains unclear. Although parathyroid hormone concentrations are variable, they are typically elevated in response to the hypocalcemia.

Hypocalcemia is also very common in critically ill or postsurgical patients. Sepsis and severe burns can also be associated with clinically important hypocalcemia. These patients frequently also have hypoalbuminemia, lactic acidosis, and hypomagnesemia. The cause appears to be a combination of impaired secretion of parathyroid hormone coupled with reduced calcitriol production and end-organ resistance to the action of parathyroid hormone. The probable underlying mechanisms include hypomagnesemia and actions of inflammatory cytokines on the parathyroid glands, kidneys, and bone.

Hypocalcemia can also occur during or following surgery, most often in patients who received large volumes of blood, because the citrate used as an anticoagulant chelates calcium. In these cases, total calcium is normal while ionized calcium is reduced as a result of citrate binding. In addition, it can also occur during and following major surgery in the absence of blood transfusions as the result of volume expansion and hypoalbuminemia. However, these changes, which are proportional to the severity of the surgery/anesthesia procedure, generally subside within hours.

Disorders of magnesium, both hypo- and hypermagnesemia can cause hypocalcemia. Hypomagnesemia results in a syndrome characterized by hypocalcemia, hypomagnesemia, and hypokalemia. It typically requires a rather severe degree of hypomagnesemia (serum magnesium <0.8 mEq/L) for all of the manifestations to be observed. As noted, magnesium deficiency has multiple effects, including reduction of parathyroid hormone release, inhibition of parathyroid action on bone, and possibly blocks bone resorption that may be unrelated to changes in parathyroid hormone. These abnormalities rapidly resolve if with correction of the hypomagnesemia, but calcium administration does not correct the hypocalcemia until serum magnesium levels are restored to normal. Malabsorption, chronic alcoholism, prolonged parenteral fluid administration, diuretic therapy, and the administration of aminoglycosides are common causes of hypomagnesemia. Severe hypermagnesemia, a very rare disorder, can also cause hypocalcemia by suppressing parathyroid hormone secretion. This requires a serum magnesium concentration generally above 6 mg/dL, a concentration encountered only when magnesium is given such as to pregnant women with eclampsia. Symptomatic hypocalcemia is rare in these patients, most likely due to its short duration and the antagonistic neuromuscular effects of hypermagnesemia.

There are several drugs that can cause hypocalcemia. Substances such as citrate (used to inhibit coagulation in blood or plasma), lactate, foscarnet, and sodium ethylenediaminetetraacetic acid (EDTA) chelate calcium in serum, thereby reducing serum ionized calcium concentrations but not serum total calcium concentrations. Symptomatic hypocalcemia during transfusion of citrated blood or plasma is rare as normal subjects rapidly metabolize citrate in the liver and kidney. However, a clinically important fall in serum ionized calcium concentration can occur if citrate metabolism is impaired due to hepatic or renal failure or if large quantities of citrate are given rapidly, for example during plasma exchange, leukapheresis, or massive blood transfusion. Bisphosphonates, generally used to treat osteoporosis, inhibit bone resorption and may cause significant hypocalcemia when used in high doses as well as in patients with vitamin D deficiency or impaired renal function. Denosumab, a fully human monoclonal antibody to the receptor activator of nuclear factor kappa-B ligand (RANKL), an osteoclast differentiating factor that is used to treat osteoporosis as well as hypercalcemia associated with malignancies. It inhibits osteoclast formation, decreases bone resorption, increases bone mineral density (BMD), and reduces the risk of fracture. It transiently causes hypocalcemia and hyperparathyroidism in most patients, however, in patients with conditions that predispose to hypocalcemia, such as chronic kidney disease, malabsorption syndromes, or other causes of vitamin D deficiency, or hypoparathyroidism, symptomatic hypocalcemia may occur. The calcimimetic agents, cinacalcet (oral preparation that has been available for many years), and etelcalcetide (parenteral preparation recently approved) are used to help control secondary hyperparathyroidism of renal failure cause about 8–10% decrease in serum calcium and may result in symptomatic hypocalcemia.

Hypocalcemia can also occur in patients treated with some chemotherapeutic drugs. Among them, cisplatin is probably most common. It causes hypocalcemia by causing hypomagnesemia. Combination therapy with 5-fluorouracil and leucovorin decrease production and have been shown to cause hypocalcemia.

Complications

The predominant complications associated with hypocalcemia are either neuromuscular or cardiovascular. Neuromuscular irritability may progress from tetany to seizures, laryngospasm, and bronchospasm. Whereas cardiovascular complications include prolonged QT interval which may lead to arrhythmias, as well as heart failure and hypotension. Acute hypocalcemia may also result in papilledema. Complications from chronic hypocalcemia may result in neuropsychiatric manifestations, including mental retardation in children or dementia and other psychiatric syndromes including depression and anxiety in adults. Rarer complications include Parkinsonian syndrome. Other manifestations of chronic hypocalcemia may include subcapsular cataracts, dry skin, osteopenia/osteoporosis, and abnormal dentition. Death from hypocalcemia is rare but has been reported.

Treatment

Treatment of hypocalcemia depends on the cause, the severity, the presence of symptoms, and how rapidly the hypocalcemia developed. Hypocalcemia generally results from another disease process, thus identify the cause of the hypocalcemia is important so that disease process could be appropriately managed. In patients with mild hypocalcemia, who may or may not have symptoms, need to correct the underlying cause. Parenteral calcium is generally not indicated and may proceed with oral repletion. The recommended dose of elemental calcium in otherwise healthy adults is 1–2 g/day. If appropriate, vitamin D deficiency should be corrected, depending on the severity may require 1000–5000 IU/day, or 50,000 IU/wk.

In patients with severe and symptomatic hypocalcemia, supportive treatment (ie, IV fluid replacement, oxygen, cardiac monitoring) often is required prior to directed treatment of hypocalcemia. Most appropriate treatment for patients with symptomatic hypocalcemia, either acute or chronic, is intravenous calcium, in the form of 100–200 mg of elemental calcium (preferably calcium gluconate) over 10–20 minutes. Since this bolus should last 1–2 hours, it should be followed by a slow infusion of calcium. The dose of the slow infusion should be started at 0.5–1.0 mg/kg/h as 10% calcium gluconate (90 mg of elemental calcium per 10-mL ampoule). Calcium should be monitored every 4–6 hours and the infusion can be titrated up to 2 mg/kg/h as needed to maintain serum calcium concentrations at 8–9 mg/dL. In patients with cardiac arrhythmias or patients on digoxin therapy need continuous electrocardiographic monitoring during calcium replacement because calcium potentiates digitalis toxicity. Patients with post-parathyroidectomy hungry bone disease, especially those with osteitis fibrosa cystica, can present with a dramatic picture of hypocalcemia and may require therapy for many days or even weeks. Oral calcium should be started, up to 3–4 g/day, as well as active vitamin D analogs, such as calcitriol that can be dosed from 0.25 μg daily to 2 μg twice daily.

Treatment of chronic hypocalcemia depends on the cause of the disorder. Patients with hypoparathyroidism and pseudohypoparathyroidism can be managed initially with oral calcium supplements. The hypercalcemic effects of thiazide diuretics may offer some additional benefits. This is especially important in subjects who develop hypercalciuria as they would be at increased risk of kidney stones. In patients with severe hypoparathyroidism, vitamin D treatment may be required, generally 50,000 units (1–3 times weekly) however, since PTH deficiency impairs the conversion of vitamin D to calcitriol, the most efficient treatment is the addition of 0.5–2 μg of calcitriol. In patients who have severe hypocalcemia with hypoparathyroidism, recombinant human parathyroid hormone (Natpara) is available and can be used as an adjunct to calcium and active vitamin D.

While hypocalcemia is highly prevalent in patients with CKD, symptomatic hypocalcemia is rare. The approach to hypocalcemia in renal failure is primarily to lower serum phosphorus with phosphate binders and supplement patients with oral calcium and active forms of vitamin D. In dialysis patients, the dialysate calcium concentration can be increased.

If hypomagnesemia is the cause of hypocalcemia, 2 g of magnesium sulfate should be infused as a 10% solution over 10 minutes, followed by 1 g in 100 mL of fluid per hour until serum magnesium remains normal. In patients with hypocalcemia and severe acute hyperphosphatemia from tumor lysis syndrome, correction of the hyperphosphatemia with either phosphate binders or even hemodialysis will typically ameliorate hypocalcemia.

▶ When to Refer/Admit

All patients with severe or symptomatic hypocalcemia should be admitted and treated appropriately.

KEY READINGS

Cooper MS, Gittoes NJ: Diagnosis and management of hypocalcaemia. BMJ 2008;336:1298.

Goltzman D, Cole DEC: Hypoparathyroidism. In: *Primer on the Metabolic Bone Diseases and Disorders of Bone Metabolism*, 6th ed. Favus MJ (editor). American Society of Bone and Mineral Research, Washington, DC. 2006. p. 216.

Hannan FM, Thakker RV: Investigating hypocalcaemia. BMJ 2013;346:f2213.

Steele T et al: Assessment and clinical course of hypocalcemia in critical illness. *Crit Care* 2013;17:R106.

HYPERCALCEMIA

ESSENTIALS OF DIAGNOSIS

- ▸ Hypercalcemia generally presents as a mild increase in serum calcium, although more severe forms may present as hypercalcemic emergencies.

- ▸ Symptoms associated with sustained hypercalcemia are generally nonspecific.

- ▸ Combination of neuropsychiatric complaints such as depression, anxiety, cognitive dysfunction, headache, fatigue, and even organic brain syndrome.

- ▸ Renal problems including polyuria, nocturia, polydipsia, nephrogenic diabetes insipidus, nephrolithiasis, and either acute or chronic renal failure.

- ▸ Gastrointestinal complaints such as constipation, peptic ulcer disease, or acute pancreatitis.

- ▸ Hypercalcemia is frequently identified from routine laboratory testing.

- ▸ The signs and symptoms associated with the underlying disease causing hypercalcemia may dominate the clinical picture.

▶ General Considerations

Hypercalcemia is a relatively common clinical problem. Primary hyperparathyroidism and malignancy are the most common causes, accounting for greater than 90% of cases.

It is generally not difficult to differentiate hyperparathyroidism from malignancy. Malignancy is often clinically evident by the time hypercalcemia develops. Patients with hypercalcemia of malignancy usually have higher serum calcium concentrations with relatively low parathyroid hormone concentrations and are more symptomatic from hypercalcemia than individuals with primary hyperparathyroidism. Although hypercalcemia in otherwise healthy outpatients is usually due to primary hyperparathyroidism and malignancy is more often responsible for hypercalcemia in hospitalized patients, other potential causes of hypercalcemia must be considered.

▶ Pathogenesis

Hypercalcemia can result from increased bone resorption, decreased renal excretion, or increased gastrointestinal absorption. However, bone resorption and intestinal hyperabsorption of calcium are the predominant causes of hypercalcemia. Impaired renal function may further facilitate hypercalcemia as decreased glomerular filtration rate will result in decreased renal excretion of calcium. Typically, the mechanism underlying hypercalcemia is complex and multifactorial. In primary hyperparathyroidism, all three components come into play. Increased parathyroid hormone concentrations induce bone resorption, increase renal tubular reabsorption of calcium, and stimulate the production of calcitriol causing increased gastrointestinal calcium absorption. Parathyroid hormone is the master hormone regulating overall calcium metabolism. Parathyroid hormone is a constitutively produced hormone whose production and secretion increases in response to a fall in serum ionized calcium concentration. Parathyroid hormone raises serum calcium levels by stimulating osteoclastic bone resorption and increasing renal tubular resorption of calcium. It also increases the renal production of calcitriol, which indirectly raises serum calcium levels by increasing gastrointestinal calcium absorption. Parathyroid hormone also induces renal phosphate excretion, which helps to enhance the rise in serum calcium as phosphate tends to cryoprecipitate with calcium and block the effects of parathyroid hormone on bone as well as facilitating the deactivation of calcitriol.

In primary hyperparathyroidism, there is a fundamental dysregulation of parathyroid hormone secretion. Normally, the calcium sensing receptor on the surface of parathyroid cells senses serum calcium and inhibits parathyroid hormone release and production as the serum calcium increases. There is a sigmoidal relationship between the ionized serum calcium and parathyroid hormone concentrations. In primary hyperparathyroidism this relationship is altered, such that it takes a higher serum calcium to suppress parathyroid hormone secretion and production.

Vitamin D is a steroid hormone that may be ingested with the diet but is also produced in the skin by the action of sunlight on metabolic antecedents of vitamin D. Calcitriol, the active form of vitamin D, is derived from the hydroxylation of cholecalciferol, which is first hydroxylated in the liver to calcidiol (25-hydroxyvitamin D), then in the kidneys to calcitriol (1,25-dihydroxyvitamin D). Vitamin D has a plethora of actions, including altering the growth dynamics of many cell types. Its actions to increase serum calcium are complex and include an increase in the transport of calcium across the gastrointestinal tract and an increase in calcium release from bone during PTH-induced bone resorption. In the absence of parathyroid hormone, the gastrointestinal effect in concert with adequate dietary calcium can maintain normal serum calcium levels and with pharmacologic doses of vitamin D, even induce hypercalcemia. Furthermore, parathyroid cells also have the vitamin D receptor and calcitriol also acts to inhibit parathyroid hormone release and production.

Malignancy-associated hypercalcemia may occur from many different cancers, both solid tumors and leukemias. Serum calcium values above 13 mg/dL are less commonly seen in primary hyperparathyroidism and, in the absence of another apparent cause, are more likely due to malignancy. The mechanism of increased bone resorption with malignancy depends upon the type of cancer. In patients with bone metastases, direct induction of local osteolysis by the tumor cells is common. Cytokines such as tumor necrosis factor and interleukin-1 appear to play an important role by stimulating the differentiation of osteoclast precursors into mature osteoclasts. In patients with multiple myeloma, hypercalcemia is similarly due to the release of osteoclast activating factors such as lymphotoxin, interleukin-6, hepatocyte growth factor, and receptor activator of nuclear factor kappa-B ligand (RANK ligand). A common cause of hypercalcemia in patients with nonmetastatic solid tumors is secretion of parathyroid hormone-related protein (PTHrP). Another mechanism of malignancy-induced hypercalcemia is from increased extrarenal production of calcitriol by activated mononuclear cells (particularly macrophages) in patients with lymphoma. Although rare, there are reports of nonparathyroid cancers that ectopically secret parathyroid hormone.

▶ Prevention

The key to prevention is to identify the underlying cause of hypercalcemia. Treatment should be aimed both at lowering the serum calcium concentration and, if possible, treating the underlying disease. Effective treatments reduce serum calcium by inhibiting bone resorption, increasing urinary calcium excretion, or decreasing intestinal calcium absorption.

▶ Clinical Findings

A. Signs and Symptoms

The most common outpatient cause of hypercalcemia is primary hyperparathyroidism, which is generally asymptomatic and frequently found during routine laboratory screening. Symptoms, when present, may include nephrolithiasis with renal colic, bone pain, pathologic fractures, and proximal muscle weakness. Other nonspecific symptoms such as depression, lethargy, constipation, fatigue, and vague aches and pains are frequently reported. Rarely, full-blown psychiatric disorders may be seen. In more severe hypercalcemia, usually calcium concentrations greater than 13.0 mg/dL, symptoms including polyuria, polydipsia, dehydration, anorexia, nausea, peptic ulcer disease, muscle weakness, changes in sensorium, confusion, coma, bradycardia, hypertension, acute or chronic renal failure, and acute pancreatitis may develop.

B. Laboratory Findings

The primary goal of the laboratory evaluation is to differentiate hyperparathyroidism from nonparathyroid hormone-mediated hypercalcemia, such as malignancy, vitamin D intoxication, or other causes. Thus, once hypercalcemia is confirmed, the next step is measurement of serum intact parathyroid hormone level. There appears to be a higher incidence of primary hyperparathyroidism in patients with malignancy than in the general population, thus, it is reasonable to order an intact parathyroid hormone as part of the routine evaluation for hypercalcemia even in a patient with known malignant disease. An elevated parathyroid hormone concentration in the setting of hypercalcemia is likely the result of primary hyperparathyroidism, even in the presence of an underlying malignancy that is associated with hypercalcemia.

High normal to minimally elevated parathyroid hormone concentrations in the presence of hypercalcemia is also consistent with the diagnosis of primary hyperparathyroidism, since it is inappropriately high considering the presence of hypercalcemia. However, the diagnosis of familial hypocalciuric hypercalcemia (FHH) also should be ruled out by measuring urinary calcium excretion (24-hour urinary calcium or calcium-to-creatinine ratio). In FHH, you have a low urinary calcium, less than 100 mg/24 hours.

A low or low-normal serum intact parathyroid hormone concentration (<20 pg/mL) is most consistent with nonparathyroid hormone mediated hypercalcemia. In the presence of low-serum parathyroid hormone concentrations, parathyroid hormone-related protein and vitamin D metabolites should be measured to assess for hypercalcemia of malignancy and vitamin D intoxication. If parathyroid hormone-related protein and vitamin D metabolites are also low, another source for the hypercalcemia must be considered. Additional laboratory data (including serum protein electrophoresis [SPEP] for possible multiple myeloma, thyroid-stimulating hormone) will often lead to the correct diagnosis.

Serum concentrations of the vitamin D metabolites, 25-hydroxyvitamin D (calcidiol) and 1,25-dihydroxyvitamin D (calcitriol), should be measured if there is no obvious malignancy and parathyroid hormone is not elevated. An elevated serum concentration of calcidiol is indicative of vitamin D intoxication due to the ingestion of either vitamin D or calcidiol itself. Although the serum concentration of calcidiol at which hypercalcemia typically occurs is undefined, most experts define vitamin D intoxication as a value greater than 150 ng/mL. On the other hand, increased concentrations of calcitriol may be induced by direct intake of this metabolite, extrarenal production in granulomatous diseases or lymphoma, or increased renal production that can be induced by primary hyperparathyroidism but not by parathyroid hormone-related peptide.

C. Imaging Studies

Plain skeletal radiographs may be helpful in evaluating the severity of hyperparathyroidism. Radiographs may demonstrate findings of increased bone resorption, described as subperiosteal resorption and brown tumors, which are evident on skull, clavicular, hand, and pelvic films. In patients with elevated calcitriol concentrations, chest radiograph or CT scan should be performed looking for malignancy or sarcoidosis. Patients with granulomatous disease or lymphoma generally have widespread pulmonary and extrapulmonary disease. Other imaging techniques that may be useful include either a bone or a CT-PET scan.

In patients with hyperparathyroidism, localization of the parathyroid adenoma could be ascertained with either a radionuclide sestamibi scan, ultrasound, CT, or MR scanning of the neck. Other radiologic testing to evaluate for complications would include bone mineral densitometry to evaluate for osteoporosis, and renal ultrasound or noncontrast CT scan to evaluate for kidney stones.

D. Special Tests

In patients in which multiple myeloma is suspected, a bone marrow biopsy should be performed.

▶ Differential Diagnosis

The various disorders that result in hypercalcemia are listed in Table 6–2. The most common causes of hypercalcemia are hyperparathyroidism and malignancy; thus these disorders should be initially ruled out. Primary hyperparathyroidism causes hypercalcemia by activation of osteoclasts leading to increased bone resorption. In addition, intestinal calcium absorption is elevated. Primary hyperparathyroidism is most often due to a parathyroid adenoma. Patients typically have only small elevations in serum calcium concentrations (<11.5 mg/dL), and many have mostly high-normal values with intermittent hypercalcemia. Thus, when one suspects primary hyperparathyroidism, it may be necessary to obtain a series of serum calcium and parathyroid hormone measurements to detect hypercalcemia with an inappropriately elevated parathyroid hormone concentration. In patients with advanced CKD and secondary hyperparathyroidism usually have low or normal serum calcium concentrations, but with prolonged disease, may develop hypercalcemia. The rise in plasma calcium most often occurs in patients with adynamic bone disease and markedly reduced bone turnover. In such patients, hypercalcemia is due to a marked reduction in the bone uptake of calcium after a calcium load, as with calcium containing phosphate binders. In other patients with advanced renal failure, hypercalcemia is due to progression from inappropriate parathyroid hyperplasia to autonomous overproduction of parathyroid hormone, a disorder called tertiary hyperparathyroidism.

Table 6–2. Major causes of hypercalcemia.

Parathyroid Mediated	Nonparathyroid Mediated	Medications	Miscellaneous
Primary hyperparathyroidism	Vitamin D intoxication	Vitamin D • Calcitriol	Hyperthyroidism
Inherited • MEN syndromes • Familial isolated hyperparathyroidism	Malignancy • Osteolytic bone lesions • Parathyroid related peptide • Calcitriol production	Thiazide diuretics	Milk-alkali syndrome
Familial hypocalciuric hypercalcemia	Chronic granulomatous diseases • Calcitriol production	Lithium	Immobilization
Tertiary hyperparathyroidism • Renal failure		Excessive vitamin A	

Malignancy-associated hypercalcemia occurs in patients with many different types of cancer, both solid tumors and leukemias. The mechanism of increased bone resorption with malignancy depends upon the cancer as previously discussed.

Hypervitaminosis D, defined as increased concentrations of either calcidiol or calcitriol, can cause hypercalcemia by increasing calcium absorption and bone resorption. Intestinal transport of calcium is primarily regulated by calcitriol, which is more potent than calcidiol. However, hypercalcemia does occur in patients with markedly elevated serum calcidiol, though levels generally have to be higher than 150 ng/dL, for example, those who ingest high doses of either vitamin D (which is converted to calcidiol in the liver) or calcidiol. High-serum calcitriol concentrations are usually due to ingestion of calcitriol as treatment for hypoparathyroidism or for the hypocalcemia and secondary hyperparathyroidism of renal failure. Calcitriol-induced hypercalcemia usually lasts only 1–2 days because of the relatively short biologic half-life of calcitriol. Hypercalcemia caused by vitamin D or calcidiol lasts longer. Hypercalcemia can also be caused by increased endogenous production of calcitriol with malignant lymphoma (as previously discussed), chronic granulomatous disorders.

Hypercalcemia may occur in most granulomatous disorders. Hypercalcemia is seen in about 10% of patients with sarcoidosis; hypercalciuria is about three times more frequent. Tuberculosis, fungal diseases, including histoplasmosis, coccidioidomycosis, and berylliosis, are other conditions that are associated with hypercalcemia. These abnormalities of calcium metabolism are due to production of calcitriol by activated macrophages either in pulmonary alveoli or in other sites of granulomatous inflammation. Macrophages have the enzymatic capacity to convert calcidiol to calcitriol. As this condition is associated with suppressed parathyroid hormone concentrations, hypercalciuria is a common feature of this form of hypercalcemia.

Thyrotoxicosis may cause mild hypercalcemia occurs in up to 15–20% of thyrotoxic patients, due to a thyroid hormone-mediated increase in bone resorption. It typically resolves following correction of hyperthyroidism. If the hypercalcemia persists after the restoration of euthyroidism, serum parathyroid hormone should be measured to assess for concomitant hyperparathyroidism.

The milk-alkali syndrome became rare with the advent of modern gastric ulcer therapy. However, the growing popularity of the use of calcium carbonate as an antacid or as calcium supplementation to prevent osteoporosis has led to a reappearance of this problem. Patients with this syndrome typically ingest massive quantities of calcium and absorbable alkali resulting in mild alkalosis and possibly underlying mild kidney disease. The metabolic alkalosis augments the hypercalcemia by directly stimulating calcium reabsorption in the distal tubule, thereby diminishing calcium excretion. A calcium-induced further decline in renal function, due

to renal vasoconstriction and, with chronic hypercalcemia, structural injury, can also contribute to the inability to excrete the excess calcium. They generally present with the triad of hypercalcemia, metabolic alkalosis, and renal failure that is occasionally so severe that dialysis is necessary. The serum parathyroid hormone and calcitriol levels are appropriately decreased in response to the hypercalcemia. Renal function usually returns to baseline after cessation of milk or calcium carbonate intake, but irreversible injury can occur in patients who have prolonged hypercalcemia.

Immobilization leads to an increase in bone resorption and is a rare cause of hypercalcemia. Bone mineral density tests have shown evidence of bone resorption from prolonged immobilization after a variety of diseases including spinal injury and stroke. The mechanism is unknown and hypercalcemia usually develops after 4 weeks of immobilization. Hypercalciuria may result from the combination of hypercalcemia and suppressed parathyroid hormone secretion may attenuate hypercalcemia and even maintain normocalcemia. In fact, patients can have a negative calcium balance as a result of urine calcium losses, which can last for months. If an impairment in renal function occurs, however, hypercalcemia may ensue.

Hypervitaminosis A from the prolonged ingestion of high doses or the administration of retinoic acid to patients with certain tumors, as either cis-retinoic acid or all-trans retinoic acid can cause a dose-dependent increase in bone resorption, resulting in hypercalcemia. All-trans retinoic acid inhibits cell growth in part by downregulation of interleukin-6 receptors; the subsequent rise in serum interleukin-6 concentrations may be responsible for increased bone resorption and hypercalcemia.

Familial hypocalciuric hypercalcemia is a rare autosomal dominant disorder characterized by mild hypercalcemia, hypocalciuria (suggesting a contribution from increased renal tubular calcium reabsorption), normal to moderately elevated serum magnesium concentrations, and normal to slightly increased serum parathyroid hormone concentrations. The primary defect in this disorder is a loss-of-function mutation in the calcium-sensing sensor on the parathyroid cells and in the kidneys so that higher than normal serum calcium concentrations are needed to suppress parathyroid hormone release. The diagnosis is made by demonstrating low urine calcium (<100 mg/24 hours) in the presence of normal renal function, elevated serum calcium, and parathyroid hormone. The majority of these patients is asymptomatic and require no therapy. Parathyroidectomy does not correct the condition and should not be pursued, as too aggressive surgery may result in hypocalcemia.

Other rare causes of hypercalcemia include various medications. Thiazide diuretics increases renal calcium reabsorption resulting in a mild increase in serum calcium. They are frequently used to treat idiopathic hypercalciuria in patients with calcium nephrolithiasis or osteoporosis. Patients on chronic lithium therapy often develop mild hypercalcemia, most likely due to increased secretion of parathyroid hormone due to decreasing the sensitivity of the parathyroid cells to calcium thus a higher serum calcium is required to suppress parathyroid hormone secretion. The hypercalcemia usually, but not always, subsides when the lithium is stopped. Lithium can also unmask previously unrecognized mild hyperparathyroidism. Conversely, lithium can also raise serum PTH concentrations without raising serum calcium concentrations.

▶ Complications

Complications associated with hypercalcemia could be divided into either renal, gastrointestinal, musculoskeletal, neurologic, or cardiovascular. Renal manifestations range from polyuria and polydipsia, nephrogenic diabetes insipidus, renal tubular acidosis, to nephrolithiasis with nephrocalcinosis and either acute or chronic renal failure. Gastrointestinal manifestations range from anorexia, nausea, vomiting, and constipation to peptic ulcer disease and pancreatitis. Musculoskeletal manifestations range from muscle weakness, bone pain, and osteopenia/osteoporosis. Neurologic manifestations range from fatigue and confusion to stupor and coma. Cardiovascular manifestations include shortening of the QT interval, bradycardia, and hypertension.

▶ Treatment

Summary of treatment options are shown in Table 6–3. In patients with fairly acute, symptomatic, or severe hypercalcemia (>12 mg/dL) the initial approach is hydration to dilute the extracellular calcium concentration and enhance renal calcium excretion by correcting extracellular volume contraction with isotonic saline. The volume expansion will inhibit tubular sodium and calcium reabsorption. The addition of a loop diuretic should be considered after correcting the volume depletion as it will further inhibit thick ascending limb calcium reabsorption. Next line of therapy would be to add agents to suppress osteoclastic bone resorption. They may include calcitonin, a hormone with a rapid onset of action (within 2 hours) to suppress bone resorption. Unfortunately, it is effective in only 60–70% of patients and even if effective, typically induces tachyphylaxis, thus has limited utility. Other medications to inhibit bone resorption would be the use of bisphosphonates (pamidronate, alendronate, risedronate, or zoledronic acid). They have a somewhat delayed onset of action (24–48 hours) but they are highly effective and will maximally reduce calcium levels in 3–4 days and have a persisting effect for up to 1 month. Denosumab, is a monoclonal antibody to RANK ligand and thus also inhibits bone resorption. It is also useful in metastatic disease to bone. Glucocorticoids are effective at decreasing intestinal calcium absorption as well as decreasing calcitriol production and thus is very effective in granulomatous disease. The calcimimetics, cinacalcet (oral), and etelcalcetide

Table 6–3. Treatment regimens for hypercalcemia.

Treatment	Mechanism of Action
Isotonic saline hydration	Restores intravascular volume Promotes calciuria
Loop diuretics	Promotes calciuria by inhibiting calcium reabsorption in the loop of Henle
Calcitonin	Inhibits bone resorption via inhibiting osteoclastic activity
Bisphosphonates	Inhibits bone resorption via inhibiting osteoclastic recruitment and activity
Denosumab	Inhibits osteoclastic activity via inhibition of RANK ligand
Glucocorticoids	Inhibits gastrointestinal calcium absorption Decreases extrarenal calcitriol production
Calcimimetics	Calcium sensing receptor mimetic, thus inhibits parathyroid release and production at a lower ionized calcium
Dialysis	Directly removes calcium from the circulation
Surgery	Removal of parathyroid adenoma or decreasing hypertrophied parathyroid tissue

(parenteral) are effective in decreasing parathyroid hormone release and reducing serum calcium by making parathyroid cells more sensitive to the ionized calcium concentration. In those patients with severe renal insufficiency, especially with symptomatic severe hypercalcemia (>13 mg/dL) it may be necessary to remove calcium directly from the blood by hemodialysis.

In patients with chronic hypercalcemia, the specific underlying disease or cause for the hypercalcemia should also be treated or corrected if possible. For those with primary hyperparathyroidism, therapy of choice for symptomatic disease (ie, renal stones, renal disease, neuromuscular symptoms, bone fractures) is surgical removal of a parathyroid adenoma or removal of a large fraction of parathyroid tissue if there is diffuse parathyroid hyperplasia.

▶ When to Refer/Admit

All patients with severe or symptomatic hypercalcemia should be admitted and treated appropriately.

KEY READINGS

Alexander A et al: Imaging in chronic kidney disease-metabolic bone disease. Semin Dial 2017;30:361.
Lafferty FW: Differential diagnosis of hypercalcemia. J Bone Miner Res 1991;6:S51.

Meng QH, Wagar EA: Laboratory approaches for the diagnosis and assessment of hypercalcemia. Crit Rev Clin Lab Sci 2015;52:107.

Shane E, Dinaz I: Hypercalcemia: pathogenesis, clinical manifestations, differential diagnosis, and management. In: *Primer on the Metabolic Bone Diseases and Disorders of Mineral Metabolism*, 6th ed. Favus MJ (editor). Philadelphia: Lippincott, Williams, and Wilkins. 2006;26:176.

Shinall MC Jr, Dahir KM, Broome JT: Differentiating familial hypocalciuric hypercalcemia from primary hyperparathyroidism. Endocr Pract 2013;19:697.

Žofková I: Hypercalcemia. Physiological aspects. Physiol Res 2016;65:1.

■ CHAPTER REVIEW QUESTIONS

1. A 78-year-old Caucasian man with a history of hypertension presents to the emergency department after a fall. His wife reports that he has been especially fatigued and confused over the last few days. He has lost 15 lb over the last couple of months and has been complaining of low back pain, anorexia, polyuria, and polydipsia for several weeks. History significant for a 50-pack-year history of smoking. Currently taking Lisinopril, Metoprolol, Hydrochlorothiazide, Tums 500 mg daily and Ergocalciferol 50,000 units weekly. Significant laboratory data as noted.

   Hgb 10.9 g/dL
   WBC 8900
   Plts 124,000
   Sodium 135 mEq/L
   Potassium 4.1 mEq/L
   Chloride 110 mEq/L
   CO_2 22 mEq/L
   Creatinine 1.9 mg/dL
   BUN 28 mg/dL
   Glucose 94 mg/dL
   Calcium 14.1 mg/dL
   Phosphorus 4.2 mg/dL
   Albumin 2.9 g/dL

   The most likely cause for his hypercalcemia would be
   A. Vitamin D toxicity
   B. Multiple myeloma
   C. Primary hyperparathyroidism
   D. Hydrochlorothiazide
   E. Prostate cancer

2. Which of the following conditions would not be associated with the development of hypocalcemia?
   A. Acute kidney injury
   B. Hypomagnesemia
   C. Metabolic acidosis
   D. Acute pancreatitis
   E. Rhabdomyolysis

3. A 32-year-old female patient has been having troubles getting pregnant and is undergoing a medical evaluation. She feels perfectly fine with no complaints. Other than seasonal allergies, she has no past medical history, the only medications she takes is a daily multivitamin with both 500 mg of calcium carbonate and 2000 IU units of vitamin D_3. Routine laboratories demonstrate

   Hgb 13.1 g/dL
   WBC 6400
   Plts 185,000
   Sodium 139 mEq/L
   Potassium 4.1 mEq/L
   Chloride 106 mEq/L
   CO_2 24 mEq/L
   Creatinine 0.7 mg/dL
   BUN 13 mg/dL
   Glucose 94 mg/dL
   Calcium 10.6 mg/dL
   Albumin 3.9 g/dL

   Which of the following statements would be correct?
   A. A serum parathyroid hormone concentration of 85 pg/dL would confirm the diagnosis of primary hyperparathyroidism.
   B. A serum phosphorus concentration of 2.8 mg/dL would confirm the diagnosis of primary hyperparathyroidism.
   C. A vitamin D concentration of 16 ng/mL would confirm the diagnosis of secondary hyperparathyroidism.
   D. A serum magnesium concentration should be obtained.
   E. A 24-hour urine calcium measurement should be obtained.

4. A 78-year-old Caucasian male patient was referred because of fatigue and weight loss. He has a past medical history of coronary heart disease, undergoing a coronary artery bypass graft (CABG) 1 year ago, prostate cancer treated with surgery and has been in remission for 10 years and hypertension. Current medications include Nifedipine, Metoprolol, and Hydrochlorothiazide. His initial laboratories demonstrate

Hgb 11.1 g/dL
WBC 5400
Plts 148,000
Sodium 141 mEq/L
Potassium 3.9 mEq/L
Chloride 105 mEq/L
CO_2 25 mEq/L
Creatinine 2.0 mg/dL
BUN 25 mg/dL
Glucose 99 mg/dL
Calcium 12.6 mg/dL
Phosphorus 4.0 mg/dL
Albumin 3.9 g/dL
Total protein 6.9 g/dL

Serum protein electrophoresis normal
Prostate specific antigen 1.4 ng/mL
Parathyroid hormone 15 pg/mL

Further testing should include
A. Angiotensin converting enzyme (ACE) level
B. Vitamin D level
C. Calcitriol (1,25-dihydroxycholecalciferol level)
D. A and B
E. A and C

5. Which of the following statements concerning calcium homeostasis is true?
A. The use of thiazide diuretics frequently cause hypocalcemia.
B. The hungry bone syndrome is accompanied by severe hypercalcemia.
C. Hypoalbuminemia will result in an increase of the ionized calcium.
D. In normal individuals about 15–25% of the ingested calcium is absorbed in the GI tract.
E. Hypercalcemia is an indicator of total body calcium overload.

Disorders of Phosphorus Balance: Hyperphosphatemia and Hypophosphatemia

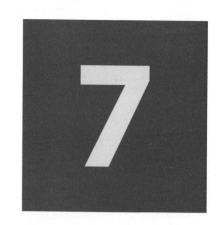

Robert F. Reilly, MD

INTRODUCTION

Approximately 80–85% of phosphorus in the body is contained in bone, 14% in cells and soft tissues, and 1% in the extracellular fluid. A very small fraction of the intracellular pool is inorganic and available for synthesis of high-energy phosphorus-containing molecules. Neutral phosphate balance is maintained with dietary intakes over a wide range from 800 to 1500 mg/day. Phosphorus homeostasis is dependent upon the interaction of three organ systems: the gastrointestinal (GI) tract, bone, and kidney. A general overview of phosphorus metabolism is shown in Figure 7–1.

Normal plasma phosphorus concentration is about 2.5–4.5 mg/dL. Approximately 85–90% of plasma phosphorus is freely filtered by the glomerulus. The small amount that is nonfilterable is due to protein binding. Normally, renal tubules reabsorb 80–97% of the filtered load so that only 3–20% of filtered phosphate appears in urine. The proximal convoluted tubule reabsorbs nearly 80% of filtered phosphate. Another 10% is reabsorbed in the distal convoluted tubule by unclear mechanisms. Phosphate reabsorption in the proximal tubule occurs by a transcellular route. Phosphate traverses the apical cell membrane via a Na^+/PO_4 cotransporter (Figure 7–2). Energy for this process is supplied by the basolateral Na^+/K^+ ATPase, which maintains intracellular Na^+ concentration low, thus providing a favorable gradient for inward Na^+ movement. There is a variety of different sodium phosphate cotransporters expressed in kidney. Types IIa and IIc mediate the majority of phosphate transport in proximal tubule, while the role of PiT-2 is still being actively investigated. Parathyroid hormone (PTH) and fibroblast growth factor (FGF)-23 decrease transporter activity via an endocytic retrieval process whereby the proteins are removed from the luminal membrane and degraded in the lysosomal compartment. This leads to an increase in phosphorus excretion.

FGF-23 is a 251 amino acid protein secreted by osteocytes and osteoblasts in response to hyperphosphatemia, high phosphorus intake, and 1,25-dihydroxyvitamin D_3. It inhibits PTH synthesis and secretion and results in removal of sodium-phosphate cotransporters from the proximal tubular luminal membrane. It decreases 1,25-dihydroxyvitamin D_3 concentration due to downregulation of 1α-hydroxylase and upregulation of 24-hydroxylase. FGF-23 can be detected in the circulation of healthy people, indicating that it may play a role in normal phosphate homeostasis.

Several lines of evidence suggest that FGF-23 is important in the feedback regulation of 1,25-dihydroxyvitamin D_3 concentration. FGF-23 knockout mice have elevated 1,25-dihydroxyvitamin D_3 levels. When injected into animals, FGF-23 reduces 1,25-dihydroxyvitamin D_3 concentration within 3 hours (a result of a combination of decreased synthesis and increased degradation). This is followed several hours later by a decrease in NaPi-IIa and phosphaturia. Injection of 1,25-dihydroxyvitamin D_3 into animals increases FGF-23 concentration. Klotho binds to several FGF23 receptors (FGFR1c, FGFR3c, and FGFR4) and acts as a cofactor that is required for FGF23 binding.

HYPERPHOSPHATEMIA

▶ Pathophysiology

A. Decreased Renal Excretion

1. Reduction in glomerular filtration rate (GFR)—The most common cause of hyperphosphatemia is advanced chronic kidney disease (CKD). About 15% of CKD stage 4 patients will have hyperphosphatemia and this increases to 50% in those with CKD 5 predialysis. In order to maintain phosphorus homeostasis as GFR declines single nephron phosphate excretion must increase. The increase in renal phosphate excretion is mediated by an early increase in FGF-23 levels, a decrease in 1,25-dihydroxyvitamin D_3 concentration, and a rise in PTH levels that lead to decreased expression of sodium phosphate cotransporters in the lumen

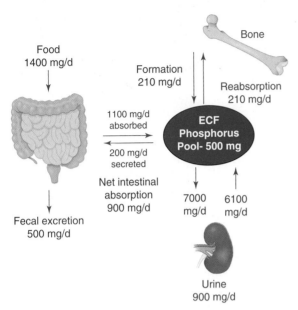

▲ Figure 7–1. Total body phosphorus homeostasis and phosphorus metabolism for a normal human in neutral phosphorus balance.

of the proximal tubule. With further declines in GFR, FGF-23 resistance develops likely due to reduced expression of Klotho, the coreceptor for FGF-23. Once renal phosphate reabsorption is maximally inhibited, phosphate concentration must rise until a new steady state is reached where intake matches excretion, albeit at the expense of hyperphosphatemia.

2. Increased proximal tubular phosphate reabsorption— Further insights into the mechanism of action of FGF-23 were provided by the study of the rare autosomal recessive disorder tumoral calcinosis. Reduced levels or effect of FGF-23 characterizes tumoral calcinosis. The full length

FGF-23 molecule is the active form, and when cleaved into amino- and carboxy-terminal fragments is inactive. Tumoral calcinosis is associated with hyperphosphatemia and soft tissue calcium deposition caused by mutations in three genes. First mutation is an inactivating mutation in GALNT3, encoding a glycosyltransferase involved in O-linked glycosylation. Lack of glycosylation increases cleavage of full length FGF-23. The second mutation was in the FGF-23 gene and involves a serine residue thought to be involved in FGF-23 glycosylation by GALNT3. This mutation increases cleavage of full length FGF-23. The third mutation was described in the Klotho gene. Klotho binds to several FGF-23 receptors and acts as a cofactor that is required for FGF-23 binding (Figure 7–3).

Other causes of hyperphosphatemia related to increased renal reabsorption of phosphate include: hypoparathyroidism-reduced PTH levels; and acromegaly-increased levels of insulin-like growth factor 1 stimulate phosphate transport.

Hypoparathyroidism can be the result of a variety of inherited or acquired disorders that result from decreased PTH synthesis or release, or resistance to PTH action. The most common cause of idiopathic primary hypoparathyroidism is polyglandular autoimmune syndrome type I. In addition to hypoparathyroidism these patients also develop mucocutaneous candidiasis and primary adrenal insufficiency. These clinical findings tend to present in a characteristic order, mucocutaneous candidiasis in early childhood, followed a few years later by hypoparathyroidism, adrenal insufficiency usually develops last in adolescence. The disease is a result of mutations in the AIRE gene (autoimmune regulator gene). Genetic disorders can cause PTH end-organ resistance (pseudohypoparathyroidism). In type I, the mutation is in the G_s-α_1 protein of the adenylate cyclase complex, although PTH binds to its receptor it cannot activate adenylate cyclase. The mutation in type II pseudohypoparathyroidism has yet to be identified. In these patients, there is a resistance to the intracellular effects of cyclic adenosine monophosphate (cAMP).

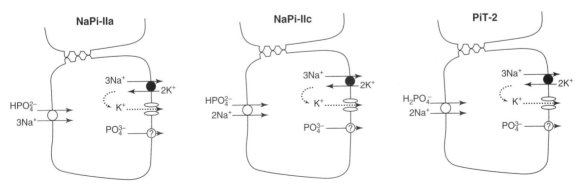

▲ Figure 7–2. Proximal tubule Na/P_i cotransport.

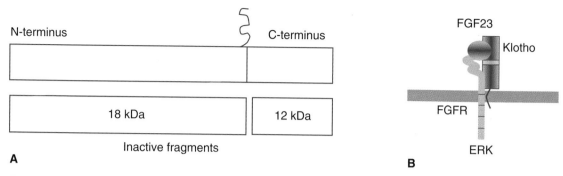

▲ **Figure 7–3.** Familial tumoral calcinosis (FTC) and FGF-23. **A.** Only the full length FGF-23 fragment is active and mutations can reduce the activity or effect of FGF-23. Three mutations result in FTC: GALNT3—a defect in O-linked glycosylation increases cleavage by SPC, FGF-23 mutations—increase cleavage. **B.** The third mutation is in Klotho a cofactor required for FGF receptor activation by FGF-23.

B. Acute Phosphorus Addition to the ECF

1. Endogenous—Phosphorus can be released from cells as a result of tumor lysis syndrome, rhabdomyolysis, or hemolysis. Tumor lysis syndrome is often accompanied by other laboratory abnormalities including hypocalcemia, hyperkalemia, hyperuricemia, and acute kidney injury.

2. Exogenous—Exogenous phosphorus loads include: phosphorus-containing laxatives and enemas, solvent-detergent-treated fresh-frozen plasma, and high-dose liposomal amphotericin. Of these laxatives and enemas are most common. They contain large amounts of phosphorus. A 90-mL bottle contains 16.2 g of dibasic phosphate and 43.2 g of monobasic phosphate. Case series of acute kidney injury due to calcium phosphate precipitation in the distal nephron have been reported with their use, as well as case reports of severe hyperphosphatemia and even death (serum phosphorus concentration: 17.8 mg/dL). Hyperphosphatemia as a result of these agents may be more common than previously recognized. In one study, as many as 37% of patients with a creatinine clearance more than 70 mL/min had serum phosphorus concentrations above 8.0 mg/dL. Those on diuretics, more than 55 years of age and with impaired gastrointestinal motility may be at particularly high risk. These agents should be avoided in patients with CKD and a polyethylene glycol based solution used.

C. Pseudohyperphosphatemia

A variety of conditions can spuriously elevate the serum phosphorus concentration including paraproteinemias, hyperbilirubinemia, hyperlipidemia, and hemolysis. With paraproteinemia the assay may need to be run with sulfosalicylic acid deproteinized serum.

▶ **Clinical Findings**

Clinical findings are largely the result of hypocalcemia. The point at which symptoms occur depends not just on the degree of hypocalcemia but also on the rate of decline of serum calcium concentration, as well as pH and whether or not hypomagnesemia and hypokalemia are also present. Symptoms that patients present with are the result of increased neuromuscular activation and include circumoral paresthesias, carpopedal spasm, seizures, and mental status changes. On physical exam bradycardia, hypotension, and laryngospasm may be present. One can also test for Trousseau and Chvostek signs. Although there are case reports of congestive heart failure with very low serum calcium concentrations that reverse with correction, this is very rare.

It is commonly thought that when the calcium-phosphorus product exceeds 72 mg^2/dL^2 vascular soft tissue calcification occurs. The original studies upon which this assumption is based are difficult to locate and this is clearly an oversimplification of the soft tissue and vascular calcification process. In the short term an acute phosphorus load does not cause hypocalcemia from calcium-phosphorus precipitation but is a result of decreased calcium flux from bone to the extracellular fluid. In patients with CKD and end-stage renal disease (ESRD) vascular calcification is common and associated with increased all cause and cardiovascular mortality. The vascular calcification process is a balance between factors that inhibit calcification and those that promote calcification (Figure 7–4). Elevations in serum phosphorus concentration are associated with a biomineralization process in which vascular smooth muscle cells undergo transdifferentiation into bone forming cells with upregulation of Runx2, osteopontin, and alkaline phosphatase. They produce a collagen matrix and form calcium and phosphorus-rich matrix vesicles.

▶ **Treatment**

The clinician most commonly treats hyperphosphatemia in the setting of CKD and ESRD. Current Kidney Disease: Improving Global Outcomes (KDIGO) and Kidney Disease

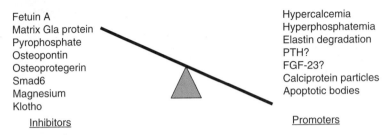

Inhibitors   Promoters

Fetuin A   Hypercalcemia
Matrix Gla protein   Hyperphosphatemia
Pyrophosphate   Elastin degradation
Osteopontin   PTH?
Osteoprotegerin   FGF-23?
Smad6   Calciprotein particles
Magnesium   Apoptotic bodies
Klotho

▲ **Figure 7–4.** Pathophysiology of vascular calcification.

Outcomes Quality Initiative (KDOQI) recommendations are shown in Table 7–1.

Phosphorus concentration in dialysis patients is difficult to control for multiple reasons and there is little margin for error. Reasons for this include hemodialysis is not very efficient at removing phosphorus; dietary phosphorus restriction is challenging; and the lack of an ideal phosphorus binder. The majority of phosphorus removal with hemodialysis occurs in the first 2 hours and is related to the predialysis phosphorus concentration. Since phosphorus is released slowly from intracellular compartments one can only increase phosphorus removal either by increasing the frequency (daily) or duration (nocturnal) of the sessions.

It is difficult to restrict dietary phosphorus without also restricting dietary protein. If we prescribe the recommended 1.2 g of protein per kilogram recommended, dietary phosphorus intake will be high, since about 70% of dietary phosphorus intake is from protein sources. The protein source is important, since phosphorus present in plants is in the form of phytates, which is much less bioavailable than phosphorus derived from meats. The target phosphorus to protein ratio should be about 10. Egg whites have one of the lowest phosphorus-to-protein ratios: 1.4, while dairy products, which commonly have ratios greater than 30, have to be virtually excluded from the diet. Estimates of phosphorus content uniformly underestimate the amount of phosphorus in the diet. This is likely the result of a common practice in the food industry to add phosphorus to foods in order to improve the shelf life, appearance, and taste. In one study, 44% of grocery products contained added phosphorus. More than half of prepared frozen foods, packaged meats, and baked goods contain added phosphorus. Medications are also another unrecognized source of dietary phosphorus, for example, a 40-mg paroxetine tablet, manufactured by GlaxoSmithKline, contains 111.5 mg of phosphorus.

There are no randomized controlled trials of patients with CKD in which treatment of hyperphosphatemia with a specific intervention is compared to placebo, nor will one likely ever be conducted. As a result, we must draw conclusions regarding potential benefits of therapy from observational studies. Perhaps, the most intriguing is the COSMOS (Current Management of Secondary Hyperparathyroidism in a Multicenter Observational Trial) trial. This was a 3-year prospective cohort study involving 6797 hemodialysis patients from 20 European countries. It examined changes in mortality associated with changes in strata of serum phosphorus, calcium, and PTH concentrations. Moving from a baseline serum phosphorus concentration of greater than 5.2 mg/dL to a lower phosphorus level was associated with decreased mortality. Patients prescribed phosphate binders had a 29% lower mortality regardless of the type of binder prescribed.

More than 90% of hemodialysis patients take phosphorus binders. The selection depends on the CKD stage, level of serum calcium, other therapies and side effects. Many advocate avoiding calcium-containing binders in those with persistent or recurrent hypercalcemia, arterial calcification, low PTH levels, or adynamic bone disease. Some recommend limiting elemental calcium intake to 1500–2000 mg/day. The ideal phosphorus binder would be effective, inexpensive, have minimal systemic absorption, a low pill burden, and few GI side effects. No currently available binder meets all of these criteria. A comparison of commonly prescribed binders is shown in Table 7–2. Aluminum-containing binders are rarely prescribed due to concerns regarding dementia, osteomalacia, and anemia. Whether noncalcium-containing binders are associated with lower mortality remains unclear.

Another consequence of hyperphosphatemia is parathyroid hyperplasia, secondary hyperparathyroidism, and renal osteodystrophy. Treatment of secondary hyperparathyroidism should be based on serum phosphorus and calcium levels. In the setting of hyperphosphatemia, cinacalcet is often employed. Cinacalcet increases sensitivity of the PTH receptor to calcium and decreases PTH synthesis and secretion.

Table 7–1. Treatment of hyperphosphatemia—clinical practice guidelines.

	KDOQI	KDIGO
Serum phosphorus	CKD 3 and 4: 2.7–4.6 mg/dL CKD 5: 3.5–5.5 mg/dL	CKD 3–5 normal range CKD 5D: lower toward the normal range

Table 7–2. Commonly prescribed phosphate binders.

	Aluminum Hydroxide	Calcium Acetate 667 mg	Calcium Carbonate 1 g	Sevelamer Carbonate 800 mg	Lanthanum Carbonate 750 mg	Sucroferric Oxyhydroxide 500 mg
Elemental calcium	None	169 mg	400 mg	None	None	None
Phosphorus bound	22.3 mg/ 5 mL	33 mg/tab	44 mg/tab	26 mg/tab	86 mg/tab	NA
Pros	Effective, low cost	Effective, low cost	Effective, low cost	Effective, calcium free, decreases low-density lipoprotein (LDL)	Effective, calcium free	Calcium free, potential to increase transferrin, iron and hemoglobin
Cons	Osteomala-cia, anemia, central nervous system (CNS) side effects, limit use to 4 wk	Hypercalcemia vas-cular calcification, ADB disease	Hypercalcemia vascular calcifica-tion, ADB disease	Swallowing disorders, interferes with vitamin D and K absorption	GI side effects, about 6 y experience	? Iron accumulation long term, short track record
Pill burden	Liquid	High	High	High	Low	Low
Cost per pill	–	$0.18	$0.02	$1.02	$1.32	$6.46

It lowers PTH levels even in those with severe secondary hyperparathyroidism. In one study, cinacalcet lowered PTH by 47% and serum phosphorus concentration by 7%. In the EVOLVE trial, comparing cinacalcet to placebo, there was no effect on the primary composite endpoint of death, myocardial infarction (MI), hospitalization for unstable angina, heart failure, or a peripheral vascular event. The secondary endpoint of an adjusted intention to treat analysis did show a beneficial effect of cinacalcet. Parathyroidectomy was reduced 57%, as was the incidence of calciphylaxis. This study suffered from a high crossover rate between groups. In the placebo group 19.8% were on cinacalcet before a primary event. Patients randomized to cinacalcet were also slightly older. Age is an extremely important risk factor for almost all adverse outcomes in the dialysis population.

KEY READINGS

Block GA et al: Association of serum phosphorus and calcium x phosphate product with mortality risk in chronic hemodialysis patients: a national study. Am J Kidney Dis 1998;31:607.

Chertow GM et al: Effect of cinacalcet on cardiovascular disease in patients undergoing dialysis. N Engl J Med 2012;367:2482.

Fernandez-Martin JL et al: Improvement of mineral and bone metabolism markers is associated with better survival in haemodialysis patients: the COSMOS study. Nephrol Dial Transplant 2015;30:1542.

Kaye M et al: Hypocalcemia after an acute phosphate load is secondary to reduced calcium efflux from bone: studies in patients with minimal real function and varying parathyroid activity. J Am Soc Nephrol 1995;6:273.

Mucsi I et al: Control of serum phosphate without any phosphate binders in patients treated with nocturnal hemodialysis. Kidney Int 1998;53:1399.

Oenning LL et al: Accuracy of methods estimating calcium and phosphorus intake in daily diets. J Am Diet Assoc 1988;88:1076.

O'Neil WC: The fallacy of the calcium-phosphorus product. Kidney Int 2007;72:792.

Leon JB et al: The prevalence of phosphorus-containing food additives in top-selling foods in grocery stores. J Renal Nutr 2013;23:265.

Sherman RA et al: A dearth of data: the problem of phosphorus in prescription medications. Kidney Int 2015;87:1097.

HYPOPHOSPHATEMIA

Pathophysiology

Hypophosphatemia occurs as a result of one or more of three pathophysiologic processes: increased renal excretion, decreased net intestinal absorption, or a shift of phosphorus from the extracellular fluid (ECF) to the intracellular fluid (ICF) shown in Table 7–3. These three basic pathophysiologic processes can be separated based on an analysis of urinary phosphate excretion using fractional excretion, 24-hour urine or $TmPO_4/GFR$ (Figure 7–5). With cellular shift or decreased net intestinal absorption the kidney will appropriately reabsorb phosphate; however, when the disease process is centered in the kidney, urinary phosphate excretion is inappropriately high. If increased renal excretion is the cause then 24-hour urinary phosphate excretion will be more than or equal to 100 mg, fractional excretion of phosphate

Table 7–3. Etiologies of hypophosphatemia.

Shift from extracellular to intracellular fluid
Respiratory alkalosis
Correction of respiratory acidosis in chronic obstructive pulmonary disease (COPD) patients
Diabetic ketoacidosis
Hungry bone syndrome
Decreased GI absorption
Decreased dietary intake
Phosphate binders
Alcoholism
Sorafenib
Increased renal excretion
PTH-related
Primary hyperparathyroidism
Secondary hyperparathyroidism—vitamin D deficiency
FGF-23 or phosphatonin related
X-linked dominant hypophosphatemic rickets
Autosomal dominant hypophosphatemic rickets
Autosomal recessive hypophosphatemic rickets
Tumor-induced osteomalacia
Fibrous dysplasia of bone or McCune Albright syndrome
Other processes
Partial hepatectomy
Fanconi syndrome
Osmotic diuresis

more than or equal to 5%, or $TmPO_4/GFR$ greater than 2.1 mg/dL. Those patients with inappropriately elevated urinary phosphate excretion can be further subdivided based on examination of serum calcium concentration, urinary glucose and amino acid excretion, and levels of vitamin D, PTH, or FGF-23 as warranted by the clinical presentation, as illustrated in Figure 7–5.

A. Cellular Shift

Shift of phosphorus from the ECF to the ICF can occur in a variety of conditions. It can result from increases in insulin levels as in the treatment of diabetic ketoacidosis (DKA) and with refeeding. The first known description of the refeeding syndrome occurred during the Roman's siege of Jerusalem. The onset of hypophosphatemia depends on the degree of malnutrition, the caloric load of the refeeding, and the amount of phosphorus in the refeeding formulation. In undernourished patients it develops in 2–5 days and it can occur with enteral feeding, as well as parenteral feeding. The fall in serum phosphorus concentration may be more marked in patients with cirrhosis. Carbohydrate repletion and insulin release enhance the intracellular uptake of phosphorus, glucose, and potassium. In glycolysis, four molecules of phosphorus are utilized for each molecule of glucose that enters the cell. The combination of total body phosphorus depletion from decreased intake and the intracellular uptake of phosphorus

with refeeding can result in severe hypophosphatemia. It has been reported in patients that were nil per os (NPO) for periods as short as 48 hours.

One of the more common causes is respiratory alkalosis, which occurs as a result of stimulation of glycolysis. This can be seen in normals but is also observed in patients with chronic obstructive pulmonary disease (COPD) after intubation. An early report by Mostellar et al in 11 healthy adults aged 20–40 years showed a decline in serum phosphorus concentration to less than 1.0 mg/dL in 90 minutes with voluntary hyperventilation to a pCO_2 of 13–20 mm Hg. This was associated with a marked reduction in urinary phosphate excretion. In COPD patients after intubation, as respiratory acidosis corrects, the serum phosphorus concentration falls. This occurs with rises of pH to normal and does not require alkalemia. It is also seen in hungry bone syndrome, although hypocalcemia is more important in this setting.

B. Decreased Intestinal Absorption

Decreased oral intake as the sole cause of hypophosphatemia is uncommon. In order to develop hypophosphatemia, decreased GI intake needs to be associated with increased GI losses as with diarrhea or phosphate binder use. Lotz and Bartter were the first to show that hypophosphatemia was associated with reversible symptoms. They studied a group of normal volunteers on a low-phosphorus diet combined with phosphate binders. A decline in urinary phosphate within 5–7 days, negative phosphorus balance after 14–21 days, and severe hypophosphatemia after 75–100 days was observed. Subjects developed weakness, bone pain, malaise, and anorexia that reversed with phosphorus repletion.

Other intestinally related causes may include steatorrhea and malabsorption, although in these conditions phosphorus loss also occurs in urine due to secondary hyperparathyroidism as a result of calcitriol deficiency. The association of sorafenib, a drug commonly used in patients with advanced renal cell carcinoma, and hypophosphatemia is thought to be related to decreased intestinal absorption.

C. Increased Renal Excretion

Increased renal phosphate excretion occurs most commonly as a result of the effects of increased PTH levels from either primary hyperparathyroidism or secondary hyperparathyroidism in the presence of normal renal function, overproduction of FGF-23 or other "phosphatonins", drugs, partial hepatectomy, and Fanconi syndrome.

PTH as discussed above, after binding to its receptor in proximal tubule, activates an endocytic retrieval process resulting in removal of phosphate transporters from the luminal membrane and an increase in renal phosphate excretion. However, because of extrarenal actions of PTH, hypophosphatemia is often mild to moderate in severity (1.5–2.4 mg/dL). PTH increases phosphate and calcium

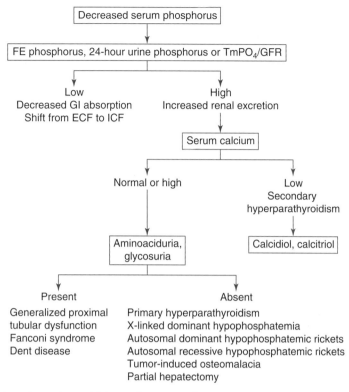

```
                    ┌─────────────────────────────────┐
                    │   Decreased serum phosphorus     │
                    └─────────────────────────────────┘
                                   │
                    ┌──────────────────────────────────────────────┐
                    │ FE phosphorus, 24-hour urine phosphorus       │
                    │ or TmPO₄/GFR                                   │
                    └──────────────────────────────────────────────┘
                        │                              │
                       Low                           High
              Decreased GI absorption        Increased renal excretion
              Shift from ECF to ICF                   │
                                              ┌────────────────┐
                                              │ Serum calcium  │
                                              └────────────────┘
                                       │                          │
                                 Normal or high                  Low
                                       │                      Secondary
                                       │                   hyperparathyroidism
                                       │                          │
                            ┌────────────────────┐     ┌──────────────────────┐
                            │   Aminoaciduria,   │     │ Calcidiol, calcitriol│
                            │     glycosuria     │     └──────────────────────┘
                            └────────────────────┘
                             │                    │
                          Present               Absent
```

Decreased serum phosphorus

FE phosphorus, 24-hour urine phosphorus or TmPO$_4$/GFR

Low — Decreased GI absorption / Shift from ECF to ICF

High — Increased renal excretion

Serum calcium

Normal or high

Low — Secondary hyperparathyroidism

Aminoaciduria, glycosuria

Calcidiol, calcitriol

Present
Generalized proximal tubular dysfunction
Fanconi syndrome
Dent disease

Absent
Primary hyperparathyroidism
X-linked dominant hypophosphatemia
Autosomal dominant hypophosphatemic rickets
Autosomal recessive hypophosphatemic rickets
Tumor-induced osteomalacia
Partial hepatectomy

▲ **Figure 7–5.** Approach to the patient with hypophosphatemia.

release from bone, as well as increases intestinal phosphorus absorption indirectly by activating 1α-hydroylase and stimulating production of 1,25-dihydroxyvitamin D$_3$, which to some degree offset the renal effects of PTH. Secondary hyperparathyroidism from vitamin D deficiency may also cause renal phosphate wasting via a similar mechanism provided renal function remains relatively preserved.

The term "phosphatonin" was introduced in 1994 to describe a circulating phosphaturic factor, yet to be isolated, in a patient with tumor-induced osteomalacia (TIO). TIO is characterized by hypophosphatemia, inappropriate renal phosphate wasting, reduced levels of 1,25 dihyroxyvitamin D$_3$, and osteomalacia. The tumor was commonly a small hemangiopericytoma that was often difficult to localize, and the syndrome resolved with tumor removal. FGF-23 production by the tumor was the most common pathophysiologic mechanism although other "phosphatonins" have been described, such as matrix extracellular phosphoglycoprotein (MEPE), secreted frizzle-related protein 4 (sFRP-4), and dentin matrix protein-1. Unlike PTH, which increases 1,25 dihydroxyvitamin D$_3$ concentration, FGF-23 reduces 1,25-dihydroxyvitamin D$_3$ levels (Figure 7–6). As a result, disease states that are associated with increased circulating

FGF-23 levels are often characterized by severe hypophosphatemia (serum phosphorus concentration ≤1.0 mg/dL) because increased renal phosphate excretion is combined with reduced intestinal phosphorus absorption.

Several rare hereditary diseases result in increased FGF-23 activity, including X-linked dominant hypophosphatemic rickets (XLH), autosomal dominant hypophosphatemic (ADHR) rickets, and autosomal recessive hypophosphatemic rickets types 1–3 (ARHR). These diseases are inherited and generally manifest in childhood. Affected patients present with rickets, in addition to severe hypophosphatemia and renal phosphate wasting. These disorders have provided insight on how FGF-23 is regulated.

ADHR results from a gain of function mutation at the subtilisin-like proprotein convertase (SPC) proteolytic cleavage site. This mutation results in an FGF-23 molecule that is more resistant to proteolytic cleavage. Since it is full-length FGF-23 that is biologically active and its concentration is increased— the characteristic phenotype of excess FGF-23 activity results.

XLH is due to a loss of function mutation in the phosphate-regulating gene with homology to endopeptidases (PHEX). PHEX is a member of the M13 family of metalloproteases and is most highly expressed in osteocytes, osteoblasts, and

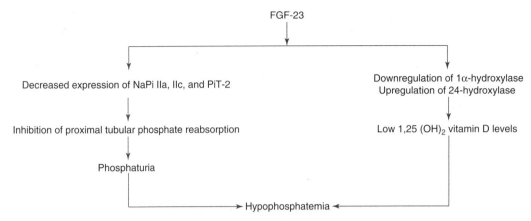

▲ **Figure 7–6.** Pathophysiology of FGF-23-induced hypophosphatemia.

odontoblasts. The interaction between PHEX and FGF-23 must be indirect given that FGF-23 is not a PHEX substrate. In experimental animals FGF-23 mRNA expression in bone is increased and there is a differentiation defect in osteocytes although the molecular mechanism is unclear. It has been postulated that the PHEX mutation alters biologic sensing of phosphate, although a phosphate sensing protein has yet to be identified.

A mutation in the dentin matrix protein-1 (DMP-1) gene results in ARHR type I. DMP-1 is a member of the Small Integrin-Binding Ligand, N-linked glycoprotein (SIBLING) family and is also highly expressed in osteocytes. Loss of function of DMP-1 also leads to a defect in osteocyte maturation and an increase in FGF-23 levels. Type 2 ARHR is due to a loss of function mutation in the ectonucleotide pyrophosphatase/phosphodiesterase-1 (ENPP1) gene. ENPP1 hydrolyzes adenosine triphosphate (ATP) to pyrophosphate, which is an inhibitor of mineralization. There is a defect in osteoblast differentiation and an increase in FGF-23 levels. It has been speculated that the ratio of pyrophosphate to inorganic phosphate may play a role in regulation of FGF-23 production.

Loss of function mutations in the FAMily with sequence similarity 20, member C (FAM20c) and the dentin matrix protein-4 gene were described in patients with ARHR type 3. FAM20c is an atypical kinase that is located in the endoplasmic reticulum/trans Golgi network. FGF-23 is a direct substrate for this kinase. FGF-23 phosphorylation in vitro by FAM20c on residue S180 prevents GALNT3-mediated glycosylation of T178. This results in an FGF23 protein that is more susceptible to proteolysis by SPC. It would logically follow that a loss of function of this protein would result in increased FGF-23 levels.

Fibrous dysplasia of bone and the McCune–Albright syndrome (MAS) result from a postzygotic gain of function mutation in the α subunit of a stimulatory G protein (GNAS). In MAS mutations occur early in development and involve multiple organs. Clinical presentation varies depending on

the tissue(s) expressing the mutation. In fibrous dysplasia of bone the mutation can result in monostotic or polyostotic fibrous dysplasia. Fibrous bone cells produce FGF-23, although the mechanism remains unclear. There is a correlation between burden of bone disease and the degree of hypophosphatemia and renal phosphate wasting.

Transient, reversible hypophosphatemia was recently described in women treated with ferric carboxymaltose for iron deficiency anemia. In a study by Wolf et al, iron deficiency was associated with a normal intact but an increased C-terminal FGF-23 level at baseline. Women were then randomly divided into two groups and repleted with either iron dextran or ferric carboxymaltose. C-terminal FGF-23 levels fell markedly in both groups while intact FGF-23 levels increased only in the iron carboxymaltose-treated group. The authors speculated that iron decreases FGF-23 transcription, as previously described in experimental animals; however, the carbohydrate portion of the iron preparation inhibited FGF-23 degradation. This interesting phenomenon suggests that FGF-23 levels are regulated by interplay between production (transcription) and susceptibility to degradation. The latter is governed by the relative activities of GALNT3 (glycosylation inhibits cleavage) and SPC cleavage (cleaved FGF-23 is not biologically active).

Renal phosphate wasting has also been observed postoperatively after partial hepatectomy. In experimental animals there is downregulation of sodium phosphate cotransporters in kidney and intestine. This is not a result of either PTH or FGF-23 but rather due to abnormal nicotinamide metabolism. Markedly increased eNampt (extracellular nicotinamide phosphoribosyltransferase) was not a phosphaturic factor but iNampt-mediated nicotinamide metabolism reduced expression of renal sodium phosphate cotransporters. This was attenuated by the Nampt specific inhibitor FK866.

Fanconi syndrome is characterized by aminoaciduria, glycosuria with a normal serum glucose concentration, proximal renal tubular acidosis (RTA), and renal phosphate wasting. It can be either inherited or acquired. Inherited causes include: Lowe syndrome, Wilson disease, cystinosis, and hereditary fructose intolerance. Acquired causes include renal transplantation, multiple myeloma, and drugs. Ifosfamide, tetracyclines, streptozosin, valproic acid, ranitidine, cidofovir, tenofovir, and adefovir have all been implicated. Over the counter medications can also cause Fanconi syndrome, the most notable being the Chinese herb Boui-ougi-tou, which has been used for the treatment of obesity. Patients with Dent disease, an X-linked inherited disorder most commonly caused by a mutation in the gene encoding the $2Cl^-/H^+$ exchanger CLCN-5, present with some but not all the features of full blown Fanconi syndrome. Hypercalciuria, nephrolithiasis, nephrocalcinosis, and progressive loss of renal function are characteristic findings, in addition to rickets, renal phosphate wasting, and low molecular weight proteinuria.

Clinical Findings

Clinical consequences of hypophosphatemia vary depending on its severity. A phosphorus concentration between 1.0 and 2.4 mg/dL is considered moderate hypophosphatemia, while a concentration less than 1.0 mg/dL is considered severe.

Moderate hypophosphatemia increases insulin resistance but this appears to be of minimal clinical relevance. Impaired cardiac contractility has not been described in patients with moderate hypophosphatemia. However, patients with moderate hypophosphatemia and acute respiratory failure did show improved diaphragmatic function after phosphate repletion. In eight intubated patients a short-term phosphorus infusion increased serum phosphorus concentration from 1.72 to 4.16 mg/dL on average and increased transdiaphragmatic pressure in all subjects. In a cross-sectional study of ventilated patients a serum phosphorus concentration of less than 2.4 mg/dL was associated with a 20% increase in weaning failure from the ventilator compared to those with a normal serum phosphorus concentration. In 321 patients on continuous dialytic therapy, 27% developed a serum phosphorus concentration less than 2.0 mg/dL, which was associated with an increased risk of prolonged respiratory failure requiring tracheostomy. Taken together, although uncontrolled, these studies argue that moderate hypophosphatemia is associated with impaired diaphragmatic contractility and impaired ventilator weaning.

Severe hypophosphatemia is clearly associated with morbidity. In the 1970s and 1980s, there were multiple case reports of difficult to wean patients from the ventilator that were extubated shortly after severe hypophosphatemia was corrected. Severe hypophosphatemia increased the length of time patients were ventilated (10.5 versus 7.1 days), and increased their hospital stay (12.1 versus 8.2 days) in one study. Similar findings were reported in patients after cardiac surgery. Severe hypophosphatemia impairs myocardial contractility and response to pressors. Correction improves myocardial contractility on average by about 20% although the response is highly variable. Hemolytic anemia has been reported in two patients with very low-serum phosphorus concentrations (0.1 and 0.2 mg/dL). Severe hypophosphatemia reduces red cell 2,3 diphosphoglycerate levels and shifts the red cell-oxygen dissociation curve to the left but the clinical relevance of this is uncertain. Evidence linking severe hypophosphatemia to rhabdomyolysis is weak in humans. A serum phosphorus concentration less than 0.5 mg/dL results in impaired white cell function (chemotaxis, phagocytosis, and bacterial killing), whether this predisposes to infection is not clear.

Treatment

Other than in the mechanically ventilated patient there is little evidence to support the treatment of moderate hypophosphatemia. If in the judgment of the clinician it is warranted, oral repletion should be considered first. A variety of available preparations are listed in Table 7–4. Oral phosphorus administration may be limited by diarrhea and caution should be used in patients with CKD.

The presence of symptoms or severe hypophosphatemia should be treated. Again caution must be utilized in those with reduced GFR. Intravenous phosphate repletion can be complicated by hypocalcemia and hyperphosphatemia. A variety of rapid repletion protocols have been reported in critically ill patients (Table 7–5). These should not be used in patients with hypocalcemia or stage 4 or 5 CKD. In general, sodium phosphate preparations should be employed except in patients who also require potassium supplementation. If the intravenous route is chosen, blood chemistries must be monitored closely including calcium, phosphorus, potassium, and magnesium. After serum phosphorus concentration increases to greater than 1.0 mg/dL an oral preparation is preferred, with the possible exception of those on mechanical ventilation.

Dipyridamole at doses of 75 mg TID-QID was shown in both short- and long-term studies to reduce renal phosphate losses and increase serum phosphorus concentration. It has been used in patients with hypophosphatemia from increased renal excretion and in renal transplant recipients. An intravenous infusion of dipyridamole in one study increased the $TmPO_4/GFR$ by 24%. Postulated mechanisms of action include a reduction of adenosine uptake in the proximal tubule resulting in reduced intracellular concentration of cyclic AMP or inhibition of P-glycoprotein.

In the severely malnourished patient, refeeding should be accomplished slowly and phosphorus and potassium concentrations monitored closely. These patients should be placed on telemetry as sudden death has been reported in patients with anorexia nervosa when refed. Caution must also be used in the setting of a recent kidney transplant. Transplant patients often have severe secondary and tertiary hyperparathyroidism. High PTH levels in the setting of a phosphate load can result in phosphate nephropathy and allograft loss.

Table 7–4. Phosphate preparations.

Preparation	Contents	Phosphorus	Sodium	Potassium
K-phos-neutral	Dibasic Na phosphate Monobasic Na phosphate Monobasic K phosphate	250 mg/tab	13 mEq/tab	1.1 mEq/tab
K-phos original	Monobasic K phosphate	114 mg/tab	–	3.7 mEq/tab
Fleets phospho-soda	Monobasic Na phosphate Dibasic Na phosphate	129 mg/mL	4.8 mEq/mL	–
Neutra-phos-K	Monobasic K phosphate Dibasic K phosphate	250 mg/cap	–	13.6 mEq/cap
Neutra-phos	Monobasic and dibasic Na and K phosphates	250 mg/cap	7.1 mEq/cap	6.8 mEq/cap
IV Na phosphate	Monobasic Na phosphate	93 mg/mL	4.0 mEq/mL	–
IV K phosphate	Monobasic K phosphate	93 mg/mL	–	4.4 mEq/mL

KEY READINGS

Lotz M et al: Evidence for a phosphate depletion syndrome in man. N Engl J Med 1968;278:409.

Mostellar ME et al: The effects of alkalosis on plasma concentration and urinary excretion of inorganic phosphate in man. J Clin Invest 1964;43:138.

Reilly RF et al: Hypophosphatemia: an evidence-based approach to its clinical consequences and management. Nat Clin Pract Nephrol 2006;2:136.

Reilly RF et al: Hereditary disorders of renal phosphate wasting. Nat Rev Nephrol 2010;6:657.

Storm TL. Severe hypophosphatemia during recovery from acute respiratory acidosis. Br Med J 1984;289:456.

White KE el al: Hypophosphatemic rickets: revealing novel control points for phosphate homeostasis. Cur Osteoporosis Rep 2014;12:252.

Wolf M et al: Effects of iron deficiency and its treatment on fibroblast growth factor 23 and phosphate homeostasis in women. J Bone Miner Res 2013;28:1793.

Table 7–5. Rapid phosphate repletion protocols in the critically ill patient.

Author	Dose	Degree of Hypophosphatemia
Rosen	15 mmol over 2 h Q6h, no >45 mmol/d total	Moderate
Vannatta	9 mmol Q12h for 48 h	Severe
Vannatta	0.32–0.48 mmol/kg Q12 h for 48 h	Severe
Kingston	0.25 mmol/kg over 4 h ([P]: 0.5 mg/dL–1.0 mg/dL) 0.50 mmol/kg over 4 h ([P]: <0.5 mg/dL)	Severe
Perreault	15 mmol over 3 h ([P]: 1.27 mg/dL–2.48 mg/dL) 30 mmol over 3 h ([P]: <1.24 mg/dL)	Moderate Severe
Charron	30 mmol over 2–4 h ([P]: 1.25 mg/dL–2.03 mg/dL) 45 mmol over 3–6 h ([P]: <1.25 mg/dL)	Moderate Severe
Taylor	10 mmol: 40–60 kg, 15 mmol: 61–80 kg, 20 mmol: 81–120 kg ([P]:1.8 mg/dL–2.2 mg/dL) 20 mmol: 40–60 kg, 30 mmol: 61–80 kg, 40 mmol: 81–120 kg ([P]: 1.0–1.7 mg/dL) 30 mmol: 40–60 kg, 40 mmol: 61–80 kg, 50 mmol: 81–120 kg ([P]: <1.0 mg/dL) Infusions given over 6 h	Mild Moderate Severe

IV, intravenous; [P], serum phosphorus concentration.

■ CHAPTER REVIEW QUESTIONS

1. Prior to rounding on your dialysis shift you are stopped by the dietician in the hall. She recently met with one of your patients and shows you their laboratory results: serum calcium concentration 10.5 mg/dL, serum phosphorus concentration 7.5 mg/dL, and PTH level 40 pg/mL. The patient is currently on calcium acetate two tablets with meals three times a day. She asks what you would like to do to better control the hyperphosphatemia. Which of the choices below is the best answer?
   A. Start paricalcitol
   B. Begin cinacalcet
   C. Shorten the patient's dialysis time
   D. Discontinue calcium acetate and start sevelamer hydrochloride
   E. Order a dose of alendronate

2. A 35-year-old woman was previously well until 5 years previously when she began to develop a series of fractures with minimal or no trauma. Laboratory evaluation revealed a serum phosphorus concentration of 0.8 mg/dL with a markedly elevated fractional excretion of phosphate and a normal serum calcium concentration. Which of the following tests would you order next?
   A. PTH
   B. PTHrP
   C. FGF-23
   D. $1,25(OH)_2$ vitamin D_3
   E. Bone biopsy

3. A 72-year-old man with ESRD secondary to diabetic nephropathy has had trouble controlling his serum phosphorus concentration. On this month's laboratory studies you inform him that his serum albumin concentration has fallen from 4.1 to 3.7 g/L. He asks you for dietary advice on how he can best raise his serum albumin concentration without worsening his phosphorus control. Which protein source listed below would best achieve this goal?
   A. Cheese
   B. Egg whites
   C. Chicken
   D. Beef
   E. Peanut butter

4. A 35-year-old weight lifter presents with the acute onset of chest pain, shortness of breath, and circumoral numbness. There are no findings on physical examination. An arterial blood gas on room air reveals—pH: 7.56, pO_2: 95 mm Hg, pCO_2: 20 mm Hg, and calculated bicarbonate concentration: 20 mEq/L. Which of the following laboratory abnormalities is the patient most likely to have?
   A. Hyperkalemia
   B. Hypercalcemia
   C. Hyponatremia
   D. Hypomagnesemia
   E. Hypophosphatemia

5. You are asked to see a 65-year-old man with the following laboratory results—serum sodium concentration: 141 mEq/L, serum chloride: 115 mEq/L, serum potassium: 2.9 mEq/L, serum bicarbonate: 18 mEq/L, BUN: 12 mg/dL, creatinine: 1.1 mg/dL, calcium: 9.5 mg/dL, phosphorus: 1.3 mg/dL, and glucose: 98 mg/dL. Urinalysis dipstick is positive for glucose. Arterial blood gases are as follows—pH: 7.35, pCO_2: 36 mm Hg, and calculated bicarbonate: 19 mEq/L. Which medication may have caused this problem?
   A. Tenofovir
   B. Lisinopril
   C. Hydrochlorothiazide
   D. Levofloxacin
   E. Ferric carboxymaltose

8

Disorders of Magnesium Balance: Hypomagnesemia and Hypermagnesemia

Sidney Kobrin, MD

DISORDERS OF MAGNESIUM BALANCE

▶ General Considerations

Magnesium is the second most abundant intracellular cation and the fourth most common cation in the human body. It plays an essential role in a variety of cellular processes, including enzyme activities involving adenosine triphosphate (ATP), energy metabolism, nucleic acid and protein synthesis, regulation of ion channels, and stabilization of membrane structures. The importance of magnesium in the body is reflected in the diverse clinical effects that accompany disorders of magnesium homeostasis. The average-size adult contains approximately 24 g (1 mol, 2000 mEq) of magnesium. It is predominantly stored in bone (55–60%) and the intracellular compartments of muscle (20%) and soft tissues (20%), and it exchanges very slowly with extracellular magnesium. Therefore, skeletal and intracellular magnesium is an ineffective buffer in the setting of acute extracellular magnesium loss.

Approximately 1% of total body magnesium is in the extracellular fluid (ECF) and is composed of three fractions: 60–65% is free, ionized, and physiologically active; 30% is protein bound; and the balance is complexed to citrate, phosphate, and other anions. In clinical practice, magnesium status is assessed by measurement of total serum magnesium.

Laboratories use different units of measurement in the United States (mg/dL and mEq/L) and other countries (mmol/L). The following equations illustrate the relationship among these units:

$$\text{mEq/L} = \text{mmol} \times \text{valence}$$

$$\text{mmol/L} = [\text{mg/dL} \times 10] \div \text{molecular weight (MW)}$$

$$\text{mEq/L} = \text{mmol/L} \times \text{valence}$$

The MW of magnesium is 24.3 and the valence is +2. Therefore, 1 mEq/L = 0.50 mmol/L = 1.2 mg/dL.

Serum magnesium concentrations normally average 1.7–2.3 mg/dL (1.4–2.1 mEq/L, 0.7–1.05 mmol/L). Given the intracellular nature of this cation, serum magnesium concentrations poorly reflect total body status.

Daily magnesium intake in the typical American diet averages 300–360 mg/day. Food sources of magnesium include green vegetables, nuts, and whole grains, as well as some meats and seafood. Of dietary magnesium 30–40% is absorbed in the gut, primarily by the small intestine, with smaller amounts being absorbed in the colon. There is some magnesium in intestinal secretions (approximately 20–40 mg/day), but under normal circumstances their contribution to overall magnesium elimination is minimal. However, these losses can become quite substantial in diarrheal states or with biliary fistulas.

The kidney is the main organ responsible for magnesium homeostasis. Approximately 70–80% (2.4 g/day) of the total serum magnesium is filtered by the kidneys. Under normal circumstances 95–97% is reabsorbed by the tubules. The plasma magnesium concentration is the most important determinant of renal magnesium excretion. Less than 5% (120 mg) is normally excreted in urine. However, hypomagnesemia results in conservation of magnesium by normal kidneys leading to a fractional excretion of less than 0.5% (<12 mg/day). Conversely, the kidneys increase excretion of magnesium to approximate the filtered load during periods of increased intake or excess magnesium administration.

In contrast to many of the other electrolytes (ie, Na^+, K^+, and Ca^{2+}), control of magnesium reabsorption does not appear to be tightly regulated by a specific hormone. Parathyroid hormone, calcitonin, vitamin D, glucagon, antidiuretic hormone, aldosterone, sex steroids, and β-adrenergic agonists can affect magnesium handling in experimental studies, but it is not known if these effects have an important role in humans.

While the proximal tubule is the major site of reabsorption of other ions, only a small percentage (15–25%) of the filterable magnesium is reabsorbed in this segment. Here, magnesium transport is passive, driven by bulk flow, and depends on sodium reabsorption. Factors that affect sodium reabsorption (ie, volume expansion) can also affect magnesium reabsorption. The majority of magnesium reabsorption (60–70%) occurs in the cortical thick ascending limb (TAL) of the loop of Henle. Here again, magnesium reabsorption is a passive, paracellular process and depends on sodium reabsorption. The driving force for the reabsorption of magnesium (and calcium) is the lumen-positive electrical potential generated by sodium chloride reabsorption via the $Na^+/K^+/2Cl^-$ cotransporter in concert with the coordinated activity of the basolateral $Na^+ - K^+$-ATPase, a chloride channel, and an apical membrane potassium channel. Disturbances of this coordinated activity at any site (such as with loop diuretics or inherited defects/Bartter syndrome) will abolish the lumen positive gradient needed to drive magnesium reabsorption and, thus, result in magnesium wasting.

The potassium channel can be secondarily inhibited by the activation of the Ca^{2+}/Mg^{2+} sensing receptor (CaSR). The CaSR binds both magnesium and calcium. This accounts for the observed magnesium wasting seen in the setting of hypercalcemia that augments activation of this receptor. If the positive transepithelial gradient is ultimately generated, the paracellular reabsorption of magnesium (and calcium) occurs passively, facilitated by a complex of two tight junction proteins, claudin-16 (also known as paracellin-1) and claudin-19. The fact that both calcium and magnesium travel in parallel through the same channel in this part of the nephron explains why disturbances resulting in hypermagnesuria will simultaneously cause hypercalciuria.

Although the distal nephron accounts for only approximately 5–10% of magnesium reabsorption, it does play an important role in determining the final urinary concentration of magnesium. On the luminal side, magnesium enters the cells passively via the magnesium channel transient receptor potential cation channel 6 (TRPM6). This process is driven by the electrochemical gradient generated by potassium flux from the cell into the lumen. The mechanism for basolateral exit of magnesium from the cell is poorly understood. Magnesuria associated with thiazide diuretics and Gitelman syndrome is likely due to downregulation of TRPM6 expression.

HYPOMAGNESEMIA

Hypomagnesemia is a common problem being found in 12% of hospitalized patients and up to 60% of critically ill intensive care unit (ICU) patients.

ESSENTIALS OF DIAGNOSIS

▸ Serum magnesium level <1.5 mg/dL.

▸ A normal serum magnesium level does not exclude the diagnosis of total body magnesium depletion.

▸ Hypomagnesemia is a relatively common disorder, occurring in 12% of hospitalized patients and in up to 60–65% of intensive care unit (ICU) patients.

▸ Evidence suggests that the presence of hypomagnesemia in the ICU patient population is associated with increased morbidity and mortality.

▸ There are conflicting data regarding the benefits of preventing hypomagnesemia, possible preventive treatment strategies, and even the level of hypomagnesemia that should prompt supplementation.

▸ **Clinical Findings**

A. Symptoms and Signs

The diversity of the cellular processes in which magnesium has been shown to take part is reflected by the diversity of symptoms attributed to magnesium deficiency (Table 8–1). Hypomagnesemia may be asymptomatic, particularly if it is mild and if it develops slowly. Severe hypomagnesemia, particularly if it develops rapidly, can be associated with signs and symptoms related to cardiovascular, neuromuscular, and central nervous system (CNS) dysfunction.

Magnesium regulates several cardiac ion channels including the calcium channel and outward potassium currents. Lowering myocardial cytosolic magnesium can

Table 8–1. Summary of main clinical manifestations of hypomagnesemia.

General	Apathy, Depression, Confusion, Anorexia
Cardiovascular	Cardiac arrhythmias (torsades de pointes, ventricular and supraventricular) Increased digitalis sensitivity Electrocardiogram (ECG) changes: widening of QRS, prolonged PR/QR intervals, T-wave changes
Neuromuscular	Chvostek and Trousseau signs Muscle fasciculations and cramps Tetany Seizures Muscle weakness Obtundation
Electrolyte abnormalities	Hypokalemia Hypocalcemia

lead to shortening of the action potential and an increased susceptibility to tachyarrhythmias, particularly of ventricular origin (including torsades de pointe, monomorphic ventricular tachycardia, and ventricular fibrillation). This is particularly true in acutely ill patients and in the setting of acute myocardial infarction, congestive heart failure, or after cardiopulmonary bypass surgery. Hypomagnesemia can magnify digitalis cardiotoxicity as both the cardiac glycoside and magnesium depletion reduce intracellular potassium by inhibition of the Na^+-K^+-ATPase. The ECG changes associated with hypomagnesemia include progressive widening of the QRS complex, prolongation of the PR interval, and abnormalities of T-wave morphology.

Hypomagnesemia augments skeletal muscle contraction and delays muscle relaxation. Therefore, affected patients can develop signs of neuromuscular hyperexcitability, including tremor, muscle twitching, muscle cramps, respiratory muscle weakness in critically ill patients, involuntary movements, Trousseau and Chvostek signs, and frank tetany. These signs may be exacerbated by a coexistent electrolyte abnormality such as hypocalcemia. Patients may also present with delirium, coma, or seizures. Severe magnesium deficiency may result in vertical nystagmus.

Electrolyte disturbances associated with symptomatic magnesium depletion include hypokalemia and hypocalcemia, both of which can be refractory to treatment unless the underlying magnesium deficit is corrected. The hypokalemia that frequently accompanies hypomagnesemia may be due to (1) a direct effect of hypomagnesemia on potassium channels in the loop of Henle (and perhaps the cortical collecting tubule) due to impairment of the Mg-dependent Na^+-K^+-ATPase leading to renal potassium wasting; and (2) the underlying disorders (ie, diarrhea, diuretics) that simultaneously cause magnesium and potassium loss. The hypocalcemia that often accompanies severe magnesium depletion (usually <1.2 mg/dL) is due to the suppressive effect of hypomagnesemia on parathyroid secretion as well as skeletal resistance to parathyroid hormone (PTH). In addition, low-plasma levels of calcitriol (1,25-dihydroxyvitamin D) have been noted in hypomagnesemic states and can contribute to the fall in calcium concentrations.

Observational studies have shown an association between hypomagnesemia and several other medical conditions, including insulin resistance, the metabolic syndrome, new-onset diabetes mellitus after solid organ transplantation, migraine headaches, asthma, hypertension, and increased mortality in dialysis patients. It remains unclear as to whether correction of hypomagnesemia results in improvement of these disorders.

Normomagnesemic magnesium depletion (total body magnesium depletion in normomagnesemic patients) should be considered in patients at risk for magnesium depletion who have clinical features consistent with magnesium depletion, such as unexplained hypocalcemia or hypokalemia.

B. Laboratory Findings

The terms hypomagnesemia and magnesium deficiency tend to be used interchangeably. However, because only a small fraction of magnesium is extracellular, the serum magnesium level is not a reliable way to assess total body magnesium depletion. The total body may be markedly depleted before the serum level drops. Hence, a normal magnesium level does not rule out the possibility of a magnesium deficit. Clues to the diagnosis of true magnesium depletion despite normal measured levels include persistent, unexplained hypocalcemia or hypokalemia, which is refractory to treatment with calcium or potassium. The magnesium retention test, which measures urinary excretion of magnesium in response to an intravenous magnesium load, has been used to assess total body magnesium status in patients suspected of having hypomagnesemia. When magnesium stores are deficient, more of the infused magnesium will be reabsorbed and, thus, less will be excreted in the urine. If less than 50% of the infused magnesium is recovered in the urine, magnesium deficiency is likely. However, this test is not in routine use as its utility is questionable and several conditions (ie, impaired renal function and renal magnesium wasting) and drugs can lead to invalid results.

If laboratory tests confirm hypomagnesemia, the next step is to distinguish between renal and extrarenal (gastrointestinal causes or redistribution of extracellular magnesium into the intracellular compartment) causes of hypomagnesemia. A review of the clinical history can often provide this information (ie, chronic diarrhea causing excessive gastrointestinal magnesium losses). If the cause is not readily apparent, quantitative assessment of urinary magnesium excretion with a 24-hour urine collection or the calculation of the fractional excretion of magnesium (FE_{Mg}) on a random urine specimen can provide insight. In the setting of magnesium depletion, conservation of magnesium by normal kidneys can decrease the usual fractional excretion of magnesium from 3% (approximately 100 mg/day) to very low levels (ie, sometimes <0.5% or 12 mg/day). Therefore, demonstrating an inappropriately high rate of renal magnesium excretion in the setting of hypomagnesemia confirms the diagnosis of renal magnesium wasting. Table 8–2 summarizes the urine tests and the criteria used for renal magnesium wasting.

▶ Etiology & Differential Diagnosis

There are multiple causes of hypomagnesemia (Table 8–3). When the cause is not obvious from the clinical history and examination, it is often helpful for the clinician to try to ascertain whether the cause is due to redistribution of extracellular magnesium into the intracellular compartment, a gastrointestinal source, urinary magnesium wasting, or "complex causes."

Table 8–2. Differentiating renal versus nonrenal causes of hypomagnesemia.

Test	Criteria for Renal Magnesium Wasting
24-hour urine collection for magnesium	>10–30 mg Mg/24 hours
Fractional excretion of magnesium[a] (FE$_{Mg}$)	>2%
$\dfrac{\text{Urine Mg} \times \text{plasma Mg}}{(0.7 \times \text{plasma Mg}) \times \text{Urine Cr}} \times 100$	

[a]Plasma magnesium concentration is multiplied by 0.7, since only 70% of the circulating magnesium is filtered because it is free (not bound to albumin).

A. Redistribution of Extracellular Magnesium into the Intracellular Compartment

Low measured serum magnesium is usually an indication of total body depletion. However, sometimes redistribution of extracellular magnesium into the intracellular compartment can lead to a decreased serum magnesium level. By itself, redistribution is an uncommon cause of significant hypomagnesemia, but it can unmask or exacerbate hypomagnesemia in patients with preexisting marginal stores. It can be encountered in a few settings. Sequestration of magnesium into the bone compartment may cause hypomagnesemia (in addition to profound hypocalcemia) in some patients with hyperparathyroidism and severe bone disease following parathyroidectomy. The sudden removal of excess PTH in this setting is believed to result in cessation of bone resorption with a continued high rate of bone formation. Insulin can also serve to drive magnesium (like potassium) into cells. Therefore, hypomagnesemia can be seen as part of the refeeding syndrome, where overzealous administration of parenteral feeds to a malnourished patient results in a surge of endogenous insulin. Similarly, exogenous administration of insulin in the treatment of diabetic ketoacidosis can have the same effect.

Hypomagnesemia can result from chelation of the magnesium ion. This can be seen after massive blood transfusions (ie, >10 U/24 hours) due to the chelating effects of citrate, particularly when citrate clearance is diminished by renal or hepatic disease. It also may contribute to the hypomagnesemia seen following surgery, where the postsurgical increase in circulating free fatty acids chelates magnesium. Hypomagnesemia may also accompany the acute hypocalcemia seen in acute pancreatitis and is presumably due to saponification of both cations in necrotic fat. Other causes of extracellular to intracellular magnesium redistribution include metabolic alkalosis and high catecholamine states.

B. Gastrointestinal Causes

If redistribution is ruled out and the urine findings are consistent with appropriate renal magnesium conservation, the gastrointestinal tract is the usual culprit. Induction of magnesium deficiency by inadequate dietary intake is not frequent because nearly all foods contain sufficient amounts of magnesium and renal conservation is so efficient. Nevertheless, magnesium deficiency of nutritional origin can be seen in a few clinical settings. It has been described in children with protein–calorie malnutrition (although usually in combination with gastrointestinal losses such as vomiting and diarrhea). It can be seen in hospitalized patients receiving only intravenous fluids or prolonged administration of magnesium-free parenteral nutrition. Therefore, addition of 4–12 mmol of magnesium per day to total parenteral nutrition (TPN) has been recommended to prevent hypomagnesemia. This is especially true in patients with marginal magnesium stores such as those with debilitating illnesses, anorexia, or with chronic alcohol use.

Although there is only a small amount of magnesium lost (approximately 40 mg/day) in intestinal secretions on a daily basis, enteric losses of magnesium can be substantial in patients with gastrointestinal fistulas, small bowel bypass surgery, or diarrheal illnesses. This is particularly true if the chronic diarrhea is associated with fat malabsorption syndromes in which free fatty acids within the intestinal lumen may combine with magnesium, forming unreabsorbable soaps. This saponification limits magnesium absorption.

Decreased intestinal absorption can also be caused by a rare inherited disorder termed *primary intestinal hypomagnesemia*. This disease typically presents in the neonatal period with hypomagnesemia and hypocalcemia that is responsive to magnesium administration. Both autosomal recessive (with linkage to chromosome 9) and X-linked recessive inheritance have been described. The autosomal recessive form is caused by mutations in the TRPM6 gene that encodes a protein which is expressed both by intestinal epithelia and by the renal distal convoluted tubule and functions as an apical magnesium entry channel. Patients with this disorder have impaired magnesium absorption as well as inappropriate renal magnesium wasting.

In recent years, case reports and large population studies have described an association between hypomagnesemia and chronic use of proton pump inhibitors (PPIs). A 2015 meta-analysis of nine observational studies with a total of 109,798 patients included in the data analysis showed that the relative risk of hypomagnesemia in patients with PPI use was 1.43 and remained significant after the sensitivity analysis only included studies with high-quality score (pooled relative risk of 1.63). The risk of hypomagnesemia is higher in patients taking concomitant diuretics. Impaired absorption of magnesium by intestinal epithelial cells due to

Table 8–3. Causes of hypomagnesemia.

High Urine Magnesium	Low Urine Magnesium
1. Polyuric states Diabetic ketoacidosis Postacute tubular necrosis (ATN) Postobstructive diuresis Postrenal transplant	1. Decreased intake or absorption Hereditary intestinal hypomagnesemia Proton pump inhibitors Malabsorption syndromes Protein–calorie malnutrition Chronic alcoholism Administration of Mg-free nutrition or fluids
2. Extracellular fluid (ECF) volume expansion Aggressive intravenous normal saline infusion Primary hyperaldosteronism	2. Gastrointestinal losses Diarrhea Fistulas Small bowel resection

3. Acquired tubular dysfunction
Postacute tubular necrosis
Postobstructive diuresis
Postrenal transplant
Chronic interstitial disease
	3. Redistribution
	Hungry bone syndrome
	Acute pancreatitis
	Refeeding syndrome
	Catecholamines
	Chelation
	    Transfusion
	    Free fatty acids after surgery
	After thyroidectomy for hyperthyroidism

4. Inherited renal Mg wasting disorders (see Table 8–4)	4. Lactation
5. Medications Diuretics (loop and chronic thiazide use) Cisplatin Aminoglycosides Amphotericin B Calcineurin inhibitors (tacrolimus, cyclosporine) Pentamidine Foscarnet Antibodies that target the epidermal growth factor receptor (cetuximab, matuzumab, panitumumab)	5. Burns
6. Alcohol (multifactorial)	
7. Hypercalcemia	

PPI-induced inhibition of TRPM6 and TRPM7 channels is the presumed mechanism for the hypomagnesemia.

Discontinuation of PPI therapy generally results in resolution of the hypomagnesemia. Some, but not all studies have suggested that H2-blockers are not associated with hypomagnesemia. If PPIs need to be continued, high-dose oral magnesium supplementation may correct the hypomagnesemia. The Federal Drug Administration has recommended periodic surveillance of serum magnesium in patients on long term PPI therapy.

C. Renal Magnesium Wasting

If redistribution and gastrointestinal causes are excluded, and renal magnesium wasting is confirmed based on laboratory findings, hypomagnesemia is due to inappropriate renal losses of magnesium.

Loop and thiazide diuretics frequently cause renal magnesium wasting. The degree of hypomagnesemia induced by the loop and thiazide diuretics is generally mild, in part because of the associated volume contraction that tends to increase proximal sodium, water, and magnesium reabsorption.

Numerous other drugs have also been shown to cause impairment in the renal tubular reabsorption of magnesium. Cisplatin, widely used as a chemotherapeutic agent for solid tumors, causes magnesium wasting in more than 50% of treated patients and the incidence increases with the cumulative dose. Renal magnesuria continues after the cessation of the drug for several months but can persist for years. The occurrence of magnesium wasting does not correlate with cisplatin-induced acute renal failure. Aminoglycosides such as gentamicin can induce magnesuria soon after the onset of therapy. The aminoglycoside-associated magnesuria is dose dependent, and is usually reversible upon withdrawal. Calcineurin inhibitors (especially Tacrolimus) are frequently associated with hypomagnesemia. When compared to cyclosporine, tacrolimus was four times more likely to cause hypomagnesemia. Foscarnet, pentamidine, amphotericin B and antibodies that target the epidermal growth factor receptor also cause renal magnesium wasting. Since the bulk of the filtered magnesium is linked to sodium chloride reabsorption, it is not surprising that factors that increase urinary excretion of sodium will also promote the urinary excretion of magnesium. Mild hypomagnesemia can occur in states of sustained ECF volume expansion as might be seen in patients receiving large amounts of intravenous normal saline. It also accounts for the hypomagnesemia that can sometimes be observed in patients with primary hyperaldosteronism. In addition, any condition that gives rise to high urine flow rates can lead to magnesium wasting. High urine flow rates can contribute to hypomagnesemia in uncontrolled hyperglycemic states with glycosuria, the recovery polyuric phase of acute tubular necrosis, postobstructive diuresis, and after renal transplantation. In the latter conditions, the residual tubule reabsorptive defects that persist from the primary renal injury likely also play an important role in inducing renal magnesium wasting.

Magnesium handling can also be affected by other electrolytes. Hypercalcemia, hypokalemia, and phosphate depletion can all lead to magnesuria by inhibiting tubular magnesium reabsorption.

Several rare hereditary renal magnesium-wasting disorders have been described and the genetic basis for many of them has recently been characterized. They represent a heterogeneous group of disorders that can usually be distinguished from each other on the basis of the clinical presentation and biochemical profile that is summarized in Table 8–4. A helpful clue to the localization of the defect is the pattern of the calcium excretion in relation to the magnesium excretion, that is, the combination of hypermagnesuria and hypocalciuria is the finding pathognomonic of disturbed DCT function. Demonstrating high urinary magnesium excretion in the absence of any other apparent cause establishes the diagnosis of these inherited disorders.

D. Complex Causes

Chronic alcoholics often have hypomagnesemia due to a combination of several factors including dietary deficiency, gastrointestinal losses (diarrhea, vomiting), and renal losses. The renal losses are a direct effect of the alcohol that can induce reversible tubular dysfunction leading to inappropriate magnesium excretion that can persist for weeks after abstinence. Alcoholics are also susceptible to acute pancreatitis, which in turn may contribute to the hypomagnesemia as a result of redistribution of magnesium as described above. Similarly, patients with insulin-dependent diabetes mellitus may have hypomagnesemia secondary to complex causes, particularly in the setting of diabetic ketoacidosis. Renal magnesium wasting accompanies the osmotic diuresis induced by hyperglycemia and rapid correction of hyperglycemia with insulin therapy drives magnesium into cells. Furthermore, magnesium deficiency may impair glucose disposal and aggravate insulin resistance.

▶ Treatment

Whenever possible the underlying cause of the hypomagnesemia should be corrected. The route and rate of magnesium repletion depend on the severity of the clinical manifestations. Since plasma magnesium is the major regulator of magnesium reabsorption in the loop of Henle, an abrupt elevation in the plasma magnesium concentration following a bolus partially removes the stimulus for magnesium reabsorption resulting in up to half of a bolus infusion being lost in the urine. In addition, uptake of magnesium by cells is slow and intracellular repletion requires sustained correction of the hypomagnesemia.

A. Severe Hypomagnesemia

If hypomagnesium is severe (<1 mg/dL) or accompanied by symptoms such as cardiac arrhythmias, neuromuscular irritability, or seizures, parenteral magnesium therapy should be administered. Magnesium sulfate 1–2 g (8–16 mEq) can be given over 15 minutes. A continuous infusion should be given after the initial bolus, that is, with $MgSO_4$ 4–8 g/24 hours (32–64 mEq). In asymptomatic patients, this dose can be repeated as necessary to maintain the plasma magnesium level greater than 1 mg/dL. Magnesium repletion should continue for at least 1–2 days after serum magnesium normalizes because the added extracellular magnesium equilibrates slowly with the intracellular compartment.

Adverse effects associated with intravenous magnesium repletion include facial flushing, loss of deep tendon reflexes (DTR), hypotension, atrioventricular block, and hypocalcemia. Since the major route of magnesium excretion is via the kidney, the above doses should be reduced by 50% and magnesium levels should be closely monitored in patients with a glomerular filtration rate (GFR) less than 30 mL/min. If the underlying cause of the hypomagnesemia persists once the acute emergency has been corrected, oral magnesium replacement may be necessary.

B. Mild Hypomagnesemia

Given that significant wasting of magnesium occurs in the setting of rapid parenteral magnesium administration,

Table 8–4. Inherited disorders of magnesium handling associated with hypomagnesemia.

Disorder	Inheritance	Defect	Serum			Urine		Other
			Mg	Ca	K	Mg	Ca	
Familial hypomagnesemia with hypercalciuria	AR	Paracellin-1, CLDN16 Occasionally due to mutations in CLDN-19	↓	↓	↓ or nl	↑	↑	Presents in early childhood; associated with polyuria, NDI, dRTA, nephrocalcinosis, recurrent nephrolithiasis, renal insufficiency Claudin-19 mutations may be associated with ocular manifestations (myopia, nystagmus, macular colobomata)
Bartter syndrome	AR	Na$^+$/K$^+$/2Cl$^-$, ROMK-1, CLC-Kb, Barttin	↓ or nl	↓	↓	↑ or nl	↑	Presents in infancy or early childhood; blood pressure normal or low; hypomagnesemia is seen in only one-third of patients due to compensatory reabsorption by other nephron segments and effects of volume depletion; Barttin defect associated with deafness
Autosomal dominant hypoparathyroidism/hypocalcemia	AD	Activating CaSR mutation	↓	↓	nl	↑	↑	
Gitelman syndrome	AR	SLC12A3 gene encoding NCCT	↓	nl	↓	↑	↓	Later age of onset than Bartter syndrome; hypomagnesemia more severe
Isolated dominant hypomagnesemia	AD	γ-Subunit of Na$^+$-K$^+$-ATPase. Genetic defect mapped to chromosome 11q23	↓	nl	nl	↑	↓	Associated with generalized convulsions
Isolated recessive hypomagnesemia	AR	Point mutation in pro-EGF resulting in ↓ EGF	↓	nl	nl	↑	Nl	↓EGF results in ↓ activation of TRPM6 leading to ↓reabsorption of magnesium
Voltage-gated potassium channel (Kv1.1) related hypomagnesemia	AD	Mutation in the gene KCNA1 that encodes the Kv1.1 channel	↓	nl	nl	↑	nl	Identified in a large Brazilian family. Kv1.1 controls TRPM6 magnesium reabsorption

AD, autosomal dominant; AR, autosomal recessive; CaSR, calcium-sensing receptor; DCT, distal convoluted tubule; dRTA, distal renal tubular acidosis; EGF, Epidermal growth factor; NCCT, sodium chloride cotransporter; NDI, nephrogenic diabetes insipidus; nl, normal.

treatment with oral magnesium salts is the more efficient way to replenish magnesium stores in patients who are asymptomatic or who require maintenance therapy due to chronic magnesium losses. The slower rise in the serum magnesium level that results from oral therapy provides a more favorable gradient for renal magnesium reabsorption. Sustained release preparations are preferable. There are several such preparations currently available, for example, Slow-Mag and Mag Delay containing magnesium chloride and Mag-Tab SR containing magnesium lactate. These orally administered magnesium preparations are given in divided doses to decrease their cathartic effect. Two to four tablets daily may be sufficient for mild asymptomatic disease whereas six to eight tablets daily may be required for severe magnesium depletion. Magnesium oxide may also be used but is more rapidly absorbed necessitating higher doses as compared to sustained release preparations. Diarrhea is a frequent adverse effect associated with magnesium oxide due to the need for higher doses. Table 8–5 summarizes some of the commonly prescribed oral magnesium preparations.

Table 8–5. Magnesium preparations.

Preparation	Elemental Mg Content/Pill
Mg chloride: Slo-Mag 535 mg	64 mg
Mg lactate: Mag Tab SR	84 mg
Mg oxide: Mag-Ox 400	242 mg
Mg gluconate: Magonate (500 mg)	27 mg

If renal magnesium wasting persists despite high dose oral magnesium replacement (as in the inherited magnesium wasting disorders, cisplatin toxicity, etc), addition of potassium-sparing diuretics such as amiloride may be beneficial. These drugs decrease magnesium excretion by increasing its reabsorption in the convoluted collecting tubule.

In some situations associated with asymptomatic mild hypomagnesemia (eg, patients who cannot take oral medications in the postoperative setting), intravenous repletion may be necessary.

> **Prevention**

Given the observed relationship between this electrolyte disorder and possible complications, it is important to recognize which patients are at increased risk of developing symptomatic hypomagnesemia and the clinical settings in which hypomagnesemia is frequently encountered. For example, patients in the ICU often have several etiologies of hypomagnesemia acting simultaneously, that is, poor nutrition, excessive gastrointestinal losses from PPI administration, diarrhea or vomiting, excessive renal losses from multiple medications such as diuretics, and antibiotics, coexisting electrolyte and acid–base disturbances that exacerbate the losses, and therapeutic interventions that can redistribute magnesium. All these factors may be superimposed on a state of chronic magnesium depletion. In addition, many of these patients have underlying cardiac disease that may increase the risk of sudden death from hypomagnesemia. As such, these patients warrant more frequent monitoring of magnesium levels and systematic repletion if the disorder is discovered.

KEY READINGS

Cheungpaisitporn W et al: Proton pump inhibitors linked to hypomagnesemia: a systematic review and meta-analysis of observational studies. Ren Fail 2015;37:1237.

Knoers NV et al: Genetic renal disorders with hypomagnesemia and hypocalciuria. J Nephrol 2003;16:293.

Margreiter R: Efficacy and safety of tacrolimus compared with ciclosporin microemulsion in renal transplantation: a randomised multicenter study. Lancet 2002;359:741.

Mouw DR et al: Clinical inquiries. What are the causes of hypomagnesemia? J Fam Pract 2005;54:174.

Noronha JL, Matuschak GM: Magnesium in critical illness: metabolism, assessment, and treatment. Intensive Care Med 2002;28:667.

Topf JM, Murray PT: Hypomagnesemia and hypermagnesemia. Rev Endocr Metab Disord 2003;4:195.

HYPERMAGNESEMIA

ESSENTIALS OF DIAGNOSIS

▸ Serum magnesium concentrations >2.5 mg/dL

▸ Occurs almost exclusively in patients with renal insufficiency and is often iatrogenic

> **General Considerations**

Hypermagnesemia is a relatively infrequent laboratory finding and symptomatic hypermagnesemia is even less common. However, severe hypermagnesemia is a serious and potentially fatal condition. The kidney has a remarkable capacity to increase magnesium excretion in states of body magnesium excess. This explains why hypermagnesemia primarily occurs in two settings: impaired renal function and excess magnesium intake at a rate that exceeds the renal excretion capacity.

In patients with chronic kidney disease, the serum magnesium levels are generally well maintained until the GFR falls less than 20 mL/min because the remaining functioning nephrons are able to significantly increase the fractional excretion of magnesium. At lower levels of GFR (<10 mL/min), mild to moderate levels of hypermagnesemia may be present (2.4–3.6 mg/dL). These patients are typically asymptomatic, but are particularly vulnerable to severe and potentially fatal, symptomatic hypermagnesemia when exposed to exogenous magnesium in the form of magnesium-containing bowel preparation regimens, antacids, or laxatives, even in the usual therapeutic doses. Similarly, patients with acute renal failure are susceptible to severe hypermagnesemia.

While much less common, there are situations in which hypermagnesemia can occur in the absence of significant renal insufficiency. Hypermagnesemia is induced deliberately in pregnant women with severe preeclampsia or eclampsia to decrease neuromuscular excitability. Such regimens, with large doses given rapidly and continuously (ie, Mg sulfate loading dose of 4–6 g, maintenance 2–3 g/h continuous infusion), can overwhelm the renal excretory capacity, achieving serum magnesium levels in the range of 6–8.4 mg/dL, or higher. Severe hypermagnesemia in the setting of normal renal function has also occasionally been described with massive oral ingestions (eg, accidental poisoning with Epsom salts in children; and in an adult who used large doses of an Epsom salt gargle for halitosis), in chronic laxative abusers, or in patients receiving large amounts of magnesium sulfate per rectum. An elevation of serum magnesium due to ingestion of magnesium-containing medications is more likely in the presence of gastrointestinal disorders that may enhance magnesium absorption. This phenomenon has been reported in patients with active ulcer disease, gastritis, inflammatory bowel disease, and intestinal obstruction. A geographically unique cause of severe hypermagnesemia has been described in Jordan due to near drowning in the Dead Sea. The magnesium concentration in the Dead Sea averages 400 mg/dL. Interestingly, since the Dead Sea also has very high levels of calcium, the resulting hypercalcemia may be somewhat protective against the cardiac toxicity associated with hypermagnesemia.

Mild hypermagnesemia, unrelated to renal insufficiency or disorders of the gastrointestinal tract, may rarely be seen in a variety of clinical settings. The causes of hypermagnesemia are listed in Table 8–6.

► Clinical Findings

A. Symptoms and Signs

Signs and symptoms of hypermagnesemia are generally not apparent until the serum magnesium concentration exceeds 4 mg/dL. Concomitant hypocalcemia may exacerbate the symptoms of hypermagnesemia at any level. Neuromuscular and cardiovascular manifestations dominate the clinical picture. High levels of magnesium decrease transmission of neuromuscular messages by inhibiting acetylcholine at the neuromuscular endplate. This ultimately leads to decreased deep tendon reflexes, muscle weakness progressing to flaccid skeletal muscle paralysis, respiratory depression, and apnea. Urinary retention and intestinal ileus due to smooth muscle dysfunction may also occur. High levels of magnesium may also cause signs and symptoms of CNS depression, including drowsiness and eventually coma. Fixed dilated pupils, induced by parasympathetic blockade, and masquerading as a central brain stem herniation syndrome, has been described. Parasympathetic blockade, vasodilation of vascular smooth muscle, and inhibition of norepinephrine release by sympathetic postganglionic nerves account for cutaneous flushing and hypotension. Hypermagnesemia also depresses the conduction system of the heart, which can manifest as lengthening of the QRS complex, PR or QT intervals, heart block, bradycardia, and eventually cardiac arrest. Hypocalcemia may be present at moderate levels of hypermagnesemia (>6 mg/dL, 5 mEq/L) due to the suppressive effects of high magnesium on PTH secretion. Hyperkalemia has been described in two hypermagnesemic patients. The mechanism is unclear, but may be related to decreased urinary excretion of potassium as a result of hypermagnesemia, inducing blockade of renal potassium channels. Hypermagnesemia may decrease the anion gap, although this appears not to occur with infusion of magnesium sulfate, as retention of the anionic sulfate moiety counterbalances the unmeasured cation. Hypermagnesemia may play a role in the development of pruritus in dialysis patients.

The magnesium levels at which the symptoms and signs of hypermagnesemia manifest are presented in Table 8–7.

B. Laboratory Findings

Elevated serum magnesium levels greater than 2.5 mg/dL are usually diagnostic. Hypocalcemia may be present at moderate levels of hypermagnesemia (>6 mg/dL, 5 mEq/L).

► Treatment

The initial assessment should focus on identifying and discontinuing the source of exogenous magnesium. In patients

Table 8–6. Causes of hypermagnesemia.

Decreased renal excretion
Acute renal failure (oliguric)
Chronic kidney disease (glomerular filtration rate [GFR] <30 mL/min)
Lithium intoxication
Increased magnesium load (usually in association with decreased GFR)
  Endogenous
   1. Diabetic ketoacidosis
   2. Severe tissue injury—burns
   3. Tumor lysis
   4. Rhabdomyolysis
  Exogenous
   Gastrointestinal: Mg-containing laxatives and antacids
   Parenteral: management of preeclampsia of pregnancy
   Dead Sea drowning
Increased renal magnesium absorption
  Familial hypocalciuric hypercalcemia (FHH)
  Hypothyroidism
  Mineralocorticoid deficiency/adrenal insufficiency
  Hyperparathyroidism

Table 8–7. Symptoms and signs of hypermagnesemia.

Magnesium Level	Signs/symptoms
4–6 mEq/L (4.8–7.2 mg/dL)	Hyporeflexia—deep tendon reflexes disappear Nausea/vomiting/flushing/lethargy/drowsiness
6–10 mEq/L (7.2–12 mg/dL)	Respiratory compromise/apnea Mental status changes/somnolence Hypotension ECG changes: prolonged PR, QRS, and QT intervals Hypocalcemia
>10 mEq/L (12 mg/dL)	Flaccid paralysis, complete heart block, coma, cardiac arrest/asystole

Table 8–8. Treatment of symptomatic hypermagnesemia.

Therapy	Dose	Rationale and Effects
Calcium Ca chloride (central line)	5 mL of 10% solution over 5–10 min	If life-threatening complications are present; antagonizes effect of Mg
Ca gluconate (peripheral line)	100–200 mg elemental Ca in 150 mL D_5W over 10 min; 10 mL of 10% solution (= 1 g)	
Intravenous fluids Normal saline	1–2 L	If volume depleted and can tolerate fluids; increases Mg excretion
Loop diuretics Furosemide Bumex	40–80 mg 0.5–2 mg	Inhibits reabsorption of Mg in ascending loop of Henle
Hemodialysis or peritoneal dialysis	Low magnesium bath; 3–4 hours of hemodialysis; more prolonged course of peritoneal dialysis	In patients with renal failure; removes magnesium

with preserved renal function and mild manifestations of magnesium toxicity, cessation of exogenous magnesium administration may be the only treatment required. In the event of symptomatic, life-threatening hypermagnesemia associated with cardiovascular, neurologic, or respiratory complications, immediate administration of intravenous calcium can serve to temporarily antagonize the effects of magnesium until more definitive therapies can be initiated and take effect (Table 8–8). In patients who are not volume overloaded and in whom some renal function is preserved, volume expansion with intravenous normal saline may enhance renal magnesium excretion. The addition of loop diuretics can further augment the magnesuria by inhibiting magnesium reabsorption in the thick ascending limb of the loop of Henle. However, this therapy warrants monitoring of the calcium levels. It can result in hypercalciuria with hypocalcemia that can intensify the clinical signs of hypermagnesemia. If the aforementioned therapies are not feasible due to renal failure, hemodialysis against a low-magnesium bath is the only way to effectively eliminate the excess body magnesium.

▶ **Prevention**

Most cases of symptomatic hypermagnesemia can be prevented by anticipation. It is important to avoid magnesium-containing medications in patients with acute or chronic kidney disease as well as those with active gastrointestinal diseases. Patients receiving high doses of parenteral magnesium should be closely monitored.

KEY READINGS

Birrer RB et al: Hypermagnesemia-induced fatality following Epsom salt gargles(1). J Emerg Med 2002;22:185.

Saris NE et al: Magnesium. An update on physiological, clinical and analytical aspects. Clin Chim Acta 2000;294:1.

Topf JM, Murray PT: Hypomagnesemia and hypermagnesemia. Rev Endocr Metab Disord 2003;4:195.

Touyz RM: Magnesium in clinical medicine. Front Biosci 2004;9:1278.

Weng YM et al: Hypermagnesemia in a constipated female. J Emerg Med 2013;44:e57.

■ CHAPTER REVIEW QUESTIONS

1. A 35-year-old man receives a course of cisplatinum for testicular cancer. One month after his last dose of cisplatinum, he presents to his primary physician complaining of palpitations and is noted to have frequent premature ventricular complexes. His laboratory tests reveal: serum potassium 3 mEq/L, serum magnesium 1 mg/dL, 24-hour urine potassium 60 mEq/day. Despite treatment with eight Slow Mag pills/day and 80 mEq of potassium chloride/day for 1 month, his serum magnesium remains low at 1.2 mg/dL and his serum potassium increases only slightly to 3.2 mEq/L.

Which one of the following medications is effective as an adjuvant therapy to correct the chronic hypomagnesemia?
A. Chlorthalidone
B. Acetazolamide
C. Amiloride
D. Furosemide
E. Omeprazole

2. What is the most likely mechanism of the hypomagnesemia-induced hypokalemia in the above patient?
A. Hypomagnesemia inhibits the NKCC2 transporter in the thick ascending limb of the loop of Henle.
B. Hypomagnesemia results in potassium to shift from the extracellular to the intracellular compartment.
C. Hypomagnesemia impairs normal function of the renal outer medullary potassium (ROMK) channels.
D. Hypomagnesemia causes secondary hyperaldosteronism leading to renal potassium secretion.
E. Hypomagnesemia impairs intestinal absorption of potassium.

3. A 64-year-old woman has been receiving weekly cetuximab infusions for the past 3 months to treat her metastatic colon cancer. She had a witnessed grand mal seizure. Imaging of her brain was normal. Her serum magnesium was low at 0.4 mg/dL. Which of following is the most likely explanation for the hypomagnesemia?

A. Competitive inhibition of epidermal growth factor receptor (EGFR)
B. Laxative abuse
C. Impaired Na^+-K^+-ATPase activity due to decreased HNF1B expression
D. Impaired paracellular Mg^{2+} transport via claudin-16
E. Transcellular shifting of magnesium from the extracellular space to the intracellular space

4. A 25-year-old patient with a history of anorexia nervosa presents to the emergency room with muscle weakness. Serum potassium is 2.3 mEq/L and the magnesium level is low at 1 mg/dL. Which of the following tests is most likely to confirm whether the hypomagnesemia is due to surreptitious laxative abuse or diuretic abuse?
A. 24-hour urine calcium
B. A spot urine test to determine the fractional excretion of sodium
C. Urine pH
D. A spot urine test to determine the fractional excretion of magnesium
E. Stool pH

5. A 36-year-old G1P0 woman is at 35 weeks' gestation and is undergoing induction of labor for preeclampsia. She has blurry vision, severe headache, and a blood pressure of 178/126 mm Hg.

Over the past 10 hours, she has been receiving oxytocin and intravenous magnesium sulfate at 2 g/h. During the past 2 hours she has become oliguric and her respiratory rate has decreased to 10 breaths/min (it was 22 breaths/min 10 hours prior). What is the likely diagnosis in this patient?
A. Severe hypokalemia
B. Anemia
C. Respiratory alkalosis
D. Magnesium toxicity
E. Hypercalcemia

Acute Kidney Injury

Muhammad Sohail Yaqub, MD

Bruce A. Molitoris, MD

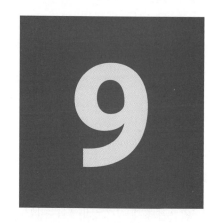

9

ESSENTIALS OF DIAGNOSIS

▸ Acute increase in blood urea nitrogen (BUN) and serum creatinine.

▸ May be associated with oliguria or normal urine output.

▸ Symptoms and signs depend on etiology and comorbidities.

▸ General Considerations

Acute kidney injury (AKI) is a life-threatening disease process occurring in approximately 5% of all hospitalized patients and up to 30% admissions to intensive care units. AKI is preferred to acute renal failure as both kidney and injury are more patient appropriate terms. Patients with AKI, regardless of their associated comorbid conditions, have greater than fivefold increased mortality rate. The hallmark for AKI is a reduction in the glomerular filtration rate (GFR), resulting in retention of nitrogenous wastes (creatinine, blood urea nitrogen [BUN], and other molecules that are not routinely measured). Early in the course of AKI patients are often asymptomatic and the condition is only diagnosed by observed elevations of BUN and serum creatinine levels or oliguria.

In 2002, the Acute Dialysis Quality Improvement Initiative (ADQI) proposed the first consensus definition scheme (RIFLE) of AKI. Since then, the Acute Kidney Injury Network (AKIN Criteria) proposed a modification of the RIFLE classification that includes the Risk, Injury, and Failure criteria with the addition of a greater than or equal to 0.3 mg/dL increase in the serum creatinine to the criteria that define risk (Table 9–1). Finally, KDIGO has modified these classification schemes.

Oliguria (urine output <400 mL/24 hours or 15 mL/h in adults) occurs commonly in AKI and may be an important indicator of renal dysfunction. However, urine output cannot be solely used as a measure of kidney function. Patients with nonoliguric AKI usually have a better prognosis primarily due to less severe injury and or a higher incidence of nephrotoxic-induced AKI in the nonoliguric group. Unfortunately, there has been little improvement in survival from AKI since the advent of hemodialysis (HD), and the mortality remains greater than 50% in many studies.

KEY READINGS

Bellomo R et al: Acute renal failure—definition, outcome measures, animal models, fluid therapy and information technology needs: the Second International Consensus Conference of the Acute Dialysis Quality Initiative (ADQI) Group. Crit Care 2004;8:R204.

KDIGO Clinical Practice Guideline for Acute Kidney Injury. Kidney Int Suppl 2012;2:1.

Mehta RL et al: Acute Kidney Injury Network: report of an initiative to improve outcomes in AKI. Crit Care 2007;11:R31.

Morgan DJ, Ho KM: A comparison of nonoliguric and oliguric severe acute kidney injury according to the risk injury failure loss end-stage (RIFLE) criteria. Nephron Clin Pract 2010;115:c59.

Schrier RW et al: Acute renal failure: definitions, diagnosis, pathogenesis, and therapy. J Clin Invest 2004;114:5.

Star RA et al: Treatment of acute renal failure. Kidney Int 1998;54:1817.

Thadhani R et al: Acute renal failure. N Engl J Med 1996;334:1448.

▸ Etiology

The etiology of AKI is best divided into prerenal, intrarenal, and postrenal causes.

A. Prerenal Azotemia

Prerenal azotemia is the single most common cause of AKI, accounting for 30–50% of all cases and is characterized by a diminished renal blood flow, primarily due to decreased

Table 9–1. KDIGO criteria for AKI.

Stage	Serum Creatinine	Urine Output
1	1.5–1.9 times baseline OR $\geq$0.3 mg/dL (26.5 μmol/L) increase	<0.5 mL/kg/h for 6–12 h
2	2.0–2.9 times baseline	<0.5 mL/kg/h for $\geq$12 h
3	3.0 times baseline OR Increase in serum Cr to $\geq$4.0 mg/dL($\geq$353.6 μmol/L) OR Initiation of renal replacement therapy OR In patients <18 y, decrease in estimated glomerular filtration rate (eGFR) to <35 mL/min/1.73 m^2	<0.3 mL/kg/h for $\geq$24 h OR Anuria for $\geq$12 h

effective arterial blood flow (Table 9–2). By definition, prerenal azotemia is a rapidly reversible process if recognized early and the underlying cause of reduced renal blood flow is corrected.

Table 9–2. Causes of prerenal azotemia.

Etiology	Mechanism	Extracellular Fluid Volume

Hemorrhage
Burns
Diuretics
Dehydration
Gastrointestinal losses
  Vomiting
  Diarrhea
  Pancreatitis
  Nasogastric suctioning
  Enteric fistula
	True intravascular volume depletion	Reduced

Congestive heart failure Cardiac tamponade Aortic stenosis Cirrhosis with ascites Nephrotic syndrome	Decreased effective circulating volume	Increased
Angiotensin-converting enzyme inhibitors Nonsteroidal anti-inflammatory drugs Renal artery stenosis Renal vein thrombosis	Impaired renal blood flow	Normal
Sepsis Vasodilatory drugs Anesthetic agents	Systemic vasodilation	Normal

Prerenal azotemia occurs when there is a reduction in the effective arterial blood flow to the kidney, either from an absolute reduction in the volume of extracellular fluid (eg, hypovolemia) or in conditions in which the effective circulating volume is reduced despite a normal total extracellular fluid volume (eg, congestive heart failure). Effective arterial blood flow is the amount of arterial blood perfusing vital organs. The determinants of effective arterial blood flow include the actual arterial volume, cardiac output, and vascular resistance. It is important to realize that the extracellular fluid (ECF) volume and or venous volume may have no relationship to effective arterial volume. Although venous and ECF volumes can be accessed by careful physical examination, effective arterial volume cannot. Therefore, in certain circumstances clinicians must rely on additional information beyond the physical examination to ascertain a measure of organ perfusion. Invasive cardiac monitoring and determination of the renal fractional excretion of Na$^+$ (FENa$^+$) are the useful estimates of the effective arterial circulatory volume.

The fractional excretion of sodium is calculated as follows:

$$FENa^+ = \frac{Urine\ sodium/Serum\ sodium}{Urine\ creatinine/Serum\ creatinine}$$

A FENa$^+$ of less than 1%, in the setting of oliguria, an increasing serum creatinine or BUN is generally indicative of prerenal azotemia as the reduced, renal blood flow results in a sodium avid state. In patients with prerenal azotemia, proximal tubule cells are undamaged and continue to function appropriately to avidly reabsorb Na$^+$ and water. Due to increased proximal reabsorption of Na$^+$ there is decreased distal delivery of Na$^+$ leading to increased renin secretion. This mediates enhanced aldosterone synthesis, resulting in increased distal Na$^+$ reabsorption. The end result is a low FENa$^+$ (<1%). Exceptions to this rule, resulting in a high FENa$^+$ with prerenal azotemia, include use of diuretics within the previous 24 hours, glycosuria, metabolic alkalosis with high urinary bicarbonate, obligatory loss of Na$^+$, and chronic kidney disease with a high baseline Na$^+$ excretion. A low FENa$^+$ is also seen in the early stages of acute glomerulonephritis, urinary obstruction, pigment nephropathy, and AKI induced by radiocontrast agents.

Low effective arterial volume states also stimulate antidiuretic hormone (ADH) release, leading to increased distal urea and water reabsorption. A low fractional excretion of urea nitrogen (<35%) can be especially useful in states of high urinary flow when prerenal azotemia occurs as in cases of high solute administration, such as in burn and trauma patients. The BUN to serum creatinine ratio, which is usually 10:1, also increases (>20:1) as filtered urea is reabsorbed and creatinine is excreted in prerenal azotemia.

The primary pharmacologic agents causing prerenal azotemia include angiotensin-converting enzyme (ACE) inhibitors, angiotensin receptor blockers (ARBs), and non-steroidal anti-inflammatory drugs (NSAIDs), including Cox-2 inhibitors. ACE inhibition results in a decreased GFR due to dilatation of the efferent arteriole and a reduction in glomerular filtration pressure. In certain patients (eg, those with bilateral renal artery stenosis) the GFR is particularly dependent on the effects of angiotensin II. If these patients take an ACE inhibitor, their GFR decreases even though renal blood flow is not reduced. NSAIDs cause prerenal azotemia by blocking the intrarenal vasodilatory effect of prostaglandins. Their use should be avoided in patients with a reduced effective arterial volume including patients with congestive heart failure, liver disease, nephrotic syndrome, and preexisting renal dysfunction.

B. Subclinical AKI

Subclinical AKI consists of tubular damage biomarker positivity without dysfunction. An early diagnosis of AKI can be made by using tubular damage biomarkers preceding filtration function. Some studies have shown evidence that there is an additional value of new biomarkers not only because they allow a diagnosis to be made earlier but also because they allow a kidney injury to be diagnosed even in the absence of subsequent dysfunction.

KEY READINGS

Blantz RC et al: Pathophysiology of pre-renal azotemia. Kidney Int 1998;53:512.
Liano F et al: Outcomes in acute renal failure. Semin Nephrol 1998;18:541.
Ronco C et al: Subclinical AKI is still AKI. Crit Care 2012;16:313.

C. Intrarenal Causes of Acute Kidney Injury

Intrinsic AKI is subdivided into four categories: tubular disease, glomerular disease, interstitial disease, and vascular disease (Table 9–3).

1. Acute tubular necrosis—Acute tubular cell injury is the most common cause of intrinsic AKI accounting for approximately 90% of all hospital acquired AKI. Acute tubular necrosis (ATN) is the common term used for this type of AKI, which is usually induced by ischemia, sepsis, or toxins. However, acute tubular dysfunction resulting from tubular cell injury is far more common than true cellular necrosis. ATN is usually reversible to some extent unless the ischemia was severe enough to cause cortical necrosis, which is associated with severe oliguria or anuria and is rare.

Tubular cell injury and death are important contributors to alterations in GFR following ischemic injury through several mechanisms. A variety of biochemical changes may play a role in cell injury in AKI. These include mitochondrial dysfunction, adenosine triphosphate (ATP) depletion,

Table 9–3. Common causes of intrinsic acute kidney injury.

Etiologies	Examples
Tubular ischemia and inflammation (moderate to severe)	Shock, sepsis, bypass surgery, trauma
Nephrotoxins	Aminoglycosides, cisplatin, NSAIDs hemepigments, NSAIDs radiocontrast agents, tacrolimus, cyclosporine
Small vessel vasculitis	Pauci immune glomerulonephritis, hemolytic uremic syndrome, thrombotic thrombocytopenic purpura
Acute glomerular nephritis	Rapidly progressive glomerulonephritis, infective endocarditis
Interstitial nephritis	Methicillin, NSAIDs, any drug
Tubular obstruction	Uric acid, methotrexate, acyclovir, sulfonamides

phospholipid degradation, elevation in cytosolic-free calcium, lysosomal changes, and the production of oxygen-free radicals. Sloughed cellular material results in cast formation in the tubular lumen causing obstruction, which leads to increased tubular pressures and decreased single nephron GFR of the obstructed tubule. Tubular fluid back leaks from the lumen to the blood via the paracellular route further decreases GFR. Finally, loss of tubule cell surface membrane polarity results in several transporters and channels, such as Na^+, K^+ ATPase, dissociating from their surface membrane location and redistributing into the cytoplasm, and the alternate surface membrane domain. This impairs vectorial sodium transport and decreases sodium reabsorption. This in turn results in high solute and water delivery to the macula densa and initiates afferent arteriole vasoconstriction and the resulting decrease in GFR.

The hallmark of ischemic cell injury is cellular ATP depletion. This occurs in multiple cell types within the ischemic kidney. Activation of endothelial cells, with release of vasoactive mediators, and an imbalance between endothelial-derived nitric oxide and endothelin may also contribute to decreased regional blood flow in the kidney. Following restoration of the effective arterial volume, activated white blood cells release cytokines, reactive oxygen species, proteases, elastases, myeloperoxidase, and other enzymes. Leukocyte-endothelial interactions, mediated by adhesion receptors, result in capillary obstruction and persistent reduced blood flow that contributes to persistent ischemia and hypoxia after the initial insult. This is especially true in the cortical-medullary region, or outer medullary stripe of the previously ischemic kidney.

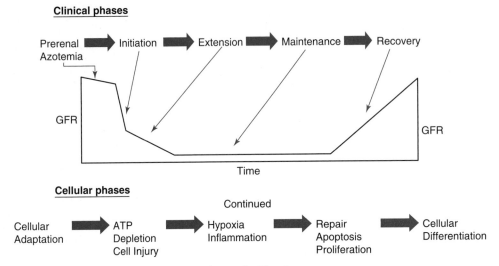

Clinical phases

Prerenal Azotemia → Initiation → Extension → Maintenance → Recovery

GFR

Time

GFR

Cellular phases

Cellular Adaptation → ATP Depletion Cell Injury → Continued Hypoxia Inflammation → Repair Apoptosis Proliferation → Cellular Differentiation

▲ **Figure 9–1.** Phases of acute kidney injury. GFR, glomerular filtration rate.

Figure 9–1 outlines the pathophysiology and clinical phases of ischemic AKI. In the initiation phase of AKI, there is ATP depletion, resulting in proximal tubule, endothelial and smooth muscle injury, and apoptosis. The extension phase of AKI occurs with persistent ischemia, vascular congestion, and ongoing hypoxia. Endothelial damage and activation result in an imbalance in vasoactive mediators and persistent vasoconstriction, particularly in the outer medulla. These mediators and endothelial damage lead to an increase permeability, which increases interstitial pressure and decreases capillary blood flow. This results in continued hypoxia during reperfusion and enhanced tubular cell injury and cell death via apoptosis in this area. The end result of these various pathophysiologic processes is further worsening of the GFR. The extension phase is followed by a prolonged maintenance phase in which BUN and creatinine continued to rise. If there is no further injury than the recovery phase begins in 1–2 weeks depending on the extent of injury. Apoptosis occurs in all phases leading to remodeling of injured tubules and facilitating their return to a normal structural and functional state. Most cells recover by cellular repair. However, some epithelial cells dedifferentiate, replicate, and migrate to fill the epithelial cell defect left along the tubule. Thereafter they spread out, become attached to the tubular membrane, and reestablish their polarized differentiated structure.

A. AKI AND SEPSIS—AKI occurs in approximately 19% of patients with moderate sepsis, 23% with severe sepsis, and 51% with septic shock when blood cultures are positive. The combination of AKI and sepsis is associated with a 70% mortality, as compared with a 45% mortality among patients with AKI alone. Thus, the combination of sepsis and AKI constitutes a particularly serious medical problem. The cytokine-mediated induction of nitric oxide synthesis that occurs in sepsis decreases total systemic vascular resistance. This arterial vasodilatation predisposes patients with sepsis to AKI, the need for mechanical ventilation, and ultimately, increased mortality. There is experimental evidence that early in sepsis-related AKI, the predominant pathogenetic factor is renal vasoconstriction with intact tubular function, as demonstrated by increased reabsorption of tubular sodium and water. Thus, intervention at this early stage may prevent progression to AKI and cell injury. Plasma concentrations of catecholamines and activation of the renin–angiotensin–aldosterone system are known to be heightened in cases of sepsis and septic shock. Another pressor hormone that has been observed to be elevated in sepsis is endothelin, a potent vasoconstrictor. Renal vasoconstriction in sepsis seems to be due, at least in part, to the ability of tumor necrosis factor to release endothelin. Endothelial damage occurs during sepsis and may be associated with microthrombi and an increased concentration of von Willebrand factor in the circulation. The vasodilatory effect of constitutive endothelial nitric oxide synthase within the kidney might be expected to lessen the renal vasoconstriction induced by norepinephrine, angiotensin II, and endothelin during sepsis. However, the results of in vitro studies showed that the increase in the plasma nitric oxide concentration, stimulated by inducible nitric oxide synthase during endotoxemia, downregulated endothelial nitric oxide synthase within the kidney. Endotoxemia is known to be associated with the generation of oxygen radicals and thus may contribute to the early vasoconstrictor phase of AKI.

Several chemokines are also expressed during endotoxemia in association with neutrophil and macrophage attachment to the endothelium. Complement pathways are activated during sepsis by bacterial products such as lipopolysaccharide, C-reactive protein, and other stimuli. Complement C5a that is generated during sepsis seems to have procoagulant properties, and blocking C5a receptor in a rodent model of sepsis has been shown to improve survival. Sepsis can also be viewed as a procoagulant state that leads to disseminated intravascular coagulation with consumptive coagulopathy, thrombosis, and ultimately, hemorrhage. Disseminated intravascular coagulation has been associated with glomerular microthrombi and AKI. Since the early vasoconstrictor phase of sepsis and AKI is potentially reversible, it should be an optimal time for intervention. However, clinical studies performed in patients up to 72 hours after admission to the intensive care unit, in which attempts were made to optimize hemodynamics and monitor the patients with a pulmonary-artery catheter, not only were negative, but showed increased mortality among patients with sepsis. In contrast, a randomized study of 263 patients with a mean serum creatinine concentration of 2.6 mg/dL (230 μmol/L) on admission to the emergency department showed that early goal-directed therapy during the first 6 hours after admission was effective. The central venous oxygen saturation was continuously monitored as goal-directed therapy was instituted; in patients assigned to such interventions, the multiorgan dysfunction score decreased significantly and in-hospital mortality decreased (30.5%, as compared with 46.5% in the control patients, who received standard care; $P = 0.009$). The goal-directed approach included early volume expansion and administration of vasopressors to maintain mean blood pressure at or above 65 mm Hg and transfusion of red cells to increase the hematocrit to 30% or more if central venous oxygen saturation was less than 70%. If these interventions failed to increase central venous oxygen saturation to greater than 70%, then therapy with dobutamine was instituted.

KEY READING

Schrier RW: Acute renal failure and sepsis. N Engl J Med 2004; 351:159.

B. NEPHROTOXINS—Nephrotoxins induce tubular cell injury by several primary mechanisms, including direct cellular injury, vasoconstriction, and tubular obstruction.

(1) Exogenous nephrotoxins

(a) Antibiotics—Nephrotoxins like aminoglycosides, amphotericin, heavy metals, foscarnet, pentamidine, and cisplatin cause direct tubular cell injury. The most important manifestation of aminoglycoside nephrotoxicity is AKI secondary to ATN, which occurs in 3–5% of patients receiving aminoglycosides. Maintaining blood levels in the therapeutic range reduces but does not eliminate the risk of nephrotoxicity. Risk factors for developing nephrotoxic nephropathy include use of high or repeated doses or prolonged therapy, advanced age, volume depletion, a reduced effective arterial volume and the coexistence of renal ischemia or other nephrotoxins. Again, patients with a reduced effective arterial volume are at a markedly increased risk for nephrotoxin-induced AKI. This synergistic interaction may raise the incidence of AKI from a nephrotoxin as much as a factor of 10.

AKI caused by aminoglycosides is usually nonoliguric. It is manifested by an increase in BUN and creatinine after about 1 week of therapy, although in patients with concurrent renal hypoperfusion it can occur within 48 hours. Patient may develop polyuria and hypomagnesemia. Once-daily dosing of aminoglycosides is as effective as more frequent dosing and may result in less nephrotoxicity, but should not be used in patients with chronic kidney disease (CKD).

Cyclosporin and tacrolimus nephrotoxicity is usually dose dependent. High blood levels may help to predict renal failure. In many cases, a kidney biopsy may be necessary to distinguish between toxicity and other causes. Renal function usually improves after decreasing the dose or discontinuing the drug.

(b) Radiographic contrast media (see also Chapter 12)—Radiocontrast agents cause both vasoconstriction and direct cellular injury. Contrast nephropathy typically presents as an acute decline in GFR within 24–48 hours following administration. Individuals with reduced baseline kidney function, diabetic nephropathy, severe cardiac failure, volume depletion, advanced age, those receiving a large dose of contrast and concomitant exposure to other nephrotoxins appear particularly vulnerable and should be volume expanded prior to the study. In a meta-analysis, a favorable outcome was reported for patients receiving low-osmolar agents. Iodixanol, a nonionic, iso-osmolar contrast media, has been shown to be beneficial in preventing contrast nephropathy in high-risk patients.

(c) Intratubular obstruction—AKI may occur in patients with malignancies with a high rate of tumor cell turnover. Such cell turnover may occur either spontaneously or after chemotherapy. There may be an increase in uric acid production and hyperuricosuria, causing uric acid nephropathy. The peak uric acid level is often greater than 20 mg/dL. Prevention of AKI involves establishing a urine output greater than 3–5 L/24 hours and initiating treatment with allopurinol before institution of chemotherapy. Allopurinol blocks uric acid production by inhibiting xanthine oxidase. Urinary alkalization also increases the solubility of xanthine and enhances its excretion. More rapid declines in uric acid levels are seen following the intravenous administration of urate oxidase (uricase, rasburicase), which converts uric acid to allantoin, a much more soluble metabolite. It should not be used in place of allopurinol and hydration if the latter is all that is required in a particular patient (eg, uric acid <9 mg/dL, no renal failure, and tumor lysis not expected).

Tubular obstruction has been implicated as a central event in the pathophysiology of ATN induced by some therapeutic agents such as acyclovir, sulfonamides, methotrexate, triamtrene, ethylene glycol, and myeloma light chains. To minimize possible nephrotoxicity from these agents, hydration and a high urine flow rate should be maintained in these patients during therapy.

(d) AKI due to cancer treatment—Several new drugs have been in use for the treatment of various cancers.

The use of cytotoxic or targeted chemotherapy can lead to renal injury. In this setting, tubulointerstitial injury and thrombotic microangiopathy (vascular injury) are more common than other forms of kidney injury, including glomerular. Tyrosine kinase inhibitors and monoclonal antibodies that block the vascular endothelial growth factor pathway are most commonly associated with thrombotic microangiopathy.

Immune checkpoint inhibitors (CPIs), monoclonal antibodies that target inhibitory receptors expressed on T cells, represent an emerging class of immunotherapy used in treating solid organ and hematologic malignancies.

CPI-induced AKI is a new entity that presents with clinical and histologic features similar to other causes of drug-induced acute tubulointerstitial nephritis, though with a longer latency period. Glucocorticoids appear to be a potentially effective treatment strategy.

KEY READINGS

Cortazar FB et al: Clinicopathological features of AKI associated with immune checkpoint inhibitors. Kidney Int 2016;90: 638.
Troxell ML et al: Antineoplastic treatment and renal injury: an update on renal pathology due to cytotoxic and targeted therapies. Adv Anat Pathol 2016;23:310.

(e) Ethylene glycol—Ingestion of ethylene glycol, usually in the form of antifreeze, produces severe metabolic acidosis with an elevated anion gap and osmolar gap. Ethylene glycol is metabolized by alcohol dehydrogenase to glycolic and oxalic acid, which are toxic to the renal tubules. Hypocalcaemia is a prominent feature that occurs as a result of the deposition of calcium oxalate in multiple tissues. Calcium oxalate crystals are typically found in the urine sediment. Aggressive intervention with intravenous sodium bicarbonate to increase excretion of glycolate through ion tapping along with intravenous ethanol or fomepizole to block the metabolism of ethylene glycol should be done. In many cases emergent hemodialysis is needed to remove ethylene glycol, glycolate and to correct metabolic acidosis.

(2) Endogenous nephrotoxins

(a) Pigments—Myoglobinuria as a consequence of rhabdomyolysis is a frequent cause of AKI. The release of large amounts of myoglobin from necrotic muscle tissue in the setting of volume depletion results in ATN. Patients with rhabdomyolysis will frequently complain of muscle pain and have elevated levels of creatine phosphokinase (CPK). Beside trauma some other metabolic derangements that can cause rhabdomyolysis include hypokalemia and hypophosphatemia. Cocaine use, neuroleptic malignant syndrome, and the use of HMG-CoA reductase inhibitors in the treatment of hypercholesterolemia also contribute or cause rhabdomyolysis. The urine will appear dark brown. The urine dipstick, even in the absence of red blood cells, will be positive for blood because of presence of myoglobin. Hyperkalemia, hyperphosphatemia, hyperuricemia, and hypocalcemia, followed by hypercalcemia are other clinical features associated with rhabdomyolysis. The most important aspect of management is rapid volume repletion. Experience from recent disasters has shown that early aggressive hydration and urinary alkalinazation are capable of preventing myoglobinuric AKI.

Massive intravascular hemolysis can be seen in severe transfusion reactions and snake bites and may cause significant hemoglobinuria and ATN. The renal injury in this setting is due to the obstruction by intratubular heme pigment casts and concurrent volume depletion and renal ischemia. In contrast to other forms of acute tubular necrosis, the fractional excretion of sodium is often less than 1%, a finding that may reflect the primacy of tubular obstruction rather than tubular necrosis.

2. Glomerular disease—Glomerulonephritis (GN) is characterized by hypertension, proteinuria, and hematuria. Glomerulonephritis that causes AKI is referred to as rapidly progressive glomerulonephritis (RPGN). RPGN can occur in systemic lupus nephritis, Wegener granulomatosis, polyarteritis nodosa, Goodpasture syndrome, Henoch-Schonlein purpura, immunologic glomerulonephritis due to infection, and hemolytic uremic syndrome. Together these account for less than 5% of AKI cases.

3. Interstitial nephritis—Many drugs can induce interstitial nephritis by an idiosyncratic immune-mediated mechanism. This is often associated with fever, maculo-papular rash, and eosinophils in the urine. Many drugs can cause acute interstitial nephritis but the most common are NSAIDs, penicillins, cephalosporins, sulfonamides, diuretics, and allopurinol. In the hospital setting AKI is often multifactorial and it is very important to carefully analyze the hospital course and the medication history of every patient.

4. Vascular disease—Atheroembolic disease due to cholesterol emboli is another important cause of AKI, especially in elderly patients. It may present 1 day to several weeks after undergoing an invasive vascular procedure or major trauma. Patients classically present with lower extremity rash, livedo reticularis, and eosinophils in the urine. Unfortunately, there is no specific treatment. The patients blood pressure should be controlled and further intra-arterial procedures should be limited.

D. Postrenal Acute Kidney Injury

The primary causes of postrenal AKI include benign prostatic hypertrophy, prostate cancer, cervical cancer, retroperitoneal fibrosis, retroperitoneal lymphoma, metastatic carcinoma, and nephrolithiasis. Blood clots within the urinary tracts can also present with obstruction. Hydronephrosis detected on renal ultrasound examination is the major signal that obstruction is present. False-negative ultrasound examinations can occur if the obstruction is very early or retroperitoneal fibrosis is present.

KEY READINGS

Beauchamp GA et al: Toxic alcohol ingestion: prompt recognition and management in the emergency department. Emerg Med Pract 2016;18:1.
Xavier B et al: Rhabdomyolysis and acute kidney injury. N Engl J Med 2009;361:62.

▶ Clinical Findings

A. Symptoms and Signs

Unfortunately, the signs and symptoms are limited, nondiagnostic, and often go unrecognized. The symptoms of AKI include those related to azotemia generally and those due to underlying cause. Suggestive symptoms include a decrease in urine output, dark and cola-colored urine. Azotemic patients often complain of anorexia, nausea, malaise, metallic taste in the mouth, itching, confusion, fluid retention, and hypertension. Physical examination may reveal signs of volume overload, pericardial friction rub or asterxis. This is why aggressive laboratory surveillance in high-risk patients is necessary.

B. Laboratory Findings

The diagnosis of AKI is made by documenting elevations of the BUN and serum creatinine. Serum cystatin C is also a useful marker of AKI, and may detect AKI 1–2 days earlier than serum creatinine. Cystatin C is a 13kD endogenous cysteine protease inhibitor produced by nucleated cells at a constant rate. Cystatin C is freely filtered at the glomerulus, reabsorbed, and catabolized, but it is not secreted by tubules.

Classifying intrinsic AKI into one of the histological sites is in large part dependent upon the urinalysis. For example, in ischemic or nephrotoxin induced AKI the urinalysis shows mild proteinuria and often pigmented granular casts. However, in acute GN there is a higher degree of proteinuria, white blood cells, erythrocytes, and cellular casts. In interstitial nephritis, urinalysis shows mild to moderate proteinuria, leukocytes, erythrocytes, and eosinophils. The presence of heme postivity on the urine dipstick in a freshly voided sample, and no erythrocytes suggest the presence of myoglobin or free hemoglobin, indicating either rhabdomyolysis or hemolysis. The presence of eosinophilis is suggestive of acute interstitial nephritis, but can also be seen in renal atheroembolism or pyelonephritis. Specific urinary crystals can also be indicative causes of AKI. For example, calcium oxalate crystals are seen in cases of ethylene glycol ingestion, and uric acid crystals are seen in cases of tumor lysis syndrome. Urinary diagnostic indices should be sent in any case where prerenal azotemia is in the differential diagnosis. Glomerulonephritis and acute interstitial nephritis require kidney biopsy for diagnosis. Table 9–4 lists the urine findings suggestive of specific etiologies of AKI.

Table 9–4. Urinary findings in acute kidney injury.

Etiology	Sediment	FENa$^+$	FE-Urea	Proteinuria
Prerenal azotemia	Few hyaline casts	<1	<35	None or trace
Ischemia	Epithelial cells, muddy-brown casts pigmented granular casts	>2	>50	Trace to mild
Acute interstitial nephritis	White blood cells, WBC cast, eosinophils, RBC, epithelial cells	>1		Mild to moderate
Acute glomerulonephritis	Dysmorphic RBCs, RBC cast,	<1 early		Moderate to severe
Post renal	Few hyaline casts, possible RBC	<1 early >1 late		None or trace
Tumor lysis	Uric acid crystals			None or trace
Arterial/venous thrombosis	RBCs			Mild to moderate
Ethylene glycol	Calcium oxalate crystals			Trace to mild

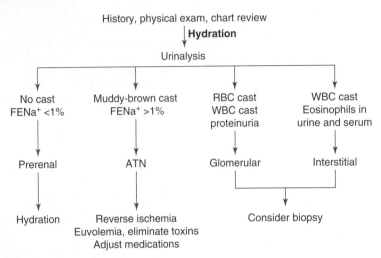

▲ **Figure 9–2.** Stepwise approach to the common causes of acute kidney injury. FENa+, fractional excretion of Na+; RBC, red blood cells; WBC, white blood cells; ATN, acute tubular necrosis.

It is important to remember that a very high serum creatinine does not preclude the diagnosis of prerenal azotemia. A low FENa+, less than 1%, is generally indicative of prerenal azotemia as the etiology of AKI. If the patient had existing CKD, prior to developing AKI, a high FENa+ may not indicate ATN. In CKD patients adaptation to volume depletion may take days, not hours, and a FENa+ may be falsely high. An ultrasound is done to evaluate for obstruction. If the clinical situation dictates evaluation of renal vasculature with isotope scans, Doppler flow studies or angiography should be utilized. Figure 9–2 outlines the clinical approach to the common causes of AKI.

BioMarkers: The search for AKI biomarkers began more than a decade ago; many potential urinary biomarkers have been studied in prospective studies. These biomarkers included lipocalin, Interleukin 18, fatty acid binding protein, kidney injury molecule 1 (KIM-1), and others. Recently, the US Food and Drug Administration (FDA), the European Medicines Agency, and the Japanese Pharmaceutical allowed marketing of the NephroCheck test (Astute Medical, San Diego, CA), which helps to determine if certain critically ill patients are at risk of developing moderate-to-severe AKI within 12 hours following testing. NephroCheck measures urinary levels of TIMP-2 (tissue inhibitor of metalloproteinase 2) and IGFBP7 (insulin-like growth factor binding protein 7), implicated in G1 cell cycle arrest. These biomarkers have increased sensitivity over serum creatinine leading to the diagnosis of biomarker positive creatinine negative AKI. This has been termed "subclinical AKI" and has a worse prognosis than no AKI, but a better prognosis than clinical or creatinine positive AKI.

KEY READINGS

Schaub AJ et al: Biomarkers of acute kidney injury and associations with short- and long-term outcomes. Version 1. F1000Res. 2016;5: F1000 Faculty Rev-986.
Steven G et al: TRIBE-AKI Consortium. Urinary biomarkers of AKI and mortality 3 years after cardiac surgery. J Am Soc Nephrol 2014 May;25:1063.

▶ Complications

A. Hyperkalemia

In patients with AKI the serum potassium rises rapidly especially in the presence of cell lysis such as occurs with muscle injury, hemolysis, gastrointestinal ischemia, tumor lysis syndrome, high fever, or blood transfusions. Hyperkalemia is further aggravated by metabolic acidosis as potassium is shifted from the intracellular to the extracellular compartment. The serum potassium concentration can be temporarily lowered by the administration of glucose and insulin, bicarbonate, inhaled β_2-agonists, and potassium binding resins. However, if renal failure persists hyperkalemia will continue to reoccur and will ultimately only respond to renal replacement therapy (RRT). As AKI patients are more prone to the cardiotoxic side effects of hyperkalemia, the serum potassium level should be lowered to nontoxic levels as soon as possible. Potassium is a small molecule and is easily dialyzable. Even at a blood flow of 200 mL/min, dialysate potassium concentration of 1 mmol/L and a starting serum potassium concentration of 6 mmol/L, about 60 mmol of potassium are removed per hour.

B. Metabolic Acidosis

The severity of metabolic acidosis cannot usually be explained by the normal production rate of 1 mEq/kg/day of hydrogen ions. Patients with AKI are often in a hypercatabolic state (fever, trauma, sepsis) and in addition lactic acidosis may also occur because of anaerobic metabolism (hypoperfusion). The addition of respiratory acidosis, secondary to CO_2 retention, to metabolic acidosis can result in severe acidemia (pH <7.1) that may have severe negative inotropic and metabolic effects. Correction of a metabolic acidosis with administration of intravenous (IV) sodium bicarbonate is limited by the risk of hypervolemia and/or hypernatremia. Since bicarbonate is the commonly used buffer in hemodialysis dialysate, dialysis will result in reasonable control of metabolic acidosis and removal of organic acids. Continuous forms of dialysis have also been shown to be effective in the correction of severe acidosis. However, if lactate is used as a buffer, hyperlactatemia and lactic acidosis might possibly be induced. This is particularly relevant in patients with liver failure, as the liver accounts for 53% of lactate metabolism. Failure to convert lactate to bicarbonate can result in accumulation of lactic acid with worsening of metabolic acidosis. Acetate containing dialysate solutions can also be used as acetate is metabolized in the body and converted to bicarbonate. However, plasma bicarbonate levels may not increase, or may even fall slightly, during the first hour of dialysis due to diffusive loss of bicarbonate from blood to dialysate along with delayed metabolism of acetate to bicarbonate. Acetate is also a vasodilator and is associated with hypotension in some patients. This is why bicarbonate is the generally preferred anion used in RRT.

C. Fluid Overload

Volume overload is a major problem in oliguric AKI (urine output <400 mL/day). Critically ill patients are at high risk of developing hypervolemia, as fluid restriction is not always feasible because of the need for intravenous administration of drugs, nutrition, blood, and blood products. In addition, patients often receive aggressive fluid resuscitation in the early phase of their illness. This may result in pulmonary and peripheral edema when this fluid is redistributed later during their illness.

The most useful therapy for volume overload is loop diuretics. Furosemide or other such diuretics can be given intravenously as a bolus or by continuous infusion. If started in the early stages of AKI this intervention, along with fluid restriction, can be very beneficial in preventing or minimizing volume overload. When using diuretics one must be careful to avoid volume depletion as the lack of renal autoregulation during AKI leaves the kidney vulnerable to additional hypotensive insults.

Hemofiltration, both by hemodialysis and continuous renal replacement therapy (CRRT), removes fluid and small molecular weight solute by convection and is the treatment modality of choice for fluid removal in hemodynamically stable patient. Ultrafiltration rates of 2–3 L/h can be achieved with high flux dialyzers. In oliguric patients with a degree of fluid overload, who are about to receive large amounts of fluids for therapeutic purposes, RRT should be initiated early on with the aim of preventing clinically important pulmonary edema. Episodes of hypotension should be avoided as renal functional recovery may be retarded because of recurrent ischemia and cell injury.

D. Hyponatremia

Hyponatremia is usually associated with volume overload. The clinical manifestations of hyponatremia are primarily neurologic in nature. Symptomatic hyponatremia should be treated aggressively but also with caution as rapid correction of low sodium level can lead to central pontine myelinolysis if the duration of electrolyte imbalance has been longer than 48 hours. The targeted range of change of sodium level should be 1–2 mEq/L/h until symptoms resolve or until the serum sodium level increases to 120 mEq/L.

E. Anemia

Anemia is very common in patients with AKI. There are several mechanisms leading to anemia in patients with AKI. The most common cause of anemia associated with AKI is inadequate production of erythropoietin and decreased responsiveness to erythropoietin play a role. There is also an increase in the rate of destruction of RBCs as a result of increased erythrocyte fragility. Furthermore, patients with AKI have an increased tendency to bleed from various sites due to platelet dysfunction secondary to azotemia. Platelet dysfunction may respond to conjugated estrogens or infusion of dDAVP dosed at 0.3 mcg/kg.

Subcutaneous or intravenous erythropoietin is increasingly being used in the acute setting to improve hemoglobin and to help minimize transfusions. The efficacy of this therapy in correcting anemia in AKI is still not clear.

F. Hyperphosphatemia

Hyperphosphatemia is common in patients with AKI. The main mechanism is a decrease in renal excretion, tissue destruction, and shifts from intracellular to extracellular space. If patients can ingest food, hyperphosphatemia should be treated with phosphate binders like calcium carbonate, calcium acetate, sevelamer HCL, or lanthanum carbonate. If the calcium × phosphorous product is high (>70) or the phosphate concentration exceeds 5.5 mEq/L a non–calcium-based binder like sevelamer or lanthanum should be used.

G. Other Electrolyte Imbalance

Hypocalcemia, although common, rarely requires treatment. The factors responsible for hypocalcemia include hypomagnesemia, hyperphosphatemia, resistance to parathyroid hormone, lack of active vitamin D, calcium sequestration in tissues, use of blood products that have been stored in citrate and the use of sodium bicarbonate infusions. Rarely patients may have hypercalcemia if the underlying disorder is malignancy or multiple myeloma. Hypercalcemia can also occur in AKI due to rhabdomyolysis.

▶ **Treatment**

A. Prerenal Azotemia

By definition, prerenal azotemia is rapidly reversible on restoration of renal perfusion. Hypovolemia caused by hemorrhage is ideally corrected with packed red blood cells if the hematocrit is dangerously low. There is compelling evidence that aggressive intravascular volume expansion dramatically reduces the incidence of ATN after major surgery or trauma, burns, and cholera. In the absence of active bleeding isotonic saline may be sufficed. However, if large volumes of normal saline are required using an anion like lactate of bicarbonate in place of chloride helps minimize the occurrence or worsening of hyperchloremic metabolic acidosis. The routine use of colloids has recently been associated with adverse outcomes and this has been called into question. Serum potassium and acid–base status should be monitored in all subjects. Cardiac failure may require aggressive management with positive inotropics, preload- and or afterload-reducing agents, and mechanical aids such as an intra-aortic balloon pump. Fluid management is particularly challenging in patients with cirrhosis, requiring careful monitoring to avoid increased ascites formation.

B. Acute Tubular Necrosis

Management of ATN is usually supportive. Attempts to convert oliguric to nonoliguric AKI may be attempted by giving a loop diuretic like furosemide. However, one must be certain to avoid volume depletion as a result of the diuretic. Use of mannitol should be avoided as it may precipitate congestive heart failure due to intravascular volume expansion if urine output remains low. In oliguric AKI, once vascular volume has been normalized, management consists of restricting fluids to match measurable insensible losses, potassium restriction, and limitation of phosphorous intake.

There are no prospective clinical data to support the use of low-dose dopamine for the protection or improvement of renal function in patients with ATN or AKI. In a multicenter study comparing dopamine with placebo, dopamine was not found to improve survival or eliminate the need for dialysis.

Several small studies suggested that fenoldopam could reduce the incidence of AKI in high-risk clinical situations; however, a subsequent larger randomized trial comparing fenoldopam to standard hydration in patients undergoing invasive angiographic procedures found no benefit in regard to decreasing the incidence of contrast-induced AKI.

KEY READING

Jakob SM et al: Prevention of acute renal failure—fluid repletion and colloids. Int J Artif Organs 2004;27:1043.

C. Role of RRT in AKI

Dialysis is the only FDA-approved treatment of AKI, and hemodialysis was started for this purpose in early 1960s. Although hemodialysis is the standard modality in hemodynamically stable patients with AKI, both continuous renal replacement therapies and peritoneal dialysis are also used in selected cases. The determining factors of which modality is chosen include the catabolic state, hemodynamic stability, and whether the primary goal is solute removal (uremia, hyperkalemia), fluid removal, or both.

1. Indications for dialysis—The indications of RRT in patients with AKI include refractory fluid overload, hyperkalemia, severe metabolic acidosis, azotemia, signs of uremia, such as pericarditis, neuropathy, or an otherwise unexplained decline in mental status, over dose with a dialyzable drug/toxin. In an attempt to minimize morbidity, dialysis should generally be started prior to the onset of complications due to renal failure. Nephrologists often initiate renal replacement therapy even in the absence of the above mentioned indications when the BUN reaches 60–80 mg/dL to prevent complications from AKI. Currently, peritoneal dialysis (PD) is rarely performed in adults as a treatment modality for AKI. This modality can be used in selective patient populations with access difficulties, contraindication to anticoagulation or patients who are hemodynamically unstable.

2. Hemodialysis—Frequent hemodialysis is required to control metabolic abnormalities and volume status in AKI. Hypercatabolic patients require more aggressive dialysis to maintain acceptable or optimal steady-state or time-averaged concentrations of solutes. In a recent study daily hemodialysis resulted in better control of uremia, fewer hypotensive episodes during hemodialysis, and more rapid resolution of AKI than did conventional hemodialysis. The mortality rate, according to the intention-to-treat analysis, was 28% for daily dialysis and 46% for alternate-day dialysis.

The impact of frequency of intermittent hemodialysis (IHD) was also evaluated in the VA/NIH Acute Renal Failure Trial Network (ATN) study.

Patients randomized to the less-intensive treatment strategy received hemodialysis on a thrice weekly (alternate-day except Sunday) schedule while patients randomized to the intensive arm received six times per week (daily except Sunday) IHD. Although the study was not designed to evaluate outcomes by individual modality of RRT, there were no differences in mortality between groups when evaluated based on percentage of time treated using IHD. Based on these results, it does not appear that there is further benefit to routinely increasing the frequency of IHD treatments beyond three times per week so long as the delivered Kt/V_{urea} is at least 1.2 per treatment.

In hemodialysis, solute removal occurs primarily by diffusion from the plasma into the dialysate during dialysis and, to a much lesser degree, by convection during ultrafiltration as solvent drag carries small and intermediate-sized solutes with the water. The rate of solute diffusion is determined by the surface area and unit solute permeability of the dialysis membrane, blood and dialysate flow rate, duration of dialysis, and transmembrane pressure gradient.

3. Continuous renal replacement therapies—Continuous renal replacement therapies (CRRTs) involve either dialysis (diffusion-based solute removal) or filtration (convection-based solute and water removal) treatments that operate in a continuous mode. The various forms of CRRTs include continuous venovenous hemofiltration (CVVH), continuous venovenous hemodialysis (CVVHD), continuous arteriovenous hemodialysis (CAVHD), continuous venovenous hemodiafiltration (CVVHDF), slow continuous ultrafiltration (SCUF), and sustained low-efficiency dialysis (SLED).

CRRTs have several theoretical advantages over intermittent hemodialysis in critically ill patients with AKI. These include accurate continuous control of volume, increased delivered dose of dialysis, hemodynamic stability, the ability to provide aggressive nutritional support, gradual and continuous removal of fluid and solutes, and a possible anti-inflammatory effect. Patients with multiorgan failure or sepsis require large amounts of volume in the form of blood products, vasopressors, and parentral nutrition. In these settings, continuous therapies provide an ability to remove fluid, which in most patients achieves an optimal volume balance. The possible elimination of inflammatory mediators is another advantage of CRRT. Many proposed mediators of sepsis have a molecular weight below the cutoff point of hemofilters and thus are filterable. CRRT may also be more beneficial in patients with increased intracranial pressure and combined fulminant hepatic failure and AKI.

Although several studies have suggested that CRRT is associated with improved rates of recovery of kidney function in surviving as compared to IHD, all of these studies are notable for higher mortality rates in the CRRT group. When analyzed across studies in which there were no differences in mortality, rates of recovery of kidney function do not appear to be impacted by modality of RRT.

However, the superiority of CRRT in terms of patient outcomes is still controversial.

CRRT also has some disadvantages. Transport of patients for technical investigations becomes far more complicated and many times a new set of disposable tubing have to be used to restart dialysis. Anticoagulation is needed on a continuous basis during CRRT and thus the risk of bleeding is greater in CRRT than HD.

KEY READINGS

Bagshaw SM et al: Continuous versus intermittent renal replacement therapy for critically ill patients with acute kidney injury: a meta-analysis. Crit Care Med 2008;36:610.
Palevsky PM et al: Intensity of renal replacement therapy in acute kidney injury: perspective from within the Acute Renal Failure Trial Network Study. Crit Care 2009;13:310.

▶ **Prevention**

The underlying principles of identification of high-risk patients, use of preventative measures, and aggressive surveillance are of key importance. Prevention of AKI is of paramount importance. Certain risk factors that have been identified to enhance the likelihood of AKI are listed in Table 9–5. These include volume depletion or hypoperfusion, preexisting renal failure, and exposure to vasoconstricting drugs such as NSAIDs. Prevention of AKI primarily involves recognition of the high-risk patient and correction of volume depletion. Persistent volume depletion leads to a prolonged "extension phase" resulting in worsening ATN. Aggressive restoration of intravascular volume dramatically reduces the incidence of acute tubular necrosis after major surgery or trauma. The mortality of AKI is higher if it develops in the hospital. Therefore, it is imperative to prevent AKI, particularly that is associated with nephrotoxic drugs and interventional procedures. Correction of hypovolemia (normalizing the effective arterial volume) before radiocontrast administration and surgical procedures and nephrology consultation in patients with even minimally decreased renal function, may decrease the frequency of AKI. For the prevention of contrast induced nephropathy, prophylactic infusion of half-normal saline (1 mL/kg for 12 hours before and after procedure) appears more effective in preventing AKI than other commonly used agents such as mannitol and furosemide. N-acetylcysteine was been found to be beneficial in the prevention of contrast induced nephropathy in the initial trial. Several recent clinical trials of oral and IV N-acetylcysteine have yielded conflicting findings.

More recently, clinical trials have compared isotonic sodium bicarbonate with isotonic sodium chloride and

Table 9–5. Patients at risk.

Elderly patients
Diabetes mellitus
Volume depletion
Vascular surgery
Chronic kidney disease
Multiple antibiotics
Multiple insults
Congestive heart failure

have yielded conflicting results. As a result, isotonic fluid comprised of either sodium bicarbonate or sodium chloride is considered the standard of care for the prevention of contrast-induced AKI. For hospitalized patients, a regimen of isotonic saline or sodium bicarbonate at 1 mL/kg/h administered for 12 hours prior to and 12 hours following the procedure is recommended. An alternative regimen that may be more feasible in the outpatient setting is 3 mL/kg/h for 1 hour prior to the procedure followed by 1–1.5 mL/kg/h for 6 hours following the procedure.

Trials of other pharmacologic interventions, including furosemide, dopamine, fenoldopam, calcium channel blockers, and mannitol have failed to demonstrate significant benefit and, in some cases, have been associated with an increased risk of AKI.

Allopurinol is useful for limiting uric acid generation in patients at high risk for tumor lysis syndrome if administered days in advance of chemotherapy. Finally, since many cases of ischemic or nephrotoxic AKI result from sepsis or use of nephrotoxic antibiotics, respectively, limiting infection and careful monitoring for infections are important strategies.

KEY READING

Eng G et al: Comparative effect of contrast media type on the incidence of contrast-induced nephropathy: a systematic review and meta-analysis. Ann Intern Med 2016;164:417.

▶ Nutrition in AKI

Recent evidence indicates more attention should be paid to the nutritional aspect of patients with both chronic renal failure (CRF) and AKI. Excessive catabolism caused by shock, sepsis, burns, or rhabdomyolysis is common. During sepsis cytokines, including interleukins and tumor necrosis factor, are stimulated and in turn increase skeletal muscle breakdown. Severe net protein catabolism may accelerate the rate of rise in plasma concentrations of potassium, phosphorous, nitrogenous metabolites, and non–nitrogen-containing acids. Acute uremia is associated with increased gluconeogenesis and protein degradation as well as reduced protein synthesis. Insulin resistance, secondary hyperparathyrodisim, increased glucagon concentrations and metabolic acidosis also contributes to the malnutrition in AKI.

RRT itself can cause increased metabolism through several mechanisms. Inevitable losses of nutrients during RRT also cause increase catabolism. If high flux membranes are used the losses of amino acids increases by 30% as compared to low-flux membranes. The losses of amino acids may range between 7 and 50 g/day with CRRT. This unavoidable removal of nutrients predisposes the AKI patient to negative nitrogen balance. In addition to increased catabolism, AKI patients also have a diminished utilization of available nutrients. Abnormalities in the growth hormone-insulin like growth factor 1 (IGF-1) axis prevent optimal utilization of available nutrients. Although the plasma concentration of growth hormone increases in renal failure, there is growth hormone resistance at the cellular level. Also, many patients are unable to eat adequately because of anorexia or vomiting. Malnutrition is a predictor of outcomes in AKI patients.

Protein intake should be around 1.2–1.4 g/kg and 20–25% of daily calories should be provided by lipids. Glucose is usually administered in a 70% solution. The estimated energy requirements for patients with AKI usually fall between 30 and 40 kcal/kg normal body weight/day. Urinary urea nitrogen (UUN) may be measured and higher calories and daily protein may be prescribed for the patients who have a higher UUN. This estimation cannot be done in anuric patients. Higher energy intakes generate more carbon dioxide from the catabolized carbohydrates and fat and can promote hypercapnia if pulmonary function is impaired. Vitamin and mineral requirements have not been well defined for patients with AKI. However, water soluble vitamins should be supplemented, as these are lost during RRT. Controlled studies are needed as nutrition requirements for HD versus CRRT may be different.

KEY READINGS

Casaer MP et al: Nutrition in the acute phase of critical illness. N Engl J Med 2014;370:1227.
Fiaccadori E et al: Specific nutritional problems in acute kidney injury, treated with non-dialysis and dialytic modalities. NDT Plus 2010;3:1.

▶ Prognosis

The outcome of patients with AKI has consistently been at a 50% survival rate, despite improved technology. The prognosis for hospitalized patients with AKI depends largely on the site (ICU or ward). In hospitalized patients with AKI caused by ATN, the oliguric phase of ATN typically lasts for 1 to 2 weeks, but it can persist for 4 to 6 weeks. It is followed by diuretic phase. Although uremia and volume overload can be controlled with dialysis, AKI and its complications worsen patient outcomes. Survival after AKI is dramatically influenced by the severity of the underline illnesses and number of failed organs. The mortality rate of patients with AKI on a ventilator is about 80% and the mortality dramatically increases with increasing number of failed non-respiratory organs. Mortality among patients who developed AKI following cardiac surgery was 63.7% compared with 4.3% of patients who underwent cardiac surgery and did not develop renal failure. Oliguric AKI, developing in a surgical setting or in older patients, carries a higher mortality than other forms of AKI. It has been noted that after discharge from a hospitalization that included AKI, a substantial fraction of patients required renal replacement therapy in long-term care facilities.

Large population-based studies have demonstrated that patients who survive an episode of AKI are at considerable risk for progressing to advanced stages of chronic kidney disease. Patients with AKI who required dialysis and then recovered were at especially high risk for progression to CKD. Hence, the severity of AKI is a robust predictor of progression to CKD.

In summary, AKI remains a medical challenge to clinicians and researchers. Recognition of patients at risk, institution of preventive measures and aggressive surveillance, and early treatment of AKI will be much more effective than treatment of established AKI with RRT.

KEY READINGS

Coca SG et al: Chronic kidney disease after acute kidney injury: a systematic review and meta-analysis. Kidney Int 2012;81:442.

Pannu N et al: Association between AKI, recovery of renal function, and long-term outcomes after hospital discharge. Clin J Am Soc Nephrol 2013;8:194.

■ CHAPTER REVIEW QUESTIONS

1. A 58-year-old Caucasian female patient develops oliguric AKI after a motor vehicle accident. She is mechanically ventilated and requires pressor therapy with 0.2 mcg/kg/min of norepinephrine to maintain a mean arterial BP of 75 mm Hg.

   Which ONE of the following statements regarding renal replacement therapy in this setting is evidence based?
   A. Intermittent hemodialysis is associated with decreased mortality as compared to continuous renal replacement therapy.
   B. Intermittent hemodialysis should be prescribed to deliver a single-pool Kt/V of 1.3 on a three-times-per-week schedule.
   C. Continuous renal replacement therapy will provide greater volume control with less hemodynamic instability than intermittent hemodialysis.
   D. Continuous renal replacement therapy should be prescribed to deliver an effluent flow rate of 16 mL/kg/h.
   E. Continuous renal replacement therapy leads to better survival.

2. A 77-year-old African–American man undergoes coronary artery bypass and aortic valve replacement. His past medical history includes type 2 diabetes mellitus, hypertension, congestive heart failure, and chronic kidney disease stage 4 (baseline serum creatinine 2.7 mg/dL). He receives perioperative therapy with dopamine (3 mcg/kg/min) to prevent acute-on-chronic kidney disease.

   Which ONE of the following statement regarding the use of low-dose dopamine (<3 mcg/kg/min) to prevent or treat AKI in is CORRECT?
   A. It reduces AKI.
   B. It decreases the duration of dialysis dependence.
   C. It increases the risk of atrial fibrillation.
   D. It decreases mortality.
   E. It improves urine output.

3. A 31-year-old Hispanic man with HIV admitted with high-grade fever, cough, and an infiltrate on chest X-ray. He was diagnosed with *Pneumocystis jirovecii* pneumonia and started on high dose sulfamethoxazole-trimethoprim for pneumocystis. BUN/creatinine on admission 13/1.0, potassium 4, and after 4 days BUN/creatinine 17/1.8 and serum potassium increased to 6.3.

   The etiology of the elevated serum potassium and creatinine is best explained by which of the following mechanisms?
   A. HIV-induced AKI
   B. Intratubular obstruction from trimethoprim crystals
   C. Sulfamethoxazole-trimethoprim-induced acute interstitial nephritis
   D. Sepsis causing AKI
   E. Trimethoprim-mediated blockade of collecting duct apical Na channels and increase in serum creatinine

4. A 59-year-old man with diabetes mellitus and hypertension and stage 3 chronic kidney disease (estimated GFR, 37 mL/min) presents with acute MI. Coronary angiography demonstrated severe 3 vessel disease. Coronary artery bypass grafting was recommended.

Which ONE of the following treatments decreases the risk of AKI after coronary artery bypass grafting?
A. Furosemide
B. Off-pump bypass grafting
C. N-acetylcysteine
D. Normal saline
E. Dopamine

5. A 32-year-old construction worker fell from 10 ft and had his body pinned under a pile of rubble in a construction accident. Upon arrival in the emergency room he is found to have a creatinine

Phosphokinase of 40,000 U/L and a serum creatinine of 3.2 mg/dL.

Which ONE of the following treatments can decrease the risk of AKI?
A. Intravenous furosemide
B. N-acetylcysteine
C. Renal dose dopamine
D. Intravenous normal saline
E. Norepinephrine

Hepatorenal Syndrome

Florence Wong, MD, FRACP, FRCP(C)

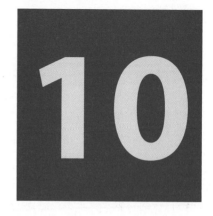

General Considerations

Renal dysfunction is a common and serious problem in patients with advanced liver cirrhosis, estimated to occur in 20% of hospitalized patients with cirrhosis, and even more commonly at 54% in the outpatient setting. Renal dysfunction in cirrhosis has always been regarded as being related to the hemodynamic changes of systemic arterial vasodilatation and paradoxical renal vasoconstriction peculiar to cirrhosis without any structural changes in the kidneys. Such cases of renal dysfunction are known as functional renal failure and the prototype is hepatorenal syndrome (HRS). However, it is now recognized that many liver conditions such as alcoholic cirrhosis or hepatitis C can cause structural renal diseases, and yet the same patients can also develop hemodynamic abnormalities as cirrhosis advances, predisposing them to functional renal failure. Therefore, the demarcation between functional and structural renal diseases is no longer as clear as once thought. Furthermore, many common systemic conditions such as diabetes can cause both cirrhosis and nephropathy, once again blurring the separation between structural and functional renal diseases. Therefore, the concept of renal dysfunction in cirrhosis has been evolving, and that also includes redefining HRS, especially in light of recent changes in the definition of acute kidney injury (AKI) by the nephrology community.

The Concept of Acute Kidney Injury

The term AKI was adopted in the early 2000s to describe cases of acute kidney dysfunction that were trivial and therefore could not be termed renal failure, and yet they could lead to permanent structural damage in those patients who survived the insult. For example, it was observed in patients who underwent cardiac surgery that a rise in serum creatinine by 0.3 mg/dL (26.4 μmol/L) was associated with a negative effect on patient survival. There followed a flurry of

academic activities reassessing the need for redefining renal dysfunction. Various definitions and diagnostic criteria of AKI, starting with the RIFLE criteria, then the Acute Kidney Injury Network (AKIN) criteria, then the Kidney Disease Improving Global Outcome (KDIGO) criteria appeared in the literature, with each set of criteria improving over the previous one. In order to conform to the changing concept of renal dysfunction in other patient populations, the hepatology community also felt that there was a need to redefine renal dysfunction in cirrhosis. The International Ascites Club, together with the Acute Dialysis Quality Initiative group, first proposed to define AKI in cirrhosis in 2011 as an increase in serum creatinine by 0.3 mg/dL (26.4 μmol/L) in less than 48 hours, or a 50% increase in serum creatinine from baseline, defined as a stable serum creatinine within the previous 6 months (Table 10–1), irrespective of the final serum creatinine level. This would allow the diagnosis of AKI at an earlier stage of renal dysfunction, thereby allowing earlier therapeutic intervention. The concept of chronic kidney disease (CKD) was also introduced, and acute on chronic kidney disease defined (Table 10–1). The International Ascites Club further clarified the definition of AKI in cirrhosis in 2015, setting out guidelines for staging of AKI and definitions for baseline renal function as well as response to treatments for AKI (Table 10–2).

The Diagnosis of Hepatorenal Syndrome

The International Ascites Club defined HRS as the development of renal failure in patients with advanced liver failure (acute or chronic) in the absence of any identifiable causes of renal pathology. It is divided into two types: acute or type 1 HRS and chronic or type 2 HRS. It is a diagnosis of exclusion after all other causes of renal failure have been excluded. The diagnostic criteria for type 1 HRS require that there has to be doubling of serum creatinine in less than 2 weeks, with the final serum creatinine reaching at least 2.5 mg/dL

Table 10–1. The International Ascites Club and Acute Dialysis Quality initiative's proposed definition for renal dysfunction in cirrhosis.

Diagnosis	Definition
Acute kidney injury	Rise in serum creatinine of ≥50% from baseline, or a rise of serum creatinine by ≥0.3 mg/dL (≥26.4 µmol/L) in <48 h. HRS type 1 is a specific form of acute kidney injury
Chronic kidney disease	Glomerular filtration rate of <60 mL/min for >3 months calculated using MDRD6 formula. HRS type 2 is a specific form of chronic kidney disease
Acute-on-chronic kidney disease	Rise in serum creatinine of ≥50% from baseline, or a rise of serum creatinine by ≥0.3 mg/dL (≥26.4 µmol/L) in <48 h in a patient with cirrhosis whose glomerular filtration rate is <60 mL/min for >3 months using MDRD6 formula

HRS, hepatorenal syndrome, MDRD6, Modification in Diet in Renal Disease using 6 parameters (patient's age, gender, ethnicity, serum creatinine, blood urea nitrogen and albumin). (Adapted from Wong F et al: Gut 2011;60:702 with permission.)

Table 10–2. New International Club of Ascites' Revised Consensus Diagnostic Criteria for Acute Kidney Injury in cirrhosis.

Parameter	Definition
Baseline SCr	Stable SCr ≤3 mo. If not available, a stable SCr closest to current one. If no previous SCr at all, use admission SCr
Definition of AKI	↑ SCr ≥0.3 mg/dL (≥26.4 µmol/L) in <48 h, or ↑ 50% from baseline
Staging	Stage 1: ↑ SCr ≥0.3 mg/dL (≥26.4 µmol/L) or ↑ SCr ≥1.50–2.0 X from baseline. Stage 2: ↑ SCr >2.0–3.0 X from baseline. Stage 3: ↑ SCr >3.0 X from baseline or SCr ≥4.0 mg/dL (≥352 µmol/L) with an acute ↑ ≥0.3 mg/dL (≥26.4 µmol/L) or initiation of renal replacement therapy
Progression	Progression of AKI to a higher stage, or need for renal replacement therapy
Regression	Regression of AKI to a lower stage
Response to treatment	None: No regression of AKI. Partial: Regression of AKI stage with a ↓ in SCr to a value ≥0.3 mg/dL above baseline. Complete: ↓ SCr to <0.3 mg/dL from baseline

AKI, acute kidney injury; SCr, serum creatinine. (Adapted from Angeli P et al: Gut 2015;64:531 with permission.)

Table 10–3. Diagnostic criteria for acute kidney injury—hepatorenal syndrome.

Cirrhosis and ascites
Stage 2 or 3 AKI
No improvement of serum creatinine (decrease of serum creatinine to within 0.3 mg/dL of baseline serum creatinine) after ≥48 h of diuretic withdrawal and volume expansion with albumin (1 g/kg b.w. × 2 days)
Absence of hypovolemic shock or severe infection requiring vasoactive drugs to maintain arterial pressure
No current or recent treatment with nephrotoxic drugs
Proteinuria <500 mg/day and no microhematuria (<50 RBC/high power field)

AKI, acute kidney injury; b.w.: body weight; RBCs, red blood cells. (Adapted from Angeli P et al: Gut 2015;64:531 with permission.)

(233 µmol/L). However, adhering to these strict diagnostic criteria means that many patients may have very advanced renal failure before treatment can be started, especially in the context of a clinical trial. Furthermore, for patients without a previous serum creatinine measurement who present to hospital in renal failure, the diagnosis of type 1 HRS may be very difficult to make, since there is no baseline serum creatinine to compare with. Therefore, the International Ascites Club further refined the diagnosis of type 1 HRS by renaming the condition as acute kidney injury-hepatorenal syndrome (AKI-HRS), so to recognize that type 1 HRS is a very special form of AKI. The diagnosis of AKI-HRS still requires that there is a doubling of serum creatinine without setting a rigid time frame of 2 weeks (Table 10–3). In other words, as long as patients develop at least stage 2 AKI, and fulfilling all other diagnostic criteria of HRS, then a diagnosis of AKI-HRS can be made. Stage 2 AKI can be reached by either doubling of the serum creatinine from a baseline measurement within 48 hours, or from a stable baseline serum creatinine measurement within the past 3 months. Furthermore, the threshold serum creatinine of 2.5 mg/dL (233 µmol/L) required for diagnosis of HRS has been removed, thus making it possible for patients to receive treatment at an earlier stage of their renal dysfunction. The term AKI-HRS will be used to mean acute or type 1 HRS throughout the chapter.

KEY READINGS

Angeli P et al: Diagnosis and management of acute kidney injury in patients with cirrhosis: revised consensus recommendations of the International Club of Ascites. Gut 2015;64:531.
Salerno F et al: Diagnosis, prevention and treatment of hepatorenal syndrome in cirrhosis. Gut 2007;56:1310.
Wong F: The evolving concept of acute kidney injury in patients with cirrhosis. Nature Rev Gastroenterol Hepatol 2015;12:711.
Wong F et al: Working Party proposal for a revised classification system of renal dysfunction in patients with cirrhosis. Gut 2011;60:702.

Pathophysiology

The pathophysiology of AKI-HRS is complex. The hallmark of the condition is one of renal hypoperfusion, which is due to a reduction in the renal perfusion pressure as well as to active renal vasoconstriction. This leads to a decrease in the renal blood flow and a reduction in the glomerular filtration rate.

A. The Peripheral Arterial Vasodilatation Hypothesis

Traditionally, the hemodynamic changes of advanced cirrhosis are thought to be responsible for the development of AKI-HRS in cirrhosis. The Peripheral Arterial Vasodilatation Hypothesis proposed that in cirrhosis, there is significant arterial vasodilatation, especially in the splanchnic circulation, related partly to an increase in sheer stress on the splanchnic vessels, and partly to an increased release of vasodilators such as nitric oxide from the vascular endothelium. The systemic circulation becomes vasodilated when these excess vasodilators are transferred from the splanchnic to the systemic circulation through collateral channels. Although there has been no loss of intravascular volume, this state of splanchnic and systemic arterial vasodilatation means that there has been a reduction in the effective arterial blood volume. The homeostatic response is to increase the cardiac output, and to activate various vasoconstrictor systems, including the renin–angiotensin system, the sympathetic nervous system, and arginine vasopressin in order to counteract the vasodilatory effects of the vasodilators and to direct the kidneys to retain sodium and water in order to maintain hemodynamic stability. As cirrhosis progresses, systemic arterial vasodilatation increases. Clinically, we recognize these changes as gradual worsening of systemic hypotension, and the patient has a hyperdynamic circulation with tachycardia, wide pulse pressure, and warm peripheries. At some point, the renal perfusion pressure will fall. When combined with increasing levels of the systemic vasoconstrictors, total renal blood flow gradually decreases. When the production of endogenous renal vasodilators cannot keep pace with the fall in renal blood flow, renal failure ensues.

B. The Systemic Inflammation Hypothesis

Cirrhosis is known to be associated with the development of systemic inflammation, as indicated by increased white cell count, C-reactive protein, the presence of various inflammatory cytokines, and oxidative stress. The extent of inflammation seems to parallel the degree of liver dysfunction and the severity of decompensation. The source of inflammation in cirrhosis is likely increased bacterial translocation whereby both viable bacteria as well as various bacterial products (known as pathogen associated molecular patterns or PAMPs) pass through an anatomically intact intestinal barrier from the intestinal lumen to mesenteric lymph nodes, and then to other extra-intestinal organs and sites. This is related to intestinal bacterial overgrowth, structural abnormalities in the intestinal mucosa, and reduced intestinal mucosal immune function, features that are common in cirrhosis. Once translocated, the presence of excess bacteria and bacterial products are recognized by various pattern recognition receptors (PRRs) such as toll like receptors (TLRs) on the cells of the host's innate immune system. This leads to the activation of an inflammatory response by stimulating genes in the immune cells that encode for molecules responsible for inflammation such as various inflammatory cytokines including tumor necrosis factor alpha (TNF-α), interleukins, interferon γ, and nitric oxide. These in turn can impair the effective circulation by enhancing arterial vasodilatation. The fact that anti-TNF antibodies can attenuate the hyperdynamic circulation in an animal model of cirrhosis suggests that inflammation is involved in the pathogenesis of the hemodynamic changes of cirrhosis. The fact that the systemic inflammatory response syndrome is present in approximately 40% of cirrhotic patients with renal dysfunction including AKI-HRS with or without infection is another piece of evidence supporting the role of inflammation in inducing renal dysfunction in cirrhosis. The use of selective intestinal decontamination with norfloxacin in patients with cirrhosis can partially reverse the hyperdynamic circulation, associated with a reduction in endotoxin levels, provides a further link between bacterial translocation, inflammation, and vascular changes in cirrhosis.

In addition to contributing to the arterial vasodilatation of cirrhosis, excess inflammation can also cause direct tissue damage, a process known as immunopathology. This is because cells in the immune systems such as neutrophils, monocytes, and various activated T cells that are recruited by the inflammatory process can cause direct cellular apoptosis and necrosis. This in turn will release tissue debris known as damage associated molecular patterns or DAMPs. These particles are also recognized by PRRs, a process that will trigger further inflammation, and the process becomes an ongoing vicious cycle.

C. The Role of Tubular Injury

The fact that renal dysfunction in cirrhosis is not just a vasomotor nephropathy has been recognized by the hepatology community. Renal tubular injury is increasingly being accepted as being involved in the pathogenesis of AKI-HRS. Toll like receptors are a family of PRRs that can recognize molecules from microbes. Their overexpression has been linked to various renal injuries including ischemic kidney injury and sepsis-related renal failure. Increased TLR4 expression has been found in the proximal renal tubules in patients with cirrhosis, likely the result of increased bacterial translocation from the gut, associated with renal cell injury and deterioration in renal function. In an animal model of cirrhosis, decontamination of the gut with norfloxacin resulted in attenuation of TLR4 expression, together with improvements in renal histology and renal function. Other findings of renal tubular injury include the increased urinary excretion of β_2-microglobulin, a marker of renal tubular injury, in patients with AKI-HRS compared to controls. In addition, cirrhotic patients with AKI-HRS were found to have increased levels of plasma and urinary neutrophil gelatinase-associated lipocalin, a protein expressed by the renal tubules and upregulated in renal tubular injury, when compared to stable cirrhotic patients without AKI-HRS. Therefore, the long-held concept that the kidneys of patients with AKI-HRS are structurally intact will need to be revisited. Indeed, features of acute tubular necrosis have been identified in patients with AKI-HRS with electron microscopy examination. The upregulation of TLR4 receptors can also increase the production of proinflammatory cytokines, thereby setting up a vicious cycle of further exaggeration of the hyperdynamic circulation, with further compromise of the renal circulation. Inflammation within the kidneys can also cause direct tubular injury, including apical vacuolization, loss of tight junctions, and apoptosis of renal tubular cells. Renal tubular cell damage can in turn impair the glomerulotubular feedback mechanism, and induce afferent arteriolar vasoconstriction. Therefore, hemodynamic abnormalities, inflammation, and renal tubular damage are all intertwined to produce AKI-HRS in cirrhosis.

D. Other Contributing Factors

Patients with cirrhosis and ascites have been documented to have altered renal autoregulation, related to their sympathetic overdrive. Autoregulation refers to the ability of the kidneys to maintain a fairly constant renal blood flow despite fluctuations in the systemic blood pressure, and hence the renal perfusion pressure. In cirrhotic patients, the autoregulation curve is shifted to the right, that is, for any given mean arterial pressure; the renal blood flow is reduced compared to normal individuals. This right shift of the autoregulation curve is more pronounced the more advanced the cirrhotic stage and more severe the ascites. Therefore, the patient is predisposed to develop renal failure by virtue of the fact that advanced cirrhosis is present, especially when accompanied by refractory ascites.

The presence of portal hypotension also contributes to the development of renal failure in cirrhosis. In a cohort of cirrhotic patients who have had their portal hypertension eliminated via the insertion of a transjugular intrahepatic portosystemic shunt, the instant recreation of portal hypertension by insertion of an angioplasty balloon, thereby blocking the shunt, was associated with a significant reduction of renal blood flow. This returned to baseline upon release of the angioplasty balloon, with elimination of the portal hypertension.

Cirrhotic cardiomyopathy is a condition peculiar to cirrhosis, consisting of diastolic dysfunction, systolic incompetence under conditions of stress (pharmacological or physiological), and electrophysiological abnormalities in the absence of ischemic or valvular heart disease. Krag and colleagues have reported that the presence of baseline reduced cardiac output, a reflection of the presence of cirrhotic cardiomyopathy with systolic incompetence, was associated with reduced renal blood flow and glomerular filtration rate in cirrhosis with ascites. Forty-three percent of these patients developed AKI-HRS during follow-up compared to 5% in those with normal baseline cardiac output. In cirrhotic patients with spontaneous bacterial peritonitis, those patients who went on to develop AKI-HRS despite clearance of the peritonitis had further reduction of their mean arterial pressure at AKI-HRS diagnosis, supporting the role of cardiomyopathy in contributing to the development of AKI-HRS.

Figure 10–1 describes the current concept in the pathogenesis of AKI-HRS in cirrhosis.

KEY READINGS

Adebayo D et al: Renal dysfunction in cirrhosis is not just a vasomotor nephropathy. Kidney Int 2015;87:509.

Bernardi M et al: Mechanisms of decompensation and organ failure in cirrhosis: from peripheral arterial vasodilation to systemic inflammation hypothesis. J Hepatol 2015;63:1272.

Gomez H et al: A unified theory of sepsis-induced acute kidney injury: inflammation, microcirculatory dysfunction, bioenergetics, and the tubular cell adaptation to injury. Shock 2014;41:3.

Shah N et al: Increased renal expression and urinary excretion of TLR4 in acute kidney injury associated with cirrhosis. Liver Int 2013;33:398.

Thabut D et al: Model for end-stage liver disease score and systemic inflammatory response are major prognostic factors in patients with cirrhosis and acute functional renal failure. Hepatology 2007;46:1872.

▶ Precipitating Factors

The aforementioned pathophysiological changes in advanced cirrhosis predispose these patients to the development of AKI-HRS. Any additional perturbation of the hemodynamics or exaggeration of the inflammation can further compromise the renal circulation, resulting in AKI-HRS.

A. Bacterial Infections

In a cohort of 62 patients who developed AKI-HRS while wait-listed for liver transplantation, 42 patients (68%) had infection as the precipitating factor for the development of their AKI-HRS, with urinary tract infection, bacteremia, and spontaneous bacterial peritonitis as the most common infections. It has been proposed that amplification of the inflammation associated with the bacterial infection can cause oxidative stress in renal tubular cell. Together with exposure of the renal tubular cells to DAMPS and PAMPS, which can cause renal tubular cell damage and microvascular changes,

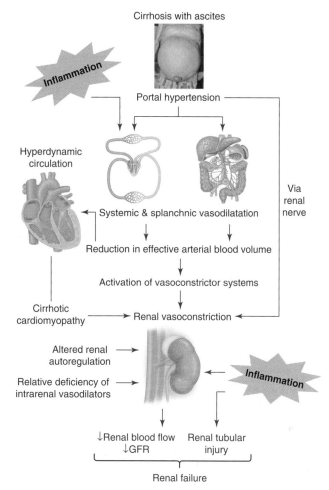

Cirrhosis with ascites

Inflammation

Portal hypertension

Hyperdynamic
circulation

Via
renal
nerve

← Systemic & splanchnic vasodilatation

Reduction in effective arterial blood volume

Activation of vasoconstrictor systems

Cirrhotic
cardiomyopathy → Renal vasoconstriction ←

Altered renal →
autoregulation

Relative deficiency of →
intrarenal vasodilators

← Inflammation

↓Renal blood flow   Renal tubular
↓GFR   injury

Renal failure

▲ **Figure 10–1.** The current concept in the pathogenesis of acute kidney injury—hepatorenal syndrome in cirrhosis. GFR, glomerular filtration rate.

the kidneys are primed for the development of AKI-HRS. Infections also induce the production of various cytokines and endotoxins, which in turn stimulates the production of nitric oxide and other vasodilators, causing further arterial vasodilatation. Therefore, bacterial infections exaggerate the reduction in the effective arterial blood volume and increase the risk of further deterioration of the systemic hemodynamics, further compromising the renal function in patients who may already have infection-related renal damage.

B. Diuretic Therapy

Diuretic therapy, by decreasing the intravascular volume, further exaggerates the reduction in effective arterial blood volume, and predisposes the patient to the development of AKI-HRS. Clinicians have a tendency to increase the diuretic doses when there is an inadequate diuretic and

natriuretic response, despite rising serum creatinine levels. Cirrhotic patients with refractory ascites typically excrete approximately 500 mL of urine per day even in the presence of a "normal" serum creatinine level. Therefore, when increasing doses of diuretics do not result in an increased urine volume or urinary sodium excretion, further increases in the diuretic doses will increase the likelihood of developing AKI-HRS in these patients. Conversely, decreasing the diuretic doses in a patient with refractory ascites and rising serum creatinine may reverse the renal dysfunction.

C. Gastrointestinal Bleed

Acute gastrointestinal blood loss will contract the intravascular volume, with reduction in the effective arterial blood volume, which is compensated by further activation of various vasoconstrictor systems, potentially worsening the renal circulation. Significant contraction of the blood volume can also cause acute tubular necrosis. Patients with decompensated cirrhosis and gastrointestinal bleeding commonly develop a systemic inflammatory syndrome, manifesting as an increase in temperature, tachycardia, tachypnea, and leukocytosis with or without an infection, associated with the activation of many cytokines. Once again, these cytokines can stimulate the production of nitric oxide and other vasodilators. Thus, the patient with gastrointestinal bleeding is predisposed to further exaggeration of the systemic arterial vasodilatation by virtue of excess inflammation. This, in the presence of a contracted blood volume, makes the cirrhotic patient much more vulnerable to the development of AKI-HRS. Gastrointestinal bleeding also predisposes the cirrhotic patient to the development of infection, which in turn predicts rebleeding after control of the initial bleeding episode. The presence of infection in a cirrhotic patient with gastrointestinal bleeding adds to the inflammatory response and to cytokine production, thereby increasing the likelihood of developing AKI-HRS. To support this hypothesis, the routine use of prophylactic antibiotics in cirrhosis with gastrointestinal bleeding has led to a significant reduction in the incidence of AKI-HRS associated with the bleeding episode.

D. Large Volume Paracentesis

The removal of more than 5 L of ascitic fluid initially leads to an increase in the venous return following the reduction of intra-abdominal pressure. This has the effect of exaggerating the systemic vasodilatation within the first 24 hours. This is followed by activation of various vasoconstrictor systems at about 1 week after the large volume paracentesis. This phenomenon is known as postparacentesis circulatory dysfunction, and is associated with renal dysfunction in 20% of patients. This phenomenon can be obviated with the use of intravenous albumin due to its oncotic properties. However, albumin does not prevent every case of renal dysfunction associated with large volume paracentesis. In general, the larger the volume of the paracentesis, the more likely is the chance for developing AKI-HRS even with albumin infusion.

E. Acute on Chronic Liver Failure

Renal failure is common in patients with acute-on-chronic liver failure, a newly recognized syndrome that describes a stage in decompensated cirrhosis, when patients deteriorate rapidly with liver failure, usually following some precipitating event. Renal failure is not common in cases of acute on chronic liver failure that are related to direct hepatocellular insult such as a flare of viral hepatitis, or drug-induced liver failure. However, in cases where the liver injury also involves significant inflammation such as alcoholic hepatitis, renal failure including AKI-HRS is common. Inflammatory

mediators can cause sluggish flow within the renal microcirculation and induce direct renal tubular damage, thereby causing renal failure. The fact that an anti-inflammatory agent such as pentoxifylline has been shown to prevent the development of AKI-HRS in patients with alcoholic cirrhosis supports this contention. AKI-HRS in patients with acute-on-chronic liver failure is more likely to have evidence of structural renal damage, more likely to be prolonged, and more likely to progress to a more severe stage of renal dysfunction than other causes of renal failure in cirrhosis.

It must be emphasized that the most common precipitant of AKI-HRS is bacterial infection, whereas all the other precipitants comprise of approximately 5–6% each of all cases of AKI-HRS. In a small number of cases of AKI-HRS, no precipitant can be found.

▶ Clinical Findings

Hepatorenal syndrome used to be divided into two types, acute or type 1 HRS and chronic or type 2 HRS. The current thinking is that rather than regarding type 1 and type 2 HRS as two distinct entities, the two conditions should be regarded as part of the same continuum of kidney disease in cirrhosis, as there is so much overlap in the pathophysiology of the two types of HRS. Furthermore, type 1 HRS should be regarded as a special form of AKI, and type 2 HRS as a special form of CKD.

Clinically, type 1 or AKI-HRS is characterized by a rapid and progressive deterioration of renal function. The patient is usually ill with severely decompensated liver cirrhosis, jaundice, and hyponatremia. Oliguria and rising creatinine develop over the course of a few days. Type 2 or CKD-HRS is characterized by a steady increase in serum creatinine over a period of months, usually in a patient with cirrhosis and refractory ascites. With the etiologies of cirrhosis slowly evolving over the past decade due to an increased prevalence of diabetes, together with associated nonalcoholic steatohepatitis, and the gradual elimination of hepatitis C infection, metabolic syndrome-related CKD will be on the rise. Thus the scenario of an obese patient with cirrhosis from fatty liver disease who develops AKI-HRS superimposed on underlying CKD from diabetic nephropathy will becoming increasingly common.

▶ Differential Diagnosis

The clinician needs to recognize that renal dysfunction may be present despite a normal serum creatinine. This may be due to two factors: (1) cirrhotic patients are often wasted with a reduced muscle mass and hence lower normal serum creatinine levels, and (2) a high bilirubin level may interfere with the creatinine assay. A creatinine greater than 1 mg/dL (88 μmol/L) in a patient with cirrhosis should alert the clinician to the presence of renal dysfunction.

AKI-HRS represents only a small portion of all causes of renal failure in decompensated cirrhotic patients with ascites. It is a diagnosis of exclusion. To arrive at a diagnosis of AKI-HRS, the circulation of the patient has to be full and there has to be no clear evidence of organic kidney disease.

A. Prerenal Renal Failure

Events that tend to reduce the intravascular volume further such as gastrointestinal bleeding, large volume paracentesis without volume replacement, overzealous diuretic use, or excessive lactulose doses causing diarrhea are likely to lead to prerenal azotemia. To confirm prerenal azotemia, patients should be challenged with a fluid load, preferably with monitoring of their central venous blood pressure filling up to 10 cm of water. Therefore, resuscitation following gastrointestinal bleeding should be as complete as possible. Patients who receive large volume paracentesis of greater than 5 L should receive intravascular volume replacement in the form of a colloid solution, as crystalloids tend to be distributed directly to the peritoneal cavity as ascites and not be retained in the circulation. The International Ascites Club recommends 1 g of albumin/kg of body weight, up to a maximum of 100 g/day, although no formal dose response study on albumin has ever been conducted. It is very tempting to increase the diuretic doses in patients who have large ascites and an inadequate urine output. The end result may be further reduction in renal function as the intravascular volume is further depleted. Often, by reducing the diuretic doses or eliminating the diuretics altogether, the serum creatinine may decrease, accompanied by an improvement in urine output. Significant fluid loss can also result from the gastrointestinal tract with lactulose use in patients who are encephalopathic. These patients should have the lactulose dose reduced and the hepatic encephalopathy managed with the addition of rifaximin. Patient with prerenal azotemia should respond to these measures with the serum creatinine slowly decreasing as the circulation is gradually refilled.

B. Intrinsic Renal Disease

To diagnose intrinsic renal diseases as a cause of AKI, one needs to assess the urine for casts and cellular sediment, a 24-hour urine collection may reveal significant proteinuria of greater than 500 mg/day, or the abdominal ultrasound may show small echogenic kidneys suggesting parenchymal renal disease. Acute tubular necrosis can sometimes be difficult to distinguish from AKI-HRS. Typically, urine sodium of less than 10 mmol/L occurs in AKI-HRS, while a urine sodium of greater than 20 mmol/L is typical for acute tubular necrosis due to impaired reabsorption of sodium from damaged renal tubules. There may be tubular casts in the urine. However, this feature is not always reliable, especially in the late stage of AKI-HRS, acute tubular necrosis can also occur. Acute tubular necrosis should be considered when AKI develops abruptly following hypovolemia, septic shock, or exposure to nephrotoxins, but some of these conditions

can also precipitate AKI-HRS. The recent application of various renal damage biomarkers has helped to differentiate between acute tubular necrosis and AKI-HRS. Renal damage biomarkers are biological parameters that are usually absent in the urine. However, their levels rise significantly with renal tubular damage. When a panel of tubular damage biomarkers is used, the more biomarkers that are positive, the more accurate is the diagnosis of acute tubular necrosis. Unfortunately, these biomarkers currently are still research tools and are not yet widely available for clinical use.

KEY READINGS

Gines P et al: Hepatorenal syndrome. Lancet 2003;362:1819.
Salerno F et al: Diagnosis, treatment and survival of patients with hepatorenal syndrome: a survey on daily medical practice. J Hepatol 2011;55:1241.

▷ Treatment of Acute Kidney Injury— Hepatorenal Syndrome

Figure 10–2 describes the algorithm for the management of AKI-HRS in cirrhosis.

A. General Measures

The first step in the management of AKI-HRS in cirrhosis is to recognize that it has occurred. This requires at least doubling of the serum creatinine within 48 hours or from a stable baseline value within the past 3 months, and the increase is presumed to have occurred within the past 7 days. The next step is to assess for the presence of bacterial infections by culturing all possible sites including blood, urine, ascites, sputum, as well as inspecting the skin surfaces for cellulitis. The threshold for starting antibiotics should be low if the index of suspicion for the presence of infection is high, and antibiotics can be stopped if all cultures subsequently prove to be negative. Simultaneously, one needs to exclude as best as possible the presence of parenchymal renal disease by examining the urine for proteinuria, hematuria, and various casts. The use of recent nephrotoxic drugs or radiographic dyes also needs to be excluded. Once all of these conditions are excluded, the patient is likely to have functional AKI, and a trial of fluid challenge should be given. The recommended fluid is albumin to be given at a dose of 1 g/kg of body weight up to a maximum dose of 100 g/day for at least 48 hours. Patients who have been on diuretics or nephrotoxic drugs should have these withdrawn. Gastrointestinal blood loss should have the blood volume replaced. Often, the AKI will resolve once the precipitating event is removed and volume replacement given. These are cases of volume responsive AKI and most likely represent prerenal azotemia. In those patients whose renal function does not return to baseline levels despite these measures are said to have volume non-responsive AKI, and are likely to have AKI-HRS. Further

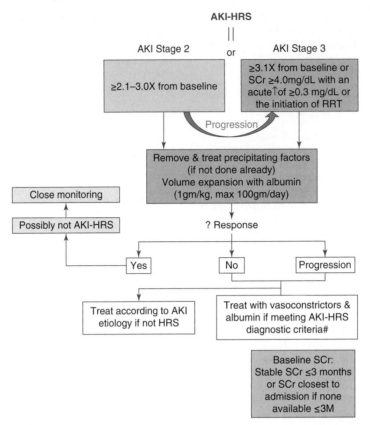

▲ **Figure 10–2.** A suggested algorithm for the management of acute kidney injury—hepatorenal syndrome in cirrhosis. AKI, acute kidney injury; HRS, hepatorenal syndrome; M, months; RRT, renal replacement therapy; SCr, serum creatinine; #, acute kidney injury—hepatorenal syndrome diagnostic criteria as outlined in Table 10–3.

manipulation of splanchnic and systemic hemodynamics with vasoconstrictors will be required.

B. Albumin

Albumin is a negatively charged molecule; it attracts sodium, which in turn retains water, thereby providing its oncotic property. Albumin also has antioxidant and scavenging properties, and therefore is useful in absorbing many unwanted molecules such as proinflammatory cytokines, bacterial products, and reactive oxygen species. Often, the cirrhotic patient's own native albumin exhibits post-transcriptional changes, related to the proinflammatory state of advanced cirrhosis, with the albumin molecule existing in an oxidized form, thereby reducing its ability to perform its scavenger and detoxification functions. Therefore, it is preferable to transfuse some albumin from healthy donors, so that it can assume all of the functions of native albumin.

Albumin is used for both the diagnosis of AKI-HRS, as well as an adjunct therapy to vasoconstrictor treatment in

the treatment of AKI-HRS, as the addition of albumin seems to enhance the beneficial effects of vasoconstrictors. Apart from using albumin as a volume expander to improve the effective arterial blood volume, an endothelial stabilizing function of albumin has also been suggested as a contributor to the improvement of renal function in patients in AKI-HRS, as there has been a correlation observed between the reduction in endothelial activation and improvement in renal blood flow with albumin infusion. Furthermore, a recent meta-analysis showed a dose-dependent increase in survival up to 180 days with albumin infusion in patients with AKI-HRS when used in conjunction with vasoconstrictors. Therefore, albumin is now recommended as an integral part of the management of patients with AKI-HRS.

C. Vasoconstrictors

Vasoconstrictors are the mainstay of treatment for patients with AKI-HRS. Terlipressin is a vasopressin V1 receptor agonist, which acts on the V1 receptors in the splanchnic vasculature by causing vasoconstriction in the dilated splanchnic vessels, thereby transferring some of the splanchnic volume to the central circulation, improving the effective arterial blood volume with consequent reduction in the systemic vasoconstrictor activities, leading to reduced renal vasoconstriction. Norepinephrine and midodrine are systemic vasoconstrictors. They directly act on the systemic circulation, improving the mean arterial pressure and hence the renal perfusion pressure.

1. Terlipressin—In 3 clinical trials, totaling 354 patients with AKI-HRS, terlipressin has been given in bolus doses of 1 mg every 6 hours intravenously, increasing to 2 mg every 6 hours for suboptimal response on day 4, versus either albumin alone or placebo with or without albumin for up to 14 days. Reversal of AKI-HRS was only observed between 24% and 44% of patients, with no significant difference between placebo and terlipressin when individual trials were assessed separately. However, when the results of the two larger North American trials were combined, there were significant more patients who achieved reversal of their AKI-HRS with terlipressin than with placebo (Figure 10–3). These findings have been confirmed by a recent meta-analysis. However, the benefits of terlipressin over placebo for improved survival are less clear.

Terlipressin is generally considered to be safe and well tolerated. It can be administered in the general ward. However,

it is associated with ischemic side effects in approximately 30% of patients. Patients can develop abdominal cramps or pain associated with diarrhea, possibly representing splanchnic ischemia. Other signs and symptoms of ischemia include cyanosis in digits, and occasionally arrhythmia, indicating cardiac ischemia, although myocardial infarcts are rare. The use of a continuous infusion of terlipressin rather than bolus doses has allowed for a lower total daily dose with significant less side effects. A high-serum bilirubin of more than 10 mg/dL (170 μmol/L) and a high-baseline serum creatinine of greater than 5 mg/dL (440 μmol/L) are predictors of poor renal response to terlipressin. In contrast, a sustained rise in the mean arterial pressure by 5 mm Hg during treatment was predictive of a positive renal response. In North America, terlipressin is only available in the context of a clinical trial.

2. Norepinephrine—To date, there are four studies assessing the efficacy of norepinephrine versus terlipressin with concomitant albumin in the treatment of AKI-HRS. However, only two studies had a homogeneous population totaling 86 patients with true AKI-HRS, whereas the other two studies had mixed populations of both AKI-HRS and CKD-HRS patients. Despite this, all studies showed that norepinephrine was equally efficacious as terlipressin in reversing AKI-HRS. Patients treated with norepinephrine had a similar 30-day mortality as those treated with terlipressin, but with significantly less severe ischemic side effects. Most hospitals will require norepinephrine to be administered in the intensive care unit, which adds to the cost of using norepinephrine to treat AKI-HRS. However, given the fact that terlipressin is not commercially available North America, norepinephrine may be a useful alternative for the treatment of AKI-HRS.

3. Midodrine—Midodrine is an α-agonist. It is indicated for the treatment of postural hypotension. However, it has been used off label as a means of improving mean arterial pressure and hence renal perfusion pressure in patients with AKI-HRS. Many studies, both prospective and retrospective, have assessed the combination of midodrine, octreotide, and albumin as a treatment for AKI-HRS. The overall consensus is that the combination can improve renal function, albeit rather slowly. A recent clinical trial comparing terlipressin plus albumin versus midodrine, octreotide plus albumin reported that 70.4% of patients who received terlipressin and albumin had reversal of their AKI-HRS, compared to 28.6% in the midodrine, octreotide, and albumin group. The patients who had reversal of their AKI-HRS had an improved survival. The combination of midodrine, octreotide, and albumin is still widely used in North America, as terlipressin is not commercially available.

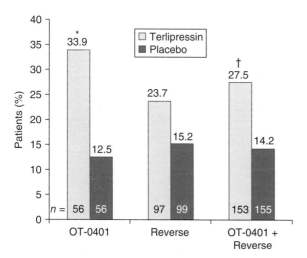

▲ **Figure 10–3.** Incidence of hepatorenal syndrome reversal in the pooled analysis and in the individual OT-0401 (Sanyal AJ et al: Gastroenterology 2008;134:1360) and REVERSE (Boyer TD et al: Gastroenterology 2016;150:1579) studies. *P = 0.008 versus placebo; †P = 0.004 versus placebo. (Adapted from Sanyal AJ et al: Aliment Pharmacol Ther 2017;45:1390 with permission.)

D. Nonpharmacologic Therapies

There is no role for the use of transjugular intrahepatic portosystemic stent shunt, or albumin dialysis in the management of AKI-HRS.

Renal replacement therapy should not be given to patients with cirrhosis and AKI-HRS, unless there is a reversible component of the liver failure, or the patient is listed for liver transplant. For patients who have an indication for renal replacement therapy, continuous dialysis allows for the slower correction of serum sodium and provides greater cardiovascular stability compared to standard intermittent hemodialysis. Otherwise, patients with AKI-HRS are hemodynamically very unstable, and starting renal replacement therapy will only prolong the inevitable dismal outcome.

E. Liver Transplantation

Liver transplantation is the definitive treatment for AKI-HRS. It eliminates portal hypertension and liver dysfunction; the two pivotal pathogenetic mechanisms for the development of AKI-HRS. Hemodynamics improves in the weeks following liver transplantation, together with recovery of renal function. However, renal recovery is not universal, as we now know that prolonged renal ischemia can lead to structural renal damage. Therefore, patients who have AKI-HRS should receive a timely liver transplant, especially in those who do not respond to vasoconstrictor therapy. The United Network for Organ Sharing organization in the United States has recommended that patients with AKI-HRS who have had dialysis for more than 8 weeks in the pretransplant period should be considered for a combined liver-kidney transplant (CLKT), indicating the unlikely event of reversal of renal dysfunction with liver transplant alone.

The European guidelines have similarly recommended a dialysis period of more than 8–12 weeks as the indication for CLKT. In addition, they have also suggested that patients with renal biopsy revealing more than 30% fibrosis and glomerulosclerosis should receive CLKT. A recent retrospective study consisting of a homogeneous cohort of cirrhotic patients with AKI-HRS showed that a dialysis period of more than 14 days was predictive of renal nonrecovery in the post-transplant period. In fact, for every additional day of renal dialysis in the pretransplant period, there is an additional 6% risk of nonreversal of renal dysfunction post-transplant. Survival post-liver transplant for those who reverse their AKI-HRS is excellent at 90% at 1 year. This contrasts with 60% 1-year survival for those who do not reverse their AKI-HRS with liver transplantation (Figure 10–4). The use of living donor liver transplant provides the same excellent results as cadaveric liver transplant in experienced hands. Therefore, this should expand the donor pool available for these patients.

KEY READINGS

Cavallin M et al: Terlipressin plus albumin versus midodrine and octreotide plus albumin in the treatment of hepatorenal syndrome: a randomized trial. Hepatology 2015;62:567.

Gifford FJ, Morling JR, Fallowfield JA: Systematic review with meta-analysis: vasoactive drugs for the treatment of hepatorenal syndrome type 1. Aliment Pharmacol Ther 2017;45:593.

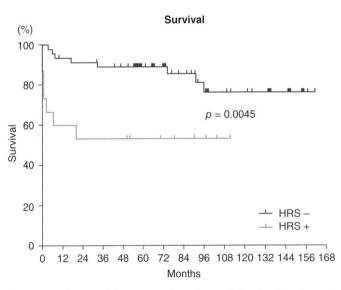

▲ **Figure 10–4.** Survival of patients with type 1 hepatorenal syndrome following liver transplantation. HRS–: patients who recovered from their type 1 hepatorenal syndrome following liver transplantation; HRS+: patients who did not recover from their type 1 hepatorenal syndrome following liver transplantation. (Adapted from Wong F et al: Liver Transpl 2015;21:300 with permission.)

Martin P et al: Evaluation for liver transplantation in adults: 2013 practice guideline by the American Association for the Study of Liver Diseases and the American Society of Transplantation. Hepatology 2014;59:1144.

Salerno F, Navickis RJ, Wilkes MM: Albumin treatment regimen for type 1 hepatorenal syndrome: a dose-response meta-analysis. BMC Gastroenterol 2015;15:167.

Wong F, Angeli P: New diagnostic criteria and management of acute kidney injury. J Hepatol 2017;66:860.

Wong F et al: Outcomes of patients with cirrhosis and hepatorenal syndrome type 1 treated with liver transplantation. Liver Transpl 2015;21:300.

► Prevention

As AKI-HRS is usually precipitated by some factors that either reduces the effective arterial blood volume or increases the inflammatory state of cirrhosis, avoiding these precipitating factors can potentially prevent the development of AKI-HRS.

A. Judicious Use of Diuretics and Lactulose

Diuretic-induced renal impairment occurs in 20% of patients with ascites. This happens when the rate of diuresis exceeds the rate of ascites reabsorption, resulting in reduction in the effective arterial blood volume. The renal failure is nearly always reversible with cessation of the diuretics. Patients with ascites and no edema are only able to mobilize maximally 700 mL of ascitic fluid per day. Any diuresis of more than 700 mL/day will occur at the expense of plasma volume contraction and the risk of renal insufficiency. Patients with peripheral edema appear to be protected from these effects because of the preferential mobilization of edema and therefore may safely undergo diuresis at a more rapid rate (>2 kg/day) until edema disappears.

Lactulose is the mainstay of treatment for hepatic encephalopathy. Its side effect is diarrhea. Excess diarrhea with greater than 4 loose bowel movements a day occurs in about 8% of patients, and this can lead to dehydration and azotemia. With the availability of rifaximin as an adjunctive therapy for the prevention of recurrent hepatic encephalopathy, it is advisable to reduce the lactulose dose and add rifaximin in order to prevent this complication.

B. Prophylaxis against Circulatory Dysfunction

Large volume paracentesis of greater than 5 L without volume replacement is associated with the development of postparacentesis circulatory dysfunction, and this is associated with an increased risk for ascites recurrence, hyponatremia, the development of renal failure and mortality. A meta-analysis in infected cirrhotic patients undergoing large volume paracentesis showed that the use of albumin was able to reduce the incidence of renal impairment and mortality when compared to no albumin, with an odds ratio of 0.34. A recent study in noninfected cirrhotic patients showed that

the use of 6–8 g of albumin with large volume paracentesis, restricting the volume removed to 8 L, was able to prevent the development of renal dysfunction over a mean follow-up period of nearly 2 years. An older meta-analysis suggests that albumin infusion with large volume paracentesis may also provide a survival benefit. However, this has not been confirmed by a more recent meta-analysis.

C. The Use of Albumin in Patients with Proven Bacterial Infections

Albumin infusions, in addition to antibiotic, have been proven to improve renal function and survival in patients with spontaneous bacterial peritonitis in various randomized controlled trials. In the first study, albumin infusions plus cefotaxime prevented the rise in renin, decreased the incidence of renal failure, and improved mortality from 29% to 10% when compared to cefotaxime alone. In that particular study, the patients who benefited the most were those with elevated baseline urea, a bilirubin of greater than 4 mg/dL (68 μmol/L) or a Protime of less than 60% of control at baseline. It was unclear whether albumin infusions were necessary in patients without any of these parameters, as their mortality rate was only 4% without albumin versus 0% with albumin. A subsequent meta-analysis of these four studies have confirmed the benefit of albumin in patients with spontaneous bacterial peritonitis by reducing the risk from 30.6% to 8.3% for the development of renal failure, defined as either a rise in serum creatinine to a final value of greater than 1.5 mg/dL (133 μmol/L), or by 50% if there was baseline renal impairment. In addition, there was also a reduction in mortality in the albumin group. In fact, the pooled odds ratio for renal failure with albumin was 0.21, and that for mortality was 0.34. The subgroup analysis did not show that patients with higher bilirubin or creatinine derived more advantage with the use of albumin when compared to patients without these parameters.

The benefits of albumin in the prevention of renal failure in infections other than spontaneous bacterial peritonitis are less clear. In two randomized controlled trials enrolling a total of 303 such cirrhotic patients, the addition of albumin either delayed the onset of renal failure of reduced the incidence insignificantly without a survival benefit at 3 months. Therefore, the routine use of albumin in cirrhotic patients with infections other than spontaneous bacterial peritonitis cannot be recommended at present.

D. Antibiotic Prophylaxis against Infection

For cirrhotic patients with ascites who have never developed spontaneous bacterial peritonitis, significant predictive factors for its occurrence include a low ascites protein levels (<15 g/L), advanced liver failure with a Child-Pugh score of greater than or equal to 9, and serum bilirubin of greater than or equal to 3 mg/dL (51 μmol/L) or impaired renal function as indicated by a serum creatinine level greater than or equal to 1.2 mg/dL (105 μmol/L). Primary prophylaxis with norfloxacin 400 mg daily in these patients has been shown to significantly reduce the likelihood of the first ever occurrence of spontaneous bacterial peritonitis and AKI-HRS.

Cirrhotic patients with gastrointestinal bleeding have a high incidence of bacterial infections, estimated to be 22–40% within 48 hours after admission. Since infections, whether occult or proven, are the triggers for renal failure in cirrhosis, it is recommended that patients with gastrointestinal bleeding be given antibiotic prophylaxis of norfloxacin 400 mg twice daily for 7 days. The alternative is to use intravenous ciprofloxacin, especially in patients who have to remain fasting because of the bleeding, or in patients with advanced liver cirrhosis. This has been proven to be successful in reducing bacterial infections and renal failure, especially in patients with advanced cirrhosis.

E. In Patients With Alcoholic Hepatitis

Alcoholic hepatitis is a condition whereby there is intense acute inflammation of the liver superimposed on chronic alcoholic liver disease. It is a known precipitant of acute-on-chronic liver failure and often associated with multiorgan failure, including renal failure. The hepatic inflammation from the excess alcoholic presents clinically as liver failure with jaundice, coagulopathy, and encephalopathy. The use of corticosteroid as an anti-inflammatory agent in alcoholic hepatitis has been proven useful in improving survival in certain subset of patients with alcoholic hepatitis. In patients who have contraindications to corticosteroids, the use of a TNF-α antagonist was able to yield a reduction in short-term mortality by preventing the development of AKI-HRS. However, a subsequent more robust multicenter, double-blind, randomized controlled trial including more than 1000 patients with alcoholic hepatitis showed that pentoxifylline, whether used alone or in combination with prednisone, was no better than placebo in terms of improving mortality or preventing renal dysfunction. A more recent meta-analysis of 25 well-designed randomized controlled trials showed that the combination of pentoxifylline and corticosteroids decreased the incidences of HRS or AKI with an odds ratio of 0.47 and the infection risk with an odds ratio of 0.63, and these were significantly better than corticosteroid monotherapy. Corticosteroids alone were able to improve the 1-month survival, but there was no improvement on medium- or long-term survival with either corticosteroids alone or with the combination. However, the use of corticosteroids in patients with severe alcoholic hepatitis was associated with increased susceptibility to infection and infection-related mortality. Therefore, the use of combination therapy needs to be considered carefully in patients with severe alcoholic hepatitis.

F. Avoidance of Nephrotoxic Drugs

Nonsteroid anti-inflammatory drugs (NSAIDs) inhibit formation of intrarenal prostaglandins, which are vasodilatory compounds that counteract the effects of various vasoconstrictors on the renal circulation, and therefore should not be given to cirrhotic patients with ascites. The incidence of renal failure is 33% compared with 3–5% in the general population, although in most cases, the renal dysfunction is transient and renal function recovers upon withdrawal of the NSAID, but in at least one-third of the patients, the renal impairment can be permanent, associated with a reduced 3-month survival. Short-term COX-2 inhibitors appear to be safe, but the effect of long-term use on renal function in cirrhosis is unknown. Patients with cirrhosis and ascites are predisposed to acute tubular necrosis with the use of aminoglycosides and these should be avoided. Monitoring urinary β_2-microglobulin has proven to be not useful in the prediction of acute tubular necrosis in these patients. Angiotensin converting enzyme inhibitors and angiotensin II blockers result in arterial hypotension and predispose cirrhotic patients to the development of renal failure, and therefore should not be prescribed.

KEY READINGS

Chen TA et al: Effect of intravenous albumin on endotoxin removal, cytokines, and nitric oxide production in patients with cirrhosis and spontaneous bacterial peritonitis. Scand J Gastroenterol 2009;44:619.

Kwok CS et al: Albumin reduces paracentesis-induced circulatory dysfunction and reduces death and renal impairment among patients with cirrhosis and infection: a systematic review and meta-analysis. Biomed Res Int 2013;2013:295153.

Thursz MR et al: Prednisolone or pentoxifylline for alcoholic hepatitis. N Engl J Med 2015;372:1619.

Vergis N et al: In patients with severe alcoholic hepatitis, prednisolone increases susceptibility to infection and infection-related mortality, and is associated with high circulating levels of bacterial DNA. Gastroenterology 2017;152:1068.

▶ Prognosis

Fifteen years ago, the development of AKI-HRS in patients with cirrhosis and ascites was almost universally fatal if not treated. This was because patients were frequently diagnosed late in the course of the illness, and the treatment options were very limited. The definitive treatment of AKI-HRS, liver transplantation, was a very limited resource that was available to only a selected few. However, many changes have taken place in the intervening years. The introduction of the new diagnostic criteria of AKI-HRS in cirrhosis means that many patients with renal dysfunction can now be diagnosed earlier in the natural history of the renal failure, with earlier institution of treatment. The improved understanding of the pathophysiology of AKI-HRS means that new treatment strategies can now be tailored to correct the abnormal physiology that has led to the development of renal failure. This is particular true in the understanding that inflammation plays a significant role in the pathogenesis of AKI-HRS. Therefore, any interventions that can reduce the extent of inflammation in cirrhosis will certainly help. Vasoconstrictors have been the mainstay of treatment for AKI-HRS. Survival following AKI-HRS reversal without renal replacement therapy or liver has now increased to 76%, especially with refinements to infusion protocol and careful patient selection. The availability of living related liver donation means that the donor pool for patients with cirrhosis and AKI-HRS is expanding, further improving the prospects of these patients. Therefore, the overall prognosis of AKI-HRS is improving. The onus is on the treating physicians to recognize the onset of AKI-HRS and to initiate prompt treatment. We also need to educate our patients in the prevention of comorbid conditions such as hypertension and diabetes, so to reduce the likelihood of CKD development, a known predisposing factor for AKI-HRS.

■ CHAPTER REVIEW QUESTIONS

1. A 62-year-old woman with nonalcoholic steatohepatitis induced cirrhosis and ascites underwent insertion of a transjugular intrahepatic portosystemic shunt (TIPS) as a definitive treatment of refractory ascites. One month later, an abdominal ultrasound revealed that the TIPS had become stenosed at the portal venous end. So it was organized for her to undergo an interventional radiological procedure to dilate the TIPS. Her serum creatinine immediately after TIPS insertion was 0.84 mg/dL, which was the similar to her serum creatinine for the previous 3 months. However, at the time that the TIPS revision was organized 1 month later, her creatinine was 1.26 mg/dL.
   A. The patient had developed acute kidney injury (AKI) because her serum creatinine had risen by greater than or equal to 50% from a stable baseline in the previous 3 months.
   B. The patient did not developed AKI because her serum creatinine increase did not occur within 48 hours.
   C. We cannot make a diagnosis of AKI without having given her a fluid challenge to determine whether the rise in serum creatinine would return to baseline.
   D. We cannot diagnose AKI without knowing the urine output, urinalysis, or urine microscopy.
   E. The patient may have had a creatinine increase, but the change is too trivial to be of any clinical importance. It is best to repeat the serum creatinine to confirm the rise in serum creatinine.

2. Repeat serum creatinine the next day showed it to be 1.38 mg/dL. Patient reported that her urine output had decreased, and her ascites had not gone down as she had expected. What should be done next?
   A. Urinalysis, urine microscopy, mid-stream urine.
   B. Monitor her blood pressure to ensure that her mean arterial pressure was adequate.
   C. Enquire about diuretic use or other medications prescribed by other physicians.
   D. Perform a large volume paracentesis to relieve the abdominal pressure.
   E. Give her a fluid challenge in the form of albumin.

3. Her electrolytes showed her serum sodium to be 139 mmol/L, serum potassium to be 4.0 mmol/L, serum bicarbonate to be 19 mmol/L. Urinalysis showed her to have a urine glucose concentration of 100 mg/dL, trace of ketones, trace of blood, specific gravity greater than 1.030 and small bilirubin. There was no protein in the urine. Urine culture was negative. Her random blood glucose was 128 mg/dL. What should be done next?
   A. Rehydrate her with normal saline.
   B. Rehydrate her with albumin.
   C. Make a referral to the diabetic clinic.
   D. She needs a glucose tolerance test.
   E. She needs education about a diabetic diet.

4. This patient's serum creatinine continued to climb despite interventions. It reached a reading of 2.17 mg/dL 12 days after it was noted to rise.
   A. The patient did not have acute hepatorenal syndrome because her serum creatinine had not reached the threshold of 2.5 mg/dL yet.
   B. The patient had developed AKI-HRS.
   C. The patient had not developed AKI-HRS because her serum creatinine had not increased by twofold within 14 days.
   D. She should be admitted for fluid challenge and monitoring of blood pressure.
   E. She should have her TIPS revised, as this will improve filling of her central circulation by having some of the splanchnic volume transferred to the central compartment with opening up of her TIPS.

5. The patient was admitted into hospital for further management. Her liver function has remained somewhat compromised, with her serum bilirubin at 5.29 mg/dL, and her international normalized ratio at 1.84. The respective values before her TIPS insertion were 1 mg/dL and 1.41. However, her liver enzymes have remained normal. You suggested

A. Start her on a combination of midodrine, octreotide, and albumin, as she now has established acute or type 1 hepatorenal syndrome.

B. Enquire whether there is terlipressin available through a clinical trial, as that is the best treatment option for acute or type 1 hepatorenal syndrome.

C. Transfer her to intensive care unit to start norepinephrine infusion.

D. Obtain a liver transplant consult as this patient's condition is deteriorating.

E. Obtain a nephrology consult, as this patient may need dialysis in the near future, since her rise in serum creatinine has been very rapid.

Rhabdomyolysis

Sana F. Khan, MD

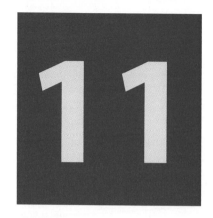

11

▸ Elevated creatine kinase (CK) levels greater than five times upper limit of normal.

▸ Muscle pain, tenderness, or weakness.

▶ General Considerations

Rhabdomyolysis is a clinical disorder characterized by skeletal muscle breakdown and release of intracellular contents (myoglobin, electrolytes, intracellular enzymes) into the circulation. Approximately 26,000 cases occur annually in the United States. The common clinical presentation includes muscle pain, weakness, tea- or dark-colored urine (myoglobinuria), and elevation of creatine kinase (CK) greater than five times upper limit of normal. Myoglobin is readily filtered by the glomerulus, and in high levels it can lead to renal tubular injury and acute kidney injury (AKI). The severity of illness ranges from asymptomatic elevations in CK to life-threatening electrolyte imbalances, intravascular volume depletion, and complications from AKI.

▶ Pathogenesis

Table 11–1 lists common causes of rhabdomyolysis.

The manifestations of rhabdomyolysis are a result of muscle cell death. The mechanisms involved include direct muscle injury (trauma) or muscle adenosine triphosphate (ATP) depletion. Trauma leading to muscle compression has been described in several situations. Crush injuries sustained in earthquakes and accidents are a common cause of rhabdomyolysis. Similar prolonged muscle compression is seen during prolonged surgical procedures as well as vascular occlusion (tourniquet use). Effects of muscle compression are also evident in prolonged immobilization,

resulting in limb compression. Normal individuals are noted to have developed rhabdomyolysis following intense physical exertion. Several cases of rhabdomyolysis have been noted in extreme conditioning programs involving repetitive, high-intensity exercise. Studies have demonstrated that these participants have concomitant significant fluid losses and elevation of body temperature. Sickle cell trait has also been associated with a significantly high risk of exertional rhabdomyolysis. Besides direct muscle injury, decreased muscle energy stores are thought to be contributory to development of rhabdomyolysis. Injury threshold is also lowered in strenuous activity in physically untrained individuals, during fasting states and extremely hot conditions. Certain pathologic states including grand mal seizures and delirium tremens can lead to rhabdomyolysis in normal individuals.

Recurrent episodes of rhabdomyolysis usually reflect an underlying inherited defect in muscle metabolism. The mechanism of muscle breakdown is assumed to be insufficient ATP in the muscle cells. These genetic defects include disorders of glycolysis or glycogenolysis, lipid metabolism, and mitochondrial disorders. Examples include carnitine palmitoyltransferase deficiency and myophosphorylase deficiency. Specific diagnostic tests can identify these abnormalities.

Rhabdomyolysis has also been associated with various electrolyte and endocrine disorders. During exercise, potassium release mediates local vasodilation and increased muscle blood flow. Profound hypokalemia (<2.5 mEq/L) has been shown to decrease blood flow and contribute to ischemic damage. Severe hypophosphatemia has been associated with rhabdomyolysis in alcoholic patients as well as refeeding syndrome. Hyponatremia has also been reported with rhabdomyolysis in some athletes although a direct pathophysiological link is uncertain. Hypothyroidism, as well as electrolyte disorders accompanying diabetic ketoacidosis, and hyperglycemic hyperosmotic states have also been associated with rhabdomyolysis.

Table 11-1. Causes of rhabdomyolysis.

Category	Common Causes
Traumatic	Crush injuries, multiple trauma, immobilization, vascular or orthopedic surgery
Exertion/hyperkinetic states	Strenuous exercise, presence of sickle cell trait, seizures, delirium tremens
Genetic defects	Disorders of glycolysis or glycogenolysis Disorders of lipid metabolism Mitochondrial disorders Malignant hyperthermia
Metabolic disorders	Hypokalemia, hypophosphatemia, acute hyponatremia, diabetic ketoacidosis, hyperosmotic states
Infections	HIV, Coxsackie virus, influenza A and B *Clostridium perfringens, Legionella, Staphylococcus aureus, Streptococcus pyogenes*
Drugs and toxins	Statins, fibrates, alcohol, heroin, cocaine, ecstasy Carbon monoxide, snake venom, bee sting, Haff disease

HIV, human immunodeficiency virus.

Several drugs cause rhabdomyolysis. Common drugs of abuse that have been implicated include heroin, lysergic acid diethylamide (LCD), cocaine, ecstasy, and amphetamine derivatives. Drug-induced agitation and hyperthermia (overstimulation of β_3-adrenergic receptors in muscle) have been shown to be the mechanism of rhabdomyolysis. Prescription drugs most commonly causing muscle breakdown have been noted to be antipsychotics, 3-hydroxy-3-methylglutaryl coenzyme A (HMG-Co-A) reductase inhibitors (statins), selective serotonin reuptake inhibitors (SSRIs), and colchicine, among others. Rhabdomyolysis due to prescription drugs has been noted to be due to direct toxicity (statins, colchicine) or drug interactions leading to elevated levels of toxic substances. Statin-induced toxicity is potentiated by macrolide antibiotics, fibrates, and cyclosporine, via increased statin concentrations due to competition for the CYP3A4 enzyme system.

Several infections (see Table 11-1) are known to be associated with rhabdomyolysis. Acute viral infections have been shown to by myotoxic, whereas several bacterial infections are also well known causes of rhabdomyolysis. In patients without direct muscle infection, toxicity may be caused by toxins or associated hyperthermia and dehydration.

Other exposures may also result in rhabdomyolysis via direct toxicity in addition to effecting muscle energy production. Examples include carbon monoxide, snake venom, bee stings, ingestion of fish toxins (Haff disease), and mushroom poisoning.

Disorders associated with hyperthermia are known to be associated with rhabdomyolysis. Malignant hyperthermia is a rare genetic abnormality of the ryanodine receptor. Manifestations include rhabdomyolysis, acidosis, hypoxia, and muscle contraction occurring during anesthesia, and are precipitated by succinylcholine and volatile anesthetics. Similarly, neuroleptic malignant syndrome (fevers, rigidity, dystonia) has been known to occur after exposure to neuroleptic drugs.

▶ Prevention

There is an increase in popularity of extreme conditioning programs promoting high-intensity functional training. Such extreme repetitious exercise in untrained individuals has been shown to result in muscle injury. For all exercise, a gradual increase in training would allow individuals to be safely conditioned, and avoid serious complications. Additionally, extreme heat conditions, as well as water and electrolyte depletion, should be avoided. Recreational drugs used for enhancing performances (cocaine, amphetamines) should be avoided. Prevention of rhabdomyolysis in patients using offending prescription medications is a more difficult issue. Statin discontinuation is recommended in symptomatic patients, as well as those with 10-fold rise in CK levels.

▶ Clinical Findings

A. Symptoms and Signs

The clinical presentation of rhabdomyolysis has marked variations, with more than half of all patients being asymptomatic, whereas others may experience severe myalgias. The classic symptoms associated with rhabdomyolysis are muscle pain, weakness, and the presence of dark-colored urine. Additionally, local stiffness and edema may be present. Muscle pain is prominent in proximal muscle groups, as well as lower back and calves. Patients with resulting AKI may also present with oliguria and anuria.

B. Laboratory Findings

The hallmark of rhabdomyolysis is an elevation in CK levels. The CK is generally entirely the CK-MM isoform (dominant in skeletal muscle). Serum CK levels at presentation may range from five times upper limit of normal to over 100,000 IU/L. CK levels usually peak at 24–72 hours following muscle injury. The $t_{1/2}$ of CK is approximately 48 hours, and levels decline by 40–50% each consecutive day. Additional lab abnormalities include elevated lactate dehydrogenase (LDH), aspartate aminotransferase (AST), and alanine aminotransferase (ALT) levels.

Release of organic acids from muscle breakdown results in an anion gap acidosis. Additionally, the release of intracellular nucleosides results in hyperuricemia. Elevation of creatinine levels is often seen, and it results from conversion of creatine (released from nonviable muscle cells).

Creatinine levels also rise in those individuals with AKI. Additional metabolic derangements include hyperkalemia and hyperphosphatemia. Hyperkalemia is more pronounced in patients with AKI. Additionally, hypocalcemia may occur due to calcium sequestration in damaged muscle during early rhabdomyolysis. Hypercalcemia may be evident in the recovery phase, due to release from injured muscle.

Myoglobin (a heme-containing protein) is released from damaged muscle and subsequently excreted in the urine, resulting in red to brown urine. However, due to its rapid rate of metabolism, routine urine testing may be negative for myoglobinuria.

▶ Differential Diagnosis

Myoglobinuria (though not always present) causes reddish-brown discoloration of urine. Differentials for such discoloration include hematuria, hemoglobinuria, and drug metabolites. Urine microscopy (which will not show red blood cells in patients with rhabdomyolysis) in addition to serum hemolysis (such as LDH and haptoglobin) laboratory tests can help distinguish these conditions. Additionally, serum CK levels are unlikely to be elevated in such cases (except for traumatic rhabdomyolysis with concurrent trauma to urinary tract).

Serum CK levels may be elevated in myocardial infarction. The CK-MM isotype is elevated, in addition to other specific cardiac enzymes. Moreover, rhabdomyolysis is unlikely to present with symptoms and electrocardiographic (ECG) changes consistent with myocardial infarction. Patients with inflammatory myopathies often present with elevated CK levels, myoglobinuria, and myalgias. These patients can be differentiated from patients with rhabdomyolysis due to chronicity of disease, presence of auto-antibodies, and other systemic features.

▶ Complications

AKI is the most serious complication of rhabdomyolysis, and its incidence ranges between 10% and 50%. AKI as a complication of rhabdomyolysis represents approximately 7–10% of all cases of AKI in the United States. Intravascular volume depletion due to muscular fluid sequestration, tubular cast formation, and myoglobin-induced tubular toxicity are pathophysiologic mechanisms of AKI. Though directly nephrotoxic, myoglobin rarely causes AKI in the absence of predisposing volume depletion, ischemia, and acidosis. Myoglobin becomes concentrated along the tubules and precipitates and causes obstructive cast formation, more so in acidic urine. Additionally, high uric acid generation and urinary excretion result in additional tubular obstruction due to uric acid casts. CK levels are not a predictor of AKI in rhabdomyolysis, though development of kidney injury is less likely if serum levels are less than 5000 U/L. A prediction score (McMahon score) for composite outcome for renal replacement therapy or in-hospital

Table 11–2. McMahon risk prediction score.

Variable	Score
Age	
>50 to ≤70 years	1.5
>70 to ≤80 years	2.5
≥80 years	3.0
Female sex	1
Initial creatinine	
1.4–2.2 mg/dL	1.5
>2.2 mg/dL	3.0
Initial calcium <7.5 mg/dL	2.0
Initial CK >40,000 U/L	2.0
Initial phosphate	
4–5.4 mg/dL	1.5
>5.4 mg/dL	2.0
Underlying cause other than seizures, syncope, exercise, statins, or myositis	3.0
Initial serum bicarbonate <19 mEq/L	2.0

mortality has been developed and validated in small studies. Significant predictors of the composite outcome were age, female sex, cause of rhabdomyolysis, initial creatinine, CK, phosphate, calcium, and bicarbonate levels. Variables with assigned scores are listed in Table 11–2. Using this prediction model, patients with a score less than 5 were found to have low risk (<3%) for severe AKI or death, whereas patients with a score greater than 10 were at a higher risk (>59%).

Additional concurrent complications include hypovolemia due to muscle fluid sequestration. As mentioned in laboratory findings, electrolyte abnormalities are a result of muscle necrosis. Severe hyperkalemia, metabolic acidosis, and hypocalcemia may lead to cardiac arrhythmias.

Compartment syndrome is another potential complication of rhabdomyolysis. Increased muscle edema in a closed space may be more evident after fluid resuscitation, resulting in worsening limb ischemia.

Rarely, severe rhabdomyolysis may be associated with disseminated intravascular coagulation due to systemic release of intramuscular prothrombotic substances.

▶ Treatment

Treatment of the underlying cause of muscle injury is the first component of rhabdomyolysis management. In addition to management of causative insult, prevention of AKI and associated metabolic abnormalities are the cornerstone of rhabdomyolysis treatment.

Intravenous (IV) fluid replacement is essential in rhabdomyolysis management. Capillary damage and fluid leakage result in a state of volume depletion, which needs rapid correction. The goal of fluid management is to increase renal perfusion and urinary flow rate, thereby minimizing tubular cast formation and increasing potassium excretion. The optimal fluid and rate of repletion are unclear. Types of IV fluids used in studies have varied from 5% dextrose with 0.45% normal saline, lactated Ringer solution, normal saline, and normal saline with varying concentrations of sodium bicarbonate. Rate of infusions has been reported as an hourly rate of 200–400 mL/h as well as daily total volume of 4–8 L/day. No studies have directly compared the efficacy of different types and rates of fluid administration. In certain studies, fluids are titrated to maintain urine output of 200–300 mL/h. Patients with serum CK levels less than 5000 to 10,000 U/L are thought to be at low risk for development of AKI and do not require aggressive IV fluids. In patients with CK greater than 5000 U/L, fluid resuscitation is continued until plasma CK levels decrease to less than 5000 U/L.

Forced alkaline diuresis to achieve urine pH greater than 6.5 is thought to decrease myoglobin toxicity. The use of bicarbonate infusion for prevention of AKI is based on the concept of decreasing myoglobin cast formation in an alkaline urine environment. Despite this theoretical benefit, there is no clear data on an alkaline diuresis being superior to saline diuresis in AKI prevention. Additionally, potential risks from alkalinization include worsening hypocalcemia, reduced ionized calcium levels, and promoting calcium phosphate deposition.

Use of loop diuretics and mannitol to increase urinary flow has also been debated in the prevention of AKI; however, the benefit has not been established and these therapies cannot be routinely recommended. Retrospective studies have yielded conflicting results.

The use of dialysis and extracorporeal therapy to remove myoglobin and uric acid in order to prevent AKI has not been shown. However, renal replacement therapy is indicated in severe AKI complicated by volume overload, hyperkalemia, metabolic acidosis, and uremia.

In addition to prevention of AKI, therapeutic goals also involve correction of metabolic abnormalities including hyperkalemia, hypocalcemia, hyperphosphatemia, and hyperuricemia. Hyperkalemia is the only anomaly requiring rapid correction for prevention of cardiac arrhythmias. Hypocalcemia correction with calcium chloride or calcium gluconate needs to be more judicious, given concern for hypercalcemia as well as leading to a rise in the calcium × phosphorus product with the risk of ectopic calcification. Thus, calcium replacement should be reserved unless patients are symptomatic or with severe hyperkalemia associated with ECG changes.

▶ **Prognosis**

The overall prognosis of patients with rhabdomyolysis-induced AKI is favorable, with most patients recovering to normal or near-normal renal function. Some studies have shown increased association of mortality and rhabdomyolysis, with the effect on mortality mediated by AKI rather than rhabdomyolysis. A recent study has reported an 8% incidence of 30-day death or dialysis. Patients with initial estimated glomerular filtration rate (eGFR) greater than 60 mL/min/1.73 m^2 appeared to be at low risk of these outcomes.

KEY READINGS

Altintepe L et al: Early and intensive fluid replacement prevents acute renal failure in the crush cases associated with spontaneous collapse of an apartment in Konya. Ren Fail 2007; 6:737.

Aynardi MC, Jones CM: Bilateral upper arm compartment syndrome after a vigorous cross-training workout. J Shoulder Elbow Surg 2016;3:e65.

Bagley WH, Yang H, Shah KH: Rhabdomyolysis. Intern Emerg Med 2007;2:210.

Banhidy NF, Banhidy FP: Sickle cell trait and rhabdomyolysis among US army soldiers. N Engl J Med 2016;375:1695.

Bosch X, Poch E, Grau JM: Rhabdomyolysis and acute kidney injury. N Engl J Med 2009;361:62.

Bouchama A, Knochel JP: Heatstroke. N Engl J Med 2002;346:1978.

Brogan M et al: Freebie rhabdomyolysis: a public health concern. Spin class induced rhabdomyolysis. Case reports and review of literature. Am J Med 2017;130:484.

Brown CV et al: Preventing renal failure in patients with rhabdomyolysis: do bicarbonate and mannitol make a difference? J Trauma 2005;56:1191.

Cho YS, Lim H, Kim SH: Comparison of lactated Ringer's solution and 0.9% saline in the treatment of rhabdomyolysis induced by doxylamine intoxication. Emerg Med J 2007;24:276.

Giannoglou GD, Chatzizisis YS, Misirli G: The syndrome of rhabdomyolysis: pathophysiology and diagnosis. Eur J Intern Med 2007;18:90.

Grunau BE et al: Characteristics and thirty-day outcomes of emergency department patients with elevated creatine kinase. Acad Emerg Med 2014;6:631.

Gunal AI et al: Early and vigorous fluid resuscitation prevents acute renal failure in the crush victims of catastrophic earthquakes. J Am Soc Nephrol 2004;7:1862.

Hohenegger M: Drug induced rhabdomyolysis. Curr Opin Pharmacol 2012;12:335.

Holt SG, Moore KP: Pathogenesis and treatment of renal dysfunction in rhabdomyolysis. Intensive Care Med 2001;27:803.

Huerta-Alardin AL, Varon J, Marik PE: Bench-to-bedside review: rhabdomyolysis—an overview for clinicians. Crit Care 2005; 9:158.

Iraj N et al: Prophylactic fluid therapy in crushed victims of Bam earthquake. Am J Emerg Med 2011;7:738.

Kalil MA, Saab BR: Resistance exercise-induced rhabdomyolysis. Need for immediate intervention and proper counseling. Aust Fam Physician 2016;45:898.

Knochel JP: Hypophosphatemia and rhabdomyolysis. Am J Med 1992;92:455.

Landau ME et al: Exertional rhabdomyolysis: a clinical review with a focus on genetic influences. J Clin Neuromuscul Dis 2012;13:122.

McMahon GM, Zeng X, Waikar SS: A risk prediction score for kidney failure or mortality in rhabdomyolysis. JAMA Intern Med 2013;19:1821.

Mehmet SS et al: Disaster nephrology: a new concept for an old problem. Clin Kidney J 2015;8:300.

Melli G, Chaudhry V, Cornblath DR: Rhabdomyolysis: an evaluation of 475 hospitalized patients. Medicine (Baltimore) 2005;84:377.

Olson SA, Glasgow RR: Acute compartment syndrome in lower extremity muscular trauma. J Am Acad Orthop Surg 2005;13:436.

Oshima Y: Characteristics of drugs-associated rhabdomyolysis: analysis of 8610 cases reported to the US Food and Drug Administration. Intern Med 2011;50:845.

Pariser JJ et al: Rhabdomyolysis after major urologic surgery: epidemiology risk factors and outcomes. Urology 2015; 6:1328.

Paul V et al: Rhabdomyolysis after fish consumption: Haff's disease. QJM 2014;107:67.

Sauret JM, Marinides G, Wang GK: Rhabdomyolysis. Am Fam Physician 2002;65:907.

Simpson JP et al: Rhabdomyolysis and acute kidney injury: creatine kinase as a prognostic marker and validation of the McMahon Score in a 10-year cohort: a retrospective observational evaluation. Eur J Anaesthesiol 2016;12:906.

Stewart IJ et al: Rhabdomyolysis among critically ill combat casualties: associations with acute kidney injury and mortality. J Trauma Acute Care Surg 2016;3:492.

Torres PA et al: Rhabdomyolysis: pathogenesis, diagnosis and treatment. Oschsner J 2015;15:58.

Van Staa TP et al: Predictors and outcomes of increases in creatine phosphokinase concentrations or rhabdomyolysis risk during statin treatment. Br J Clin Pharmacol 2014;78:649.

Vanholder R et al: Rhabdomyolysis. J Am Soc Nephrol 2000;11:1553.

Warren JD, Blumbergs PC, Thompson PD: Rhabdomyolysis: a review. Muscle Nerve 2002;25:332.

■ CHAPTER REVIEW QUESTIONS

1. A 22-year-old woman presents to the emergency department with severe upper arm pain, red urine, and generalized weakness. She recently underwent a high-intensity-resistance training workout 48 hours prior to presentation. She has no history of prescription or other drug use.

   Evaluation reveals blood pressure 130/70 mm Hg and pulse 110 beats/min. Physical examination is positive for tenderness to palpation over proximal arms bilaterally.

   Laboratory data

CBC	Normal
Creatinine	1.5 mg/dL
Sodium	135 mEq/L
Potassium	5.2 mEq/L
Chloride	110 mEq/L
Bicarbonate	21 mEq/L
Phosphorous	5.4 mEq/L
Urinalysis	3+ blood, negative protein, 0 red blood cell count per high-power field (RBC/hpf)

   What is the most likely diagnosis?
   A. Polymyositis
   B. Rhabdomyolysis
   C. IgA nephropathy
   D. Acute glomerulonephritis

2. A 68-year-old man with a history of diabetes, hypertension, and coronary artery disease presents for evaluation of generalized fatigue and myalgias. One month ago he was hospitalized for angina, during which high-dose atorvastatin was added on discharge. Other medications include aspirin, metoprolol, amlodipine, lisinopril, and insulin. The patient reports compliance with all medications.

   Examination reveals blood pressure 140/70 mm Hg and heart rate 65 beats/min. Physical examination is positive for generalized muscle tenderness.

   Laboratory data

CBC	Normal
Sodium	138 mEq/L
Potassium	4.5 mEq/L
Chloride	112 mEq/L
Bicarbonate	22 mEq/L
Creatinine	1.0 mg/dL
CK	3000 U/L

   What is the next best step in this patient's management?
   A. Discontinuation of atorvastatin
   B. Normal saline infusion at 500 mL/h
   C. Cardiology evaluation for possible acute coronary syndrome (ACS)
   D. Sodium bicarbonate infusion

3. A 13-year-old boy is brought to the emergency department with myalgias, fatigue, and reddish-brown urine. Myalgias and fatigue started 15 minutes into soccer practice. Similar situations have occurred during the past two practices. The patient is new to playing field sports. He shows no history of prescription or other medication use. He has remained asymptomatic between these episodes.

Examination reveals blood pressure 110/60 mm Hg and heart rate 90 beats/min. Physical examination is positive for generalized tenderness to palpation.

Laboratory data

Blood glucose	160 mg/dL
Sodium	136 mEq/L
Potassium	5.2 mEq/L
Chloride	110 mEq/L
Bicarbonate	22 mEq/L
Creatinine	0.8 mEq/L
CK	4000 U/L
Urinalysis	3+ blood, negative protein, urine microscopy 0 RBC/hpf

What is the next step in diagnostic workup?
A. Cortisol stimulation test
B. Enzyme studies and muscle biopsy
C. Thyroid function test
D. Glucose tolerance test

4. A 55-year-old man is trapped following a motor vehicle collision. Emergency crews at the scene manage to extricate the patient after 2 hours. The patient has severe crush injuries to his torso and legs. Blood pressure at extrication is 90/60 mm Hg. What is the best step to prevent rhabdomyolysis-induced AKI?
A. Rapid infusions of albumin
B. Wide open boluses of 0.9% normal saline
C. Lactated Ringer infusion at 100 mL/h
D. Application of tourniquet to reduce blood loss

5. A 22-year-old college student with a history of alcohol and drug abuse is brought to the emergency department after being found down. Duration of current presentation is unknown. Initial workup reveals the patient testing positive for cocaine. Blood pressure is noted to be 180/100 mm Hg and pulse 110 beats/min. On examination, the patient is drowsy but arousable, with dry mucus membranes. Foley catheter is placed, with reddish-brown urine output.

Laboratory data

Sodium	148 mEq/L
Potassium	6.7 mEq/L
Chloride	118 mEq/L
Bicarbonate	16 mEq/L
Creatinine	2.5 mg/dL
CK	35,000 U/L
Urinalysis	3+ blood, trace protein, microscopy with several granular casts, 0 RBC/hpf

What is the most appropriate next step to reduce myoglobin-induced AKI?
A. Continuous renal replacement therapy
B. Initiation of normal saline boluses
C. Initiation of sodium bicarbonate infusions
D. Use of mannitol to increase urinary flow

Contrast-Induced Nephropathy

Blaise Abramovitz, DO

Anushya Jeyabalan, MD

Michael R. Rudnick, MD, FACP, FASN

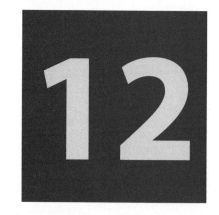

ESSENTIALS OF DIAGNOSIS

- ▶ Rise of serum creatinine of ≥0.5 mg/dL or ≥25% baseline within 48 hours after parenteral contrast administration.

- ▶ Peak in serum creatinine usually occurs within 3–5 days with complete resolution in 7–10 days for most patients.

- ▶ Oliguria and need for dialysis are unusual and are primarily seen in patients with diabetes with severe chronic kidney disease (CKD).

▶ General Considerations

Contrast-induced nephropathy (CIN) is a reversible form of nonoliguric acute kidney injury (AKI) brought about by iodinated contrast. It typically occurs within 24–48 hours after intravascular administration of contrast. Contrast-induced nephropathy is a common cause of AKI whose incidence is expected to grow as the population ages with more chronic kidney disease (CKD) along with an increased incidence of diabetes mellitus (DM). Observational retrospective studies have demonstrated that patients incurring CIN had significantly higher in-hospital and late mortality than counterparts who did not develop CIN, particularly so if they went on to need a dialysis. Multivariate regression analysis, adjusting for baseline differences in comorbidities, strongly suggests that CIN is, in fact, an independent predictor of mortality. Other observational studies suggest CIN may result in CKD or worsening of preexisting CKD.

There are a number of patient-related risk factors for the development of CIN of which the most important is that of underlying CKD. The majority of patients developing CIN have baseline CKD with higher incidences of CIN seen with more severe CKD. Another risk factor is that of DM,

but only if this disease is present concomitantly with CKD. Patients with underlying CKD and DM are at the highest risk for the development of CIN and oliguric CIN. Patients with a similar magnitude of CKD without DM are at lower risk and DM without CKD is associated with minimal or no increased risk. Other risk factors for the development of CIN include congestive heart failure, older age, and a volume-depleted state all of which are probably markers for a low glomerular filtration rate. An additional risk factor may include the concurrent use of nephrotoxic agents, such as nonsteroidal anti-inflammatory drugs. Multiple myeloma has traditionally been considered a risk factor for CIN. However, recent studies using modern contrast agents indicate that patients with multiple myeloma are not at a greater risk, provided that they are volume replete at the time of contrast exposure.

Procedure-related factors will also influence the likelihood of CIN. Most studies suggest that exposure to larger volumes of parenteral contrast causes greater predisposition to CIN. A precise "safe" volume of contrast cannot be recommended since risk of CIN depends on multiple risk factors in addition to volume. Formulas to calculate low-risk volumes rely heavily on the magnitude of underlying CKD. In the past, choice of contrast media, specifically high-osmolar contrast media has been shown to increase CIN risk compared to low-osmolar or iso-osmolar contrast media. However, high-osmolar contrast media is no longer used for studies which require intravascular imaging. Currently, the risk of CIN from low-osmolar and iso-osmolar contrast media is felt to be equivalent. In general, the incidence of CIN is higher with intra-arterial compared to intravenous contrast administration. Recent observational studies suggest that the risk of CIN following intravenous contrast is very low and may not exceed the risk of AKI in similar patients who do not get intravenous contrast. Given the limitations of observational studies, we suggest that patients with estimated glomerular filtration rates (eGFRs) less than 45 mL/min/ 1.73 m² who require intravenous contrast still be considered at risk for CIN.

KEY READING

James MT et al: Contrast-induced acute kidney injury and risk of adverse clinical outcomes after coronary angiography: a systematic review and meta-analysis. Circ Cardiovasc Interv 2013;6:37.

▶ Pathogenesis

Several mechanisms have been proposed to explain the pathogenesis of CIN. Measures aimed to prevent CIN (see Prevention below) are based on these mechanisms. Renal ischemia is currently considered the primary mechanism for CIN. It is known that the outer renal medulla has an extremely low oxygen tension (Po₂ 10–20 mm Hg), as the result of countercurrent oxygen exchange and removal between vasa rectae and utilization of oxygen by active tubular transport of sodium by the ascending loop of Henle. Administration of contrast media has been shown to selectively further reduce oxygen tension in this area of the kidney by a two-pronged mechanism. The first is reduction in renal blood flow, mediated by release of vasoconstrictive compounds such as endothelin and adenosine, an effect that is magnified by blockade or reduction of vasodilatory compounds such as nitric oxide and prostaglandins. The second is increased oxygen utilization caused by increased work of active transport in response to an osmotic diuresis induced by contrast media in the renal tubule. A summary of these effects is depicted in Figure 12–1.

Hyperosmolarity may itself be etiologic in the development of CIN. Intratubular hyperosmolality may activate tubuloglomerular feedback or increase intratubular hydrostatic pressure, either of which could reduce glomerular filtration. Hyperosmolality may also increase tubular cell apoptosis. However, this effect may only be present with very high osmolalities (high-osmolar contrast media) since, as stated previously, low-osmolar contrast media, which are still hyperosmolar with osmolalities of 600–800 mOsm/kg, have clinically not been found to be more nephrotoxic than iso-osmolar contrast media.

There is also evidence to suggest that generation of oxygen-free radicals contributes to the pathogenesis of CIN. This theory would explain the possible ability of N-acetylcysteine (NAC), a free radical scavenger, and sodium bicarbonate, which inhibits the enzymatic formation of free radicals, to prevent CIN (see Prevention below).

Finally, there is evidence to suggest that contrast media cause direct cellular toxicity. Contrast media have been shown to cause proximal tubule cell vacuolization, interstitial inflammation, and cellular necrosis both in experimental animals and in isolated nephron segments.

▶ Prevention

Multiple preventive strategies for CIN have been studied (Table 12–1). A number of these have been proven to

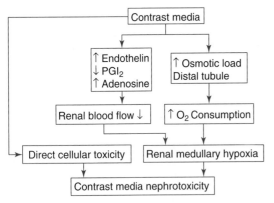

▲ **Figure 12–1** Mechanism for contrast-induced nephropathy. (Adapted with permission from Heyman SN et al: Radiocontrast nephropathy: a paradigm for the synergism between toxic and hypoxic insults in the kidney. Exp Nephrol 1994;2:153.)

Table 12–1. Strategies for the prevention of contrast-induced nephropathy.

Strategies that do not work
Mannitol
Furosemide
Dopamine
Atrial natriuretic factor
Fenoldopam
Hemodialysis
Strategies that may work
Isotonic sodium bicarbonate
N-acetylcysteine
Theophylline
Hemofiltration
Calcium channel blockers
Ascorbic acid
Discontinuation of ACE inhibitors or ARBs
Statins
Remote ischemic preconditioning
RenalGuard diuresis
Current recommended strategies
Employ noniodinated contrast studies
Avoid nonsteroidal anti-inflammatory agents
Spacing between multiple contrast administrations
Minimize contrast volume
Hydration with isotonic saline or bicarbonate
Low-osmolar or iso-osmolar contrast media

be ineffective in well-designed, randomized control trials. Among this group are diuretics, mannitol, dopamine, atrial natriuretic peptide, endothelin receptor antagonists, and fenoldopam. Other strategies have proven more successful and are discussed below.

Extracellular fluid (ECF) volume expansion has traditionally been considered the primary therapeutic intervention to prevent CIN. Correction of volume contraction with ECF expansion is expected to diminish vasoconstrictive responses that contribute to renal ischemia and decrease contact time and concentration of contrast media within the renal tubules. Early clinical studies using historic controls suggested a beneficial role for ECF expansion. Following these studies, volume expansion quickly became the standard of care, although no prospective, randomized, placebo-controlled studies have been conducted to evaluate its efficacy, probably for ethical concerns. Randomized trials comparing various protocols for prophylactic ECF expansion have not been performed. The limited literature suggests that intravenous volume expansion is superior to oral and that isotonic fluids are superior to hypotonic fluids. It remains unclear if longer courses or parenteral fluid administration are superior to shorter courses. In recent years, several studies have demonstrated that isotonic bicarbonate expansion is superior to isotonic saline for the prevention of CIN, but studies of bicarbonate's value have been inconsistent. In our opinion, either fluid is acceptable for CIN prevention. A common protocol for parenteral fluid administration, which we endorse, is as follows. Among outpatients, give 3 mL/kg of isotonic saline or bicarbonate over 1 hour preprocedure and 1–1.5 mL/kg/h during and for 4–6 hours postprocedure. Among inpatients, give 1 mL/kg/h of isotonic saline for 6–12 hours preprocedure, intraprocedure, and for 6–12 hours postprocedure. Studies currently in progress which are adequately powered hopefully will resolve the saline versus bicarbonate controversy.

NAC was first reported in the late 1990s to be a viable prophylactic strategy for CIN. The most commonly employed doses of NAC are 600 or 1200 mg by mouth twice daily the day prior to and the day of contrast administration. Initially, this finding was greeted with widespread enthusiasm, and the use of NAC quickly became common in clinical practice. Subsequent studies of its efficacy have been mixed, as have meta-analyses of those studies. To date, it remains uncertain if NAC is an effective preventive measure, but it is nonetheless often used in clinical practice, based on its safety, simplicity, and low cost. Similar to bicarbonate versus saline, large powered studies of NAC's effectiveness are currently underway.

Reduction in contrast volume is a well-established and reliable means of diminishing the occurrence of CIN in high-risk azotemic patients. When possible, alternative means of radiologic imaging without iodinated contrast should be used to avoid CIN in high-risk azotemic patients.

Unfortunately gadolinium-based magnetic resonance imaging is not an option due to risks of nephrogenic systemic fibrosis in patients with very severe CKD or end-stage renal disease (ESRD). If gadolinium is absolutely required in this population, we recommend using agents whose chelates have high affinity binding for gadolinium (ionic and/or cyclic chelates) in the smallest dose. In patients with ESRD on dialysis or severe CKD with a functional dialysis access, we recommend postgadolinium procedure hemodialysis (HD) to remove gadolinium, although the value of this practice has not been confirmed in scientific trials. If iodinated contrast media must be given to patients with severe CKD, techniques such as use of intravascular ultrasound, automated injectors, dilution of contrast with saline, and CO_2 angiography should be used to minimize the contrast dose.

Because of the high clearance of contrast media by HD and hemofiltration (HF), studies investigating the value of both renal replacement therapies in prevention of CIN have been conducted. The studies which have used HD have shown no reduction in CIN occurrence or any long-term clinical outcomes. Studies which use HF have not been effective when HF is started postprocedure. However, a few studies have demonstrated that if HF is started preprocedure and continued during and after the procedure, there was a reduction in CIN compared to saline hydration alone. Despite this, we do not recommend either HD or HF for CIN prevention due to lack of efficacy and/or limitation of studies evaluating these modalities, the logistic problems with employment and cost, and the potential risks of access placement. Somewhat related are clinical issues with giving iodinated contrast media in an established HD patient. Similar to patients with CKD, intravascular iodinated contrast should be avoided if possible in these patients due to potential negative effects of loss of fluid elimination and small and middle molecule solute clearance due to a loss of residual renal function. Furthermore, there is a common misconception that if intravascular iodinated contrast is given to an HD patient, urgent postprocedure HD to remove the contrast is required. There is no evidence to support this practice, and observational studies indicate that hemodialysis can be safely delayed until the next scheduled dialysis treatment within 24–48 hours.

There are many other CIN prophylactic strategies which have been proposed and are currently under investigation. Included in this group are administration of HMG-CoA reductase inhibitors or "statins," remote ischemic preconditioning, withholding of angiotensin-converting enzyme (ACE) inhibitors or angiotensin receptor blockers (ARBs), and creating large-volume diuresis while maintaining euvolemia with a technology known as RenalGuard. Currently studies of these prophylactic measures have involved small numbers of patients, many of whom are not at high risk for CIN, or have other methodological limitations preventing us at this time from recommending any of these measures.

KEY READINGS

Bernstein EJ, Schmidt-Lauber C, Kay J: Nephrogenic systemic fibrosis: a systemic fibrosing disease resulting from gadolinium exposure. Best Pract Res Clin Rheumatol 2012;26:489.

Briguori C et al: RenalGuard system in high-risk patients for contrast-induced acute kidney injury. Am Heart J 2016;173:67.

Eng J et al: Comparative effect of contrast media type on the incidence of contrast-induced nephropathy. Ann Intern Med 2016;164:417.

Mariani J et al: Intravascular ultrasound guidance to minimize the use of iodine contrast in percutaneous coronary intervention. JACC Cardiovasc Interv 2014;7:1287.

Rosenstock JL et al: The effect of withdrawal of ACE inhibitors or angiotensin receptor blockers prior to coronary angiography on the incidence of contrast-induced nephropathy. Int Urol Nephrol 2008;40:749.

Susantitaphong P, Eiam-Ong S: Nonpharmacological strategies to prevent contrast-induced acute kidney injury. BioMed Res Int 2014;2014:1.

Trivedi HS et al: A randomized prospective trial to assess the role of saline hydration on the development of contrast nephrotoxicity. Nephron Clin Pract 2004;93:c29.

Wang N, Qian P, Yan TD, Phan K: Periprocedural effects of statins on the incidence of contrast-induced acute kidney injury: a systematic review and trial sequential analysis. Int J Cardiol 2016;206:143.

Weisbord SD, Palevsky PM: Iodinated contrast media and the role of renal replacement therapy. Adv Chronic Kidney Dis 2011;18:199.

Xu R et al: Effectiveness of N-acetylcysteine for the prevention of contrast-induced nephropathy: a systematic review and meta-analysis of randomized controlled trials. J Am Heart Assoc 2016;5:e003968.

Zhang B et al: The efficacy of sodium bicarbonate in preventing contrast-induced nephropathy in patients with pre-existing renal insufficiency: a meta-analysis. BMJ Open 2015;5:e006989.

▶ Clinical Findings

A. Symptoms and Signs

Most patients will display no symptoms or signs that would clue one into the diagnosis of CIN. A small subset of patients may develop symptoms or physical examination findings related to uremia or presence of volume overload secondary to the presence of oliguria.

B. Laboratory Findings

The majority of patients who develop CIN will have an elevation in serum creatinine within 24–48 hours after intravascular contrast media exposure. Creatinine will peak within 3–5 days with return to baseline levels within 7–10 days. If urine studies are obtained, urine sodium typically is noted to be low. Evaluation of urine sediment may reveal coarse granular casts and renal tubular epithelial cells, which would be characteristic of findings seen with acute tubular necrosis related to CIN, although these sediment findings are neither sensitive nor specific to the diagnosis. In more severe cases of CIN, creatinine may not peak until 5–10 days. Such severe cases are more likely to be seen in patients with significant CKD. Uncommonly, this subset of patients may require renal replacement therapy.

C. Imaging Studies

Imaging of the kidneys provides no value in the diagnosis of CIN. If there is concern for another etiology of patient's oliguric AKI, imaging studies such as a renal ultrasound to rule out obstructive uropathy may be beneficial.

▶ Differential Diagnosis

The differential diagnosis for CIN includes other causes for AKI, such as ischemic acute tubular necrosis, acute interstitial nephritis, renal atheroemboli, obstructive uropathy, and prerenal changes caused by the addition of or dose adjustments in diuretics and ACE inhibitors or ARBs in the postcontrast period.

Renal atheroembolism is a distinct cause of AKI following contrast exposure that needs to be distinguished from CIN. This complication may arise in any patient who receives contrast media through an intra-arterial route, regardless of whether the contrast was administered for a diagnostic procedure or for an interventional therapeutic indication. Renal atheroembolism is suggested when the rise in serum creatinine begins more than 48 hours after contrast exposure but can also present within 48 hours following contrast administration. On physical examination, the physician should look for livedo reticularis, digital ischemia (purple/blue toe syndrome), retinal embolization (Hollenhorst plaque), or other signs of systemic embolization, which would suggest atheroembolism. Patients with atheroembolism may demonstrate urine or peripheral blood eosinophilia and/or hypocomplementemia on laboratory analysis, abnormalities not found with CIN.

▶ Complications

Complications related to the development of CIN may include progression of an oliguric AKI and may ultimately require, if indicated, renal replacement therapy. This complication, uncommon in its incidence, would most likely be seen in a patient with both severe CKD and DM.

KEY READING

Rudnick M, Feldman H: Contrast-induced nephropathy: what are the true clinical consequences? Clin J Am Soc Nephrol 2008;3:263.

▶ Treatment

There is no specific therapy for CIN once it occurs. The best strategy is one of prevention. Preemptive nephrology consultation to ensure that optimal prophylactic strategies are provided may be of value in certain high-risk azotemic patients.

Once a patient develops CIN, care should be taken to judiciously manage fluid and electrolytes and adjust medications that are renally eliminated. Regular monitoring of electrolytes, blood urea nitrogen (BUN), and creatinine is recommended since it is not possible to predict which patients with CIN will have a short, transient, and asymptomatic course of AKI or demonstrate more clinically severe AKI. Patients developing oliguria, severe electrolyte or acid–base abnormalities, or volume overload may require HD.

Prognosis

Complete recovery of renal function is expected in most patients who have developed CIN. Some patients, of whom the percentage is unknown, will have a permanent decrease in renal function, although not severe enough to require dialysis. Multiple studies have shown that in-hospital and long-term mortality is increased in patients with CIN, especially so when CIN requires renal replacement therapy. Whether this increased mortality can be attributed solely to CIN or other associated comorbidities has yet to be determined.

When to Refer/When to Admit

For a select population of high-risk patients, a preemptive consultation with a nephrologist may be indicated to ensure optimal prophylactic strategies are provided to minimize risk of CIN.

As discussed in the previous "General Considerations" section, there have been many risk factors that have been identified, most important of which is existing CKD. There are some well-validated risk stratification tools to identify this group of patients. However, an eGFR below 60 mL/min/1.73 m² has been identified to be an acceptable CIN risk threshold for contrast administration. Since the risk of CIN is less in patients who receive intravenous contrast media, the risk threshold for these patients is an eGFR below 45 mL/min/1.73 m². For patients who require contrast and are at risk for CIN, intravenous hydration before and after contrast load along with close monitoring of renal function postcontrast load is recommended. Limited periods of intravenous fluid expansion can be achieved in an outpatient setting, especially in patients undergoing coronary angiography. For patients with severe CKD who require intravascular contrast, admission for prolonged intravascular hydration may be necessary.

■ CHAPTER REVIEW QUESTIONS

1. A 52-year-old woman with past medical history of type 2 diabetes mellitus, hypertension, hyperlipidemia, and chronic kidney disease presents with acute onset of chest discomfort, dyspnea, and diaphoresis while gardening. In the emergency department, serum troponin is noted to be elevated with ST depression noted in the lateral leads of an electrocardiogram (EKG). On examination, vital signs are blood pressure of 140/94 mm Hg, pulse rate 92 beats/min, and oxygen saturation of 99% on room air. Physical examination is unremarkable aside from decreased breath sounds noted at the bases bilaterally.

Lab work is notable for creatinine of 2.2 mg/dL and an eGFR of 35 mL/min/1.73 m². The patient is to be admitted and made nothing by mouth after midnight in preparation for left heart catheterization in the morning. What should be your next step in the medical management of this patient?
   A. Begin oral *N*-acetylcysteine.
   B. Provide prophylactic hemodialysis prior to the procedure.
   C. Begin therapy with a statin.
   D. Provide volume expansion with intravenous isotonic normal saline.

2. A 56-year-old man with past medical history of type 2 diabetes mellitus and chronic kidney disease presents to the hospital with complaint of chest tightness and worsening dyspnea on exertion. The patient is diagnosed with ST-elevation myocardial infarction and undergoes emergent left-sided heart catheterization. He had percutaneous coronary intervention with bare metal stent placement for 99% lesion of the left anterior descending artery. Two days after the procedure, he is noted to have abnormal lab work. Basic metabolic panel reveals creatinine of 2.2 mg/dL (admission creatinine of 1.6 mg/dL). Urinalysis is obtained and shows trace protein, 0–1 red blood cells and 0–1 white blood cells. Urine sediment is evaluated and shows muddy brown granular casts. What of the following is the correct diagnosis?
   A. Acute interstitial nephritis
   B. Contrast-induced nephropathy
   C. Prerenal injury
   D. Cholesterol crystal embolism

3. A 48-year-old man was admitted to the hospital with acute onset of dyspnea and found to have pulmonary embolism after computed tomography (CT) of the chest with intravenous contrast. The patient has a medical history significant for type 2 diabetes mellitus, chronic kidney disease (baseline creatinine 1.9 mg/dL), hypertension, hyperlipidemia, peripheral artery disease, and stage II colon cancer. Two days into his admission, he develops an acute kidney injury. Five days after admission, he is discharged for home after creatinine has plateaued and has begun decreasing. Which of the following is considered the major risk factor(s) in this patient associated with the development of contrast-induced nephropathy?
   A. Peripheral artery disease
   B. Chronic kidney disease
   C. Hypertension
   D. Chronic kidney disease and diabetes mellitus

4. A 65-year-old woman is evaluated during a hospital admission for chest pain with ultimate diagnosis of non–ST-elevation myocardial infarction. She is scheduled for an inpatient cardiac catheterization in 24 hours. Her other previous comorbidities include hypertension, type 2 diabetes mellitus, and chronic kidney disease (stage III). On physical examination, blood pressure is 135/95 mm Hg, pulse rate is 75 beats/min, and pulse oximetry shows an oxygen saturation of 99% on room air. The remainder of the examination is unremarkable.

   Laboratory studies show a serum creatinine level of 1.3 mg/dL (estimated glomerular filtration rate of 50 mL/min/1.73 m^2). Urine dipstick demonstrates no hematuria and trace proteinuria. A spot urine protein-creatinine ratio is 40 mg/g. A transthoracic echocardiogram shows normal ejection fraction and no wall motion abnormalities. Which of the following is the most appropriate management to reduce her risk of contrast-induced nephropathy?
   A. Administer N-acetylcysteine
   B. Administer theophylline
   C. Start intravenous fluids 6 hours prior to cardiac catheterization
   D. No intervention necessary at this time

5. A 70-year-old man with history of severe peripheral artery disease is evaluated during a hospital admission with angiography. Three days after the radiologic procedure, serum creatinine began to rise and he became oliguric by the fifth day postcontrast exposure. On physical examination, blood pressure is 187/102 mm Hg, and pulse rate is 68 beats/min. The distal phalanges of both the feet were mottled and dusky. The remainder of the examination is unremarkable.

   Laboratory studies show a serum creatinine level of 7.6 mg/dL with a preoperative serum creatinine of 2.1 mg/dL, and a white blood cell count demonstrated 10% eosinophilia. Urine dipstick demonstrates no blood or protein. Which of the following is the most likely cause of the acute kidney injury?
   A. Allergic interstitial nephritis
   B. Contrast induced nephropathy
   C. Acute glomerulonephritis
   D. Atheroembolic renal disease

Tumor Lysis Syndrome

Mandana Rastegar, MD, EdM

Anushree Shirali, MD

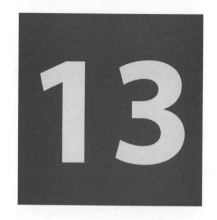

ESSENTIALS OF DIAGNOSIS

▸ Due to tumor cell lysis (TLS), commonly in high-risk hematologic malignancies and/or tumors with large cellular burden.

▸ Results when intracellular contents of nucleic acids, potassium, phosphorus are rapidly released into the bloodstream.

▸ Characterized by laboratory findings of hyperuricemia, hyperkalemia, hyperphosphatemia, and/or hypocalcemia with clinical manifestations of renal, cardiac, and/or neurologic dysfunction.

▸ Knowledge of risk factors of TLS and early detection of TLS are imperative to implementing preventive and therapeutic strategies to reduce morbidity and mortality.

▸ General Considerations

Tumor lysis syndrome (TLS) is a common emergency in clinical oncology. TLS describes a constellation of metabolic abnormalities resulting from the release of intracellular contents into the bloodstream, either spontaneously or more commonly during chemotherapy-induced tumor cell lysis. Cell lysis ultimately results in the characteristic findings of TLS which include hyperuricemia, hyperkalemia, hyperphosphatemia, and hypocalcemia. Clinically, these metabolic derangements can present as acute kidney injury (AKI), cardiac arrhythmias, seizure, and lead to significant morbidity and mortality.

The classification of TLS is divided into laboratory and clinical TLS (Table 13–1). These schemas were first defined by Hande and Garrow in 1994 and were modified and expanded 10 years later by Cairo and Bishop. Cairo and Bishop define laboratory TLS as the presence of two

or more of the classic metabolic abnormalities (hyperuricemia, hyperkalemia, hyperphosphatemia, and hypocalcemia) within 3 days before, or up to 7 days following the administration of chemotherapy, despite adequate volume expansion and the use of hypouricemic agents. The specific values which fulfill diagnostic criteria of laboratory TLS are provided in Table 13–1. Clinical TLS is defined by laboratory TLS accompanied by renal, neurologic, or cardiac dysfunction which is not a direct result of chemotherapy itself. Cairo and Bishop also provide a grading system to assess the severity of TLS based on a 0–5 scale, taking into account the severity of the clinical manifestations (Table 13–2). In 2011, Howard et al. offered modifications to the standard Cairo–Bishop definition of TLS, specifying the simultaneous presence of two or more metabolic abnormalities at the time of diagnosis for the definition of laboratory TLS. They also challenge the criterion of 25% increase from baseline as it may not always be clinically relevant if the baseline value is normal. Last, they also propose that symptomatic hypocalcemia should be included in the definition of clinical TLS. Various groups have objected that the Cairo and Bishop criteria exclude spontaneous TLS, potentially limiting the recognition of severe metabolic disturbances that have the potential for severe patient morbidity. Others have debated that the Cairo–Bishop definition of renal dysfunction of creatinine greater than 1.5 times the upper limit of normal should be replaced with an increase of 0.3 mg/dL in creatinine or a relative 50% increase in baseline creatinine, to better reflect standardized definitions of AKI.

Risk factors for the development of TLS can be divided into intrinsic features related to the tumor and extrinsic features related to the patient's clinical presentation. First, the type of cancer is an important predictor for TLS. A risk classification system based on expert opinion has been developed, incorporating the type and extent of malignancy (see Table 13–2). TLS is most often seen with high-grade hematologic malignancies such as Burkitt lymphoma, acute

Table 13–1. The Cairo–Bishop definition of laboratory and clinical tumor lysis syndrome.

TLS Type	Diagnostic Criteria	
	Electrolyte or Metabolic Product	Absolute Value or Change from Baseline
Laboratory TLS	Potassium	≥6 mEq/L or 25% increase from baseline
	Phosphorous	≥4.5 mg/dL (adults; in children, ≥6.5 mg/dL) or 25% increase from baseline
	Calcium	25% decrease from baseline
	Uric acid	≥8 mg/dL or 25% increase from baseline
Clinical TLS	Laboratory TLS and one or more of the following: 1. AKI: Serum creatinine ≥1.5x ULN 2. Seizure 3. Cardiac arrhythmia or sudden death	

AKI, acute kidney injury; TLS, tumor lysis syndrome; ULN, upper limit of normal.

lymphocytic and lymphoblastic leukemia, and acute myeloid leukemia. TLS has also been reported to a lesser degree in various solid tumor malignancies, including small-cell carcinoma of the lung, breast carcinoma, endometrial cancer, hepatocellular carcinoma, and germ cell tumor. Second, an increased tumor burden, as determined by an elevated lactate dehydrogenase (LDH) two times the upper limit of normal prior to therapy, a white blood cell (WBC) count greater than 50×10^9/L, tumor bulk of greater than 10 cm, extensive metastases, organ infiltration, or bone marrow involvement, also carries a high risk for TLS. Another important tumor-specific feature that increases risk of TLS is its potential for cell lysis, as characterized by a high tumor proliferation rate

and increased sensitivity to chemotherapy. Patient-related features that are associated with elevated risk of TLS include advanced age, male sex, preexisting chronic kidney disease (CKD) with baseline creatinine of greater than 1.4 mg/dL, serum uric acid greater than 7.5 mg/dL prior to any treatment, volume depletion, acidic urine, and concomitant use of nephrotoxic drugs.

▶ Pathogenesis

TLS is the direct result of cell lysis with rapid release of intracellular contents into the bloodstream. In particular, the expulsion of potassium, phosphorus, cytokines, and nucleic

Table 13–2. Risk assessment for TLS includes specific malignancy type, disease extent, and evidence for kidney dysfunction.[a]

Low	Intermediate	High
Solid tumors	CLL treated with biological agent	Burkitt-type lymphoma (early stage and LDH >2x ULN)
Multiple myeloma	Burkitt-type lymphoma (early stage and LDH < 2x ULN)	Burkitt-type lymphoma at advanced stage
CML	Lymphoblastic lymphoma (early stage and LDH < 2x ULN)	Burkitt-type leukemia
CLL treated with alkylating agent	DLBCL, adult T cell, blastoid mantle cell (LDH > ULN and nonbulky disease)	Lymphoblastic lymphoma (early stage and LDH > 2x ULN or advanced stage)
Anaplastic large cell	AML (if WBC = $25–100 \times 10^9$/L or <25×10^9/L and LDH >2x ULN)	DLBCL, adult T cell, blastoid mantle cell (LDH > ULN and bulky disease)
Hodgkin lymphoma	ALL (if WBC <100×10^9/L and LDH <2x ULN)	ALL (if WBC >100×10^9/L or <100×10^9/L and LDH >2x ULN)
Small lymphocytic lymphoma		
Follicular		
Marginal zone B cell		
MALT		
AML (if WBC <25×10^9/L and LDH <2x ULN)		
ALL		
DLBCL, adult T cell, blastoid mantle cell (LDH normal)		

Presence of renal dysfunction alone changes any low risk to intermediate risk and intermediate risk to high risk.
If UA is abnormal or phosphorous or potassium is more than ULN, intermediate risk becomes high risk.

ALL, acute lymphoblastic leukemia; CML, chronic myeloid leukemia; CLL, chronic lymphocytic leukemia; DLBCL, diffuse large B-cell lymphoma; LDH, lactate dehydrogenase; MALT, mucosa-associated lymphoid tissue; UA, urine analysis; ULN, upper limit of normal.
[a]Criteria for pediatric patients may be different than above.

acids which are converted to uric acid, combined with impaired renal, hepatic, and/or phagocytic clearance of these products relative to the high serum burden, is the hallmark of TLS pathophysiology.

Prevention

Because the incidence of TLS varies widely, early recognition of patients at risk of developing TLS is critical, as preventive measures must be implemented prior to treatment initiation. The two key measures are administration of intravenous (IV) fluids for volume expansion and provision of hypouricemic agents, such as rasburicase or allopurinol. Aggressive crystalloid volume expansion is recommended to maintain a urine output of 2 mL/kg/h, typically 3L/day in adults, while monitoring for clinical signs of fluid overload. The initial IV fluid should be isotonic fluid in the form of 0.9% normal saline. Volume expansion reduces the risk of developing AKI by supporting adequate intravascular volume and renal blood flow. Furthermore, targeting high urinary flow rates reduces the risk of uric acid or calcium-phosphate crystal formation, and increases the excretion of potassium, uric acid, and phosphorous. Urinary alkalinization should not be pursued. While increasing urine pH may increase solubility of uric acid, it also favors urinary precipitation of calcium phosphate. Furthermore, IV alkaline fluid may exacerbate the tendency to develop hypocalcemia.

The prophylactic use of allopurinol is recommended for patients at low or intermediate risk of developing TLS. Allopurinol, via its active metabolite, oxypurinol, acts as a xanthine oxidase inhibitor, which impairs the formation of new uric acid, thereby reducing complications of hyperuricemia, detailed later in this chapter (Figure 13–1). Treatment with allopurinol should start 24–48 hours prior to chemotherapy. Depending on the clinical setting, both oral and IV formulations are available and dose adjustments are required in patients with CKD or AKI. A hypersensitivity syndrome has been ascribed to allopurinol. Though rare, it is manifested by fever, rash, and eosinophilia, and it requires discontinuation of the drug. In such cases, febuxostat, a xanthine oxidase inhibitor without the hypersensitivity profile of allopurinol, may be considered. However, decreased availability and higher cost compared to allopurinol have limited its widespread use.

Rasburicase is recommended for patients with intermediate or high risk of developing clinical TLS, and in patients with pretreatment uric acid level of greater than 7.5 mg/dL. Rasburicase is a recombinant urate-oxidase enzyme that promotes the conversion of uric acid to carbon dioxide, hydrogen peroxide, and allantoin, all of which are highly soluble and readily excreted when compared to uric acid. Rasburicase significantly reduces uric acid levels within 4 hours of administration. The Food and Drug Administration (FDA)-recommended dose is 0.2 mg/kg once daily for

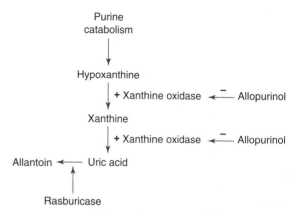

▲ **Figure 13–1.** Diagram of purine metabolism. Purines are converted to uric acid via a series of steps that include the intermediate water-insoluble metabolites, hypoxanthine and xanthine. These steps are stimulated by xanthine oxidase which is negatively regulated by allopurinol. Uric acid is converted to the water-soluble allantoin by urate oxidase, an enzyme that humans lack. Clinically, this is achieved by use of rasburicase, a recombinant form of urate oxidase.

up to 5 days with length of treatment depending on plasma uric acid levels. There are alternative dose recommendations based on TLS risk stratification. Rasburicase should not be used in patients with glucose 6 phosphate dehydrogenase deficiency, due to the high risk of hemolysis and methemoglobinemia triggered by the increased formation of hydrogen peroxide. In conjunction with these preventive measures, patients should be taken off concurrent medications that may have the potential for nephrotoxicity, hyperkalemia, or hyperphosphatemia.

Clinical Findings

A. Symptoms, Signs, and Laboratory Findings

The clinical presentation of TLS is associated with specific laboratory derangements, as outlined below, and may include mild, nonspecific symptoms such as nausea and muscle cramps or severe manifestations such as tetany, seizure, oliguria/hematuria, or cardiac dysrhythmias. Therefore, depending on where in this wide spectrum a particular patient presents, a high clinical suspicion for prompt laboratory investigation is needed for the following electrolytes.

1. Hyperkalemia—Since intracellular potassium concentrations are as high as 120 mEq/L, cell lysis may result in an exuberant release of potassium into the extracellular space. When this overwhelms the normal capacity of muscle and liver cells to uptake potassium, significant hyperkalemia (potassium >6.0 mEq/dL) occurs, particularly if there is impaired renal clearance of potassium in the setting of reduced glomerular filtration rate (GFR). One important consideration when noting an elevated potassium level in a patient with a hematologic malignancy is pseudohyperkalemia, which occurs when blood from patients with severe leukocytosis (WBC >120 × 10^9/L) lyses during phlebotomy or in collection tubes. In true hyperkalemia, patients may endorse mild neuromuscular complaints such as lethargy, muscle cramps, paresthesias, or manifest severe complications, such as cardiac arrhythmias.

2. Hyperphosphatemia and hypocalcemia—Intracellular phosphorus concentrations of malignant hematologic cells may be four times higher than nonmalignant cells. This may rapidly exceed renal capacity for phosphorous excretion and result in severe hyperphosphatemia (phosphorus ≥6.5 mg/dL), especially in the setting of preexisting or concomitant reduction in GFR. As a result, increased serum phosphorous anions may complex with calcium cations, leading to hypocalcemia (serum calcium ≤7 mg/dL) as well as formation of insoluble calcium-phosphate crystals that can result in end-organ damage. Clinical symptoms of hypocalcemia include paresthesias, muscle cramps, seizure, or cardiac arrhythmias such as prolongation of the QT interval.

3. Hyperuricemia—Uric acid is the water-insoluble metabolic end product of the purine nucleic acids, adenine and guanine, that gets converted into hypoxanthine and xanthine via xanthine oxidase. Humans lack the enzyme urate oxidase, which converts uric acid to the soluble allantoin, resulting in a sudden and detrimental rise in serum uric acid levels. Uric acid is freely filtered at the glomerulus, and further handling occurs at the proximal tubule. In TLS, the renal capacity to handle high levels uric acid is overwhelmed, leading to crystallization of uric acid within the tubular lumen. Factors which favor crystallization include low urine volume and acidic urine pH. Uric acid impairs kidney function by both crystal-dependent and crystal-independent mechanisms. Crystal-dependent mechanisms include direct tubular injury from obstruction which stimulates influx of inflammatory cytokines. Crystal-independent renal injury due to uric acid has been attributed to hemodynamic changes such as elevated peritubular capillary pressures, increased vasoconstriction, and reduced renal blood flow.

4. AKI—AKI results from either one or a combination of the following mechanisms: (1) hyperphosphatemic nephrocalcinosis causing tubulointerstitial damage, (2) acute urate nephropathy leading to intratubular obstruction and inflammation, and (3) hyperuricemia causing derangements in renal hemodynamics. A rise in serum creatinine, a rise in blood urea nitrogen, and oliguria are the associated laboratory findings. The spectrum of clinical symptoms may vary from asymptomatic azotemia to gross uremia, causing vomiting, altered mental status, and seizures.

B. Other Studies

Tumor lysis is diagnosed in the appropriate clinical setting with the aforementioned laboratory findings; however, several additional studies can support the diagnosis, especially to guide timely therapy and intervention.

1. Electrocardiogram (ECG)—Hyperkalemia and hypocalcemia can lead to serious cardiac conduction defects and arrhythmias, requiring immediate recognition. Hyperkalemia can manifest as peaked T waves, prolongation of the PR and QRS interval, atrioventricular blocks, or ventricular arrhythmias. ECG changes in hypocalcemia most often present as widened QT interval.

2. Urinalysis—Microscopic examination of the urine may reveal concentrated urine with a high specific gravity, hematuria, and uric acid crystals. Uric acid crystals take on a variety of shapes such as rosettes, rhomboids, needles, or hexagonal plates.

▶ Differential Diagnosis

The differential diagnosis of electrolyte abnormalities and AKI in cancer patients is broad and complex, especially in the setting of cancer treatment and hospitalization. Patients at risk for TLS are often hospitalized, and the two most common causes of AKI in this setting include prerenal azotemia and acute tubular necrosis (ATN). Patients may be volume depleted due to poor oral intake from nausea or from increased gastrointestinal (GI) losses with chemo-associated vomiting and diarrhea. Increased insensible losses from fever and/or sweats may be an additional factor. Prolonged volume depletion may result in ATN, and cancer patients also have additional risk factors for developing ATN. For example, they are more susceptible to infection and, therefore, ATN from septic shock or cytokine release. Additionally, IV contrast for computed tomography (CT) imaging and drugs, such as aminoglycosides, amphotericin B, or platinum-based chemotherapy, are frequently used in cancer patients and may lead to toxic ATN. Other reported etiologies of AKI in hospitalized cancer patients include obstructive uropathy from a compressing tumor or lymphadenopathy, acute interstitial nephritis from immune checkpoint inhibitors or tyrosine kinase inhibitors, and thrombotic microangiopathy with antiangiogenesis drugs, mitomycin C, gemcitabine, and cisplatin.

These broad etiologies of AKI in cancer patients may reduce GFR and cause electrolyte disturbances which mimic the electrolyte disturbances seen in TLS. Therefore, knowing the clinical circumstance, understanding the risks related to the development of TLS, and having high suspicion in the right clinical setting are imperative for early and accurate diagnosis of TLS.

Complications

The clinical complications of TLS include renal, cardiac, and neurologic dysfunction and death and result from a constellation of abnormal laboratory findings. The specific complications of TLS are detailed as follows.

1. **Potassium.** Hyperkalemia may be sudden and severe in TLS, resulting in cardiac arrhythmias. ECG abnormalities include peaked T waves, PR and QRS prolongation, atrioventricular conduction blockade, and, ultimately, cardiac arrest.

2. **Phosphorus and calcium.** The major complication of extracellular phosphorus release during TLS is the rapid chelation of serum calcium by phosphorous, resulting in marked hypocalcemia. The sequelae of hypocalcemia include cardiac arrhythmias, depressed cardiac contractility, hypotension, and death. Furthermore, deposition of calcium-phosphorus complexes in various tissues causes organ injury. In the kidney, nephrocalcinosis may occur and contribute to AKI.

3. **Uric acid.** Elevated uric acid levels may result in AKI by crystal-dependent and crystal-independent mechanisms. Crystal-dependent AKI occurs when hyperuricemia overwhelms the handling of uric acid in the proximal tubule. This leads to formation of uric acid crystallization, particularly when urine pH is acidic, and results in AKI when uric acid crystals obstruct the tubular lumen. Furthermore, uric acid crystals promote the release of various cytokines (MCP-1, MIF, TNF-α) associated with inflammatory kidney injury. Crystal-independent mechanisms of AKI attributed to soluble uric acid revolve around impaired autoregulation, increased peritubular capillary pressures, and reduced renal blood flow. In addition, elevated uric acid levels have independently been demonstrated to impede recovery from AKI due to impaired proximal tubule cell proliferation.

Treatment

Given the significant morbidity associated with TLS, prevention is the most important step in the management of patients at high risk of TLS. As outlined previously, the two major preventive measures include volume expansion with crystalloids to encourage high urine flow rates and use of hypouricemic agents such as allopurinol to inhibit uric acid formation and rasburicase to degrade serum uric acid. If preventive measures fail in avoiding TLS, specific measures are necessary to treat complications such as electrolyte abnormalities.

Of the electrolyte derangements, hyperkalemia commands immediate attention as a delay in diagnosis and treatment carries high risk of mortality. Treatment for hyperkalemia focuses on transcellular shifts or elimination. Transcellular shifts of potassium from the extracellular space to the intracellular compartment may be achieved by use of insulin and/or inhaled high-dose β-agonist therapy. IV calcium may be added to prevent cell membrane depolarization, but it does not directly affect serum potassium levels. These are temporizing measures to address critical hyperkalemia and are susceptible to significant rebound unless elimination methods are instituted. Potassium elimination from the body is dependent on GI and renal excretion. Use of ion exchange resins such as sodium polystyrene sulfonate (SPS) is effective in facilitating GI excretion. SPS binds intestinal potassium in exchange for sodium and is removed via fecal elimination. SPS is generally safe but should be avoided in patients with bowel disease, as it has been associated with colonic necrosis when used in conjunction with sorbitol. Newer orally administered potassium-binding resins such as patiromer may also be options. Loop diuretics are potent drugs in promoting renal potassium excretion and work quickly via IV dosing. If GFR is affected by AKI related to TLS or preexisting CKD, larger doses may be required for effective diuresis and clearance of potassium.

Treatment of hyperphosphatemia focuses on limiting dietary intake and intestinal absorption. The latter requires use of phosphate binders with meals. The choice of binders depends on serum calcium, as hypocalcemia may require calcium supplementation. For severe hyperphosphatemia (serum levels >8 mg/dL), aluminum-containing binders are acceptable for short-term use.

Hypocalcemia should not routinely be treated unless there are demonstrated signs cardiovascular and/or neuromuscular irritability. Calcium replacement in the setting of hyperphosphatemia may encourage formation and tissue deposition of calcium-phosphate crystals. Thus, calcium repletion should be limited to severe, symptomatic cases.

In some cases of TLS, the treatment measures discussed so far are not sufficient to keep pace with ongoing cell lysis and the resulting metabolic abnormalities, particularly when AKI is present and further exacerbates these abnormalities. In such cases, renal replacement therapy (RRT) will be required, usually in the form of intermittent hemodialysis (IHD). If rebound of serum potassium and phosphate occurs despite initiation of IHD, continuous dialysis modalities may be required.

Prognosis

TLS carries a high morbidity and mortality burden. While these data are confounded by many factors, the presence of AKI is specifically associated with higher hospital as well as longer term mortality.

When to Refer/When to Admit

As detailed earlier, the complications of TLS can be fatal, and therefore any patient presenting with an abnormal laboratory value consistent with TLS or is at any degree of risk of developing clinical TLS should be hospitalized for close laboratory monitoring and initiation of preventive and therapeutic maneuvers. Due to the potential of rapid progression into fulminant clinical TLS, nephrology consultation should be sought at the earliest stages of laboratory TLS and/or at the presence of AKI or oliguria.

KEY READINGS

Adeani E, Shirali AC: Chapter 4: Tumor Lysis Syndrome. Onco-Nephrology Curriculum. Retrieved from http://www.asn-online.org/education/distancelearning/curricula/onco/.

Cairo MS, Bishop M: Tumour lysis syndrome: new therapeutic strategies and classification. Br J Haematol 2004;127:3.

Cairo MS et al: Recommendations for the evaluation of risk and prophylaxis of tumour lysis syndrome (TLS) in adults and children with malignant diseases: an expert TLS panel consensus. Br J Haematol 2010;149:578.

Coiffier B et al: Guidelines for the management of pediatric and adult tumor lysis syndrome: an evidence-based review. J Clin Oncol 2008;26:267.

Darmon M et al: Prognostic significance of acute renal injury in acute tumor lysis syndrome. Leuk Lymphoma 2010;51:221.

Howard SC, Jones DP, Pui C: The tumor lysis syndrome. N Engl J Med 2011;64:1844.

Lopez-Olivo MA et al: Rasburicase in tumor lysis syndrome of the adult: a systematic review and meta-analysis. Am J Kidney Dis 2013;62:481.

Mirrakhimov AE et al: Tumor lysis syndrome: a clinical review. World J Crit Care Med 2015;4:130.

Mirrakhimov AE et al: Tumor lysis syndrome in solid tumors: an up to date review of the literature. Rare Tumors 2014;6:68.

Wilson FP, Berns JS: Onco-nephrology: tumor lysis syndrome. Clin J Am Soc Nephrol 2012;7:1730.

Wilson FP, Berns JS: Tumor lysis syndrome: new challenges and recent advances. Adv Chronic Kidney Dis 2014;21:18.

■ CHAPTER REVIEW QUESTIONS

1. Which of the following electrolyte disturbances are seen in TLS?
   A. Hyperkalemia, hypercalcemia, hyperphosphatemia
   B. Hyperkalemia, hypocalcemia, hyperphosphatemia
   C. Hypokalemia, hypocalcemia, hyperphosphatemia
   D. Hyperkalemia, hypocalcemia, hypophosphatemia

2. A 70-year-old man presents to the emergency department (ED) with fatigue, ecchymoses, and gum bleeding for 2 days. Vital signs are stable, and physical examination is notable for gingival hyperplasia, gum bleeding, splenomegaly, and petechiae on the lower extremities. Complete blood cell count (CBC) revealed WBC 150 × 10^9/L, hemoglobin of 8 g/dL, and platelets of 12,000/μL. Other notable laboratory data include sodium 134 mmol/L, potassium 5.6 mmol/L, bicarbonate 16 mmol/L, creatinine 1.2 mg/dL, calcium 6.9 mg/dL, phosphorus 8.2 mg/dL, and uric acid 13.4 mg/dL. Peripheral smear reveals the majority of cells are blasts. The patient is diagnosed with acute lymphoblastic leukemia (ALL). ECG does not reveal any abnormalities. Which of the following therapies should be initiated prior to chemotherapy?
   A. Crystalloid IVF and Kayexalate
   B. Crystalloid IVF and rasburicase
   C. Crystalloid IVF, allopurinol, and Kayexalate
   D. Crystalloid IVF, allopurinol, rasburicase, and hemodialysis

3. The patient in question 2 was given 3 L of 0.9% normal saline in the ED and given rasburicase at 0.2 mg/kg. He was admitted to the intensive care unit (ICU) for close monitoring, started on ½ NS + 2 amps bicarbonate at 75 cc/h, the following morning (6 hours later) he was to start chemotherapy; however, nursing noticed that his urine output started to drop less than 50 cc/h, and a chemistry panel revealed sodium 138 mmol/L, potassium 6.1 mmol/L, bicarbonate 18 mmol/L, creatinine 1.9 mg/dL, calcium 5.9 mg/dL, phosphorus 9.8 mg/dL, and uric acid 5 mg/dL. The patient is now on RRT. What is the most likely primary etiology of this patient's AKI?
   A. Acute urate nephropathy
   B. ATN
   C. Hyperphosphatemic nephrocalcinosis

4. Rasburicase catalyzes the conversion of uric acid to which of the following water-soluble products?
   A. Hypoxanthine
   B. Xanthine
   C. Allantoin

5. Which of the following cancers is associated with the highest risk for developing TLS?
   A. Breast cancer
   B. Multiple myeloma and renal injury
   C. ALL with WBC < 100 × 10^9/L and normal LDH
   D. Leukemia, Burkitt type

Acute Kidney Injury from Therapeutic Agents

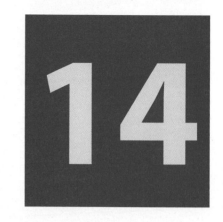

Ali J. Olyaei, PharmD

Joseph B. Lockridge, MD

William M. Bennett, MD

ESSENTIALS OF DIAGNOSIS

- Acute renal failure occurs in 4.9% of hospitalized patients with renal insufficiency.

- Fifty percent of patients experience nonoliguric acute renal failure.

- Antibiotics, analgesics, nonsteroidal anti-inflammatory drugs (NSAIDs), contrast media, and angiotensin-converting enzyme (ACE) inhibitors are the most common causes of acute renal failure.

- Impaired renal function, decreased volume status, exposure to contrast media, and aminoglycosides account for 79% of all cases of renal failure.

▶ General Considerations

Although most therapeutic agents infrequently cause community-acquired kidney injury, a number of diagnostic and therapeutic agents can produce kidney injury and kidney failure among hospitalized patients. These kidney injuries may be caused either directly or indirectly by drugs or metabolites of these agents. Recent data suggest that kidney adverse effects caused by pharmaceutical agents may contribute to approximately 30% of acute kidney injury (AKI) incidents in hospitalized patients. Antibiotics, analgesics, nonsteroidal anti-inflammatory drugs (NSAIDs), contrast media, and angiotensin-converting enzyme (ACE) inhibitors/angiotensin receptor blockers were the most commonly reported causes of AKI. A number of factors make the kidneys more susceptible to drug toxicity. First, the kidneys receive a high fraction (20–25%) of cardiac output relative to their weight, so drugs transit to the kidneys in large amounts. The kidneys represent only 0.4% of the body weight but receive 25% of resting cardiac output;

therefore, kidneys are exposed to a significant concentration of therapeutic agents. Second, the kidneys are very sensitive to reductions in blood perfusion and oxygen deprivation. Third, the renal concentrating mechanisms also concentrate drugs and chemicals within the filtered tubular fluid. Thus, local concentrations of these substances in contact with renal epithelia may exceed that in peripheral blood. Finally, most drug-induced AKI occurs in patients with subclinical preexisting kidney dysfunction.

AKI associated with drug-induced nephropathy can be classified into six categories based on pathophysiologic injuries. These injuries include prerenal failure, acute tubular necrosis (ATN), acute tubulointerstitial disease (ATID), tubular obstruction (crystal-induced ARF), hypersensitivity (glomerulonephritis), and thrombotic microangiopathy. A list of common therapeutic agents associated with each of these injuries is provided in Table 14–1.

Histologically, acute interstitial nephritis (AIN), most commonly known as tubulointerstitial disease, is differentiated from other injuries by infiltration and proliferation of inflammatory cells within the interstitium. The most frequent etiologies of AIN include drug-induced AIN, infection, and autoimmune disorders. Patients with drug-induced AIN usually present with nonspecific symptoms and an increase in serum creatinine, and decrease in kidney function are usually present. Nausea and vomiting, malaise, and/or anorexia may be present. Patients with NSAID-induced AIN usually present with renal dysfunction 8–12 months following exposure. The clinical features of AIN include a low-grade fever, rash, and eosinophilia. In AIN, the reduction of kidney function appears as a result of infiltration of inflammatory cells within the kidney interstitium. Although fibrosis is not very common initially, patchy fibrotic lesions will ultimately develop in the kidney cortex and medullocortical sections. The most common causes of drug-induced AIN include NSAIDs, penicillins and cephalosporins, rifampin, sulfonamides (including

Table 14–1. Classification of various drugs based on pathophysiologic categories of acute renal failure.

1. Prenal failure
   NSAIDs, ACE inhibitors, cyclosporine, norepinephrine, angiotensin receptor blockers, diuretics, interleukins, cocaine, mitomycin C, tacrolimus, estrogen, quinine
2. Acute tubular necrosis
   Antibiotics: Aminoglycosides, cephaloridine, cephalothin, amphotericin B, rifampicin, vancomycin, foscarnet, pentamide
   NSAIDs, contrast media, acetaminophen, cyclosporine, cisplatin, intravenous immunoglobulin, dextran, maltose, sucrose, mannitol, heavy metals
3. Acute interstitial nephritis
   Antibiotics: Ciprofloxacin, methicillin, penicillin G, ampicillin, cephalothin, oxacillin, rifampicin
   NSAIDs, contrast media, sulfonamides, thiazides, phenytoin, furosemide, allopurinol, cimetidine, omeprazole, phenindione
4. Tubular obstruction
   Sulfonamides, methotrexate, methoxyflurane, triamterene, acyclovir, ethylene glycol, protease inhibitors
5. Hypersensitivity reaction
   Penicillin G, ampicillin, sulfonamides
6. Thrombotic microangiopathy
   Mitomycin C, cyclosporine, oral contraceptives

ACE, angiotensin-converting enzyme; ADA, adalimumab; NSAIDs, nonsteroidal anti-inflammatory drugs.

medications that include sulfa moieties such as furosemide, bumetanide, and thiazide-type diuretics), cimetidine, allopurinol, ciprofloxacin, 5-aminosalicylates (eg, mesalamine), proton pump inhibitors, and, to a lesser degree, other quinolone antibiotics. There is strong evidence that suggests hypersensitivity and immunologically mediated mechanisms play an important role in the etiology of drug-induced AIN. The presence of cytotoxic T cells, helper T cells, T-cell-mediated cell injury, and B-cell involvement suggests activation of an immune cascade following exposure to an offending agent. Clinically, these histopathologic reactions are infrequently accompanied by fever, skin rash, eosinophilia, and arthralgia. Supportive care, withdrawal of nephrotoxins, and discontinuation of any suspected offending agents are the initial steps in the treatment of AIN. Drug-induced AIN is often reversible and patients usually improve without any long-term sequelae. In more serious cases, systemic corticosteroid therapy leads to rapid improvement.

Crystal nephropathy defines a prototype of kidney injury associated with crystal deposition and tubular obstruction in the kidneys. Drugs that may cause crystal nephropathy include acyclovir, sulfonamides, methotrexate, vancomycin, and indinavir. Risk factors for drug-induced crystal nephropathy include age, kidney impairment, volume depletion, liver failure, and decreased effective circulating volume. The patient's risk factors influence kidney blood flow and ultimately drug tubular flow. Many cases of drug-induced crystal nephropathy have occurred after prolonged administration of causative agents or large doses without adjustment of the dose for impaired kidney function. Certain drugs (methotrexate, sulfonamides, and triamterene) are eliminated more readily in an alkaline environment, and lowering of the urine pH may place these patients at a higher risk of crystal nephropathy. In contrast, the severity of crystal nephropathy by indinavir is influenced by alkaline urine.

The mechanism of drug-induced glomerulonephritis involves several different pathways. In most cases, the exact pathway is unknown, but several theories have been proposed. Drugs that have been reported to cause drug-induced glomerular disease are listed in Table 14–1. Drugs that induce glomerular disease can be classified according to the immunologic reaction they induce or by acting as a hapten and activating antigen–antibody complex formation. Some agents have a dose-dependent effect on glomerular structures. Although the signs and symptoms of drug-induced glomerular disease are highly variable, most patients with glomerular disease usually present with sudden loss of glomerular filtration rate (GFR) and proteinuria.

KEY READINGS

Bellomo R et al: Acute kidney injury in sepsis. Intensive Care Med 2017;43:816.
Goldstein SL: Medication-induced acute kidney injury. Curr Opin Crit Care 2016;22:542.
Mas-Font S et al: Prevention of acute kidney injury in Intensive Care Units. Med Intensiva 2017;41:116.
Pazhayattil GS, Shirali AC: Drug-induced impairment of renal function. Int J Nephrol Renovasc Dis 2014;7:457.
Raghavan R, Shawar S: Mechanisms of drug-induced interstitial nephritis. Adv Chronic Kidney Dis 2017;24:64.

▼ ANTIBIOTICS & ANTI-INFECTIVE AGENTS

AMINOGLYCOSIDES

▶ Incidence & Risk Factors

Aminoglycosides have important antibacterial properties and are highly effective for the treatment of gram-negative infections. These agents have shown a concentration-dependent bactericidal property against most gram-negative bacteria. The major dose and duration-limiting factors related to toxicity of aminoglycosides are nephrotoxicity and ototoxicity. Although a single large dose may cause reversible kidney dysfunction, most studies correlate nephrotoxicity with prolonged use in patients at risk for aminoglycoside toxicities. According to a number of studies, the incidence of aminoglycoside-induced nephrotoxicity is in the range of 5–15%. Patients over 70 years of age and patients with preexisting kidney impairment, intravascular volume depletion, hepatorenal syndrome, and septic patients have a higher incidence of kidney dysfunction following exposure to aminoglycosides. Even with aggressive monitoring and when peak and trough serum concentrations are kept within the desired therapeutic range, aminoglycoside-induced kidney dysfunction is still a possibility in high-risk populations. Various risk factors that predispose to the development of aminoglycoside nephrotoxicity have been identified.

Aminoglycoside-induced nephrotoxicity manifestations have varied from a mild and reversible increase in blood urea nitrogen (BUN) and serum creatinine, to serious but infrequent end-stage renal disease (ESRD) requiring lifelong dialysis. The onset of aminoglycoside-induced nephrotoxicity is usually after 7–10 days of therapy. However, a rapid onset of nephrotoxicity after even one dose of aminoglycosides has been reported. In most patients, serum creatinine and BUN return to normal levels 2–3 weeks after discontinuation of aminoglycosides. Nonoliguric kidney insufficiency is the most common manifestation of aminoglycoside nephrotoxicity. Less common manifestations include various isolated tubular syndromes, for example nephrogenic diabetes insipidus, Fanconi syndrome, and kidney potassium or magnesium wasting. Fortunately, severe oliguric kidney failure requiring dialysis is rare from aminoglycosides alone. A drug-induced concentrating defect characterized by polyuria and secondary thirst stimulation precedes the detectable rise in BUN and serum creatinine and occurs in as many as 30% of hospitalized patients given more than 5–7 days of aminoglycoside treatment. Granular casts and mild proteinuria occur frequently but are not diagnostic. In addition, in patients who satisfy the clinical criteria for aminoglycoside nephrotoxicity, cellular autophagocytosis has been observed with electron microscopy.

Loading doses should be sufficient to achieve high peak levels to maximize bacterial killing. Because the elimination half-life of aminoglycosides is markedly prolonged as kidney function falls, maintenance-dose intervals should be carefully adjusted in patients with existing kidney dysfunction when aminoglycosides are required. Extending the interval between doses is safer than reducing the size of individual doses in patients with kidney insufficiency. Correctable risk factors should be minimized. Among the clinically available aminoglycosides, the spectrum of nephrotoxicity is gentamicin > tobramycin > amikacin > netilmicin. Monitoring of peak serum levels will ensure efficacy, whereas elevation of the trough level, showing drug accumulation, will often precede a rise in the serum creatinine measurements. Once-daily aminoglycoside dosing may be less nephrotoxic for a given total daily dose.

Pathogenesis

A number of mechanisms have been proposed for nephrotoxicity of aminoglycosides. Most data suggest that aminoglycosides accumulate in the kidney cortex. These findings have been reported in animal and human studies. Megalin is an endocytotic receptor expressed and located at the brush-border membrane. Following binding to this receptor, aminoglycosides are taken up into the proximal tubular cells. The concentration of aminoglycosides in the proximal tubule is approximately 10- to 100-fold higher than the plasma concentration. At this concentration, aminoglycosides may interfere with protein synthesis in proximal tubular cells and lead to ATN.

Once-a-day gentamicin dosing or once every 36-hour dosing has become common in recent years. This method is particularly common when patients are at risk of nephrotoxicity or ototoxicity. A number of meta-analyses of randomized clinical trials and single-center reports with the use of a once-a-day dosing schedule suggest a reduced incidence of aminoglycoside nephrotoxicity. Compared to conventional three times a day administration, once-daily dosing may result in a 10–50% lower incidence of serious adverse reactions. This paradoxic finding can be explained in part by the saturable nature of aminoglycoside transport across the brush-border membrane of proximal tubular cells. During once-daily dosing, only a limited quantity (15 mg/dL) of aminoglycosides can cross during the initial high plasma concentration. This method of administration allows for a prolonged exposure to a low plasma concentration of aminoglycosides below the saturable threshold.

► Prevention & Treatment

Therapeutic drug monitoring plays an important role in the treatment of serious infections with aminoglycosides. Several studies have demonstrated that therapeutic drug monitoring with appropriately applied pharmacokinetic principles reduces the nephrotoxicity and other adverse drug reactions related to use of aminoglycosides. Table 14–2 provides dosing recommendations for the use of aminoglycosides in the treatment of various infections.

Aminoglycoside nephrotoxicity may occur despite therapeutic drug monitoring, use of once-daily dosing, and/or short-term treatment. Progression of nephrotoxicity can occur after discontinuation of the last dose. Most patients recover, but it may take several months before recovery is complete. Permanent kidney impairment leading to chronic kidney disease or ESRD requiring dialysis may occur.

KEY READINGS

Ahmed RM et al: Gentamicin ototoxicity: a 23-year selected case series of 103 patients. Med J Aust 2012;196:701.

Lopez-Novoa JM et al: New insights into the mechanism of aminoglycoside nephrotoxicity: an integrative point of view. Kidney Int 2011;79:33.

Table 14–2. Adult once-a-day aminoglycoside (gentamicin and tobramycin) dosing guidelines.

Dosing
For dosing weight, use adjusted IBW
Use IBW to calculate dose
  Male = 50 kg + 2.3 (height in inches – 60)
  Male = 45.5 kg +2.3 (height in inches – 60)
  Obese = IBW + 0.4 (actual BW – IBW)

A. Calculate CrCl
   Males: [(140 – Age) × IBW]/[SrCr × 72]
   Female: [(140 – Age) × IBW]/[SrCr × 72] × 0.85
B. Gentamicin/tobramycin dosing
   Dose according to estimated CrCl
   CrCl ≥60 mL/min = 5 mg/kg/24 h
   CrCl 40–60 mL/min = 5 mg/kg/36 h
   CrCl 40–20 mL/min = 1–1.5 mg/kg/q12h or consult pharmacist
   CrCl <20 mL/min ARF = consult clinical pharmacist

Round dose to the nearest 25 mg. For patients <35 kg, do not need to round.

Labs
For once daily dosing, please order serum creatinine/BUN every day or every 2 days.
Random level (12 h before the next dose). Note: Level should not be drawn from the same line from which it is administered. Repeat every 5 days or as needed while in hospital.

Dosage increases
If random level (drawn 12 h before the next dose) is undetectable, consider increasing the aminoglycoside dosage to 7 mg/kg/day. Repeat random level on new dosage.
If random level is >3, check a 24-h level; if it is >0.5 mg/dL, consider extending the dosing interval. Repeat random level on new dosage.

ARF, acute renal failure; BUN, blood urea nitrogen; BW, body weight; CrCl, creatinine clearance; IBW, ideal body weight; SrCr, serum creatinine.

Plajer SM et al: Gentamicin and renal function: lessons from 15 years' experience of a pharmacokinetic service for extended interval dosing of gentamicin. Ther Drug Monit 2015;37:98.
Samiee-Zafarghandy S, van den Anker JN: Nephrotoxic effects of aminoglycosides on the developing kidney. J Pediatr Neonat Individual Med 2013;2:1.

VANCOMYCIN

▶ Incidence & Risk Factors

Vancomycin is a commonly used antibiotic for the treatment of gram-positive bacterial infections resistant to penicillin and cephalosporins. The reported incidence of vancomycin-induced nephrotoxicity varies widely depending on the criteria used to define nephrotoxicity and generally ranges between 0 and 35%.

The relationship between therapeutic plasma monitoring (trough levels) of vancomycin and nephrotoxicity is uncertain. Since vancomycin is excreted mainly through the kidneys, kidney dysfunction would predispose patients to elevated serum vancomycin concentrations. It is not clear whether high serum vancomycin levels and nephrotoxicity are linked. Recent studies indicate a relationship between the combination of vancomycin and piperacillin-tazobactam with high nephrotoxicity rates

▶ Pathogenesis

Most histologic examinations of the kidneys indicate that vancomycin might cause marked destruction of proximal tubules. The hallmark of vancomycin-induced renal dysfunction is destruction of glomeruli and necrosis of proximal tubules. It has been suggested that oxidative stress is the underlying pathogenesis of vancomycin-induced nephrotoxicity. However, more recent data suggest that vancomycin may form obstructing crystals in the tubules. The factors independently associated with vancomycin kidney impairment are vancomycin level greater than 40, end-stage liver disease, and prolonged exposure to vancomycin.

▶ Prevention & Treatment

Vancomycin-induced nephrotoxicity is a largely unpredictable event. However, if patients are at risk for kidney dysfunction, a number of measures can be taken to prevent overt kidney failure. When treating a serious bacterial infection, all therapeutic options should be considered and vancomycin should be utilized only when medically necessary. In patients who require vancomycin treatment, consideration should be given to volume status, baseline kidney function, prolonged treatment course (over 10 days), concomitant use of aminoglycosides and/or other nephrotoxic agents, and advanced age. Frequent monitoring of kidney function is highly recommended, particularly in patients with preexisting kidney dysfunction. If kidney toxicity is observed, the vancomycin dose should be adjusted according to kidney function (Table 14–3). A doubling of the baseline serum creatinine is indicative of serious nephrotoxicity.

KEY READINGS

Lacave G et al: Incidence and risk factors of acute kidney injury associated with continuous intravenous high-dose vancomycin in critically ill patients: a retrospective cohort study. Medicine (Baltimore) 2017;96:e6023.
Rutter WC et al: Acute kidney injury in patients treated with vancomycin and piperacillin-tazobactam: a retrospective cohort analysis. J Hosp Med 2017;12:77.

ACYCLOVIR

▶ Incidence & Risk Factors

Over the past decade, there has been an increased use of antiviral agents to treat local and severe systemic viral infections

Table 14–3. Initial and adjusted vancomycin dose determination in adults.

Initial Maintenance Dose[a]	
Estimated CrCl (mL/min)	**Initial Dosing Regimen**
Continuous renal replacement (eg, CVVH, CVVHD)	1000 mg intravenously q24h
<20 and/or intermittent hemodialysis	1000 mg intravenously q72h
20–29	1000 mg intravenously q48h
30–39	1500 mg intravenously q48h or 750 mg intravenously q24h
40–55	1000 mg intravenously q24h
56–99	1000 mg intravenously q12h
100–120, age >65	1000 mg intravenously q12h
100–120, age <65	1250 mg intravenously q12h
≥120 and/or hypermetabolic state[b]	1000 mg intravenously q8h

CVVH, continuous venovenous hemofiltration; CVVHD, continuous venovenous hemodialysis.
[a]Consider loading doses in obese patients: Obese = actual body weight >120% ideal body weight. Give 1500 mg loading dose for obese patients weighing 85–109 kg. Give 2000 mg loading dose for obese patients weighing >110 kg.
[b]Hypermetabolic states include trauma and burn patients.

Adjusted Dose		
Trough Serum Concentration[a]	**Dose Adjustment Recommended**	**Follow-up/Monitoring[b]**
<3.5 mg/L	Shorten dose interval to next standard interval: If q48h → q24h If q24h → q12h If q12h → q8h If q8h → q6h	Draw trough level 30 min prior to third dose of new dosing regimen
3.5–4.9 mg/L	Increase dose by 250–500 mg at same time interval; if improvement in renal function,[c] consider shortening interval	Draw trough level ~30 minutes prior to third dose of new dosing regimen
5–15 mg/L	No change in therapy[d]	No further trough levels to be drawn unless Duration of therapy is >7 days; if therapy >7 days, check trough level every 5–7 days Patient status declines Serum creatinine in increases >0.5 mg/dL from baseline
15.1–19.9 mg/L	Decrease dose by 250 mg at same time interval	Draw trough level ~30 min prior to third dose of new dose regimen therapy
≥20 mg/L and dose ≥1000 mg	Decrease dose by 500 mg at same time interval or If decline in renal function,[c] hold dose(s) and check another level in 12–24 h; when trough is therapeutic, restart at lower dose and/or extend interval, based on patient-specific clearance	Draw trough level ~30 min prior to third dose of new dose regimen therapy

(Continued)

Table 14–3. Initial and adjusted vancomycin dose determination in adults. (*Continued*)

	Adjusted Dose	
Trough Serum Concentration[a]	Dose Adjustment Recommended	Follow-up/Monitoring[b]
≥20 mg/L and dose <1000 mg	Extend dose interval to next standard interval: If q6h → q8h If q8h → q12h If q12h → q24h If q24h → q48h or If decline in renal function,[c] hold dose(s) and check another level in 12–24 h; when trough is therapeutic, restart at lower dose and/or extend interval, based on patient-specific clearance	Draw trough level ~30 min prior to third dose of new dose regimen therapy

[a]Higher trough concentrations may be necessary for some types of patients/infections. Examples include, but are not limited to, meningitis, endocarditis, and osteomyelitis.

[b]Serum creatinine levels should also be monitored daily in patients with decreased renal function and/or increased risk of nephrotoxicity.

[c]Changes in serum creatinine of ±50% from baseline may signify change in renal function.

[d]Maximum serum trough level in patients with increased risk for nephrotoxicity is 12 mg/L, particularly patients on concomitant nephrotoxins (eg, aminoglycosides, amphotericin B, cisplatin, cyclosporin, foscarnet, ganciclovir, loop diuretics, nonsteroidal anti-inflammatory drugs, radio-contrast dye, tacrolimus, vasopressors).

in immunocompromised patients. Most antiviral agents appear to be safe and do not cause nephrotoxicity. AKI is an important dose-limiting toxicity of acyclovir.

Acyclovir is primarily eliminated through the kidney with a small amount being metabolized in the liver. Many cases of acyclovir nephrotoxicity have been reported in the medical literature over the past 15 years. These reports have increased awareness and concern of acyclovir's nephrotoxic potential. Kidney dysfunction most commonly occurs within the first few days of initiation of intravenous acyclovir therapy. Patients who receive high-dose bolus intravenous therapy, those who are volume depleted, and patients with preexisting kidney insufficiency are at the greatest risk of developing kidney injury. AKI has been reported in as many as 5% of patients who receive high-dose bolus intravenous therapy but is rare in patients receiving oral therapy. The most common symptoms include nausea, vomiting, abdominal pain, and/or back pain. Patients may, however, be asymptomatic. A moderate rise (1–3 mg/dL) in serum creatinine from baseline may be seen while oliguria is uncommon. Urinalysis may show trace protein-urea, pyuria, and microscopic hematuria. Birefringent needle-shaped crystals may be seen free or within white blood cells in the urine sediment.

Pathogenesis

The pathogenesis of acyclovir-induced AKI is unclear and may involve an obstructive nephropathy from intratubular precipitation of acyclovir and/or immune hypersensitivity reaction. Acyclovir is moderately insoluble in the urine. The

maximum solubility of acyclovir is 2.5 mg/mL. Low urine output and a high rate of intravenous infusion of a large dose (500 mg/mm^2) of acyclovir may lead to intratubular precipitation by raising the intratubular concentration above the solubility threshold.

Prevention & Treatment

The most effective means of preventing acyclovir nephrotoxicity is to administer adequate intravenous fluid (normal saline [NS] 0.9%) to induce a urinary output of 100–150 mL/h. Acyclovir-induced nephropathy may also be prevented by avoiding rapid bolus infusion. Acyclovir should be administered at a rate of 60 minutes for every 500-mg dose. Approaches to treatment of acyclovir-induced nephropathy are similar to those caused by other agents. Discontinuation of acyclovir therapy, increased hydration, or dose reduction/interval extension allows most patients to return to normal kidney function within a few days to 2 weeks. Temporary dialysis is usually unnecessary. However, for severe complications of kidney failure associated with acyclovir, hemodialysis could be utilized to decrease plasma acyclovir levels by 40–60%.

KEY READINGS

Fleischer R, Johnson M: Acyclovir nephrotoxicity: a case report highlighting the importance of prevention, detection, and treatment of acyclovir-induced nephropathy. Case Rep Med 2010;2010:pii: 602783.

Gunness P et al: Acyclovir-induced nephrotoxicity: the role of the acyclovir aldehyde metabolite. Transl Res 2011;158:290.

FOSCARNET

▶ Incidence & Risk Factors

Foscarnet is a virostatic agent used in HIV-infected and other immunocompromised patients to prevent or treat serious cytomegalovirus (CMV) infections and acyclovir-resistant mucocutaneous herpes simplex infections. Foscarnet exhibits poor oral absorption necessitating intravenous therapy. As foscarnet is a phosphate analog, it can chelate calcium and be deposited in bone. Biotransformation does not occur, and up to 28% is excreted unchanged in the urine. Foscarnet induces a rather unique form of kidney failure. Kidney impairment occurs in varying degrees in the majority of patients. The exact incidence of foscarnet-induced nephropathy is not known. The rates of AKI from foscarnet vary in patients from 27% to 66%. Risks for kidney failure have not been well defined but include impaired kidney function, age, concomitant administration with other nephrotoxic agents, and dehydration.

▶ Pathogenesis

The pathogenesis of foscarnet-induced kidney failure remains speculative with a number of hypotheses being suggested. AKI appears to be caused by the formation of a foscarnet/ionized calcium complex that precipitates in renal glomeruli causing a crystalline glomerulonephritis. The salt crystals may also precipitate in renal tubules causing tubular necrosis. Fluid and electrolyte imbalances have been reported with foscarnet therapy. Polyuria, nephrogenic diabetes insipidus, hypokalemia, hypomagnesemia, hypophosphatemia or hyperphosphatemia, and hypocalcemia have been observed in patients treated with foscarnet. Hypocalcemia is the most frequently encountered and most serious imbalance. Although the total calcium levels remain unaffected, the ionized calcium decreases substantially. Patients with low ionized calcium levels may experience paresthesias, tingling, numbness, seizures, and death. Foscarnet therapy has been able to be resumed in some patients after restoration of electrolyte or mineral abnormalities. Ionized hypocalcemia may primarily be a result of foscarnet complexing with ionized calcium. However, kidney dysfunction may also contribute to these electrolyte abnormalities.

▶ Prevention & Treatment

Minimization of foscarnet-induced nephrotoxicity can be accomplished through vigorous hydration prior to therapy. Use of foscarnet with other nephrotoxins increases the likelihood of developing AKI. Intermittent infusion, as opposed to continuous infusion, may reduce foscarnet-induced nephrotoxicity. AKI is usually reversible; however, recovery may be gradual. Azotemia may worsen and last for several days before resolving. Continuation of foscarnet in patients who develop mild azotemia may be possible with reduced doses. Temporary dialysis may be necessary. Patients with preexisting kidney insufficiency may require several months to recover full kidney function following discontinuation of foscarnet.

CIDOFOVIR, ADEFOVIR, & TENOFOVIR

▶ Incidence & Risk Factors

Cidofovir, adefovir, and tenofovir belong to a newer class of antiviral agents structurally described as acyclic nucleoside phosphonates. Cidofovir is an analog of the monophosphate of cytosine. When activated, these agents appear to interfere with synthesis and/or degradation of cellular membrane phospholipids. Cidofovir exhibits broad activity against the herpes viruses. It is primarily used to treat CMV retinitis in patients who have failed other treatments as well as adenoviral infections in transplant recipients. Adefovir is an analog of adenine that interferes with a variety of ATP-dependent processes once it undergoes phosphorylation within cells. It is used to treat active or chronic hepatitis B infections in patients intolerant to other antiviral therapies. However, it is rarely used. Tenofovir, a newer nucleotide analog, is a reverse-transcriptase inhibitor approved to treat HIV infection. Nephrotoxicity is a major dose-dependent and dose-limiting toxicity of both cidofovir and adefovir. In clinical trials, approximately 25% or more of patients receiving intravenous cidofovir 3 mg/kg or more developed AKI related to renal proximal tubular injury. Associated abnormalities included proteinuria, increased serum creatinine, Fanconi syndrome with tubular proteinuria, and evidence of proximal tubular injury including glucosuria, hypophosphatemia, urinary bicarbonate wasting, and, rarely, chronic interstitial nephritis and nephrogenic diabetes insipidus. Upon discontinuation of cidofovir, kidney function parameters return toward baseline. Proximal tubular injury was reported in 22–50% of HIV-positive patients infected with hepatitis B virus receiving doses of adefovir at greater than 30 mg/day for 72 weeks. The role of adefovir at doses of 10 mg/day inducing any kidney or tubular dysfunction is rare, and no case reports were found in a recent literature search. Toxicity appeared to be mild to moderate and accompanied by changes in serum potassium, bicarbonate and uric acid levels, proteinuria, and glucosuria. The incidence of these abnormalities appeared to be dose related. Tenofovir alafenamide is a novel tenofovir formulation with a significant lower rate of kidney injury and a better safety profile compared with tenofovir disoproxil.

▶ Pathogenesis

Cidofovir and adefovir (>30 mg/day) have been noted to have significant nephrotoxicity. These potent drugs cause injury to proximal tubular epithelia. Proximal tubular cells express an organic anion transporter that actively takes up a variety of acyclic nucleotide analogs, including cidofovir and adefovir. These agents concentrate in tubular cells, interfere with various cell processes, and are then actively secreted into the tubular lumen. Renal clearance of these agents exceeds creatinine clearance, suggesting that active tubular secretion contributes to renal clearance. Probenecid, an inhibitor of organic anion transport, decreases renal toxicity of these agents by reducing cellular uptake. A spectrum of injuries ranging from isolated proximal tubular defects (Fanconi-like syndrome) to severe ATN requiring renal replacement therapy has been observed with cidofovir and adefovir. Tenofovir, like cidofovir and adefovir, appears to accumulate in proximal tubular epithelial cells. However, based on clinical trials to date, tenofovir appears to have lower nephrotoxic potential.

▶ Prevention & Treatment

In a recent study, switching from tenofovir disoproxil fumarate to tenofovir alafenamide was associated with a significant improvement in proteinuria, albuminuria, proximal renal tubular function, and bone mineral density. In early evidence of kidney impairment, patients should be switched from tenofovir disoproxil fumarate to tenofovir alafenamide. The following guidelines should be employed to reduce or avoid kidney injury caused by cidofovir and adefovir: pretreatment intravascular volume expansion with intravenous fluids, appropriate dosing for the level of kidney function, avoidance in patients with significant kidney dysfunction, avoidance of administration with recent use of any potentially nephrotoxic drug, and co-administration with probenecid. Recent use of other nephrotoxic agents, preexisting kidney impairment, and the development of proteinuria or other proximal tubular abnormalities during treatment may result in severe AKI. Kidney failure may require dialysis. Despite drug discontinuation, proximal tubular damage and resulting kidney failure may be partially reversible or irreversible.

KEY READINGS

Arribas JR et al: A randomized, double-blind comparison of tenofovir alafenamide (TAF) vs. tenofovir disoproxil fumarate (TDF), each coformulated with elvitegravir, cobicistat, and emtricitabine (E/C/F) for initial HIV-1 treatment: week 144 results. J Acquir Immune Defic Syndr 2017;75:211.

Raffi F et al: Long-term (96-week) efficacy and safety after switching from tenofovir disoproxil fumarate (TDF) to tenofovir alafenamide (TAF) in HIV-infected, virologically suppressed adults. J Acquir Immune Defic Syndr 2017;75:226.

INDINAVIR

▶ Incidence & Risk Factors

Protease inhibitors share common adverse drug reaction profiles. Each agent, however, has its own unique toxicity. Compared with other protease inhibitors, a lower incidence of nausea, vomiting, abdominal discomfort, and taste disturbances have been reported with the use of indinavir. Indinavir is considered safe, although 4% of patients experienced flank pain with or without hematuria associated with nephrolithiasis during phase II/III clinical studies. However, it was not clear that indinavir or its metabolites were responsible for the formation of crystals in the urine. Nephrolithiasis or crystal precipitation has not been associated with other protease inhibitors. Subsequent studies have clearly demonstrated that indinavir may form intratubular crystals and stones. Two distinct patterns of crystalluria have been reported in HIV-positive patients: symptomatic and asymptomatic crystalluria. Asymptomatic crystalluria is more common than actual nephrolithiasis with symptomatic renal colic. In addition to nephrolithiasis, some patients develop crystalluria and dysuria with evidence of intrarenal sludge.

Several risk factors may influence the incidence of indinavir-induced urolithiasis. The incidence of first episode or recurrence of urolithiasis may increase during warmer temperatures. This finding may correlate with a higher incidence of dehydration or lack of compliance with fluid replacement during high environmental temperatures. HIV-positive patients with hepatitis C virus (HCV) coinfection and hemophilia or receiving trimethoprim-sulfamethoxazole (TMP/SMX) may incur greater risk of indinavir-associated urolithiasis.

▶ Pathogenesis

Indinavir stones are usually considered radiolucent. These stones include calcium oxalate and calcium phosphate. Therefore, they may present as partly radiopaque. Kidney biopsy documentation of acute indinavir-induced interstitial nephritis and obstructive AKI has been described in several HIV-positive patients. Renal biopsy showed evidence of interstitial nephritis/fibrosis and tubular atrophy. The medullary collecting tube was filled with crystals associated with histiocytes and giant cells. The exact mechanism of indinavir-induced AKI has not been elucidated. A high incidence of asymptomatic crystalluria or urolithiasis suggests the possibility of intrarenal obstruction due to precipitation of indinavir and/or its metabolites in the urinary collecting system.

▶ Prevention & Management

Management and prevention in patients with indinavir-induced kidney dysfunction may include discontinuation of indinavir, dose reduction, and hydration. Most patients can be treated for indinavir-associated nephrolithiasis with aggressive hydration and pain control. Patients should be advised to ingest at least 48 oz of fluid throughout the day. The urine output should be 1500 mL/day to limit indinavir urine concentrations. Patients with indinavir stones may be treated with hydration, but surgical intervention may be needed for the treatment of both obstruction and pain.

KEY READINGS

Cattaneo D, Gervasoni C: Novel antiretroviral drugs in patients with renal impairment: clinical and pharmacokinetic considerations. Eur J Drug Metab Pharmacokinet 2017;42:559.

Jafari A, Khalili H, Dashti-khavidaki S: Tenofovir-induced nephrotoxicity: incidence, mechanism, risk factors, prognosis and proposed agents for prevention. Eur J Clin Pharmacol 2014;70:1029.

Koklu S et al: Differences in nephrotoxicity risk and renal effects among anti-viral therapies against hepatitis B. Aliment Pharmacol Ther 2015;41:310.

Post FA: Managing chronic kidney disease in the older adults living with HIV. Curr Opin Infect Dis 2017;30:4.

PROTON PUMP INHIBITORS

▷ Incidence & Risk Factors

Proton pump inhibitors (PPIs) are one of the most prescribed drugs worldwide. Their efficacy in acid-related gastrointestinal (GI) diseases and the very low number of side effects have contributed to their massive prescription. The interval between drug initiation and the onset of kidney abnormalities can vary between 1 month and few years with most commonly reported time period of approximately 6 months. As in other types of drug-induced AIN, leukocyturia, hematuria, and non-nephrotic proteinuria are commonly observed, but the classic triad of fever, skin rash, and eosinophilia has been found in less than 10% of patients. PPI-induced AIN had less severe AKI than antibiotic-induced cases, but the probability of recovery by 6 months was significantly lower.

▷ Pathogenesis

PPIs have been suggested as a potential cause of drug-induced AIN. PPI users have been reported to be four to five times more likely to experience AIN compared to nonusers. Clinicians should therefore maintain a high index of suspicion for AIN in patients on a PPI who have a change in kidney function, especially during the first 6 months following PPI. Baseline and monitoring of kidney function may be appropriate.

▷ Treatment

Kidney impairment caused by PPIs is usually reversible if detected early in the course of the treatment. The PPI use should be terminated, but delays in diagnosis can lead to the development of chronic kidney disease.

KEY READINGS

Lazarus B et al: Proton pump inhibitor use and the risk of chronic kidney disease. JAMA Intern Med 2016;176:238.

Perazella MA, Luciano RL: Review of select causes of drug-induced AKI. Expert Rev Clin Pharmacol 2015;8:367.

INTRAVENOUS IMMUNOGLOBULIN & HYDROXYETHYLSTARCH

▷ Incidence & Risk Factors

Intravenous immunoglobulin (IVIG) is used to treat a variety of autoimmune disorders. Since IVIG is prepared from pooled plasma from thousands of donors, it contains a range of antibodies. The majority of the antibodies are unmodified immunoglobulin (Ig) G (95%). The pharmacologic effect of IVIG includes blockade of macrophage Fc receptor, anti-inflammation by inhibiting the generation of membrane attack complex, neutralization of autoantibody, inhibition of cell proliferation, and regulation of apoptosis. The side effects of IVIG include infusion reaction (fever, chills, and facial flush), tachycardia, palpitation, anaphylaxis AKI, thrombosis, and aseptic meningitis. The Food and Drug Administration (FDA) has received over 100 reports of adverse kidney events related to IVIG use. Most of these serious adverse events have occurred in older patients with diabetes with previous kidney impairment. Kidney dysfunction usually occurs within 7 days of IVIG administration, with mean peak serum creatinine levels in the range of 6 mg/dL. Approximately 40% of patients required dialysis and 15% mortality was reported despite renal replacement therapy. The mean time to recover kidney function in surviving patients is 10 days. Histologic evidence of extensive vacuolation of the proximal tubules has been reported in patients with IVIG-induced kidney dysfunction. This histologic finding is consistent with osmotic nephrosis associated with administration of a high load of sucrose. Since 90% of the cases were reported in patients receiving sucrose-containing IVIG, sucrose was thought to be the culprit in IVIG-induced nephrotoxicity. Between nonsucrose products, amino-acid-stabilized formulations are associated with less tubular toxicity than carbohydrate-stabilized IVIG.

Kidney failure has been reported in a small number of patients exposed to hydroxyethyl starch following surgery. Osmotic nephrosis has been reported in these patients. Due to the concerns regarding the excess risk of AKI with hydroxyethyl starch, this medication is no longer recommended as a volume replacement therapy.

▷ Pathogenesis

IVIG-induced nephrotoxicity is largely related to the preparation of the product. Factors such as volume load, sugar, and sodium content, and osmolarity of the product should be considered. Sugar, such as sucrose, is often used as a stabilizer to prevent the aggregation of IgG. Sucrose is a disaccharide of glucose and fructose. It is reabsorbed in the proximal convoluted tubule (PCT) after being filtered. Unfortunately, the human kidney lacks the enzyme to hydrolyze sucrose. The accumulation of sucrose inside the PCT cells increases the osmolarity and draws the fluid into the cells. Kidney failure occurs as a result of cell swelling, vacuolization, and tubular luminal occlusion from swollen tubular cells.

Different preparations contain varied amounts of sucrose. The incidence of AKI does not seem to correlate with the amount of sucrose, so it has been proposed that small amounts of sucrose may be sufficient to induce renal impairment or IVIG itself may be contributing to or causing renal failure.

▶ Prevention & Management

Patients should be adequately hydrated prior to IVIG administration. The concurrent use of IVIG, NSAIDs, and radiocontrast agents should be avoided because of the synergistic effect on kidney function. For sucrose-containing products, the infusion rate should not exceed 3-mg sucrose/kg/min. Baseline serum creatinine, BUN, and urine output should be obtained and monitored closely during the course of IVIG therapy. In patients at an increased risk of AKI, use of non–sucrose-containing IVIG products is highly recommended.

KEY READINGS

Luque Y et al: Renal safety of high-dose, sucrose-free intravenous immunoglobulin in kidney transplant recipients: an observational study. Transpl Int 2016;29:1205.

Orbach H, Tishler M, Shoenfeld Y: Intravenous immunoglobulin and the kidney—a two-edged sword. Semin Arthritis Rheum 2004;34:593.

AMPHOTERICIN B

▶ Incidence & Risk Factors

Amphotericin B is a polyene antibiotic with activity against a broad spectrum of fungi. However, kidney function becomes impaired in approximately 80% of patients given amphotericin B. This nephrotoxicity is dose related and probably inevitable when the cumulative dose exceeds 3 g in adults. Patients at high risk include elderly patients, particularly those with depleted extracellular volume.

▶ Pathogenesis

The usual clinical presentation of amphotericin B nephrotoxicity is characterized by defects in renal tubular function. Occasionally, this condition will progress to nonoliguric AKI. Modest proteinuria associated with a relatively normal urinary sediment is the initial finding. Frank azotemia is preceded by hypokalemia, renal tubular acidosis, and impaired urinary concentrating capacity. In addition, the presence of a magnesium-wasting syndrome is a prominent feature of amphotericin nephrotoxicity. Repetitive courses of amphotericin B may cause permanent impairment of kidney function.

Histologic changes associated with the administration of amphotericin B are surprisingly minimal. These changes are seen in the glomerulus and renal tubule. Amphotericin B has been shown to cause acute renal vasoconstriction and damage to the distal tubular epithelium. Although the exact mechanism causing nephrotoxicity is unclear, amphotericin B may bind to membrane sterols in renal vasculature cells and renal tubular epithelial cells altering membrane permeability. This event may initiate sequelae of other events that alter kidney function. These events may include activation of second messengers, activation of renal homeostatic mechanisms, and/or release of mediators. Frequent monitoring of serum creatinine is recommended. If toxicity occurs, the amphotericin dosage can be reduced, interrupted for 2 days, or a double dose can be given on alternative days. Consideration of stopping amphotericin B in patients with kidney toxicity should occur. A doubling of the baseline serum creatinine is indicative of serious nephrotoxicity.

▶ Prevention & Treatment

Sodium supplementation in the form of intravenous saline can be used as a safe and effective means of reducing the risk of amphotericin nephrotoxicity to approximately 10% of patients. Sodium (150 mEq/day) can be administered as follows: 500 mL 0.9% NS 30 minutes before amphotericin B administration and a second 500 mL given during the 30 minutes after completion of the amphotericin infusion. The goal is to achieve a urinary sodium excretion of 250–300 mmol/day. Liposomal amphotericin B may allow for larger doses to be administered with a higher therapeutic index. Several different lipid-based amphotericin B preparations have been introduced in the market recently. These formulations have a lower rate of nephrotoxicity when compared to the standard formulation of amphotericin B. Administration-associated adverse drug reactions (fever, chills) are significantly lower with lipid-based amphotericin B. Among all lipid-based amphotericin B formulations, liposomal amphotericin (AmBisome) is significantly less nephrotoxic. Fewer patients require a dose reduction/discontinuation with AmBisome for the treatment of invasive mycoses due to adverse drug reactions when compared to other lipid-based amphotericin B formulations (ABLC, Abelcet, and ABCD, Amphotec).

Patients should be premedicated with diphenhydramine 25 mg intravenously/orally and acetaminophen 650 mg orally before receiving amphotericin to minimize infusion-related reactions. To protect the kidneys, patients should be well hydrated and should receive sodium loading.

Voriconazole, posaconazole, and isavuconazole are pharmacokinetically and therapeutically superior to amphotericin B in many respects and should be substituted for amphotericin for the treatment of disseminated aspergillosis infections. These are a potent inhibitor of cytochrome

P450-3A4 hepatic metabolism. Therefore, plasma concentrations of cyclosporine/tacrolimus should be monitored closely to avoid potential toxicities. Echinocandin is also an excellent choice for the management of invasive *Candida* infection.

KEY READINGS

Karimzadeh I et al: Frequency and associated factors of amphotericin B nephrotoxicity in hospitalized patients in hematology-oncology wards in the southwest of Iran. Nephrourol Mon 2016;8:e39581.
Steimbach LM et al: Efficacy and safety of amphotericin B lipid-based formulations—a systematic review and meta-analysis. Mycoses 2017;60:146.

ACE INHIBITORS & ANGIOTENSIN RECEPTOR BLOCKERS

Incidence & Risk Factors

ACE inhibitors and ARBs are frequently used in the treatment of hypertension. Emerging evidence suggests that treatment of hypertension and concomitant lowering of intraglomerular pressure has a renoprotective effect in patients with diabetes and nondiabetic nephropathy. ACE inhibitors have become the antihypertensive therapeutic class of choice when the first evidence of microalbuminuria is detected in patients with diabetes.

ACE inhibitors and ARBs selectively dilate the efferent arteriole affecting renal hemodynamics. Dilation of the efferent arteriole rarely compromises the GFR in patients with normal renal perfusion. However, AKI can occur if atherosclerotic vascular disease is present in major renal arteries, when high-grade bilateral renal artery stenosis or stenosis in a single kidney (renal transplant recipients) exists, or in any condition or drug-induced condition in which renal hemodynamics maintained by the renin/angiotensin system is altered (Figure 14–1).

Pathogenesis

Several conditions including volume depletion from diuretic therapy, concomitant administration with agents that cause vasoconstriction (NSAIDs, cyclosporine), chronic kidney insufficiency of any cause (eg, congestive heart failure [CHF], hypertension], or during development of illnesses that decrease circulatory volume (vomiting, diarrhea, worsening CHF) put patients at greater risk of kidney impairment. These patients depend on efferent arteriolar vasoconstriction to maintain adequate glomerular filtration. Initiation of ACE inhibitors or ARBs may result in a rapid fall in the GFR and a rise in serum creatinine. This usually occurs within 2 weeks of initiation of these agents and can be more pronounced in patients with documented risk factors. Clinicians should ensure that patients are not hypovolemic and therapy should begin with a low dose that is slowly titrated. A chemistry panel should be obtained on all patients prior to and within 5–7 days of initiation of drug therapy. This is critical, especially in elderly patients and those with known preexisting risk factors. Patients at risk of developing AKI with initiation of ACE inhibitors or ARBs can be identified early in therapy if cautious monitoring occurs (Figure 14–2).

Prevention & Treatment

AKI caused by ACE inhibitors is usually reversible. If kidney dysfunction occurs, reduction in dosage or reduction in the dosage of any concomitantly administered diuretic usually results in improved renal hemodynamics. Restoration of fluid and electrolyte balance, withdrawal of any interacting drugs, and, if necessary, temporary dialysis may be indicated. Substitution with an ARB almost always elicits the same effect and should be avoided.

Hyperkalemia is often present with ACE inhibitor–induced AKI, especially in elderly patients with CKD or patients receiving selective aldosterone inhibitors. The rise in plasma potassium concentration is usually modest. Often, ACE inhibitors offset hypokalemia, which occurs with many diuretics. Concomitant administration with potassium-sparing diuretics or potassium supplements increases the risk of developing hyperkalemia. If potassium levels above 6 mEq/L do not decline upon restoration of fluid balance, treatment with a potassium-binding resin may be indicated. Substitution with an ARB may reduce the incidence of hyperkalemia if potassium is less than 5.5 mEq/L. Upon discontinuation of ACE inhibitors/ARBs, kidney function usually improves within a few days provided tubular damage has not occurred. Correction of risk factors for developing ACE inhibitor– or ARB-induced AKI may allow continuation of therapy unless renal vascular disease or CKD is the cause of ACE inhibitor- or ARB-associated ARF. In patients with CKD, up to a 20–30% rise in serum creatinine can be anticipated. This rise indicates that the drug is exerting its desired effect, reversing glomerular hyperfiltration. If the rise in serum creatinine does not exceed 20–30%, the ACE inhibitor or ARB should be continued. As surviving nephrons adapt, stabilization of serum creatinine usually ensues. A 50% reduction in dosage can be attempted when serum creatinine rises above 30%. If the rise in serum creatinine does not stabilize within 4 weeks, the ACE inhibitor or ARB should be discontinued (Figure 14–3).

KEY READINGS

Awdishu L, Mehta RL: The 6R's of drug induced nephrotoxicity. BMC Nephrol 2017;18:124.
Paueksakon P, Fogo AB: Drug-induced nephropathies. Histopathology 2017;70:94.

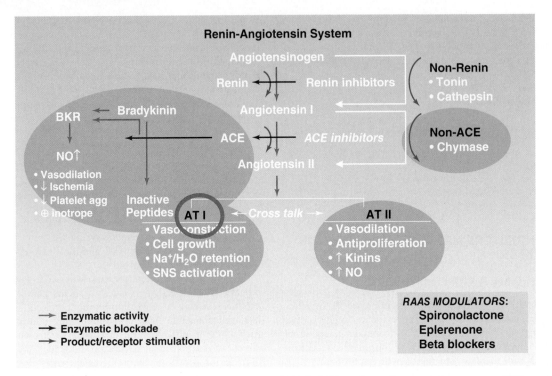

▲ **Figure 14–1.** The renin–angiotensin–aldosterone system (RAAS). ACE, angiotensin-converting enzyme; SNS, sympathetic nervous system.

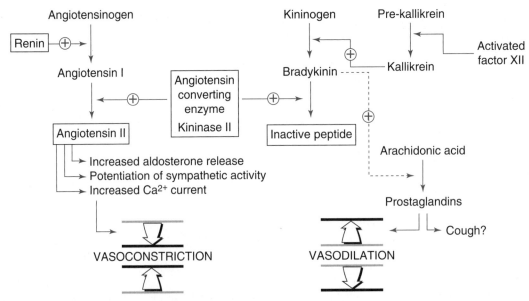

▲ **Figure 14–2.** Inhibition of the angiotensin-converting enzyme or kinase II.

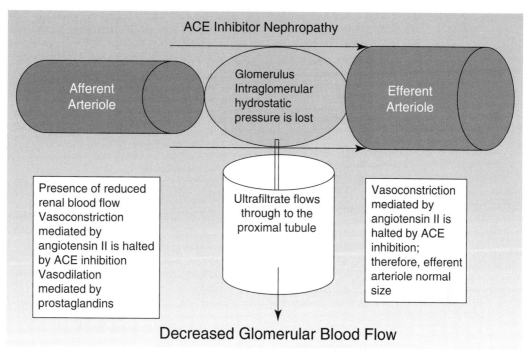

▲ **Figure 14–3.** Angiotensin-converting enzyme (ACE) inhibitor nephropathy.

CISPLATIN & CARBOPLATIN

▶ Incidence & Risk Factors

Cisplatin and carboplatin are among the most widely used antineoplastic agents. Both agents exhibit a dose-related effect against a variety of solid tumor types. Cisplatin inhibits DNA synthesis through formation of DNA intrastrand cross-links, denatures the double helix, binds covalently to DNA bases, and disrupts DNA function. It also binds to RNA and proteins. Nephrotoxicity is the primary dose-limiting toxicity of cisplatin. Carboplatin was subsequently developed to avoid the nephrotoxicity of cisplatin while maintaining the antitumor effect. Carboplatin has since been shown to possess nephrotoxicity comparable to cisplatin. The epidemiology of nephrotoxicity varies between different cancer treatment regimens. Loss of 30–50% of GFR is a common reported adverse reaction with the use of platins. Use of other nephrotoxic agents, volume depletion, larger doses, co-administration with other nephrotoxic agents, and/or diuretics increased the risk of nephrotoxicity following exposure to platin analogues.

▶ Pathogenesis

The majority of cisplatin is excreted largely unchanged in the urine. Platinum binds extensively to plasma proteins.

Unbound cisplatin is freely filtered at glomeruli and may be secreted. Excreted platinum is mutagenic and may be responsible for secondary malignancies that arise after cisplatin therapy. Cisplatin accumulates in renal tubular cells via transport or binding to components of the organic base transport system. Autoradiographic studies have shown that radiolabeled cisplatin accumulated primarily in the S3 segment of proximal tubules, which is also the site of cisplatin-induced renal cell toxicity. Several suspected intracellular targets have been identified, including those involved in renal tubule energy production and DNA synthesis. Upon entry into renal cells, cisplatin undergoes biotransformation. Cisplatin binds cell macromolecules while a large portion of total cell platinum exists in a form with a molecular weight below 500 Da and exhibits a different chromatographic behavior than cisplatin.

Polyuria, reduced glomerular filtration, and electrolyte disturbances are frequently observed in cisplatin-treated patients. Polyuria occurs in two phases. During the first 24–48 hours after administration, urine osmolality falls while the GFR remains unchanged. Early polyuria often improves spontaneously. A second phase of polyuria occurs between 72 and 96 hours following cisplatin administration. This phase is accompanied by a disruption of glomerular filtration. A 20–40% sustained reduction in the GFR is common. Cisplatin-induced alteration of cellular respiration may lead to an incomplete distal tubule acidosis, causing disturbances in magnesium, potassium, hydrogen, and calcium balance. Hypomagnesemia is a frequent complication of treatment with cisplatin. Repletion of serum magnesium levels and magnesium supplementation reduce the risk of adverse effects from hypomagnesemia. ATN and AIN have also been reported with cisplatin treatment.

▶ Prevention & Management

Several strategies have been employed to reduce cisplatin-induced nephrotoxicity. Prehydration with hypertonic salts may reduce cisplatin-induced ARF. A high urinary chloride concentration following saline-based hydration may reduce conversion of cisplatin to toxic metabolites. Diuretics (furosemide) have also been utilized to decrease cisplatin transit time thorough renal tubules and to maintain adequate urinary output during vigorous hydration therapy. Although diuresis is commonly used, several clinical studies have shown it to be of no clinical benefit. Administering cisplatin as a continuous infusion or divided daily dose over 3–5 days is as effective therapeutically as a bolus dose. Avoidance of a large bolus dose decreases the intensity of renal drug exposure and may reduce cisplatin-induced nephrotoxicity. Co-administration with mannitol is thought to confer a protective effect by dilution of cisplatin within renal tubules due to urine volume expansion. Co-administration with nephrotoxic drugs such as aminoglycosides, NSAIDs, or iodinated contrast media should be avoided. Cisplatin and carboplatin should be used with caution in patients at risk for kidney dysfunction.

KEY READING

Arany I, Safirstein RL: Cisplatin nephrotoxicity. Semin Nephrol 2003;23:460.

LITHIUM

▶ Incidence & Risk Factors

Lithium was discovered in 1817 and has been used since 1949 for the treatment of bipolar disorder. Following oral administration, lithium is absorbed completely from the gastrointestinal (GI) tract. Lithium is not protein bound and distributes in all human tissues. It is eliminated largely unchanged through renal excretion without any metabolism. A higher lithium half-life has been reported in bipolar patients compared to others. The most common side effects reported with lithium are kidney toxicities, thyroid toxicosis, weight gain, somnolence, and cardiovascular abnormalities. Lithium-induced nephropathy is slow but progressive and is characterized by chronic interstitial nephritis, including fibrosis, tubular atrophy, cystic tubular lesions, and glomerular sclerosis.

The true incidence of lithium-induced nephropathy is largely unknown. Kidney dysfunction secondary to exposure to lithium occurs in up to 20% of the patients receiving lithium for any psychiatric disorder. The reported incidence ranged from 1% to 30%. Renal biopsy information obtained from psychiatric patients without exposure to lithium has shown similar renal injuries and histologic patterns. This finding suggests that renal injury can be from other etiologic processes independent of exposure to lithium. The prevalence, incidence, and severity of lithium-induced kidney failure depend on the plasma concentration as well as the patient's kidney function.

▶ Pathogenesis

Lithium toxicities appear to be dose and concentration dependent. Serum concentrations between 1 and 1.5 mEq/L will most likely cause impaired concentration, lethargy, irritability, muscle weakness, tremor, slurred speech, and nausea. Plasma concentrations greater than 2.5 mEq/L have been associated with kidney failure. At therapeutic plasma concentrations, lithium impairs the acidification ability of distal collecting tubules, which leads to renal tubular acidosis but not systemic metabolic acidosis. In the collecting tubule, lithium inhibits production of cyclic AMP (cAMP), downregulates the aquaporin-2 channel, decreases antidiuretic hormone (ADH) receptor density, and leads to ADH resistance and impairment of collecting duct concentrating capacity, which leads to polyuria, polydipsia, and nephrogenic diabetes insipidus. Because of the need for long-term lithium therapy in bipolar patients, CKD manifesting as chronic tubulointerstitial nephropathy (CTIN) is often seen. Kidney biopsy reveals tubular atrophy and interstitial fibrosis either associated with cortical and medullary tubular cysts and dilation. CTIN is predominantly found in the distal and collecting tubule. Lithium also directly affects the glomerulus. Focal segmental glomerulosclerosis and global glomerulosclerosis are also seen, and they tend to parallel in severity the underlying tubulointerstitial disease. This finding explains the reduced GFR and proteinuria in patients with chronic lithium therapy.

Despite the discontinuation of the lithium, many patients who had serum creatinine greater than 2.5 mg/dL progressed to ESRD.

▶ Prevention & Management

Bipolar patients usually require long-term lithium treatment. Lithium has a narrow therapeutic range (1–1.5 mEq/L during acute episode therapy and 0.6–1.2 mEq/L during maintenance therapy). Chronic and acute poisoning can occur in patients whose lithium dosage has been increased or in those with a decreased effective circulating volume. Therefore, close monitoring of serum levels is important to prevent acute and chronic renal failure. Patients should be instructed to drink 8–12 glasses of liquid every day during lithium therapy. Because low sodium intake could promote lithium reabsorption, patients should maintain a regular non–low-salt diet. To avoid dehydration, prolonged exposure to the sun is discouraged and physicians should be contacted immediately if fever, diarrhea, or vomiting develops. Diuretics, especially thiazides, should be avoided with lithium concomitantly if possible. Thiazide diuretics contract extracellular volume; therefore, lithium reabsorption is increased in the proximal tubule. In addition, medications that potentially increase serum lithium levels such as cyclosporine and NSAIDs (except low-dose aspirin) or drugs with nephrotoxic properties such as aminoglycosides should be avoided (Table 14–4).

Fluid restoration is essential to manage lithium-induced nephrotoxicity. AKI usually occurs in association with severe dehydration, and adequate fluid replacement rapidly restores kidney function. Loop diuretics can acutely abolish the lithium reabsorption process in the loop of Henle and increase lithium excretion; hence, furosemide (up to 40 mg/h)

Table 14–5 Management of lithium intoxication.

1. Protect oral airway if consciousness is impaired
2. Volume resuscitation
3. Gastric lavage, whole bowel irrigation with polyethylene glycol to prevent continued absorption of lithium
4. Lithium removal
   Serum lithium level >3.5–4 mEq/L: Most patients require hemodialysis
   Serum lithium level 2–4 mEq/L: Unstable patients and patients with severe nephrologic signs of renal insufficiency require hemodialysis
   Serum lithium level 1.5–2.5 mEq/L:
   Hemodialysis indicated for patient with renal failure or if patient fails to reach a lithium level below 1 mEq/L
   Fluid therapy or forced diuresis treatment should be recommended in patients with early signs of lithium intoxication and normal renal function, and when it is known that lithium levels have been elevated for only a few days

can be used in case of lithium toxicity. However, such treatment cannot take place unless a large volume of fluids will be used to replace the loss of sodium and water induced by furosemide. In addition, lithium retention can occur following the discontinuation of furosemide due to its short duration of action and the reestablishment of intra- and extracellular lithium equilibrium. Acetazolamide combined with sodium bicarbonate can also be used instead of furosemide because acetazolamide inhibits the reabsorption of lithium by the proximal tubules.

Electrolyte supplements, especially sodium and potassium, should be given at the same time as management of lithium-induced nephrotoxicity because hyponatremia and hypokalemia are often seen in these patients. When patients cannot be managed medically or when kidney function is severely impaired, hemodialysis is the most efficient way to decrease lithium levels because lithium is entirely dialyzable. Lithium leaves the cells rather slowly and serum levels can rebound if hemodialysis stops too soon. Therefore, hemodialysis should take place for a longer period or at frequent intervals (Table 14–5).

NONSTEROIDAL ANTI-INFLAMMATORY DRUGS

▶ Incidence & Risk Factors

NSAIDs are frequently used to treat chronic inflammatory conditions and for amelioration of acute and chronic pain. Widespread access and over-the-counter availability of these agents lead to the frequent impression that these drugs are safe and relatively devoid of toxicity. Unfortunately, NSAIDs or even aspirin use can pose a substantial risk to a large number of patients, especially when used chronically. Kidney toxicity of the NSAIDs is discussed in Chapter 15.

Table 14–4. Drug interactions with lithium.

Drug	Effect on Serum Lithium Concentration
Thiazide diuretics	Increase
Acetazolamide and other carbonic anhydrase inhibitors	Decrease[a]
Osmotic diuretics	Decrease
K+-sparing diuretics	Minimal decrease or no effect
Methyl xanthine inhibitors	Decrease
Loop diuretics	Decrease[a]
ACE inhibitors	Increase
NSAIDs	
Indomethacin	Increase
Ibuprofen	Increase
Mefenamic acid	Increase
Naproxen	Increase
Sulindac	No effect
Aspirin	No effect

ACE, angiotensin-converting enzyme; NSAIDs, nonsteroidal anti-inflammatory drugs.
[a]When given acutely for lithium intoxication.

■ CHAPTER 14 REVIEW QUESTIONS

1. A 29-year-old man with ITP and complex PMHx was diagnosed with nonischemic cardiomyopathy that required emergent biventricular and heart transplantation. His perspective cross-match was positive donor-specific antibodies. He was started on plasmapheresis and IVIG. His serum creatinine increased from 1 to 1.9. Explain the possible mechanism for the kidney injury.
   A. Sucrose stabilizer causes increased osmolarity and leads to cell swelling and vacuolization of cells.
   B. Immune globulin alters the apoptotic pathways in tubular epithelial cells, which can cause inappropriate cell death in certain kidney tissue.
   C. IVIG can cause alteration of regional blood flow and lead to ischemic AKI.
   D. IVIG is not harmful to the kidney, and the patient's problem is likely prerenal.
   E. None of the above.

2. A 72-year-old woman was seen at clinic for increasing complaining of shortness of breath on exertion. She was started on frusemide 40 mg in the morning about 1 year ago for lower extremity edema and diclofenac 50 mg twice daily for the management of osteoarthritis. Her last Echo indicated left ventricular systolic dysfunction. And ACE inhibitor (lisinopril) was started. The patient serum creatinine increased from 1 to 1.3 mg/dL with normal K level after 72 hours. How should you proceed?
   A. Check patients potassium and add spironolactone for hyperkalemic.
   B. Decrease dose of lisinopril by 50%.
   C. Switch to ARB.
   D. Stop NSAIDs and observe patient.
   E. Discontinue ACE inhibitor/ARB therapy and change to different class of antihypertensive agent.

3. A 62-year-old man with a PMHx of leukemia with cytostatics and several adjuvant drugs, including pantoprazole, ciprofloxacin, fluconazole, furosemide, amphotericin B lipid complex, gentamicin, and vancomycin. Four days later, the patient's serum creatinine was 1.8 mg/dL (baseline value 0.6 mg/dL). Treatment with

piperacillin, vancomycin, and amphotericin B were stopped. By day 8, serum creatinine rose to a maximum of 3.6 mg/dL. Two days later, pantoprazole therapy was stopped and serum creatinine began to normalize. Explain the mechanism of PPI-induced nephropathy.
   A. Acute tubular necrosis
   B. Acute interstitial nephritis
   C. Drug-induced thrombotic microangiopathy
   D. Crystal nephropathy
   E. Osmotic nephrosis

4. A 40-year-old woman is receiving tenofovir disoproxil for HIV/HBV but experiencing renal dysfunction. Her serum creatinine was 0.6 mg/dL before initiation of HIV/HBV treatment and today it is 1.4 mg/dL. You are concerned about renal complications of tenofovir disoproxil. What would be the best approach in management of her infections?
   A. Coadminister mannitol to reduce OAT uptake into proximal tubule cells.
   B. Do nothing, as the AKI will resolve on its own in 2–3 days.
   C. Switch to tenofovir alafenamide.
   D. Give IV NaCl to replenish fluid load.
   E. Adjust dosing to every other day to account for accumulation due to decreased clearance.

5. A 48-year-old woman presents for evaluation of abdominal pain and fever. She was started on both vancomycin and piperacillin-tazobactam. After 3 days, her renal function worsened and serum creatinine was 6.1 mg/dL (baseline of 0.8 mg/dL). Last vancomycin level was therapeutic at 10.1. Explain the potential mechanism of AKI, which vancomycin and piperacillin-tazobactam might cause.
   A. Acute tubular necrosis
   B. Acute interstitial nephritis
   C. Crystal nephropathy
   D. A and B
   E. Unknown mechanism

NSAIDs and the Kidney: Acute Kidney Injury

Mark A. Perazella, MD, FACP

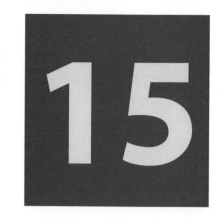

▶ General Considerations

A. Epidemiology of Nonsteroidal Anti-inflammatory Drug Use

NSAIDs are employed widely to treat pain, fever, and inflammation. Other potential uses for these drugs include treatment and prevention of colonic polyposis and Alzheimer-type dementia. The first NSAID discovered was sodium salicylate in 1763. In 1950, phenylbutazone was introduced into clinical practice. It was efficacious, but its use faded due to bone marrow toxicity. Subsequently, indomethacin entered the market in the 1960s. More than 20 NSAIDs from seven major classes, including the selective cyclooxygenase (COX)-2 inhibitors (Table 15–1), are available in the United States. In addition to prescription NSAIDs, a large percentage of the general population consumes over-the-counter NSAIDs. Annually, more than 50 million patients ingest these drugs on an intermittent basis, while some 15–25 million people in the United States use an NSAID on a regular basis. Importantly, the elderly patients who are at risk for multiple complications of NSAID therapy constitute a growing population that has a prevalence of NSAID use as high as 15–20%.

B. Epidemiology of Nonsteroidal Anti-inflammatory Drug-Associated Acute Kidney Injury

Unfortunately, the price paid for these therapeutic benefits include a number of gastrointestinal (GI) complications and, to a lesser degree, adverse renal effects. It has been estimated that from 5% to 7% of admissions to the hospital occur due to toxicity of NSAIDs, with the major organs involved being the GI tract, kidneys, and nervous system. The nephrotoxicity of NSAIDs, in particular hemodynamic acute kidney injury (AKI), is a relatively uncommon but important problem. It has been estimated that anywhere from 1% to 5% of patients who ingest NSAIDs will develop nephrotoxicity. Some calculations approximate that 500,000 persons are likely to develop some form of NSAID-associated adverse renal impairment (Table 15–2). In a study of 121,722 new NSAID users older than 65 years, the adjusted relative risk (RR) for AKI was 2.05. Current and recent NSAID use had an adjusted RR of 1.62. A dose response for these drugs in causing AKI was also observed.

Exposure to NSAIDs has been noted to double the risk of hospitalization for AKI in patients with chronic kidney disease (CKD). Patients with a history of heart failure and hypertension, as well as those treated with diuretics, are at greatest risk of NSAID-induced AKI. The effect also appeared to be dose related with AKI occurring with higher NSAID

Table 15–1. Classes of nonsteroidal anti-inflammatory drugs.

Class	Trade Name	Total Dose/Day (Dosing Interval)
Carboxylic acids		
Aspirin	Aspirin	2.4–6.0 g (qid)
Salsalate	Disalcid	1.5–3.0 g (bid)
Choline magnesium	Trilisate	1.5–3.0 g (bid–tid)
Diflunisal	Dolobid	0.5–1.5 g (bid)
Acetic acids		
Indomethacin	Indocin	75–150 mg (bid–qid)
Tolmetin	Tolectin	400–2400 mg (bid–tid)
Sulindac	Clinoril	200–400 mg (bid)
Diclofenac	Voltaren, Cataflam Arthrotec	100–150 mg (bid) 100 mg (bid)
Etodolac	Lodine	400–1200 mg (bid–qid)
Ketorolac	Toradol	Oral 40 mg (qid) Intravenous 60–120 mg (qid)
Propionic acids		
Ibuprofen	Motrin, Rufen	800–3200 mg (qid)
Naproxen	Naprosyn, Anaprox Alleve	500–1000 mg (bid) 450 mg (bid)
Ketoprofen	Orudis	225 mg (tid)
Flurbiprofen	Ansaid	200–300 mg (bid–tid)
Fenoprofen	Nalfon	1200–2400 mg (qid)
Oxaprozin	Daypro	1200 mg (qd)
Enolic acids		
Piroxicam	Feldene	10–20 mg (qd)
Phenylbutazone	Butazolidin	300–600 mg (tid)
Fenamates		
Mefenamic acid	Ponstel	1000 mg (qid)
Meclofenamate	Meclomen	150–400 mg (tid–qid)
Naphthylkanones		
Nabumetone	Relafen	1000–1500 mg (bid–tid)
COX-2 inhibitors		
Celecoxib	Celebrex	100–400 mg (qd–bid)

Table 15–2. Renal syndromes associated with nonsteroidal anti-inflammatory drugs.

Acute kidney injury
Metabolic disturbances
   Hyponatremia
   Hyperkalemia
   Metabolic acidosis
Hypertension
Edema
Acute interstitial nephritis
Chronic interstitial nephritis
Glomerular disease (minimal change disease, membranous nephropathy)
Papillary necrosis
Uroepithelial malignancy

dose. Hospitalized patients are at even higher risk. Of the cases of drug-induced AKI that develop in the hospital, it is estimated that nearly 16% are due to NSAID therapy. The number of NSAID-related cases of AKI and the associated clinical and metabolic complications increases further when these drugs are combined with other medications such as the renin-angiotensin-system (RAS) antagonists and diuretics. In one study, the adjusted rate ratio for AKI was highest with the three combined drug groups (1.31, 1.12–1.53; 95% confidence interval [CI]) versus NSAIDs plus diuretics or NSAIDs plus RAS antagonists.

As will be discussed in more detail, the healthy general population is at less risk for AKI as compared with patients who possess multiple risk factors associated with NSAID nephrotoxicity. The majority of adverse renal effects are attributable to inhibition of renal prostaglandins (PGs) by NSAIDs. The selective COX-2 inhibitor, celecoxib appears to have a renal profile similar to other NSAIDs. Therefore, the term *NSAIDs* will refer to both nonselective NSAIDs and the selective COX-2 inhibitors. Electrolyte and acid–base disorders that occur with these drugs (hyperkalemia, hyponatremia, metabolic acidosis), hypertension that develops or is exacerbated by NSAIDs, and disturbances in sodium balance (edema formation, exacerbation of heart failure) will also be reviewed briefly in the context of AKI.

▶ **Pathogenesis**

A. Prostaglandin Synthesis

It is essential to review the pathway of prostaglandin (PG) production to facilitate an understanding of NSAID efficacy and toxicity. PGs, the major products of COX enzyme metabolism, are produced throughout the body and act at the local organ level in an autocrine and paracrine fashion. The initial step in PG synthesis is the liberation of arachidonic acid from cell membrane phospholipids. This reaction is mediated by phospholipase A_2, which is triggered by a number of hormones and mechanical factors. Arachidonic acid is the substrate for COX. Following synthesis, PGs promptly exit the cell to bind PG receptors found on parent or neighboring cells, thereby modulating cellular functions (Figure 15–1).

Two isomers of COX, COX-1 and COX-2, catalyze the synthesis of PGs. These isomers share a similar amino acid sequence and catalytic function. Differences in gene regulation between the COX isomers provide a molecular basis for their purported roles as "constitutive" (COX-1) and "inducible" (COX-2) enzymes. These labels accurately describe the synthesis of COX in most tissues, where COX-1, but not COX-2, is expressed in appreciable levels at baseline. In contrast, abundant expression of COX-2 is demonstrated in macrophages

and other cell types in response to inflammatory mediators. However, it is now known that COX-2 is also constitutively expressed and upregulated in the kidney, and it plays an important role in renal physiologic processes. It is probable that the nephrotoxicity of selective and nonselective NSAIDs results from the inhibition of COX-2 rather than COX-1.

B. Role of Prostaglandins in Renal Physiology

PG synthesis is of minimal importance in the kidney of healthy individuals with normal volume status. As such, it is not a primary regulator of renal function. Rather, eicosanoids locally modulate the effects of both systemic and locally produced vasoconstrictor hormones. A variety of

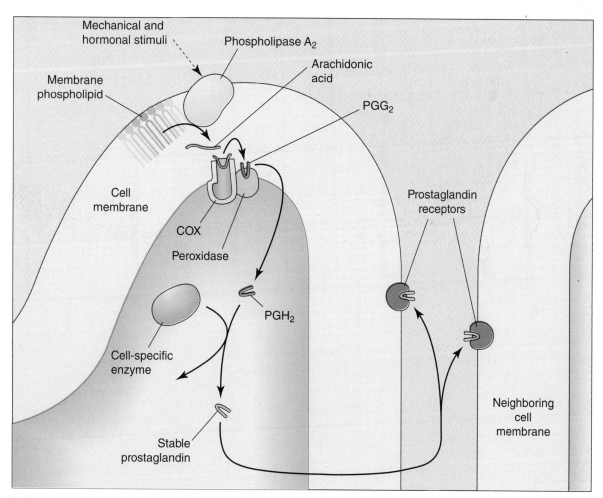

▲ **Figure 15–1.** Pathway of prostaglandin biosynthesis. Arachidonic acid is released from membrane phospholipids, modulated by cyclooxygenase (COX) and cell-specific enzymes to form prostaglandins (PGs). Prostaglandins then produce their effect by binding receptors on parent and neighboring cells. (Reproduced, with permission, from Perazella MA: COX-2 inhibitors and the kidney. Hosp Pract 2001;36:43.)

PGs are synthesized within distinct anatomic locations in the kidney, including PGI_2, PGE_2, thromboxane A_2 (TXA_2), and $PGF_{2\alpha}$ (Figure 15–2). PGI_2 and PGE_2 are the predominant mediators of physiologic activity in the kidney. Functionally, PGI_2 and PGE_2 induce vasodilation in interlobular arteries, afferent and efferent arterioles, and glomeruli. There is also an effect of PGs to maintain peritubular capillary perfusion and tubular cell health, reducing ischemic tubular injury.

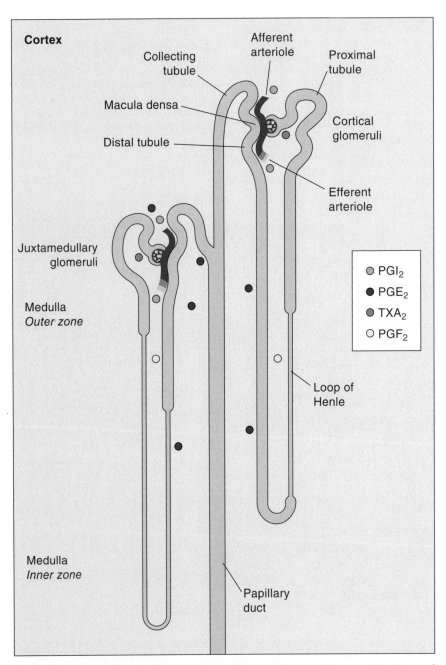

▲ **Figure 15–2.** Anatomic locations of prostaglandin (PG) synthesis within the kidney and their sites of action. TXA_2, thromboxane A_2. (Reproduced, with permission, from Perazella MA: COX-2 inhibitors and the kidney. Hosp Pract 2001;36:43.)

In the loop of Henle and distal nephron, PGE_2 decreases cellular transport of sodium chloride in thick ascending limb cells and collecting duct cells, respectively. An increase in renal sodium excretion and a decrease in medullary tonicity are the direct result of PGE_2 action in these nephron segments. PGE_2 and PGI_2 also stimulate renin secretion in the juxtaglomerular apparatus, ultimately leading to increased angiotensin II and aldosterone synthesis, enhancing sodium retention and potassium excretion in the distal nephron. Finally, PGE_2 and PGI_2 also inhibit cyclic adenosine monophosphate (cAMP) synthesis and oppose the action of antidiuretic hormone (ADH), facilitating water excretion.

C. Risk Factors for Nonsteroidal Anti-inflammatory Drug-Associated Acute Kidney Failure

Since basal PG production is low in healthy persons, the risk of NSAID-associated AKI is negligible. There are, however, risk factors (Table 15–3) that render the kidney PG dependent and, therefore, place patients at risk for the development of AKI when they use NSAIDs. PGs have their major role in the preservation of renal function when pathologic states supervene and compromise physiologic kidney processes. The development of "true" intravascular volume depletion, as seen with vomiting, diarrhea, and diuretic therapy, stimulates PG synthesis to optimize renal blood flow. "Effective" decreases in renal blood flow as seen with congestive heart failure (CHF), cirrhosis, and nephrotic syndrome also stimulate compensatory PG production. PGI_2 and PGE_2 antagonize the local effects of circulating angiotensin II, endothelin, vasopressin, and catecholamines that would normally maintain systemic blood pressure at the expense of the renal circulation. Specifically, these eicosanoids preserve glomerular filtration rate (GFR) by antagonizing arteriolar vasoconstriction and blunting mesangial

Table 15–3. Risk factors for NSAID-associated acute kidney injury.

"True" intravascular volume depletion
Vomiting
Diarrhea
Diuretics
"Effective" intravascular volume depletion
Congestive heart failure
Cirrhosis
Nephrotic syndrome
Kidney disease
Acute kidney injury
Chronic kidney disease
Medications
Angiotensin-converting enzyme inhibitors
Angiotensin receptor blockers
Old age

and podocyte contraction induced by these endogenous vasopressors. A significant reduction in GFR can occur following administration of an NSAID to a patient with any of these underlying disease states (Figure 15–3).

PG production is also increased in CKD. Upregulation of PG synthesis in CKD is induced by intrarenal mechanisms activated to increase perfusion of remnant nephrons. As a result, impairment of PG production with an NSAID is associated with acute reductions in renal blood flow and GFR. Certain medications, such as drugs that antagonize the RAS such as angiotensin-converting enzyme (ACE) inhibitors and angiotensin receptor blockers (ARBs), increase the risk for AKI when an NSAID is administered. This is typically a problem in patients with true or effective intravascular volume depletion or underlying CKD. In the absence of underlying kidney disease, AKI rarely develops when these patients are euvolemic. Finally, the elderly patients are at risk for AKI because of unrecognized CKD, intravascular volume depletion, and hypoalbuminemia (which increases levels of free NSAID in the circulation). Excessive free serum levels increase the nephrotoxic effects of these drugs.

▶ Clinical Findings

A. Symptoms and Signs

In the absence of severe AKI, most patients with NSAID-associated prerenal azotemia are asymptomatic. The underlying risk factor that predisposes the patient to AKI often determines the clinical presentation. For example, patients with "true" intravascular volume depletion will present with uremic manifestations such as anorexia, nausea and vomiting, weakness, fatigue, inability to concentrate, and possibly GI dyspepsia (from NSAID gastropathy). They will not be hypertensive or edematous. In contrast, patients with "effective" intravascular volume depletion such as CHF, cirrhosis, or nephrotic syndrome will manifest volume overload. In the CHF patient, this can manifest as lung crackles, elevated jugular venous pulsations, and an S3 cardiac gallop from pulmonary edema, as well as peripheral pitting edema. Increased abdominal girth from ascites and worsened peripheral edema can develop in the patient with cirrhosis. Increased peripheral edema and anasarca may develop in the patient with nephrotic syndrome. Patients with CHF and nephrosis will often be hypertensive, whereas the patient with cirrhosis does not develop an increase in blood pressure.

Patients with underlying hypertension, especially when under therapy with antihypertensive medications, will often manifest a destabilization of blood pressure and present with worsened hypertension. The patient with CKD will develop acute uremia, severe hypertension, increased peripheral edema, and CHF. Muscle weakness and cardiac arrhythmias (from hyperkalemia) can occur in CKD patients who receive NSAIDs. In addition, patients treated with medications

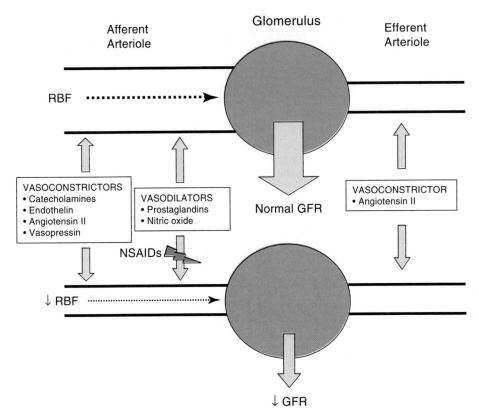

▲ **Figure 15–3.** Renal prostaglandins maintain RBF and GFR by balancing the vasoconstrictor effects of various endogenous factors during "true" or "effective" volume depletion. NSAIDs blunt prostaglandin production and tip the balance in favor of vasoconstriction, resulting in reduced RBF and GFR, manifesting clinically as acute renal failure. GFR, glomerular filtration rate; NSAIDs, nonsteroidal anti-inflammatory drugs; RBF, renal blood flow.

that impair potassium homeostasis (ACE inhibitors, ARBs, spironolactone, eplerenone, calcineurin inhibitors, heparin) may also develop these adverse effects when an NSAID is added to their regimen. The elderly patient can present with any number of these clinical symptoms and signs.

B. Laboratory Findings

AKI associated with NSAIDs is hemodynamic, and therefore the laboratory parameters typically reflect a "prerenal" state. Both serum and urine tests support this. BUN and serum Cr concentrations are both elevated; however, the BUN concentration typically increases more than the serum Cr concentration. In general, the BUN/Cr ratio is greater than 20, although this does not occur in all patients. Not uncommonly, several electrolyte disturbances may also be present. They include hyponatremia (serum [Na+] <135 mEq/L) from impaired renal water excretion and hyperkalemia (serum [K+] >5.5 mEq/L) with or without a nonanion gap metabolic acidosis. NSAID-induced

hyporeninemic hypoaldosteronism underlies the hyperkalemia and nonanion gap metabolic acidosis. Importantly, these electrolyte and acid–base disturbances can develop even with minimal AKI as they are caused via direct effects of the NSAID on various tubular segments in the nephron.

Urine testing also points to a prerenal state of AKI. The urine-specific gravity (SG) is typically greater than 1.015. Urine [Na+] is often less than 10–20 mEq/L. Calculation of the fractional excretion of sodium (FE_{Na^+} = [urine Na+ × serum Cr] ÷ [serum Na+ × urine Cr]) reveals a value less than 1% (Table 15–4). This contrasts with a value greater than 3%, which would characterize acute tubular necrosis (ATN). Rarely, the specific gravity and FE_{Na^+} may be suggestive of ATN (SG ≤1.015, FE_{Na^+} >3.0%) in patients with NSAID-associated AKI. This represents a situation in which some level of ischemic ATN develops, probably due to hypotension and severe renal hypoperfusion. Hyperkalemia is evaluated by calculating the transtubular potassium gradient

Table 15–4. Urine findings noted in NSAID-associated acute renal failure and acute tubular necrosis.

SG	Urine [Na$^+$]	FE$_{Na^+}$	Sediment
NSAID >1.020	<10–20 mEq/L	<1.0%	Bland, acellular, hyaline casts
ATN ± 1.015	>20 mEq/L	>3.0%	RTE cells, RTE cell casts, granular casts
AIN ± 1.015	>20 mEq/L	>3.0%	WBCs, RBCs, rare eosinophils, WBC casts

AIN, acute interstitial nephritis; ATN, acute tubular necrosis; NSAID, nonsteroidal anti-inflammatory drug; RBCs, red blood cells; RTE, renal tubular epithelial; SG, specific gravity; WBCs, white blood cells.

(TTKG). TTKG is calculated as follows: TTKG = [urine K$^+$ ÷ (urine osmolality/serum osmolality)] ÷ serum K$^+$. A TTKG less than 6 in the setting of hyperkalemia reflects impaired renal potassium excretion due to hypoaldosteronism and is consistent with a diagnosis of NSAID nephrotoxicity.

Microscopic examination of the urine in patients with NSAID-associated AKI generally reveals a bland sediment with no cellular elements and sometimes a few hyaline casts or mixed hyaline/finely granular casts. This is consistent with the prerenal azotemia that develops in this setting. Rarely, a few renal tubular epithelial (RTE) cells, RTE cell casts, and granular casts may be present if ischemic tubular injury has also developed. It is uncommon to view red blood cells, white blood cells, or casts containing these cellular elements unless another renal disease coexists. Their presence suggests superimposition of NSAID nephrotoxicity on another renal process, such as acute interstitial nephritis (AIN).

Imaging tests are normal in the absence of another concurrent disease process in the kidneys. Renal ultrasonography reveals normal-sized kidneys with normal echotexture and no evidence of hydronephrosis. Computerized tomography (CT) scan and magnetic resonance imaging (MRI) are also normal in pure NSAID-associated AKI. Due to the concern for NSF, gadolinium, even with the newer chelate agents, should be avoided in AKI to assess for renovascular stenosis. An ACE inhibitor renal perfusion scan would show bilateral decreased uptake of tracer by the kidneys, consistent with prerenal azotemia.

Differential Diagnosis

AKI that develops in the setting of NSAID therapy needs to be differentiated from other prerenal states, as well as various intrinsic renal processes such as ATN and AIN. As with other causes of ARF, obstructive uropathy also needs to be considered in the differential diagnosis.

Since both "true" and "effective" intravascular volume depletion cause prerenal AKI and also are risk factors for NSAID-associated AKI, it is very difficult to ascribe renal injury to either alone. This is because the addition of an NSAID can potentially worsen underlying CHF and cirrhosis, making them appear as poorly compensated disease

states. Regardless, discontinuation of the drug and therapy directed at the underlying clinical disease are required. Ischemic ATN can develop from the underlying clinical problem (ie, hypotension, sepsis) as well as from the effect of NSAID on renal hemodynamics, which further worsens renal perfusion and GFR in these settings. The urine data distinguish NSAID-associated AKI from ATN as an SG of 1.015 or less, urine [Na$^+$] greater than 20 mEq/L, FE$_{Na^+}$ greater than 3%, and urine sediment with RTE cells, RTE cell casts, and granular casts generally characterize ATN.

AKI from AIN may also develop from an NSAID. Patients who do not recover within several days of stopping the NSAID should be evaluated for AIN. Although not always the case, AIN usually is associated with eosinophilia, tubular proteinuria (<1 g/day), pyuria (± eosinophiluria), and hematuria (see Table 15–4). AIN from NSAIDs, however, is often devoid of the classic findings of AIN and can present with a bland urine sediment. Finally, AKI from partial urinary tract obstruction can be confused with NSAID-associated AKI because the urine sediment can also be unremarkable. However, the urine SG and electrolytes more often reflect tubular injury and are similar to those seen with ATN.

Complications

As with any drug that induces AKI, a number of uremic, metabolic, and intravascular volume-related complications can develop. Severe AKI may be associated with several uremia-related problems. These include central nervous system dysfunction (confusion, agitation, seizure), bleeding from platelet dysfunction, increased infection risk, malnutrition from a catabolic state, and inflammation of serosal surfaces (pericarditis, pleuritis). Hyponatremia, hyperkalemia, and nonanion gap metabolic acidosis can develop from AKI or from direct effects of the NSAID. Hyperkalemia can be more severe than expected for the level of renal dysfunction due to the state of hyporeninemic hypoaldosteronism promoted by the NSAID. Volume overload with pulmonary edema and peripheral edema can complicate NSAID-associated nephrotoxicity in cardiac patients. Precipitation of hepatorenal syndrome is a potentially devastating complication of NSAID therapy in cirrhotic patients. Also, diuretic resistance can develop in patients with CHF and nephrotic syndrome. Increased risk for adverse cardiovascular events has been noted with both selective and nonselective NSAIDs.

▶ Treatment

The mainstay of therapy is discontinuation of the NSAID. Additional measures include correction of the underlying process that predisposed to nephrotoxicity. In some cases, intravenous normal saline rapidly repairs volume status and facilitates renal recovery in patients with intravascular volume depletion. High-dose intravenous diuretics, sometimes in combination, may be required in cardiac patients with AKI complicated by CHF and in nephrotic patients with severe edema and anasarca. Life-threatening hyperkalemia mandates intravenous calcium gluconate (stabilize cardiac tissue), intravenous insulin plus glucose, high-dose nebulized β_2-agonists to shift K^+ into cells, and diuretic therapy to enhance renal excretion in patients who maintain reasonable kidney function. It is unusual for metabolic acidosis to be severe enough to warrant sodium bicarbonate administration. Severe AKI complicated by advanced uremia or other life-threatening complications (pulmonary edema, metabolic disturbances) that does not recover within a few days of stopping NSAID therapy requires renal replacement therapy.

▶ Prognosis

Fortunately, discontinuation of the NSAID is often associated with recovery of renal function. In general, renal function returns to baseline within 2–5 days; however, recovery may be delayed in patients with decompensated heart disease, cirrhosis, and underlying CKD. It is extremely unusual that a patient does not recover kidney function. The failure to do so should elicit an evaluation for other causes of AKI such as ATN, AIN, and obstructive uropathy.

KEY READINGS

Bouvy ML et al: Effects of NSAIDs on the incidence of hospitalizations for renal dysfunction in users of ACE inhibitors. Drug Safety 2003;26:983.

Eras J, Perazella MA: NSAIDs and the kidney revisited: are selective cyclooxygenase-2 inhibitors safe? Am J Med Sci 2001;321:181.

Gambaro G, Perazella MA: Adverse renal effects of antiinflammatory agents: evaluation of selective and non-selective cyclooxygenase inhibitors. J Intern Med 2003;253:643.

Huerta C et al: Nonsteroidal anti-inflammatory drugs and risk of ARF in the general population. Am J Kidney Dis 2005;45:531.

Perazella MA: Drug-induced hyperkalemia: old culprits and new offenders. Am J Med 2000;109:307.

Perazella MA, Tray K: Selective COX-2 inhibitors: a pattern of nephrotoxicity similar to traditional nonsteroidal anti-inflammatory drugs. Am J Med 2001;111:64.

Schneider V et al: Association of selective and conventional nonsteroidal antiinflammatory drugs with acute renal failure: a population-based, nested case-control analysis. Am J Epi 2006;164:881.

Sturmer T et al: Nonsteroidal anti-inflammatory drugs and the kidney. Curr Opin Nephrol Hypertens 2001;10:161.

■ CHAPTER REVIEW QUESTIONS

1. A 69-year-old man with hypertension, chronic obstructive pulmonary disease (COPD), osteoarthritis, CAD, and gout develops 3 days of nausea and diarrhea. In addition, he developed a gout flare during this time and took indomethacin to reduce the pain and inflammation. Other medications include atenolol, acetaminophen, inhaler, aspirin, and allopurinol. He sees his primary care physician who notes a serum creatinine concentration of 1.9 mg/dL (baseline 1 mg/dL). He advises the patient to stop the indomethacin, and the serum creatinine declines to 1.1 mg/dL on the blood draw 5 days later.

Which of the following made the patient prostaglandin dependent for renal perfusion and GFR?
A. Hypertension
B. Gout
C. Aspirin
D. Diarrhea
E. Allopurinol

2. A 55-year-old woman with underlying congestive cardiomyopathy (ejection fraction [EF] 25%) from alcohol abuse injures her shoulder after a fall. She takes over-the-counter naproxen twice daily for the pain. Ten days later, she presents to the emergency department (ED) with worsening dyspnea and lower extremity edema. Exam reveals blood pressure (BP) 120/65 mm Hg, pulse rate 90 beats/min with bilateral lung crackles, S_3 cardiac gallop, and 2+ lower extremity pitting edema. Laboratory report reveals the following: Na 127 mEq/L, K 5.7 mEq/L, HCO_3 19 mEq/L, BUN 44 mg/dL, and serum Cr 2.1 mg/dL.

In this patient, which of the following are associated with naproxen therapy?
A. Hypervolemia
B. Hyponatremia
C. Hyperkalemia
D. AKI
E. All of the above

3. A 49-year-old woman with stage 4 CKD develops acute kidney injury following 7 days of ibuprofen. Her BP is 145/80, and exam reveals 1+ pedal edema. Electrolytes reveal Na 130 mEq/L, K 5.3 mEq/L, HCO_3 19 mEq/L, BUN 88 mg/dL, and serum Cr 5.8 mg/dL. Ibuprofen is discontinued, and her serum Cr returns to baseline after 5 days.

Which of the following urine studies would you expect to see in this patient?
A. SG-1.010; FeNa-2.5%; protein-negative; blood-negative; sediment-granular casts
B. SG-1.020; FeNa-0.5%; protein-negative; blood-negative; sediment-hyaline casts
C. SG-1.015; FeNa-1.5%; protein-2+; blood-2+; sediment-dysmorphic RBCs
D. SG-1.012; FeNa-1.3%; protein-1+; blood-trace; sediment-many WBCs, few RBCs
E. SG-1.020; FeNa-0.9%; protein-3+; blood-negative; sediment-oval fat bodies

4. Which of the following is a non–dose-related adverse effect of NSAIDs?
A. Ischemic acute tubular injury
B. Prerenal azotemia
C. Acute interstitial nephritis
D. Hyponatremia
E. Hyperkalemia

5. A 76-year-old woman with stage 3a CKD, hypertension, and congestive cardiomyopathy asks her primary care physician for an analgesic for her back and knee pain from osteoarthritis. She requests celecoxib as she has seen ads on television for this drug.

What would be your recommendation to this patient?
A. Celecoxib is less nephrotoxic as compared with nonselective NSAIDs and is okay to use for pain control.
B. Celecoxib is more nephrotoxic than nonselective NSAIDs and should be avoided.
C. Celecoxib and nonselective NSAIDs are equally nephrotoxic, and either can be used.
D. Celecoxib and nonselective NSAIDs are equally nephrotoxic, and neither should be used in this patient due to high risk for adverse renal effects.

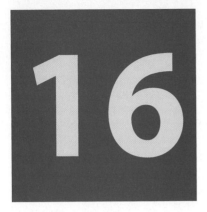

Obstructive Uropathy

Beckie Michael, DO, FASN

▶ Urinary tract obstruction should be included in the differential diagnosis of acute or chronic kidney disease.

▶ The diagnosis of obstructive uropathy usually requires the presence of hydronephrosis, hydroureter, and/or bladder distention.

▶ Ultrasound is the imaging study of choice to determine if obstructive uropathy is present.

▶ General Considerations

Urinary tract obstruction is not uncommon and can present at any age, although it is more commonly encountered in the elderly. Obstructive uropathy is defined as the blockage of urine drainage from the kidney, ureter, or bladder. While lower urinary tract symptoms may be present when bladder or urethral causes of obstruction exist, upper urinary tract obstruction may be asymptomatic. Urinary tract obstruction can lead to acute and chronic kidney disease. Urinary tract imaging should be included in the evaluation of individuals who present with impaired renal function.

▶ Prevention

Individuals at high risk of urine retention should be screened for symptoms and examined for bladder distention. These include patients with diabetes, Guillain–Barré syndrome, peripheral neuropathy and older males. Medications associated with urine retention include sympathomimetics, anticholinergics, antihistamines, and muscle relaxants and these medications should be avoided in those with risk factors for urine retention. If urinary tract infection has been excluded, urodynamic testing can be performed to determine the best treatment option for those with lower urinary tract symptoms.

Patients with a history of kidney stones should undergo metabolic evaluation to determine the cause and appropriate treatment if an abnormality is found. Unless contraindicated, all patients with a history of kidney stone should increase water intake to greater than 2.5 L daily. Temporary placement of ureter stents should be considered in individuals undergoing renal transplant or complex pelvic surgeries to reduce the risk of ureter-related complications.

▶ Clinical Findings

A. Symptoms and Signs

Individuals with obstructive uropathy may present with lower urinary tract symptoms, including frequency, nocturia, incontinence, dysuria, hesitancy, weak stream, or straining to void. Incomplete obstruction can result in fluctuating urine output. Acute obstruction can result in pain due to distention of the bladder and/or collecting system or renal capsule. Renal colic due to calculi is often sudden and severe, with pain beginning in the flank and radiating into the groin. This can be accompanied by nausea, vomiting, and/or hematuria. Patients with renal colic prefer to be in motion, compared to patients with peritonitis, whose pain is worsened with movement. Occasionally, patients may develop a superimposed urinary tract infection due to the blockage and stasis of urine flow. In this case, patients may have fever or even present with sepsis.

A distended bladder or the presence of a flank or abdominal mass on physical examination is suggestive of obstruction. Hypertension can occur in obstructive uropathy due to volume expansion and activation of the renin–angiotensin–aldosterone system. Patients with obstruction of a solitary kidney or bilateral obstruction may present with acute oligoanuric renal failure.

B. Laboratory Findings

Table 16–1 lists the common laboratory abnormalities in obstructive uropathy. The kidney loses its ability to

Table 16–1. Common laboratory findings in obstructive uropathy.

Elevated blood urea nitrogen (BUN)
Elevated serum creatinine
Ratio of BUN:Cr > 10:1
Normal anion gap metabolic acidosis (distal renal tubular acidosis)
Normal potassium or hyperkalemia
Hematuria and/or pyuria

concentrate urine early in obstruction. Later, it cannot concentrate or dilute urine well, resulting in isosthenuria (urine specific gravity similar to plasma). Defects in distal urinary acidification result in hyperchloremic metabolic acidosis (distal renal tubular acidosis). This can be accompanied by hyperkalemia. Blood urea nitrogen (BUN) and serum creatinine are often elevated if there is bilateral obstruction or obstruction of a solitary functioning kidney. The ratio of BUN to serum creatinine is often greater than 10:1 due to increased urea reabsorption throughout the collecting system, but this finding is neither sensitive or specific. Patients with partial obstruction may develop nephrogenic diabetes insipidus (resistance to antidiuretic hormone) and hypernatremia. Patients may have polycythemia due to excess erythropoietin production, or may be anemic with more advanced renal impairment. Urine stasis can result in urinary tract infections, particularly with urease-producing bacteria like *Proteus* or *Klebsiella*, which increase ammonia production. This results in an alkaline urine pH, which can cause struvite (magnesium ammonium phosphate) calculi.

C. Imaging Studies

1. Abdominal X-ray—Abdominal X-ray is useful in identifying radiopaque calculi; however, it will not detect obstruction. Patients suspected of having renal colic often proceed directly to noncontrast CT imaging for diagnosis.

2. Ultrasound—Ultrasound is very sensitive and specific for detecting hydronephrosis, defined as a dilated renal pelvis and calyces (Figure 16–1). It is the imaging study of choice to evaluate for urinary tract obstruction because it can be performed quickly and avoids exposure to ionizing radiation. Ultrasound can also detect urine flow from the ureter into the bladder, known as the urinary jet. The absence of a urinary jet can indicate obstruction. Ultrasound can be falsely negative early in obstruction, if there is volume depletion, or if the ureters are involved in a retroperitoneal process like retroperitoneal fibrosis. Ultrasound can detect radiolucent stones missed on X-ray, but is less likely than CT to detect small stones or stones in ureters. An extrarenal pelvis may be mistaken for proximal hydroureter on ultrasound.

Bladder ultrasound is often performed with measurement of postvoid residual (PVR) to detect incomplete

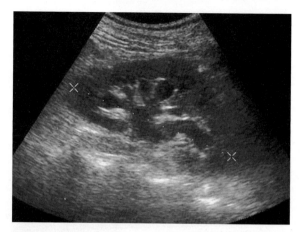

▲ **Figure 16–1.** Ultrasound demonstrating hydronephrosis. Longitudinal sonogram of a hydronephrotic left kidney shows dilatation of the minor and major calyces and the pelvis. (Reproduced with permission from Zeidel ML, O'Neill WC: Clinical manifestations and diagnosis of urinary tract obstruction and hydronephrosis. In: UpToDate, Post TW (editor), UpToDate, Waltham, MA. (accessed on February 8, 2017.) Copyright © 2017 UpToDate, Inc. For more information visit http://www.uptodate.com.)

bladder emptying. Normal PVR is less than 30 mL, but clinically significant urine retention is considered when PVR is greater than 200 mL. Bladder ultrasound can identify signs of bladder damage due to chronic urine retention. These findings may include increased bladder wall thickness (>2.9 mm), diverticuli, trabeculations, and calculi.

3. CT and CT urogram—CT without contrast is the imaging study of choice for detecting renal stones and can also readily detect obstruction. CT is now being performed with limited radiation exposure. A CT urogram is helpful in determining the exact location of obstruction and can detect ureteric neoplasms, but should be avoided in patients at risk of contrast-induced nephropathy. Figure 16–2 shows a contrast-enhanced CT scan, demonstrating hydronephrosis of the left kidney.

4. Magnetic resonance urography—Magnetic resonance urography (MRU) can be performed with or without the use of contrast (gadolinium) and therefore is beneficial in patients who cannot receive iodinated contrast required for CT urogram. It is less sensitive than CT in detecting calculi.

5. Radionuclide scanning—Radionuclide scanning requires injection of a radioisotope (Tc-99mMAG3), often with furosemide, and is helpful in differentiating obstructive from nonobstructive hydronephrosis. It also can be used to determine the function of each kidney or to test for reflux via voiding cystourethrogram.

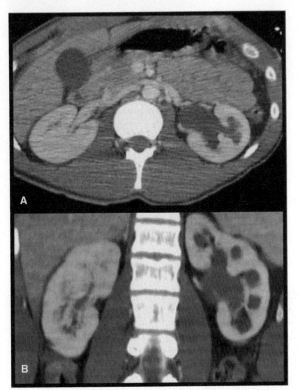

▲ **Figure 16–2.** Hydronephrosis: contrast-enhanced CT scan. Transverse **(A)** and coronal reconstruction **(B)** from a contrast-enhanced scan (corticomedullary phase) showing dilated calyces, pelvis, and proximal ureter on the left side. (Reproduced with permission from Zeidel ML, O'Neill WC: Clinical manifestations and diagnosis of urinary tract obstruction and hydronephrosis. In: UpToDate, Post TW (editor), UpToDate, Waltham, MA. (accessed on [date].) Copyright © 2017 UpToDate, Inc. For more information visit http://www.uptodate.com.)

6. Intravenous pyelography—Intravenous pyelography (IVP) should be avoided in patients with renal impairment due to the risk of worsening renal function after intravenous contrast administration. Prior to the availability of CT, IVP was used to determine the location of obstruction and was helpful in identifying papillary necrosis. The use of IVP has been largely replaced by contrast-enhanced CT, which has been found to be more sensitive than IVP in determining the cause of obstruction.

KEY READINGS

Galosi AB et al: Modifications of the bladder wall (organ damage) in patients with bladder outlet obstruction: ultrasound parameters. Arch Ital Urol Androl 2012;84:263.

Guzel O et al: Can bladder wall thickness measurement be used for detecting bladder outlet obstruction? Urology 2015;86:439.
Riddell J et al: Sensitivity of emergency bedside ultrasound to detect hydronephrosis in patients with computed-tomography-proven stones. West J Emerg Med 2014;15:96.

D. Special Examinations

If a bladder scanner is not available, bladder catheterization can be performed to determine if urine retention is present. Rectal and pelvic examinations are performed to determine the presence of a mass (cervix, uterus, ovary, rectum, or prostate) and the size of the prostate. Cystoscopy with retrograde ureterogram avoids systemic contrast administration and is not only a diagnostic procedure but can result in interventions to relieve obstruction. Percutaneous nephrostomy can also be performed to relieve obstruction.

▶ Differential Diagnosis

Obstructive uropathy should be considered in the differential diagnosis of acute or chronic kidney disease. Table 16–2 lists the common causes of obstructive uropathy according to location. The most common causes of bilateral obstruction are bladder outlet obstruction and neurogenic bladder (from diabetes, spinal cord injury, multiple sclerosis, or Guillain–Barré syndrome).

Table 16–2. Etiologies of obstructive uropathy.

Upper tract obstruction
Intrinsic
Stone
Papillary necrosis
Blood clot
Transitional cell carcinoma
Valve/polyp
Ureteropelvic junction obstruction
Extrinsic
Retroperitoneal fibrosis
Aortic aneurysm
Retroperitoneal or pelvic adenopathy or malignancy
Masses of uterus/ovary
Endometriosis
Ureter ligation
Lower tract obstruction
Urethral stricture
Posterior urethral valve
Prostate disease
Bladder, cervix, colon cancer
Bladder stones
Blood clot
Neurogenic bladder

In men, bladder outlet obstruction due to prostate disease or urethral stricture is the most common cause of lower urinary tract obstruction and is easily diagnosed by assessing post void urine residual by ultrasound or catheterization. In women, cervical cancer, uterine prolapse, and pregnancy are common causes of obstructive uropathy.

Stones are a common cause of unilateral upper tract obstruction. Urine flow is usually obstructed due to the presence of stones at one of three locations: the ureteropelvic junction, where the ureter crosses over the iliac vessels, or at the ureterovesicular junction. Papillary necrosis occurs when there is sloughing of renal papillae, often due to ischemia or toxins. The sloughed papillae can cause ureteric obstruction. These patients often present with hematuria. Ketamine-induced uropathy can also cause hydronephrosis.

Pathologic processes in the retroperitoneal space, including radiation injury, fibrosis, trauma, infection, and granulomatous diseases, can cause ureter obstruction. Retroperitoneal fibrosis can encase the ureters and result in obstructive uropathy without the presence of hydronephrosis on ultrasound. A contrast-enhanced imaging study reveals external compression of the ureter.

Urinary tract dilation can occasionally be seen without obstruction. A classic example is pregnancy, when high levels of progesterone reduce ureter peristalsis and tone, resulting in hydroureter. Right hydroureter occurs in 60–80% of pregnant women, and left hydroureter in 30%. The greater right ureter involvement is likely due to external compression from the gravid uterus. Hydronephrosis may not resolve for 6–12 weeks postpartum. Vesicoureteral reflux can also result in hydroureter without obstruction.

KEY READING

Huang LK et al: Evaluation of the extent of ketamine-induced uropathy: the role of CT urography. Postgrad Med J 2014;90:185.

▶ **Complications**

Urinary tract obstruction results in increased intratubular pressure, decreased renal blood flow, and decreased glomerular filtration rate. Renal injury also occurs independent of pressure due to ischemia and influx of inflammatory cells, which release substances that cause tubular injury and fibrosis. Urinary tract obstruction can lead to permanent renal injury and end stage renal disease. Obstruction is often complicated by urinary tract infection. Postobstructive diuresis can occur after relief of chronic obstruction and may result in volume and/or electrolyte depletion. Postobstructive diuresis is thought to predict renal recovery and may be an appropriate response to volume expansion which occurred during obstruction. If intravenous fluid replacement is used, the volume should be less than urine output unless the patient is volume depleted. This will prevent continued diuresis due to intravenous fluid administration.

KEY READING

Hamdi A et al: Severe post-renal acute kidney injury, postobstructive diuresis and renal recovery. BJU Int 2012;110:1027.

▶ **Treatment**

Obstructive uropathy complicated by acute kidney injury, hyperkalemia, or infection requires emergent intervention. The procedure of choice is dependent on the cause and location of obstruction. Bladder outlet obstruction is relieved with a transurethral or suprapubic catheter. Patients with otherwise untreatable neurogenic bladder or bladder outlet obstruction require chronic intermittent catheterization or suprapubic catheter. Ureteric obstruction can be relieved with cystoscopy and retrograde ureteroscopy with stent placement or with percutaneous nephrostomy. The underlying cause of obstruction should be identified and treated. For patients with gynecologic malignancy, predictors of ureteric stent failure include ureter obstruction greater than 3 cm. These patients may have a better outcome with placement of a percutaneous nephrostomy tube. Stones that are less than 5–6 mm often pass spontaneously and can be observed. These patients are treated with increased fluid intake, analgesics, and an α-blocker like tamsulosin. Treatment for larger stones, or those that do not pass with conservative therapy, includes ureteroscopic stone extraction, shock wave lithotripsy, percutaneous nephrolithotomy, and laparoscopic stone removal. The gold standard treatment for ureteropelvic junction obstruction is now minimally invasive robot-assisted laparoscopic pyeloplasty (RALP).

KEY READINGS

Hopf HL, Bahler CD, Sundaram CP: Long-term outcomes of robot-assisted laparoscopic pyeloplasty for ureteropelvic junction obstruction. Urology 2016;90:106.

Song Y, Fei X, Song Y: Percutaneous nephrostomy versus indwelling ureteral stent in the management of gynecological malignancies. Int J Gynecol Cancer 2012;4:697.

▶ **Prognosis**

Relief of complete obstruction lasting less than 1 week often results in full recovery of renal function, whereas there is little to no improvement in renal function after relief of complete obstruction lasting for greater than 8–12 weeks. Obstruction lasting greater than 2 weeks often results in chronic kidney disease and hypertension.

KEY READING

Lucarelli G et al: Delayed relief of obstruction is implicated in the long-term development of renal damage and arterial hypertension in patients with unilateral ureteral injury. J Urol 2013;189:960.

▶ **When to Refer/When to Admit**

Obstructive uropathy often requires referral to urology and/or nephrology. Patients with obstructive uropathy complicated by acute kidney injury, hyperkalemia, or infection require hospitalization.

■ **CHAPTER REVIEW QUESTIONS**

1. A 64-year-old female patient presents to the emergency department with severe right flank pain and fever. These symptoms have worsened over the past 3 days. Her past medical history includes diabetes and hypertension. Her temperature is 101.8°F, BP 90/50, pulse 110 beats/min. Urinalysis shows many WBCs and bacteria. A renal ultrasound shows severe right hydronephrosis. In addition to intravenous antibiotics, which is the most appropriate next step for this patient?
   A. Placement of right percutaneous nephrostomy
   B. Observation
   C. Extracorporeal shockwave lithotripsy
   D. CT urogram

2. An 83-year-old male patient reports new onset urine incontinence and frequency. Vital signs are stable. A distended bladder is detected during abdominal examination. He has no peripheral edema. A Foley catheter is placed with some difficulty and initial urine output is 1800 mL. Over the next 4 hours, urine output is 1000 mL. The best option at this time is
   A. Replace hourly urine output with intravenous fluids
   B. Replace urine output with intravenous fluid 0.5 mL/mL urine output
   C. Administer DDAVP (desmopressin acetate injection)
   D. Observation

3. A 46-year-old male patient complains of left flank pain radiating into his groin. A urinalysis shows 2+ blood and 15 RBC/HPF. CT stone study shows a 4-mm stone in the distal left ureter and mild left hydronephrosis. The most appropriate initial treatment for this patient is

   A. Increased fluid intake, pain medication, and tamsulosin
   B. Extracorporeal shockwave lithotripsy
   C. Ureteroscopic stone extraction
   D. Percutaneous nephrostomy

4. A 32-year-old gravid female patient reports urine frequency. Urinalysis is normal. An abdominal ultrasound shows moderate right and mild left hydronephrosis. The most appropriate recommendation for this patient is
   A. Begin antibiotic
   B. Monthly renal ultrasound until delivery
   C. Renal ultrasound 2–3 months postpartum
   D. Induce labor when fetus is viable

5. A 64-year-old female patient undergoes CT abdomen for evaluation of abdominal pain. In addition to findings consistent with diverticulitis, there is severe hydronephrosis of the right kidney which appears to originate at the ureteropelvic junction. The right renal cortex is thin and echogenic. Her basic metabolic panel results are normal except serum creatinine is 1.4 mg/dL. Which of the following statements is most correct?
   A. Percutaneous nephrostomy will result in significant improvement in function of right kidney.
   B. Regardless of the intervention, there is little likelihood that renal function of right kidney will improve.
   C. Right nephrectomy should be performed.
   D. Radionuclide scanning should be performed to assess function of right kidney.

The Kidney in Malignancy

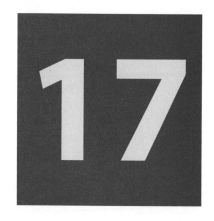

Rimda Wanchoo, MD

Nishita Parikh, MD

Kenar D. Jhaveri, MD

Onconephrology is a new and evolving subspecialty that focuses on all aspects of kidney disease in cancer patients. Given that up to a quarter of patients with a cancer diagnosis will develop some form of kidney impairment, a discipline that aims to understand and manage the overlapping fields of nephrology and oncology is needed. Topics considered to be part of onconephrology are electrolyte disorders of malignancy, secondary glomerular diseases of cancer, chemotherapy and targeted therapy-related kidney complications, paraproteinemias, thrombotic microangiopathies, hematopoietic stem cell transplant (HSCT)-related kidney diseases, tumor lysis syndrome, and acute kidney injury (AKI) in the cancer patient. Other topics include the ethics of providing dialysis in a dying cancer patient, postnephrectomy kidney disease and obstructive nephropathy, dosing of chemotherapy in chronic kidney disease (CKD) patients, and renal cell cancer. This chapter serves as an overview of key onconephrology topics.

Acute Kidney Injury in the Cancer Patient

The overall incidence of cancer is rising in the United States. The overall incidence of both acute and CKD in cancer patients is unknown. AKI is thought to be fairly common in cancer patients. Based on a Danish population study, the 1-year risk of AKI in patients with cancer, defined as a greater than 50% rise in serum creatinine, is 17.5% with a 27% risk over 5 years. Unfortunately, many cancer patients are left with CKD following AKI episodes.

Four salient features that can be deduced from major studies are (1) the incidence of AKI among hospitalized cancer patients (12%)is higher than that of patients without cancer; (2) acutely ill cancer patients admitted to the ICU have a higher risk of AKI; (3) some cancers are associated with higher risk of AKI than others (kidney, gall bladder, liver, myeloma, and pancreas); and (4) treatment with HSCT, especially myeloablative allogenic HSCT, further raises the risk of AKI associated with malignancies.

AKI in patients with cancer may occur by at least two mechanisms; as a complication of a particular cancer treatment (eg, tumor lysis syndrome, drug-induced nephropathy, post-transplant-related kidney diseases, and surgical procedures) or related to the neoplasm itself (eg, renal cell cancer, anatomic obstruction due to a metastatic lesion or obstructing mass, and myeloma/amyloid affecting the kidney). The cancer patient developing AKI has a worse prognosis than one without kidney impairment. Table 17–1 summarizes the prerenal, intrinsic, and postrenal causes of AKI in the cancer patient.

Chronic Kidney Disease in the Cancer Patient

Data on the incidence and prevalence of CKD in cancer patients are limited. Some of the identified risk factors for developing CKD in patients treated for cancers during childhood are (1) post nephrectomy, (2) history of abdominal radiation, (3) high-dose ifosfamide exposure, and (4) high-dose cisplatin exposure.

Management of patients with CKD who develop cancer is complex. These patients carry a higher mortality risk as compared to the general population. Two large studies demonstrated that men with CKD stage 3 or higher had an increased risk of cancer. In addition, this risk increased by 29% for every 10 cc/min decrease in glomerular filtration rate (GFR) at filtration rates of 55 cc/min per 1.73 m^2 or less. The major cancers involved were primarily of urinary origin and lung cancers. In many other large studies, CKD was significantly associated with liver cancer, kidney cancer, and urinary tract cancers. In patients with kidney and urological cancers, lower estimated GFR was associated with a higher mortality from kidney and urological cancers. In addition, CKD may itself be a risk factor for worse outcomes in patients with cancer. CKD following cancer can be a result of the cancer, leading to acute tubular necrosis (ATN), tumor infiltration, and vascular, tubular, interstitial, or glomerular

Table 17–1. Prerenal, intrinsic, and postrenal causes of AKI in the cancer patient.

Prerenal	Intrinsic	Postrenal
Renal hypoperfusion due to sepsis, ascites, and effusions	Acute tubular necrosis due to	Obstruction due to
Volume depletion (↓ oral intake, diarrhea, overdiuresis)	- *Protracted ischemia*	-*Primary or metastatic abdominal*
Impaired cardiac output	- *Nephrotoxic agents: eg, IV contrast,*	*or pelvic malignancy*
Hepatic sinusoid obstructive syndrome	*ifosfamide, cisplatin, aminoglycosides*	-*Retroperitoneal fibrosis*
Hypercalcemia	Lymphomatous infiltration of the kidney	-*Crystals (acyclovir, urate, methotrexate)*
Nonchemo drugs (NSAIDS, ACEI/ARB, calcineurin inhibitors)	Acute interstitial nephritis	
Capillary leak syndrome (eg, due to IL2)	Tumor lysis syndrome	
Chimeric antigen receptor (CAR) T-cell therapy	Cast nephropathy	
	Thrombotic microangiopathy	
	Calcineurin inhibitor toxicity	

ACEI, angiotensin converting enzyme inhibitor; ARB, angiotensin receptor blocker; NSAIDs, nonsteroidal anti-inflammatory drugs.

toxicities of chemotherapy agents. The toxicities from chemotherapy are the most common causes of CKD in cancer patients. In addition, because many of these patients are living longer, they are not immune from getting CKD from more common causes such as hypertension and/or diabetes mellitus.

Paraneoplastic Glomerular Diseases

Membranous nephropathy (MN) remains the most common glomerular pathology reported in patients with solid tumors. The true prevalence of malignancy with MN is unknown. Minimal change disease (MCD) is the most common glomerular disease associated with hematologic malignancies. Figure 17–1, shown below, summarizes the published list of paraneoplastic glomerular diseases that are seen with various types of cancers. It has been recently identified that circulating autoantibodies to podocyte transmembrane glycoprotein M-type phospholipase A2 receptor (PLA2R) are seen in a majority of cases of adult primary MN. These autoantibodies were not found in cases of secondary MN such as those associated with cancer. Table 17–2 depicts how clinicians can differentiate primary MN from secondary MN associated with cancer.

Recent studies have identified the molecule thrombospondin type 1 domain containing 7A(THSD7A) as a pathogenic antigen identified in cancer-associated membranous GN. In a large study, the authors screened more than 1200 patients by Western blot analysis for THSD7A. Within this cohort, the investigators identified 40 patients with THSD7A-associated MN, eight of whom developed a malignancy within a median time of 3 months from diagnosis of MN. Patients with THSD7A-associated MN differ in their clinical characteristics from patients with PLA2R-associated MN. These findings suggest that a more intensive screening for the presence of malignancies may be warranted in those with THSD7A-associated MN.

▶ Kidney Diseases Associated with Hematopoietic Stem Cell Transplantation

AKI is a well-established complication of HSCT. The exact incidence of AKI reported in the literature varies among studies due to different criteria used to define AKI. The incidence of AKI depends on the type of transplant performed (autologous versus allogeneic), and the consolidation regimen administered (fully ablative versus reduced intensity). An incidence as high as 60% is seen in myeloablative allogeneic transplants, and as low as 12% in autologous stem cell transplants. Many different etiologies of AKI in HSCT patients have been identified (Table 17–3).

CKD after HSCT is estimated to affect up to 60% of HSCT survivors and can be clinically evident as early as 6 months after transplantation. Older age, female gender, hypertension, baseline kidney dysfunction, nonrecovery from episodes of AKI, fludarabine exposure, use of unfractionated total body irradiation, and graft versus host disease (GHVD) have all been implicated in the development of CKD after HSCT. Table 17–4 lists the potential causes of CKD in the HSCT patient population.

Nephrotic syndrome after HSCT is considered to represent a kidney manifestation of GVHD. In a case series of patients with nephrotic syndrome after HSCT, the most common etiology identified was membranous nephropathy followed by minimal change disease and close to half of these patients developed the nephrotic syndrome concurrently with onset of GVHD in another organs. A diagnosis of minimal change disease should prompt the nephrologist to rule out relapse of a primary hematologic malignancy.

Unlike idiopathic membranous nephropathy, patients who develop MN post HSCT are rarely anti-PLA2R antibody positive. The mainstay of treatment varies on the pathology noted. Treatment options described in the literature varies and ranges from high-dose steroids, calcineurin inhibitors (CNIs) mycophenolate mofetil, or rituximab.

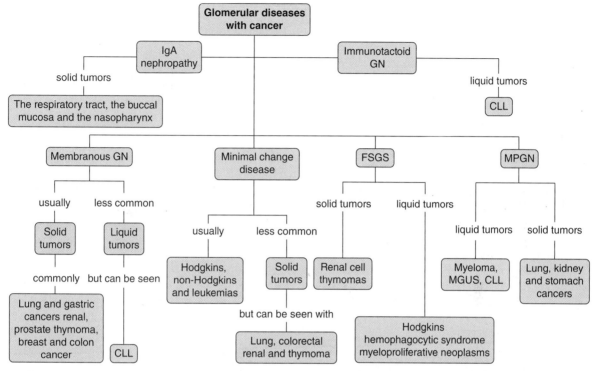

▲ **Figure 17–1.** Glomerular diseases associated with solid tumors and hematologic malignancies. C3GN, complete C3 glomerulonephritis; CLL, chronic lymphocytic leukemia; FSGS, focal segmental glomerulosclerosis; GI, gastrointestinal; GN, glomerulonephritis; HSP, Henoch–Schonlein purpura; IgAN, IgA nephropathy; MCD, minimal change disease; MGUS, monoclonal gammopathy of unclear significance; MN, membranous nephropathy; MPGN, membranoproliferative glomerulonephritis; TMA, thrombotic microangiopathy. (Adapted from Jhaveri KD: http://www.nephronpower. com/2015/01/concept-map-glomerular-diseases-seen.html, with permission.)

Thrombotic microangiopathy (TMA) in HSCT patients can present early (<6 months) as well as late (>6 months) after the stem cell transplant. It is more prevalent in allogenic HSCT as compared to autologous transplants. The pathological hallmark of TMA is endothelial injury which in turn leads to activation of the coagulation system/ complement and fibrin/platelet accumulation. Risk factors for endothelial injury include the particular conditioning regimen (chemotherapy and radiation), CNIs, presence of GVHD and infections (human herpes virus (HHV)6, adenovirus, cytomegalovirus (CMV), BK, and parvovirus). In terms of treatment, several different approaches have

Table 17–2. Clinical pathologic features differentiating primary from malignancy associated MN.

Clinicopathologic Parameters	Primary MN	Solid Tumor Associated MN
Historical clues	No history of smoking	Age over 65 years, smoking for more than 20 pack years
Serological testing	Presence of circulating anti-PLA2R autoantibodies in serum	Absence of circulating anti-PLA2R autoantibodies in serum
Pathological findings	Predominance of glomerular IgG4 deposition, enhanced glomerular PLA2R staining, presence of less than 8 inflammatory cells per glomeruli	Predominance of IgG1,2 deposition, normal glomerular PLA2R staining, presence of more than 8 inflammatory cells per glomeruli

IgG, immunoglobulin G; MN, membranous nephropathy; PLA2R, phospholipase A2 receptor.

Table 17–3. Common causes of AKI in HSCT patients.

Prerenal
Ischemic ATN (sepsis, hypotension)
Toxic ATN (antibiotics, antifungals, antivirals, chemotherapy)
Contrast nephropathy
Interstitial nephritis (medications, viruses such as BK, CMV, adenovirus)
TMA (medication induced, or related to total body irradiation, viruses, GVHD)
Hepatic veno-occlusive disease (VOD) leading to hepatorenal syndrome
Obstructive uropathy
Bladder outlet obstruction (BK cystitis)

AKI, acute kidney injury; ATN, acute tubular necrosis; CMV, cytomegalovirus; GVHD, graft versus host disease; HSCT, hematopoietic stem cell transplants; TMA, thrombotic microangiopathy.

been described. These include plasmapheresis, stopping CNIs, and the use of rituximab, defibrotide, or eculizumab. Of note, although there is no randomized data to favor one approach over another, eculizumab a complement inhibitor

Table 17–4. Chronic kidney diseases in HSCT patients.

TMA (calcineurin inhibitor related, GVHD related, radiation nephropathy)
Glomerular diseases (membranous nephropathy, minimal change diseases, focal segmental glomerulosclerosis)
Other causes (chronic disease from prior AKI, viruses, medications)

AKI, acute kidney injury; GVHD, graft versus host disease; TMA, thrombotic microangiopathy.

has shown benefit in small published case series. Figure 17–2 summarizes renal diseases seen with HSCT patients.

▶ Kidney Toxicities Associated with Traditional Chemotherapy Agents

Chemotherapeutic agents can lead to a variety of kidney-specific toxicities. While most of these agents cause intrinsic renal injury (Table 17–5), notable exceptions exist. For example, Interleukin -2(IL-2) and chimeric antigen receptor (CAR) T-cell therapy are associated with capillary leak

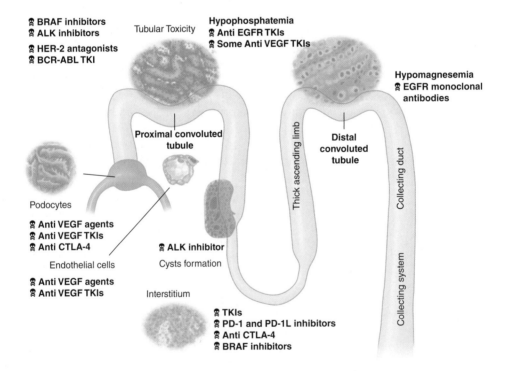

▲ **Figure 17–2.** Summary of renal adverse events noted with targeted therapies. ALK, anaplastic lymphoma kinase; BCR-ABL, breakpoint cluster region–abelson; CTLA-4, cytotoxic T lymphocyte antigen-4; EGFR, epidermal growth factor receptor; HER-2, human epidermal growth factor-2; PD, programmed cell death; TKI, tyrosine kinase inhibitors; VEGF, vascular endothelial growth factor. (Adapted from Jhaveri KD et al: Renal effects of novel targeted oncologic agents, a narrative review. Kidney Int Rep 2017;2:108, with permission.)

Table 17–5. Chemotherapeutic agents associated with AKI and other forms of kidney injuries.

Chemotherapeutic Agent	Mechanism of Injury	Clinical Presentation
Azacytidine	Proximal and distal tubular injury	Fanconi syndrome, and polyuria
Bisphosphonate (pamidronate, zoledronate)	Acute tubular injury, collapsing FSGS, MCD	AKI, proteinuria
Cisplatin	Toxic damage to renal tubule	AKI, hypomagnesemia, diabetes insipidus, Fanconi syndrome
Clofarabine	ATN, FSGS	Sudden onset AKI
Cyclophosphamide	Increased ADH activity	Hyponatremia, hemorrhagic cystitis
Gemcitabine (cell cycle-specific pyrimidine antagonist)	TMA	HTN, proteinuria, and AKI +/– edema
Ifosfamide	Proximal +/– distal tubular injury	ATN (often subclinical), type 2 RTA with Fanconi syndrome, severe electrolyte disarray, nephrogenic diabetes insipidus
Interferon (alpha, beta, or gamma)	Podocyte injury resulting in MCD or FSGS	Nephrotic syndrome, AKI
Interleukin-2	Renal hypoperfusion due to capillary leak, renal vasoconstriction	AKI, hypotension, proteinuria, pyuria, edema
Methotrexate	Tubular obstruction by precipitation of methotrexate and 7-hydroxymethotrexate	AKI (nonoliguric)
Mitomycin C	TTP and HUS (associated with cumulative dose >60 mg)	AKI, proteinuria, hypertension
Nitrosoureas	Glomerular sclerosis and tubulointerstitial nephritis	Insidious, often irreversible renal injury

AKI, acute kidney injury; ATN, acute tubular necrosis; CrCl, creatinine clearance; FSGS, focal segmental glomerulosclerosis; GFR, glomerular filtration rate; HTN, hypertension; MCD, minimal change diseases; TMA, thrombotic microangiopathy.

syndrome, which can cause intravascular volume depletion and prerenal azotemia. Postrenal injury is rare with chemotherapy agents but case reports have linked cyclophosphamide to bladder outlet obstruction from vesicular thrombi in the setting of hemorrhagic cystitis. Intrinsic causes can be further divided into glomerular diseases/TMA, tubular and interstitial toxicities.

▶ Kidney Toxicities Associated with Targeted Therapies

In the past decade, advances in cell biology have led to the development of anticancer agents that target-specific molecular pathways. The National Cancer Institute (NCI) defines targeted therapies as "drugs or substances that block the growth and spread of cancer by interfering with specific molecules involved in tumor growth and progression." Targeted therapies are now commonly used in cancer treatment and it is vital that their kidney toxicities be recognized and investigated. Early reports suggest that targeted therapies are associated with a range of toxicities from hypertension to AKI. Table 17–6 and Figure 17–3 summarize the renal effects of targeted therapies.

Vascular endothelial growth factor (VEGF) is produced by glomerular podocytes and tubular epithelial cells in the kidney and binds to the VEGF receptors (a tyrosine kinase receptor) located in the mesangium, glomerular endothelial cells, and peritubular capillaries. VEGF is involved in proliferation, differentiation, and survival of mesangial and endothelial cells. It plays a vital role in the development of endothelial fenestration, vascular permeability, endothelial cell health, and maintenance of structure and function of the glomerular filtration barrier. Anti-VEGF therapy includes drugs such as bevacizumab, which is a recombinant humanized monoclonal antibody to VEGF. In general, highly vascular tumors with high levels of VEGF expression and a high density of VEGF receptors are responsive to anti-VEGF therapy. Tyrosine kinase inhibitors of the VEGFR such as sorafenib, sunitinib, axitinib have anti-VEGF properties as they inhibit the downstream signaling cascade once VEGF binds to its receptors. VEGF antagonism leads to hypertension, proteinuria, TMA, and interstitial nephritis/acute kidney injury. TMA related to anti-VEGF therapy is usually limited to the kidney although some patients will also present with extra renal manifestations of thrombocytopenia

Table 17–6. Known renal side effects of various targeted therapies.

Name of Agent	Mechanism of Action of the Targeted Therapy	Reported Nephrotoxicities
Bevacizumab	VEGF inhibitor	HTN, proteinuria, nephrotic syndrome, preeclampsia like syndrome, renal limited TMA
Aflibercept	VEGF inhibitor	HTN, proteinuria
Sunitinib	Multikinase TKI	HTN, proteinuria, MCD/FSGS, AIN, chronic interstitial nephritis
Pazopanib	Multikinase TKI	HTN, proteinuria
Axitinib	Multikinase TKI	HTN, proteinuria
Sorafenib	Multikinase TKI	HTN, proteinuria, MCD/FSGS, AIN, chronic interstitial nephritis, hypophosphatemia
Imatinib	Cellular TKI (BCR-ABL)	ATN, HTN, hypocalcemia, hypophosphatemia
Dasatinib	Multikinase TKI	Proteinuria
Nilotinib	Multikinase TKI	HTN
Ponatinib	Multikinase TKI	HTN
Cetuximab	EGFR inhibitor	Hypomagnesemia, hypokalemia, AKI, hyponatremia, glomerulonephritis
Panitumumab	EGFR inhibitor	Hypomagnesemia, AKI, hypokalemia
Erlotinib	EGFR inhibitor	AKI, hypomagnesemia
Afatinib	EGFR inhibitor	AKI, hyponatremia
Gefitinib	EGFR inhibitor	AKI, hypokalemia, fluid retention, minimal change disease, proteinuria
Vemurafenib	B-RAF inhibitor	AIN, ATN, hypophosphatemia, Fanconi syndrome
Dabrafenib	B-RAF Inhibitor	AIN, ATN, hypophosphatemia, nephrotic syndrome (in combination with MEK inhibitor)
Crizotinib	ALK inhibitor	ATN, renal cysts
Ipilimumab	CTLA-4 inhibitor	AIN, MN, MCD, hyponatremia, TMA
Nivolumab	PD-1 Inhibitor	AIN
Pembrolizumab	PD-1 Inhibitor	AIN
Temsirolimus	mTOR inhibitor	ATN, FSGS
Carfilzomib	Proteasome inhibitor	Prerenal, ATN, TMA
Bortezomib	Proteasome inhibitor	TMA
Lenalidomide	Immunomodulators	Fanconi syndrome, AIN, MCD
Trametinib	MEK inhibitor	AKI, nephrotic syndrome (in combination with BRAF)

AIN, acute interstitial nephritis; AKI, acute kidney injury; ALK, anaplastic lymphoma kinase; ATN, acute tubular necrosis; BCR-ABL, breakpoint cluster region–abelson; CTLA-4, cytotoxic T lymphocyte antigen-4; EGFR, epidermal growth factor receptor; FSGS, focal segmental glomerulosclerosis; HTN, hypertension; MCD, minimal change disease; MEK, mitogen-activated protein kinase; MN, membranous nephropathy; PD, programmed cell death; TKI, tyrosine kinase inhibitor; TMA, thrombotic microangiopathy; VEGF, vascular endothelial growth factor.

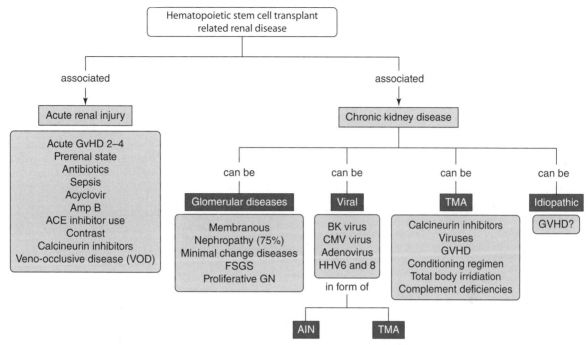

▲ **Figure 17–3.** Summary of renal diseases seen with hematopoietic stem cell transplant patients. ACE, angiotension converting enzyme; CMV, cytomegalovirus; FSGS, focal segmental glomerulosclerosis; GVDH, graft versus host disease; HHV, human herpes virus; TMA, thrombotic microangiopathy; GN, glomerulonephritis; AIN, acute interstitial nephritis. (Adapted from Jhaveri KD: http://www.nephronpower.com/2017/03/concept-map-hsct-related-renal-disease.html, with permission.)

and schistocytosis. Furthermore, kidney function remains preserved with control of blood pressure and withdrawal of the drug. These findings help differentiate TMA caused by this class of drugs from other causes of TMA. For example, TMA induced by gemcitabine and/or mitomycin is more aggressive, causes greater hematological abnormalities and affects both the glomerulus and arterioles. It is also associated with worse kidney survival despite the discontinuation of the drug.

Immune check-point inhibitors include the anticytotoxic T lymphocyte associated protein 4 (CTLA-4) antibody as well as antiprogram death antibodies (PD-1). These antibodies serve to enhance the innate anti-tumor T-cell immunity, leading to tumor regression as well as stabilization of some solid tumors. Acute interstitial nephritis is the most common biopsy finding reported with PD-1 inhibitors. Ipilimumab, a CTLA-4 inhibitor, is also associated with AIN; however podocytopathies such as MN, minimal change disease, and TMA have also been reported. Hyponatremia related to hypophysitis is also seen with CTLA-4 antagonists. The time of onset usually differs in the two drugs. CTLA-4 antagonist-mediated injury usually occurs earlier, within the first 2–3 months of use, while PD-1 inhibitor-mediated injury is usually seen later, within 2–10 months into treatment. Treatment usually involves interruption of therapy and treatment with high dose steroids.

Chemotherapy Dosing in CKD

The kidneys are one of the major routes of elimination for most chemotherapy agents and hence dose adjustments are required when they are administered to patients with CKD. Many chemotherapy-based trials exclude patients with severe CKD, as a result accurate dosing guidelines are lacking and patients with CKD receive either too little or too much chemotherapy (or may be excluded from receiving a medication). In addition, the method of calculating dose adjustments in patients with CKD and extrapolating from pharmacokinetic data may not always coincide with what is done in clinical practice. CKD status and uremic milieu can also lead to altered hepatic metabolism of drugs. Many of the dosing guidelines are opinion-based, or based upon case series or institutional experience. A list of common chemotherapy agents requiring dose adjustments is presented in Table 17–7.

Electrolyte Abnormalities in Cancer Patients

Electrolyte disorders in patients with cancer are common. They could be as a result of the cancer, chemotherapeutic agent, or other patient-related factors. Hyponatremia and hypercalcemia are the most common electrolyte abnormalities noted.

Table 17–7. Chemotherapy dose adjustments in CKD patients.

Chemotherapy Agents	Dose Adjustment Required for eGFR 10–50 mL/min (%)	Dose Adjustment Required When eGFR <10 mL/min (%)	Evidence Level
Capecitabine	75	50–75	B
Cisplatin	75	50, avoid if possible	A
Carboplatin	50 (AUC based)	50	D
Chlorambucil	75	50	B
Ifosfamide	100	75	B
Cyclophosphamide	100	75	D
Cytarabine	50	10	D
Dacarbazine	75 for eGFR 45–60 mL/min	70	D
Doxorubicin	100	100	D
Daunorubicin	100	100	D
Epirubicin	100	100	D
Etoposide	75	50	B
Carmustine	75 for eGFR 30–60 mL/min	Avoid if eGFR <30 mL/min	D
Lomustine	70 for eGFR 30–60 mL/min	Avoid if eGFR <30 mL/min	B
Semustine	70 for eGFR 30–60 mL/min	Avoid if eGFR <30 mL/min	B
Streptozocin	75	50	D
Mitomycin C	100	75	B
Mithramycin	75	50	B
Azacitidine	100	100	B
Gemcitabine	100	100	B
Cytarabine	100	100	D
Methotrexate	50	Avoid	A
Pentostatin	60 for eGFR 30–60 mL/min	Avoid when eGFR <30 mL/min	B
Fludarabine	75	50	D
Cladribine	75	50	D
5-Fluorouracil	100	100	B
Melphalan	75	50	B
Oxaliplatin	100	50	A
Paclitaxel	100	100	A
Pemetrexed	100 if GFR 45–79 mL/min with oral folic acid and vit B_{12}	Avoid with eGFR <45 mL/min	B

(Continued)

Table 17–7. Chemotherapy dose adjustments in CKD patients. (*Continued*)

Chemotherapy Agents	Dose Adjustment Required for eGFR 10–50 mL/min (%)	Dose Adjustment Required When eGFR <10 mL/min (%)	Evidence Level
Temozolomide	100	100	B
Topotecan	75	50	A
Vincristine	100	100	B
Vinblastine	100	100	B
Sunitinib	100	100	B
Sorafenib	50	50	D
Erlotinib	100	100	B
Gefitinib	100	100	B
Imatinib	100	50	A

AUC, area under the curve. Strength of evidence: A: human trials, B: human case studies, C: in vitro data, D: clinical opinion.

Other electrolyte abnormalities such as hypernatremia, hypomagnesemia, hypophosphatemia, hyperphosphatemia, hyperkalemia, and hypokalemia are also encountered. Figure 17–4 summarizes the known electrolyte disorders with chemotherapy and targeted therapy agents.

A. Hypercalcemia in Malignancy

Hypercalcemia of malignancy is caused by two mechanisms:

1. Osteolytic release of calcium from bone that is involved by cancer cells, as seen in skeletal metastasis of solid tumors of breast, lungs, kidneys, and multiple myeloma. The release of calcium from the bone is mediated by the RANK (receptor activator of nuclear factor kappa B) and RANK-L (receptor activator of nuclear factor kappa B ligand) interaction. RANK-L is produced by the bone marrow stromal cells and osteoblasts. The binding of RANK, present on osteoclast progenitor cells to its ligand results in osteoclast activation, proliferation, and bone resorption resulting in release of calcium. The neoplastic environment with activated T cells, inflammatory cytokines (IL-6, IL-1B0, TNF alpha) all promote the RANK-L driven bone resorption and disturb the RANK/RANK-L/osteoprotegerin (OPG) balance.

2. Stimulation of osteoclast activity by release of tumor-derived endocrine factors (paraneoplastic). In these cases: parathyroid-related hormone (PTHrP) and 1,25-dihydroxyvitamin D play an important role. PTHrP is secreted by the squamous cell carcinoma of the lung, head, and neck cancers, renal cell cancer, ovarian, breast, and esophageal cancers. PTHrP causes stimulation of osteoclasts, increases calcium absorption in the loop of Henle and distal convoluted tubule. Another mechanism involves activated 1,25-dihydroxyvitamin D which can be secreted by lymphoma, or tumor-associated macrophages that possess 1-alpha hydroxylase activity.

The primary goal in the management of hypercalcemia is to enhance the urinary excretion of calcium and to decrease the osteoclast mediated bone resorption. The first goal is achieved by aggressive volume repletion with intravenous fluids with a goal urine output of 100–150 cc/h. Furosemide should only be used once adequately volume replete and only in the setting of volume overload. Calcitonin inhibits bone resorption and osteoclast maturation and acts quickly within 4–6 hours of administration. Tachyphylaxis prevents its long-term use. In volume, overloaded or anuric patients, dialysis with a low dialysate calcium may be needed.

Bisphosphonates, such as zoledronate or pamidronate have become the cornerstone of treatment of hypercalcemia of malignancy. Bisphosphonates reduce the osteoclast activity by preventing the osteoclasts to adhere to the bone surface and also prevents the production of their proteins which are responsible for continued bone resorption. They also result in decreased osteoclast progenitor development and promote their apoptosis. RANKL inhibitors such as denosumab may have a role in the management of bisphosphonate resistant hypercalcemia of malignancy.

B. Hyponatremia

Syndrome of inappropriate antidiuretic hormone (SIADH) is the most common cause of hyponatremia in cancer

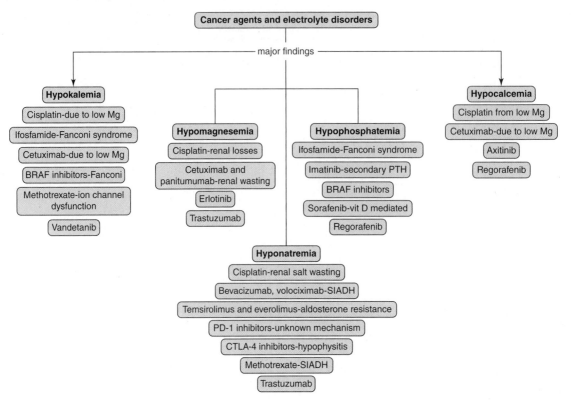

▲ **Figure 17–4.** Electrolyte disorders with anticancer agents. CTLA-4, cytotoxic T lymphocyte antigen-4; EGFR, epidermal growth factor receptor; HER-2, human epidermal growth factor-2; PD, programmed cell death; SIADH, syndrome of inappropriate diuretic hormone; TKI, tyrosine kinase inhibitors; VEGF, vascular endothelial growth factor. (Adapted from Jhaveri KD: http://www.nephronpower.com/2016/10/concept-map-electrolyte-disorders-and.html, with permission.)

patients, especially among patients with small cell lung cancer (SCLC) and head and neck cancers. The other potential causes of SIADH include pain, nausea, and certain medications (cisplatin, cyclophosphamide, vinblastine, and vincristine).

Cisplatin and ifosfamide can also injure renal tubular cells, impairing renal sodium absorption leading to renal salt wasting. Current treatment recommendations (similar to noncancer patients) are that the serum sodium should not be corrected more than 10 mEq/L within the first 24 hours. In a patient who is severely symptomatic, presenting with seizures, impaired mental status, or coma 3% saline should be administered along with frequent neurological and serum sodium monitoring.

In minimally symptomatic or asymptomatic patients with euvolemic hyponatremia, patients should be asked to limit their water intake to 1–1.5 L/day. Patients who can tolerate diuretics may be administered loop diuretics to increase free water loss in the urine along with salt tablets to replace renal sodium losses. The above measures can hinder the quality of

life of cancer patients and thus aquaretics which inhibit the vasopressin type 2 receptor (V2-R) in the collecting duct and inhibit water reabsorption can be considered for the management of hyponatremia secondary to SIADH in cancer patients. In a small study of cancer patients, tolvaptan was shown to be safe and have superior efficacy in controlling hyponatremia when compared with standard therapy using fluid restriction, diuretics, and salt tablets.

C. Hypophosphatemia

A relatively common cause of hypophosphatemia in cancer patients is the redistribution of phosphate from the extracellular to intracellular space. This happens in the setting of administration of enteral or parenteral nutrition in a malnourished cancer patient. In these cases, there is a massive shift of electrolytes/phosphorous to the intracellular compartment due to increased requirement of phosphorous during tissue anabolism resulting in profound hypophosphatemia. This is also seen in stem cell transplant recipients at the time of hematopoietic reconstitution as well as in leukemic patients who have a rapid cell turnover.

Renal phosphate wasting is another important cause of hypophosphatemia. This may be a as a result of the Fanconi syndrome. Common drugs implicated in causing the Fanconi syndrome are cisplatin, ifosfamide, imatinib, lenalidomide, and pamidronate. Monoclonal gammopathies are also an important cause for hypophosphatemia due to this mechanism.

Tyrosine kinase inhibitors such as imatinib, sorafenib, regorafenib, and sunitinib have also been associated with hypophosphatemia. A very rare cause of renal phosphate wasting is tumor-induced oncogenic osteomalacia, which is characterized by high levels of FGF-23. This leads to phosphaturia, hypophosphatemia, and osteomalacia. Malignancies associated with this are hemangiopericytoma, osteoblastoma, and giant cell tumors.

D. Hypomagnesemia

The two cancer agents causing hypomagnesemia are the platinum drugs (mostly cisplatin) and the epidermal growth factor receptor (EGFR) inhibitors such as cetuximab and panitumumab. EGFR inhibitors block the translocation of the transient receptor potential membrane 6 (TRPM 6) channel to the apical membrane of the distal convoluted tubule (DCT), resulting in decreased magnesium absorption and hypomagnesemia.

Hypomagnesemia related to EGFR inhibitors usually improves with cessation of therapy; however, that related

to cisplatin tends to be permanent and does not improve despite withdrawing treatment. Treatment of severe hypomagnesemia often involves intravenous repletion of 6–10 g daily or two times per week.

▶ Tumor Lysis Syndrome

Tumor lysis syndrome (TLS) is the most common oncologic emergency with an incidence as high as 26% in high-grade B-cell acute lymphoblastic leukemia. TLS results from rapid release of intracellular contents of dying cancer cells into the bloodstream either spontaneously or in response to cancer therapy (Figure 17-5). It is biochemically characterized by hyperuricemia, hyperkalemia, hyperphosphatemia, and hypocalcemia. Table 17-8 discusses the various electrolyte disorders and their presentations in TLS. Cardiac arrhythmias, seizures, and superimposed AKI are common clinical presentations. Table 17-9 summarizes the Cairo-Bishop definition of laboratory tumor lysis syndrome and clinical tumor lysis syndrome. This is the classic definition used in diagnosing of TLS. Certain cancers are more prone to TLS than others. Table 17-10 lists the various cancers and their known risk in development of TLS (low, intermediate, or high). The pathophysiology of TLS-mediated AKI involves intratubular obstruction and inflammation by precipitation of crystals of uric acid, calcium phosphate, and/or xanthine. Preexisting renal dysfunction favors intratubular crystal precipitation (Figure 17-5). Consensus recommendations for TLS prophylaxis include volume expansion for all risk groups, use of allopurinol in medium- and high-risk groups,

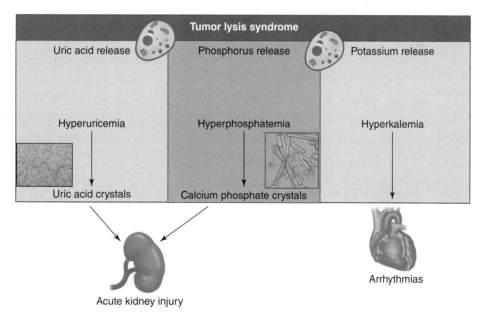

▲ **Figure 17-5.** Pathophysiology of tumor lysis syndrome.

Table 17–8. Electrolyte disorders associated with tumor lysis syndrome and their treatment options.

Electrolyte	Pathophysiology	Clinical Consequences	Treatment Options
Potassium	Rapid expulsion of intracellular potassium into the circulation	Skeletal and cardiac manifestations (arrhythmias, weakness, paresthesias)	Insulin/glucose, sodium bicarbonate, β-agonists, resins, calcium gluconate, dialysis
Phosphate	Release of phosphate due to cell lysis and renal injury	Muscle cramps, tetany, seizures	Phosphate binders, dialysis
Calcium	Precipitation of calcium phosphate complex leading to hypocalcemia	Muscle cramps, tetany, seizures, renal injury (nephrocalcinosis)	Calcium gluconate, dialysis
Uric acid	Increased purine nucleic acids from cell lysis lead to increased circulation of uric acid	Acute renal injury (uric acid nephropathy)	Hydration, xanthine oxidase inhibitors, alkalization of urine, urate oxidase, dialysis

and use of recombinant urate oxidase (rasburicase) in high-risk groups. The utility of diuretics and urine alkalization are variable and their efficacy is debatable.

Kidney Involvement with Plasma Cell Dyscrasias

Multiple myeloma can present in the kidney in various forms (Table 17–11). Figure 17–6 is a schematic of how free light chains can pathologically effect the different compartments of the kidney.

Multiple myeloma is traditionally associated with tubular and glomerular renal disease; however, there are increased associations of renal diseases with monoclonal gammopathy of undetermined significance (MGUS), monoclonal B-cell lymphocytosis (MBL), smoldering myeloma, Waldenstrom macroglobulinemia, and low-grade lymphoma. When renal disease is seen with the later, it is defined as monoclonal gammopathy of renal significance (MGRS).

Table 17–11 summarizes the renal diseases associated with paraproteinemias (multiple myeloma or MGRS). In this section, we will discuss the three most common tubular

and glomerular disorders associated with paraproteinemias. Detailed discussion of each entity is beyond the scope of this chapter. Figure 17–7 summarizes the known renal presentations of MGRS.

1. Tubular disorders—Myeloma cast nephropathy, also known as light chain cast nephropathy or myeloma kidney, commonly presents as AKI. It is one of the most common kidney manifestations of multiple myeloma. Urinalysis detects non-nephrotic range proteinuria because most of the proteinuria is primarily due to light chains (Bence Jones protein).

Table 17–10. Types of cancers and their risks of developing tumor lysis syndrome.

Type of Cancer	Risk of Tumor Lysis Syndrome
Solid tumor	Low
Myeloma	Low (unless transforming to plasmablastic leukemia or treatment-induced carfilzomib can cause tumor lysis syndrome)
Chronic leukemia (myeloid of lymphoid)	Low
Burkitt lymphoma	High if advanced stage, early and intermediate stage-intermediate
Non-Burkitt lymphoma	Low
Lymphoblastic lymphoma	High
Hodgkin disease	Low
Adult T-cell lymphoma	Low but if disease burden is bulky high
Diffuse large B-cell lymphoma	Low but if disease burden is bulky high
Burkitt leukemia	High
Acute myeloid leukemia	Intermediate

Table 17–9. Cairo-Bishop definition of laboratory tumor lysis syndrome and clinical tumor lysis syndrome.

Electrolyte Disorder	Criterion
Potassium	≥6 mEq/L or 25% increase from baseline
Phosphorus	≥4.5 mg/dL or 25% increase from baseline
Calcium	>25% decrease from baseline
Uric acid	≥8 mg/dL or 25% increase from baseline

Clinical criteria: Laboratory criteria and one or more of the following: (1) creatinine × ≥1.5 upper limit of normal, (2) seizures, and (3) cardiac arrhythmia or sudden death.

Table 17–11. Paraproteinemia-related renal diseases.

Tubular disorders
Myeloma cast nephropathy
Acute interstitial nephritis
Infiltration of plasma cells
Thrombotic microangiopathy (paraprotein or treatment related)
Acute tubular necrosis (paraprotein or treatment related)
Proximal tubulopathy (including Fanconi syndrome)

Glomerular diseases
Monoclonal immunoglobulin deposition disease (light chain/heavy chain)
Amyloidosis
Fibrillary glomerulonephritis
Immunotactoid glomerulopathy
C3 glomerulonephritis
Proliferative glomerulonephritis with monoclonal deposits
Cryoglobulinemic glomerulonephritis
Monoclonal crystalline glomerulonephritis
Membranous like glomerulopathy with masked IgG k deposits

Electrolyte disorders
Hypercalcemia
Fanconi syndrome
Pseudo-electrolyte disorders (sodium, phosphate, bicarbonate)
Tumor lysis syndrome

The patient might have an identifiable precipitating factor for AKI, such as volume depletion, hypercalcemia, diuretics, nephrotoxins, or infections. Kidney biopsy is necessary to confirm the diagnosis. The casts can lead to obstruction and cause direct toxicity to the tubules. The casts appear eosinophilic with hematoxylin and eosin (H&E) stain, pale or negative on PAS stain, and are polychromatic (red and blue) on the trichrome stain. The most effective treatment is chemotherapy (especially bortezomib); other treatments include, increasing fluid intake and avoiding nephrotoxic agents (NSAIDS, ACEI/ARB, diuretics, contrast dye), especially when the free light chain burden is high. The use of plasmapheresis for cast nephropathy is controversial, with three randomized trials with mixed results. Two of the trials, including the largest one, were negative; however, some of the largest limitations were that serum-free light chains (FLC) were not used as a marker of response in any of the trials and a kidney biopsy was not used to confirm the diagnosis of cast nephropathy. A single center report found high rate of renal recovery (86%) when plasmapheresis was combined with a bortezomib-based therapy, but other studies have found nearly as high rates of renal recovery with bortezomib-based therapy alone. More recently, high-cutoff (HCO) dialysis membranes with molecular cutoffs as high as 45 kDa have been used to remove FLC. Extended hemodialysis with a HCO dialyzer permits continuous and safe removal of FLC in large amounts (1.7 kg of FLC was removed from one patient over a period of 6 weeks).

Randomized trials are currently being conducted with HCO dialyzers in cast nephropathy and preliminary data have shown mixed results.

2. Glomerular diseases—Renal lesions in the glomerulus can be classified based on the ultrastructural characteristics of the deposit. Patients usually present with proteinuria, nephrotic syndrome, microscopic hematuria, hypertension, and deterioration of renal function.

- Organized deposits include AL amyloidosis, fibrillary glomerulonephritis, type 1 and 2 cryoglobulinemic GN, immunotactoid GN

- Nonorganized deposits include monoclonal immunoglobulin deposition disease (MIDD), proliferative GN with monoclonal Ig deposits (PGNMID), C3GN with monoclonal gammopathy

- Thrombotic microangiopathy with no immune complex present.

A. AL AMYLOIDOSIS (ORGANIZED DEPOSITS)—The most common form of systemic amyloidosis is light chain amyloid (AL amyloid) with an incident rate in the US of 6.1–10.5 patients per million person-years. AL amyloidosis is caused by a neoplastic plasma cell or B cell clone which synthesizes abnormal amounts of a specific immunoglobulin. Certain amino acid sequences within the light chain predisposes them to form amyloid. It is the uptake of these light chains by the mesangial cells that is critical in forming the amyloid structure.

AL amyloidosis in the kidney can result in proteinuria, nephrotic syndrome, hematuria, and renal impairment. Amyloid can also involve other organs, causing cardiomyopathy, hepatomegaly, or neuropathy. A person who presents with any one of these clinical findings should undergo a biopsy of the involved organ to detect the amyloid deposits. Identification and quantification of the light chain clone is with serum and urine electrophoresis and immunofixation and serum-free light chain assay. Fat pad biopsy with congo red staining is a reliable test that identifies amyloid in 78% of the patients. If a monoclonal protein is detected, patients should also undergo a bone marrow biopsy to evaluate for myeloma or another lymphoproliferative disorder. In the kidney biopsy, diagnosis is made confirming the congo red stain which reveals apple green birefringence. Immunofluorescence (IF) reveals staining for one type of light chain (usually lambda) and electron microscopy shows randomly oriented fibrils 8–12 nm in thickness.

The goal of treatment is to reduce the monoclonal paraprotein to prevent further toxicity as well as improve organ function. Most low risk patients are offered chemotherapy followed by an autologous HSCT. Patients with high risk disease who are not suitable for HSCT are offered chemotherapy with supportive care. Use of proteosome inhibitors such as bortezomib has improved the outcome

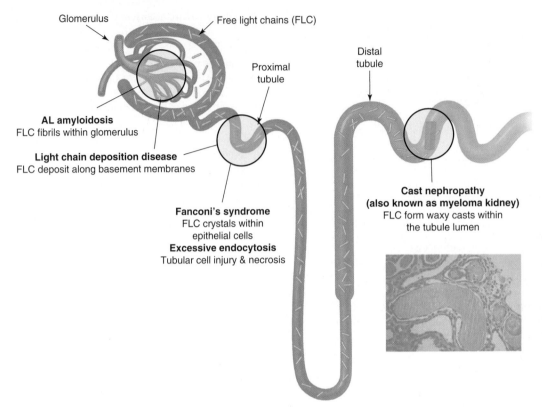

▲ **Figure 17–6.** Paraproteinemia and their effects on various parts of the kidney. (Reproduced from The Binding Site Group Ltd, Birmingham, UK, with permission.)

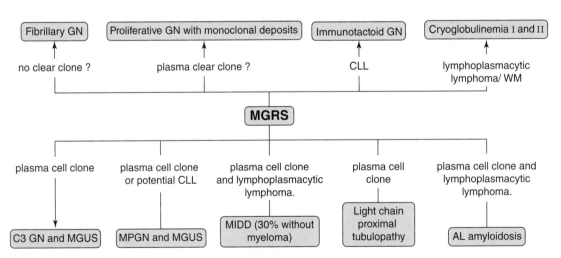

▲ **Figure 17–7.** Renal pathology seen with monoclonal gammopathy of renal significance (MGRS). GN, glomerulonephritis; MGUS, monoclonal gammopathy of undetermined significance. (Adapted from Jhaveri KD: http://www.nephronpower. com/2013/04/concept-map-monoclonal-gammopathy-of.html, with permission.)

of these patients. Other drugs used include bendamustine, thalidomide, lenalidomide, pomalidomide, and melphalan. Management of edema in patients with concurrent cardiac/autonomic nervous system involvement is usually difficult as they are very susceptible to fluid shifts and hypotension. The benefit of angiotensin converting enzyme inhibitors to reduce proteinuria has not been established in these patients. Renal transplantation can be offered to patients who are in complete remission.

B. Monoclonal immunoglobulin deposition disease (nonorganized deposits)—Renal impairment, microscopic hematuria, hypertension, and proteinuria are commonly seen in patients with monoclonal immunoglobulin disease (MIDD). Histologically, the most recognizable lesion of MIDD is nodular mesangial sclerosis similar to diabetic nephropathy. The diagnosis is made on immunofluorescence where the monoclonal light chain stains in a linear pattern along the basement membrane (glomerular, tubular, and vascular). Complement staining for C3 may also be seen. Electron microscopy reveals electron dense or amorphous deposits in the same compartments as in IF. Sometimes, one can see monoclonal immunoglobulin deposition disease along with myeloma cast nephropathy. Treatment of MIDD is based on treating the clone responsible for the production of the monoclonal protein. If a patient with MIDD is found to have myeloma or chronic lymphocytic leukemia, treatment of the underlying malignancy should be pursued. In patients who do not have a malignant clone, treatment should still be offered in order to preserve renal function. In the era of novel antimyeloma agents, such as bortezomib, renal outcomes and overall survival of patients with MIDD have improved.

▶ Conclusion

Onconephrology is a rapidly growing subspecialty area within nephrology. This area of subspecialization combines the unique knowledge and efforts of a number of specialists which include nephrologists, oncologists, urologists, pharmacologists, and intensivists. Nephrologists seeing patients with cancer and complications must master an understanding of the pathophysiology of kidney disease that develops in patients with various malignancies, the treatment rendered for the particular cancer, as well as the clinical approach to diagnosis and management of the particular type of kidney injury. Acquiring this knowledge and clinical skills will allow the general and onconephrologists to treat the cancer patient with kidney diseases.

KEY READINGS

Bridoux F et al: Diagnosis of monoclonal gammopathy of renal significance. Kidney Int 2015;87:698.

Doshi M et al: Paraprotein-related kidney disease: kidney injury from paraproteins—what determines the site of injury? Clin J Am Soc Nephrol 2016;11:2288.

Finkel KW et al: Paraprotein-related kidney disease: evaluation and treatment of myeloma cast nephropathy. Clin J Am Soc Nephrol 2016;11:2273.

Flombaum CD: Metabolic emergencies in the cancer patient. Semin Oncol 2000;27:322.

Gurevich F, Perazella MA: Renal effects of anti-angiogenesis therapy: update for the internist. Am J Med 2009;122:322.

Jhaveri KD et al: Glomerular diseases seen with cancer and chemotherapy: a narrative review. Kidney Int 2013;84:34.

Jhaveri KD et al: Renal effects of novel targeted oncologic agents, a narrative review. Kidney Int Rep 2017;2:108.

Lam AQ, Humphreys BD: Once-nephrology: AKI in the cancer patient. Clin J Am Soc Nephrol 2012;7:1692.

Motwani SS et al: Paraprotein-related kidney disease: glomerular diseases associated with paraproteinemias. Clin J Am Soc Nephrol 2016 Dec 7;11:2260.

Perazella MA: Onco-nephrology: renal toxicities of chemotherapeutic agents. Clin J Am Soc Nephrol 2012;7:1713.

Rosner MH: Onconephrology. The pathophysiology and treatment of malignancy associated hypercalcemia. Clin J Am Soc Nephrol 2015;7:1722.

Salahudeen AK et al: Incidence rate, clinical correlates, and outcomes of AKI in patients admitted to a comprehensive cancer center. Clin J Am Soc Nephrol 2013;8:347.

■ CHAPTER REVIEW QUESTIONS

1. You are referred a patient for evaluation of hypomagnesemia on cetuximab therapy. The patient is a 59-year-old male patient with metastatic colon cancer previously treated failed FOLFOX therapy and now started on cetuximab. He has been complaining of fatigue and muscle weakness. His electrolytes reveal a potassium level of 3.2 mg/dL and magnesium of 0.9 mg/dL. He has a high fractional excretion of magnesium. What are the risk factors for the development of hypomagnesemia with cetuximab therapy?
   A. Duration of therapy
   B. Race (African–American)
   C. Elderly
   D. Chronic kidney disease
   E. A and C

2. An elderly gentleman who has CLL comes for a route clinic visit. He has no complaints. His blood work reveals a WBC of 190,000/μL and mild thrombocytopenia. The serum potassium level is 8.5 mEq/L. The patient is sent to emergency room for evaluation. The repeat potassium is 2.5 mEq/L. There are no ECG changes and physical examination and history are unremarkable. What should be done next?
   A. Admit for IV potassium repletion
   B. Request a plasma K level
   C. Give sodium polystyrene and place on low K diet
   D. Admit to telemetry floor

3. A 65-year-old male patient with history of AML s/p allogenic nonmyeloablative HSCT 4 years ago is referred to you for nephrotic syndrome. His spot urine protein creatinine ratio is 23 g. His serum albumin is 2 g/dL and serum creatinine 1 mg/dL. A kidney biopsy is performed. The figure shows the electron microscopy findings. The most likely diagnosis is
   A. Membranous nephropathy
   B. Minimal change disease
   C. IgA nephropathy
   D. Thrombotic microangiopathy

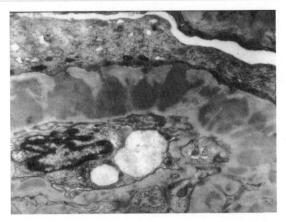

Electron microscopy reveals electron dense subepithelial deposits.

4. A 56-year-old male patient with elevated serum creatine of 2.3 mg/dL for last 1 year presents now with worsening proteinuria. A spot urinary protein/creatinine ratio reveals 13 g of proteinuria. Serum-free light chain reveals a kappa/lambda ratio of 45 and serum immunofixation confirms IgG kappa predominance. The patient has normal blood pressure, S4 on heart examination and 3+ pitting edema. The bone marrow confirms IgG kappa multiple myeloma. The kidney biopsy most likely is going to show:
   A. Monoclonal immunoglobulin deposition disease (MIDD)
   B. AA amyloidosis
   C. C3 Glomerulonephritis
   D. Minimal change disease

5. A 56-year-old male patient with melanoma presents with new onset renal injury in the last few weeks. His baseline renal function was normal and now it is 3 mg/dL. For his melanoma, he was started on nivolumab 3 months ago. His urinalysis is bland. He is not on any other medication except antinausea medications. His BP is normal and he has no edema on examination. Which is the most likely mechanism of injury of acute kidney injury in this patient?
   A. Acute tubular necrosis
   B. Acute interstitial nephritis
   C. Thrombotic microangiopathy (TMA)
   D. Hydronephrosis

Chronic Renal Failure and the Uremic Syndrome

Gregorio T. Obrador Vera, MD, MPH

ESSENTIALS OF DIAGNOSIS

▸ Abnormally elevated serum creatinine for more than 3 months

▸ Calculated glomerular filtration rate (GFR) less than 60 mL/min/1.73 m^2 for more than 3 months

▸ Clinical manifestations of the uremic syndrome in patients with advanced kidney failure

▶ General Considerations

The Kidney Disease: Improving Global Outcomes (KDIGO) Clinical Practice Guideline for the Evaluation and Management of Chronic Kidney Disease (CKD) has defined CKD as abnormalities of kidney structure or function, present for more than 3 months, with implications for health. Structural or functional abnormalities may manifest by markers of kidney damage and/or glomerular filtration rate (GFR) less than 60 mL/min/1.73 m^2 of body surface area. Markers of kidney damage include albuminuria greater than or equal to 30 mg/24 h (or ≥30 mg/g by albumin/creatinine ratio), urine sediment abnormalities (ie, microscopic hematuria), electrolyte and other abnormalities due to tubular disorders (ie, renal tubular acidosis), abnormalities detected by histology (ie, chronic glomerulonephritis) or imaging studies (ie, polycystic kidneys), or history of kidney transplantation. GFR can be estimated from serum creatinine or cystatin C with a formula, preferably the chronic kidney disease-epidemiology collaboration (CKD-EPI) equation. Persistence of abnormalities for more than 3 months is important to distinguish between acute and chronic kidney disease, and has implications for health to exclude benign conditions (ie, a simple renal cyst is a structural abnormality of the kidney but with minimal health risks for the individual).

According to KDIGO, CKD can be classified based on the level of GFR (G1–G5), the degree of albuminuria (A1–A3), and the likely cause of CKD (Table 18–1). Whereas the definition of CKD stages G3–G5 is solely based on a level of GFR less than 60 mL/min/1.73 m^2, CKD stages G1 and G2 require that the level of GFR greater than 60 mL/min/1.73 m^2 be accompanied by a marker of kidney damage (typically, moderately, or severely increased albuminuria). As an example, a patient with an estimated GFR of 40 mL/min/1.73 m^2, albuminuria of 380 mg/g by ACR, and likely diabetic nephropathy would be classified as G3b, A3, and diabetic nephropathy as the cause.

CKD is a syndrome that results from the progressive decline of GFR, typically over months to years and is due to an irreversible destruction of nephrons independent of the cause. Since it is usually asymptomatic until advanced stages, most often it is recognized by laboratory abnormalities in serum and urine. The uremic syndrome refers to a constellation of symptoms and signs that occur in patients with kidney failure (GFR <10–15 mL/min/1.73 m^2) and reflects generalized organ dysfunction. At this stage, kidney replacement therapy with dialysis or transplantation becomes necessary to sustain life. End-stage renal disease (ESRD) is an administrative term based on conditions for payment of healthcare by the Medicare ESRD program for patients treated by dialysis and transplantation in the United States.

The estimated global CKD prevalence is between 11% and 13% with the majority in stage 3. In 2010, about 2.6 million people were receiving renal replacement therapy (RRT) worldwide, and at least 2.3 million people were in need but had no access to RRT. In the United States, approximately 8.3 million Americans have an eGFR less than or equal to 60 mL/min/1.73 m^2. The prevalence of CKD in the adult US population has increased from 13.9% to 14.8% between the periods of 1999–2002 and 2011–2014, respectively. In the year 2014 alone, 120,688 patients began kidney replacement therapy, and 678,383 were receiving chronic dialysis (70%) or had a functioning kidney transplant (30%) in the United States. The crude incidence and prevalence rates of treated ESRD

Table 18–1. Classification of chronic kidney disease and management recommendations.[a]

Stage	Description (at increased risk)	GFR (mL/min/1.73 m²) (>90 [CKD risk factors])	Management (screening CKD risk reduction)
1	Kidney damage with normal or ↑ GFR	>90	Diagnosis and Rx CVD risk reduction
2	Mild ↓ GFR	60–89	Estimating progression
3	Moderate ↓ GFR	30–59	Evaluating and treating complications
4	Severe ↓ GFR	15–29	Preparation for kidney replacement therapy
5	Kidney failure	<15 or dialysis	Replacement, if uremia is present

CKD, chronic kidney disease; CVD, cardiovascular disease; GFR, glomerular filtration rate.
[a]Recommendations by the National Kidney Foundation–Kidney Disease Outcomes Quality Initiative (NKF-K/DOQI).
Source: Reproduced with permission from *Am J Kid Dis*. 2002;39(Suppl):S46.

were 370 and 2067 cases per million population, respectively. Diabetes mellitus remains the most frequent cause of ESRD, accounting for nearly 45% of cases; together with systemic hypertension, which is the second leading cause, explain over two-thirds of the cases of treated ESRD. African–Americans are more susceptible to ESRD secondary to hypertension. Genetic predisposition due to apolipoprotein L1 (APOL1) polymorphisms appears to explain at least some of the increased risk.

▶ **Pathogenesis**

The progressive nephron and GFR loss associated with progressive CKD leads to (1) abnormalities in water, electrolyte, and pH balance, (2) accumulation of waste products that are normally excreted by the kidney, and (3) abnormalities in the production and metabolism of certain hormones (ie, erythropoietin, active vitamin D, insulin). Fortunately, as the GFR declines, some compensatory mechanisms are activated, of which the most important is glomerular hyperfiltration in the remaining functioning nephrons. Due to this compensatory mechanism, a patient may be totally asymptomatic despite having lost more than 70% of kidney function. However, glomerular hyperfiltration is associated with the development of glomerulosclerosis in the remaining functioning nephrons, which contributes to further nephron loss. Other factors that contribute to nephron loss include (1) ongoing activity of the primary cause of CKD, (2) proteinuria, (3) development of tubulointerstitial lesions, (4) hyperlipidemia, and (5) acute superimposed renal insults (ie, contrast nephropathy, aminoglycoside toxicity), among others.

▶ **Prevention**

Primary prevention involves reducing risk factors for development, early detection, and adequate control of diseases that may lead to CKD (ie, diabetes, hypertension, obesity).

Secondary prevention aims at identification of CKD among asymptomatic individuals and early implementation of interventions that prevent or slow the progression of CKD. Screening is only cost-effective in people at high risk for CKD, particularly those with diabetes and hypertension. Screening tests should include a first morning or a random "spot" urine sample for albumin or protein to creatinine ratio, and serum creatinine level for estimation of GFR using an accepted prediction equation.

▶ **Clinical Findings**

A. Symptoms and Signs

Patients are usually asymptomatic until kidney failure is advanced. When the GFR falls to approximately 10–15 mL/min, nonspecific symptoms such as general malaise, weakness, insomnia, inability to concentrate, and nausea and vomiting begin to appear. Eventually, other symptoms and signs that reflect generalized organ dysfunction develop as part of the uremic syndrome (Table 18–2).

1. Skin manifestations—The skin is often pale (due to anemia) and hyperpigmented (due to increased production of β-melanocyte-stimulating hormone [β-MSH] and retention of carotenes and urochromes). Pruritus is common and can be accompanied by scratching lesions. Ecchymoses and hematomas are often seen as a result of bleeding diathesis. Uremic frost is a fine white powder visible on the skin surface that results from crystallization of urea after sweat evaporates; it is now uncommon because of earlier initiation of dialysis. Other infrequent but clinically relevant abnormalities include skin necrosis due to vessel calcification (calciphylaxis) and bullous lesions.

2. Cardiovascular manifestations—Cardiovascular manifestations are the most common cause of morbidity and mortality among patients with progressive CKD and include

Table 18–2. Clinical and laboratory manifestations of the uremic syndrome.

System	Clinical Manifestations
Skin	Paleness and hyperpigmentation Echymosis and hematomas Pruritus Skin necrosis (calciphylaxis) Bullous lesions
Cardiovascular	Volume overload and systemic hypertension Accelerated atherosclerosis and ischemic heart disease Left ventricular hypertrophy Heart failure Rhythm disturbances Uremic pericarditis
Neurologic	Cerebrovascular accidents Encephalopathy Seizures Peripheral and autonomic neuropathy
Gastrointestinal	Anorexia Nausea and vomiting Malnutrition Uremic fetor Inflammatory and ulcerative lesions Gastrointestinal bleeding
Hematologic	Anemia Leukocyte and immune system dysfunction (tendency to infections) Platelet dysfunction (bleeding diathesis)
Bone	Renal osteodystrophy Growth retardation in children Muscle weakness Amyloid arthropathy secondary to β_2-microglobulin deposition
Endocrine	Sexual dysfunction Infertility in women Glucose intolerance due to insulin resistance Hyperlipidemia
Laboratory	Hyponatremia (if excessive water intake) Hyperkalemia Hyperphosphatemia Hypocalcemia Hypermagnesemia Hyperuricemia Metabolic acidosis

volume overload, edema, systemic hypertension, ischemic heart disease, left ventricular hypertrophy, heart failure, rhythm disturbances, and uremic pericarditis. Systemic hypertension is primarily due to volume overload; other contributing

factors are hyperreninemia and erythropoietin therapy. Patients with chronic kidney failure (CKF) have accelerated atherosclerosis due to a high prevalence of "traditional" (ie, hypertension and hyperlipidemia) and "nontraditional" risk factors (those associated with the hemodynamic and metabolic abnormalities of CKF, such as volume overload, anemia, glucose intolerance, and hyperparathyroidism). Left ventricular hypertrophy is seen in 65–75% of patients with advanced CKF, and both arterial hypertension and anemia contribute to its development. Heart failure is usually multifactorial, with volume overload, hypertension, anemia, ischemic heart disease, and uremic cardiomyopathy as the main contributing factors. Rhythm disturbances are often precipitated by electrolyte abnormalities, metabolic acidosis, calcification of the conduction system, ischemia, and myocardial dysfunction. Uremic pericarditis occurs in 6–10% of patients with advanced uremia, just before initiation of dialysis or immediately after. Typical features include high blood urea levels (>60 mg/dL), an absence of the diffuse ST- and T-wave elevations observed in patients with other causes of acute pericarditis, and hemorrhagic pericardial effusion in at least 50% of cases.

3. Neurologic manifestations—Cerebrovascular accidents are common in these patients due to accelerated atherosclerosis. Uremic encephalopathy occurs in patients with advanced uremia and is characterized by insomnia, sleep pattern changes, inability to concentrate, memory loss, confusion, disorientation, emotional lability, anxiety, depression, and occasionally hallucinations. Without treatment, the encephalopathy progresses to generalized seizures, coma, and death. Other manifestations may include dysarthria, tremor, and myoclonic movements, and in advanced stages, hyperreflexia, clonus, and the Babinski sign. The electroencephalogram shows a diffuse slowing of cortical activity. Dialysis improves most of the manifestations of uremic encephalopathy. Another complication is peripheral neuropathy, which typically presents insidiously as a mixed symmetric polyneuropathy of the lower extremities. It may also affect the upper extremities but only after the lower extremities have been involved. Sensory abnormalities include the restless leg syndrome and a burning sensation on the feet, which may be severe enough to prevent ambulation. Motor abnormalities occur after the sensory abnormalities and include extremity weakness, unsteady gate, decreased deep tendon reflexes, and occasionally paraparesis and even paralysis. Autonomic nerves can also be affected, which may result in orthostatic hypotension, sweating abnormalities, impotence, and an abnormal response to the Valsalva maneuver.

4. Gastrointestinal manifestations—Anorexia, nausea, and vomiting are typical manifestations of advanced kidney failure. Anorexia usually occurs earlier, can be intermittent, and is occasionally referred to some types of food such as meat. Nausea initially presents in the morning. The combination of these symptoms together with abnormalities in protein and energy metabolism, other comorbid conditions (ie, gastroparesis in diabetic patients), and side effects of medications often leads to malnutrition. Uremic fetor is a uriniferous odor of the breath that results from the breakdown of urea to ammonia in saliva and is often associated with an unpleasant metallic taste sensation. Other manifestations include a higher frequency of inflammatory and ulcerative lesions at all levels of the digestive tract and gastrointestinal bleeding.

5. Hematologic manifestations—A normochromic, normocytic anemia almost invariably develops in patients with CKF. It is mainly due to a deficiency in the production of erythropoietin by the diseased kidneys. Other factors may also contribute, including hyporesponsiveness of progenitor cells to erythropoietin, accelerated hemolysis secondary to uremia, vitamin deficiencies (ie, folic acid), and iron losses associated predominantly with gastrointestinal bleeding. The white blood cell count is usually normal and increases in response to infections; however, leukocyte and immune system functions are abnormal, which predisposes to more frequent and severe infections. The platelet count is also normal, but the function is abnormal, which results in a prolonged bleeding time and a tendency to bleed.

6. Bone manifestations—According to KDIGO, CKD-Mineral and Bone Disorder (CKD-MBD) refers to a clinical syndrome that encompasses mineral, bone, and calcific abnormalities that develop as a complication of CKD. The term renal osteodystrophy should be restricted to describing the various types of bone lesions that occur in patients with progressive CKD. Mineral abnormalities include hyperphosphatemia, hypocalcemia, hyperparathyroidism, and low levels of vitamin D (calcidiol and calcitriol). Bone lesions include secondary hyperparathyroidism, osteomalacia, adynamic bone disease, and growth retardation in children. Calcifications can also occur in subcutaneous tissue, joints, vessels, and viscera. Although secondary hyperparathyroidism is the most common type of renal osteodystrophy, patients often have a predominant lesion or a combination of mixed lesions. Although close to 100% of patients have abnormalities in a bone biopsy, radiologic abnormalities occur in only 40% of patients, and clinical manifestations, such as bone pain or fractures, in less than 10% of patients. Renal osteodystrophy can be prevented or attenuated with appropriate management of calcium and phosphate metabolism.

7. Endocrine and metabolic manifestations—Sexual dysfunction is common in patients with progressive CKD. Impotence, infertility and decreased libido occur as a result of primary hypogonadism. Hyperprolactinemia also contributes to amenorrhea and galactorrhea in women. Total

T4 and T3 and free T3 may be low, but free T4, reverse T3, and thyroid-stimulating hormone (TSH) are normal, suggesting a normal thyroid state. In early CKD, there is insulin resistance and glucose intolerance (azotemic pseudodiabetes), whereas in advanced CKD hypoglycemic episodes are common due to the longer half-life of insulin secondary to decreased renal catabolism and reduced renal gluconeogenesis (as well as decreased clearance of some hypoglycemic medications such as sulfonylureas). Lipid abnormalities include elevated triglycerides and very low-density lipoprotein (VLDL) and decreased high-density lipoprotein (HDL); total cholesterol is normal and lipoprotein A may be elevated. Abnormalities of protein metabolism include decreased synthesis and increased catabolism.

B. Laboratory Findings

In addition to an elevated blood urea nitrogen (BUN) and serum creatinine, which are a reflection of a decreased GFR, patients with progressive CKD develop other laboratory abnormalities, particularly if they do not comply or are not given appropriate dietary instructions as the GFR declines. Typical abnormalities include hyponatremia (due to excessive water intake), hyperkalemia, hyperphosphatemia, hypocalcemia, hypermagnesemia, and hyperuricemia. Metabolic acidosis, usually with an elevated anion gap, is also common (see Table 18–2). Except for hypocalcemia, these fluid and electrolyte disturbances result from an imbalance between intake and output by the progressively diseased kidneys.

C. Imaging Studies

Renal ultrasound is especially useful for diagnosing some cases of CKD (ie, polycystic kidney disease [PKD], obstructive uropathy) and for distinguishing acute from CKD. The presence of symmetrically small (particularly if <8.5 cm) kidneys supports the diagnosis of CKD, whereas the occurrence of normal-sized kidneys favors an acute rather than a chronic process. There are exceptions, however, as some causes of CKD are associated with normal-sized or even enlarged kidneys, including diabetes, PKD, and amyloidosis. Other imaging studies may help determine the cause of CKD. Duplex Doppler ultrasound of the renal arteries, renal scintigraphy, and magnetic resonance angiography are useful in patients in whom renovascular ischemic disease is suspected. Voiding cystourethrography is helpful to rule out reflux nephropathy. Computed tomography allows for assessment of kidney stone activity and evidence of papillary necrosis.

D. Special Tests

Kidney biopsy should be reserved for patients with near-normal kidney size, in whom a clear-cut diagnosis cannot be made by less invasive means, and when a potentially treatable cause is suspected.

Treatment

Conservative treatment, usually with diet and medications, is indicated in all CKD stages. Kidney replacement therapy with dialysis or transplantation eventually becomes necessary in CKD stage 5. The goals of conservative treatment are to (1) treat the cause of CKD if possible and also to detect and treat any reversible cause of decreased kidney function, such as volume depletion, urinary tract infection, obstructive uropathy, use of nephrotoxic agents, accelerated or uncontrolled hypertension, and reactivation or flare of the original underlying etiologic disease process, (2) implement interventions to prevent or slow progression of CKD, (3) prevent or treat complications of CKD, (4) prevent or treat complications associated with other comorbid conditions, particularly diabetes and cardiovascular disease, and (5) prepare the patient and family for kidney replacement therapy (Figure 18–1). Also, periodic review of medications is recommended; nephrotoxic agents should be avoided, and dose adjustments should be made for drugs that are excreted by the renal route. Vaccinations against influenza, pneumococcus, and hepatitis B are also recommended. Patients with CKD should be referred to a nephrologist when the eGFR is less than 30 mL/min (stage 4), as this allows enough time for adequate preparation for kidney replacement therapy; for earlier stages of CKD, joint management between the primary care physician and the nephrologist is appropriate.

A. Interventions to Slow Progression of CKD

It has been shown that some interventions slow the progression of CKD, including blood pressure control, use of angiotensin-converting enzyme (ACE) inhibitors or angiotensin receptor blockers (ARBs), and glycemic control in diabetic patients. These interventions are most effective if they are implemented early in the course of CKD. Blood pressure control is essential not only to delay progression of CKD but to reduce the risk of developing coronary artery disease and left ventricular hypertrophy. Treatment includes a low-salt diet and antihypertensive medications. ACE inhibitors and ARBs are the antihypertensive agents of choice particularly in patients with albuminuria greater than 30 mg/g because they reduce glomerular hypertension by a dual mechanism: lowering of systemic blood pressure and predominant vasodilation of the efferent arteriole; also, they improve glomerular membrane permeability and decrease the production of fibrogenic cytokines. ARBs have fewer side effects than ACE inhibitors, such as cough or hyperkalemia; however, due to their higher cost, they are usually recommended for patients who do not respond to or tolerate ACE inhibitors. Recent studies indicate that the combination of ACE inhibitors and ARBs is not more effective to slow the progression of CKD than either agent alone, and it is associated with more side effects, such as acute kidney injury and hyperkalemia. Also, the combination of ARBs and direct renin inhibitors (ie, aliskiren) is not recommended. Although somewhat controversial, KDIGO recommends a target blood pressure less than 130/80 in patients with albuminuria greater than 30 mg/g and less than 140/90 in those with albuminuria less than 30 mg/g. ACE inhibitors and ARBs have also been shown to be renoprotective in patients with normal blood pressure and proteinuria, particularly those with type 1 diabetes. Strict glycemic control

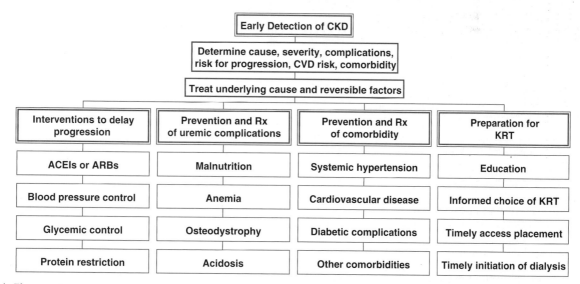

▲ **Figure 18–1.** Early detection of chronic kidney disease (CKD). ACEIs, angiotensin-converting enzyme inhibitors; ARBs, angiotensin receptor blockers; CVD, cardiovascular disease; KRT, kidney replacement therapy; Rx, treatment.

is another intervention that reduces the risk of developing nephropathy, particularly if it is initiated early in the course of diabetes and diabetic nephropathy (stage of normal to mildly or moderately increased albuminuria). The benefit of strict glycemic control in patients with diabetes and overt nephropathy (severely increased albuminuria >300 mg/g) is unclear. KDIGO recommends a target hemoglobin A_{1c} of approximately 7%, although this may be extended above 7% in individuals with comorbidities or limited life expectancy and risk of hypoglycemia. Dietary protein restriction is another intervention that may slow the progression of CKD. KDIGO suggests lowering protein intake to 0.8 g/kg/day in patients with or without diabetes and GFR less than 30 mL/min/1.73 m^2; stricter low-protein diets must be individualized, and patients should receive appropriate education and follow-up by a dietician. Other interventions, such as treatment of hyperuricemia and metabolic acidosis, may slow the progression of CKD, but further evidence is still needed. Since patients with CKD are at increased risk for acute kidney injury (AKI), every effort should be made to prevent AKI episodes in these patients.

B. Prevention and Treatment of Uremic Complications

As CKD becomes more severe, appropriate dietary changes must be made to prevent or treat water, electrolyte, and acid–base disorders. A low-salt diet (2 g of sodium or 5 g of sodium chloride per day) and loop diuretics are recommended for volume overload. Thiazide diuretics are ineffective when the GFR is less than 30 mL/min. Hyponatremia can be avoided by reducing water intake (eg, to 1.5 L/day). To prevent hyperkalemia, a low potassium diet (40–60 mEq/day) is recommended; also, exogenous sources of potassium should be avoided, including blood transfusions, salt substitutes, and certain medications (nonsteroidal anti-inflammatory drugs and potassium-sparing diuretics). Although ACE inhibitors and ARBs may cause hyperkalemia and acute kidney failure, they can be used in patients with progressive CKD because of their renoprotective effect, but with careful monitoring of serum potassium and creatinine. Hyperuricemia rarely leads to symptomatic gout, and thus treatment of this complication with low-dose allopurinol is not necessary unless it becomes a recurrent problem. To reduce the risk of developing hypermagnesemia, magnesium-containing antacids and cathartics should be avoided. Serum bicarbonate should be maintained at greater than or equal to 22 mEq/L with the administration of sodium bicarbonate, particularly in symptomatic patients and to prevent growth retardation in children. Last, therapeutic options for severe pruritus include an adequate control of calcium and phosphorus metabolism, correction of anemia, ultraviolet light, and symptomatic treatment with H$_1$ antihistamines and topical analgesics.

Regarding cardiovascular complications, management of volume overload and hypertension includes a low-salt diet, loop diuretics, and antihypertensive agents (see above). Risk factors for atherosclerotic complications should be aggressively treated. Uremic pericarditis is an indication for initiation of dialysis; a short course of corticosteroids or nonsteroidal anti-inflammatory drugs is sometimes needed for pain control; pericardiocentesis is indicated if tamponade is present. Neurologic complications such as encephalopathy are an indication for initiation of dialysis; neuropathy also improves with dialysis and more consistently with kidney transplantation. Gastrointestinal complications such as anorexia, nausea, and vomiting improve with dialysis; in the evaluation of nausea and vomiting, it is important to exclude nonuremic causes, for example, diabetic gastroparesis, peptic ulcer disease, or side effects of medications. Follow-up by a qualified dietician is recommended to avoid malnutrition; protein and energy intake of 0.8 g/kg/day and 30–35 kcal/kg/day, respectively, is recommended.

Regarding hematological complications, anemia of CKD requires initial treatment with oral or IV iron followed by short- or long-acting erythropoiesis-stimulating agents (ie, erythropoietin alfa or beta, darbepoetin alfa, continuous erythropoiesis receptor activator [CERA]). Erythropoiesis-stimulating agents may worsen hypertension and should be used with caution if at all in patients with a history of cerebrovascular accident and those with prior or current malignancy. KDIGO recommends starting therapy when the hemoglobin level is less than 10 g/dL and maintain it between 10 and 11.5 g/dL. Unless there is a clear indication, it is preferable not to use blood transfusions, particularly in potential kidney transplant patients. Treatment of platelet dysfunction is indicated in patients with active bleeding and before a surgical procedure; appropriate measures include (1) correction of anemia with erythropoietin or blood transfusion, (2) administration of desmopressin or cryoprecipitate for rapid correction, (3) conjugated estrogens for long-term correction, and (4) reduction of azotemia with dialysis if indicated.

CKD-MBD requires control of hyperphosphatemia with a low-phosphorus diet and phosphate-binding agents. Calcium-containing phosphate binders (ie, calcium carbonate or calcium acetate) are cheap and effective, but its use may be associated with the development of hypercalcemia. Noncalcium containing phosphate binders (ie, sevelamer, lanthanum carbonate) are a better option to control hyperphosphatemia in patients with hypercalcemia, low PTH, adynamic bone disease, or vascular calcifications. Aluminum-containing phosphate binders are generally not recommended because of the risk of aluminum accumulation and toxicity. Vitamin D (ergocalciferol) should be supplemented if the 25-hidroxicalciferol level is less than 30 ng/mL. Active vitamin D supplementation with cholecalciferol or alfacalcidol will eventually be needed to suppress PTH, although the optimal PTH level is not known. Selective vitamin D receptor activators, such as paricalcitol, are also effective and may reduce the risk of hypercalcemia. Calcimimetics can be used in patients with CKD 5 on dialysis but not in predialysis patients because of the risk of inducing severe hypocalcemia. Parathyroidectomy is indicated in patients with severe hyperparathyroidism that is refractory to medical treatment.

C. Prevention and Treatment of Comorbid Conditions

Since cardiovascular complications are the leading cause of death in patients with CKD, appropriate management of risk factors and established heart disease is of the utmost importance. Diabetic complications should also be managed appropriately.

D. Preparation for Kidney Replacement Therapy

An adequate preparation for kidney replacement therapy or renal conservative care includes (1) information on the different treatment modalities, (2) education regarding preservation of forearm veins for future vascular access placement for hemodialysis, (3) referral to social services to assess transportation needs to the dialysis unit, continuation of work in some cases, rehabilitation, and participation in support groups, and (4) placement of a permanent vascular access, preferably an arteriovenous fistula, when the estimated time for initiation of dialysis is 6 months (or 3–6 weeks if an arteriovenous graft is chosen); peritoneal dialysis catheters should be placed 2–4 weeks before dialysis initiation. Renal conservative and palliative care is a therapeutic option particularly suited for patients older than 75 years of age with significant comorbidities. It encompasses comprehensive medical treatment of CKD except for dialysis, active management of pain and other symptoms, and psychological, social, and family support. Although further evidence is needed, survival of conservative care compared to dialysis is similar in older patients with significant comorbidities.

► Prognosis

CKD is associated with high morbidity and mortality. Compared to the general population, the number of hospitalizations and days spent in the hospital per year are three times greater in patients with CKD stages 2–4, and six to seven times higher in patients with ESRD receiving dialysis. One-, two-, and five-year survival for dialysis patients are 80, 65, and 38%, respectively. The expected remaining lifetimes of white dialysis patients are only one-fourth to one-sixth those of the general population. Last, cardiovascular mortality is 10–30 times higher in ESRD patients treated with dialysis compared to those in the general population. These poor outcomes underscore the importance of early detection and appropriate management of CKD long before dialysis is required.

KEY READINGS

Davison SN et al: Executive summary of the KDIGO Controversies Conference on Supportive Care in Chronic Kidney Disease: developing a roadmap to improving quality care. Kidney Int 2015;88:447.

Fried LF et al: Combined angiotensin inhibition for the treatment of diabetic nephropathy. N Engl J Med 2013;369:1892.

Jha V et al: Chronic kidney disease: global dimension and perspectives. Lancet 2013;382:260.

Ketteler M et al: Revisiting KDIGO clinical practice guideline on chronic kidney disease-mineral and bone disorder: a commentary from a Kidney Disease: Improving Global Outcomes controversies conference. Kidney Int 2015;87:502.

Kidney Disease: Improving Global Outcomes (KDIGO) CKD Work Group. KDIGO 2012 Clinical Practice Guideline for the Evaluation and Management of Chronic Kidney Disease. Kidney Int Suppl 2013;3:1.

Pfeffer MA et al: A trial of darbepoetin alfa in type 2 diabetes and chronic kidney disease. N Engl J Med 2009;361:2019.

► Websites

Centers for Disease Control and Prevention's Chronic Kidney Disease (CKD) Surveillance Project: https://nccd.cdc.gov/ckd/. Provides epidemiological data on the burden of CKD in the United States and public health strategies for promoting kidney health.

Kidney Disease: Improving Global Outcomes: http://www.kdigo.org. Provides access to KDIGO guidelines.

National Kidney Foundation-Kidney Disease Outcomes Quality Initiative (NKF-K/DOQI): http://www.kidney.org/professionals/kdoqi/index.cfm. Provides access to the GFR calculator and the NKF-K/DOQI Clinical Practice Guidelines.

United States Renal Data System: http://www.usrds.org. Provides epidemiologic data on CKD and ESRD in the United States.

■ CHAPTER REVIEW QUESTIONS

1. Which of the following cases does NOT fulfill KDIGO criteria for chronic kidney disease?
   A. A 28-year-old male patient with a persistently elevated serum creatinine of 6 mg/dL over the past 4 months.
   B. A 67-year-old male patient with two simple cysts in the right kidney, without albuminuria or hematuria, and an estimated GFR of 68 mL/min.
   C. A 58-year-old female patient with a 15-year history of diabetes, albumin-to-creatinine ratio of 258 mg/g, and an estimated GFR of 54 mL/min and declining over the past year.
   D. A 70-year-old male patient with a history of poorly controlled chronic hypertension, a slowly rising serum creatinine over the past several years, and symptoms felt to be due to uremia.

2. Which of the following factor(s) contribute to the pathophysiology of anemia of chronic kidney disease?
   A. Decreased production of erythropoietin by the kidneys
   B. Accelerated hemolysis due to uremia
   C. Iron and folic acid deficiencies
   D. All of the above are correct

3. The following statements regarding secondary prevention of chronic kidney disease are true, EXCEPT:
   A. It involves early detection of CKD among asymptomatic individuals.
   B. Screening tests should include an albumin-to-creatinine ratio in a morning or random urine sample, and a serum creatinine to estimate GFR with an accepted equation.
   C. CKD screening is cost-effective when applied to the general population.
   D. Early detection should be followed by interventions to slow the progression of CKD.

4. A 57-year-old female patient, with a 15-year history of moderately well-controlled diabetes and hypertension, is seen for the first time in your office. After appropriate evaluation, you make the diagnosis of CKD G2, A2, and diabetic nephropathy as the most likely cause. Which of the following interventions would be indicated to slow the progression of CKD in this patient?
   A. Administer both ACE inhibitors and angiotensin-receptor antagonists.
   B. Administer both direct renin inhibitors (aliskiren) and angiotensin-receptor antagonists.
   C. Achieve adequate glycemic control with a target hemoglobin A_{1c} of ~7%.
   D. Target a blood pressure of <140/90.

5. The most frequent cause of treated end-stage kidney disease in the United States is
   A. Diabetes mellitus
   B. Glomerulonephritis
   C. Polycystic kidney disease
   D. Systemic hypertension

Anemia and Chronic Kidney Disease

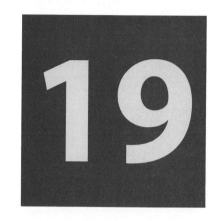

Robert Provenzano, MD, FACP, FASN

ESSENTIALS OF DIAGNOSIS

▸ Anemia is a comorbidity of progressive chronic kidney disease (CKD).

▸ Anemia of CKD results from the inability of the kidney to produce significant quantities of erythropoietin.

▸ Decreased red blood cell survival and iron deficiency are cofactors.

▸ General Considerations

Since the initial observations by Richard Bright in 1836 on the relationship of anemia to renal inefficiency, anemia has remained as an ever-present comorbidity of progressive chronic kidney disease (CKD). The Kidney Disease Outcomes Quality Initiatives (K/DOQI) clinical practice guidelines for CKD first published in 2002 helped focus attention on CKD and its comorbidities, specifically anemia.

Recent data support the direct relationship of anemia to cardiovascular disease and to patient mortality in end-stage renal disease (ESRD). Anemia of CKD is generally caused by the inability of the kidneys to produce significant quantities of erythropoietin, but other factors are frequently involved including decreased red blood cell survival and iron deficiency. Despite the clinical introduction of recombinant human erythropoietin (rHuEPO) in 1989, there is still an estimated 1.5 million individuals with anemia in the United States. Additionally, anemia (hemoglobin <12 mg/dL) is present in greater than 75% of dialysis patients.

The availability of rHuEPO revolutionized our understanding of uremia and quickly became a major tool in the armamentarium of nephrologists to improve symptoms previously thought to be due to the "uremic syndrome." Correction of anemia in these patients resulted in an improved sense of well-being, improved energy levels, a significant improvement in sleep disturbances, improved cognitive function, and an improvement in the ability to perform tasks of daily living. More significantly, improved hemoglobin levels in CKD patients have been correlated with decreased left ventricular hypertrophy (LVH) and improved cardiovascular outcomes.

Although debate continues on the proper "target" hemoglobin, the FDA directed use of erythropoiesis-stimulating agents (ESAs) to avoid the need for transfusion has been generally accepted.

▸ Pathogenesis

Under normal homeostatic conditions, the kidney very precisely regulates plasma volume through the reabsorption or excretion of salt and water. Hemoglobin levels are maintained in response to the production of erythropoietin to tissue hypoxia.

Erythropoietin is known to be a multifunctional tropic factor with effects on not only the bone marrow but on the central nervous system where studies have shown both neurotrophic and neuroprotective functions. Its primary target although is the pluripotent hematopoietic stem cells of the bone marrow. This cell line is capable of forming erythrocytes, leukocytes, and megakaryocytes. Erythropoietin is produced by specialized fibroblasts in the interstitium of the kidney in response to hypoxia (Figure 19–1).

As renal function declines, anemia becomes more common. The majority of patients with a GFR less than 60 mL/min/1.73 m^2 (K/DOQI stage 3) have insufficient erythropoietin production to maintain the hemoglobin level greater than 12 g/dL. This results in the typical normochromatic normocytic anemia present in CKD and ESRD. However, anemia of CKD often has etiologies other than insufficient erythropoietin levels. Iron deficiency, chronic inflammation, and EPO resistance are common and need to be considered in the identification and treatment of anemia of CKD.

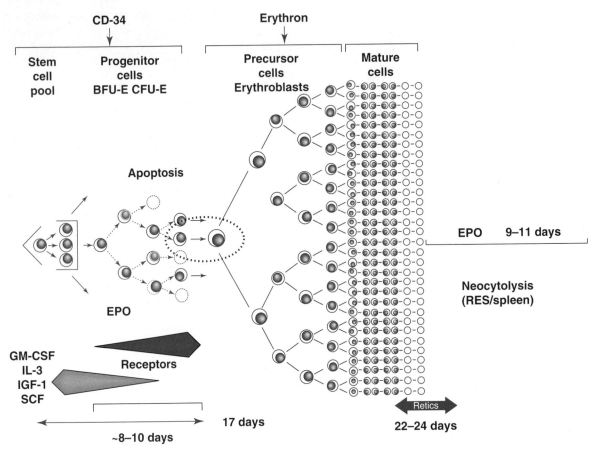

▲ **Figure 19–1.** Erythropoiesis is divided into two stages. Erythropoietin (EPO) is needed in the first stage (from multipotential to progenitor cells in the burst-forming unit erythroid) but not in the second precursor cell stage. The site of action of EPO and other growth factors is shown. Dashed circles indicate potential apoptosis of progenitor cells. (Adapted with permission from Erslev AJ et al: Erythropoietin in the pathogenesis of the anemia of chronic renal failure. Kidney Int 1997;51:623.)

▶ Treatment

A. Historical Perspective

Prior to the clinical introduction of cloned erythropoietin (rHuEPO) in 1989, the world of nephrology was very different. There was no focus on CKD, little focus on treating anemia, but considerable focus on improving the adequacy of dialysis (delivered amount of dialysis). The continued evolution of dialysis equipment including volumetric dialysis machines and dialyzer membrane biocompatibility with improvement of uremic symptoms was of paramount importance. Our ability to more accurately measure the amount of delivered dialysis added to these endeavors.

At that time, anemia was managed in two ways: severe anemia with hemoglobin less than 8 g/dL was treated with blood transfusions. Less critical management of anemia, viewed as "maintenance management," involved the use of anabolic steroids. Iron deficiency was rarely a problem; indeed, iron overload from frequent blood transfusions was a much greater problem occasionally resulting in secondary hemochromatosis.

The introduction of erythropoietin and the correction of anemia resulted in the elimination of many symptoms previously thought to be due to uremia. The avid production of new red blood cells consumed the additional iron stores and secondary hemochromatosis soon became a historical footnote along with the use of steroids and their inherent side effects.

B. Cardiovascular Disease and Anemia

See Chapter 20, on cardiovascular disease.

C. Current Management of Anemia of CKD

Despite the availability of recumbent erythropoietin, approximately 30% of patients with CKD are treated with erythropoietin and these numbers have decreased since the FDA warning on higher hemoglobin targets and may be less than 10%. It is well accepted that transitional CKD patients (CKD 4 and 5) have improved 90 days morbidity and mortality on dialysis with higher hemoglobin levels (>10 g). Although there is great debate about why so many patients remain untreated (barriers by insurers, FDA regulations, fragmentation of care, late referrals, etc.), studies looking at the logistics of management of anemia in nephrology offices suggest that a lack of an organized methodology to treat anemia is still missing in most nephrology clinical settings.

An organized methodology of identification, evaluation, treatment, and maintenance of anemia has now become a critical requirement in all nephrology practices. Although this will vary from practice to practice, algorithms (Figure 19–2) help define the minimum steps necessary to identify the majority of patients with anemia and guide them toward treatment solutions.

Providing all patients upon introduction to the CKD clinic with information on anemia and the fact that they may become anemic is critical. Checking their hemoglobin at each visit will ensure a focus on one of the major comorbidities of their disease.

1. Iron supplementation—The K/DOQI guidelines recommend baseline iron studies prior to initiation of erythropoietin therapy (serum iron, transferrin, and ferritin levels).

Although some controversy exists as to the best methods of continually accessing adequate iron stores and iron delivered to the bone marrow, the most universally available test remains transferrin saturation and serum ferritin. If iron deficiency is identified, an appropriate workup including evaluation for gastrointestinal sources of blood loss (gastritis or malignancy) must be initiated.

The USRDS Dialysis Morbidity and Mortality (UDMM) Study showed that up to 50% of patients receiving epoetin were iron deficient, making this the most common cause of "erythropoietin resistance." Although multiple normograms exist for the replacement of iron, two important points need to be made concerning oral iron. First, oral iron can rarely be

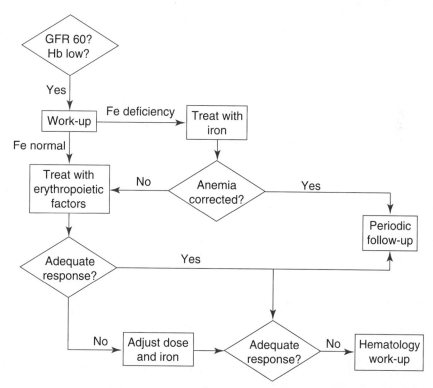

▲ **Figure 19–2.** Anemia assessment flowchart. (Adapted with permission from National Kidney Foundation: K/DOQI clinical practice guidelines for anemia of chronic kidney disease. Am J Kidney Dis 2001;37:S182.)

given in doses high enough to compensate for iron requirements in patients receiving erythropoietin therapy. Second, oral iron is rarely well tolerated and can cause gastric upset, which can easily be misidentified as uremic symptoms. The use of oral iron with gastrointestinal upset may further demoralize patients and dissuade them from compliance with other medications important to their care, which they may believe to be the cause of their gastric upset. Therefore in the United States the standard route for iron replacement remains the intravenous route.

Most protocols established for iron repletion are predicated on the iron requirements of ESRD patients. The goals, however, remain the same, achieving a TSAT of greater than 20% and a ferritin greater than 100 ng/mL. Approximately 1 g of iron is required to increase the hematocrit 10% over a 3-month period. Currently available commercial iron products are listed in Table 19–1. It should be noted that intravenous iron dextrin (INFeD) has been associated with fatal anaphylactic reactions and must be preceded by a test dose. Newer preparations such as iron gluconate (Ferrlecit) and iron sucrose (Venofer) have substantially lower rates of anaphylactic reactions and do not require test dosing. Recently Venofer has been approved by the U.S. Food and Drug Administration (FDA) for use in CKD patients. Rapid administration of high doses of iron (>500 mg) has recently been made possible by the introduction of ferumoxytol. As compared to currently available iron formulations, this product is isotonic and has very low free iron levels which may account for its very low incidence of anaphylactoid reactions.

During active administration of erythropoietin most protocols recommend reevaluating iron stores every three months as patients vary in their ability to utilize iron.

2. Erythropoietin therapy—There are currently three commercially available erythropoietic agents to treat anemia: epoetin-alfa, darbepoetin-alfa, and methoxy polyethylene glycol-epoetin beta. Epoetin-alfa is manufactured and sold under two brand names, Epogen (Amgen, Inc.) and Procrit (Ortho-Biotech, Johnson & Johnson). Both these products are biologically and structurally identical.

Epoetin-alfa is immunologically and biologically indistinguishable from endogenous erythropoietin. Darbepoetin-alfa (AraNESP) structurally differs from endogenous erythropoietin by having additional oligosaccharide chains and a rearranged amino acid sequence. It has a higher molecular weight then epoetin-alfa resulting in a longer half-life, estimated to be approximately three times that of epoetin-alfa (8 hours versus 25 hours).

Methoxy polyethylene glycol-epoetin beta; Mircera (manufactured by Roche), was approved for use by the FDA for anemia treatment in patients receiving and not receiving dialysis. In terms of its structure, Mircera is similar to the previous synthetic EPO drugs, except that it is connected to a chemical called polyethylene glycol (PEG), which extends its half-life. Micera lasts up to six times longer than darbepoetin-alfa and up to 20 times longer than epoetin and is generally administered SQ monthly.

Although there have been no randomized controlled studies comparing the efficacy of any of these products to the other, they all have been shown to effectively treat anemia of CKD. Drug selection is predicated upon the comfort level of the clinical nephrologist and cost.

Although higher initial doses of erythropoietic agents may result in a more rapid increase in hemoglobin, this is rarely necessary (rapid correction) and should be avoided as higher costs and potential target hemoglobin overshoots will result.

Recent studies, CHOIR and CREATE, have suggested that targeting higher hemoglobin levels (generally >12.5 g/dL) may result in higher cardiovascular events. Reanalysis of the CHOIR data though, has linked these adverse events to patients receiving higher doses of epoetin-alfa and not reaching their target hemoglobins. Those patients achieving higher target hemoglobins did not show increased risk of cardiovascular events.

Given these concerns, the FDA has warned that the use of all ESAs should target transfusion avoidance rather than a prespecified hemoglobin goal.

3. Adverse effects—The common side effects from the use of epoetin-alfa, darbepoetin-alfa and methoxy polyethylene glycol-epoetin beta are generally mild and transient. Approximately 5% of patients will experience flu-like symptoms and 12–15% will experience headaches. The relationship between administration of epoetin-alfa and hypertension has been well documented and occurs in approximately 23% of patients. Therefore, increases in blood pressure should be closely monitored following initiation of therapy. This hypertension appears to be related to an imbalance between endothelin and proendothelin resulting

Table 19–1. Administration of intravenous iron.[a]

Iron Compound	Maximum Single Dose	Recommended Dosage
Iron dextran	1000 mg	100 mg x 10 doses
Iron gluconate	125 mg	125 mg x 8 doses
Iron sucrose	100 mg	100 mg x 10 doses

[a]One gram of iron is required to increase the hematocrit from 25% to 35% and to maintain iron stores over a 3-month period. The recommended dose is less than 1 g.

Source: Reproduced, with permission, from National Kidney Foundation: K/DOQI clinical practice guidelines for anemia of chronic kidney disease. Am J Kidney Dis 2000;37:S182 and Van Wyck D et al: Safety and efficacy of iron sucrose in patients sensitive to iron dextran: clinical trial. Am J Kidney Dis 2000;36:88.

in increased responsiveness to the vasoconstricting actions of norepinephrine and decreased responsiveness to the vasodilatory effects of nitric oxide. This affect (hypertension) is seen most frequently when the route of administration is intravenous.

Recently approximately 100 cases of pure red blood cell aplasia have been reported in Europe. This has been linked to the European formulation of epoetin-alfa (Eprex), with patients producing neutralizing antiepoetin antibodies. This appears to be linked to a different immunogenicity of Eprex. No cases of red cell aplasia have been reported to date in patients using darbepoetin-alfa.

4. Resistance to epoetin—Resistance to epoetin-alfa is seen primarily in patients with ESRD receiving dialysis, but is now being observed in CKD patients. Resistance is defined as the need for greater than 150 units/kg of epoetin-alfa three times per week or the development of refractiveness to a previous stable dose allowing the hemoglobin level to fall below the targeted hemoglobin range. Although reports vary, approximately 5–10% of all patients with ESRD can be categorized as resistant. It is not known how many patients with CKD fall into this category. However, the numbers may be higher due to the persistent chronic "inflammatory" state in which these patients exist.

5. Newer agents—The discovery of the hypoxia inducible factor (HIF) pathway and its regulation via HIF prolyl hydroxylase enzymes in the context of erythropoiesis and iron metabolism has led to an exciting new area of focus in the management of anemia of CKD. Several agents have been developed, four of which are in active clinical trials. The rationale for targeting this pathway in treating anemia is that endogenous EPO is stimulated while simultaneously hepcidin production is suppressed and transferrin synthesis increased. The latter permits enhanced transport of iron. In a number of phase 2 clinical trials, these agents have been found to be effectively correct and maintain Hb in CKD-associated anemia.

D. Resistance to Erythropoietin

1. Iron deficiency—Iron deficiency is the most common cause of resistance as previously mentioned. Serum iron saturation, ferritin, and transferrin should be checked frequently to avoid this condition. Ensuring adequate iron stores also allows epoetin-alfa to be administered in a cost-effective manner.

2. Infection and inflammation—Infection and inflammation are the second most common conditions resulting in hyporesponsiveness to epoetin-alfa. Mediators of inflammation (tumor necrosis factor [TNF] and interleukin-1 [IL-1]) directly cause hyporesponsiveness to epoetin. Patients should be carefully scrutinized for conditions that result in chronic inflammatory processes.

3. Hyperparathyroidism—Although a much less common cause of resistance in the era of multiple vitamin D analogs and cinacalcet (Sensipar) availability, severe untreated hyperparathyroidism can result in fibrosis of the bone marrow. Unfortunately, the relationship between serum PTH levels does not directly correlate with the required epoetin dose and resistance.

4. Hemoglobinopathies—Sickle cell disease accounts for the majority of patients with resistance who have a hemoglobinopathy. High-dose epoetin-alfa therapy has mixed results with this disorder, often not reaching target hemoglobin goals.

5. Thalassemia—Thalassemia accounts for the remainder of resistant hemoglobinopathies and does respond to high-dose epoetin-alfa therapy.

6. Cofactor deficiency and malnutrition—Cofactor deficiency and malnutrition should cause close scrutiny on the part of the physician, who should then consider the initiation of dialytic therapy, particularly in the elderly who may down-play their uremic symptoms. Anorexia is an early, subtle, symptom of uremia. Falling serum albumin levels and/or the development of folate or vitamin B_{12} deficiencies necessitate close observation and treatment (dialysis) as they are directly related to dialytic mortality.

▶ Prognosis

As expectations of care continue to evolve on both the payer and patient side, closer scrutiny will be made of those disorders whose treatment results in improved outcomes. The more actionable a treatment parameter, the more likely physicians will be held accountable for its identification and management. There is considerable literature concerning the relationship of anemia to CKD, the growing population of patients with CKD and anemia, and the relationship of anemia to cardiovascular mortality. This knowledge, coupled with the availability of highly effective erythropoietic-stimulating factors and dosing strategies, makes the identification and treatment of anemia in CKD of paramount importance in the management of this at-risk population. Additionally, the potential availability of HIF-PHI agents offer an exciting, and potentially more physiologic, option for anemia management.

KEY READINGS

Bonomini M et al: Uremic toxicity and anemia. J Nephrol 2003;16:21.

Locatelli F et al: Targeting hypoxia-inducible factors for the treatment of anemia in chronic kidney disease patients. Am J Nephrol 2017;45:187.

■ CHAPTER REVIEW QUESTIONS

1. A 68-year-old white male patient with a 35-year history of type 2 diabetes and known CKD stage 3 (serum creatinine 2.5 mg/dL, eGFR 35 cc/min) comes for his routine clinic visit. His renal function remains stable but you notice his previously stable hemoglobin has decreased from approximately 11–7.8 g. Your next steps are
   A. Evaluate a complete CBC.
   B. Order an iron panel (serum iron, TIBC, and ferritin).
   C. Check for GI occult blood loss.
   D. All of the above.

2. In the management of patients with established CKD and anemia you should:
   A. Treat all patient with hemoglobin greater than 12 g females or greater than 14 g males.
   B. Only treat "symptomatic" patients irrespective of their hemoglobin levels.
   C. Treat patients to a target hemoglobin level of 11–12 g.
   D. None of the above.

3. A 45-year-old obese, African–American female patient with CKD stage 4, secondary to poorly controlled hypertension and ASHD presents with slowly progressive anemia measured at today clinic visit at hemoglobin 7.5 g. She complains of fatigue and increased SOB even though she is clinically euvolemic. In anticipation of starting ESA therapy you have measured her iron studies (all normal), but notice today a chronic nonhealing 4 cm non-healing ulcer on her left lower extremity due to chronic venous insufficiency. She tells you she is under the care of a vascular surgeon. Your next steps are

   A. Since the iron studies are normal and she has symptomatic anemia-initiate ESA therapy.
   B. She has an active inflammatory process and you should avoid ESA therapy and wait until her ulcer heals.
   C. Order a blood transfusion.

4. Your patient, a 60-year-old Hispanic male, with asymptomatic CKD stage 5 has had his anemia managed at your clinic with epoetin-alpha 10,000 U SQ every other weeks for 6 months with a stable hemoglobin of approximately 10 g. His routine labs today show the following: Hgb 8.9 g. Serum iron 12 µg/dL, TIBC 10%, Ferritin 90 ng/mL. Your next steps are
   A. Stop epoetin-alpha and institute aggressive iron replacement therapy.
   B. Initiate aggressive IV iron replacement and continue epoetin-alpha.
   C. Check for GI occult blood losses.
   D. Both A and C.

5. Your patient is a 20-year-old native African male with CKD stage 2 (eGFR 80 cc/min) secondary to type 1 diabetes. He presents with normal serum iron studies and hemoglobin of 9 g. You should initiate ESA treatment.
   A. True
   B. False

Cardiovascular Disease in Chronic Kidney Disease

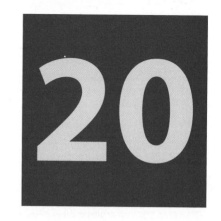

20

Georges N. Nakhoul, MD

Joseph V. Nally, MD

ESSENTIALS OF DIAGNOSIS

- ▶ Cardiovascular disease (CVD) is highly prevalent among patients with chronic kidney disease (CKD) and is the most common cause of death in this population.

- ▶ The manifestations of CVD in CKD are variable and include left ventricular hypertrophy, ischemic heart disease, heart failure, atrial fibrillation, sudden cardiac death, and peripheral vascular disease.

- ▶ Traditional and nontraditional (or "uremia-related") cardiac risk factors are common in CKD.

- ▶ Clinicians should maintain a high index of suspicion for the presence of CVD in patients with CKD, even when the presentation is atypical.

- ▶ An aggressive approach to diagnosis and treatment of CVD is recommended in patients with CKD.

▶ General Considerations

Cardiovascular disease (CVD) is highly prevalent among patients with CKD with both diseases sharing a strong association: CKD is considered to be an independent cardiovascular risk factor and CVD is independently associated with kidney function decline and with the development of kidney disease. CVD is also the most common cause of death in the CKD population. Importantly, patients with impaired kidney function are more likely to die from CVD than to progress to end-stage renal disease (ESRD) requiring renal replacement therapy and those who do reach dialysis have a staggering mortality rate of about 20% per year. In dialysis patients of all ages, the mortality rate from CVD far exceeds that observed in the general population (Figure 20–1). Dialysis has the greatest impact on younger patients, whose mortality rate from CVD is more than 100 times greater than that of their counterparts with normal kidney function. The burden of CVD begins to accumulate long before patients reach ESRD and continues to progress on dialysis. For example, left ventricular (LV) hypertrophy (LVH) increases in prevalence with declining renal function to reach a striking prevalence of 75% in patients beginning dialysis, and continues to progress on chronic dialysis. Ischemic heart disease (IHD) and heart failure also develop early, and are present in 40% and 35% of incident dialysis patients, respectively. Numerous publications across different populations have demonstrated a profound impact of a reduced glomerular filtration rate (GFR) below 60 mL/min on cardiovascular event rates.

In recent years both the National Kidney Foundation (NKF) and the American Heart Association (AHA) have recommended that patients with CKD be placed in the highest risk group for the development of CVD. However, while recognition of their high-risk status has improved, evidence from clinical trials evaluating the benefit of interventions aimed at reducing CVD risk in the CKD population is still largely lacking.

Recommendations by the NKF for the evaluation and treatment of CVD in dialysis patients recommend that an aggressive approach to diagnosis and treatment is warranted in patients with ESRD due to the high risk of CVD in this patient group.

The spectrum of CVD in CKD is wide, and includes abnormalities of the heart and blood vessels, such as LVH, congestive heart failure (CHF), valvular heart disease, pericarditis, cardiac arrhythmias, IHD, and peripheral vascular disease (PVD). Those disorders that are most common and account for the majority of the morbidity and mortality in patients with CKD will be the focus of this chapter: LVH, IHD, heart failure, and PVD. In this chapter, the term CKD is used generically to refer to patients with all degrees of kidney dysfunction, including those on dialysis. Comments pertaining to a particular subgroup of patients (eg, predialysis patients or ESRD patients) are specified as such.

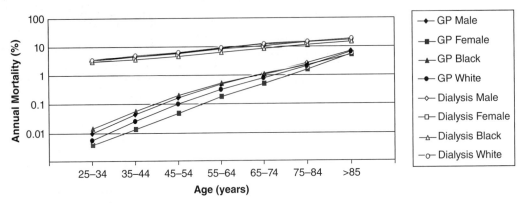

▲ **Figure 20–1.** Cardiovascular disease mortality for patients on dialysis, by age, gender, and race, in comparison to the general population. (Reproduced with permission from Foley RN et al: The clinical epidemiology of cardiovascular disease in chronic renal disease. Am J Kidney Dis 1998;32:S112.)

KEY READINGS

Elsayed EF et al: Cardiovascular disease and subsequent kidney disease. Arch Intern Med 2007;167:1130.

Go AS et al: Chronic kidney disease and the risks of death, cardiovascular events, and hospitalization. N Engl J Med 2004;351:1296.

Keith DS et al: Longitudinal follow-up and outcomes among a population with chronic kidney disease in a large managed care organization. Arch Intern Med 2004;164:659.

Navaneethan SD et al: Cause-specific death in non-dialysis-dependant CKD. J Am Soc Nephrol 2015;26:2512.

Thompson S et al: Cause of death in patients with reduced kidney function. J Am Soc Nephrol 2015;26:2504.

▶ Pathogenesis

A. Cardiovascular Risk Factors in Chronic Kidney Disease

Traditional and nontraditional risk factors have been discussed in the literature as contributors to the high rate of CVD in CKD (Table 20–1). Certainly, traditional cardiac risk factors are highly prevalent in these patients. These include advanced age, diabetes mellitus, hypertension, low high-density lipoprotein (HDL), and LVH. However, the complexity of the relationship between some traditional cardiovascular risk factors and overall mortality in ESRD must be appreciated. For example, the association between LDL-C levels and atherosclerotic CVD events is weaker for adults with nondialysis-dependent CKD compared to the general population. This was shown by data from a cohort of 800,000 adults (the Alberta Kidney Disease Network), whereas high CVD risk was observed in patients with advanced CKD stages and low cholesterol levels, possibly on the account of inflammation and malnutrition. Consequently, the CVD risk prediction equations in adults with CKD perform poorly.

A "reverse epidemiology" or "U-shaped" mortality curve has also been observed in regards to blood pressure, whereby ESRD patients with low blood pressure paradoxically have an increased mortality. This increase in mortality is

Table 20–1. Traditional and nontraditional cardiovascular risk factors in chronic kidney disease.

Traditional Risk Factors	Nontraditional Risk Factors
Older age	Albuminuria
Male gender	Homocysteine
Hypertension	Lipoprotein (a) and apo (a) isoforms
Higher LDL cholesterol	Lipoprotein remnants
Lower HDL cholesterol	Anemia
Diabetes	Abnormal calcium/phosphate metabolism
Smoking	Extracellular fluid volume overload
Physical inactivity	Electrolyte imbalance
Menopause	Oxidative stress
Family history of cardiovascular disease	Inflammation (C-reactive protein)
Left ventricular hypertrophy	Malnutrition
	Thrombogenic factors
	Sleep disturbances
	Altered nitric oxide/endothelin balance

hypothesized to reflect underlying advanced cardiomyopathy. Thus, the benefits of strategies traditionally used to combat CVD in the general population, such as lowering of cholesterol and blood pressure, may be questioned in the setting of kidney disease.

Furthermore, numerous studies across populations of different ethnicities showed that a reduced GFR per se is an independent risk factor for CVD. It may be that lower GFR is associated with, or marks for, nontraditional or "uremic" risk factors. These nontraditional risk factors, outlined in Table 20–1, include anemia, abnormalities of calcium and phosphate metabolism, inflammation, prothrombotic factors, oxidative stress, and perhaps also hyperhomocysteinemia, and elevated levels of lipoprotein(a). However, despite strong associations between these factors and CVD in epidemiologic studies, a causal relationship has not been proven, nor have interventional studies been conducted that

demonstrate changes in outcomes with treatment of these abnormalities.

In patients with nondialysis CKD, the issue of proteinuria and cardiovascular risk merits specific comment. First, moderately increased albuminuria (previously referred to as microalbuminuria) is associated with an increased risk of all-cause mortality and cardiovascular events (Figure 20–2) in both diabetic and nondiabetic subjects, even in the absence of renal insufficiency. While patients with moderately increased albuminuria often have an increased prevalence of traditional cardiac risk factors, it is also thought that moderately increased albuminuria may be a marker of generalized endothelial dysfunction or inflammation. Second, individuals with the nephrotic syndrome are known to have an increased risk of myocardial infarction (MI). Among the potential explanations for this are that hyperlipidemia, hypercoagulability, and hypertension are common

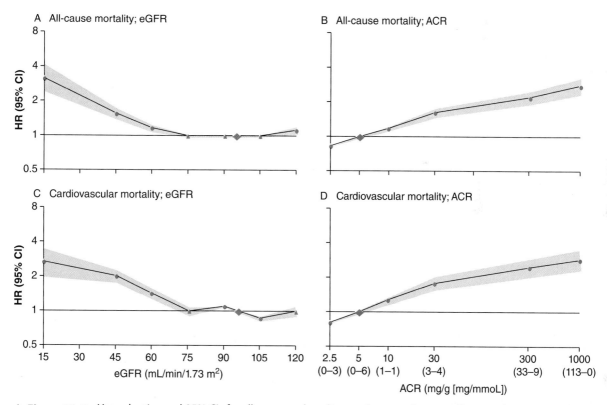

▲ **Figure 20–2.** Hazard ratios and 95% CIs for all-cause and cardiovascular mortality according to spline estimated glomerular filtration rate (A, C) and albumin-to-creatinine ratio (B, D) adjusted for each other, age, sex, ethnic origin, history of cardiovascular disease, systolic blood pressure, diabetes, smoking, and total cholesterol. The reference (diamond) was eGFR 95 mL/min/1.73 m² and ACR 5 mg/g (0·6 mg/mmol), respectively. Circles represent statistically significant and triangles represent not significant. (Reproduced with permission from Matsushita K et al: Association of estimated glomerular filtration rate and albuminuria with all-cause and cardiovascular mortality in general population cohorts: a collaborative meta-analysis. Lancet 2010; 375:2073.)

in the nephrotic syndrome and these may contribute to the increased risk of IHD. In addition, several publications describe clear associations between proteinuria and increased rates of CVD at all levels of kidney dysfunction.

Given the documented burden of CVD in CKD, the association with adverse outcomes in patients where the two coexist, and the biologically plausible explanations as to the impact of traditional and nontraditional risk factors in CKD populations, it is important for the practicing clinician to understand the complexity of this area, what is known and where gaps in our knowledge base exist.

B. Left Ventricular Hypertrophy

Left ventricular hypertrophy (LVH) is very common in CKD and constitutes an independent risk factor for mortality in all CKD patients, independent of dialysis status. From a physiology standpoint, the work performed by the LV in each cardiac cycle is equal to the product of the ventricular pressure and stroke volume. In kidney disease, the work of the left ventricular (LV) is increased due to both pressure and volume overload. Hypertension, arteriosclerosis, and aortic stenosis contribute to pressure overload, while volume overload occurs as a result of factors such as increased extracellular fluid volume and the presence of arteriovenous fistulas. CKD-specific factors also play a major role in the development of LVH. These are related to the "uremic milieu" and include hyperparathyroidism, alterations in electrolyte balance, oxidative stress, inflammation, and others. LVH is particularly associated with anemia and a fall in hemoglobin to less than 12.8 g/dL is associated with LV growth in people with CKD.

The LVH that occurs initially as an adaptive response to physiologic stimuli (pressure or volume) eventually becomes maladaptive. At the cellular level, the metabolically active myocytes begin to experience an energy deficit, partly due to ischemia, resulting in cell death. In addition, cardiac fibroblasts proliferate, expanding the extracellular matrix of the myocardium and causing myocardial fibrosis. From a functional point of view, the hypertrophied ventricle becomes stiff, impairing relaxation and resulting primarily in diastolic dysfunction, at least initially. These changes may partially explain the high prevalence of heart failure in this patient group.

C. Heart Failure

Heart failure is common in CKD and is present in about one-third of incident dialysis patients. Patients may have systolic dysfunction, diastolic dysfunction, or both. The pathogenesis of heart failure is multifactorial with contributions from LVH, IHD, valvular heart disease, and other abnormalities specific to the uremic state such as chronic extracellular fluid volume expansion, disturbances in divalent ion metabolism, anemia, and the presence of arteriovenous (AV) fistulas.

D. Atrial Fibrillation

Atrial fibrillation is very common in patients with kidney disease and its rate is several folds higher than that of the general population. Stroke is also a frequent complication of kidney disease regardless of the presence of atrial fibrillation. The risk of stroke is compounded by the presence of both CKD and atrial fibrillation and appears to increase as the renal function declines. Indeed, in a post-hoc analysis on the ROCKET AF trial, reduced creatinine clearance was a strong, independent predictor of stroke and systemic embolism, second only to prior stroke or transient ischemic attack. Unfortunately, patients with CKD are also at increased risk of bleeding, and the rate of major hemorrhagic events in patients on anticoagulation increases significantly with declining renal function. This has major implications on the preventive treatment of stroke in patients with atrial fibrillation and CKD and will be discussed in further detail in the treatment section.

E. Sudden Cardiac Death

Sudden cardiac death (SCD) is defined as "death from an unexpected circulatory arrest occurring within an hour of the onset of symptoms" and is usually due to a ventricular tachyarrhythmia. The risk of SCD increases as the renal function worsens and the estimated glomerular filtration rate appears to be independently associated with SCD. In dialysis patients, SCD accounts for about one-fourth of the deaths.

The pathophysiology of SCD in CKD is multifactorial and revolves around a high prevalence of coronary artery disease, structural heart disease (such as ischemic cardiomyopathy with reduced systolic function or left ventricular hypertrophy with diastolic dysfunction) and rapid shifts in fluids and electrolytes following exposure to low potassium/calcium dialysates, volume removal on dialysis and predialysis hyperkalemia.

F. Vascular Disease: Atherosclerosis and Arteriosclerosis

There are two general types of arterial vascular disease in CKD: atherosclerosis and arteriosclerosis. Atherosclerosis is a disease of the intima and is characterized by plaques and vessel occlusion. The most common vessels affected are the medium-sized arteries, such as the coronary, femoral, and carotid arteries. There are many contributors to atherosclerosis, including the high prevalence of cardiac risk factors such as advanced age, dyslipidemia, hypertension, and the metabolic syndrome.

Patients with CKD also have a high prevalence of arteriosclerosis, or stiffening of the arteries; this may occur in the presence or absence of significant atherosclerosis. Although it normally occurs with aging, the process appears to be accelerated in kidney disease. The intima and media of the large, elastic arteries such as the aorta and the common carotid are affected in particular. The vessel wall is remodeled and becomes thickened and stiff, reducing compliance. These stiff vessels contribute to hemodynamic changes, including an increase in systolic blood pressure, a decrease in diastolic blood pressure, and as a result, a widened pulse pressure and increased pulse wave velocity. The raised systolic blood pressure increases LV afterload and contributes to the development of LVH, while the reduced diastolic pressure compromises coronary artery perfusion and contributes to myocardial ischemia. Recent data from both dialysis and predialysis patients have confirmed the association among an elevated pulse pressure, a clinical manifestation of arterial stiffness, and adverse outcomes.

A contributor to the arterial stiffening in kidney disease that has recently been given some attention is calcification of the intimal and medial layers of these vessels. It has been observed that this calcification is a key feature of the arterial disease in CKD, especially in ESRD. The calcification is more extensive and is observed much earlier in ESRD than in the general population. Abnormalities of bone mineral metabolism, including elevations in serum phosphorus, calcium, parathyroid hormone, and fibroblast growth factor 23 (FGF 23) among other factors, are intimately involved in promoting vascular calcification, decreasing vascular compliance, and have been associated with death and cardiovascular events. For example, in the Multi-Ethnic Study of Atherosclerosis (MESA), increase in serum phosphate concentration was associated with a greater prevalence of coronary artery, thoracic, aortic valve, and mitral valve calcification.

This unique contribution of specific factors to arterial calcification and measured arterial stiffness, in conjunction with anemia (also common in CKD), may explain in part the high prevalence of CVD in CKD patients.

KEY READINGS

Adeney KL et al: Association of serum phosphate with vascular and valvular calcification in moderate CKD. J Am Soc Nephrol 2009;20:381.

Cerasola G et al: Epidemiology and pathophysiology of left ventricular abnormalities in chronic kidney disease: a review. J Nephrol 2011;24:1.

Floege J et al: Serum iPTH, calcium and phosphorus and the risk of mortality in a European haemodialysis population. Nephrol Dial Transplant 2011;26:1948.

Go AS et al: Hemoglobin level, chronic kidney disease, and the risks of death and hospitalization in adults with chronic heart failure: the Anemia in Chronic Heart Failure: Outcomes and Resource Utilization (ANCHOR) Study. Circulation 2006;113:2713.

Gutierrez OM et al: Fibroblast growth factor 23 and mortality among patients undergoing hemodialysis. N Engl J Med 2008;359:584.

Hemmelgarn BR et al: Relation between kidney function, proteinuria, and adverse outcomes. JAMA 2010;303:423.

Markossian T et al: Controversies regarding lipid management and statin use for cardiovascular risk reduction in patients with CKD. Am J Kidney Dis 2016;67:965.

Olesen JB et al: Stroke and bleeding in atrial fibrillation with chronic kidney disease. N Engl J Med 2012;367:625.

Piccini JP et al: Renal dysfunction as a predictor of stroke and systemic embolism in patients with nonvalvular atrial fibrillation: validation of the R(2)CHADS(2) index in the ROCKET AF (Rivaroxaban once-daily, oral, direct factor Xa inhibition compared with vitamin K antagonism for prevention of stroke and embolism trial in atrial fibrillation) and ATRIA (Anticoagulation and risk factors in atrial fibrillation) study cohorts. Circulation 2013;127:224.

Pun PH et al: Chronic kidney disease is associated with increased risk of sudden cardiac death among patients with coronary artery disease. Kidney Int 2009;76: 652.

Pun PH et al: Modifiable risk factors associated with sudden cardiac arrest within hemodialysis clinics. Kidney Int 2011;79:218.

Robinson BM et al: Blood pressure levels and mortality risk among hemodialysis patients in the Dialysis Outcomes and Practice Patterns Study. Kidney Int 2012;82:570.

Soliman EZ et al: Chronic kidney disease and prevalent atrial fibrillation: the chronic renal insufficiency cohort (CRIC). Am Heart J 2010;159:1102.

Tonelli M et al: Association between LDL-C and risk of myocardial infarction in CKD. J Am Soc Nephrol 2013;24:979.

USRDS 2010 Annual Data Report: Atlas of Chronic Kidney Disease & End-Stage Renal Disease in the United States, National Institutes of Health, National Institute of Diabetes and Digestive and Kidney Diseases, Bethesda, MD.

▶ Clinical Findings

A. Symptoms and Signs

1. Left ventricular hypertrophy—LVH may be asymptomatic or patients may present with diastolic dysfunction, which is discussed in further detail in the next section.

On physical examination, hypertension is common. Particular attention should be paid to the pulse pressure as a surrogate measure of arterial stiffness, where "normal values" are within 40–60 mm Hg. Precordial palpation may reveal a left ventricular heave and a sustained and diffuse cardiac apical impulse. On auscultation, a fourth heart sound may be heard.

Due to the lack of sensitivity of symptoms and physical examination findings, echocardiography is usually used for diagnosis and clinical follow-up of patients with LVH.

2. Heart failure—Heart failure may occur as a result of systolic dysfunction, diastolic dysfunction, or both. It may be asymptomatic or patients may present with shortness of breath, orthopnea, paroxysmal nocturnal dyspnea, reduced exercise tolerance, and progressive extracellular fluid volume expansion. In addition, patients with LV dysfunction on hemodialysis often tolerate dialysis treatments poorly and episodes of intradialytic hypotension may occur.

On physical examination, the signs of heart failure include pulmonary vascular congestion such as jugular venous distention and crackles due to pulmonary edema. LVH is the most common cause of diastolic dysfunction in CKD and these patients would be expected to have the cardiac findings discussed under that section. However, findings in patients with predominantly systolic heart failure include cardiomegaly, manifested by an inferiorly and laterally displaced apical pulsation, and the presence of a third heart sound on auscultation.

Due to the insensitivity of the physical examination, echocardiography is usually used for the diagnosis of heart failure. In addition to evaluating left ventricular function and geometry, echocardiography also has the advantage of providing other useful information, such as the presence of valvular heart disease, which may also contribute to left ventricular dysfunction.

3. Ischemic heart disease—The main symptom of cardiac ischemia is angina, which may be accompanied by symptoms of CHF. In CKD, the high proportion of patients with a concomitant diagnosis of diabetes mellitus means that atypical presentations of cardiac ischemia, such as shortness of breath without chest pain, may occur. In addition, patients with CKD may experience episodes of silent cardiac ischemia. For example, asymptomatic ST segment depression has been observed during hemodialysis treatments.

Findings on physical examination of acute cardiac ischemia may be relatively few. Signs of left and/or right heart failure may be observed depending on the size and location of the vascular territory affected. In general, the diagnosis of an acute coronary syndrome (ACS) relies on laboratory findings, including serial cardiac enzyme determinations and an electrocardiogram (ECG).

In the CKD population, a number of factors may interfere with the timely diagnosis of IHD, including diabetes, atypical presentations, and the relative lack of utility of specific tests in dialysis patients. Thus, a high index of suspicion in patients at high CVD risk is imperative.

4. Peripheral vascular disease—PVD, also a result of the atherosclerotic process, is common in CKD. The symptoms and signs depend on the vascular territory affected. Carotid artery disease causes neurologic changes during a transient ischemic attack or stroke. When the arteries supplying the lower extremities are affected, intermittent claudication with exertion may result. However, given the poor tolerance to exercise in the CKD population in general, this symptom probably lacks sensitivity. Chronic ischemia of the legs results in skin changes, hair loss, and muscle atrophy. Other signs include pallor, reduced or absent pulses, and bruits. Without treatment, skin ulceration and gangrene can occur when ischemia becomes critical.

The key to the diagnosis of PVD is serial assessment of peripheral arterial function through clinical examination

and laboratory investigations. Reluctance to evaluate PVD in a timely manner may have led to an increase in morbidity and mortality in this particular cohort of patients.

B. Laboratory Findings

1. Cardiac disease

A. CARDIAC BIOMARKERS

(1) Cardiac troponins—Troponins comprise part of the contractile apparatus of myocytes in both cardiac and skeletal muscle. They consist of three subunits: troponin C, troponin T, and troponin I. While cardiac and skeletal troponin C are identical, cardiac troponin T (cTnT), and I (cTnI) are encoded by genes different from their skeletal counterparts, and the molecules are also different. The assays currently in use for detection of cTnT and cTnI are specific for troponin released from the heart muscle. They are also highly sensitive to even small amounts of myocardial damage. Because of their high sensitivity and their near absolute specificity, they are considered to be the gold biochemical standard for the diagnosis of myocardial infarction. Additionally, the degree of troponin elevation in patients presenting with a suspected ACS provides important prognostic information, even in the presence of renal dysfunction. Indeed, abnormal troponin measurements have been linked to an increased risk of major cardiac events and the levels of cTnT prior to commencing renal replacement is a significant independent predictor of survival. For these reasons, cTnT and cTnI are the preferred markers for the diagnosis of acute cardiac injury.

Interpretation of cardiac troponin concentration in the setting of ESRD is complicated by the fact that the levels, particularly of cTnT, may be elevated in apparently asymptomatic individuals. The reasons for elevations in troponin in the absence of cardiac symptoms and the significance of the levels are still debated but increased levels of cTnT are associated cardiac structural abnormalities, including LVH and left ventricular systolic dysfunction. This suggests that chronic elevation of troponin levels may be an indicator of heart failure rather than atherosclerosis or ischemia. However, the finding of an elevated troponin concentration in a patient with ESRD cannot necessarily be dismissed as a false-positive result even if unaccompanied by cardiac symptoms.

What is even less clear is why asymptomatic troponin elevations in ESRD are observed more frequently with cTnT than with cTnI. Proposed explanations for this include differences in release patterns from damaged cardiac myocytes, circulating half-life, and dialyzability, in addition to the particular characteristics of the assays themselves.

Because of these controversies, management strategies of ACS in people with CKD are uncertain. However, these biochemical markers can be useful when interpreted in the clinical context. Patients with advanced CKD suspected of having an ACS should be followed with serial cardiac troponin assessments. A troponin level rising over time suggests an acute injury, especially if accompanied by other cardiac symptoms or ECG changes. A positive but unchanging level may not indicate acute damage, but it has prognostic implications in ESRD patients nonetheless. On the other hand, obtaining serial "normal" or "negative" results has an excellent negative predictive value and is therefore useful for excluding an ACS.

(2) Brain natriuretic peptide (BNP)/N-terminal-proBNP (NT-proBNP)—Natriuretic peptides belong to a family of circulatory peptides that impact salt and water handling and pressure regulation. Both atrial natriuretic peptide (ANP) and brain natriuretic peptide (BNP) and released from the heart muscle in response to volume expansion and increased wall stress. ANP is primarily released from the atria while BNP is primarily released from the ventricles. The active BNP hormone is cleaved from the C-terminal end of its prohormone, pro-BNP. The remainder of the molecule, N-terminal pro-BNP (NT-proBNP) is also released into the circulation. In patients with left ventricular dysfunction and heart failure, and as a result of elevated filling pressures and myocardial stretch, ventricular cells are recruited to secrete both ANP and BNP. As a result, the plasma concentration of ANP, BNP, and NT-proBNP will be increased, which allows their use a diagnostic tool for heart failure. However, the kidneys contribute to the clearance of BNP and NT-proBNP, which means that the concentration of BNP and NT-proBNP can be elevated in patients with CKD whether or not they have clinical heart failure. Even though the prevalence of fluid overload and heart failure increases with CKD, natriuretic peptides becomes less reliable predictors of fluid overload and heart failure and should be interpreted with caution in this patient population.

B. CARDIAC IMAGING STUDIES

(1) Electrocardiography—All patients suspected of having an ACS should be evaluated with an ECG. However, the interpretation can be complicated by preexisting abnormalities on the baseline tracing. In the absence of acute cardiac ischemia, ST-T segment morphology can be altered by LVH, electrolyte disturbances, and medications such as digoxin. In a patient presenting with possible cardiac ischemia, obtaining an old ECG for comparison can be extremely helpful. Aside from abnormalities of the baseline study, ischemic changes are expected to have an appearance the same as in individuals without kidney disease.

(2) Exercise treadmill testing—In screening for coronary artery disease (CAD), detection of exercise-induced ischemia with exercise treadmill testing is of limited utility in patients with advanced CKD and ESRD. Patients are often unable to attain their target heart rate for reasons that include poor exercise tolerance, autonomic neuropathy, and use of medications that impair the chronotropic response to exercise, such as β-blockers and calcium channel blockers.

Abnormalities of the resting ECG further compromise the sensitivity and specificity of this test. For these reasons, pharmacologic stress testing is generally preferred in advanced kidney disease.

(3) Echocardiography—Two-dimensional echocardiography has multiple uses in the CKD population. It can be used to assess for abnormalities of cardiac structure, such as LVH and valvular heart disease, and also provides a good estimate of systolic and diastolic LV function. Ideally, patients on dialysis should be as close to their estimated dry weight as possible at the time of this study or at least have studies performed at the same time in their dialysis cycle for comparison purposes.

Dobutamine stress echocardiography (DSE) can be used as a noninvasive screening test for ischemic heart disease. Studies in the renal failure population are limited in number and comparisons between studies are difficult because of inconsistencies in methodology. Overall, DSE appears to be a useful, but imperfect, screening test for CAD in CKD.

(4) Nuclear scintigraphy—Nuclear scintigraphy has uses similar to echocardiography in patients with kidney disease: assessment of ventricular function, screening for CAD, and prediction of future cardiac events.

To screen for myocardial ischemia, a radionuclide is injected and fixed or reversible perfusion defects are detected by comparing cardiac single-photon emission computed tomography (SPECT) images at rest and following stress (exercise or pharmacologic). Dipyridamole is a pharmacologic agent that acts by blocking the cellular reuptake of adenosine, thereby increasing its levels and causing vasodilation. In patients with markedly impaired kidney function, baseline levels of adenosine are increased, thus a reduced vasodilatory response to exogenously administered dipyridamole may occur, thereby potentially producing a false-negative result.

Additionally, people with CKD are underrepresented in studies evaluating the diagnostic sensitivities and specificities of perfusion tests: while in the general population, abnormalities on myocardial perfusion studies correlate well with the presence of CAD, their performance is more variable in patients with renal diseases with sensitivities ranging from as low as 37% to as high as 90%. Nonetheless, results from myocardial perfusion studies have prognostic value and appear to be linked to an increased risk of cardiac events and cardiac death.

Currently, there is no literature to guide the choice between nuclear scintigraphy and DSE in screening for CAD in CKD, as there are no studies directly comparing the two modalities. Therefore, it is reasonable to consider local expertise, availability, and cost to guide test selection.

(5) Computerized tomography scanning—Electron beam computerized tomography (EBCT) and helical CT scanning

methods can be used to assess the degree of coronary artery calcification (CAC). In the general population, where calcification occurs in the intima in association with atherosclerotic deposits, CAC scores have been found to correlate with angiographic plaque burden and to predict future cardiac events. However, their utility in CKD populations is less clear.

Vascular calcification of both the intimal and medical layers is common in renal failure. The CAC scores of ESRD patients in particular are often several times greater than those found in the general population. However, CT scanning cannot distinguish between intimal and medial calcification, and there are conflicting reports as to whether there is a correlation between CAC scores and atherosclerotic plaque burden. Furthermore, while data demonstrate an association between higher CAC scores and mortality in ESRD, debate still exists as to the utility of this test in routine clinical care or as an endpoint in clinical trials. Until the appropriate long-term and interventional studies are undertaken, CT scanning is not recommended as a screen for CAD in the CKD population.

(6) Percutaneous coronary angiography—While IHD is most commonly a result of atherosclerotic CAD, a substantial proportion of patients with CKD may experience cardiac ischemia without significant coronary artery stenosis. It is likely that these patients, particularly those with LVH, have microvascular insufficiency that limits myocardial perfusion and causes ischemia.

The gold standard for diagnosis of CAD is angiography; however, the cost and the potential for morbidity make it impractical as a screening test. In general, it is reserved for patients whose noninvasive screening tests are positive, those who present with an ACS, or those with known CAD who have developed recurrent symptoms despite optimal management.

In predialysis patients, angiography may worsen renal function by causing contrast nephropathy or cholesterol embolization. Invasive examinations should be undertaken only after careful consideration of their necessity, and whether the results will alter patient management. Contrast nephropathy generally produces a transient and reversible decline in renal function and in the modern era, with low osmolality contrast dyes, improved technology, and some evidence of renoprotective effects of specific agents, the risk may be lower than previously described. On the other hand, the decline in renal function caused by cholesterol emboli is usually permanent and can render patients with earlier stages of CKD dialysis dependent.

(7) Peripheral vascular disease—In general, the initial approach to investigating PVD is with noninvasive testing, as is done in the general population. An ankle–brachial index (ABI) (at rest plus or minus postexercise) is a simple test that can be performed in the physician's office to confirm the suspicion of PVD. An ABI of less than 0.90 suggests PVD and further investigations with segmental limb pressures, plethysmography, and various ultrasound techniques or magnetic resonance angiography are indicated.

Conventional angiography is generally performed in patients with significant ischemia as part of the workup for a revascularization procedure in suitable candidates.

KEY READINGS

Covic A et al: Vascular calcification in chronic kidney disease. Clin Sci (Lond) 2010;119:111.

De Lemos JA et al: Association of troponin T detected with a highly sensitive assay and cardiac structure and mortality risk in the general population. JAMA 2010;304:2503.

Hayashi T et al: Cardiac troponin T predicts occult coronary artery stenosis in patients with chronic kidney disease at the start of renal replacement therapy. Nephrol Dial Transplant 2008;23:2936.

Iwanaga Y et al: B-type natriuretic peptide strongly reflects diastolic wall stress in patients with chronic heart failure: comparison between systolic and diastolic heart failure. J Am Coll Cardiol 2006;47:742.

Maisel A et al: State of the art: using natriuretic peptide levels in clinical practice. Eur J Heart Fail 2008;10:824.

Mueller C et al: B-type natriuretic peptide for acute dyspnea in patients with kidney disease: insights from a randomized comparison. Kidney Int 2005;67:278.

Roberts MA et al: Understanding cardiac biomarkers in end-stage kidney disease: frequently asked questions and the promise of clinical application. Nephrology (Carlton) 2011;16:251.

Wong CF et al: Technetium myocardial perfusion scanning in prerenal transplant evaluation in the United Kingdom. Transplant Proc 2008;40:1324.

▶ Prevention and Treatment

A. Left Ventricular Hypertrophy

LVH is an independent predictor of morbidity and mortality in patients with ESRD. LV growth begins early in CKD and is associated with a number of potentially modifiable risk factors, such as anemia and hypertension. Partial regression of LVH has been associated with reduced mortality in observational studies, but randomized studies have yet to convincingly demonstrate this. It may be that primary prevention of LVH by earlier treatment of risk factors is a better approach; however, there is a paucity of randomized data supporting this as well. The following sections will outline the current evidence for the prevention and treatment of LVH with a focus on treatment of anemia and hypertension.

1. Anemia—In observational studies of patients with advanced CKD and ESRD, declining hemoglobin, particularly less than 10–11 g/dL, is associated with the development of LVH and increased cardiovascular mortality. Uncontrolled studies have also shown that treatment of anemia is associated with partial regression of LVH and reduced mortality.

Unfortunately, the data available from randomized controlled trials are less convincing. Treatment of renal anemia with erythropoietin stimulating agents was investigated in several large trials with disappointing results. While it may lead to improvement in the quality of life and exercise capacity, there is little evidence to suggest further benefit. As a matter of fact, in the CREATE cohort, patients randomized to normal hemoglobin targets had significantly worse cardiovascular outcomes. In a meta-analysis of 15 trials, LV mass was reduced by anemia correction but only in patients with severe disease (hemoglobin <10 g/dL) who were treated to a lower target hemoglobin level (<12 g/dL). The treatment of renal anemia follows the recommendations of the general KDIGO guidelines (detailed below) independently of the LVH status.

2. Hypertension—In the general population with essential hypertension, lowering blood pressure is associated with a regression of LVH. A meta-analysis evaluating the relative efficacy of various antihypertensive agents found that the reduction in LVMI was greatest with angiotensin II receptor blockers (ARBs), followed by angiotensin-converting enzyme (ACE) inhibitors and calcium channel blockers. Diuretics and β-blockers were least effective. In addition, it has recently been shown that ARBs can reduce the myocardial fibrosis observed in LVH, indicating that these medications have a direct effect on the myocardium, beyond their ability to lower blood pressure.

Data are limited in kidney disease, but some small studies support regression of LVH when hypertension is treated with pharmacologic inhibition of the rennin–angiotensin–aldosterone system (RAAS), although this has not been an entirely consistent finding. In most studies, it is difficult to ascertain how much of the effect is due to blood pressure reduction per se and how much is related to a specific effect of RAAS blockade. Nonetheless, because of the clinical and basic science evidence demonstrating that ACE inhibitors and ARBs are associated with delay of progression of kidney disease and fibrotic processes as well as other cardiovascular benefits, they are recommended as first-line antihypertensives in the CKD population.

Finally, blood pressure control has been associated with regression of LVH in observational studies of hemodialysis patients receiving either nocturnal or short daily hemodialysis compared to standard three times weekly hemodialysis.

B. Ischemic Heart Disease

1. Primary prevention—There have been few randomized controlled trials conducted in the CKD population addressing primary prevention of ischemic heart disease. In addition, elevated serum creatinine is often a criterion for exclusion from interventional studies of the general population, which further contributes to the scarcity of data in patients with kidney disease. Nonetheless, given

that CKD patients are in the highest risk group for development of CVD, it seems reasonable to apply the same general treatment recommendations applied for other patients at similar CV risk. This includes lifestyle modification, such as smoking cessation, exercise, and maintenance of ideal body weight. Glycemic control in diabetic patients and treatment of hypertension to a target blood pressure of less than 130/80 mm Hg are also recommended by the Kidney Disease Outcomes Quality Initiative (K/DOQI) group for CV risk reduction in CKD.

Aspirin has been recommended for primary prevention of myocardial infarction in the general population when CVD risk is high. However, these recommendations are based on the CV benefits outweighing the risk of major (intracranial or gastrointestinal) bleeding events. In the CKD population, the data is sparse and the KDIGO clinical practice guidelines for the evaluation and management of chronic kidney disease do NOT recommend the use of aspirin for primary prevention. Nonetheless, this recommendation is somewhat controversial: although individuals with CKD have a propensity for bleeding, in the recently published First United Kingdom Heart and Renal Protection (UK-HARP-1) Study, only an increased risk of minor, not major, bleeding episodes was observed with use of low-dose aspirin in CKD. It is worthy to note that patients with advanced CKD, who would be expected to be at highest risk of bleeding complications, represented a minority of patients in this study. In their post hoc analysis of the Hypertension Optimal Treatment (HOT) trial, Jardine et al. reported preventing 76 major cardiovascular events and 54 all-cause deaths for every 1000 persons with eGFR less than 45 mL/min/1.73 m^2 treated with aspirin for 3.8 years while only reporting 27 excess major bleeds. This suggests that the benefits of aspirin outweigh the risk of major bleeding events. Well-conducted clinical trials in heterogeneous populations of both dialysis and predialysis populations need to be performed before aspirin can be adopted into clinical practice for primary prevention on a routine basis. Note that KDIGO does recommend aspirin for second prevention.

3-Hydroxy-3-methylglutaryl coenzyme A (HMG-CoA) reductase inhibitors (statins) appear to be safe and effective in reducing LDL cholesterol levels in renal failure. However, statins have not been shown to be beneficial for the primary prevention of CVD in dialysis patients. Indeed, the association between levels of LDL-C and adverse outcomes in dialysis patients appears to follow a U-shaped curve, whereas both the highest and lowest levels of LDL-C are associated with increased risk of CV events. This paradoxical association has been attributed to protein energy wasting, inflammation, and malnutrition, all of which are common in dialysis patients. The AURORA study was a double-blinded trial that randomized 2776 hemodialysis patients to either rosuvastatin 10 mg daily or a placebo. After a median follow up of 3.8 years, the trial concluded that rosuvastatin did not reduce the risk of death from cardiovascular causes, nonfatal MI, or nonfatal stroke, nor of all-cause mortality (HR 0.96; 95% CI 0.86–1.07; p = 0.51). The SHARP trial was another double-blinded randomized controlled trial that compared a combination of Simvastatin 20 mg plus ezetimibe 10 mg daily to placebo in 9270 patients with CKD and followed them over a period of 5 years. Thirty-three percent of participants were receiving dialysis at randomization. Statin plus ezetimibe therapy was associated with a significant 17% RR reduction of the primary outcome of major atherosclerotic events (coronary death, MI, nonhemorrhagic stroke, or any revascularization) compared with placebo (HR 0.83; 95% CI 0.74–0.94). However, combination treatment did not significantly reduce the risk of the primary outcome in the subgroup of over 3000 patients treated with dialysis at baseline. These findings suggests that statins are not effective in the primary prevention of CVD in dialysis patients but that they are of benefit in the nondialysis CKD population.

Whereas the association between levels of LDL-C and adverse outcomes in dialysis patients follows a U-shaped curve, in CKD patients, this relation appears to be more linear. As eGFR declines, the magnitude of the excess risk associated with increased low-density lipoprotein cholesterol (LDL-C) decreases. The relation between LDL-C and the risk of hospitalization for MI per eGFR level is shown in Figure 20–3. At LDL-C above 2.6 mmol/L (100 mg/dL), the relation between LDL-C and the risk of MI is linear and appears weaker in patients with lower levels of kidney function. Indeed, the hazard ratio (HR) of MI associated with each 1 mmol/L (39 mg/dL) increase in LDL-C above 2.6 mmol/L (100 mg/dL) is 1.48, 1.33, 1.26, 1.20, and 1.13 among people with eGFR of 90, 60, 45, 30, and 15 mL/min/1.73 m^2, respectively. This again suggests a theoretical benefit of statin therapy in the primary prevention of CVD in the nondialysis CKD population.

Based on the above studies as well as several others, the KDIGO clinical practice guidelines for lipid management in CKD recommend treating nondialysis CKD patients above age 50 with either a stain or a combination of statin/ezetimibe. Adults below 50 years of age with nondialysis CKD should be treated based on the assessment of their individual risk. For adults with dialysis dependent CKD, the KDIGO practice guidelines recommend against initiation of lipid-lowering treatment.

2. Acute coronary syndromes—CKD patients presenting with an ACS should be managed in the same way as the general population, recognizing that patients with severe renal insufficiency have generally been excluded from most trials of therapy. Patients with CKD and acute coronary syndromes appear less likely to receive evidence-based therapies and have substantially higher mortality rates. Additionally, these patients require dose adjustments of potentially life-saving medications and have a higher risk of drug-related

adverse events. For example, the clearance of low-molecular-weight heparin (LMWH) is primarily renal, therefore elimination is slower and less predictable, and bleeding complications may be increased. Thus, unfractionated heparin is generally preferred in patients with significant renal disease. Patients with CKD seem to have a higher risk of drug-related adverse effects: there are some reports of an increased risk of bleeding with the use of GPIIb-IIIa antagonists; however, their use is still generally recommended in appropriate individuals. Dose adjustments may be necessary for some of the preparations as their excretion is partially renal. The discovery and marketing of new oral anticoagulants such as the factor Xa inhibitor apixaban and the direct thrombin inhibitor dabigatran offers promising prospects but have yet to be studied in patients with advanced CKD and ESRD.

3. Secondary prevention—According to the KDIGO clinical practice guidelines and because of a lack of evidence specific to the renal failure population, patients with CKD should receive the same secondary prevention measures employed in the general population. This includes lifestyle modification (smoking cessation, exercise, and maintenance of ideal body weight), aspirin, β-blockers, statins, ACE inhibitors, and revascularization procedures in suitable candidates.

Anemia can contribute to exercise-induced ischemia and exacerbation of angina in CKD. The target hemoglobin currently recommended by KDIGO is 10–11.5 g/dL in patients with IHD. In those patients, targeting normal or near-normal hemoglobin values has been associated with an increased rate of cardiovascular events in several randomized controlled trials (CHOIR, CREATE, TREAT) and KDIGO recommends against the use of erythropoiesis-stimulating agents to intentionally increase the hemoglobin levels above 13 g/dL.

Coronary revascularization with percutaneous coronary intervention (PCI) or coronary artery bypass grafting (CABG) is sometimes necessary in suitable candidates with CAD. When CKD patients are compared to the general population with CAD, patients with renal failure are more likely to experience postprocedure hemorrhagic complications, and they have higher rates of in-hospital mortality as well as poorer long-term survival with both PCI and CABG. In addition, PCI restenosis rates appear to be increased with angioplasty alone, but are likely improved if accompanied by stenting. Moreover, CKD does not appear to mitigate the angiographic benefits observed with drug-eluting stents. Finally, while there are no prospective randomized studies guiding the choice of revascularization method in CKD, a retrospective analysis of data from the United States Renal Data System (USRDS) favors CABG over PCI in dialysis patients, particularly in those with diabetes. Ideally, prospective studies are needed to answer this question.

In general, the decision for revascularization must be individualized and assessed on a case-by-case basis.

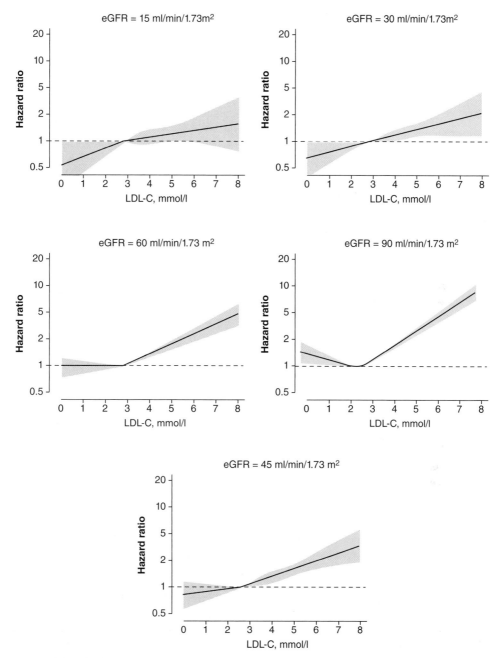

▲ **Figure 20–3.** Adjusted relation between LDL-C and HR of myocardial infarction by eGFR as a continuous variable. Data are adjusted hazard ratios for MI during a median follow-up period of 48 months. Data are from 836,060 participants in the Alberta kidney disease cohort and have been adjusted for age, sex, diabetes, hypertension, aboriginal status, socioeconomic status, proteinuria categories, statin use, and the Charlson comorbidities (cancer, cerebrovascular disease, congestive heart failure, chronic pulmonary disease, dementia, metastatic solid tumor, MI, liver disease, hemiplegia/paraplegia, peptic ulcer disease, peripheral vascular disease, and rheumatic disease). eGFR, estimated glomerular filtration rate; HR, hazard ratio; LDL-C, low-density lipoprotein cholesterol; MI, myocardial infarction. (Reproduced from Tonelli M et al: Association between LDL-C and risk of myocardial infarction in CKD. J Am Soc Nephrol 2013;24:979.)

Unfortunately, current decision making often reflects a pervasive therapeutic nihilism on the part of the general medical community toward patients with renal failure, which may lead to a postponement of testing and interventions and ultimately adversely impact the long-term outcomes of this group of patients.

C. Heart Failure

The two variants of heart failure, diastolic and systolic, can coexist in patients with CKD. Those CKD patients with predominantly diastolic heart failure often have significant LVH. In this case, attention should be focused on potentially modifiable contributing factors, which include hypertension and anemia.

Systolic heart failure has been studied extensively in the general population, but much less so in CKD patients. Thus studies in the general population are the only basis upon which to guide treatment in CKD. Salt restriction and diuresis are the mainstays of therapy to attain euvolemia. While loop diuretics are the diuretics of choice, a thiazide may be added to potentiate diuresis in resistant patients. Drug dose modification is often necessary in those with GFR less than 60 mL/min. The dose of loop diuretics must often be increased while medications that rely on renal excretion, including certain β-blockers (eg, atenolol) and digoxin, require a dose reduction. Close follow-up is required for potentially dangerous complications that may be more common in CKD, such as hyperkalemia with the use of ACE inhibitors, ARBs, or aldosterone antagonists, and cardiac toxicity with digoxin. In addition, sotalol has been recognized as a particularly problematic antiarrhythmic in CKD patients and should probably be avoided.

While patients with CKD are underrepresented in studies of heart failure, recent observational studies seem to indicate that patients with CHF and mild to moderate CKD derive a mortality benefit from medications including ACE inhibitors and β-blockers.

Finally, while correction of anemia to a target of 10–11.5 g/dL is important, current evidence suggests that further normalization of hemoglobin may be associated with adverse outcomes, at least in hemodialysis patients with CHF.

D. Atrial Fibrillation

In the general population of nonvalvular atrial fibrillation patients, the benefit of oral antithrombotic therapy for the prevention of stroke and peripheral embolism usually outweighs the risk of increased bleeding. However, in patients with renal disease, the clinical decision is more complex as these patients are at increased risk of both strokes and major bleeding events. Additionally, anticoagulation therapy in these patients has been associated not only with a reduced risk of stroke but also an increased risk of bleeding when compared to the general population.

Patients with stage III CKD and an estimated glomerular filtration rate (eGFR) of 30–59 mL/min/1.73 m² appear to derive similar benefit from anticoagulation than the general population and should generally be anticoagulated unless their CHADS₂ score is zero. Compared with warfarin, non-vitamin K oral anticoagulants (NOACs) such as dabigatran, apixaban, and rivaroxaban appear to have equal efficacy and safety among patients with stage III CKD. In patients with stage IV and V CKD and corresponding eGFRs of 15–29 mL/min/1.73 m² and less than 15 mL/min/1.73 m², respectively, there is little evidence to recommend for or against anticoagulation. Indeed, these patients constitute a very small percentage of the population studied in clinical trials and the limited data is insufficient to make informed decisions. These patients can be treated based on individual risk/benefit assessment. The 2014 American Heart Association/American College of Cardiology/Heart Rhythm Society (AHA/ACC) atrial fibrillation guidelines give a weak recommendation for anticoagulation in these patients. When anticoagulation is desired, warfarin is preferred over NOACs due to the wide clinical experience available with warfarin in these patients and also to the fact that patients with an eGFR of less than 30 mL/min/1.73 m² were almost entirely excluded from the randomized trials of the NOAC agents.

In patients with ESRD, the clinical conundrum is even greater as retrospective analyses have raised concerns percolating to the efficacy of anticoagulation. Indeed, use of anticoagulation has been associated with an increased risk of mortality and a paradoxical increase in the risk of strokes. Based on those findings, the KDOQI guidelines recommend against the routine use of anticoagulation for primary prevention of stroke in dialysis patients who develop atrial fibrillation, and suggest anticoagulation for secondary prevention with careful monitoring based upon individual risk–benefit profile. The AHA/ACC guidelines offer only a weak recommendation that the use of anticoagulation be individualized based on shared decision making after discussing the risks of stroke and bleeding on a case-by-case basis. There is insufficient data to support the use of NOAC in dialysis patients and they are typically avoided.

E. Sudden Cardiac Death

There are few effective therapies to prevent SCD in patients with kidney disease. Avoiding rapid fluid and electrolyte shifts is supported by observational data, but randomized-controlled trials assessing the benefits of intensive/daily dialysis are lacking. There is no data on the prevention of SCD in renal patients using antiarrhythmic therapy. Implantable cardioverter-defibrillators (ICDs) are well studied in the general population but their potential benefit in the dialysis population is mitigated by a fivefold increase in postimplant complications. A recent study used propensity matching to compare patients who had ICDs placed to those without

ICDs across different CKD stages. It showed that the use of ICDs was associated with a survival benefit in patients with eGFR greater than or equal to 30 mL/min/1.73 m² but not in patients with eGFR less than 30 mL/min/1.73 m². Randomized-controlled trials are needed in order to accurately identify the benefits of ICD placement in the CKD population. Whether wearable defibrillators or leadless subcutaneous devices can impact survival while reducing complication rates remains to be seen.

F. Peripheral Vascular Disease

PVD is a significant source of morbidity in CKD patients. The medical management of PVD generally focuses on treatment of cardiovascular risk factors such as sedentary lifestyle, smoking, diabetes, hypertension, and dyslipidemia. Revascularization, either with percutaneous intervention or with bypass surgery, is often required and amputations are common. There are no RCTs comparing percutaneous versus surgical revascularization techniques in patients with CKD and PVD but outcome studies all suggest that CKD confers an increased risk of adverse outcome, regardless of the revascularization technique employed.

Given that calcification is a key feature of the vascular pathology of CKD, attempts to reduce this should theoretically be of benefit in attenuating the progression of vascular disease. This is currently an area of active research. Perhaps rigorous attention to bone mineral metabolism and maintenance of appropriate levels of serum calcium, phosphorus, and parathyroid hormone through judicious use of calcium and non-calcium-containing phosphate binders, vitamin D, and calcimimetics will attenuate the progression of vascular calcification and may improve clinical outcomes in CKD.

KEY READINGS

Aggarwal A et al: Clinical characteristics and in-hospital outcome of patients with end-stage renal disease on dialysis referred for implantable cardioverter-defibrillator implantation. Heart Rhythm 2009;6:1565.

Baigent C et al: The effects of lowering LDL cholesterol with simvastatin plus ezetimibe in patients with chronic kidney disease (Study of Heart and Renal Protection): a randomised placebo-controlled trial. Lancet 2011;377:2181.

Baigent C et al: First United Kingdom Heart and Renal Protection (UK-HARP-I) study: biochemical efficacy and safety of simvastatin and safety of low-dose aspirin in chronic kidney disease. Am J Kidney Dis 2005;45:473.

Besarab A et al: The effects of normal as compared with low hematocrit values in patients with cardiac disease who are receiving hemodialysis and epoetin. N Engl J Med 1998;339:584.

Chan KE et al: Anticoagulant and antiplatelet usage associates with mortality among hemodialysis patients. J Am Soc Nephrol 2009;20:872.

Chan KE et al: Warfarin use associates with increased risk for stroke in hemodialysis patients with atrial fibrillation. J Am Soc Nephrol 2009;20:2223.

Charytan DM et al: Long-term clinical outcomes following drug-eluting or bare-metal stent placement in patients with severely reduced GFR: results of the Massachusetts Data Analysis Center (Mass-DAC) State Registry. Am J Kidney Dis 2011;57:202.

Drüeke TB et al: CREATE Investigators. Normalization of hemoglobin level in patients with chronic kidney disease and anemia. N Engl J Med 2006;355:2071.

Fellstrom BC et al: Rosuvastatin and cardiovascular events in patients undergoing hemodialysis. N Engl J Med 2009;360:1395.

Fox CS et al: Acute Coronary Treatment and Intervention Outcomes Network registry. Use of evidence-based therapies in short-term outcomes of ST-segment elevation myocardial infarction and non-ST-segment elevation myocardial infarction in patients with chronic kidney disease: a report from the National Cardiovascular Data Acute Coronary Treatment and Intervention Outcomes Network registry. Circulation 2010;121:357.

Harel Z et al: Comparisons between novel oral anticoagulants and vitamin K antagonists in patients with CKD. J Am Soc Nephrol 2014;25:431.

Herzog CA et al: Cardiovascular disease in chronic kidney disease. A clinical update from Kidney Disease: Improving Global Outcomes (KDIGO). Kidney Int 2011;80:572.

January CT et al: 2014 AHA/ACC/HRS guideline for the management of patients with atrial fibrillation: a report of the American College of Cardiology/American Heart Association Task Force on practice guidelines and the Heart Rhythm Society. Circulation 2014;130:e199.

Jardine MJ., et al: Aspirin is beneficial in hypertensive patients with chronic kidney disease: a post-hoc subgroup analysis of a randomized controlled trial. J Am Coll Cardiol 2010;56:956.

Kidney Disease: Improving Global Outcomes (KDIGO) Anemia Work Group. KDIGO Clinical Practice Guideline for Anemia in Chronic Kidney Disease. Kidney Int Suppl 2012;2:279.

Kidney Disease: Improving Global Outcomes (KDIGO) Blood Pressure Work Group. KDIGO Clinical Practice Guideline for the Management of Blood Pressure in Chronic Kidney Disease. Kidney Int Suppl 2012;2:337.

Kidney Disease: Improving Global Outcomes (KDIGO) Lipid Work Group. KDIGO Clinical Practice Guideline for Lipid Management in Chronic Kidney Disease. Kidney Int Suppl 2013;3:259.

Kidney Disease: Improving Global Outcomes (KDIGO) CKD Work Group. KDIGO 2012 Clinical Practice Guideline for the Evaluation and Management of Chronic Kidney Disease. Kidney Int Suppl 2013;3:1.

Krane V et al: Association of LDL cholesterol and inflammation with cardiovascular events and mortality in hemodialysis patients with type 2 diabetes mellitus. Am J Kidney Dis 2009;54:902.

Nakhoul GN et al: Implantable cardioverter-defibrillators in patients with CKD: a propensity-matched mortality analysis. Clin J Am Soc Nephrol 2015;10:1119.

O'Hare AM et al: Renal insufficiency and use of revascularization among a national cohort of men with advanced lower extremity peripheral arterial disease. Clin J Am Soc Nephrol 2006;1:297.

Parfrey PS et al: Erythropoietin therapy and left ventricular mass index in CKD and ESRD patients: a meta-analysis. Clin J Am Soc Nephrol 2009;4:755.

Patel UD et al: Hospital performance and differences by kidney function in the use of recommended therapies after non-ST-elevation acute coronary syndromes. Am J Kidney Dis 2009;53:426.

Pfeffer MA et al: TREAT Investigators. A trial of darbepoetin alfa in type 2 diabetes and chronic kidney disease. N Engl J Med 2009;361:2019.

Shlipak MG et al: Cardiovascular mortality risk in chronic kidney disease: comparison of traditional and novel risk factors. JAMA 2005;293:1737.

Singh AK et al: Correction of anemia with epoetin alfa in chronic kidney disease. N Engl J Med 2006;355:2085.

Tonelli M et al: Effect of pravastatin on cardiovascular events in people with chronic kidney disease. Circulation 2004;110:1557.

Wanner C et al: Deutsche Diabetes-Dialyse-Studie (4D) study group. Randomized controlled trial on the efficacy and safety of atorvastatin in patients with type 2 diabetes on hemodialysis (4D study): demographic and baseline characteristics. Kidney Blood Press Res 2004;27:259.

Washam JB et al: Pharmacotherapy in chronic kidney disease patients presenting with acute coronary syndrome: a scientific statement from the American Heart Association. Circulation 2015;131:1123.

▶ Summary

The prognosis for CKD patients with CVD is uniformly poor whenever it has been studied. For example, the mortality rate of dialysis patients is an astounding 20% per year, with CVD representing the most common cause. LVH is an independent risk factor for mortality in ESRD. Declining GFR is associated with increased mortality following an acute myocardial infarction. Patients with an estimated GFR greater than 75 mL/min had a 3-year mortality rate from MI of 14% compared to almost 46% in patients with an estimated GFR less than 45 mL/min. The outcome for patients with CHF and/or PVD in conjunction with lower GFR is also much worse than that observed in the general population.

The evidence base for treating CVD in CKD is far from complete. However, it now appears that patients with concurrent CKD and CVD likely benefit from many of the interventions implemented in individuals with CVD alone. In addition, most of these interventions can be used safely with appropriate monitoring in the CKD setting. Nonetheless, it has been consistently demonstrated that patients with CKD are less likely to receive these potentially beneficial therapies than their counterparts with normal kidney function. This has been termed "therapeutic nihilism" by some and may represent a further contribution to the poor outcomes observed with CVD in CKD.

In summary, CVD in patients with CKD is prevalent, and is likely due to a combination of both traditional and nontraditional risk factors. These factors are present to variable extents and for varying durations over the lifespan of patients with reduced GFR, and their effects are likely multiplicative rather than additive. Current data describing methods of investigation and treatment fail to give adequate direction to physicians caring for patients throughout the entire spectrum of CKD. Nonetheless, this chapter attempts to synthesize the current state of knowledge, identify gaps in the evidence base, and describe reasonable strategies based on the data available.

Given the increasing recognition of CKD as a risk factor for CVD, ongoing trials will need to explore more completely the mechanisms by which lower GFR or dialysis therapies impact the natural history of CVD. Therapeutic strategies will then be evaluated in the context of a more complete understanding of the complexity of this disease.

■ CHAPTER REVIEW QUESTIONS

1. A 61-year-old man presents to the nephrology clinic for evaluation of a recently diagnosed stage III Chronic Kidney Disease (CKD). He has a history of long-standing hypertension, gout, and diabetes. He denies history of heart disease. He had an appendectomy at age 17. He is presently asymptomatic and is in the clinic at the request of his primary care physician. His vital signs show a blood pressure (BP) of 135/72, heart rate (HR) 74, respiratory rate (RR) of 14, oxygen saturation of 99%. His physical examination is notable for clear sclera, regular heart rate with no murmurs, clear lungs, nondistended nontender abdomen and trace bilateral lower extremity edema. He takes amlodipine, allopurinol, metformin, and over the counter vitamin D. Outpatient blood work shows the following: sodium 141 mEq/L, potassium 4.2 mEq/L, chloride 97 mmol/L, CO_2 25 mmol/L, glucose 97 mg/dL, blood urea nitrogen 34 mg/dL, creatinine 1.45 mg/dL with an MDRD-estimated glomerular filtration rate (eGFR) of 55 mL/min. Urinary testing reveals a urinary albumin/creatinine ratio (UACR) of 252 mg/g. Which of the following is accurate regarding his prognosis?

    A. His mortality risk is similar to the general population because his blood pressure and diabetes are well controlled.

    B. His risk of progression to ESRD requiring dialysis is higher than his risk of death.

    C. His mortality risk is similar to the general population because his UACR is less than 300 mg/g.

    D. He should not be worried about his CKD because his eGFR is very close to 60 mL/min.

    E. His risk of progression to end-stage renal disease (ESRD) requiring dialysis is lower than his risk of death.

2. You are rounding in the dialysis unit and you meet one of your new patients. She is a 73-year-old woman with end stage renal disease secondary to hypertension and was started on dialysis a week ago. Her past medical history is notable for smoking, hypertension, coronary artery disease, congestive heart failure, atrial fibrillation, and remote stroke with residual right hemiparesis. She takes aspirin, carvedilol, losartan, atorvastatin, hydralazine, and isosorbide mononitrate. Her physical examination reveals a thin elderly woman with pale conjunctivas. Heart sounds are irregularly irregular without murmurs. She has mild ronchi at bilateral lung bases with 1+ bilateral peripheral edema. Abdomen is supple, nontender with normal bowel sounds. She has a right brachiocephalic arteriovenous fistula with good thrill and bruit and no aneurysmal dilations. Vitals: BP 157/83, HR 57, O_2 saturation 97%. Her CBC shows a hemoglobin of 8.1 g/dL. She is getting an injection of erythropoietin-stimulating agent (ESA) and she asks you about its benefits. What do you tell her?
   A. ESAs will boost her hemoglobin and increase her chance of survival.
   B. Increasing her hemoglobin above 10 g/dL will protect her from cardiovascular events.
   C. Increasing her hemoglobin above 10 g/dL will protect her from developing strokes.
   D. The benefits of ESAs are limited to decreasing transfusion need and possibly improving the quality of life.

3. A 55-year-old man presents to the outpatient clinic for follow-up of chronic kidney disease. He has a history of recurrent kidney stones complicated by several episodes of obstruction. He has required several interventions, including numerous lithotripsies and stenting of the right ureter. He denies history of hypertension, diabetes, or coronary artery disease. His family history is notable for hypertension on his father's side but with history of heart attacks or heart failure. He does not take any medications. His physical examination reveals a well-built man, clear sclera, normal heart sounds, clear lung, supple abdomen with mild right flank tenderness and no edema. Vitals: BP 110/62, HR 65, RR 12, O_2 saturation 99%. Blood work shows: sodium 139 mEq/L, potassium 4.1 mEq/L, chloride 101 mmol/L, CO_2 24 mmol/L, glucose 92 mg/dL, blood urea nitrogen 39 mg/dL, creatinine 1.94 mg/dL with an MDRD-estimated glomerular filtration rate (eGFR) of 38 mL/min.

What medications should you prescribe for the purpose of primary prevention of cardiovascular events?
   A. Start aspirin and statin.
   B. Start aspirin and check a lipid panel to see if a statin is indicated.
   C. Prescribe a statin only.
   D. He does not need primary prophylaxis because his risk of cardiovascular events is very low.
   E. Refer him to preventive cardiology for risk assessment of cardiovascular disease in CKD.

4. A 29-year-old man presents to the emergency department with chest pain. He states his pain started as soon as he finished eating a large meal. The pain is epigastric, dull and nonradiating. He states that it feels like "indigestion" and he thinks it might be his gastroesophageal reflux disease worsening because he ran out of omeprazole a few days ago. He denies nausea, vomiting or diaphoresis. His medical history is relevant for type 1 diabetes, hypertension, end-stage renal disease on hemodialysis for 3 years and hiatal hernia with gastroesophageal reflux disease. He denies history of coronary artery disease or heart failure. He takes nifedipine, lisinopril, hydralazine, and omeprazole. His physical examination reveals a well-nourished young man with clear conjunctivas. Heart sounds are regular with no murmurs. Lungs are clear to auscultation. Abdominal examination reveals mild epigastric tenderness but is otherwise unremarkable. Pulses present in all four extremities. No edema. Vitals: BP 162/93, HR 75, RR 15, O_2 saturation 98%. What is the most appropriate next step?
   A. Obtain a full evaluation for acute coronary syndrome that includes an electrocardiogram (ECG) and cardiac troponins.
   B. Obtain a full evaluation for acute coronary syndrome that includes an ECG and cardiac troponins but also give a loading dose of aspirin.
   C. Obtain an ECG only. Cardiac troponins will likely be elevated because he is on dialysis and will not provide useful clinical information.
   D. Resume his omeprazole. His chest pain is unlikely to be secondary to an acute coronary syndrome.

5. You are seeing 35-year-old African–American woman on dialysis. She has a history of hypertension, hyperlipidemia, osteoarthritis of the right hip and focal segmental glomerulosclerosis on hemodialysis for 6 months. She denies personal or family history of heart disease. Her medications include hydralazine, furosemide, rosuvastatin, sevelamer, cinacalcet and as needed Tylenol. She also gets darbepoetin and doxercalciferol in the dialysis unit. Physical examination reveal an obese woman with clear conjunctivas, normal heart sounds without murmurs, diminished breath sounds at bilateral lung bases, supple nontender abdomen and no edema. Vitals: BP 145/93, HR 82, RR 15, O_2 saturation 99%. Her hemoglobin is 14.1 g/dL. Which of the following is true regarding darbepoetin administration?

A. The darbepoetin should be continued at the same dose to maintain her hemoglobin greater than 13 g/dL.
B. The darbepoetin should be continued but the dose should be decreased to prevent further increase in the hemoglobin.
C. The darbepoetin should be stopped.
D. The darbepoetin should be decreased but only after checking iron studies and correcting an underlying iron deficiency if present.

Chronic Kidney Disease-Mineral Bone Disorder

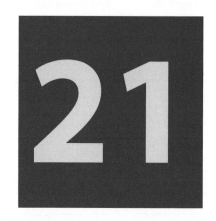

Sharon M. Moe, MD, FASN

▶ The Kidney Disease Improving Global Outcomes (KDIGO) work group defined chronic kidney disease mineral bone disorder (CKD-MBD) as a systemic disorder of mineral and bone metabolism due to CKD manifested by either one or a combination of the following:

▶ Abnormalities of blood levels of calcium, phosphorus, parathyroid hormone (PTH), and vitamin D metabolism.

▶ Abnormalities in bone turnover, mineralization, volume (which together are called renal osteodystrophy), linear growth, or strength.

▶ Vascular or other soft tissue calcification.

General Considerations

The definition of CKD-MBD was developed at an international consensus conference organized by KDIGO and meant to emphasize the importance of disordered mineral metabolism in the pathogenesis of morbidity and mortality on patients with CKD. Although not included in the original discussion, abnormalities in blood levels of fibroblast growth factor 23 (FGF-23) and α-klotho (hereafter called klotho) are considered a component of CKD-MBD. All components of CKD-MBD—abnormalities of blood levels, bone, and extraskeletal calcification—are associated with morbidity and mortality in patients with CKD as discussed throughout this chapter.

KEY READING

Moe SM et al: Chronic kidney disease-mineral-bone disorder: a new paradigm. Adv Chronic Kidney Dis 2007;14:3.

Pathogenesis

1. CKD-MBD—Abnormal Blood Levels

Blood and intracellular levels of calcium and phosphorus are tightly maintained to protect *homeostasis* and cellular function by an organized series of homeostatic feedback loops that all involve the kidney. In addition, calcium and phosphorus *balance* is maintained to ensure adequate mineral stores for bone health. The four hormones $1,25(OH)_2$-vitamin D (hereafter $1,25[OH]_2D$), PTH, FGF23, and klotho work to regulate homeostasis.

- Vitamin D is taken in through food, supplements, or sunlight, and then synthesized into 25(OH)-vitamin D (25D or calcidiol) at the liver, and to $1,25(OH)_2$-vitamin D ($1,25(OH)_2D$ or calcitriol) by the CYP27B1 (1α-hydroxylase) enzyme in the kidney and other nonrenal sites. CYP27B1 activity is increased by PTH, estrogen, low calcium and decreased by FGF23, calcitriol, and high phosphorus. The major function of $1,25(OH)_2D$ is to enhance intestinal absorption and kidney reabsorption of calcium.

- PTH is secreted from the parathyroid gland in response to hypocalcemia and hyperphosphatemia, and is inhibited by $1,25(OH)_2D$ and FGF23. The major target organs of PTH are bone where it increases calcium and phosphorus resorption, and kidney where it increases calcium reabsorption and phosphorus excretion.

- FGF23 is synthesized in osteocytes/osteoblasts of bone with the primary effect on kidney to increase phosphorus excretion; FGF23 is stimulated by $1,25(OH)_2D$, PTH, and likely hyperphosphatemia or increased dietary phosphate.

- α-Klotho is synthesized in the kidney where it serves as a coreceptor for FGF23 to enhance phosphaturia and facilitates calcium reabsorption; the extracellular klotho domain is also cleaved and circulates to act on other organs.

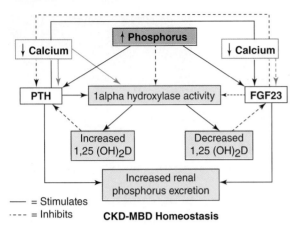

— = Stimulates
---- = Inhibits   **CKD-MBD Homeostasis**

▲ **Figure 21–1. Homeostasis of phosphorus and calcium in CKD.** As phosphorus levels increase (or there is a chronic phosphate load), both PTH and FGF23 are increased. Both the elevated PTH and FGF23 increase urinary phosphorus excretion. The two hormones differ in respect to their effects on the vitamin D axis. PTH stimulates 1α-hydroxylase (CYP27B1) activity, thereby increasing the production of 1,25(OH)$_2$D, which in turn negatively feeds back on the parathyroid gland to decrease PTH secretion. In contrast, FGF23 inhibits 1α-hydroxylase activity, thereby decreasing the production of 1,25(OH)$_2$D feeding back to stimulate further secretion of FGF23. FGF23 and PTH also regulate each other. Finally, low calcium levels stimulate PTH whereas high calcium levels stimulate FGF23. Last, there is some evidence that FGF23 also inhibits PTH secretion (solid line = stimulates; dashed line = inhibits). (Reprinted, with permission, from Moe SM, Sprague SM: Pathogenesis of CKD-MBD and renal osteodystrophy. In: Taal MW et al, eds. *Brenner and Rector's The Kidney*, 10th ed. Elsevier Saunders, 2015.)

The intersection of these homeostatic loops is shown in Figure 21–1.

HOMEOSTATIC LOOPS CONTROLLING BLOOD LEVELS

A. PTH-FGF23-1,25(OH)$_2$D Loop

PTH and FGF23 both stimulate urinary phosphate excretion. However, PTH stimulates CYP27B1 activity, thus increasing the production of 1,25(OH)$_2$D, which in turn negatively feeds back on the parathyroid gland to decrease PTH secretion. In contrast, FGF23 inhibits CYP27B1, thereby decreasing the production of 1,25(OH)$_2$D which limits further secretion of FGF23 (as normally 1,25(OH)$_2$D stimulates FGF23 production).

B. Calcium-PTH-FGF23 Loop

Hypocalcemia stimulates PTH which increases renal calcium reabsorption, increases bone resorption to release calcium from bone, and enhances 1,25(OH)$_2$D stimulation of intestinal calcium absorption with the goal of normalizing calcium levels. Hypocalcemia also appears to blunt FGF23 release. The latter would therefore "remove" both the FGF23 inhibition of PTH and the FGF23 inhibition of 1,25(OH)$_2$D synthesis during times of hypocalcemia. Hypercalcemia has opposing effects: It stimulates FGF23 (which reduces PTH and 1,25(OH)$_2$D synthesis), directly inhibits CYP27B1 and thus decreases 1,25(OH)$_2$D synthesis, and directly inhibits PTH secretion. This results in decreased intestinal calcium absorption, renal reabsorption, and bone resorption. The mechanism by which calcium may regulate FGF23 is not yet known.

C. Phosphate-PTH-FGF23-Klotho Loop

As phosphate levels increase, both PTH and FGF23 are increased. Both the elevated PTH and FGF23 (via coreceptor α-klotho) increase urinary phosphate excretion, but by different signaling mechanisms. PTH increases renal calcium reabsorption, minimizing the possibility of high calcium in the urine at the same time there is phosphaturia. PTH stimulates the secretion of FGF23 from osteocytes, and increased FGF23 inhibits PTH by decreasing both PTH gene expression and secretion, thus regulating each other.

The multiple homeostatic loops described above enable tightly controlled calcium and phosphorus blood levels and minimize the risk of calcification in soft tissue, kidney, and urine. As kidney function declines, hormone levels change as a normal homeostatic response to impaired renal handling of calcium and phosphorus. However, at some point the appropriate rise in PTH and FGF23 move from normal homeostasis to pathogenic, inducing end-organ damage in the form of bone loss, left ventricular hypertrophy (LVH), and arterial calcification. As shown in Figure 21–1, all of these homeostatic loops involve the kidney; thus it is not surprising that homeostasis is disrupted in patients with CKD. By stage 3 CKD, nearly 100% of patients have some evidence of CKD-MBD—abnormalities of calcium, phosphorus, PTH, vitamin D metabolism, and FGF-23. The earliest detectable abnormality in blood levels is a rise in FGF23.

KEY READINGS

Isakova T et al: Fibroblast growth factor 23 is elevated before parathyroid hormone and phosphate in chronic kidney disease. Kidney Int 2011;79:1370.

Kuro-O M, Moe OW: FGF23-alphaKlotho as a paradigm for a kidney-bone network. Bone 2017;100:4.

Moe SM: Calcium homeostasis in health and in kidney disease. Compr Physiol 2016;6:1781.

Wolf M: Update on fibroblast growth factor 23 in chronic kidney disease. Kidney Int 2012;82:737.

2. CKD-MBD—Abnormalities in Bone

Bone is a dynamic organ. It is resorbed by osteoclasts that originate from circulating hematopoietic cells, and unmineralized bone (osteoid) is formed by osteoblasts that originate from within the bone. The osteoid is then mineralized through incorporation of calcium and phosphorus into hydroxyapatite in a poorly understood process. This cycle of resorption–formation is termed *remodeling* and assessed as bone turnover. Renal osteodystrophy is diagnosed by bone biopsy where changes in bone turnover, mineralization, and volume can be quantified with histomorphometry by using tetracycline labeling to fluoresce the bone. The amount of bone that accumulates between florescent labels is quantified to define new bone formation which is then converted to a bone formation rate.

In the majority of patients with CKD stages 3–4, high turnover predominates. In patients on dialysis, low turnover bone predominates perhaps due to diabetes, calcium-based phosphate binders, and oversuppression of PTH with calcitriol. If the low turnover bone disease is associated with a paucity of cells, it is called *adynamic bone disease*. The reason for the paucity of cells is unknown, although recent animal studies suggest it may be due to abnormalities of osteoblast differentiation from mesenchymal cells in the bone marrow. In addition, bone mineralization is important in renal osteodystrophy. If the bone does not mineralize, newly formed bone stays in an unmineralized state called *osteoid*. The causes of impaired mineralization include aluminum overload, vitamin D deficiency, and possibly a role for FGF23. Abnormal mineralization is especially common in children. Finally, the amount of bone or bone volume is also important in bone health. Patients have multiple underlying abnormalities of bone before they develop CKD, for example postmenopausal bone loss, steroid-induced bone loss, low testosterone, and malabsorption. On top of these underlying bone problems, there can be abnormal bone formation resulting in impaired volume.

This complexity led KDIGO to change the older classification of renal osteodystrophy (high turnover, low turnover) to a TMV system where all three components are evaluated separately- turnover, mineralization, and volume. The focus in clinical practice is to manage bone health by treating secondary hyperparathyroidism, but the reality is that bone is far more complex, and that is one reason that the use of PTH alone is not very predictive of underlying bone histology. In children with CKD, there is impaired linear growth due to renal osteodystrophy and abnormalities in the insulin-like growth factor—growth hormone regulation of bone. Most importantly, in children and adults there is impaired bone strength leading to fractures. Thus, bone abnormalities are very common in patients with CKD.

KEY READINGS

Carvalho C, Alves CM, Frazao JM: The role of bone biopsy for the diagnosis of renal osteodystrophy: a short overview and future perspectives. J Nephrol 2016;29:617.
Graciolli FG et al: The complexity of chronic kidney disease-mineral and bone disorder across stages of chronic kidney disease. Kidney Int 2017;91(16):1436.
Wesseling-Perry K: Defective skeletal mineralization in pediatric CKD. Curr Osteoporos Rep 2015;13:98.

3. CKD-MBD—Vascular or Other Soft Tissue Calcification

Calcification in arteries can occur in atherosclerotic plaques and in the medial layer of arteries. Arterial calcification is a tightly regulated process that involves the de-differentiation of vascular smooth muscle cells to osteoblast-like cells, the accumulation of calcium and phosphorus into vesicles or exosomes that then are released from osteoblast-like cells and deposited on collagen and other bone proteins in the blood vessel. The balance of promineralizing factors is countered by calcification inhibitors. Unfortunately, factors stimulating calcification are increased in CKD, and the regulation of many of these inhibitors is impaired with CKD, thus shifting the balance towards calcification. In nonvascular tissues a similar process occurs, although it is less well studied.

KEY READINGS

Chen NX, Moe SM: Pathophysiology of vascular calcification. Curr Osteoporos Rep 2015;13:372.
Yamada S, Giachelli CM: Vascular calcification in CKD-MBD: roles for phosphate, FGF23, and Klotho. Bone 2017;100:87.

▶ Prevention

With the complex physiology detailed previously, it would be logical to prevent the development of the pathologic manifestations of CKD-MBD. However, to date, early administration of calcitriol, phosphate binders, or calcium have not prevented the progressive rise in PTH and FGF23. This is likely because we cannot yet determine when normal homeostatic response becomes abnormal, and thus do not know when to intervene, and because each of these treatments itself alters other components of the other homeostatic loops.

▶ Clinical Findings, Differential Diagnosis, & Complications

1. Biochemical Abnormalities

Elevated phosphorus, alkaline phosphatase, PTH, and FGF23 are all associated with mortality in patients with

CKD and end-stage renal disease (ESRD). Both low calcium and very high calcium levels are also associated with mortality. Elevated phosphorus or FGF23 are associated with the greatest risk of mortality. The population attributable risk, which takes into account both the magnitude of risk and the prevalence of the abnormality, is greater for CKD-MBD biochemistries than anemia or urea reduction ratio. In addition, these biochemical abnormalities do not move in isolation of each other, and thus co-trending helps in the assessment of the impact of biochemical abnormalities on outcomes. The mechanism by which CKD-MBD causes mortality is principally through cardiovascular disease and fractures.

KEY READINGS

Block G et al: Co-trending of parathyroid hormone and phosphate in patients receiving hemodialysis. Clin Nephrol 2016;85:142.

Gutierrez OM et al: Fibroblast growth factor 23 and mortality among patients undergoing hemodialysis. N Engl J Med 2008;359:584.

Isakova T et al: Fibroblast growth factor 23 and risks of mortality and end-stage renal disease in patients with chronic kidney disease. JAMA 2011;305:2432.

Palmer SC et al: Serum levels of phosphorus, parathyroid hormone, and calcium and risks of death and cardiovascular disease in individuals with chronic kidney disease: a systematic review and meta-analysis. JAMA 2011;305:1119.

2. Bone Abnormalities

Bone disorders are often asymptomatic, but abnormalities can be seen on plain radiographs including resorption of the cortical layer of the phalanges, resorption of the distal clavicles, and salt and peppering of skull. Impaired cortical bone will reduce strength of bone to stress resulting in fractures. The incidence of fractures is increased at all stages of CKD compared to the general population (Figure 21–2). Interestingly, the location of fracture is predominately in the cortical bone as opposed to the trabecular or cancellous bone, likely because of the importance of PTH in maintaining cortical bone. In the EVOLVE (EValuation Of Cinacalcet Hydrochloride [HCl] Therapy to Lower CardioVascular Events) study, where clinical fractures were adjudicated, 50% of fractures were in the cortical bone (wrist, clavicle, face) and these were more common than hip fractures (which are a combination of cortical and cancellous bone). Similar to the general population, low bone mineral density assessed by dual X-ray absorptiometry (DXA) is predictive of fractures. DXA underestimates the fracture risk due to abnormalities in bone quality, which cannot be assessed by DXA. Abnormal bone quality is from altered collagen and renal osteodystrophy. Furthermore, DXA at the distal radius is the most predictive of future fractures than hip or spine in patients with advanced CKD and is the preferred site to measure. This is

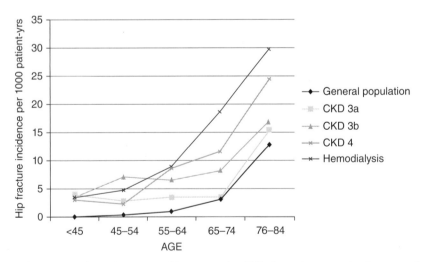

▲ **Figure 21–2.** Hip fracture incidence increases with progressive CKD. As patients age, in the general population there is an increased incidence of hip fracture. This incidence increases with progression of CKD. Data from Alem et al for dialysis patients and the general population from Olmstead Minnesota (Alem AM et al: Kidney Int 2000;58:396–399), Naylor et al for CKD stages 3–4 (Naylor KL et al: Kidney Int 2014;86:810–818) courtesy of the Canadian Institute for Clinical Evaluative Sciences (ICES). Pt-yrs = patient years. (Reprinted, with permission from, Moe SM, Nickolas TL: Fractures in patients with CKD: time for action. Clin J Am Soc Nephrol 2016;11(11):1929–1931.)

likely because the radius is most reflective of cortical bone changes.

Normal bone remodeling is important for the strength of bone but also for the metabolic function of bone as bone is the largest reservoir of calcium, phosphorus, and magnesium. If bone turnover is low, calcium and phosphorus will not be incorporated into bone; if bone turnover is high, bone resorption may overwhelm bone formation leading to net negative bone balance. This metabolic function is important, as multiple studies have demonstrated an inverse relationship between bone mineral content and vascular calcification, implying that abnormal bone metabolism may lead to excess mineral for deposition elsewhere. In addition, bone marrow is home to multiple stem cells, and there is an interaction between bone cells and other marrow cells; the importance of this relationship that is just beginning to be recognized.

With severe secondary hyperparathyroidism, pain and muscle weakness can occur. The muscle weakness is usually proximal and results in an inability to rise from a chair without using hands, difficulty climbing steps, and difficulty raising arms to comb the back of one's hair. These easily assessed symptoms are rapidly relieved with a parathyroidectomy.

KEY READINGS

Babayev R, Nickolas TL: Bone disorders in chronic kidney disease: an update in diagnosis and management. Semin Dial 2015; 28:645.

Barreto DV et al: Association of changes in bone remodeling and coronary calcification in hemodialysis patients: a prospective study. Am J Kidney Dis 2008;52:1139.

Moe SM, Nickolas TL: Fractures in patients with CKD: time for action. Clin J Am Soc Nephrol 2016;11:1929.

Ott SM: Bone strength: more than just bone density. Kidney Int 2016;89:16.

3. Extraskeletal Calcification & Cardiovascular Disease

Cardiovascular disease is the leading cause of death in patients with CKD. In early-stage CKD (grades 3 and 4), atherosclerotic disease prevails due to traditional Framingham risk factors, such as diabetes and hypertension. At this stage of CKD, studies have shown that statins are effective. However, most patients with CKD that have significant atherosclerotic disease die of a cardiovascular event prior to ever-needing dialysis. In contrast, in dialysis patients, most patients have diastolic dysfunction rather than systolic dysfunction, LVH, and high rate of sudden cardiac death. Autopsy studies of patients who were receiving dialysis have demonstrated similar quantity of atherosclerotic/intimal plaque but more calcification of plaque and more medial calcification than nondialysis patients who die a cardiac death. Calcification of the aorta results in increased pulse pressure,

with impaired diastolic blood flow and cardiac oxygenation, resulting in LVH, fibrosis, and diastolic dysfunction. These changes will usually manifest as non-ST elevation myocardial infarctions (NSTEMIs) rather than ST elevation myocardial infarctions. Thus, it is not surprising that statins are ineffective in dialysis patients in preventing cardiovascular mortality. In addition to large vessel calcification, small arteriole calcification in the heart will also lead to fibrosis and conduction abnormalities, contributing to the high rate of sudden cardiac death in patients with advanced CKD. Such small arteriole calcification can also occur in the skin epidermis, leading to necrosis of the skin called *calciphylaxis*. It is also likely that small vessel calcification may also cause other abnormalities such as impotence, increase muscle cramping, and visceral abnormalities perhaps manifesting as bowel changes.

Imaging of calcification of arteries cannot differentiate whether the calcification is in the intimal or medial layer. Computed tomography (CT)-based imaging (multislice CT, electron beam CT) can be quantified and is very useful for research studies. However, the presence of calcification in arteries on plain radiographs is also associated with mortality, and of course much less expensive.

In addition to calcification-induced LVH, FGF23 appears to have a direct effect to induce LVH. Direct injection of FGF23 into hearts in animal models induced hypertrophy, and serum FGF23 levels are higher in CKD patients with progressive LVH than those without progression.

Unfortunately, despite the likely contribution of CKD-MBD to both fractures and cardiovascular disease, there are limited studies evaluating whether CKD-MBD treatments improve mortality.

KEY READINGS

Anaya P et al: Coronary artery calcification in CKD-5D patients is tied to adverse cardiac function and increased mortality. Clin Nephrol 2016;86:291.

Bellasi A, Raggi P: Techniques and technologies to assess vascular calcification. Semin Dial 2007;20:129.

Faul C et al: FGF23 induces left ventricular hypertrophy. J Clin Invest 2011;121:4393.

Fujii H, Joki N: Mineral metabolism and cardiovascular disease in CKD. Clin Exp Nephrol 2017;21:53.

Moe SM: Calcium as a cardiovascular toxin in CKD-MBD. Bone 2017;100:94.

▶ Treatment

1. Overview of Approach to Treatment

CKD-MBD is difficult to treat because of the interrelated pathophysiology detailed previously. A treatment that might lower PTH may also alter FGF23 or calcium levels. A multipronged approach is needed to attempt to maintain normal calcium and phosphorus homeostasis and balance. This approach also changes when a patient progresses from CKD to ESRD due to the concomitant dialytic shifts of phosphorus and calcium. Unfortunately, the treatments themselves may have unwanted consequences.

Over the past 40 years there have been major changes in the treatment approach to CKD-MBD. In the 1970s, the emphasis was solely on the bone manifestations and the systemic effects of PTH. At that time, the only known regulator of PTH was calcium, and thus treatment was to increase the serum calcium through dialysis and oral calcitriol. Phosphorus was managed by aluminum-based phosphate binders until aluminum toxicity was identified at which time calcium-based phosphate binders were used. It was presumed the calcium would also add efficacy by raising the serum calcium level and suppressing PTH. In the 1990s, hypercalcemia was increasingly observed and "less calcemic" vitamin D analogues and non–calcium-containing phosphate binders were developed. In the late 1990s, data demonstrated a direct role of calcium and phosphorus on cardiovascular disease in humans, most notably vascular calcification. In the K/DOQI guidelines published in 2003, a low grade (of evidence) recommendation was to limit calcium-containing phosphate binders in the presence of vascular calcification, recognizing the importance of avoiding positive calcium balance. The 2009 KDIGO guidelines include the development of calcimimetics, additional non–calcium-containing phosphate binders such as lanthanum- and iron-based phosphate binders. This large group of choices for the treatment of the various manifestations of CKD-MBD can make clinical management difficult, and the continued development of new treatments indicates current options are suboptimal. The updated KDIGO guidelines for CKD-MBD in 2017 acknowledge continued lack of large randomized trials that can definitively guide an evidence-based approach to patient care.

In the absence of definitive clinical trials, the general approach to patients with CKD-MBD is to control total body phosphorus burden, treat elevated PTH, and in so doing maintain normal or near normal calcium balance. Each of these strategies will be discussed in the following text. The targets for phosphorus, calcium, and PTH differ across the stages of CKD (Table 21–1), although there are many nuances in understanding the rationale behind these targets as discussed in the following text.

KEY READINGS

KDIGO: Clinical practice guidelines for the management of CKD-MBD. Kidney Int Suppl 2009;76:S1.
Ketteler M et al: Executive summary of the 2017 KDIGO chronic kidney disease-mineral and bone disorder (CKD-MBD) guideline update: what's changed and why it matters. Kidney Int. 2017 Jul;92(1):26-36. doi: 10.1016/j.kint.2017.04.006.
Melamed ML, Buttar RS, Coco M: CKD-mineral bone disorder in stage 4 and 5 CKD: what we know today? Adv Chronic Kidney Dis 2016;23:262.

2. Management of Phosphorus & Calcium

A. Target Levels of Phosphorus (see Table 21–1)

Phosphorus levels should be maintained in the normal range in CKD stages 3–5 predialysis patients. As patients progress to needing dialysis, the ideal target for phosphorus is less clear. The data available from studies of patients with ESRD are based on large cohort studies looking at the relative risk or hazard ratio of mortality at various levels of phosphorus. The inflection point, the level of phosphorus at which there is a significant association with mortality, varies depending

Table 21–1. "Target" blood levels for calcium, phosphorus, and PTH.

		CKD Stage 3	CKD Stage 4	CKD Stage 5D
Phosphorus (mg/dL)	K/DOQI	2.7–4.6 mg/dL (Opinion)	2.7-4.6 mg/dL (Opinion)	2.7–5.5 mg/dL (Evidence)
	KDIGO	**Normal range (2C)**	**Normal range(2C)**	**Toward the normal range(2C)**
Calcium (mg/dL)	K/DOQI	Normal (Opinion)	Normal (Opinion)	8.4-9.5; hypercalcemia ≥10.2 (Evidence)
	KDIGO	**Normal range (2D)**	**Normal range (2D)**	**Normal range (2D)**
Intact PTH (pg/mL)	K/DOQI	35–70 pg/mL (Opinion)	70–110 pg/mL (Opinion)	150–300 pg/mL (Evidence)
	KDIGO	Ideal level unknown	Ideal level unknown	>2 and <9 times the upper limit of normal (if TREND changing within that range, adjust treatment) (2C)

K/DOQI, Kidney Disease Outcomes Quality Initiative; KDIGO, Kidney Disease Improving Global Outcomes; PTH, parathyroid hormone.
The 2003 K/DOQI guidelines rated statements as either opinion or evidence, with no clear definition of what constitutes evidence. In contracts, the 2009 KDIGO guidelines used the International GRADE System. Levels 1 and 2 indicate the strength of the recommendation, and letters A, B, C, D indicate the quality of the evidence. These grades 2C and 2D in this table indicate low level of evidence.

on the study size and the chosen reference range. In general, the phosphorus levels in dialysis patients greater than 6–6.5 mg/dL are associated with increased mortality. Other studies have looked at time averaged phosphorus levels with similar results. Unfortunately, there is no randomized trial targeting one level of phosphorus compared to a lower level that can inform an actual target level. For this reason, the KDIGO guidelines in 2009 and in the 2017 update recommend lowering the serum phosphorus in dialysis patients toward normal. The benefit of moving the phosphorus level from 9 to 7 mg/dL likely outweighs the benefit of moving the phosphorus level from 7 to 5 mg/dL. In the absence of randomized trials comparing target phosphorus levels low and high, therapy should be individualized.

B. Lower Phosphorus with Diet

The goal of dietary phosphate restriction is to reduce the overall phosphorus burden that the kidney must then excrete minimizing excessive increases in the phosphaturic hormones, PTH and FGF23. However, designing a low-phosphate diet is not straightforward as phosphate is in nearly every food, including dairy products, all sources of protein, legumes, and as a preservative in nearly all boxed and canned foods. The goal, therefore, is to choose foods that have a high protein-to-phosphate ratio and balancing these needs with other dietary requirements necessitates a renal dietician. The source of the phosphate also matters, as equivalent amounts of phosphate in the food source may not mean equivalent bioavailability due to differences in intestinal absorption. For example, meat and dairy source of phosphate is more readily absorbed than phytate-bound phosphate, approximately 70 versus 50%. The latter is found in grains and legumes, and the phosphate must be digested by phytase before release; humans lack this enzyme. At the other extreme are phosphate-containing additives in processed foods that are over 90% bioavailable. Another common culprit of phosphate intake is carbonated dark-colored soda pops. These are particularly problematic as they are often ingested away from meals and therefore away from phosphate binders.

The preservative source of phosphate is often hidden as food labels do not quantify the amount of phosphate, and these additives are currently listed as "generally safe" by the Food Labeling Division of the Food and Drug Administration (FDA) as well as other non-US food regulatory agencies. As a result, there can be differences in preparations of the same food that is not apparent on food labels. Two studies examined the result of randomizing patients to avoid food with preservatives and additives. The studies, one study in CKD and one study in dialysis patient found urinary phosphorus excretion and the serum phosphorus levels, respectively, were reduced. As is apparent by this discussion, following a low phosphate diet is not straightforward and is difficult for nearly all patients. As a provider counseling

a patient on phosphorus intake, it is most important that the patient be advised to avoid processed foods; this has the added benefit of lowering sodium intake as well. Eating freshly prepared plant- or animal-based protein sources is preferable over processed foods and eating plant-based protein is preferable over animal-based protein. Teaching patients on how to read a food label is important in lowering sodium intake. A simple recommendation is to have a patient read the food label and choose a low-sodium food, *and* then check the ingredient list to avoid foods that have any ingredient with the letters PHOS. Another suggestion is to recommend patients only shop the perimeter of a grocery store, as almost every store has the processed foods in the center.

KEY READINGS

Gutierrez OM: Sodium- and phosphorus-based food additives: persistent but surmountable hurdles in the management of nutrition in chronic kidney disease. Adv Chronic Kidney Dis 2013;20:150.

Isakova T et al: Effects of dietary phosphate restriction and phosphate binders on FGF23 levels in CKD. Clin J Am Soc Nephrol 2013;8:1009.

Kalantar-Zadeh K et al: Understanding sources of dietary phosphorus in the treatment of patients with chronic kidney disease. Clin J Am Soc Nephrol 2010;5:519.

Moorthi RN et al: The effect of a diet containing 70% protein from plants on mineral metabolism and musculoskeletal health in chronic kidney disease. Am J Nephrol 2014;40:582.

Sullivan C et al: Effect of food additives on hyperphosphatemia among patients with end-stage renal disease: a randomized controlled trial. JAMA 2009;301:629.

C. Phosphate Binders

Reducing phosphate intake from food is difficult, and thus treating hyperphosphatemia often requires the addition of phosphate binders taken with food. The best phosphate binder is the one the patient will take which may be a factor of pill size, gastrointestinal side effects, chewing versus swallowing, or coating on the pills. However, there are key differences in the available phosphate binders as shown in Table 21–2. All of the binders lower phosphorus compared to placebo in short-term studies. Some binders are more potent and thus may require fewer pills. As noted previously, calcium-based phosphate binders became the mainstay of therapy as a replacement for aluminum-based phosphate binders in the 1980s. Calcium-based binders were never subjected to rigorous clinical trials at that time.

The first non–calcium-based binder sevelamer was compared to calcium-based phosphate binders. In most, but not all, studies sevelamer reduced coronary artery calcification compared to calcium-based binders. Sevelamer has also been shown to be associated with reduced mortality by meta-analyses and has reduced incidence of adynamic bone

Table 21–2. Phosphate binders used in chronic kidney disease.

	Aluminum	Calcium Carbonate or Acetate	Magnesium	Lanthanum Carbonate	Sevelamer HCl or Carbonate	Sucroferric Oxyhydroxide	Ferric Citrate
Trade names	Alucaps	Tums, Os-Cal, and Phos-lo	MagneBind Alpharen (under study)	Fosrenol	Renagel and Renvela	Velphoro	Auryxia
Efficacy based on *in vitro* binding	✓✓✓	✓✓	✓✓	✓✓✓	✓✓	✓✓✓	✓✓✓
Absorbed across the intestine and thus potential to accumulate	Yes	Yes	Yes	Yes	No	No	Yes
Nonphosphorus biochemical effects	No	No	No	No	Yes Lowers LDL	No	Yes Increases iron levels
Studies evaluating nonbiochemical endpoints	No May increase risk of aluminum toxicity-muscle weakness, aluminum-induced osteomalacia, and seizures/dementia	Yes Calcium increases risk of low turnover bone disease and in some, but not all, studies increases vascular calcification	No	Yes Does not accumulate in bone long term	Yes Sevelamer decreases risk of low turnover bone disease and in some, but not all, studies decreases vascular calcification, mortality benefit in meta-analysis	No	No

disease on bone biopsies compared to calcium-based binders. Sevelamer may also have pleiotropic effects. However, at this time sevelamer is more expensive than calcium-based phosphate binders, and thus some physicians still prefer calcium-based binders.

Lanthanum carbonate is an alternative non–calcium-containing binder. Initially there were concerns that lanthanum may cause aluminum-like effects of osteomalacia, but this has not been proven in long-term bone-biopsy studies. Lanthanum, similar to sevelamer, has a reduced risk of adynamic bone disease compared to calcium-based binders. However lanthanum, as opposed to sevelamer, has not been the subject of long-term human trials looking at endpoints such as coronary calcification and mortality. Lanthanum is more potent than sevelamer and thus requires fewer pills. The pills must be chewed; swallowing entire pills can lead to gastrointestinal problems.

New to the market in the past few years are two iron-containing phosphate binders. These agents are effective phosphate binders and reduce pill burden compared to sevelamer. Sucroferric oxyhydroxide must be chewed and it increases iron and ferritin levels, whereas ferric citrate does not. Sucroferric oxyhydroxide does not increase iron and ferritin levels. Thus, the choice of iron-based phosphate binders would be determined by the iron needs of the individual patient. To date only biochemical endpoint studies have been conducted with iron based binders; outcome studies have not yet been done with these new agents.

KEY READINGS

Habbous S et al: The efficacy and safety of sevelamer and lanthanum versus calcium-containing and iron-based binders in treating hyperphosphatemia in patients with chronic kidney disease: a systematic review and meta-analysis. Nephrol Dial Transplant 2017;32:111.

Ketteler M, Liangos O, Biggar PH: Treating hyperphosphatemia—current and advancing drugs. Expert Opin Pharmacother 2016;17:1873.

Palmer SC et al: Phosphate-binding agents in adults with CKD: a network meta-analysis of randomized trials. Am J Kidney Dis 2016;68:691.

D. Prescribing Phosphate Binders

In patients not yet on dialysis, one of the unknowns is when to start phosphate binder therapy. In theory, starting phosphate binders early may prevent pathologic rises in PTH and FGF23. However, in the Phosphorus Normalization Trial, large doses of phosphate binders in individuals who had normal phosphorus levels with glomerular filtration rates (GFRs) between 20 and 46 mL/min failed to prevent increases in PTH and FGF23. In addition, they had no effect on coronary calcification or bone density over 9 months of treatment. The doses of phosphate binders given in that trial were large, on average of six to nine pills of the various phosphate binders with meals. Based on this study, beginning phosphate binders is not recommended until patients are hyperphosphatemic. At that point, a dietary history can determine which meal contributes the greatest dietary phosphate, and a simple treatment approach of giving one binder with the largest meal may be effective with mild CKD. Furthermore, if the patient ate a large dairy and protein meal the night before a phosphorus measurement, it is possible that you would get a spurious elevated value. In addition to dietary history, one should take into account the diurnal variation and the wide flux of phosphorus based on the previous day's intake. Phosphorus levels are highest in early morning (4–9 AM) and lowest in the early afternoon. For example, the patient comes to clinic one day in the morning and one day in the afternoon, the phosphorus level may vary as much as 1 mg/dL. Thus, only sustained hyperphosphatemia should be treated with phosphate binders due to the lack of any known efficacy of lowering phosphorus levels by any intervention on patient level outcomes in CKD not yet on dialysis. In contrast, restricting dietary phosphate intake, as long as it does not also excessively restrict protein intake, is likely safe. As noted previously, simply asking the patients to avoid processed and fast food can achieve a number of goals including reduction in phosphate and sodium intake.

KEY READINGS

Block GA et al: Effects of phosphate binders in moderate CKD. J Am Soc Nephrol 2012;23:1407.
Ix JH et al: Effect of dietary phosphate intake on the circadian rhythm of serum phosphate concentrations in chronic kidney disease: a crossover study. Am J Clin Nutr 2014;100:1392.

E. Dialytic Therapy to Remove Phosphorus

Once patients reach dialysis nearly all require phosphate binders, and the quantity of binders needed will increase with loss of residual renal function. Dialysis adds another level of complexity to managing phosphorus. The vast majority of phosphorus is not in the extracellular space. A standard hemodialysis session will lower phosphorus over the first 2 hours and thereafter plateau. After dialysis there is flux from the bone and intercellular stores of phosphorus to bring the level back up to near predialysis levels. The net amount of phosphorus removed with standard thrice weekly hemodialysis is not effective in keeping up with oral intake of phosphate and thus phosphate binders are required. In the frequent hemodialysis study, short daily hemodialysis or nocturnal dialysis, compared to thrice-weekly dialysis was more effective in lowering serum phosphorus and reduced the need for phosphate binders. Nocturnal dialysis was most effective but not directly compared to daily dialysis. Thus daily or nocturnal hemodialysis should be considered in patients in whom phosphorus seems impossible to control. Peritoneal dialysis will also remove phosphorus better than standard hemodialysis due to its more continuous nature, but not to the extent of daily or nocturnal hemodialysis.

KEY READINGS

Copland M et al: Intensive hemodialysis, mineral and bone disorder, and phosphate binder use. Am J Kidney Dis 2016;68:S24.
Sherman RA: Hyperphosphatemia in dialysis patients: beyond nonadherence to diet and binders. Am J Kidney Dis 2016;67:182.

F. Managing Calcium Levels and Balance in CKD

Blood calcium levels only represent 0.01% of total body calcium stores, and only a component of the extracellular calcium that is in the ionized form is involved in homeostatic regulation. Thus, appropriate management of calcium requires looking beyond the serum level and thinking about total body balance. As noted previously, there are two primary goals of mineral metabolism: homeostasis (maintaining normal serum and intracellular levels) and balance (appropriate calcium and phosphorus when bone is growing). In healthy individuals, peak bone mass is achieved by age 25–35 years; thereafter in both sexes there is a gradual bone loss with an accelerated bone loss in women around the time of menopause. In healthy individuals, calcium balance is appropriately positive through young adulthood, but once peak bone mass is achieved, patients are in neutral calcium balance. This implies signaling between bone and the other organs that regulate calcium, including the kidney.

In the presence of CKD, there are impairments in urinary calcium excretion that begin quite early in the course of CKD due to unclear mechanisms. In parallel, levels of $1,25(OH)_2D$ are also reduced, limiting intestinal calcium absorption with a net effect is to limit excess calcium retention. However, when patients are given calcium-based phosphate binders, calcium supplements, or calcitriol and its analogues, there is enhanced intestinal calcium absorption but no increase in urinary excretion. While some of this additional intestinal calcium absorption may go into bone, it is also likely that excess calcium goes into soft tissues and vasculature. If the patient has high turnover bone disease, this calcium would be unlikely to be incorporated into bone. Similarly, if the patient has very low turnover bone disease, the calcium would not be incorporated into bone, leading to increased risk of soft tissue or vascular calcification. Formal balance studies in patients with stages CKD 3b and 4 have demonstrated that calcium intake of levels of greater than 800–1000 mg/day (calcium pills plus diet) leads to positive calcium balance. Because of these studies, 2017 KDIGO guidelines have recommended limiting the calcium intake from binders and diet although no specific maximum intake was provided.

In patients on dialysis, calcium balance is also affected by the calcium content of the dialysate. However, formal balance studies cannot be done in patients on dialysis, as they are not in steady state due to the intermittent nature of dialysis. The total amount of calcium delivered to a patient will be determined by the serum calcium level and dialysate calcium concentration. The most common dialysate calcium concentration used is 2.5 mmol/L (= 5 mEq/L or 10 mg/dL). Thus if a patient's blood level of calcium is less than 10 mg/dL, it is likely that the patient may have net influx of calcium during dialysis. While programs exist to try to quantify the calcium delivered, the assumptions in these formulas make accuracy unlikely. Importantly, a randomized trial of high versus lower calcium dialysate (3.5 vs 2.5 mmol/L) for 1 year demonstrated that patients dialyzed against the 3.5 mmol/L dialysate had progression of coronary artery calcification assessed by CT scan compared to the 2.5 mmol/L dialysate. Importantly, this progression was greatest in patients who simultaneously had hyperphosphatemia.

The amount of elemental calcium differs in calcium acetate and calcium carbonate phosphate binders: Calcium acetate contains 167 mg of calcium per pill and calcium carbonate contains 500 mg of elemental calcium per pill. The two size pills give equivalent phosphate binding, and thus it would be prudent to use calcium acetate over calcium carbonate to minimize calcium intake from binders. Calcium carbonate also comes in multiple strengths. For example, chewable Tums is available in 300 mg calcium, 400 mg calcium, and 500 mg calcium, creating confusion as to what the patient is actually taking. The total daily calcium intake should also take into account dietary intake, which can vary widely. In general, a serving of dairy is approximately 250 mg calcium. Thus if a patient takes in two servings of dairy per day and one calcium acetate with each of three meals, the patient would have an intake of 1001 mg/day. If 500 mg calcium carbonate is given with each meal, the total calcium intake would be 2000 mg. It should be noted that the actual amount of calcium absorbed from each pill is unknown so these are only estimates. In conclusion, avoidance of excess calcium intake through either high calcium dialysate, large calcium dietary intake, or calcium-based binders seems prudent in patients with advanced CKD and those on dialysis.

KEY READINGS

Hill KM et al: Oral calcium carbonate affects calcium but not phosphorus balance in stage 3-4 chronic kidney disease. Kidney Int 2012.

Ok E et al: Reduction of dialysate calcium level reduces progression of coronary artery calcification and improves low bone turnover in patients on hemodialysis. J Am Soc Neph 2016 Aug 27:3475.

Moe SM: Confusion on the complexity of calcium balance. Semin Dial 2010;23:492.

Pun PH, Horton JR, Middleton JP: Dialysate calcium concentration and the risk of sudden cardiac arrest in hemodialysis patients. Clin J Am Soc Nephrol 2013;8:797.

Spiegel DM, Brady K: Calcium balance in normal individuals and in patients with chronic kidney disease on low- and high-calcium diets. Kidney Int 2012;81:1116.

G. Summary and Treatment Guidance for the Management of Phosphorus and Calcium

Managing phosphorus and calcium intake requires knowledge of dietary intake. This should be done in concert with a dietician, but in the absence of a dietician, the physician can ask simple questions such as processed food intake, number of meals, and dairy intake as a surrogate of calcium intake. Most patients can easily comprehend general dietary recommendations of avoiding boxed and canned food and shopping the perimeter of a grocery store. Should hyperphosphatemia persist in either CKD or dialysis patients, phosphate binders should be started. In patients with mild hyperphosphatemia, binders can be given with the largest meal, or with the meal that has the greatest phosphate content (largest protein or dairy intake). With persistent hyperphosphatemia, binders should be given with each meal. In patients poorly controlled hyperphosphatemia despite phosphate binders, the patient may need to take additional binders with snacks. The choice of phosphate binders should be the one the patient tolerates with consideration for non–phosphate-lowering effects and long-term safety profiles as listed in Table 21–1. The amount of calcium intake from diet and calcium-based binders should also be taken into consideration to avoid positive calcium balance. Finally, the frequency of dialysis should be increased in patients with refractory hyperphosphatemia.

3. Treatment of Elevated Parathyroid Hormone

PTH is a uremic toxin. This is predominantly based on animal studies and the clinical improvement in patients after a parathyroidectomy. In vivo testing in the 1980s–1990s demonstrated direct toxicity in rodent models of CKD: cardiomyopathy, vascular disease, neuropathies, and bone abnormalities. In patients post-parathyroidectomy, bone pain goes away; muscle strength improves; itching decreases;

Table 21–3. Pharmacologic agents used to lower parathyroid hormone (form, generic, and trade names).

Native vitamin D	**Vitamin D$_3$** cholecalciferol
	Vitamin D$_2$ ergocalciferol
25-hydroxlated vitamin D	**25-hydroxy-vitamin D$_3$ (calcidiol)** Calderol, Didrogyl, Dedrogyl, Hidro Ferol)
	Extended-release calcifediol (Rayaldee)
Calcitriol prodrugs	**1α(OH)D$_3$ – alfacalcidol** (Alfarol, One-alpha, EinsAlpha, Etalpha, AlphaD$_3$)
	1α(OH)D$_2$ doxercalciferol (Hectorol)
Calcitriol	**1,25(OH)$_2$D$_3$ calcitriol** (Rocaltrol, Calcijex)
Vitamin D analogues	**19-nor-1α25(OH)$_2$D$_2$ paricalcitol** (Zemplar)
Calcimimetics	**Cinacalcet** (Sensipar)—oral **Etelcalcetide** (Parsabiv)—IV

and there is improvement in anemia, neuropathy, mentation, sexual function, blood pressure, and cardiac output. However, most of these benefits were demonstrated in small series. With recent knowledge of FGF23, the potential effect of parathyroidectomy on lowering FGF23 has raised questions about whether the clinical effects observed postparathyroidectomy are direct from PTH, or indirect through changes in lowering FGF23, calcium, and phosphorus. PTH predominately affects cortical bone and can cause increased absorption and porosity resulting in impaired biomechanical instability and increased risk of fractures. Cortical bone is predominantly in the distal radius, some in the hip and very little in the lumbar spine. Thus, bone mineral densitometry should be preferably assessed at the distal radius. Resorption at the edges of the phalanges and distal clavicles can be observed with plain radiographs. Multiple treatments are available that lower PTH (Table 21–3).

KEY READING

Sprague SM, Moe SM: The case for routine parathyroid hormone monitoring. Clin J Am Soc Nephrol 2013;8:313.

A. Vitamin D and Related Compounds

1. Overview of available vitamin D compounds—Vitamin D is synthesized in the skin from ultraviolet light or can be ingested from foods in the form of vitamin D$_2$ (from plants and yeast) and vitamin D$_3$ (from fatty fish and fish oils). Vitamins D$_2$ and D$_3$ are carried to the liver through vitamin D–binding protein. In the liver, both vitamins D$_2$ and D$_3$ are activated to 25(OH)D (also known as *calcidiol*). Calcidiol is then converted to 1,25(OH)$_2$D in the kidney through the

CYP27B1 (1α-hydroxylase enzyme). This same hydroxylation step can occur in many other cells/organs other than the kidney as demonstrated by measurable 1,25(OH)$_2$D levels in anephric patients on dialysis. Both 25(OH)D and 1,25(OH)$_2$D are catabolized by CYP24A1. Recent data have shown that the catabolism by CYP24A1 is stimulated by FGF23. This finding is probably the major reason why 1,25(OH)$_2$D levels are so markedly suppressed in patients with CKD. Similarly, FGF23 stimulation of 25(OH)D catabolism may explain why 25(OH)D levels are lower in patients with CKD than expected. Measurements of 25(OH)D levels are an accurate reflection of intake and sun exposure due to prolonged half-life. However, separation of 25(OH)D$_2$ and 25(OH)D$_3$ levels is not clinically relevant. In contrast, the half-life of 1,25(OH)$_2$D is very short and the assay is expensive and thus routine measurement is not recommended.

The term "vitamin D receptor activator" is often used to differentiate calcitriol and its analogues from cholecalciferol and ergocalciferol, but in reality, all forms of vitamin D activate the receptor. Further complicating nomenclature is that the term vitamin D outside of nephrology is synonymous with cholecalciferol or ergocalciferol, whereas nephrologists generally use the term to identify calcitriol and its analogues. Thus, KDIGO recommends use of the term "nutritional" vitamin D for ergocalciferol or cholecalciferol, and the term "calcitriol and its analogues" for calcitriol, paricalcitol, and doxercalciferol.

Pharmaceutical preparations of vitamin D (see Table 21–3) include cholecalciferol (vitamin D$_3$) and ergocalciferol (vitamin D$_2$). These two vitamin D preparations have similar profiles. In the United States, vitamin D$_3$ is considered an over-the-counter supplement and is in most multivitamins (including renal vitamins), in milk, and supplemented in many foodstuffs. It is also in many "health supplements." In contrast, vitamin D$_2$, ergocalciferol, is considered a prescription drug and thus covered under most insurance plans. Ergocalciferol can be given on a weekly or monthly basis whereas cholecalciferol requires daily use. Once these drugs are converted into 25(OH)D by the liver, they are either converted by the kidney to the biologically active 1,25(OH)$_2$D, or taken up by nonkidney cells (including the parathyroid gland) and converted intracellularly to 1,25(OH)$_2$D to act on the vitamin D response element of many genes. Circulating levels of 25(OH)D are nearly 1000-fold that of 1,25(OH)$_2$D, and thus although 1,25(OH)$_2$D (calcitriol) is a more potent inhibitor of PTH than 25(OH)D calcidiol, nutritional or native vitamin D will suppress PTH.

A new vitamin D analogue, calcifediol (Rayaldee), has been developed and is 25(OH)D$_3$ that has been formulated to be extended release. The sustained levels (in contrast to intermittent dosing) suppresses CYP24A1 and thus prevents catabolism of both the 25(OH)D$_3$ and 1,25(OH)D. In a phase 3 randomized trial comparing califediol to placebo in patients with 25(OH)D levels less than 30 ng/mL and CKD stage 3 or 4, calcifediol lowered PTH, raised $1,25(OH)_2D$ levels, and had no effect of FGF23 levels. No studies have yet been done looking at surrogate or other endpoints in patients with CKD.

Early studies in the 1980s demonstrated efficacy of calcitriol to suppress PTH and improve bone pain and histology. At that time, there was no knowledge of extrarenal conversion of 25(OH)D, and thus it was assumed that calcitriol would be required in patients with kidney disease. When phosphate binders changed from aluminum- to calcium-based binders, hypercalcemia became more common and analogues of calcitriol were designed to maximize PTH suppressive effect and minimize intestinal calcium absorption. In the United States, two such analogues became FDA approved: paricalcitol and doxercalciferol. The latter is a prodrug that is then metabolized to calcitriol similar to alfacalcidol used in other countries. In preclinical studies, these drugs led to less hypercalcemia.

Studies in patients with late-stage CKD and those on dialysis demonstrated greater PTH suppressive effects with calcitriol compared to placebo. In patients on dialysis, observational studies from large dialysis provider databases demonstrated reduced mortality in patients prescribed calcitriol and its analogues compared to those who were not prescribed these drugs. Unfortunately, such studies are biased, as it is nearly impossible to control for the reason the drug was prescribed. A systematic review of these observational studies confirmed a reduction in mortality in patients receiving these agents compared to those who did not. However, to date there are no long-term randomized controlled trials demonstrating efficacy of calcitriol, paricalcitol, or doxercalciferol compared to placebo or each other on patient level endpoints such as mortality, fractures, or hospitalizations.

KEY READINGS

Duranton F et al: Vitamin D treatment and mortality in chronic kidney disease: a systematic review and meta-analysis. Am J Nephrol 2013;37:239.

Jean G, Souberbielle JC, Chazot C: Vitamin D in chronic kidney disease and dialysis patients. Nutrients 2017;9:pii: E328.

Sprague SM et al: Use of extended-release calcifediol to treat secondary hyperparathyroidism in stages 3 and 4 chronic kidney disease. Am J Nephrol 2016;44:316.

Xu C et al: Evaluation of responses to vitamin D3 (cholecalciferol) in patients on dialysis: a systematic review and meta-analysis. J Investig Med 2016;64:1050.

2. Which vitamin D to use?—The native vitamin D preparations are safe because they require conversion to $1,25(OH)_2D$ (calcitriol) by CYP27B1 for efficacy. That step is blocked by hypercalcemia, and thus it is nearly impossible to develop significant hypercalcemia on these "nutritional" vitamin D compounds. A study comparing cholecalciferol to doxercalciferol in stage 3 CKD found equivalence of

PTH suppressive effects. A recent study of 200 CKD stages 3–5 (mostly stage 3) patients found no difference in biochemical outcomes between ergocalciferol dosed weekly and calcitriol dosed daily over 33 months. In contrast, a study comparing ergocalciferol to paricalcitol in stage 4 patients found that paricalcitol was superior in suppressing PTH, and a placebo-controlled study in dialysis patients failed to demonstrate suppression of PTH with ergocalciferol. Thus, although not yet adequately studied, it appears that the efficacy of cholecalciferol and ergocalciferol in suppressing PTH decreases with progressive kidney disease. In addition to PTH-lowering effects, there is some evidence that vitamin D can reduce falls, prevent fractures, and confer an immunoprotective effect in non-CKD patients. Unfortunately, to date, we have no data demonstrating these benefits or any patient-centered outcomes in patients with kidney disease.

In patients not yet on dialysis with secondary hyperparathyroidism, there are no data on long-term effects of any PTH-lowering therapy on patient level endpoints such as mortality, fractures, or hospitalizations. Early studies clearly demonstrated improvement in bone histology in patients with severe hyperparathyroid disease treated with calcitriol, but it is unclear if that effect is observed in patients with mild disease. The data on improving bone in rodents or humans are not convincing. Vitamin D receptors are found in the myocardium, and in animal models calcitriol and other analogues decrease the development of LVH. Vitamin D receptors are also located in the kidney and many other tissues, and thus systemic effects are likely. In contrast, in animal models calcitriol can induce arterial calcification likely due to its effects on increasing intestinal calcium and phosphorus absorption.

In human studies of patients not yet on dialysis, there are relatively few comparative studies. Figure 21–3 shows the change in PTH, calcium, and phosphorus with the available treatments used in CKD stages 3 and 4 based on placebo-controlled trials. The graph demonstrates an increase in calcium and phosphorus in all studies (although not always statistically significant), which is expected given the primary role of $1,25(OH)_2D$ on intestinal absorption. Calcimimetics decrease PTH, but also induced hypocalcemia and hyperphosphatemia. The latter is due to the removal of the phosphaturic effects of PTH and is a major reason not to use these drugs in CKD stages 3 and 4. A 24-week study comparing 1 µg/day of paricalcitol versus 0.25 µg calcitriol in stages 3 and 4 CKD with an intact PTH greater than 120 pg/mL demonstrated equivalent efficacy in suppressing PTH and equivalent increases in calcium and phosphorus of 0.3–0.4 mg/dL.

There are no patient level endpoint studies such as hospitalization, mortality, or fractures in studies evaluating treatment of secondary hyperparathyroidism with vitamin D, calcitriol or its analogues, in patients with CKD not yet on dialysis, and limited surrogate endpoint studies. Two studies have evaluated the effect of paricalcitol on LVH in patients

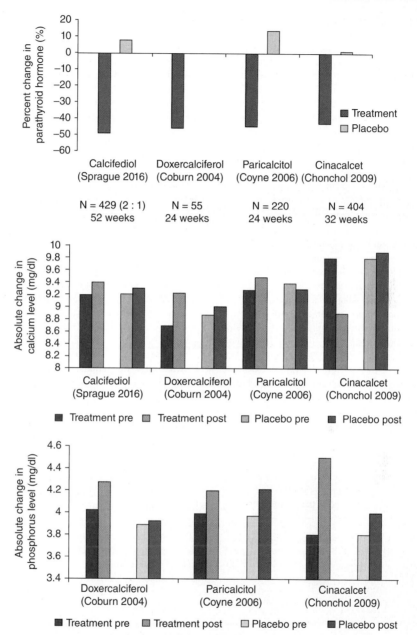

▲ **Figure 21–3.** Efficacy of treatments for elevated parathyroid hormone in patients with stage 3 and 4 CKD in placebo-controlled studies. The change in PTH (A), calcium (B), and phosphorus (C) are shown for various treatments that are available clinically. The duration, sample size, and first author and year are below the graphs. The efficacy of all treatments on PTH is similar. All of the vitamin D derivatives have slight increases in calcium and phosphorus. In contrast, cinacalcet lowers calcium but increases phosphorus. The latter occurs only in patients not yet on dialysis and is likely due to the removal of the phosphaturic effects of PTH. (Adapted, with permission, from on-line education material from the American Society of Nephrology.)

not yet on dialysis, the paricalcitol capsule benefits in renal failure-induced cardiac morbidity (PRIMO) and oral paricalcitol in stage 3–5 CKD (OPERA) studies. In both studies, there was no significant difference in the change in left ventricular mass over 1 year, and yet in both studies there was significant risk of hypercalcemia. Thus, the recent KDIGO update in 2017 noted that the efficacy of calcitriol and its analogues in patients with CKD stages 3–5, and secondary hyperparathyroidism was limited to only to biochemical changes of unclear significance. With the uncertainty of efficacy on patient level endpoints and the risk of hypercalcemia without judicious monitoring, the KDIGO update recommended not routinely giving calcitriol or its analogues in predialysis patients unless the PTH is extremely high and continuing to rise despite conservative approaches. In addition to hypercalcemia, another risk of calcitriol and its analogue therapy is stimulation of FGF23 that is associated with LVH progression in animals and patients with CKD stages 3 and 4. It appears that ER calcifediol may be different and not increase FGF23, but more studies are needed.

In patients on dialysis, radiolabeled calcium studies demonstrated less calcium absorption with paricalcitol compared to calcitriol. In randomized studies comparing intravenous formulations, there was less sustained hypercalcemia with paricalcitol (a secondary analyses of approval trials), but in recent comparisons of oral paricalcitol versus calcitriol, there was no difference in PTH suppression or the change in calcium and phosphorus levels. However, both agents increase FGF23 levels.

KEY READINGS

Coyne DW et al: A randomized multicenter trial of paricalcitol versus calcitriol for secondary hyperparathyroidism in stages 3–4 CKD. Clin J Am Soc Nephrol 2014;9:1620.

Newman CL et al: Calcitriol suppression of parathyroid hormone fails to improve skeletal properties in an animal model of chronic kidney disease. Am J Nephrol 2016;43:20.

Ong LM et al: Randomized controlled trial to compare the efficacy and safety of oral paricalcitol with oral calcitriol in dialysis patients with secondary hyperparathyroidism. Nephrology (Carlton) 2013;18:194.

Thadhani R et al: Vitamin D therapy and cardiac structure and function in patients with chronic kidney disease: the PRIMO randomized controlled trial. JAMA 2012;307:674.

Wang AY et al: Effect of paricalcitol on left ventricular mass and function in CKD—the OPERA trial. J Am Soc Nephrol 2014;25:175.

B. Calcimimetics

Calcimimetics are allosteric activators of the calcium-sensing receptor, and they suppress PTH by "mimicking" the parathyroid gland into thinking that there is elevated calcium. Calcimimetics have been shown to suppress PTH in dialysis patients, but in contrast to calcitriol and its analogues also they lower calcium (sometimes significantly), phosphorus, and FGF23 levels. The intravenous formulation of calcimimetics, etelcalcetide has recently been FDA approved. It is administered three times per week with dialysis. In head-on trials, intravenous etelcalcetide had greater efficacy in lowering PTH than oral cinacalcet, but it also had lower calcium levels. Unfortunately, the intravenous administration did not reduce the side effect of nausea, which occurred in nearly 20% of patients in the head-to-head comparison trial. However, intravenous administration of calcimimetics would improve compliance and therefore indicated in some patients.

Nonbiochemical endpoints have also been studied with cinacalcet. A randomized trial of calcimimetics versus placebo (on a background of vitamin D and phosphate binders) demonstrated no effect on the primary endpoint of vascular calcification in dialysis patients (p = 0.6). However, there was a decrease in progression of aortic valve calcification, and using a different assessment of vascular calcification showed reduced progression. The EVOLVE trial was a large international 5-year event-driven study enrolling nearly 4000 dialysis patients with PTH of greater than 300 ng/mL comparing cinacalcet versus placebo on a background of standard of care therapy, which consisted of phosphate binders in nearly 80% and calcitriol or analogues in approximately 60% of patients. The primary endpoint was a composite of time to all-cause mortality or nonfatal cardiovascular events (myocardial infarction, hospitalization for angina, heart failure, or peripheral events). Secondary endpoints were fracture, parathyroidectomy, cardiovascular death, stroke, and each individual component of the primary endpoint. The initial unadjusted intention to treat analysis was not significant. However, the a priori planned secondary analysis adjusted for usual factors was significant. Fractures were reduced with cinacalcet treatment in an adjusted analysis. Secondary analyses demonstrated greater efficacy of cinacalcet with nonatherosclerotic events compared to atherosclerotic events, and that a reduction in FGF23 by 30% or greater with cinacalcet reduced cardiovascular mortality, heart failure admissions, and sudden cardiac death. Given the primary endpoint of the EVOLVE study was negative, the KDIGO updated guidelines do not state a preference for calcimimetics or calcitriol/analogues at this time.

KEY READINGS

Block GA et al: Effect of etelcalcetide vs cinacalcet on serum parathyroid hormone in patients receiving hemodialysis with secondary hyperparathyroidism: a randomized clinical trial. JAMA 2017;317:156.

Cozzolino M et al: Paricalcitol- or cinacalcet-centred therapy affects markers of bone mineral disease in patients with secondary hyperparathyroidism receiving haemodialysis: results of the IMPACT-SHPT study. Nephrol Dial Transplant 2014;29:899.

Investigators ET et al: Effect of cinacalcet on cardiovascular disease in patients undergoing dialysis. N Engl J Med 2012;367:2482.

Moe SM et al: Effects of Cinacalcet on fracture events in patients receiving hemodialysis: the EVOLVE trial. J Am Soc Nephrol 2015;26:1466.

Wetmore JB et al: A randomized trial of cinacalcet versus vitamin D analogs as monotherapy in secondary hyperparathyroidism (PARADIGM). Clin J Am Soc Nephrol 2015;10:1031.

C. Parathyroidectomy

In patients with refractory hyperparathyroidism despite efforts at lowering PTH with pharmacologic treatments, parathyroidectomy should be considered. The exact PTH level or the duration of disease that requires a parathyroidectomy is not clear. The long-term damage to the bone and other organs with sustained hyperparathyroidism may be of more concern to a patient who will be receiving a kidney transplant, whereas the risk of the operation may be of more concern in a patient with multiple comorbidities. Using the USRDS, long-term risk of fracture and mortality is reduced in patients who underwent a parathyroidectomy compared to matched controls. However, analyses from the EVOLVE study found that patients who underwent a parathyroidectomy were younger with less comorbidities making anything but a randomized trial biased.

KEY READINGS

Kestenbaum B et al: Survival following parathyroidectomy among United States dialysis patients. Kidney Int 2004;66:2010.

Parfrey PS et al: The clinical course of treated hyperparathyroidism among patients receiving hemodialysis and the effect of cinacalcet: the EVOLVE trial. J Clin Endocrinol Metab 2013;98:4834.

Rudser KD et al: Fracture risk after parathyroidectomy among chronic hemodialysis patients. J Am Soc Nephrol 2007;18:2401.

D. Summary and Treatment Guidance for Lowering PTH

The management of CKD-MBD is difficult due to the complexity of the homeostatic system, multiple treatment options without definitive randomized trials, and the effects of each treatment on additional biochemical parameters. Unlike other treatments given to patients with CKD, there are no trials in the general population that can be extrapolated to patients with CKD.

The ideal level or "target" for PTH is controversial (see Table 21–1). In CKD stages 3–4, some PTH rise is expected to help maintain calcium and phosphorus levels. Deciding when to treat patients not yet on dialysis is not straightforward and one must take into account not only the PTH but also the stability of the kidney function. For example, one patient may have CKD due to multiple AKI episodes, and now the kidney function is stable or very slowly declining. If that patient's PTH is 100–150 pg/mL (normal 65 pg/mL) but stable for years because the kidney function is stable, treatment should be less aggressive. In contrast, in a patient with more rapid decline in kidney function, dialysis or transplant in the near future may benefit from keeping the PTH from rising further.

If an elevated PTH level is identified, it is first appropriate to ensure adequate (but not excessive) calcium intake, control of phosphorus, and consider giving cholecalciferol or ergocalciferol. These drugs are less toxic than calcitriol and its analogues because there is an additional safety step to block conversion to calcitriol in the setting of hypercalcemia and hyperphosphatemia due to inhibition of the CYP27B1. Thus, it is nearly impossible to get hypercalcemic on these precursor forms of vitamin D. Should PTH stay elevated and continue to rise, therapy with calcitriol or its analogues can be started. In most cases, starting calcitriol at 0.25 μg thrice weekly will be adequate to suppress PTH and often only 3–6 months of therapy is needed. This approach also minimizes hypercalcemia. The new calcifediol may offer an alternative, but it has not yet been compared to other available agents. Once the parathyroid gland hypertrophies, it is much harder to suppress PTH and thus the main reason to treat elevated PTH in patients with early CKD is to avoid very large glands. After kidney transplantation, the new kidney can appropriately respond to PTH resulting in hypercalcemia. While the glands eventually involute, treatment with cinacalcet may often be required in transplant patients.

In patients on dialysis, initial studies and guideline recommendations from Kidney Disease Outcomes Quality Initiative (K/DOQI) in 2003 suggested a goal of 150–300 pg/mL. This was based on an association between these levels of PTH and normal bone turnover by bone biopsy in dialysis patients. However, the PTH assay used in those studies is no longer available, and it appears that assays that are more recent demonstrate higher PTH levels are associated with normal bone turnover with considerable overlap between low and high PTH levels. Importantly, unlike many other biochemical assays, there is no PTH standard; thus each kit provides its own standard, and thus there is quite a bit of variability among various commercial kits. Thus, the most important thing is to measure PTH using the same assay/lab.

Recent studies from KDIGO and others have demonstrated that PTH levels have an area under the curve about 0.71 in terms of its prediction of bone formation rates. Additional observational studies have demonstrated associations of both markedly elevated and markedly suppressed PTH levels with mortality. The latter usually only occurs in individuals who are malnourished or have severe immobility. The KDIGO guidelines in 2009 recommend that the PTH be kept between a two- to ninefold range over the upper limit of normal for the assay, as these extremes are associated with mortality. Since most assays have an upper limit of 65 pg/mL, this range is 110 to nearly 600 pg/mL. However, the guidelines also clearly state that if the patient is within that range but the levels are rising, treatment should be initiated or increased. Similarly, if a patient has a PTH level within that range but levels are decreasing, therapy should be reduced. The addition of alkaline phosphatase can also help clinicians. In the setting of high bone turnover, the alkaline phosphatase and, more specifically, the bone alkaline phosphatase will be elevated. The choice of treatment should be based on the serum calcium and phosphorus level. In patients with hypercalcemia or hyperphosphatemia, calcimimetics would be the treatment of choice. In patients with hypocalcemia on calcimimetics, the addition of calcitriol or its analogues makes more sense than starting or increasing calcium-based binders as the goal is to lower PTH, not increase calcium balance. It is important to remember that calcimimetics shift the ionized calcium-PTH curve such that lower levels of calcium are expected and the "normal" range for calcium used by laboratories may not be valid when a patient is taking a calcimimetic. Thus, care to differentiate serum calcium level from calcium balance is needed to avoid calcium overload. In patients with well-controlled calcium and phosphorus levels, the choice of PTH lowering therapy is up to physician.

KEY READING

Sprague SM et al: Diagnostic accuracy of bone turnover markers and bone histology in patients with CKD treated by dialysis. Am J Kidney Dis 2016;67:559.

4. Treatment of Bone Loss in Chronic Kidney Disease

In patients at all stages of kidney disease, the risk of hip fracture is substantially greater than the general population. This is likely due to the abnormalities of bone remodeling (with extremes from high turnover due to secondary hyperparathyroidism to low turnover adynamic bone) but also due to changes in the bone architecture from collagen crosslinking abnormalities. Cortical bone is preferentially affected over cancellous bone in renal osteodystrophy, but both compartments are affected. If a patient has low bone mineral density by DXA, it can be assumed that they are at an increased fracture risk, and it is likely that risk is greater in patients with CKD at a given DXA score. However, KDIGO does not recommend routine DXA screening for patients with advanced CKD or those on dialysis, as there are no definitive treatments.

In patients with CKD stage 3 and no evidence of CKD-MBD (meaning normal PTH, calcium, phosphorus), patients can be treated as if they do not have CKD. In these patients, secondary analyses of randomized controlled trials suggest efficacy and safety for bisphosphonates, raloxifene, teriparatide, and denosumab. In patients with CKD stages 3–5 and elevated PTH and/or evidence of CKD-MBD, the treatment must be individualized. All of the currently available antiosteoporosis drugs suppress bone turnover so efficacy will be limited in patients with low bone turnover. The difficulty is that the knowledge of bone turnover cannot be definitively assessed without a bone biopsy. Thus if someone has a fracture in the setting of low bone turnover, reducing that remodeling further with anti-osteoporotic agents may impair bone strength or at minimum is unlikely to be effective. Bone biopsy is the only definitive way to differentiate low from high turnover, and if not available, care should be taken to trend PTH and alkaline phosphatase (preferably bone alkaline phosphatase) and to correct 25(OH) vitamin D levels prior to initiating therapy. If the decision is made to treat bone loss or fracture, there are several options.

Bisphosphonates have not been formally studied in CKD patients and these drugs will reduce bone turnover. Whether that causes adynamic bone disease (paucity of cells in addition to low bone formation rate) is controversial. Clearly in the presence of hyperparathyroid disease or high bone turnover, bisphosphonates would be safe as they principally inhibit osteoclasts. However, the problem with bisphosphonates is that they deposit in the bone and have a half-life of over 10 years, and thus effects are not easily reversible. However, post hoc analyses of large studies evaluating bisphosphonates in patients with low GFR (but not necessarily high PTH) showed similar efficacy in terms of fracture prevention and improving bone mass. Raloxifene, a selective estrogen receptor modulator, has been studied in dialysis patients and increases the bone mineral density. Recombinant PTH (teriparatide; Forteo) is given subcutaneously to simulate an acute rise in PTH as the pulsatile secretion of PTH can induce bone formation (anabolic effect) whereas continuing high levels cause bone resorption. Thus, the intermittent administration of PTH may have a positive bone on patients with CKD. However, no studies have confirmed this potential hypothesis. Studies using denosumab (Prolia) did not exclude patients with CKD. Denosumab is an antibody to the RANK-ligand and prevents RANK from activating osteoclasts. Thus, it is a decoy receptor and makes the osteoclast think that it needs to shut off. It is efficacious in the general population in improving bone density and reducing fractures and has a shorter half-life than bisphosphonates. The few patients treated with CKD also showed similar efficacy, but an increase in the severity of hypocalcemia. Clearly more research is needed in this area.

KEY READINGS

Babayev R, Nickolas TL: Bone disorders in chronic kidney disease: an update in diagnosis and management. Semin Dial 2015;28:645.

Miller PD: Bone disease in CKD: a focus on osteoporosis diagnosis and management. Am J Kidney Dis 2014;64:290.

Moe SM, Nickolas TL: Fractures in patients with CKD: time for action. Clin J Am Soc Nephrol 2016;11:1929.

Ott SM: Bone strength: more than just bone density. Kidney Int 2016;89:16.

Ott SM: Pharmacology of bisphosphonates in patients with chronic kidney disease. Semin Dial 2015;28:363.

Prognosis

Nearly all patients with CKD and estimated GFR (eGFR) less than 60 mL/min have CKD-MBD. The overall prognosis and ease of treatment of CKD-MBD therefore reflect the underlying cause and severity of CKD. Although the focus of therapy has been on biochemical endpoints, there is a major need for studies evaluating the concomitant use of multiple agents on significant patient level endpoints such as fracture and cardiovascular disease.

KEY READINGS

Chonchol M et al: A randomized, double-blind, placebo-controlled study to assess the efficacy and safety of cinacalcet HCl in participants with CKD not receiving dialysis. Am J Kidney Dis 2009;53:197.

Coburn JW et al: Doxercalciferol safely suppresses PTH levels in patients with secondary hyperparathyroidism associated with chronic kidney disease stages 3 and 4. Am J Kidney Dis 2004;43:877.

Coyne D et al: Paricalcitol capsule for the treatment of secondary hyperparathyroidism in stages 3 and 4 CKD. Am J Kidney Dis 2006;47:263.

Sprague SM et al: Use of extended-release calcifediol to treat secondary hyperparathyroidism in stages 3 and 4 chronic kidney disease. Am J Nephrol 2016;44:316.

ACKNOWLEDGMENTS

Dr. Moe is supported by a VA Merit Grant and NIH R01DK11087 and R01DK100306. She is grateful for the assistance of Deb Abbott in the preparation of this chapter.

■ CHAPTER REVIEW QUESTIONS

1. A 50-year-old patient presents with end-stage kidney disease (ESKD) secondary to diabetes on hemodialysis thrice weekly 4 hours each treatment. Her monthly laboratory tests show calcium of 9.2 mg/dL, phosphorus of 7.8 mg/dL, and PTH of 200 pg/mL and stable. She is taking four sevelamer and two calcium acetate drugs with each meal, but some days she has problems taking them due to gastroparesis. The phosphorus levels have been progressively rising despite dietary counseling and multiple phosphate binder changes. She states that she cannot cook for herself due to visual impairment and thus frequently eats processed foods. She also has difficult chewing due to loss of many teeth. Which of the following options will have the greatest impact on her serum phosphorus level?
   A. Continue dietary counseling.
   B. Change phosphate binder to lanthanum as it is a more potent binder than sevelamer.
   C. Encourage the patient to change to daily or nocturnal dialysis if her family is willing to help.
   D. Prescribe a calcimimetic.
   E. Prescribe calcitriol.

2. A 32-year-old African–American woman comes to your clinic with newly diagnosed CKD from poorly controlled hypertension and nonsteroidal anti-inflammatory drug (NSAID) use. Her estimated GFR is 25 mL/min, phosphorus is 4.9 mg/dL (NL range 3.2–4.7 mg/dL), calcium level is 9.2 mg/dL, and PTH is 90 pg/mL (NL up to 65 pg/mL). You have no previous phosphorus levels available. What do you do about the elevated phosphorus level?
   A. Begin treatment with sevelamer 800 mg po tid.
   B. Begin treatment with calcium acetate 667 mg po tid.
   C. Repeat the phosphorus level next visit.
   D. Recommend she avoid processed foods and repeat the phosphorus level next visit.

3. A 56-year-old white woman on dialysis for 8 years has monthly laboratory tests that show calcium of 10.2, phosphorus of 7.4, and PTH of 1200 pg/mL. In review of her chart, the calcium level has fluctuated between 9.7 and 11.0 mg/dL. Her PTH has been between 800 and 2000 pg/mL for 2 years. She has been tried on cinacalcet but became nauseated on the medication. She has been active on the transplant list for 5 years. What should be done about her elevated PTH?
   A. Increase the dose of oral cinacalcet.
   B. Give IV calcimimetics.
   C. Lower her dialysate calcium concentration to lower her calcium level so you can add more calcitriol or vitamin D analogue.
   D. Give her a bisphosphonate to lower the calcium level.
   E. Refer her for a parathyroidectomy.

4. A 62-year-old white female patient with CKD and eGFR of 45 mL/min and no proteinuria is seen in your clinic for routine follow-up. She had undergone a bone mineral density test by DXA ordered by her gynecologist. The result was a T-score of −3.0 at the hip, and −2.8 at the lumbar spine. Her PTH is 60 pg/mL (normal 15–65 pg/mL), her calcium and phosphorus levels are normal, and her 25(OH) vitamin D (calcidiol) level is slightly low. She drinks two glasses of milk per day. What do you recommend be done with the DXA results?

A. Do not intervene as she has CKD and the DXA is not predictive of fracture in CKD.

B. Prescribe ergocalciferol 50,000 units weekly.

C. Prescribe to take 1000 mg/day of calcium supplements.

D. Prescribe to undergo treatment with a bisphosphonate or denosumab.

E. Prescribe calcitriol 0.25 μg daily.

5. Which of the following biochemical changes are typical with treatment of calcitriol?

A. A rise in calcium, no change in phosphorus, and decrease in both PTH and FGF23.

B. A rise in both calcium and phosphorus and decrease in both PTH and FGF23.

C. A rise in both calcium and phosphorus, decrease in PTH, and rise in FGF23.

D. No change in calcium, phosphorus, and FGF23, and a decrease in PTH.

Chronic Renal Failure and the Uremic Syndrome: Nutritional Issues

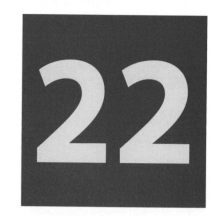

Kamyar Kalantar-Zadeh, MD, PhD, MPH

Joel D. Kopple, MD

Introduction

In patients with chronic kidney disease (CKD), as the glomerular filtration rate (GFR) declines, numerous *nutritional and metabolic disorders* develop, and the *dietary requirements* for many nutrients are altered. These disorders and alterations include, (1) diminished appetite or anorexia; (2) abnormalities in intestinal absorption of certain minerals, for example calcium, and other nutrients including some trace elements (eg, iron, selenium, zinc, and copper) and vitamins (eg, vitamin K, folic acid, riboflavin); (3) abnormalities in urinary, intestinal and dermal excretion of nutrients, including changes in microbiome; and (4) disorders of nutrient metabolism.

Patients with renal insufficiency also are prone to accumulate toxins that normally are eaten in small amounts and would readily be excreted by the kidneys, such as aluminum. There are alterations in the concentrations and/or composition of certain lipoproteins, with an abnormal proportion of individual lipids and altered structure of some apolipoproteins. Potentially toxic oxidants and reactive carbonyl compounds accumulate in plasma and tissues. Deficiencies of antioxidants may predispose to increased oxidative stress. Oxidative stress, along with the occurrence of inflammation in renal insufficiency, increases the risk of endothelial injury and atherosclerosis, leading to cardiovascular disease and higher death rates that is usually observed in patients with advanced CKD.

Additionally, in people at very high risk of CKD such as those with diabetes mellitus or hypertension or persons after cancer or donor nephrectomy, nutritional management including dietary adjustments such as balancing protein and salt intake may mitigate the risk of incident CKD. This is important given CKD pandemics that may be mitigated by nutritional interventions.

▶ Malnutrition & Protein–Energy Wasting

Patients with moderate to advanced CKD (stages 3–5) or persons with any stage of CKD and significant proteinuria (>0.3 g/kg/day) frequently suffer from *protein–energy wasting* (PEW) or at high risk of PEW. The PEW is defined as the state of decreased body protein mass with or without fat depletion or a state of diminished functional capacity due to protein–energy depletion, which is usually caused at least partly by inadequate nutrient intake relative to nutrient demand and/or which is improved by nutritional repletion. In CKD, several conditions may contribute to PEW and are discussed below. Because these conditions may be caused by factors in addition to inadequate nutrient intake, the more inclusive term "wasting" (or protein–energy wasting) should be used instead of malnutrition, which is more specific to nutrient intake and balance. It is important to recognize that in advanced CKD, that is, stages 4 and 5 CKD or estimated GFR (eGFR) less than 30 mL/min/1.73 m² of body surface area (BSA), there are different types of PEW including muscle and fat wasting and true malnutrition. In advanced CKD, malnutrition is particularly likely to occur for calcium, iron, zinc, and vitamins C, B_6, folic acid, and 1,25-dihydroxycholecalciferol.

Approximately one-third to one-half of patients with advanced CKD, including those undergoing maintenance dialysis therapy, have mild to moderate PEW, and 5–10% more have severe protein–energy malnutrition. In malnourished CKD patients, *decreased* relative body weight or body mass index (BMI, body weight [kg] divided by the square of body height in m²), skinfold thickness (an estimate of body fat), arm muscle diameter area (a reflection of muscle mass), total body nitrogen and potassium, and *increased* total body water and extracellular water (Table 22–1) are usually observed. PEW is also manifested by decreased concentrations

Table 22–1. Manifestations of PEW in patients with progressive CKD.

Decreased food intake and diminished appetite
Low body weight (BMI or standardized height-for-weight)
Decreased total body fat percent and skinfold thickness
Decreased muscle mass and arm circumference
Low growth rate in children, or failure to thrive in adults
Decreased total body nitrogen
Increased levels of acute phase proteins and proinflammatory cytokines
Decreased levels of albumin, prealbumin, transferrin, and cholesterol
Decreased levels of plasma amino acids

BMI, body mass index; CKD, chronic kidney disease; PEW, protein–energy wasting.

of many serum proteins, including albumin, prealbumin, and transferrin. Serum lipoprotein concentrations including total cholesterol may also be reduced. Low growth rates are observed in children with advanced CKD. Increased levels of proinflammatory cytokines occur frequently.

The *Modification of Diet in Renal Disease* (*MDRD*) study indicated that the dietary protein and energy intake and the nutritional status begin to decline when the GFR is about 25–38 mL/min/1.73 m². In a cross-sectional analysis of the baseline data obtained in over 1700 individuals with stages 3–5 CKD, a gradual but persistent decline in serum transferrin and albumin concentrations (Figure 22–1), body weight, mid-arm muscle circumference, and percent body fat was observed parallel the GFR reduction. A decreased energy intake was also observed when the GFR was reduced below about 25–35 mL/min/1.73 m².

KEY READINGS

Guarnieri G et al: Mechanisms of malnutrition in uremia. Kidney Int 1997;52:S41.
Kopple JD et al: Effect of dietary protein restriction on nutritional status in the Modification of Diet in Renal Disease study. Kidney Int 1997;52:778.
Obi Y et al: Latest consensus and update on protein-energy wasting in chronic kidney disease. Curr Opin Nutr Metab Care 2015;18:254.
Pupim LB, Flakoll PJ, Ikizler TA: Protein homeostasis in chronic hemodialysis patients. Curr Opin Clin Nutr Metab Care 2004;7:89.

▶ Causes of Protein–Energy Wasting in CKD

Table 22–2 lists potential causes of PEW in CKD.

A. Inadequate Nutrient Intake

Anorexia, a salient manifestation of renal insufficiency, worsens as CKD progresses and is thought to be engendered by uremic toxins. Serum *leptin* levels, a hormone known to induce anorexia, is also elevated in uremia. Several studies describe an inverse relationship between serum leptin and dietary protein intake or a direct relation between serum leptin and weight loss in dialysis patients. Elevated serum leptin levels in CKD can be caused by impaired degradation by the diseased kidney and possibly also by insulin stimulates leptin synthesis in CRI patients who are often hyperinsulinemic. *Inflammation*, which is commonly present in renal insufficiency, is associated with increased levels of proinflammatory cytokines, including interleukin-6 (IL-6) and tumor necrosis factor-α (TNF-α), each of which is known to induce anorexia. Derangements in ghrelin and adiponectin may play roles as well.

Other reasons for inadequate food intake include the debilitating effects of renal insufficiency and underlying illnesses (eg, diabetes mellitus including diabetic gastroparesis), the impact of the progressive illness on the patient's ability to eat, and emotional disorders. Whereas recommending low-protein diet (LPD) for CKD management has been blamed, it is highly unlikely that an LPD in the range of 0.6–0.8 g/kg ideal body weight per day (g/kg/day) plays any significant role. However, imposing restrictions in intake of potassium and phosphorus may lead to nutrients that are less heart healthy (eg, by restricting fresh fruits and vegetables) or less palatable to the patient and difficult to prepare.

B. Increased Losses of Nutrients

The dialysis procedure itself may promote wasting by removing nutrients. During routine hemodialysis there are losses of about 6–10 g of free amino acids when patients are postabsorptive (fasting) and about 8–10 g, when they are postprandial. Approximately 2–3 g of peptides or bound amino acids is also removed. The use of high flux polysulfone hemodialyzers may lead to greater losses of amino acids. During peritoneal dialysis (PD), about 2–3.5 g of free amino acids, 8–9 g of total protein, and 5–6 g of albumin are lost into the dialysate per day. With mild peritonitis, the quantity of protein removed increases to an average of 15 g/day; peritoneal protein losses as high as 100 g/day have been reported in severe peritonitis. Protein losses fall rapidly with antibiotic therapy but may remain elevated for many days to weeks.

Water-soluble *vitamins* and other bioactive compounds are also removed by both hemodialysis and PD. Although these vitamin losses can be theoretically replaced from the diet or by multivitamin supplementations, these measures may be suboptimal in patients with poor nutrient intake due to a myriad of clinical, social or financial barriers.

Finally, many CKD patients often lose substantial quantities of blood secondary to occult gastrointestinal bleeding, frequent blood sampling for laboratory testing, and the sequestration of blood in the hemodialyzer. Since blood

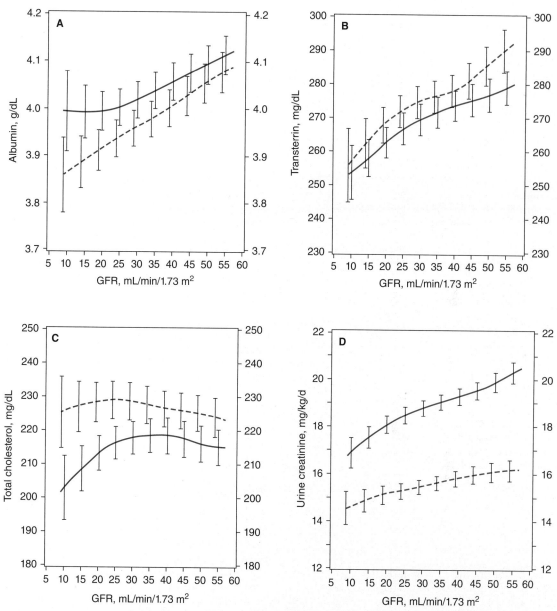

▲ **Figure 22–1.** Mean levels of biochemical measures of nutritional status as a function of GFR in MDRD study. The estimated mean levels with 95% confidence limits of biochemical nutritional markers are shown as a function of glomerular filtration rate (GFR) (males, solid line; females, dashed line) controlling for age, race, and use of protein- and energy-restricted diets. In men, the slope of the relationship was greater at GFR = 12 than GFR = 55 mL/min/1.73 m^2 for serum total cholesterol ($P = 0.014$). (A) Males, $N = 1065$ ($P = 0.004$); females, $N = 698$ ($P < 0.001$). (B) Males, $N = 1065$ ($P < 0.001$); females, $N = 698$ ($P < 0.001$). (C) Males, $N = 1063$ ($P = 0.052$); females, $N = 694$ ($P = 0.63$). (D) Males, $N = 1017$ ($P < 0.001$); females, $N = 664$ ($P < 0.001$). (Printed, with permission, from Kopple JD et al: Relationship between nutritional status and the glomerular filtration rate: results from the MDRD study. Kidney Int 2000;57(4):1688–1703.)

Table 22–2. Causes of PEW in CKD patients.

A. Inadequate nutrient intake
1. Anorexia[a]
   (a) Caused by uremic toxicity
   (b) Caused by impaired gastric emptying
   (c) Caused by inflammation with or without comorbid conditions[a]
   (d) Caused by emotional and/or psychological disorders
2. Dietary restrictions
   (a) Prescribed restrictions: low-potassium, low-phosphorus dietary regimens
   (b) Social constraints: poverty, inadequate dietary support
   (c) Physical incapacity: inability to acquire or prepare food or to eat

B. Sources of nutrient loss in dialysis patients
1. Loss through hemodialysis membrane into hemodialysate
2. Adherence to hemodialysis membrane or tubing
3. Loss into peritoneal dialysate

C. Hypercatabolism caused by comorbid illnesses
1. Cardiovascular diseases[a]
2. Diabetic complications
3. Infection and/or sepsis[a]
4. Other comorbid conditions[a]

D. Hypercatabolism associated with dialysis treatment
1. Negative protein balance
2. Negative energy balance

E. Endocrine disorders of uremia
1. Resistance to insulin
2. Resistance to growth hormone and IGF-1
3. Increased serum level of and sensitivity to glucagons
4. Hyperparathyroidism
5. Other endocrine disorders

F. Acidemia with metabolic acidosis
G. Concurrent nutrient loss with frequent blood losses
H. Inflammation (see Table 22–3)

CKD, chronic kidney disease; IGF-1, Insulin-like growth factor 1; PEW, protein–energy wasting.

[a]The given condition may also be associated with inflammation.

is rich in protein, these blood losses may contribute to additional protein wasting. For example, a person with a hemoglobin of 12 g/dL and a serum total protein of 7 g/dL will lose approximately 16.5 g of protein in each 100 mL of blood removed.

C. Increased Net Catabolism

CKD patients usually suffer from additional concurrent *comorbid conditions*, which often induce a hypercatabolic state and also may physically prevent ingestion, gastrointestinal absorption, or assimilation of foods (eg, pancreatitis, gastrointestinal surgery). Hemodialysis per se can enhance *net protein breakdown* and promote negative nitrogen balance.

More bio-*in*compatible hemodialysis membranes, such as Cuprophane, are more likely to stimulate the release of interleukins and promote net protein degradation than are more biocompatible membranes. The accumulation of endogenously formed *uremic toxins* might engender wasting more directly. In renal failure, there are increased plasma or tissue concentrations of probably hundreds of metabolic products. Some of these compounds are bioactive and may have catabolic or antianabolic actions.

Acidemia enhances decarboxylation of branched chain amino acids and engenders protein catabolism in skeletal muscle, bone reabsorption, and negative nitrogen balance. The *endocrine disorders* of uremia may also promote wasting. Resistance to the actions of insulin and insulin-like growth factor-1 (IGF-1) and hyperglucagonemia may promote protein wasting. Parathyroid hormone (PTH) increases hepatic gluconeogenesis and may lead ultimately to protein wasting. It is not clear whether fibroblast growth factor 23 (FGF-23) plays any role in PEW. The findings that 1,25 dihydroxy-cholecalciferol has pervasive effects on calcium metabolism, that vitamin D deficiency may cause a proximal myopathy, and that 25 hydroxycholecalciferol stimulates muscle protein synthesis in vitro suggest that deficiency of 1,25 dihydroxycholecalciferol might be another cause muscle protein wasting.

Exogenously derived uremic toxins and accumulated elements (eg, aluminum) may cause debility and possibly wasting. Finally, since the kidney synthesizes or degrades many biologically active compounds including certain amino acids, peptide hormones, other peptides, glucose, and fatty acids, it is possible that loss of these metabolic activities of the kidney in renal failure may disrupt the body's metabolism and promote PEW.

D. Inflammation

Advanced CKD and the dialysis treatment process may sustain inflammation and an associated acute phase response with elevation of serum acute phase proteins and reduction in negative acute phase proteins. Potential causes of inflammation in CKD patients are listed in Table 22–3. In maintenance dialysis patients, indicators of inflammation are correlated with anorexia, wasting, and malnutrition. These findings, together with the known catabolic effects of some proinflammatory cytokines, have bolstered the conclusion that inflammation promotes wasting. With inflammation, serum concentrations of negative acute phase proteins decrease; these include albumin, transferrin, retinol-binding protein, transthyretin (prealbumin), and certain lipoproteins. Most surveys suggest that the serum concentration of C-reactive protein (CRP), a marker of inflammation, is increased (>3 mg/L) in about 30–50% of American and European dialysis patients and perhaps in a lower proportion of Asian patients. It has been argued that these

Table 22–3. Possible causes of inflammation in CKD patients.

A. Causes of inflammation due to CKD or decreased GFR

1. Decreased clearance of proinflammatory cytokines
2. Volume overload[a]
3. Oxidative stress (eg, oxygen radicals)[a]
4. Carbonyl stress (eg, pentosidine and advanced glycation end products)
5. Decreased levels of antioxidants (eg, vitamin E, vitamin C, carotenoids, selenium, glutathione)[a]
6. Deteriorating protein–energy nutritional state and food intake

B. Coexistence of comorbid conditions

1. Inflammatory diseases with kidney involvement (SLE, HIV, etc)
2. Increased prevalence of comorbid conditions (CVD, DM, advanced age, etc)[a]

C. Additional inflammatory factors related to dialysis treatment

I. Hemodialysis

1. Exposure to dialysis tubing
2. Dialysis membranes with decreased biocompatibility (eg, cuprophane)
3. Impurities in dialysis water and/or dialysate
4. Back-filtration or back-diffusion of contaminants
5. Foreign bodies (eg, PTFE) in dialysis access grafts
6. Intravenous catheter

II. PD

1. Episodes of overt or latent peritonitis[a]
2. PD catheter as a foreign body and its related infections
3. Constant exposure to PD solution

CKD, chronic kidney disease; CVD, cardiovascular disease; DM, diabetes mellitus; GFR, glomerular filtration rate; HIV, human immune deficiency virus; PD, peritoneal dialysis; PTFE, polytetrafluoroethylene; SLE, systemic lupus erythematosus.
[a]Indicates that the given factor may also be associated with PEW without inflammation.

elevated cytokines may promote PEW in CKD patients both by inducing anorexia and also by engendering protein catabolism, for example by activation of proteolytic enzymes released from granulocytes or by suppressing protein synthesis. Indeed, albumin synthesis is often suppressed when serum CRP is elevated.

Both biocompatible and bioincompatible hemodialysis membranes, hemodialysis tubing, and filters, both functioning and old thrombosed arteriovenous synthetic grafts, other vascular accesses and PD catheters, hemodialysate and possibly peritoneal dialysate solutions, and low-grade infections, such as caused by chlamydia, may stimulate the inflammatory response in CKD patients by activating monocytes and/or macrophages. These inflammatory cells then release the cytokines (eg, IL-6 and TNF-α) that stimulate the

acute phase response. Finally, both *oxidants* and *carbonyl* compounds, as well as a deficiency of antioxidants, may cause tissue injury and inflammation and possibly engender a catabolic state.

KEY READINGS

Ikizler TA et al: Amino acid and albumin losses during hemodialysis. Kidney Int 1994;46:830.
Ikizler TA et al: Increased energy expenditure in hemodialysis patients. J Am Soc Nephrol 1996;7:2646.
Kalantar-Zadeh K et al: Appetite and inflammation, nutrition, anemia and clinical outcome in hemodialysis patients. Am J Clin Nutr 2004;80:299.
Kovesdy CP, Kalantar-Zadeh K: Novel targets and new potential: developments in the treatment of inflammation in chronic kidney disease. Expert Opin Investig Drugs 2008;17:451.
Stenvinkel P et al: IL-10, IL-6, and TNF-alpha: central factors in the altered cytokine network of uremia—the good, the bad, and the ugly. Kidney Int 2005;67:1216.

▶ Malnutrition–Inflammation Cachexia Syndrome & Clinical Outcome

Nutritional status is a powerful predictor of *morbidity* and *mortality* and *quality of life* in CKD patients. Low dietary protein intake, decreased body weight for a given height such as BMI, and low serum concentrations of albumin, transthyretin, urea, creatinine, cholesterol, bicarbonate, and phosphorus are also associated with higher death risk in dialysis patients. Serum albumin is probably the strongest predictor of mortality in maintenance dialysis patients with a strictly linear and incremental association with survival (Figure 22–2). Some of these measurements such as daily protein intake (DPI), (as determined by normalized protein catabolic rate [nPCR]) also known as normalized protein nitrogen appearance [nPNA]) and serum concentrations of cholesterol, phosphorus, and bicarbonate have a J- or U-curve relationship with mortality, in that both low and very high values are associated with a poor survival.

Since obesity and hypercholesterolemia are paradoxically associated with better survival and lower cardiovascular death in maintenance dialysis patients, a *reverse epidemiology* of cardiovascular risk factors has been described. This phenomenon, also known as *obesity paradox* or *lipid paradox*, is believed to be mostly due to the overwhelming effect of PEW and inflammation, both of which are common in CKD. Indeed, according to some investigators, the strong association observed between PEW and mortality in CKD patients is because of an atherogenetic role of inflammation. Because the causes and consequences of PEW and inflammation overlap considerably and many of the clinical manifestations of PEW and inflammation are identical, the term "malnutrition–inflammation cachexia syndrome" (MICS) has been suggested to indicate the close associations between

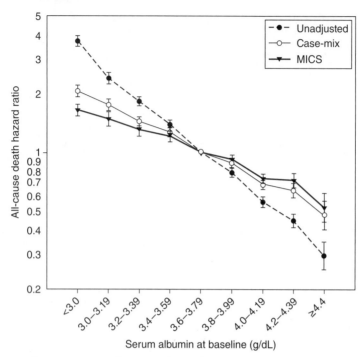

▲ Figure 22–2. Association between serum albumin and mortality in maintenance dialysis patients. MICS, malnutrition–inflammation complex syndrome.

PEW and inflammation in CKD patients and their link to clinical outcome (Figure 22–3).

The occurrence of measures indicating the presence of either PEW or inflammation in CKD or maintenance dialysis patients has become of great concern to researchers and clinicians, because there is a strong association between the markers of MICS such as hypoalbuminemia, hypocholesterolemia and underweight, and an increased death risk. This issue is of particular importance because in maintenance dialysis patients the mortality rate, especially due to cardiovascular disease, has remained inappropriately high, 10–20% per year, and because such traditional cardiovascular risk factors as hypertension, hypercholesterolemia, and obesity not only do not appear to be associated with this high death risk, but paradoxically they show a protective effect, that is, the reverse epidemiology. The *time discrepancy* between competing risk factors may play a role, in that the deleterious effects of undernutrition are usually manifested within a much shorter period of time when compared to the consequences of overnutrition, which usually requires a longer time to become manifest. According to this theory, many dialysis patients may die prematurely of undernutrition before they can experience the cardiovascular consequences of overnutrition. Hence, in patients with advanced CKD the priority management is targeting PEW rather than obesity,

whereas obesity is a cause of incident CKD, but once CKD in present and advanced, it may paradoxically confer survival advantages.

KEY READINGS

Kalantar-Zadeh K et al: Diets and enteral supplements for improving outcomes in chronic kidney disease. Nat Rev Nephrol 2011;7:369.

Kalantar-Zadeh K et al: Malnutrition-inflammation complex syndrome in dialysis patients: causes and consequences. Am J Kidney Dis 2003;42:864.

Kalantar-Zadeh K et al: The obesity paradox in kidney disease: how to reconcile it with obesity management. Kidney Int Rep 2017;2:271.

Rhee CM, Ahmadi SF, Kalantar-Zadeh K: The dual roles of obesity in chronic kidney disease: a review of the current literature. Curr Opin Nephrol Hypertens 2016;25:208.

▶ Assessment of Nutritional Status in CKD Patients

Classically, four major lines of inquiries, that is, dietary intake, biochemical measurements, body composition, and composite scores (based on measures from the prior three categories), are used to assess the protein–energy nutritional status in

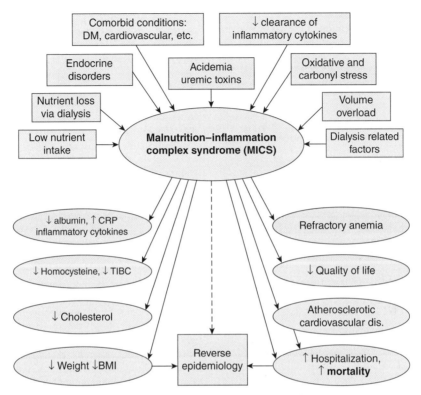

▲ **Figure 22–3.** Schematic representation of the causes and consequences of the protein–energy wasting, also known as malnutrition–inflammation complex syndrome or malnutrition–inflammation-atherosclerosis. BMI, body mass index; CRP, C-reactive protein; DM, diabetes mellitus; TIBC, total iron-binding capacity.

CKD patients as indicated in Table 22–4. The most frequently used composite scores include the *subjective global assessment of nutritional status* (SGA) and *malnutrition–inflammation score* (MIS). More technologically based nutritional measures that have been used in CKD patients include *dual energy X-ray absorptiometry* (DEXA), total body nitrogen or potassium measurements, underwater weighing, *bioelectrical impedance* analysis, and *near-infrared interactance*. Many of these nutritional assessment tools also reflect inflammation and provide a measure of its severity. Hence, the overlap between PEW and inflammation exists both at the diagnostic and at the etiologic levels. The MIS provides a numerical value between 0 and 30 and is currently among the most frequently used tools for rating the severity of PEW in CKD patients.

▶ Dietary Protein Intake in the Management of CKD

Different methods to slow the rate of progression of chronic renal insufficiency (CRI) in CKD patients are discussed in Chapters 27 and 38. LPDs are one such method. There have been primarily three types of low-nitrogen diets that have been used for the treatment of patients with CKD: (1) an LPD providing about 0.6–0.8 g protein/kg ideal body weight/day (g/kg/day); (2) a very low-protein diet (VLPD) providing approximately 16–20 g/day of protein of miscellaneous quality (ie, about 0.3–0.4 g/kg/day) supplemented with about 10–20 g/day of the nine L essential amino acids; and (3) any of the above, LPD, or VLPD, but generally supplemented with four essential amino acids histidine, lysine, threonine, and tryptophan, as well as and the keto-acid or hydroxy-acid analogues of the other five essential amino acids, and sometimes with a few other amino acids added. This is sometimes referred to as keto-diet.

In one of the study arms of the MDRD study, those prescribed the 0.6–0.8 g/kg/day diet had faster declines in GFR during the first 4 months, but thereafter, the rate of decline in the GFR in the LPD group was significantly slower than in the group ingesting a usual protein and phosphorus diet. If the trend toward slower progression of renal failure in the LPD groups that was present after month 4 until the termination of the MDRD study had persisted during a longer follow-up

Table 22–4. Systematic classification of the assessment tools for evaluation of PEW in patients with advanced CKD.

A. Nutritional intake
1. Direct: diet recalls and diaries, food frequency questionnaires[a]
2. Indirect: based on UNA: nPNA (nPCR)[a]

B. Body composition
1. Weight-based measures: BMI, weight-for-height, edema-free fat-free weight[a]
2. Skin and muscle anthropometry via caliper: skinfolds, extremity muscle mass[a]
3. Total body elements: total body potassium
4. Energy-beam–based methods: DEXA, BIA, NIR[a]
5. Other energy-beam–related methods: total body nitrogen
6. Other methods: underwater weighing

C. Scoring systems
1. Conventional SGA and its modifications (eg, DMS, MIS, CANUSA version)[a]
2. Other scores: HD-PNI, others (eg, Wolfson, Merkus, Merckman)[a]

D. Laboratory values
1. Visceral proteins (negative acute phase reactants): albumin, prealbumin, transferrin[a]
2. Lipids: cholesterol, triglycerides, other lipids and lipoproteins[a]
3. Somatic proteins and nitrogen surrogates: creatinine, SUN
4. Growth factors: IGF-1, leptin
5. Peripheral blood cell count: lymphocyte count

BIA, bioelectrical impedance analysis; BMI, body mass index; CANUSA, Canada–USA study-based modification of the SGA; CKD, chronic kidney disease; CRP, C-reactive protein; DEXA, dual-energy X-ray absorptiometry; DMS, dialysis malnutrition score; HD-PNI, hemodialysis prognostic nutritional index, IGF-1, insulin-like growth factor 1; IL, interleukin (eg, IL-1 and IL-6); MIS, malnutrition–inflammation score; NIR: near-infrared interactance; nPCR, normalized protein catabolic rate; nPNA, normalized protein nitrogen appearance; SAA, serum amyloid A; PEW, protein–energy wasting; SGA, subjective global assessment of nutritional status; SUN, serum urea nitrogen; TNF-α, tumor necrosis factor-α; UNA, urea nitrogen appearance.
[a]Indicates that the given tool also may be altered by inflammation.

period, significantly slower progression probably would have been observed with the LPD of 0.6–0.8 g/kg/day, as compared to a usual (1–1.2 g/kg/day) protein diet, in one arm of the study; and the very low protein, ketoacid-amino acid supplemented diet as compared with the 0.60 g/protein/lg/day diet in the other arm of the study. Several meta-analyses indicate that LPD is effective is slowing the rate of progression of CKD to renal replacement therapy. Thus, taken together with other published research in this field, the results of the MDRD study are interpreted to indicate that dietary protein and phosphorus restriction will retard the rate of progression of renal failure in patients with progressive renal disease. On average, this effect, although clear-cut, is not dramatic and often requires many months of treatment to become evident.

Independent of CKD progression rate, patients ingesting LPDs are reported to be started on dialysis at lower GFRs than individuals eating higher protein intakes. This is likely because LPDs lead to less generation of nitrogenous compounds and, hence, less uremic toxin accumulation. Long-term follow-up analyses of the MDRD study patients showed that the combined hazard ratio of either dialysis initiation or all-cause mortality in those assigned to the 0.6–0.8 g/kg/day diet versus those assigned to higher-protein diet was significantly lower, suggesting another benefit of LPD. A retrospective analysis of the Nurses' Health Study showed that in women with CKD stage 2, a trend toward faster fall in GFR was observed in those who described ingesting a higher dietary protein intake. In renal transplant recipients ingesting a higher-protein diets lead to greater losses of GFR as well. Taken together, the data point to the probability that LPD may not only retard the rate of CKD progression but also delay the onset of the need for maintenance dialysis therapy by mitigating uremia and independent of an effect on progression. Because LPD often engenders sufficiently lower uremic toxicity for a given level of reduced renal function, patients fed these diets may be able to defer or avoid dialysis therapy at GFR levels that would require individuals ingesting higher protein intakes to commence such therapy. Hence, LPD is the most promising method to postpone transition to dialysis treatment. We also recommend concomitant low sodium intake of less than 4 g/day, although some guidelines recommend even lower sodium intake of less than 2.3 g/day.

A. Recommended Dietary Protein Intake in CKD

For CKD stages 1 and 2 (GFR >60 mL/min) and mild proteinuria (<0.3 g/day) as well as patients at very high risk of CKD such as those with diabetes or hypertension and those after cancer or donor nephrectomy, we recommend 0.8–1 g/kg/day dietary protein intake per kg/day unless there is evidence that renal function is continuing to decline, in which case the lower level of 0.6–0.8 g/kg/day should be pursued. In patients with substantial proteinuria (>0.3 g/day) and in patients with CKD stages 3–5 not yet on dialysis, an LPD of 0.6–0.8 is recommended, which may not only retard progression but also mitigate uremic symptoms and delay dialysis initiation. At least half of the protein should be of high biologic value to ensure a sufficient intake of the essential amino acids. For advanced CKD (stages 4 and 5), the potential advantages to using an LPD are more compelling, especially since at this degree of renal failure, the LPD will generate less nitrogenous compounds that are potentially toxic both systemically and to the kidney itself. Moreover, the LPD generally contains less phosphorus and potassium, the low intake of which is usually imperative at this advance renal failure stage. An LPD of 0.6–0.8 g/kg/day will generally maintain neutral or positive nitrogen balance as long as energy intake is not deficient, that is, 30–35 cal/kg/day. Many persons with progressive CKD are willing and able to adhere to diets providing 0.6–0.8 g/kg/day protein, relatively low-salt diet less than 4 g/day, and adequate energy intake of 30–35 cal/kg/day.

Patients on maintenance dialysis without residual kidney function (urea clearance <1.5 mL/min) should receive relatively high-protein diet of 1.2–1.4 g/kg/day (see the following justification). This is of particular importance especially on dialysis days for thrice-weekly or more frequent dialysis patients. In patients who transition gradually from nondialysis to "incremental" dialysis, that is, initially only once- to twice-weekly hemodialysis sessions, some data suggest maintaining an LPD (0.6–0.8 g/kg/day) on nondialysis days, combined with a high-protein diet (1.2–1.4 g/kg/day) on the dialysis treatment days. This regimen is thought to lead to longer preservation of the residual kidney function.

In the past, in patients with stage 5 CKD (eGFR <15 mL/min/1.73m²) who did not undergo maintenance dialysis but exhibited signs of PEW despite vigorous attempts to optimize protein and energy intake, initiation of maintenance dialysis or a renal transplant was recommended. Recent data appear to be in favor of delaying the initiation of dialysis therapy as long as the patient is stable and not at high risk of adverse consequences of uremia or PEW, especially if the rate of progression of renal insufficiency is very slow, even if the eGFR may be quite low, for example in the range of 5–15 mL/min/1.73m².

Nitrogen balance studies suggest that most maintenance dialysis patients on thrice-weekly or more frequent hemodialysis or high-dose PD without substantial residual kidney function (urea clearance <1/5 mL/min) require more than 1 g/kg/day to maintain both protein balance and normal total body protein. The high protein requirement can be due to the fact that maintenance dialysis patients have increased dietary protein requirements because of the removal of amino acids and peptides by the dialysis procedure and possibly because hemodialysis appears to stimulate protein catabolism by engendering an inflammatory, catabolic response. Most guidelines currently recommend 1.2–1.4 g/kg/day for clinically stable patients undergoing full dose (thrice-weekly) maintenance hemodialysis or chronic PD.

B. Dietary Protein Intake and Its Assessment

Since the control of protein intake is central to the nutritional management of patients with renal insufficiency, it is important to accurately monitor nitrogen intake. Because urea is the major nitrogenous product of net protein and amino acid degradation, the *urea nitrogen appearance* (UNA) can be used to estimate total nitrogen output and hence nitrogen intake. UNA is the amount of urea nitrogen that appears or accumulates in body fluids and is removed in all outputs (eg, urine, dialysate, fistula drainage). In addition

to dietary interviews and assessments, in CKD patients who are not yet on dialysis, the 24-hour urine collection should be used to assess adherence to restricted protein and sodium intake. The so-called low-protein diets (LPDs) and very low-protein diets (VLPDs) usually represent a DPI of 0.6–0.8 g/kg/day and 0.3–0.4 g/kg/day, respectively. To monitor the adherence to a DPI of protein intake can be achieved by estimating it (eDPI) using 24-hour urinary urea nitrogen (UUN) where 1 g UN represents 6.25 g of protein and non-urea nitrogen excretion of 30 mg/kg/day along with urinary protein losses if greater than 5 g/day:

$$eDPI \ (g/day) = 6.25 \times UUN \ (g/day) + 0.03 \times weight \ (kg) + proteinuria \ (g/day)$$

The same 24-hour urine collection should also be used to examine 24-hour urinary creatinine (to estimate muscle mass and to calculate 24-hour creatinine clearance), potassium (target <2–3 g/day), phosphorus (target <1000 mg/day), sodium (target <4 g/day although some guidelines suggest <2.3 g/day), and fluid intake (<1.5 L/day). If the eDPI is greater than 0.8 g/kg/day, more dietary counseling including higher intake of vegetarian meals may be considered. If the intake is less than 0.6 g/kg/day or if there are signs of PEW, oral nutritional supplementation with products specially designed for CKD should be considered. Because adequate calorie intake is needed to spare protein and prevent vitamin and mineral deficiencies, it is important to ensure a dietary energy intake of at least 30–35 cal/kg/day to avoid energy malnutrition.

In dialysis-dependent patients, the *dietary protein intake* can be estimated by both dietary interviews and diaries and the nPCR, also known as the nPNA, that is, protein equivalent of total nitrogen appearance normalized to the volume of distribution of urea or some other function of body mass. Patients on maintenance dialysis without residual kidney function (urea clearance <1.5 mL/min) should receive relatively high-protein diet of 1.2–1.4 g/kg/day. This is of particular importance especially on dialysis days for thrice-weekly or more frequent dialysis patients. The nPCR can be used to monitor to this end.

KEY READINGS

Bolasco P et al: Dietary management of incremental transition to dialysis therapy: once-weekly hemodialysis combined with low-protein diet. J Ren Nutr 2016;26:352.

Eriguchi R et al: Longitudinal associations among renal urea clearance—corrected normalized protein catabolic rate, serum albumin, and mortality in patients on hemodialysis. Clin J Am Soc Nephrol 2017;12:1109.

Kalantar-Zadeh K et al: North American experience with low protein diet for non-dialysis-dependent chronic kidney disease. BMC Nephrol 2016;17:90.

Ko GJ et al: Dietary protein intake and chronic kidney disease. Current Opin Clin Nutr Metab Care 2017;20:77.

Ravel VA et al: Low protein nitrogen appearance as a surrogate of low dietary protein intake is associated with higher all-cause mortality in maintenance hemodialysis patients. J Nutr 2013;143:1084.

Shinaberger CS et al: Longitudinal associations between dietary protein intake and survival in hemodialysis patients. Am J Kidney Dis 2006;48:37.

▶ Energy Intake in CKD Patients

In nondialyzed CKD patients and patients undergoing maintenance dialysis, energy expenditure, measured by indirect calorimetry, appears to be normal during resting and sitting, following ingestion of a standard meal, and with defined exercise. Nitrogen balance studies in nondialyzed stage 5 CKD patients ingesting 0.55–0.6 g/kg/day indicate that the amount of energy intake necessary to ensure neutral or positive nitrogen balance is approximately *35 kcal/kg/day*. On the other hand, virtually every study of the dietary habits of nondialyzed stages 4 and 5 CKD patients and dialysis patients indicates that their mean energy intakes are lower than this level, usually about 24–27 kcal/kg/day. The practice guidelines currently recommend that the energy intake for nondialyzed patients with advanced CKD (eGFR <25 mL/min/1.73m²) and for maintenance dialysis patients should be *35 kcal/kg/day* for individuals who are younger than 60 years and *30–35 kcal/kg/day* for those who are 60 years or older, who are usually more sedentary (Table 22–5). The same energy intakes are recommended for people with stage 3 or 4 CKD (ie, GFR <60 mL/min/1.73 m²).

KEY READINGS

Fouque D et al: A proposed nomenclature and diagnostic criteria for protein-energy wasting in acute and chronic kidney disease. Kidney Int 2008;73:391.

National Kidney Foundation I, Kidney Disease-Dialysis Outcome Quality Initiative. K/DOQI Clinical Practice Guidelines for nutrition in chronic renal failure. Am J Kidney Dis 2000;35:S1.

▶ Management of Other Nutritional Factors in CKD

The number and magnitude of the changes in the dietary intake and restrictions for CKD patients may be so great that if they were all presented to the patient at one time, the patient could become demoralized and lose his/her motivation to comply with the diet. One therefore needs to prioritize goals for dietary treatment. Usually the importance of controlling the protein, phosphorus, sodium, energy, potassium, and magnesium intake and the need to take calcium and vitamin supplements should be emphasized. On the other hand, unless the patient has a lipid disorder or other risk factors that indicate there is a high odds ratio for adverse

Table 22–5. Recommended dietary nutrient intake for adult patients undergoing maintenance hemodialysis.

Macronutrients and Fiber	
Dietary protein intake (DPI)[a]	1.2–1.4 g/kg body weight/day for clinically stable maintenance hemodialysis (MHD) patients (at least 50% of the dietary protein should be of high biological value) >1.4 g/kg/day may be necessary for acutely ill patients
Daily energy intake (DEI)[b]	30–35 kcal/kg body weight/day for those who are aged <60 years and 30–35 kcal/kg body weight/day for individuals aged ≥60 years.
Fat intake[c]	30% of total energy intake
Total fat[c,d]	30% of total energy intake
Saturated fat[c]	Up to 10% of total energy intake
Polyunsaturated—saturated fatty acids[c]	Up to 10% of total calories
Monounsaturated fatty acids[c]	Up to 20% of total calories
Carbohydrate[c–e]	Rest of nonprotein calories
Total fiber[f]	25–30 g/day

[a]According to K/DOQI guidelines.
[b]Refers to percent of total energy intake (diet plus dialysate).
[c]Although atherosclerotic vascular disease constitutes a common and serious problem for MHD patients, these recommendations are often hard to adhere to. Moreover, there is no prospective interventional study indicating these dietary modifications are beneficial for MHD patients, although, reasonably, the potential benefits of these modifications seem valuable. They are strongly recommended only if patients adhere closely to more critical aspects of the diet (eg, sodium, water, potassium, phosphorus, protein, and energy intake), and have expressed a particular interest in these modifications or have a specific disorder that may respond to their medications.
[d]Refers to percent of total energy intake; if triglyceride levels are very high, the percentage of fat in the diet may be increased to about 35% of total calories; otherwise, 25–30% of total calories is preferable. Intake of fatty acids should be kept low because they raise LDL cholesterol (see text).
[e]Should be primarily complex carbohydrates.
[f]Less critical to adhere to the typical MHD patient.

cardiovascular events, the recommended quantity and types of dietary carbohydrate, fat and fiber are discussed with the patient, but adherence to these dietary guidelines are not as strongly emphasized. If the patient has complied well with the other, more critical elements of dietary therapy, has a specific lipid disorder that may benefit from dietary therapy, or has expressed an interest in modifying fat, carbohydrate or fiber intake, then the modification of the dietary intake of these latter nutrients is explored more intensively with the patient.

A. Lipids

Elevated serum triglyceride levels are common in stages 4 and 5 CKD. Hypertriglyceridemia is caused primarily by impaired catabolism of triglyceride-rich lipoproteins. The reduced catabolic rate leads to increased quantities of apo-B–containing triglyceride-rich lipoproteins in IDL and VLDL and reduced concentrations of HDL. Since diets for renal failure patients are usually restricted in protein, sodium, potassium, and water, it is often difficult to provide sufficient energy without resorting to intakes of purified sugars that may increase triglyceride production. In PD patients, the glucose load in the peritoneal fluid appears to further increase serum triglycerides and cholesterol. Low serum HDL-cholesterol, a common phenomenon in CKD patients, appears to be an independent risk factor for adverse coronary artery disease.

Although the treatment of altered lipid levels and the risk of cardiovascular disease are highly recommended in early stages of CKD and among renal transplant patients, it is currently somewhat controversial in advanced CRI including in maintenance dialysis patients. This is due to several considerations: (1) A *reverse epidemiology* of cardiovascular risk factors has been observed in hemodialysis patients, in that a higher cholesterol level and BMI are paradoxically associated with better survival; (2) a clinical trial known as The 4D Study (*Die Deutsche Dialyse Diabetes Studie*) did not show any survival advantage of using atorvastatin in diabetic dialysis patients; and (3) according to the lipoprotein-endotoxin hypothesis, adequate levels of lipoproteins may be needed to neutralize the proinflammatory effects of circulating endotoxins that can be prevalent among patients with heart failure or fluid overload. In general, it is believed that serum cholesterol is a marker of nutritional status and/or inflammation, so that a low serum cholesterol is associated with a poor outcome, especially among maintenance dialysis patients. Currently there are no consistent data with regard to LDL and HDL in CKD patients.

Omega-3 fatty acids (eg, eicosapentaenoic acid and docosahexaenoic acid, which are found in fish oil) lower serum triglycerides and have more variable effects on serum LDL cholesterol and HDL cholesterol. Fish oil also decreases platelet aggregation and appears to exert anti-inflammatory effects, and omega-3 fatty acids may enhance immune function.

Low-fat diets and lipid-lowering medicines may retard the rate of progression of renal failure in some but not all animal models of CKD. In humans, some research suggests that taking supplements rich in omega-3 fatty acid may lower the progression of renal failure in renal transplant patients.

A preponderance of studies suggests that omega-3 fatty acids given as fish oil may retard the rate of progression of IgA nephropathy. Racial disparities have been observed in that African–American dialysis patients appear to eat higher saturated fat than Caucasian patients.

Abnormal carnitine metabolism (see below) has also been implicated as a cause of hypertriglyceridemia in CKD. However, the many studies of treatment of hypertriglyceridemia with carnitine in CKD patients are divided between substantial numbers that show carnitine lowers serum triglycerides and substantial numbers that show no change or, rarely, a rise in serum triglycerides.

At present, there is no consensus as to what dietary fat constellation is the most appropriate for CKD patients. Whereas we recommend a *therapeutic lifestyle changes* (TLC) diet for those with mild to moderate CKD not on maintenance dialysis treatment (Table 22–6), there are no supportive data to this end, although across all stages of CKD, a

Table 22–6. Nutrient composition of the therapeutic lifestyle change (TLC) diet.

Nutrient	Recommended Intake
Saturated fat[a]	<7% of total calories
Polyunsaturated fat	Up to 10% of total calories
Monounsaturated fat	Up to 20% of total calories
Total fat	25–35% of total calories
Carbohydrate[b,c]	50–60% of total calories
Fiber	20–30 g/day
Protein[c]	Approximately 15% of total calories
Cholesterol	<200 mg/day
Total calories[d]	Balance energy intake and expenditure to maintain desirable body weight/prevent weight gain

[a]*Trans*-fatty acids are another LDL-raising fat that should be kept at a low intake.
[b]Carbohydrates should be derived predominantly from foods rich in complex carbohydrates, including grains, especially whole grains, fruits, and vegetables.
[c]Dietary content of protein and, hence, carbohydrate should be modified according to the specific needs of the MHD (ie, 1.20 g protein/kg/day) (see text).
[d]Daily energy expenditure should include at least moderate physical activity (contributing approximately 200 kcal/day).
Adapted from Executive Summary of the Third Report of the National Cholesterol Education Program (NCEP) Expert Panel on Detection, Evaluation, and Treatment of High Blood Cholesterol in Adults (Adult Treatment Panel III). JAMA 2001;285(19):2486–2497.

higher intake of poly- and mono-unsaturated fat is preferred including olive oil and cannula oil products. We treat hypertriglyceridemia by dietary modification only when serum triglycerides are greatly elevated (>200 or 300 mg/dL). In this situation, dietary fat intake should not be above 40% of total calories. A high proportion of dietary carbohydrates should be complex. These modifications often lower the palatability of the diet; therefore, the patient's total energy intake must be monitored closely to ensure that it does not fall. With high serum triglyceride values that are unresponsive to dietary therapy, a fibrate (eg, fenofibrate) may be tried. L-*Carnitine* about 500–1000 mg/day, or, for hemodialysis patients, L-carnitine, 10–20 mg/kg/day at the end of each dialysis three times weekly, may be tried if hypertriglyceridemia is severe and unresponsive to these treatments.

B. Carnitine

Carnitine is a naturally occurring compound that is essential for life. It is both synthesized in the body and ingested. Carnitine facilitates the transfer of long-chain (>10 carbon) fatty acids into muscle mitochondria. Since fatty acids are the major fuel source for skeletal and myocardial muscle at rest and during mild to moderate exercise, this activity is considered necessary for normal skeletal and cardiac muscle function. Patients undergoing maintenance dialysis do not infrequently have low serum-free carnitine and, in some but not all studies, low skeletal muscle-free and total carnitine levels. Carnitine deficiency could be due to impaired synthesis of carnitine in vivo, reduced dietary intake of carnitine, and removal of carnitine by dialysis. The weekly loss of free carnitine by dialysis is reported to be approximately equal to the normal weekly urinary excretion of carnitine. However, the finding that serum-free carnitine is normal in nondialyzed patients with stage 5 CKD and is low in maintenance dialysis patients is consistent with the thesis that dialysis of L-carnitine is the major cause of low serum carnitine in maintenance dialysis patients.

A number of clinical trials in patients with CKD, particularly those undergoing maintenance dialysis therapy, suggest that L-carnitine may provide clinical benefits, including (1) increased physical exercise capacity, (2) reduced interdialytic symptoms of skeletal muscle cramps or hypertension, (3) improvement in overall global sense of well-being or various symptoms often found in CRI patients, (4) improved response of anemia to erythropoietin treatment, (5) decrease in predialysis serum urea, creatinine and phosphorus, and (6) increase in midarm muscle circumference. However, not all clinical trials confirm these findings.

L-Carnitine can be administered to MHD or PD patients who suffer from disabling or very bothersome skeletal muscle weakness or cardiomyopathy, skeletal muscle cramps or hypotension during hemodialysis treatment, severe malaise, or anemia refractory to erythropoietin therapy and, in whom the above conditions do not respond to more standard treatment. The patient can then be given a 3- to 6-month trial of L-carnitine (up to 9 months for refractory anemia). L-Carnitine may be administered orally, intravenously or into dialysate. Oral L-carnitine is less expensive, but its intestinal absorption may be somewhat unpredictable. A dose of 20 mg/kg at the end of each hemodialysis, three times weekly, can be prescribed.

C. Sodium and Water

In both normal individuals and people with CKD, about 1–3 mEq (mmol) per day of sodium is excreted in the feces. In the absence of visible sweating, only a few millimoles per day of sodium are lost through the skin. Because both the glomerular filtration and the fractional reabsorption of sodium fall parallel to each other as renal insufficiency progresses in CKD patients, most patients with renal failure are able to maintain sodium balance with a normal sodium intake if they do not have heart or liver failure. Patients with advanced renal failure who receive large loads of sodium, particularly as sodium chloride, may be unable to excrete the quantity of sodium ingested, and they may develop edema, hypertension, and congestive heart failure. This syndrome is particularly likely to occur in stages 4 and 5 CKD with worsening isosthenuria. In these patients, hypertension often is more easily controlled when they are sodium restricted, and hypertension may be accentuated by an increased sodium intake, probably because of expanded extracellular fluid volume and possibly due to altered intracellular electrolyte composition within arteriolar smooth muscle cells that increase contractility. Moreover, the antiproteinuric effects of angiotensin-converting enzyme inhibitor (ACEIs) and probably angiotensin receptor blockers (ARBs) are substantially abrogated by even moderate sodium intakes; as urinary sodium excretion rises above about 100 mmol/day (2.3 g/day), the antiproteinuric effects abate. In most nondialyzed patients with advanced renal failure, a daily intake of 1–3 g/day of sodium (45–130 mmol/day) and 1–1.5 L/day of fluid will maintain sodium and water balance. The requirement for sodium and water varies markedly, and each patient must be managed individually. However, it is important to note that hyponatremia tends to happen more frequently in CKD and is associated with poor outcomes. Moreover, a recent large study with serial urinary sodium assessments as surrogates of dietary sodium intake suggested that a dietary sodium intake more than 4 g/day is associated with poor CKD outcomes, but no additional gains was observed with lower sodium intake. In the absence of clinical trial data, we suggest that dietary sodium intake should not exceed 4 g/day in CKD patients or in persons at very high risk of CKD. In nondialyzed CKD patients who gain excessive sodium or water despite attempts at dietary restriction, a potent loop diuretic, such as furosemide or bumetanide, may be tried to increase urinary sodium and water excretion.

Patients undergoing frequent hemodialysis (thrice-weekly or more) tend to lose their residual kidney function faster and become anuric. For hemodialysis patients, sodium and total fluid intake generally should be restricted as above. Since sodium and water can be removed easily and continuously with PD, a more liberal salt and water intake is usually allowed. Indeed, by maintaining a larger dietary sodium and water intake, the quantity of fluid removed from the CPD patient and hence the daily dialysate outflow volume can be increased. This may be advantageous, since with CPD the daily clearance of small- and middle-sized molecules is directly related to the volume of dialysate outflow. Thus for some CPD patients, a higher sodium and water intake (eg, 6–8 g/day of sodium and 3 L/day of water) may enable the patient to use more hypertonic or hyperoncotic dialysate to increase the dialysate outflow volume, thereby increasing dialysate clearances and, if hypertonic glucose is used, and energy uptake from dialysate.

D. Potassium

Approximately 90% of daily potassium intake is excreted through the kidneys. Potassium excretion occurs mostly in the cortical collecting duct and is regulated by aldosterone and distal nephron sodium delivery. Because of the relative state of fluid overload and the frequent suppression of the renin-angiotension-aldosterone axis, due to volume expression, diabetes mellitus and/or ACEIs, ARBs, and aldosterone blockers, potassium tends to be retained in advanced CKD. This is accentuated by diminished distal nephron sodium delivery in the setting of low GFR.

Fecal excretion of potassium is increased due to its enhanced intestinal secretion, and dietary restriction and anorexia can decrease intake. Nonetheless, hyperkalemia does not happen infrequently in patients with advanced CKD. Factors promoting hyperkalemia in CKD include (1) excessive intake of potassium (eg, by taking nonsodium salts or fast food with potassium based preservatives); (2) acidemia; (3) worsening oliguria, for example due to superimposed acute renal failure; (4) catabolic stress or tissue degradation; (5) possibly hypoinsulinism or hyperglycemia (solvent drag) in diabetic patients; and (6) use of medicines such as ACEIs and ARBs, aldosterone receptor blockers (eg spironolactone, eplerenone), nonsteroidal anti-inflammatory drugs, and β-receptor blockers.

Patients with stage 4 or 5 CKD (ie, GFR <30 mL/min), including those undergoing maintenance hemodialysis, should generally receive no more than 75 mEq/day (about 3 g/day) of potassium. Those with frequent hyperkalemia (>5.5 mEq/L) should restrict their potassium to less than 2 g/day if possible. However, it is important to note that many types of fresh fruits and vegetables and other healthy food contain substantial amounts of potassium. Their restriction by rigid dietary regimens deprive CKD patients, who already have a high risk of cardiovascular disease, from most important sources of antiatherogenic foods and neutraceuticals and may cause constipation, which per se is associated with poor outcomes. PD patients are an exception, since they tend to develop hypokalemia due to potassium losses in their peritoneal fluid, so that they can enjoy more liberal potassium intake.

E. Magnesium

In CKD patients, the difference between dietary intake and fecal excretion of magnesium (net absorption) amounts to about 40–50% of ingested magnesium. Since the absorbed magnesium is excreted primarily by the kidney, hypermagnesemia may occur in advanced CKD. Magnesium also commonly accrues in bone in renal failure and may play a causal role in renal osteodystrophy. The restricted diets of stage 4 or 5 CKD patients are low in magnesium (usually about 100–300 mg/day for a 40-g protein diet). Patients' serum magnesium levels are therefore usually normal or only slightly elevated unless they take substances that are high in magnesium content, such as magnesium-containing antacids and laxatives. Nondialyzed patients with stage 5 CKD require about 200 mg/day of magnesium to maintain neutral magnesium balance. The optimal dietary magnesium allowance for the maintenance dialysis patient has not been well defined. Experience suggests that when the magnesium content is about 1 mEq/L in hemodialysate or 0.50–0.75 mEq/L in peritoneal dialysate, a dietary magnesium intake of 200–300 mg/day will maintain the serum magnesium at normal or only slightly elevated levels.

F. Phosphorus

Mineral and bone disorders (MBDs) including management of renal osteodystrophy in CKD are discussed in Chapter 21. This chapter reviews the rationale for controlling dietary phosphorus and the use of gastrointestinal binders of phosphorus, hyperphosphatemia, calcium phosphorus deposition in soft tissue, and hyperparathyroidism. The dietary phosphorus intake and the use of phosphorus binders therefore are discussed here only briefly. Lower serum phosphorus levels, especially in dialysis patients without residual kidney function (urea clearance <1.5 mL/min), usually indicate severe PEW and have been shown to correlate with high risks of death in maintenance dialysis patients even after extensive multivariate adjustments for other markers of PEW. Since there is a rough correlation between the protein and phosphorus content of the diet, it is much easier to reduce phosphorus intake if a lower protein in the diet is used. However, this is at the risk of causing or worsening PEW. Since added inorganic phosphorus as preservatives is much more easily absorbable (up to 100%) as opposed to natural phosphorus (which is only 40–60% absorbable unless high vitamin D doses are given), it is important to reduce fast food or preserved food in CKD patients. Moreover, phosphorus in vegetables and fruits are in form of phytate which is hardly absorbable.

Hence, the traditional recommendation to avoid legumins, nuts, or chocolates for their high phosphorus contents has been questioned.

In dialysis patients, serum phosphorus between 3.5 and 5.5 mg/dL is often targeted. This often requires the patients to ingest a low-phosphorus diet intake of about 800–1000 mg/day or foods with lower phosphorus-to-protein ratio such as egg white which has less than 2 mg/g of phosphorus-to-protein ratio, as opposed to egg yolk that has about 25 mg/g of this ratio. The risk of PEW and hypoalbuminemia is quite high with very low amounts of protein intake among maintenance dialysis patients. Maintenance dialysis patients often require phosphorus binders to prevent more severe hyperphosphatemia unless they have substantial residual kidney function or receive frequent (daily) hemodialysis.

G. Calcium

The role of calcium in CKD associated renal osteodystrophy and the management of bone disease is discussed in detail in Chapter 21. Whereas in the past it was believed that patients with advanced CKD patients usually have an increased dietary requirement for calcium because of vitamin D deficiency and resistance to the actions of vitamin D, recent data suggest that less calcium intake is prudent given higher risk of vascular calcification and other tissue deposition of calcium. Foods high in calcium content are usually high in phosphorus (eg, dairy products) and are therefore restricted for CKD patients. For example, a 40 g of protein diet generally provides only about 300–400 mg/day of calcium, whereas the recommended dietary allowances (RDAs) for healthy, nonpregnant, nonlactating adults are about 800–1200 mg/day. Recent balance studies indicate that persons with moderate CKD should not take more than 1000 mg/day of dietary calcium, while those on maintenance dialysis are recommended not to take more than 800 mg/day. Supplemental calcium should not be given unless the serum phosphorus concentration is normal to reduce the risk of calcium phosphorus deposition in soft tissues. In addition, frequent monitoring of serum calcium is important because hypercalcemia (>10.5 mg/dL) may develop. This is especially likely to occur if the patient also has hyperparathyroidism, a common complication of chronic renal failure.

KEY READINGS

Kalantar-Zadeh K et al: Understanding sources of dietary phosphorus in the treatment of patients with chronic kidney disease. Clin J Am Soc Nephrol 2010;5:519.

Kovesdy CP et al: Hyponatremia, hypernatremia, and mortality in patients with chronic kidney disease with and without congestive heart failure. Circulation 2012;125:677.

Noori N et al: Dietary omega-3 fatty acid, ratio of omega-6 to omega-3 intake, inflammation, and survival in long-term hemodialysis patients. Am J Kidney Dis 2011;58:248.

Noori N et al: Racial and ethnic differences in mortality of hemodialysis patients: role of dietary and nutritional status and inflammation. Am J Nephrol 2011;33:157.

Rhee CM et al: Pre-dialysis serum sodium and mortality in a national incident hemodialysis cohort. Nephrol Dial Transplant 2016;31:992.

▶ Trace Elements in CKD Patients

Trace elements are those elements that are present in the body at concentrations less than 50 mg/kg. Recent advances in analytic methodology allow for accurate measurements of trace element levels in body fluids. The main source of body trace elements is diet. However, the blood and tissue levels of these elements may be affected by nondietary factors, including renal excretory function, environmental and occupational exposure, duration of renal failure, concentrations in the fresh dialysate, in flow, and, possibly, the mode of dialytic therapy. Also, many trace elements are largely protein bound. In CRI, there may be altered serum levels of binding protein levels or increased serum concentrations of compounds that compete for binding sites on these proteins; such factors may also cause major alteration in serum trace element concentrations independently of the body burden or nutritional needs for these elements. The PEW in CKD patients may lead to low serum protein concentrations and may be one of the causes of low serum zinc, manganese, and, possibly, selenium and nickel in CKD patients.

Because many trace elements are present in minuscule amounts in the plasma and are protein bound, losses during dialysis may be minimal. However, a substantial amount of bromide and zinc is removed during hemodialysis because a large proportion of the serum concentrations is not protein bound and because the levels in fresh dialysate are quite low. Conversely, the presence in the dialysate of even minute quantities of certain trace elements may lead to uptake by the body because of the avidity with which some trace elements bind to proteins. This phenomenon has been observed for lead, copper, and zinc. Table 22–7 shows the dietary recommendations for some trace elements in maintenance dialysis patients.

KEY READINGS

Kalantar-Zadeh K, Kopple JD: Trace elements and vitamins in maintenance dialysis patients. Adv Ren Replace Ther 2003;10:170.

Vanholder R et al: Trace elements metabolism in renal failure. In: Kopple JD, Massry SG (editors). *Nutritional Management of Renal Disease*, 2nd ed. Philadelphia: Lippincott, Williams & Wilkins, 2003, pp 299–314.

Table 22–7. Recommended dietary intake of trace elements for adult patients with advanced CKD.

Macronutrients	Daily Requirement in CRI	Toxicity Reported with Excessive Intake
Iron[c]	Dependent on EPO treatment and other factors	Yes
Zinc	15 mg/day	
Selenium	Not known	No data available in CKD
Copper	Not known	Yes
Aluminum	Not known	Yes

CKD, chronic kidney disease; CRI, chronic renal insufficiency; EPO, erythropoietin.

[a]Phosphate binders (aluminum carbonate or hydroxide, or calcium carbonate or acetate) often are needed to maintain normal serum phosphorus levels.

[b]These calcium intakes are commonly ingested because of the use of calcium binders of phosphate. Excess calcium intake must be avoided (see text).

[c]Iron requirements vary according to the dose of administered erythropoietin.

▶ Vitamin Requirements in CKD

CKD patients are at increased risk for deficiencies of several vitamins. The causes for vitamin deficiencies include (1) reduced total food intake due to anorexia; (2) prescription of low-phosphorus, low-potassium diets that have restrict intake of such nutritionally valuable foods as fresh fruits and vegetables, dairy products, and other items that are high in vitamins; (3) altered metabolism, as is the case for pyridoxine and possibly folate; (4) impaired synthesis (eg, for 1,25-dihydroxyvitamin D); (5) resistance to the actions of vitamins (eg, vitamin D and possibly folate); (6) decreased intestinal absorption (eg, decreased intestinal absorption of riboflavin, folate, and vitamin D have been described in rats with CRI); and (7) dialysate losses of water-soluble vitamins.

In some studies, CKD patients who did not receive vitamin supplements generally did not develop signs of vitamin deficiency when followed longitudinally. Based on these findings, some authors have questioned the need for vitamin supplementation for maintenance dialysis patients. However, recent reports continue to show that many CKD patients ingest a vitamin intake that provides less than the recommended dietary allowances, and there is a small but persistent prevalence of deficiencies for some water-soluble vitamins (as well as for 1,25—dihydroxyvitamin D) in CKD patients not taking vitamin supplements. At present, it does not seem feasible to identify, a priori, those patients

who will develop vitamin deficiencies. Since the intake of water-soluble vitamins at the proposed levels appears to be safe, we propose that these vitamins be supplemented. Table 22–8 shows the dietary recommendations for various vitamins in maintenance dialysis patients. The RDAs that are proposed for each of the water-soluble vitamins and for vitamin A are similar to those of normal individuals except for higher doses of pyridoxine HCl (10 mg/day, 8.2 mg/day of pyridoxine) and folic acid (about 1 mg/day). Vitamin C is recommended at the daily allowance levels (70 mg/day)

Table 22–8. Recommended dietary intake of selected vitamin for adult patients with advanced CKD.

Macronutrients	Daily Requirement	Toxicity Reported with Excessive Intake
Vitamin B$_1$ (thiamin)	1.1–1.2 mg/day	
Vitamin B$_2$ (riboflavin)	1.1–1.3 mg/day	
Pantothenic acid	5 mg/day	
Biotin	30 µg/day	
Niacin	14–16 mg/day	
Vitamin B$_6$ (pyridoxine)	10 mg/day	
Vitamin B$_{12}$	2.4 µg/day	
Vitamin C	75–90 mg/day	Yes
Folic acid[d]	1–10 mg/day	
Vitamin A	See text	Yes
Vitamin D	See text	Yes
Vitamin E[e]	400–800 IU (optional, see text)	
Vitamin K[f]	See text	

[a]Phosphate binders (aluminum carbonate or hydroxide, or calcium carbonate or acetate) often are needed to maintain normal serum phosphorus levels.

[b]These calcium intakes are commonly ingested because of the use of calcium binders of phosphate. Excess calcium intake must be avoided (see text).

[c]Iron requirements vary according to the dose of administered erythropoietin.

[d]At least 1 mg/day of folic acid should be given, but up to 10 mg/day may be administered to reduce elevated plasma homocysteine levels.

[e]Vitamin E, 300 or 800 IU day, may be given to reduce oxidative stress and prevent cardiovascular disease, but the value of these supplements is controversial (see text).

[f]Vitamin K supplements may be needed for patients who are not eating and who receive antibiotics.

because of the risk of increased oxalate formation at higher intakes. Some studies indicate that vitamin E has an anti-oxidant effect in chronic dialysis patients and may protect against cardiovascular events.

KEY READINGS

Chazot C, Kopple J: Vitamin metabolism in renal disease. In: Kopple JD, Massry SG (editors). *Nutritional Management of Renal Disease*, 2nd ed. Philadelphia: Lippincott, Williams & Wilkins, 2003, pp 315–356.

Kalantar-Zadeh K, Kopple JD: Trace elements and vitamins in maintenance dialysis patients. Adv Ren Replace Ther 2003;10:170.

▶ Acid-Base Management in Renal Insufficiency

CKD patients with moderate to advanced renal failure frequently develop metabolic acidosis. This is usually associated with a mild to moderate increase in anion gap because there is impaired ability of the kidney to excrete acidic metabolites. In the earlier stages of renal insufficiency, and occasionally with advanced renal failure, hyperchloremic (nongap) metabolic acidosis may also be caused by excessive renal losses of bicarbonate. Ingestion of LPDs may prevent or decrease the severity of the acidosis because the endogenous generation of acidic products of protein metabolism will be reduced. Metabolic acidemia may engender oxidation of branched chain amino acids and protein catabolism, impair albumin synthesis, increase β_2-microglobulin turnover, cause bone loss, possibly predispose to inflammation, and cause symptoms of weakness and lethargy. The acidemia-induced increased proteolysis in skeletal muscle appears to be caused by enhanced activity of the ATP-dependent ubiquitin-proteosome pathway.

Pertinent guidelines recommend that the serum bicarbonate should be measured once monthly in all maintenance dialysis patients and that the predialysis or stabilized serum bicarbonate should be maintained at or above 22 mmol/L. Because of the safety of giving bicarbonate and the potential advantages of completely eradicating acidemia, we recommend serum bicarbonate should be maintained in the 23–25 mEq/L range and arterial blood pH should be at 7.36 or higher. A similar recommendation concerning the threshold for treating low serum bicarbonate would seem appropriate for nondialyzed patients with any level of renal function.

Since in clinically stable CKD patients the rate of acid production is usually normal or below normal, alkalinizing medicines are usually very effective for preventing or treating the acidemia. Indeed there are studies to suggest that routine bicarbonate intake is associated with slower CKD progression rate. Hence, in addition to more vegetarian diet, sodium bicarbonate tablets can be given, for example 650–1300 mg of sodium bicarbonate or citrate twice daily.

If the nondialyzed CKD patient is not likely to develop edema, sodium is usually readily excreted when it is given as sodium bicarbonate or citrate. Since protein metabolism yields acidic products, an LPD (eg, 0.6–0.8 g/kg/day) will also reduce acid production and acidemia, especially if more vegetarian food is ingested. Such a diet can be nutritious for nondialyzed stages 3–5 CKD patients, but maintenance dialysis patients will require more dietary protein (see above). Calcium carbonate may correct mild acidosis, provide needed calcium, and reduce intestinal phosphorus absorption. However, the risk of soft tissue and, particularly, arterial calcification limits the amount of calcium that can be given to CKD patients (see above).

KEY READINGS

Kovesdy CP, Anderson JE, Kalantar-Zadeh K: Association of serum bicarbonate levels with mortality in patients with non-dialysis-dependent CKD. Nephrol Dial Transplant 2009;24:1232.

Wu DY et al: Association between serum bicarbonate and death in hemodialysis patients: is it better to be acidotic or alkalotic? Clin J Am Soc Neph 2006;1:70.

▶ Nutritional Management of CKD & Protein–Energy Wasting

There are four goals for the dietary treatment of CKD patients: (1) to maintain good nutritional status; (2) to reduce the risk of cardiovascular disease and to improve survival; (3) to prevent or ameliorate uremic toxicity and the metabolic disorders of renal failure; and (4), if possible, to retard the progression of renal failure. The latter two may appear to contradict the first two goals, since low protein intake is not infrequently recommended to slow the rate of progression of renal insufficiency. Dietary restrictions may remove important sources of antioxidant vitamins such as fresh fruits and vegetables, due to their rich potassium and phosphorus content; the consequences of such limitations are not yet known. Adherence to specialized diets is often a difficult and frustrating endeavor for patients and their families. Patients usually must make fundamental changes in their behavior patterns and forsake some of their traditional sources of daily pleasure. Often, they must procure special foods, prepare special recipes, usually forego or severely limit their intake of favorite foods, or eat foods that they may not desire. Demands are made on the patient's time and daily activities and on the emotional support system of the family or close associates. Therefore, it is incumbent on the physician not to prescribe radical changes in the patient's diet unless there is good reason to believe that these modifications may be beneficial.

A number of different modalities have been employed to improve the nutritional or inflammatory status in dialysis patients, as shown in Table 22–9. Animal models suggest the possibility that PEW may lead to inflammation, whereas

Table 22–9. Classification of nutritional/anti-inflammatory interventions in advanced CKD.

1. Oral interventions
   Increasing food intake
   Oral supplements
2. Enteral interventions
   Tube feeding
3. Parenteral interventions
   IDPN
   Other parenteral interventions
4. Hormonal interventions
   Androgens
   Growth factors/hormones
5. Nonhormonal medications
   Anti-inflammatory agents (see Table 22–10)
   Antioxidants (see Table 22–10)
   Appetite stimulators
   Carnitine
   Bicarbonate
6. Dietary counseling
   In-center supervision/counseling
7. Dialysis treatment related
   Dialysis dose and frequency
   Membrane compatibility

CKD, chronic kidney disease; IDPN, intradialytic parenteral nutrition.

the opposite direction is true as well; for instance, cancer cachexia is mostly engendered by inflammation and oxidative stress. Similarly, some nutritional biomarkers such as serum albumin may vary according to inflammation, whereas a recent study shows that changes in nPCR, a surrogate of dietary protein intake in dialysis patients, lead to parallel changes in serum albumin, suggesting that independent of the cause of hypoalbuminemia, serum albumin can be increased by nutritional interventions. Dietary interventions may also mitigate inflammation in CKD, as shown in several clinical trials in the general population in that dietary interventions exhibited significant modulation of inflammatory processes.

A. Nutritional Therapy in Non–dialysis-Dependent CKD

In non–dialysis-dependent CKD, a decline in protein–energy nutritional status usually develops as GFR falls to less than 25–30 mL/min, although such changes may start with a GFR as high as 55 mL/min. Enteral protein intake has not been well examined as a therapeutic strategy in this patient population; indeed, high protein intake may affect GFR through various mechanisms, including alterations of glomerular hemodynamics. Restricted protein intake, 0.6–0.8 g/kg/day or even lower in combination with oral nutritional supplements,

amino acids, or keto-analogues of amino acids, has been successfully used to delay progression of CKD in some, but not all, studies. In the MDRD study, very few patients exhibited signs of impending PEW suggesting the safety and adequacy and low protein intake in the range of 0.6–0.8 g/kg/day. There is an emerging enthusiasm about the use of keto-analogues as reflected in a recent consensus statement that mentions some beneficial effects, including decrease in uremic toxins, reduced proteinuria, and salutary effects on mineral and bone disorders and on lipid profile, in addition to potential delay in kidney disease progression and dialysis initiation with lower likelihood of engendering malnutrition.

In patients with diabetic kidney disease, although traditional concerns exist regarding the glycemic burden of nutritional interventions in diabetic patients, in approximately one-third of diabetic patients, a status of "burnt-out diabetes" is observed as the CKD progresses, in that frequent episodes of hypoglycemia necessitate a decrease or even total discontinuation of most or all diabetic medications including insulin injections and oral hypoglycemic agents. Hence, history of diabetes is not a contraindication of oral nutritional therapy in any stage of CKD and should not be a reason to withhold nutritional interventions especially among patients with hypoalbuminemia and burnt-out diabetes that is manifested by a normal to low hemoglobin A_{1c}.

B. Nutritional Management of Dialysis Patients and Intradialytic and Intraperitoneal Nutrition

In many dialysis centers in Asia and Europe, provision of meals and supplements during hemodialysis treatment is routine, whereas in North America this is practiced less frequently, likely due to concerns related to hypotension, aspiration, hygiene, and dialysis staff burden to distribute meal trays. Prevalent dialysis patients tend to eat less during hemodialysis treatment days. Among more intensive interventions, tube feeding including during dialysis therapy in the dialysis clinic has been reported to be an effective modality, particularly in pediatric, elderly, or disabled individuals. However, according to some, this modality is a cumbersome option that cannot be used in the average (stable and functional) CKD outpatient. Experience with tube feeding in adults with CKD is still limited; probably because many patients and physicians are reluctant to use tube feeding.

Whereas parenteral interventions such as intradialytic parenteral nutrition (IDPN) may be costly and employed only during dialysis treatment, they may be effective especially in patients with a serum albumin less than 3.5 g/dL (based on bromocresol green [BCG] method, or <3.2 g/dL based on bromocresol purple [BCP] method). Several studies have examined the role of IDPN in improving nutritional status and outcomes in dialysis patients, including some suggesting favorable results in correcting more severe hypoalbuminemia.

Some retrospective analyses suggest that in dialysis patients with PEW, IDPN may reduce mortality. IDPN solutions are commonly prepared from base solutions. The base solutions for amino acids, carbohydrates, and lipids can vary in concentrations. Up to 10% of essential and nonessential amino acids, 50% or 70% D-glucose and 10–20% lipids or IDPN can also be prepared lipid free. Trace elements, vitamins, and selected minerals can be included. IDPN solution can be tailored to individual patient needs.

Intraperitoneal nutrition (IPN) can be recommended to PD patients with more severe PEW including those with lower serum albumin levels, for example albumin less than 3 g/dL (using BCG method), noting that PD patients tend to have 0.2–0.3 g/dL lower serum albumin than hemodialysis patients. IPN is provided in different combinations; a more commonly used mixture includes 15 amino acids (9 essential and 6 nonessential amino acids) that are added to a peritoneal dialysate solution resulting in a 1.1% amino acid solution with reduced glucose concentration. While many studies examining the safety as well as protein synthesis and membrane characteristics showed a potential benefit, data on long-term nutritional status or anthropometric measurements are not available and there are currently no well-designed multicenter controlled studies to examine the effects and outcomes of IPN or to compare it with other types of nutritional support.

C. Appetite-Stimulating, Anti-inflammatory, and Antioxidant Modalities

It has been argued that CKD-associated anorexia is an integral component of the systemic inflammatory response as well as to other factors. Anorexia can be induced by such proinflammatory cytokines such as IL-6 and TNF-α and is correlated with all-cause and cardiovascular mortality in dialysis patients. Consequently, an exploration of the interaction between energy and protein-regulatory mechanisms and proinflammatory cytokines may lead to an effective treatment for MICS-associated anorexia.

Several appetite stimulants have been studied clinically. Among simple interventions to stimulate appetite, *hormonal* medications may be associated with many side effects such as virilism or potential for worsening atherosclerosis seen with androgens. However, some other medications, especially appetite stimulants, are often effective in increasing protein and energy intake, including megestrol acetate, dronabinol, mirtazapine, and pentoxifylline as well as modulators of leptin, ghrelin, and nystatin, among others. Among potential orexigenic agents for CKD patients, *pentoxifylline* downregulates the local proinflammatory cytokine-mediated nitric oxide synthase pathway, inhibits TNF-α production, and decreases body weight loss and muscle protein wasting in acutely ill patients.

Some pharmaceutical agents may also have anti-inflammatory/antioxidant properties (see below). It is important to note that these pharmacologic medications may be effective if there is concomitant provision of food or supplement including intradialytic nutrition. Indeed, a mere increase in energy or protein intake without the concurrent modulation of anti-inflammatory or antioxidant pathways. Therefore, it is unlikely, although not impossible, to find one single medication to correct MICS. On the contrary, oral supplements, especially if they contain a combination of several nutritional and anti-inflammatory agents, are practical and promising treatment modalities.

Although epidemiological evidence strongly links inflammation and oxidative stress to each other and to poor outcome in CKD patients, there have only been a few randomized trials that indicate an improvement in outcome with anti-inflammatory or antioxidant treatment. Other treatments (Table 22–10) have been proposed for reducing inflammation or oxidative stress in dialysis patients, but the data supporting the efficacy of these modalities are still inconclusive. One example is the administration of vitamin E, which may be associated with a decreased risk of cardiovascular mortality in dialysis patients according to some but not all reports (see above).

Table 22–10. Potential anti-inflammatory and antioxidant agents for chronic kidney disease patients.

Antioxidant vitamins
Vitamin E
Vitamin C
Vitamin A/carotenoids
Other antioxidants
Eicosanoids (fish oil)
γ-Linolenic (borage oil)
Megestrol acetate
Pentoxifylline
Steroids/adrenocorticotrophic hormone
Nonsteroidal anti-inflammatory drugs
Anti-TNF-α agents
Thalidomide
HMG-CoA reductase inhibitors (statins)
Angiotensin-converting enzyme inhibitors
Erythropoietin
n-Acetylcysteine
Glitazones
Others: dialysis technique

KEY READINGS

Foulks CJ: Intradialytic parenteral nutrition. In: Kopple JD, Massry SG (editors). *Nutritional Management of Renal Disease*, 2nd ed. Philadelphia: Lippincott, Williams & Wilkins, 2004, pp 467–476.

Heimburger O, Stenvinkel P, Lindholm B: Nutritional effects and nutritional management of chronic peritoneal dialysis. In: Kopple JD, Massry SG (editors). *Nutritional Management of Renal Disease*, 2nd ed. Philadelphia: Lippincott, Williams & Wilkins, 2004, pp 477–512.

▶ Nutritional Management of Renal Transplant Patients

Patients who undergo successful renal transplantation often develop normal or even supranormal *appetite*. Gain in body weight and fat is common. During the first year after transplantation, women may be particularly likely to increase dietary energy and protein intake and gain fat and lean body mass. Several nutritional disorders appear to be related to other factors associated with renal transplantation. These include obesity, insulin resistance and diabetes mellitus, impaired growth in children, protein wasting, altered serum lipid and homocysteine concentrations, and abnormalities in bone, mineral, and vitamin metabolism. Many of these complications are of particular concern because cardiovascular disease is the major cause of morbidity and mortality in renal transplant recipients. Indeed, unlike in dialysis patients, in whom obesity confers survival advantages, (reverse epidemiology), obesity has been shown to have strong association with increased mortality in transplanted patients; hence a so-called reversal of the reverse epidemiology is observed.

A. Lipids in Renal Transplant Patients

Renal transplant patients often have increased serum triglyceride, VLDL triglyceride, small dense LDL cholesterol, and total LDL cholesterol concentrations. HDL cholesterol is often low, and the LDL/HDL cholesterol ratio may be increased. Serum triglyceride levels correlate with the daily dose of prednisone, degree of obesity, and severity of renal insufficiency. These findings are of particular concern because several studies have found a correlation between increased serum lipids and the risk of cardiovascular disease, graft failure, and fatality in renal transplant recipients. Causes of increased serum triglycerides and cholesterol include excessive fat and energy intake, obesity, treatment with glucocorticoids, diuretics, calcineurin inhibitors or rapamycin, nephrotic range proteinuria, and underlying diseases (eg, diabetes mellitus).

A low-cholesterol, high-fiber diet with a polyunsaturated-to-saturated fatty acid ratio greater than 1.0 may lower serum total cholesterol and LDL cholesterol levels in renal transplant recipients. However, the altered lipoprotein pattern may not be affected. A combination of a similar diet with regular exercise may improve the plasma lipid pattern. Fish oil providing 3 g/day of omega-3 fatty acids for 3 months decreased serum triglycerides and VLDL cholesterol in hyperlipidemic renal transplant recipients. However, the effects of diet on the improvement in the serum lipid pattern tend to be modest, and combining dietary therapy with serum HMG-CoA reductase inhibitors (statins) is generally far more effective for reducing serum total and LDL cholesterol.

The observation that a diet low in carbohydrate and modestly restricted in calories may reduce the cushingoid appearance suggests that such individuals may be given a low carbohydrate intake (1 g/kg/day), which is limited to 28–30 kcal/kg/day. If such a low carbohydrate, moderately restricted energy intake is employed in renal transplant recipients, it should be limited to short periods of time when the prednisone dosage is very high (eg, >40 mg/day). This level of energy intake may not minimize the catabolic response during acute illness and may lead to further wasting. However, the higher protein intake with such diets (eg, 2 g protein/kg/day) may reduce PEW. Also, given the abnormalities in lipid metabolism in renal transplant recipients, such a high-fat diet should not be continued for long periods of time. In general, renal transplant patients should be encouraged to ingest a National Cholesterol Education Program TLC diet as described above for the CKD patients. Patients should be encouraged to exercise regularly and to maintain a normal or desirable body weight. For transplant recipients with superimposed catabolic illnesses, 30–40 kcal/kg/day may be prescribed. Other maneuvers to correct abnormal serum lipids are as described for the nontransplant renal failure patient (see above). For renal transplant recipients with serum LDL cholesterol levels above about 70 mg/dL, the TLC diet should be supplemented with statins.

B. Other Nutritional Issues in Renal Transplant Patients

Low serum folate levels were observed in transplant patients as long as 6 years after transplantation. Serum thiamine and vitamin B_{12} levels are generally normal in renal transplant patients. After successful renal transplantation, serum vitamin A often remains elevated for extended periods of time and may not fall to normal levels in some patients for several years.

Calcineurin inhibitors (cyclosporine A and tacrolimus) as well as sirolimus may increase serum cholesterol and cause potassium retention with hyperkalemia and urinary magnesium wasting with hypomagnesemia. Moreover, hypophosphatemia is relatively common during the first few months after the successful renal transplantation and may occur because of a condition similar to hungry bone syndrome. Hence, judicious phosphorus and magnesium supplementation is imperative to avoid the deleterious effects of hypomagnesemia and hypophosphatemia, which can be profound. Low plasma and hair zinc and hyperzincuria have also been reported often within 12 months after successful renal transplantation. On the other hand, patients who have a functioning renal transplant for more than 12 months after the surgery usually have normal plasma, hair, and urine zinc and normal taste detection and recognition thresholds.

KEY READINGS

Kasiske B et al: Clinical practice guidelines for managing dyslipidemias in kidney transplant patients: a report from the Managing Dyslipidemias in Chronic Kidney Disease Work Group of the National Kidney Foundation Kidney Disease Outcomes Quality Initiative. Am J Transplant 2004;4:13.

Kasiske BL, Adeva-Andany M: Nutritional management of renal transplantation. In: Kopple JD, Massry SG (editors). *Nutritional Management of Renal Disease*, 2nd ed. Philadelphia: Lippincott, Williams & Wilkins, 2004, pp 513–526.

Yamamoto S et al: The impact of obesity in renal transplantation: an analysis of paired cadaver kidneys. Clin Transplant 2002;16:252.

■ CHAPTER REVIEW QUESTIONS

1. What is the recommended dietary protein intake in stable nondialysis CKD patients with eGFR less than 45 mL/min?
   A. 0.3–0.4 g/kg ideal body weight per day
   B. 0.6–0.8 g/kg ideal body weight per day
   C. 0.9–1.1 g/kg ideal body weight per day
   D. 1.2–1.4 g/kg ideal body weight per day
   E. >1.5 g/kg ideal body weight per day

2. All of the following agents can be used to stimulate appetite in dialysis patients except for
   A. Megestrol acetate
   B. Dronabinol
   C. Mirtazapine
   D. Dihydroxycholecalciferol

3. What is the recommended dietary protein intake for stable maintenance (thrice-weekly) hemodialysis patients without any residual kidney function?
   A. 0.3–0.4 g/kg idea body weight per day
   B. 0.6–0.8 g/kg idea body weight per day
   C. 0.9–1.1 g/kg idea body weight per day
   D. 1.2–1.4 g/kg idea body weight per day
   E. >1.5 g/kg idea body weight per day

4. Which of the statements related to PEW in maintenance dialysis patients is not true?
   A. PEW is associated with poor outcomes including higher mortality in dialysis patients.
   B. Independent of the etiology of hypoalbuminemia, provision of high-protein diet to dialysis patients might increase serum albumin level.
   C. PD patients tend to have higher serum albumin levels than hemodialysis patients.
   D. MIS can be used to identify dialysis patients with or at high risk of PEW.

5. What statement is true about phosphorus management in CKD?
   A. Phosphorus in plant-based protein is more readily absorbable through the gastrointestinal tract than the animal-based protein.
   B. Ingesting preserved foods with added inorganic phosphorus preservatives has little impact on dietary phosphorus burden.
   C. Hyperphosphatemia (>6 mg/dL) is associated with greater survival and better outcomes.
   D. Higher protein intake is associated with higher likelihood of hyperphosphatemia.

Slowing the Progression of Chronic Kidney Disease

Edward R. Gould, MD

Julia Lewis, MD

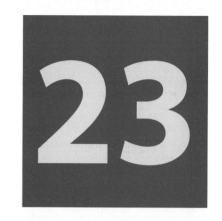

General Considerations

Caring for patients with end-stage renal disease (ESRD) and its myriad complications represents a major challenge. According to the United States Renal Data System (USRDS), there are approximately 600,000 patients with ESRD receiving renal replacement therapy (RRT) as of 2010. In the United States and globally, it is estimated that there are an estimated 2 million people currently receiving some form of RRT. Most of those patients can be found in industrialized countries with well-developed health care delivery systems. It has been suggested that this number may represent only 10% of patients globally with ESRD, with the remaining 90% of ESRD patients lacking access to maintenance RRT.

In addition to the burden that ESRD imposes on the patient, treatment of ESRD also carries a significant societal burden associated with the costs of providing such therapy. Those costs stem from the direct cost of therapy and by way of the requisite infrastructure necessary to provide chronic dialysis care. The worldwide expenditure on such care for the decade ending in 2010 is estimated to have been in excess of US $1.1 trillion. This cost grows annually, and with emerging markets and global growth of dialysis options for countries and regions that have not historically had access to them, the global cost of this care is only expected to rise.

The growing prevalence of chronic kidney disease (CKD) and ESRD associates not only with growing worldwide populations but also with the rising global rates of obesity, hypertension, and diabetes mellitus. These populations are likely to benefit from early nephrology referral with focused efforts on delaying the progression of CKD to ESRD.

Against this backdrop, it is critical to appreciate that most cases of ESRD occur as the slow progression of CKD over the course of months to years. The interval between the diagnosis of CKD and the development of ESRD offers an opportunity to meaningfully intervene, abate, or at least slow the rate of CKD progression. Interventions have varying levels of efficacy. In this chapter we briefly review the mechanisms of CKD progression and proceed to discuss the various tools and approaches directed at slowing that progression.

KEY READING

Couser WG et al: The contribution of chronic kidney disease to the global burden of major noncommunicable diseases. Kidney Int 2011;80:1258.

A. Referral to Nephrology

When, during the longitudinal management of a patient with CKD, is the appropriate time to refer a patient to a nephrologist is one of the most common questions asked by primary care providers. Individual providers differ with respect to their comfort managing CKD and its clinical manifestations. Observational data vary on the impact of early nephrology referral with respect to long-term outcomes, including rate of glomerular filtration rate (GFR) decline, time to ESRD, and overall cost of treatment.

Many professional organizations have established guidelines for management of patients with newly diagnosed CKD. Kidney Disease: Improving Global Outcomes (KDIGO) has inclusive guidelines published in the 2012 update on the issue to aid clinicians with the decision to refer (Table 23–1).

Pathogenesis

CKD should be viewed as a clinicopathologic syndrome that follows renal injury incurred by any of a variety of different kidney pathologies. While the pace of decline often associates with the nature of the initial injury, there are a number of common pathogenic pathways that engage in the setting

Table 23–1. Triggers for referral to kidney specialist care according to 2012 KDIGO recommendations.

- AKI or abrupt sustained fall in GFR
- GFR <30 mL/min/1.73 m² (CKD stages 4 and 5)
- Consistent presence of albuminuria (ACR >300 mg/g), approximately equivalent to PCR >500 mg/g (250 mg/mmol)
- Progression of CKD defined as 25% decline in GFR, or GFR loss >5 mL/min/year
- Urinary red cell casts, or microscopic hematuria (>20 RBCs/hpf) not readily explained.
- CKD and hypertension refractory to treatment with ≥4 antihypertensive agents
- Persistent abnormalities of serum potassium
- Recurrent or extensive nephrolithiasis
- Hereditary kidney disease

ACR, albumin-to-creatinine ratio; AKI, acute kidney injury; CKD, chronic kidney disease; GFR, glomerular filtration rate; hpf, high-power field; PCR, protein-to-creatinine ratio; RBC, red blood cell count.

of reduced GFR that are largely independent of the inciting insult. Decades of work in this area has identified a series of interconnected mechanisms at play in this setting and provides biologic plausibility that these pathways can be modified with available therapeutic intervention. These varied mechanisms create a vicious cycle of progressive nephron loss that leads to ESRD (Figure 23–1). For ease of discussion, we have separated them into two distinct pathways:

the glomerular hemodynamic factors and the inflammatory cascade; however, it is important to recognize that these factors are active concurrently, and the interplay between them cannot be overstated, as discussed below through discussion of specific mediators.

KEY READINGS

Kliem V et al: Mechanisms involved in the pathogenesis of tubulointerstitial fibrosis in 5/6-nephrectomized rats. Kidney Int 1996;49:666.

Lemley KV: Glomerular pathology and the progression of chronic kidney disease. Am J Physiol Renal Physiol 2016;310:F1385.

A. Glomerular Hemodynamic Factors

Early work in animal models identified that reduction in nephron mass through surgical nephrectomy would reliably produce progressive CKD. The reduction in nephron number associates with marked hemodynamic changes in the remaining glomeruli. These changes are characterized by a substantial increase in the filtration rate of each glomerulus (single nephron glomerular filtration rate [SNGFR]) that stems from an interplay between a number of distinct hemodynamic factors, including the development of higher systemic blood pressures (BPs), a decrease in afferent arteriolar tone, and an increase in efferent arteriolar tone, all conspiring to lead to an increase in glomerular capillary hydraulic pressure.

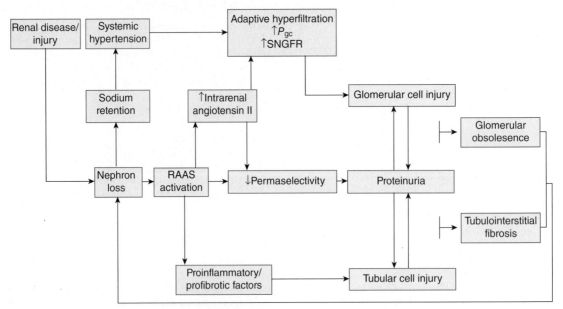

▲ **Figure 23–1.** The multiple interconnected pathways involved in progressive chronic kidney disease. P_{gc}, glomerular hydraulic pressure; RAAS, renin–angiotensin–aldosterone system; SNGFR, single nephron glomerular filtration rate.

These changes can be considered adaptive, to a point. With early renal injury, they allow for partial compensation for the loss of nephron mass. As injury progresses, though, these changes become maladaptive and lead to associated structural injuries within the glomerulus. The consequence of such injury is glomerular obsolescence and sclerosis. Many of these changes have been shown to be mediated by the renin–angiotensin–aldosterone system (RAAS). A critical breakthrough in this area of research was the demonstration that in multiple different animal models of kidney disease, including diabetic nephropathy, the inhibition of the RAAS, as opposed to treatment with other antihypertensive agents, preserved glomerular structure, and integrity as well as renal function. This is extensively discussed later in this chapter.

B. Inflammatory Factors

Inflammatory cells and their associated inflammatory mediators play an important role in the response to renal injury. They are responsible for renal healing and recovery in response to an acute insult, as well as the scarring process that follows such injuries. Delineating and favorably influencing the inflammatory process is an area of active research in preventing the progression of renal disease. Renal injury from any cause leads to an accumulation of inflammatory cells and their associated inflammatory mediators. The types of cells implicated include monocytes, lymphocytes, fibroblasts, and dendritic cells, with each contributing to the evolving extracellular milieu that promotes parenchymal scarring.

The inflammatory invasion collectively leads to activation of intrinsic renal pathways native to mesangial cells, endothelial cells, and myofibroblasts. These cells express a variety of different cytokines and chemokines, such as transforming growth factor-β (TGF-β), platelet-derived growth factor (PDGF), basic fibroblast growth factor (FGF), and tissue-type plasminogen activator. These intermediaries further recruit cells to the inflammatory response and launch matrix proliferation cascades, ultimately leading to fibroblast and myofibroblast proliferation. Those extracellular matrix-producing cells synthesize and deposit matrix proteins. These extracellular elements displace the native renal architecture leading to scarring and glomerular and tubulointerstitial sclerosis. To date, interventions targeting these inflammatory pathways have not been shown to be of benefit in modifying the progression of CKD.

C. Hemodynamic and Inflammatory Mediators

As noted previously, the loss of nephron mass seen in CKD leads to local activation of the RAAS. Whereas systemic levels of angiotensin II are normal or decreased in CKD, intrarenal angiotensin II levels are elevated. These elevated levels of angiotensin II affect intrarenal hemodynamics, increasing efferent arteriolar tone, and contributing to the increased intraglomerular hydraulic pressure that eventually becomes maladaptive. Other RAAS-mediated effects include increased glomerular permeability resulting in exacerbation of proteinuria, increased plasminogen activator inhibitor-1 production by endothelial and vascular smooth muscle cells, promotion of mesangial cell proliferation, macrophage activation and increased macrophage expression of TGF-β, and increased adrenal production of aldosterone. These factors have been shown to be mediators of fibrosis. Taken together, it is clear that angiotensin II plays a central role in the pathogenesis of progressive renal injury through multiple hemodynamic and nonhemodynamic mechanisms. Inhibition of the production or actions of angiotensin II therefore represents a single intervention that may abrogate many of these mechanisms.

D. Independent Influence of Proteinuria

Proteinuria is the result of disordered permselectivity of the glomerular filtration barrier and is therefore the hallmark of a glomerulopathy as well as a marker of disease severity. Research continues to accumulate that the presence of abnormal amounts of plasma proteins in glomerular ultrafiltrate may contribute directly to further renal damage. In the normal kidney, small amounts of low-molecular-weight proteins are present in the tubular fluid and are reabsorbed by proximal tubule cells. In vitro experiments have found that culturing renal tubule cells in the presence of high concentrations of plasma proteins induces expression of a range of proinflammatory cytokines.

In addition, in animal models of renal disease, this enhanced expression of proinflammatory chemokines and cytokines is evident on the basolateral aspect of tubule cells. These proinflammatory molecules are then secreted into the peritubular interstitium where they further contribute to the development of interstitial inflammation and fibrosis. Further experimental evidence indicates that abnormally filtered plasma proteins also accumulate within podocytes where they may contribute to glomerular injury. As discussed previously, these intertwined pathways provide a plausible mechanistic link between proteinuria from glomerular injury and progressive tubulointerstitial pathology.

▶ Prevention

A. Risk Factors

The current definitions for CKD severity are outlined in Chapter 17. There are a variety of factors that drive progressive CKD, and those factors can be divided into nonmodifiable and modifiable risk factors. Nonmodifiable risk factors include age (older age), birth weight (low birth weight), race (with non-Caucasians faring generally worse), and a variety of genetic factors that continue to be recognized as having an impact on disease progression.

The specific rate of age-related decline in GFR varies by observational cohort, but generally speaking, it accounts for a 5 to 10 mL/min decline in GFR per decade beyond the fourth decade of life. It has historically been considered a natural part of the aging process, though this remains an open controversy. Epidemiologic studies, though, have shown that this decline in GFR independently associates with worsened cardiovascular outcomes. Older patients with CKD from any specific cause fare worse than younger cohorts with that the same cause. This bears consideration while counseling patients about anticipated prognosis.

There are a number of different genetic factors that influence the risk of kidney disease progression. Some kidney diseases are associated with monogenic aberrancies; these include autosomal dominant polycystic kidney disease (ADPKD). The polycystin gene mutations leading to ADPKD—PKD1 and PKD2—lead to distinct clinical phenotypes with PKD2 mutations generally leading to a more benign clinical course than mutations in PKD1. More complex are the connections that have been identified with other genetic polymorphisms. One of the best studied examples is the *APOL1* gene, encoding for apolipoprotein L1. While the specific mechanism defining how the mutant APOL1 allele impacts the progression of renal disease has remained nebulous, it has been repeatedly observed that patients with two high-risk alleles are at a significantly higher risk of progressive CKD.

In patients of African descent who were included in the African–American Study of Kidney disease and hypertension (AASK) trial and the Chronic Renal Insufficiency Cohort Study (CRIC), *APOL1* gene variants strongly associated with increased renal risk, defined as either a doubling of serum creatinine from baseline or as progression to ESRD. Genome-wide association studies continue to identify other candidate genes that may influence the rate of CKD progression generally as well as in relation to specific underlying diseases.

Modifiable risk factors include systemic hypertension, proteinuria, dyslipidemia, hyperuricemia, smoking and obesity. These are summarized in Table 23–2 and addressed later as part of the therapeutic interventions section.

B. Primary Prevention

The myriad of diseases responsible for driving CKD, many of which occur sporadically, presents a challenge for devising an effective strategy that can be broadly applied for primary prevention of CKD.

Primary prevention of early nephropathy, as evidenced by microalbuminuria, has been best studied in diabetic nephropathy, a population well suited for such studies given that approximately 40% of diabetic patients develop nephropathy. Intensive work in this population has identified interventions that could then provide a framework for primary prevention in other diseases.

Table 23–2. Modifiable and nonmodifiable risk factors for chronic kidney disease progression.

Nonmodifiable risk factors
- Age
- Race or ethnicity
- Genetic conditions (monogenetic disease or risk alleles)
- Low birth weight

Modifiable risk factors
- High BP
- Hyperglycemia
- Cardiovascular disease
- Dyslipidemia
- Metabolic syndrome
- Hyperuricemia
- Low socioeconomic status
- Nephrotoxin exposure
- Obesity
- Smoking

In most developed countries, diabetic nephropathy is the most common cause of CKD leading to ESRD. In this case, the "at-risk" population may be readily identified making study recruitment easier than in other diseases. The landmark Diabetes Control and Complications Trial (DCCT) demonstrated that the level of glycemic control in patients with type 1 diabetes determines the risk of microvascular complications, including nephropathy. Among patients in the intensive diabetic control group, lower hemoglobin A_{1c} (HbA_{1c}) targets versus conventional therapy (goal HbA_{1c} ≤6 versus 8%) there was a 70% risk reduction for the development of microalbuminuria. However, several large randomized controlled trials done to evaluate the effects of intensive glycemic control in type 2 diabetes mellitus have failed to demonstrate a significant benefit with respect to the progression of renal disease. The UKPDS study evaluated 3867 patients with newly diagnosed type 2 diabetes. They were assigned to either intensive or standard control. At 9 years of follow-up, the intensive group had maintained an average HbA_{1c} of 7% compared to standard therapy group which had a mean of 7.9%. At the start of the study, 6.5% of patients had moderately elevated proteinuria. While not a prespecified outcome—instead being part of the larger composite outcome—at the close of the study, the intensive control group had a statistically significant lower rate of moderately elevated albuminuria (19.2 versus 25.4%), but there was no difference in the rates of macrovascular complications, including progression of CKD. Subsequent studies have led to similar findings, with no observed benefit of intensive therapy on CKD progression. Moreover, in some studies, intensive glycemic control in patients with type 2 diabetes has been associated with not only no demonstrable renal benefit, but it has also shown an increased risk of all-cause mortality—mostly attributable to increased cardiovascular risk.

The evidence, then, suggests that intensive glycemic control (HbA$_{1c}$ ≤6.0%) is important in preventing the development of CKD and other microvascular complications in type 1 diabetes mellitus. In patients with type 2 diabetes mellitus, the risk/benefit of tighter glycemic control is less clear, and it needs to be individualized.

Other interventions to prevent the development of early diabetic nephropathy have been reported with mixed results. The BENEDICT trial included 1204 patients with type 2 diabetes and hypertension that were randomized to receive an angiotensin-converting enzyme inhibitor (ACEI) with or without a calcium channel blocker (CCB), a CCB alone or placebo alone. Those patients randomized to the arms that included ACEI had a significantly lower incidence of microalbuminuria with ACEI alone (6%) or ACEI and CCB (5.7%) versus those treated with CCB (11.9%) or placebo (10%). The larger ROADMAP trial included 4447 type 2 diabetic patients randomized to receive angiotensin receptor blocker (ARB) or placebo. The studied groups used additional BP agents to achieve a target BP of less than 130/80 mm Hg. The effect size was much less dramatic in this trial with only 8.2% of the ARB-treated group developing microalbuminuria versus 9.8% in the placebo group. Although both studies demonstrated a reduction in the rate of developing microalbuminuria with inhibition of the RAAS, it is not known if that reduction translates into slower progression of CKD.

Certain cases of CKD can also be prevented through avoidance of individual acute injuries. Recurrent nephrolithiasis and its complications provide a framework for such primary prevention. Recurrent kidney stones can be avoided with appropriate metabolic evaluation and treatment, thus avoiding the episodic injuries. Certainly, some medications used chronically which have been linked to CKD should also be monitored, and—in high-risk populations—limited. Nonsteroidal anti-inflammatory drugs (NSAIDs) and the use of chronic proton pump inhibitors, both of which have associated with CKD in large epidemiologic studies, are prototypical examples of such medications; limiting use of these agents to the minimum time required for treatment may provide primary prevention of CKD. Avoiding excessive intravenous contrast exposure, episodic volume depletion, and exposure to antibiotics with known nephrotoxicity is also prudent.

Few other diseases causing CKD have a natural history that is as well described as that of diabetes; that absence of a predictable clinical course makes other nephropathies more challenging to develop randomized controlled trials for possible early primary preventative therapeutic interventions.

C. Secondary Prevention

Secondary prevention is most effective if interventions can be instituted early in the disease course. However, despite the cost of treating CKD and ESRD and the burden of disease to the individual patient, screening entire populations for early CKD, despite current guidelines, is undervalued and inconsistent. The specific screening tests used may vary according to the population studied and according to available resources. The simplest screening tool is to use dipstick urinalysis to identify abnormalities (proteinuria and/or hematuria) that could prompt more advanced investigations. For those diseases that cause CKD but that may not have any urinary findings, an estimate of renal function based on serum creatinine measurement may be done. Specific diagnostic tests and further investigations are outlined in the next section.

At a minimum, we recommend detailed screening of populations considered to be "at-risk" to increase the likelihood of early detection and to facilitate interventions aimed at slowing disease progression. Those populations would include patients with comorbidities that predispose to CKD; specific conditions to be considered "at-risk" are highlighted in Table 23–3.

KEY READINGS

Miller ME et al: Action to Control Cardiovascular Risk in Diabetes Study G; Effects of intensive glucose lowering in type 2 diabetes. N Engl J Med 2008;358:2545.

Duckworth W et al: Glucose control and vascular complications in veterans with type 2 diabetes. N Engl J Med 2009;360:129.

Group AC et al: Intensive blood glucose control and vascular outcomes in patients with type 2 diabetes. N Engl J Med 2008;358:2560.

Intensive blood-glucose control with sulphonylureas or insulin compared with conventional treatment and risk of complications in patients with type 2 diabetes (UKPDS 33). UK Prospective Diabetes Study (UKPDS) Group. Lancet 1998;352:837.

Parsa A et al: APOL1 risk variants, race, and progression of chronic kidney disease. N Engl J Med 2013;369:2183.

Ruggenenti P et al: Preventing microalbuminuria in type 2 diabetes. N Engl J Med 2004;351:1941.

▶ Clinical Findings

A. Symptoms and Signs

Early CKD is often asymptomatic. The earliest symptoms vary and may be limited to mild nocturia due to the loss of urinary concentrating ability. If nephrotic range proteinuria is present, peripheral edema may be the first symptom to develop. Patients with advanced renal failure may present with malaise, breathlessness, pruritus, loss of appetite, nausea, and vomiting.

Similarly, abnormal clinical signs are often lacking in patients with early CKD. CKD is a common cause of hypertension, and all patients who present for new-onset hypertension should be screened for CKD. If the dominant feature

Table 23–3. "At-risk" populations that warrant annual screening for chronic kidney disease (CKD).

Medical comorbidities associated with developing CKD
· Diabetes mellitus
· Hypertension
· Atherosclerotic vascular disease
· Congestive heart failure
Urologic conditions associated with increased risk of CKD
· Bladder outlet obstruction or neurogenic bladder
· Renal calculi
· Urinary diversion surgery
Multisystem disorders that may lead to renal pathology
· HIV
· Hepatitis B or C
· Systemic lupus erythematosus
· Systemic vasculitis
· Rheumatoid arthritis
· Multiple myeloma
· Amyloidosis
· Sickle cell disease
Chronic treatment with potentially nephrotoxic drugs
· Nonsteroidal anti-inflammatory drugs
· Gold, penicillamine
· Calcineurin inhibitors
· Lithium carbonate
· Aminosalicylates
· Intravenous drug use
· Proton pump inhibitors
Family members of patients affected by genetic renal diseases
First-degree relatives of patients with CKD stages 3–5
Age >65 years

of the patient's clinical syndrome is proteinuria, peripheral edema may be the initial presenting sign. Clinical pallor due to anemia may be observed in patients with CKD stages 3–5. Most (but not all) patients with more advanced CKD have urinary abnormalities detectable with standard dipstick testing. Proteinuria is a hallmark of CKD and may be accompanied by hematuria depending on the underlying pattern of renal injury.

B. Laboratory Findings

Laboratory investigations are essential for the diagnosis of CKD. As discussed previously, the diagnosis rests on the detection of impaired renal function and/or urinary abnormalities (usually proteinuria).

1. Assessment of proteinuria—Protein or albumin concentration in a spot urine specimen alone is of limited use due to variations in urine osmolality affecting concentration. The measurement of protein or albumin concentration in a 24-hour or spot urine collection normalized to urinary creatinine excretion (ie, a protein or albumin-to-creatinine—protein-to-creatinine ratio [PCR] or albumin-to-creatinine ratio [ACR], respectively) represents the most accurate method for assessment of proteinuria. While a spot PCR or ACR on a 24-hour urine collection is most representative of the total daily protein excretion due to changes in excretion observed between the supine and upright positions, patients may prefer to provide only a spot urine because of the ease of collection.

While the ACR allows detection of small amounts of increased protein in the urine, but once the proteinuria increases to the level of detection for standard protein assays, PCR testing is less expensive and as accurate to follow the status of glomerular disease.

2. Assessment of renal function—Determining the optimal method for the assessment of GFR depends on finding a method with the best compromise between accuracy and reproducibility, as well as patient convenience. Radioisotope clearance studies represent the most accurate method, but these may require a hospital attendance of several hours, water loading, and some radiation exposure, and are therefore not generally suitable for screening or for serial monitoring of renal function outside of a clinical trial setting. Creatinine clearance studies based on 24-hour urine collections were widely used in the United States until recently, but they have fallen from favor due to barriers in collection. Namely, that they are cumbersome and can be confounded by over- or undercollection. These difficulties prompted the development of a variety of formulas for estimating GFR based on serum creatinine concentration. In comparison with radioisotope, clearance studies has shown that a four-variable equation (GFR = $1.863 \times [P_{cr}$ in mg/dL$]^{1.154} \times$ [age]$^{0.203} \times 1.212$ [if black] $\times 0.742$ [if female]) derived from the Modification of Diet in Renal Disease (MDRD) study provides an accurate estimate of GFR and is now widely used in clinical practice. This equation uses age, race, and gender as surrogate markers of muscle mass to better inform the serum creatinine. Most laboratories now report an estimated GFR (eGFR) with each creatinine result. It should be noted, however, that the MDRD formula was derived from data collected in primarily Caucasian patients with eGFRs that ranged from 20 to 60 mL/min and no other major medical comorbidities, like diabetes, cancer, or cirrhosis. So the eGFR can either under or overestimate renal function in any population other than that from which it was derived; most notably, it is less accurate in patients with a GFR greater than 60 mL/min.

Alternative formulas have been developed; the Chronic Kidney Disease Epidemiology Collaboration published their formula in 2009, using a larger database of patients, including many with a GFR that was greater than 60 mL/min. The CKD-EPI formula uses the same variables as the MDRD equation, but because the analysis included a broader swath of patients, including a large cohort of individuals with higher eGFR, it is a more accurate estimate of GFR in this group. With the development of cystatin-C as an alternative to serum creatinine, even more equations have been developed to estimate GFR. None is without potential pitfalls, and application and interpretation of the estimated GFR requires attention to the characteristics of the cohort used to develop the equation and comparison of the characteristics of that cohort to the individual patient being evaluated.

KEY READINGS

Klahr S et al: The effects of dietary protein restriction and blood-pressure control on the progression of chronic renal disease. Modification of Diet in Renal Disease Study Group. N Engl J Med 1994;330:877.

Levey AS et al: A new equation to estimate glomerular filtration rate. Ann Intern Med 2009;150:604.

▶ Complications

A progressive decline in renal function and the risk of developing ESRD are the obvious complications of CKD that form the focus of this chapter. It should be noted, however, that CKD is associated with a marked increase in the risk of cardiovascular disease that in some patients exceeds the risk of ESRD. Additional complications of CKD include anemia, renal osteodystrophy, and malnutrition. Those complications are discussed in detail elsewhere.

▶ Treatment

The diagnosis of CKD is often made by primary care providers, and it precedes referral to nephrology for consideration. The initial office visit with a nephrologist sets the tone for the physician-patient relationship and provides a useful opportunity to offer education about renal function and to introduce general recommendations around conservative care. The use of pharmacologic therapies has to be carefully tailored to the individual and their disease manifestations according to the degree of renal insufficiency observed.

A. Nonpharmacologic Interventions

1. Modification of lifestyle—While true for all patients, individuals with CKD should be encouraged to adopt a healthy lifestyle as a method of reducing their cardiovascular risk. Indeed, given that patients with CKD have increased risk of adverse cardiovascular outcomes—often preceding progression to RRT—reduction of those risks has the potential to meaningfully impact patient outcomes. Multiple lines of observational evidence support lifestyle modification as a potential modifier of CKD, although large prospective

randomized multimodification studies are lacking. There is also evidence that some measures that are commonly recommended may also impact the rate of CKD progression. If overweight, patients should be encouraged to lose weight as obesity is independently associated with early glomerular hyperfiltration, proteinuria and a more rapid decline in GFR. Physical exercise should be encouraged. There is growing epidemiological evidence that smoking is associated with worse outcomes in diabetic and nondiabetic CKD as well as being a modifiable cardiovascular risk factor.

2. Dietary protein restriction—The role of dietary protein restriction in renoprotective strategies remains controversial. Protein catabolism generates metabolic byproducts known to accumulate in late-stage CKD, and those byproducts likely contribute to the uremic syndrome; further they have been shown to contribute to a more rapid GFR loss in animal models of kidney disease. Thus, dietary protein restriction as a modifier of CKD was an appealing hypothesis to evaluate. In the largest controlled clinical trial done to investigate this issue, the Modified Diet in Renal Disease (MDRD) study, very low-protein diet, defined as a restriction of 0.28 g/kg/day, was compared to low-protein diet and normal-protein diet, 0.58 g/kg/day and 1.3 g/day, respectively. Neither the low-protein nor the very low-protein diets, according to the intent-to-treat analysis, were shown to confer a slower rate of GFR decline. Though there was an observed trend toward slower GFR decline in the very low-protein diet group, the difference was not significant, and there was no difference between groups with respect to the time to ESRD by study close. However, in a small subset of patients with baseline urinary protein excretion 1 g/24 h or greater a benefit of the low-protein diet was seen. Seven years after the study was completed and the assigned protein diet was no longer being followed, there was a decreased rate of ESRD in the low-protein group. However, long-term follow-up of those patients in the very low-protein group also had a higher rate of death.

Moreover, while low-protein diets have been evaluated according to the achieved nutritional profiles and safe methods of delivery have been identified, with a restriction of about 0.7 g/kg/day being the recommendation of some large professional societies, the risk for and impact of protein energy wasting and malnutrition remains uncertain. From a practical perspective, low-protein diets are difficult to implement without frequent dietary counseling, and low-protein specialty foods. Furthermore, determining adherence also requires cumbersome monitoring with 24-hour urine collections for urea measurement. These barriers make widespread implementation challenging.

3. Avoidance of acute kidney injury (AKI)—AKI superimposed on existing CKD is an increasingly common factor in progressive loss of renal function. We recommend educating all patients about ways to avoid acute renal insults. This approach has gained increasing support as observational data continue to suggest that AKI leads to irreversible injury and contributes to a more rapid progression of underlying CKD. Patients should be counseled about avoiding certain over-the-counter therapeutic agents, both marketed pharmaceuticals like nonsteroidal anti-inflammatory drugs, fleets phosphate-based enemas, and others, as well as counseling about the risks of herbal preparations that have been linked with AKI. Patients should also be counseled about minimizing exposure to intravenous contrast whenever able, and recommend that other providers seek guidance before contrast exposure in order to allow emphasis of preexposure hydration recommendations. We also recommend avoiding prolonged periods of intravascular volume depletion—especially as most episodes of volume depletion begin at home and hemodynamic renal injuries account for most outpatient cases of AKI. This final recommendation is of increased importance because many patients followed in nephrology clinic will be treated with RAAS blockade; such treatment can—as discussed in the following text—amplify the renal consequences of intravascular volume depletion.

B. Pharmacologic Interventions

1. Control of hypertension—The treatment of hypertension remains fundamental to therapeutic interventions for slowing the progression of CKD. Early clinical studies found that even modest reductions in BP, from 180 mm Hg systolic to approximately 140 mm Hg, resulted in cardiovascular protection and suggested attenuation of the rate of decline in renal function. Two important questions raised by these early observations include what level of BP control is required for optimal preservation of renal function and what antihypertensive drugs afford the most effective renoprotection?

A. LEVEL OF BLOOD PRESSURE CONTROL—Numerous epidemiologic studies have demonstrated that lowered BP associates with better renal outcomes. In clinical trials, it has been well established that lowered therapeutic goals for BP reduction are associated with improved stroke risk and overall improved cardiovascular outcomes. Early trials evaluating lower BP targets on CKD progression were both underpowered and confounded to fully ascertain whether lower BP conferred a renal benefit. The MDRD study showed renal benefit with lower BP targets (mean arterial pressure [MAP] ≤92 mm Hg), not in the study population as a whole but only among a subset of patients who had more than 1 g/day of proteinuria at baseline. In the AASK trial, the initial intent-to-treat analysis failed to show a difference in renal outcomes between those patients assigned to an MAP goal of less than 92 mm Hg versus those assigned to less intensive control, defined as an MAP goal of 102–107 mm Hg. Despite the absence of a signal during the trial phase, 7 years after the trial was completed, after there was no longer separation in BP control between the two groups, subsequent analysis suggested that there was a slower decline of GFR in the patients initially randomized to intensive BP control. These data should be considered hypothesis generating. Recent work has offered new insights on BP targets in both the diabetic and the nondiabetic CKD populations, with the Action to Control Cardiovascular Risk in Diabetes-BP (ACCORD-BP) trial and the Systolic Blood Pressure Intervention Trial (SPRINT) offering insight.

The ACCORD-BP trial included 4733 patients with type 2 diabetes and hypertension; notably, it excluded patients with high-risk cardiovascular disease and anyone with a serum creatinine less than 1.5 mg/dL which may have led to a lower-than-expected event rate. All patients were on RAAS blockade and were randomized to either standard BP control (<140 mm Hg systolic) or intensive-therapy (<120 mm Hg systolic). The final analysis suggested that there was no benefit of the intensive goal on the prevention of either the composite cardiovascular outcome or the renal-specific outcomes; there was a trend toward reduced stroke risk (41% risk reduction), though not powered to draw firm conclusions about the veracity of that reduction.

The SPRINT was similarly designed though it targeted a nondiabetic population of patients with hypertension, cardiovascular risk factors, or the presence of CKD. It included 9361 patients who were randomized to standard BP control or intensive therapy using the same definition as that used in the ACCORD study. The trial included only patients older than 50, who also had at least one of the following: age greater than 75, a history of cardiovascular disease (CVD) *or* an intermediate to high risk for CVD, or CKD stage 3 to early 4 (eGFR 20–59 mL/min). The trial was halted after approximately 3 years because the intervention group was found to have a significant improvement in CV outcomes particularly the incidence of new-onset heart failure and CVD-associated mortality. On analysis of the effect on the decline of GFR (defined as either a 50% reduction in eGFR or progression to ESRD), the analysis was unable to demonstrate a statistically significant differences between groups, though there were few total events leaving the study underpowered to draw a definitive conclusions. The subgroup of patients enrolled with CKD did not have a statistically significant cardiovascular benefit from intensive BP control, but there is no reason to believe that the results of the primary analysis do not apply to them. However, randomization to the intensive group was associated with an increased incidence of both new CKD and of AKI. In total, the SPRINT has shifted the balance of evidence to support lower BP targets among all-comers, but those targets should still be individualized to accommodate the risk-benefit profile of specific patients.

B. Choice of antihypertensive agent—As introduced previously in pathophysiology and further discussed in detail in the following text, blockade of the RAAS affords renoprotective benefits beyond those attributable to their antihypertensive effects alone and should be regarded as first-line therapy in patients with CKD unless contraindicated. Diuretics are generally not effective as monotherapy in patients with renal failure, but they may produce a substantial additional decrease in BP if added to ACEI or ARB therapy.

Patients with CKD require, on average, three antihypertensive agents to achieve BP control. Indeed, JNC VIII recommends starting at least two antihypertensive agents simultaneously in CKD patients with newly diagnosed hypertension. Often, a CCB will be used in these patients, but there may be a difference between the effects of dihydropyridine or nondihydropyridine agents. In the Avoiding Cardiovascular Events Through Combination Therapy in Patients Living with Systolic Hypertension (ACCOMPLISH) trial, the use of ACEI with the nondihydropyridine CCB amlodipine was found to confer greater renoprotective than the use of ACEI with a thiazide diuretic. Other work has suggested that dihydropyridine CCBs may have a deleterious influence on glomerular selectivity and proteinuria. While there are insufficient data to make any definitive declarations, certainly in patients who are already being treated with RAAS blockade, and in whom there are no other clinical considerations to aid in the choice of CCB, the dihydropyridine agents may offer benefits not consistently observed with the nondihydropyridine group.

2. Inhibition of the RAAS—Multiple randomized prospective trials published over the past two decades have established a firm evidence base to support the use of ACEI or ARB therapy as the single most effective intervention for slowing the rate of progression of CKD.

A. Diabetic nephropathy—Diabetic nephropathy is the single most common underlying cause of end-stage renal failure in the developed world and is projected to increase worldwide over the next two decades. This topic is comprehensively discussed in Chapter 54, and here we review only specific aspects relevant to treatments that have been shown to slow the progression of CKD. Inhibition of the RAAS is the centerpiece of such therapy and has been demonstrated to be of benefit in both early and late diabetic nephropathy.

(1) Microalbuminuria—Microalbuminuria (urinary albumin excretion of 30–300 mg/day) represents the earliest clinically evident renal manifestation of diabetic nephropathy. Glomerular hyperfiltration, which precedes the development of microalbuminuria in the pathogenesis of diabetic nephropathy, is not sensitive or specific enough to identify those patients destined to develop progressive diabetic nephropathy and is not readily measured. The development

of microalbuminuria, then, offers an early method for identifying those patients at greatest risk for progressing to overt proteinuria, which is believed to be—as noted previously in the pathophysiology section—one of the drivers of progressive renal dysfunction. Among patients with type 1 diabetes, multiple small trials have shown benefits from treatment with an ACEI. A meta-analysis that combined the results of 12 such studies (689 individuals) found that ACEI treatment was associated with a significant reduction in the risk of progression to overt nephropathy (odds ratio 0.38). Further, in many patients—three times the frequency of those treated with alternative agents—its use led to complete normalization of microalbuminuria. Among patients with type 2 diabetes, several studies have reported a reduction in microalbuminuria or a decrease in the number of patients progressing from microalbuminuria to overt nephropathy (risk reduction 24–67%) with ACEI treatment. Importantly, multiple studies have also reported cardiovascular benefits associated with ACEI treatment. Among patients included in the Heart Outcomes Prevention Evaluation (HOPE) study, subgroup analysis of those patients with type 2 diabetes who were treated with an ACEI, there was an observed 25% reduction in the combined primary endpoint of myocardial infarction, stroke, or cardiovascular death.

Two studies have reported a clear benefit associated with ARB treatment of microalbuminuria in patients with type 2 diabetes. In the first of these, the Irbesartan Microalbuminuria Type 2 Diabetes Mellitus in Hypertensive Patients (IRMA-2), 590 patients were randomized to irbesartan treatment (at 150 versus 300 mg/day) versus placebo, there was a significant, dose-dependent reduction in the incidence of overt proteinuria (5.2% in the 300 mg group, 9.7% in the 150 mg group, and 14.9% in those treated with placebo). In a similar study, 332 patients were randomized to treatment with valsartan or amlodipine, and doses were adjusted to achieve equivalent BP control. Valsartan treatment was associated with significantly lower levels of albuminuria and more patients receiving valsartan reverted to normoalbuminuria (29.9 versus 14.5%).

In summary, there is good evidence that RAAS blockade with ACEI or ARB therapy in the setting of microalbuminuria decreases the risk of developing overt nephropathy that follows in both types 1 and 2 diabetes. Since this has been demonstrated with numerous different ACEIs and ARBs, it is likely that the specific agent used is not important. The general consensus is that ACEI and ARB can be used interchangeably between these populations. Importantly, the demonstrated dose-dependent effect seen in the IRMA-2 trial above also suggests that treatment should be escalated to the maximum approved tolerated dose of RAAS-blocking agent.

(2) Overt diabetic nephropathy—Evidence of the benefit of ACEI treatment in patients with type 1 diabetes and overt

nephropathy was provided by the landmark Captopril study, the first large randomized clinical trial to show renoprotection conferred by ACEI treatment in human CKD. In this trial, 409 patients with type 1 diabetes and proteinuria greater than 0.5 g/day, as well as a serum creatinine greater than 2.5 mg/dL, were randomized to treatment with either captopril or placebo. A systolic BP less than 140/90 mm Hg was targeted in both groups. The majority of patients in both the captopril and placebo groups required additional antihypertensive agents. After a median follow-up of 3 years, captopril treatment was associated with a 48% reduction in the risk of a doubling of serum creatinine and a 50% reduction in the incidence of the combined endpoint of death, dialysis, and renal transplantation. BP control alone did not account for this difference.

Among patients with type 2 diabetes with overt nephropathy, evidence for the use of RAAS blockade is similarly robust, though largely driven by randomized controlled trials conducted using ARB therapy. The seminal trials evaluating this question include the Irbesartan Diabetic Nephropathy Trial (IDNT) and the Reduction of Endpoints in NIDDM with the Angiotensin II Antagonist Losartan (RENAAL) trial. Both trials randomized patients with type 2 diabetes to receive treatment with an ARB agent and compared this arm to conventional antihypertensive therapy. In the IDNT trial, patients with type 2 diabetes, proteinuria 900 mg/24 h or greater, a serum creatinine between 1 (or 1.2 for men) and 3.0 mg/dL, and a BP less than 135/85 mm Hg were treated with irbesartan, amlodipine, or placebo. Patients were followed for a mean of 2.6 years; the predefined composite endpoint included doubling of baseline serum creatinine, progression to ESRD, or death. Those treated with irbesartan had a 20% lower risk than placebo and a 23% lower risk than the amlodipine group to achieve one of those endpoints. The observed decline in GFR among these patients was 21–24% slower in the irbesartan group than in the placebo and amlodipine group. The RENAAL study included patients with type 2 diabetes, urinary ACR of greater than 300 (or urinary protein excretion >0.5 g/24 h), and a serum creatinine between 1.3 and 3.0 mg/dL, and compared the addition of losartan or placebo to conventional antihypertensive therapy on the same composite endpoint used in the IDNT trial. In the group treated with losartan there was a 16% risk reduction in the composite endpoint, and a 25% and 28% risk reduction in the risk of doubling the serum creatinine or progressing to ESRD, respectively.

In summary, key data provide incontrovertible evidence for renoprotective efficacy with ACEI treatment in patients with overt nephropathy and type 1 diabetes as well as ARB treatment in type 2 diabetes. Though, again, the universal benefits seen with the myriad of RAAS inhibitors used in these and similar trials suggest that the benefits conferred stem from a class effect, and that such agents are likely interchangeable.

B. **Nondiabetic CKD**—The clear benefits of RAAS blockade in proteinuric diabetic nephropathy prompted further trials to examine potential renoprotective effects in nondiabetic patients with CKD. In the REIN study, 352 patients with nondiabetic CKD were randomized to treatment with ACEI, ramipril, or placebo. Other antihypertensive drugs were added to achieve a diastolic BP of less than 90 mm Hg in both groups.

The study was stopped early after an interim analysis and found a significantly slower rate of decline in GFR among patients who were receiving ramipril and had a pretreatment proteinuria of 3 g/day or greater (0.53 versus 0.88 mL/min/month). Further analysis showed a significant reduction in the risk of the combined endpoint of a doubling of serum creatinine or ESRD in the ramipril group (risk ratio = 1.91 for the placebo group). Among patients with pretreatment proteinuria of 1–3 g/day, ramipril treatment also significantly reduced the incidence of ESRD (relative risk for placebo group = 2.72), particularly among those with a GFR of less than 45 mL/min at baseline. Similarly in the AASK study, African–American patients with 1 g or less protein/24 h were randomized to treatment with ramipril saw a lower incidence of the composite outcome (reduction in GFR by ≥50%, progression to ESRD, or death) than those receiving amlodipine or metoprolol (risk reduction 38% and 22%, respectively). This is an important observation because ACEIs had historically been prescribed less to African–American patients due to decreased antihypertensive efficacy, a problem that can readily be overcome by combination with a diuretic. It also supports the benefit of RAAS blockade among patients with limited or no proteinuria in preventing progressive loss of GFR.

The findings of all of these studies were supported by a meta-analysis of 11 studies of nondiabetic CKD that included 1860 patients. ACEI treatment was associated with greater reductions in BP and proteinuria than other antihypertensive treatments, but even after statistical adjustment for these factors, ACEI treatment afforded a lower risk of reaching ESRD (relative risk 0.69; confidence interval [CI] 0.51–0.94). Because of the rarity of specific nondiabetic renal diseases, well-powered randomized controlled studies with RAAS blockade done within nondiabetic CKD cohorts are lacking.

C. **ACEIs versus ARBs**—Whereas ACEI and ARB both inhibit the RAAS, they act on different effector elements and, conceptually, may not necessarily produce equivalent therapeutic effects. ACEIs inhibit angiotensin-converting enzyme (ACE) and therefore block conversion of the inactive peptide angiotensin I to the potent vasoconstrictor angiotensin II. Additionally, ACE catalyzes the breakdown of bradykinin, and thus ACEI treatment is associated with elevated bradykinin levels that may mediate some of its vasodilatory effects. However, ARBs bind to and inhibit the angiotensin subtype 1 receptor (AT_1). This leaves the angiotensin subtype 2 receptor active, which may have beneficial effects. Loss of feedback inhibition with blockade of the AT_1 receptor results in elevated angiotensin II levels that may go on to exert off-target effects. Despite these conceptual considerations that suggested benefit of ARBs over ACEIs, no well-powered randomized experimental studies in humans with CKD have studied a direct comparison of ACEI versus ARB. Though in a broader sense, head-to-head trials between agents investigating the cardiovascular outcomes afforded by each class have suggested that there is no difference. In those trials, ACEIs tend to have a higher risk of drug withdrawal due to adverse effects. Based on the summation of these data, ACEI or ARB treatments probably afford similar renoprotection. An ARB should be considered as alternative therapy in patients who are ACEI intolerant, which is most often due to a cough that may affect up to 20% of patients.

D. Dual RAAS blockade—Given the observed benefits from use of ACEI or ARB alone, it had been postulated that there may be additional benefit conferred by the combination RAAS-blocking agents. Indeed, early work was suggestive of a possible benefit with respect to GFR decline in those patients treated with dual therapy. However, several large trials have since been conducted in both diabetic and nondiabetic patient populations, and collectively they suggest that there is likely a greater risk of adverse events with dual blockade with limited added benefit. While the specific conclusions of the conducted trials differ slightly, they have suggested that dual RAAS blockade in renal disease does not reliably demonstrate a statistically significant difference in the rate of GFR loss and, in fact, likely increases the potential risks of therapy, such as hyperkalemia.

E. Direct renin inhibitors (DRIs)—DRIs represent novel treatments for inhibiting the RAAS. Although not rigorously tested, they may be as effective for renoprotection as ACEI or ARB therapy as monotherapy since they similarly perturb the RAAS. Studies evaluating the effect of aliskiren as add-on therapy to ARB treatment in diabetic and nondiabetic patients had shown a reduction in proteinuria. However, the Aliskiren Trial in Type 2 Diabetes Using Cardiorenal End-points (ALTITUDE) study was a large, well-conducted trial that included 8561 patients who were already on RAAS blockade with ACEI or ARB. The addition of DRI added no benefit with respect to the measured cardiovascular or renal outcomes between the DRI-treated group and the placebo group. It also demonstrated a potential safety signal secondary to increased rates of nonfatal cerebrovascular accident, hyperkalemia, and hypotension that ultimately led to the early termination of the trial.

F. Safety considerations—Despite the proven renoprotective benefits of ACEI and ARB treatment, some physicians remain reluctant to prescribe them in patients with CKD due to concerns about their potential adverse effects. The two principal areas of concern are hyperkalemia and the precipitation of AKI, but the risk of each can be minimized by the application of simple precautions.

(1) Hyperkalemia—In large randomized trials of ACEI or ARB treatment in CKD, the risk of hyperkalemia is reported to be low and resulted in discontinuation of therapy in only 0–4% of patients. A higher risk can be anticipated in patients with more advanced CKD and in diabetic nephropathy—both of which predispose to hyperkalemia, with the risk in advanced CKD stemming from the paucity of residual nephron mass to effectively excrete a potassium load, and in diabetics stemming from the often coincident underlying type IV renal tubular acidosis that can accompany diabetic nephropathy. The mainstay of prevention is comprehensive counseling to reduce dietary potassium intake and avoidance of potassium supplements as well as potassium-sparing diuretics. Serum potassium should be measured prior to initiation of therapy and 10–14 days after the first dose and possibly also after any dose increase in patients who are felt to be at high risk.

Available options for management include the use of a cationic exchange resin including sodium polystyrene and patiromer, with sodium zirconium cyclosilicate used internationally; though it is not yet approved in the United States. These resins exchange sodium ions (or calcium ions, in the case of patiromer) for potassium ions as they move through the gastrointestinal tract—most notably in the colon—to mitigate hyperkalemia. The use of one medication to counteract the effects of another is never appealing, but given the demonstrated benefits of RAAS blockade, this approach may allow for treatment of a group of patients whose hyperkalemia had previously prohibited the use of RAAS blockade. There are studies currently being considered to explore such combinations and to evaluate the impact of their combined use.

(2) Precipitation of AKI—Without question, as illustrated in the previous sections, RAAS inhibition slows the progression of CKD. However, under certain specific circumstances they have the potential to precipitate AKI. As discussed previously, ACEI and ARB treatment results in lowering of glomerular capillary hydraulic pressure and can therefore be expected to produce an initial reduction in GFR, evidenced by a rise in serum creatinine. Analysis of data from 12 randomized trials found that, paradoxically, the extent of the reduction in renal function associated with the initiation of ACEI treatment was inversely correlated with the subsequent rate of decline in renal function over time. Thus an initial increase in serum creatinine should not prompt the discontinuation of ACEI or ARB treatment, provided the increase is not progressive and is less than 30% over the first 2 months. We recommend that serum creatinine should be

monitored 10–14 days after initiation of treatment. There are two very specific causes of AKI associated with RAAS blockade: intravascular volume depletion and ischemic renal disease. We recommend counseling patients to ensure adequate hydration while using these medications. ACEI and ARB treatments are contraindicated in patients with bilateral renal artery stenosis and should be used with careful monitoring in patients with extensive vascular disease who may have undiagnosed renovascular disease.

3. Treatment of dyslipemia—Dyslipemia, characterized by elevated triglyceride-rich lipoproteins and reduced high-density lipoprotein (HDL) cholesterol, is commonly associated with proteinuria and probably contributes to the attendant increased cardiovascular risk seen in CKD. Moreover, experimental evidence suggests that lipid abnormalities may also contribute to progressive renal injury through multiple mechanisms, including vascular changes seen in the large renal vessels and possibly at the level of the tubular capillaries. In several animal models, treatment of hyperlipidemia has been associated with attenuation of CKD progression.

Unfortunately, large-scale controlled studies evaluating the use of lipid-lowering agents in CKD patients have had mixed results. In the largest trial conducted to date, the Study of Heart and Renal Protection (SHARP) trial included more than 6000 patients with CKD (as well at >3000 with ESRD). In those patients treated with lipid-lowering agents, fewer cardiovascular outcomes were observed in the CKD but not the ESRD patients, but there was no difference in the rate of CKD progression between the treatment and the placebo group. It is our practice to recommend lipid-lowering therapy to CKD patients to modify their cardiovascular risk, though not necessarily to impact progression of their CKD. Of note, CKD is a powerful risk factor for CVD. The Kidney Disease Outcome Quality Initiative (K/DOQI) guidelines currently recommend that patients with CKD stages 1–4 should be considered to be in the highest cardiovascular risk group and managed according to guidelines published by the National Cholesterol Education Program. Current recommendations suggest that total cholesterol should be maintained at less than 200 mg/dL, and low-density lipoprotein (LDL) cholesterol should be reduced to less than 100 mg/dL.

4. Treatment of metabolic acidosis—Current recommendations for the use of alkali therapy are based on observational data or limited clinical trial data. The rationale for alkali use as adjunct therapy is largely rooted in the mitigation of CKD complications, such as bone demineralization, the risk of hyperkalemia, and suppression of protein catabolism. However, small studies have suggested a reduction in the incidence of dialysis initiation in the treated groups. While biologically plausible, the level of evidence to broadly recommend this treatment remains limited. It is our practice

to treat to maintain serum bicarbonate above 21 mmol/L. This can be accomplished with sodium bicarbonate, sodium citrate, or increasing dietary potassium citrate intake with vegetables and fruits, though the latter should be done cautiously given the previously described risk of hyperkalemia.

5. Treatment of anemia—Anemia due to decreased renal production of erythropoietin is a common complication of CKD and may have a major impact on patients' quality of life. Replacement therapy with erythropoietin-stimulating agents (ESAs) allows correction of the anemia and has been shown to result in an improved in quality of life.

Several large randomized controlled trials have been conducted to evaluate the influence of ESAs on cardiovascular outcomes and have included relevant renal outcomes as secondary endpoints. In the Cardiovascular Risk Reduction by Early Anemia Treatment with Epoetin Beta (CREATE) trial, 603 patients with an eGFR of 15–35 mL/min were randomized to receive erythropoietin to achieve either a normal or subnormal hemoglobin (13–15 versus 10.5–11.5 g/dL, respectively). There was a tendency toward increased cardiovascular risk of those treated to the higher hemoglobin goal, and suggestion that higher hemoglobin targets may also quicken the rate of CKD progression. Correction of Anemia with Epoetin Alfa in Chronic Kidney Disease (CHOIR) and The Trial of Darbepoetin Alfa in Type 2 Diabetes and Chronic Kidney Disease (TREAT) were also well-conducted randomized trials that demonstrated increased cardiovascular risk among those treated to higher hemoglobin goals, and no statistically significant difference in the rate of progression to ESRD. One large meta-analysis that included 19 smaller trials and a total of approximately 8000 patients reported no difference in the progression of CKD between those treated with ESAs and those who were not. Currently, CKD populations should be managed with ESAs to avoid transfusions and to minimize the occurrence of symptomatic anemia, but it is unlikely to be of benefit in slowing the rate of GFR decline.

6. Treatment of hyperuricemia—Uric acid is known to be a potent activator of inflammatory cascades, with evidence that treatment of hyperuricemia reduces systemic inflammatory markers. There has been significant interest in evaluating the effect of hyperuricemia treatment on progression of CKD. While many studies have been conducted, most of the randomized controlled trial data come from small, open-label trials. One of the largest trials included 113 patients with an eGFR less than 60 mL/min who were randomized to either 100 mg of allopurinol or conventional therapy. Among those treated with allopurinol, eGFR increased by 1.2 mL/min over 24 months compared to a decline in eGFR of 3.3 in the standard therapy group. A meta-analysis evaluating the efficacy of allopurinol use in delaying the rate of GFR loss included 19 trials with at least 3 months of follow-up. While the studies included were all relatively small, with a total number of included patients of only 992, the findings suggested a benefit of allopurinol with an annualized eGFR loss in the allopurinol-treated group of 3.2 mL/min less than was observed in those not treated with allopurinol.

The use of allopurinol in CKD poses certain risks, including the small risk of drug hypersensitivity that can be life threatening, manifesting as Stevens–Johnson syndrome. This risk can be mitigated by reducing the starting dose according to eGFR, by screening for high-risk alleles for hypersensitivity among high-risk populations—namely those of Asian descent—and by careful counseling at the time of initiation about this risk with specific warnings to contact a medical professional with any new fevers, rash, or other new symptoms.

An alternative to allopurinol therapy is the use of febuxostat—another xanthine oxidase inhibitor—which may have a reduced risk of hypersensitivity reactions. It has not been studied in a randomized controlled fashion among CKD patients to evaluate its effect on eGFR decline. In a study of 93 patients in a single center, those treated with febuxostat had a slower rate of GFR loss than the control group at 6 months with 38% of those treated with febuxostat having a greater than 10% decline in GFR versus 54% among those in the control group. It also remains unclear what the goal uric acid value should be in these patients.

Taken together, there is evidence suggesting that there may be benefit to treating hyperuricemia, but the limited sample size and short follow-up interval in available trials does not lend itself to a conclusive recommendation for this therapy in all patients.

7. Use of SGLT2 inhibitors—Recent work investigating the use of the sodium glucose cotransporter 2 (SGLT2) inhibitors has led to a potentially novel new pathway that may favorably impact CKD progression. Initially studied as an adjunct agent for treatment of hyperglycemia, subsequent research has demonstrated positive effect on cardiovascular outcomes among type 2 diabetics. The Empagliflozin, Cardiovascular Outcomes, and Mortality in Type 2 Diabetes (EMPA-REG) trial was designed to compare composite cardiovascular outcomes and mortality rates between patients treated with empagliflozin and those who were not. That trial demonstrated reduced risk in the primary outcome (composite of death from cardiovascular causes, nonfatal myocardial infarction, or nonfatal stroke) as well as in all-cause mortality.

Given these findings, subsequent analysis sought to investigate the impact of empagliflozin on the rate of GFR loss among treated patients found that the rate of worsening nephropathy among treated patients was significantly lower (12.7%) when compared to placebo (18.8%). This was again shown in a smaller clinical trial evaluating canagliflozin, with lower rates of both worsening GFR and proteinuria. Ongoing investigation using SGLT2 inhibitors hopes to confirm the benefit on CKD progression not only among patients with type 2 diabetes but also among patients who have *nondiabetic* renal disease.

Prognosis

Clinical trials have identified several interventions that are effective in slowing the rate of GFR decline in CKD. Whereas each affords benefit, none of them alone, or in combination, have proven able to reliably halt progression of CKD in all patients. Thus, many will still progress to ESRD, albeit at a slower rate. In light of these data, it seems logical to combine effective interventions directed at different aspects of CKD progression into a comprehensive strategy for maximizing renoprotection, though we do not yet know the full impact of combined interventions.

It should be noted that the treatments and tests required for monitoring are relatively inexpensive and are widely available. Application of a multifaceted approach should therefore be possible across a wide range of health care systems and may substantially reduce the number of patients dependent on RRT worldwide. Achieving this goal is arguably the greatest challenge facing nephrologists today.

KEY READINGS

Appel LJ et al: Intensive blood-pressure control in hypertensive chronic kidney disease. N Engl J Med 2010;363:918.

Baigent C et al: The effects of lowering LDL cholesterol with simvastatin plus ezetimibe in patients with chronic kidney disease (Study of Heart and Renal Protection): a randomised placebo-controlled trial. Lancet 2011;377:2181.

Brenner BM et al: Effects of losartan on renal and cardiovascular outcomes in patients with type 2 diabetes and nephropathy. N Engl J Med 2001;345:861.

Chawla LS et al: Acute kidney injury and chronic kidney disease as interconnected syndromes. N Engl J Med 2014;371:58.

Covic A et al: Erythropoiesis-stimulating agents (ESA) for preventing the progression of chronic kidney disease: a meta-analysis of 19 studies. Am J Nephrol 2014;40:263.

de Brito-Ashurst I et al: Bicarbonate supplementation slows progression of CKD and improves nutritional status. J Am Soc Nephrol 2009;20:2075.

Drueke TB et al: Normalization of hemoglobin level in patients with chronic kidney disease and anemia. N Engl J Med 2006;355:2071.

Effects of ramipril on cardiovascular and microvascular outcomes in people with diabetes mellitus: results of the HOPE study and MICRO-HOPE substudy. Heart Outcomes Prevention Evaluation Study Investigators. Lancet 2000;355:253.

Fried LF et al: Combined angiotensin inhibition for the treatment of diabetic nephropathy. N Engl J Med 2013;369:1892.

Goicoechea M et al: Effect of allopurinol in chronic kidney disease progression and cardiovascular risk. Clin J Am Soc Nephrol 2010;5:1388.

Group ACEIiDNT: Should all patients with type 1 diabetes mellitus and microalbuminuria receive angiotensin-converting enzyme inhibitors? A meta-analysis of individual patient data. Ann Intern Med 2001;134:370.

Group SR et al: A randomized trial of intensive versus standard blood-pressure control. N Engl J Med 2015;373:2103.

Heerspink HJ et al: Canagliflozin slows progression of renal function decline independently of glycemic effects. J Am Soc Nephrol 2017;28:368.

Investigators O et al: Telmisartan, ramipril, or both in patients at high risk for vascular events. N Engl J Med 2008;358:1547.

Jamerson K et al: Benazepril plus amlodipine or hydrochlorothiazide for hypertension in high-risk patients. N Engl J Med 2008;359:2417.

Kanji T et al: Urate lowering therapy to improve renal outcomes in patients with chronic kidney disease: systematic review and meta-analysis. BMC Nephrol 2015;16:58.

Lewis EJ et al: Renoprotective effect of the angiotensin-receptor antagonist irbesartan in patients with nephropathy due to type 2 diabetes. N Engl J Med 2001;345:851.

Lewis EJ et al: The effect of angiotensin-converting-enzyme inhibition on diabetic nephropathy. The Collaborative Study Group. N Engl J Med 1993;329:1456.

Parving HH et al: Aliskiren combined with losartan in type 2 diabetes and nephropathy. N Engl J Med 2008;358:2433.

Parving HH et al: Aliskiren Trial in Type 2 Diabetes Using Cardio-Renal Endpoints (ALTITUDE): rationale and study design. Nephrology, dialysis, transplantation: official publication of the European Dialysis and Transplant Association—European Renal Association 2009;24:1663.

Parving HH et al: Cardiorenal end points in a trial of aliskiren for type 2 diabetes. N Engl J Med 2012;367:2204.

Parving HH et al: The effect of irbesartan on the development of diabetic nephropathy in patients with type 2 diabetes. N Engl J Med 2001;345:870.

Pfeffer MA et al: A trial of darbepoetin alfa in type 2 diabetes and chronic kidney disease. N Engl J Med 2009;361:2019.

Singh AK et al: Correction of anemia with epoetin alfa in chronic kidney disease. N Engl J Med 2006;355:2085.

Sircar D et al: Efficacy of Febuxostat for slowing the GFR decline in patients with CKD and asymptomatic hyperuricemia: a 6-month, double-blind, randomized, placebo-controlled trial. Am J Kidney Dis 2015;66:945.

The GISEN Group (Gruppo Italiano di Studi Epidemiologici in Nefrologia): Randomised placebo-controlled trial of effect of ramipril on decline in glomerular filtration rate and risk of terminal renal failure in proteinuric, non-diabetic nephropathy. Lancet 1997;349:1857.

Viberti G et al: Microalbuminuria reduction with valsartan in patients with type 2 diabetes mellitus: a blood pressure-independent effect. Circulation 2002;106:672.

Wanner C, Inzucchi SE, Zinman B: Empagliflozin and progression of kidney disease in type 2 diabetes. N Engl J Med 2016;375:1801.

Zinman B, Lachin JM, Inzucchi SE: Empagliflozin, cardiovascular outcomes, and mortality in type 2 diabetes. N Engl J Med 2016;374:1094.

■ CHAPTER REVIEW QUESTIONS

1. A 61-year-old woman with a medical history notable for hypertension and diabetes mellitus type 2 presents to nephrology clinic for routine follow-up of stage 4 CKD secondary to diabetic nephropathy. She is doing well overall. Her medication regimen includes metoprolol 50 mg twice daily, lisinopril 20 mg daily, and insulin. Her BP in the office is 138/86 mm Hg, heart rate is 78 beats/min; her physical examination is otherwise unremarkable.

   Her laboratory test results reveal a stable serum creatinine of 1.87 mg/dL, potassium 4.7 mmol/L, bicarbonate 21 mmol/L, and a glucose of 178 mg/dL. She has a spot ACR of 470 mg/g. What would be the most important change to make in clinic today?
   A. Increase metoprolol dose
   B. Start sodium bicarbonate
   C. Add metformin
   D. Increase lisinopril dose

2. A 41-year-old man is seen in the office for his annual physical examination. He has a medical history that includes hypertension and gout. His only new medical problem is some anterior knee pain that started about 4 months ago. He has been treating it with ibuprofen 800 mg two to three times daily. His other daily medications include losartan, amlodipine, and allopurinol.

   His physical examination shows a BP of 151/88 mm Hg and a heart rate of 81 beats/min. His right knee is without erythema and he has no point tenderness, but pain is elicited with passive and active extension. Examination is otherwise notable for only trace peripheral edema. Including referral for imaging studies to specifically evaluate his knee pain, which of the following would also be indicated?
   A. Serum uric acid
   B. Dual-energy X-ray absorptiometry (DEXA) scan
   C. Serum creatinine
   D. Urine sodium

3. A 16-year-old girl is seen in clinic after recently being diagnosed with type 1 diabetes mellitus. She has no other medical history and presents several weeks after the initiation and of insulin therapy for counseling. In clinic her BP is 115/71 mm Hg, heart rate is 72 beats/min, and she is slender with a normal physical examination. She has a serum creatinine of 0.6 mg/dL and normal ACR.

While counseling her about potential outcomes, which of the following statements would *not* be true?
A. Tight control of blood glucose decreases microvascular (including the development of retinopathy, neuropathy, and nephropathy) outcomes.
B. Annual monitoring of microalbuminuria is important for the detection of diabetic nephropathy.
C. She should immediately begin taking a RAAS inhibitor.
D. The earliest changes of diabetic nephropathy are difficult to detect clinically.

4. A 77-year-old man is referred to nephrology for management of stage 3 CKD secondary to decades of hypertension. He is asymptomatic and has questions about his prognosis. He was started on lisinopril 80 mg as part of his antihypertensive regimen 2 years prior, and his other medications include metoprolol 25 mg twice a day, amlodipine 5 mg daily, and simvastatin 40 mg daily.

His BP is 126/72 mm Hg. His physical examination is normal. His serum creatinine was most recently 2.7 mg/dL with an eGFR of 25 mL/min. As you begin counseling him about the pathophysiology of CKD, which of the following would be considered inaccurate?
A. The cumulative loss of renal parenchyma over time is largely irreversible.
B. Changes that are considered adaptive in early CKD become maladaptive in advanced CKD.

C. The use of maximal tolerated RAAS blockade helps to block the mediators of fibrosis.
D. Avoidance of new renal injuries is of no value because progression is unavoidable.

5. A 52-year-old African–American woman presented to the clinic after being found to have new microalbuminuria. She was diagnosed with diabetes 14 years prior and had been followed by her primary care physician (PCP) annually. Two years prior to presentation, her urine microalbumin was negative. She has mild diabetic retinopathy and some peripheral neuropathy. She is on losartan 100 mg daily, amlodipine 10 mg daily, and metformin 500 mg twice daily.

Her BP is found to be 161/78 mm Hg and heart rate 72 beats/min. She has an otherwise normal physical examination. Her laboratory evaluation notes a serum creatinine of 1.3 mg/dL and a urine ACR of 637 mg/g. She follows a low-sodium diet and is adherent to her medication regimen as instructed.

Discussion and workup of her kidney disease suggest diabetic nephropathy. Plans are made in clinic to address her BP. As you are counseling her about BP control, which of the following statements is most accurate?
A. Tight BP control (systolic BP >120 mm Hg) in diabetics has been shown to improve outcomes.
B. BP control in diabetic patients is not important; she just needs to focus on glucose control.
C. Maximal RAAS blockade in patients with type 1 diabetic is critical, though in type 2 diabetics it has been shown to be less important.
D. The BP goal in her is slightly more liberal (<140 mm Hg) than in similar patients without type 2 diabetes.

Nephrotic Syndrome versus Nephritic Syndrome

James Dylewski, DO

Laura Kooienga, MD

Isaac Teitelbaum, MD

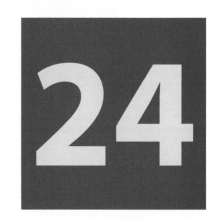

24

Glomerulonephropathies are disorders that primarily affect the structure and function of the renal glomerular apparatus. Frequently encountered in clinical practice, glomerulopathies are usually suspected from the history and the urinary findings of hematuria, red cell casts, or proteinuria. There are many different causes of glomerular disease that can be generally classified into nephrotic syndrome, nephritic syndrome, and non-nephrotic proteinuria. However, there may be considerable overlap in their clinical presentation with some diseases presenting with components of more than one syndrome.

NEPHROTIC SYNDROME

ESSENTIALS OF DIAGNOSIS

- Proteinuria >3.5 g/1.73 m^2/24 h (40–50 mg/kg/day).
- Hypoalbuminemia.
- Edema.
- Hyperlipidemia.
- Lipiduria.

▶ General Considerations

Nephrotic syndrome is defined as: more than 3.5 g of proteinuria/24 h, serum albumin less than 3 mg/dL, edema, hyperlipidemia, and lipiduria. Nephrotic syndrome may appear as a primary (idiopathic) renal disease or occur in association with any of a number of systemic conditions and hereditary diseases. The most common primary glomerular diseases include focal segmental glomerular sclerosis (FSGS), minimal change disease (MCD), membranous nephropathy, and membranoproliferative glomerulonephritis (MPGN). In the United States, the most common cause of nephrotic

syndrome is diabetes mellitus. Approximately one-third of patients with diabetes mellitus will develop nephrotic syndrome, predictably leading to kidney failure. Other systemic diseases that may lead to the nephrotic syndrome include systemic lupus erythematosus (SLE), human deficiency virus (HIV) infection, hepatitis B, hepatitis C, amyloidosis, leukemia/lymphoma, or solid organ malignancy.

▶ Pathogenesis

Nephrotic syndrome generally reflects noninflammatory damage to the glomerular capillary wall. The underlying glomerular disease results in proteinuria, which occurs from alterations in the glomerular filtration barrier. This increases glomerular permeability to plasma proteins. Albumin is the principal urinary protein lost, but other plasma proteins lost in the urine include hormone-carrying proteins such as vitamin D–binding protein, transferrin, and clotting inhibitors.

▶ Prevention

At present, we do not have means to prevent primary nephrotic syndrome. Secondary nephrotic syndromes can often be improved and sometimes completely reversed by treating and controlling the underlying disease.

▶ Clinical Findings

A. Symptoms and Signs

Nephrotic syndrome can present as asymptomatic proteinuria, but the most common symptom and sign at presentation is edema. Edema occurs initially in areas of high intravascular hydrostatic pressure, such as in the feet and ankles, as well as in areas in where tissue hydrostatic pressure is lowest, such as the periorbital and scrotal areas. If the edema becomes generalized and severe, it can present as anasarca.

B. Laboratory Findings

1. Urinalysis—Urine dipstick often demonstrates 3+ to 4+ protein, and a 24-hour urine collection will demonstrate greater than 3.5 g protein/day. Proteinuria can also be estimated from a single urine specimen by calculating the ratio of total urine protein in mg/dL to urine creatinine in mg/dL. This ratio approximates the actual 24-hour protein excretion in grams per day body surface area. Typically the urine sediment has few cells or casts. Urinary lipid may be present in the sediment and may be noted as being entrapped in casts, free in the urine, or enclosed in the plasma membrane of degenerated epithelial cells known as oval fat bodies. Under polarized light, the lipid in oval fat bodies gives it a distinctive "x" pattern and is referred to as a "Maltese cross" (Figure 24–1).

2. Blood chemistries—Fundamental laboratory abnormalities in nephrotic syndrome include decreased serum albumin concentration (<3 g/dL), decreased total serum protein concentration (<6 g/dL), and hyperlipidemia. Patients may have elevations in their blood urea nitrogen (BUN) and serum creatinine concentrations, but the glomerular filtration rate (GFR) can be normal. Some patients may also present with anemia, elevated erythrocyte sedimentation rate (ESR), hypocalcemia, and vitamin D deficiency. Other less common laboratory tests may be indicated depending on the patient's clinical presentation. These may include serum protein electrophoresis (SPEP) and urine protein electrophoresis (UPEP) to evaluate for myeloma or amyloidosis, and antinuclear antibody (ANA) to evaluate for SLE. Other tests might include hepatitis serologies, syphilis serology, HIV, complements, cryoglobulins, and thyroid function tests.

Antibodies to phospholipase-A_2 receptor (anti-PLA$_2$R) can be detected in approximately 70% of patients with primary membranous nephropathy and can be utilized for diagnosis. Anti-PLA$_2$ antibody levels can also be used to monitor treatment response since the level of the antibody tends to decrease or resolve prior to improvement in proteinuria.

C. Special Tests

Indications for kidney biopsy remain controversial, particularly in patients where diabetic nephropathy is believed to be the cause. However, biopsy is recommended when the etiology of nephrotic-range proteinuria is in doubt. Biopsy should be performed prior to beginning cytotoxic drugs or if the patient's clinical course differs from the expected. In addition to helping determine the etiology of the disease, renal biopsy can be used to aid in management decisions. Specifically, cytotoxic agents may not be appropriate if there is extensive irreversible fibrosis, making the risk of adverse effects from the medication more likely than benefit.

▶ Differential Diagnosis

The differential diagnosis in nephrotic syndrome can be narrowed significantly based on the patient's age, race, and urine evaluation. For example, minimal change accounts for the majority of cases in children. In adults worldwide, membranous nephropathy and FSGS are among the most common causes of primary nephrotic syndrome. In adults older than 50 years, membranous nephropathy is the most common cause of idiopathic nephrotic syndrome while focal glomerulosclerosis is the most common cause in African–Americans. Overall, approximately 50% of patients with nephrotic syndrome have a secondary cause, with the majority of these being secondary to diabetic nephropathy. It is important to note that about 10–20% of patients who present with membranous nephropathy older than 50 do so secondary to a malignancy and appropriate malignancy screening of these patients should be performed.

▶ Complications

A. Hyperlipidemia

Numerous alterations in lipid profiles occur in the nephrotic syndrome as a result of increased synthesis and decreased catabolism of individual lipid fractions. These include hypercholesterolemia, hypertriglyceridemia, and increased low-density protein (LDL) and very low-density protein (VLDL). These abnormalities may possibly contribute to accelerated atherosclerosis.

B. Thrombosis

Several abnormalities of the coagulation system occur in nephrotic syndrome. These abnormalities include urinary losses of antithrombin III, proteins C and S, and factors IX,

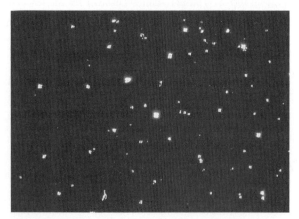

▲ **Figure 24–1.** Polarized anisotropic fat droplets. Note the "Maltese-cross" formation. (Reproduced with permission from Graff L: *A Handbook of Routine Urinalysis.* J.B. Lippincott Company, 1983.)

XI, and XII. In addition, plasma fibrinogen, tissue plasminogen activator, and platelet aggregability are all increased. These aberrations lead to an increased incidence of venous and arterial thromboemboli, especially deep venous thrombosis, pulmonary embolism, and renal vein thrombosis. Renal vein thrombosis is most common in membranous nephropathy, with as many as 20–40% of patients affected.

C. Vitamin D Deficiency and Hypocalcemia

Vitamin D–binding protein is a relatively small protein (59 kDa) that is readily filtered and hence lost in the urine. 25-Hydroxyvitamin D, which is bound to vitamin D–binding protein, is also lost in the urine in nephrotic syndrome.

D. Infection

Patients with nephrotic syndrome have urinary losses of immunoglobulins and defects in the complement cascade. This results in a higher susceptibility to infection, especially with encapsulated organisms such as *Streptococcus pneumoniae*. In addition, the immunosuppressive medications often used to treat the underlying glomerulopathy contribute to the increased risk of infection in these patients.

E. Hypoalbuminemia

Serum levels of albumin are low in nephrotic syndrome secondary to both losses in the urine and increased albumin catabolism.

F. Malnutrition

Prolonged and massive proteinuria may culminate in malnutrition as a result of negative nitrogen balance with loss of lean body mass.

G. Anemia

Urinary losses of erythropoietin (30 kDa) and transferrin may lead to an iron-resistant microcytic hypochromic anemia. If kidney function deteriorates to the point of chronic kidney disease, decreased erythropoietin production may play a role as well.

▶ Treatment

A. Underlying Systemic or Renal Disease Immunosuppressive Medications

Corticosteroids are typically used for diseases such as MCD and primary FSGS. The length of corticosteroid is typically longer with FSGS, but it depends on the patient's response to treatment. Calcineurin inhibitors have also been used in corticosteroid-sparing regimens or as a second-line agent in FSGS. Patients with primary membranous nephropathy can be treated with various immunosuppressive regimens. Most often, the combination of cyclophosphamide and steroids is

employed if there is severe clinical disease or if they fail to have a spontaneous remission. Rituximab has also been used in the treatment of primary membranous nephropathy with promising, although very limited, results.

Other treatments may consist of antimicrobial agents such as those for the treatment of secondary syphilis or tumor resection and chemotherapy for nephrotic syndrome associated with malignancy. In cases where the nephrotic syndrome is the result of a medication, such as nonsteroidal anti-inflammatory drugs (NSAIDs), discontinuation of the medication is the treatment of choice.

B. Complications of the Nephrotic Syndrome

1. Hyperlipidemia—Premature atherosclerosis and an increased incidence of myocardial infarction have been reported in patients with the nephrotic syndrome. In addition, hyperlipidemia is likely a separate risk factor for both atherosclerotic cardiovascular disease and the progression of renal disease. Hyperlipidemia typically improves after the resolution of the nephrotic syndrome. All lipid-lowering medications have been used in nephrotic syndrome to help reduce the rate of adverse coronary events. The most potent agents are the 3-hydroxy-3-methylglutaryl coenzyme A (HMG-CoA) reductase inhibitors alone or in combination with bile acid sequestrants such as cholestyramine.

2. Edema—Nephrotic syndrome results in primary renal sodium retention. This may result in peripheral and periorbital edema and, if severe and generalized, may result in anasarca with serous effusions. Goals of treatment include salt restriction and use of loop diuretics to achieve slow resolution of edema; rapid diuresis can result in hypovolemia and hypotension. Occasionally, thiazide diuretics must be added to the loop diuretics in order to block sodium reabsorption at multiple sites in the nephron. Amiloride and mineralocorticoid receptor antagonist may also be helpful in the treatment of edema by antagonizing the epithelial sodium channel, which is activated by excess levels of urinary plasmin and plasminogen (serine proteases) found in proteinuric patients.

However, it is important to monitor for hyperkalemia when amiloride or mineralocorticoid receptor antagonists are used with angiotensin-converting enzyme inhibitors (ACEIs) or angiotensin II receptor blockers (ARBs).

3. Thrombosis—Anticoagulation is indicated in patients with nephrotic syndrome and documented thrombotic events. Anticoagulation is usually continued until the patient experiences resolution of the nephrotic syndrome. Prophylactic anticoagulation and antiplatelet therapy in patients with nephrotic syndrome remain controversial. Patients with idiopathic membranous nephropathy with a serum albumin concentration less than 2–2.5 g/dL are at particularly high risk, and the benefits of anticoagulation may outweigh the risks.

4. Treatment of proteinuria

A. Angiotensin-converting enzyme inhibitors (ACEIs) or angiotensin II receptor blockers (ARBs)—These agents work by lowering intraglomerular capillary hydrostatic pressure and preventing the development of hemodynamically mediated FSGS. ARBs also decrease the formation of tumor growth factor-β_1 (TGF-β_1), which has been shown to play a role in progressive renal fibrosis.

B. Low-protein diet—A low-fat, plant-based protein diet that provides 0.7 g protein/kg/day has been demonstrated to be beneficial in decreasing urinary protein excretion and improving lipid profiles. However, protein-restricted diets, in general, may lead to malnutrition. Therefore, this treatment approach should be used under close observation to ensure adequate nutrition.

C. NSAIDs—NSAIDs work by decreasing GFR and thus decrease the amount of protein lost in the urine. Due to the risk of NSAID-induced acute kidney injury, hyperkalemia, and salt and water retention, NSAIDs are not used unless the severity of the proteinuria causes significant malnutrition and poor quality of life.

D. Dual angiotensin-converting enzyme inhibitors (ACEIs) and angiotnesin II receptor blockers (ARBs)—The combination of an ACEI and ARB simultaneously has been used and shown to be effective in reducing proteinuria. However, the risk of adverse events (namely severe hyperkalemia) has been shown to outweigh the benefits of proteinuria reduction. Thus, dual ACEI and ARB should not be used except in a very select patient population.

▶ Prognosis

The prognosis in nephrotic syndrome is typically worse in patients with heavy proteinuria, renal insufficiency, and severe hypertension. The overall prognosis depends on etiology and is related to histology. For example, MCD can have spontaneous remissions and is highly steroid responsive with an excellent prognosis. In contrast, spontaneous remission of primary FSGS is rare and the renal prognosis is relatively poor.

NEPHRITIC SYNDROME

ESSENTIALS OF DIAGNOSIS

- ▶ Hematuria.
- ▶ Red blood cell (RBC) casts.
- ▶ Variable proteinuria.
- ▶ Renal insufficiency.
- ▶ Salt retention (hypertensive nephropathy [HTN] and edema).

▶ General Considerations

Glomerulonephritis is characterized by an intraglomerular inflammatory process and renal dysfunction. It can be acute, subacute, or chronic and may or may not progress to ESRD. Nephritic syndrome is a clinical syndrome in which an individual has glomerular hematuria with or without the presence of RBC casts, variable amounts of proteinuria, renal insufficiency, and often hypertension. The nephritic syndrome is the manner in which patients with glomerulonephritis typically present; it may be caused by an intrinsic renal disease or a systemic disease process. Classic causes of the nephritic syndrome include postinfectious glomerulonephritis, immunoglobulin A (IgA) nephropathy, and lupus nephritis. IgA is the most common cause of glomerulonephritis worldwide. A subset of acute glomerulonephritis, known as rapidly progressive glomerulonephritis (RPGN), can present with severe and progressive renal failure. RPGNs are typically subdivided into one of three broad categories: (1) antiglomerular basement membrane (anti-GBM) disease (including Goodpasture syndrome); (2) immune complex diseases such as postinfectious, immunoglobulin A vasculitis (as known as Henoch–Schönlein purpura), and certain MPGN; and (3) Pauci-immune disease including polyarteritis nodosum, microscopic polyangiitis, and granulomatosis with polyangiitis (formerly known as Wegener granulomatosis). A clinical approach whereby to evaluate the cause of an RPGN is outlined in Figure 24–2.

▶ Pathogenesis

Nephritic syndrome is characterized by an inflammatory process. The degree of glomerular inflammation in part determines the severity of renal dysfunction and associated clinical manifestations. Immunologic perturbations underlie many of the glomerulopathies. Two basic mechanisms of antibody-mediated glomerular injury exist. The first involves antibodies that bind to a structural component or other material implanted in the glomeruli. For example, circulating antibodies may form and be directed against the glomerular basement membrane (GBM) as in Goodpasture disease. The second mechanism involves formation of circulating antigen–antibody complexes that escape the reticuloendothelial system and are deposited in the glomerulus. Examples include DNA-nucleosome complexes in lupus nephritis and cryoglobulins in mixed cryoglobulinemic vasculitis

Other diseases, such as postinfectious glomerulonephritis, involve deposition of an antigen in the glomeruli with subsequent activation of complement. This can result in direct tissue injury or result in an inflammatory reaction with proliferation of the intrinsic glomerular cells such as the mesangial, endothelial, and epithelial cells. In severe cases, obliteration of the glomerular capillary lumens can occur in addition to rupture of the glomerulus into Bowman's space resulting in crescent formation.

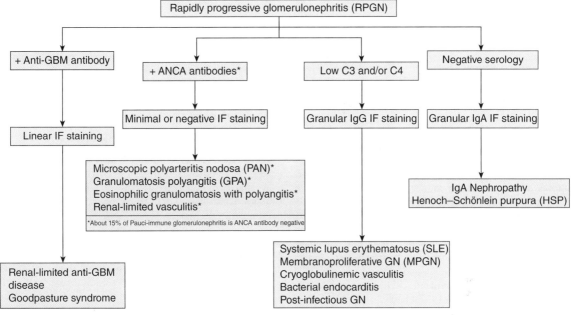

▲ **Figure 24–2.** Clinical approach to rapidly progressive glomerulonephritis.

Prevention

It is not yet known how to protect against intrinsic renal diseases or systemic diseases that cause the nephritic syndrome such as IgA nephropathy or lupus nephritis. Hence, the focus in this area is aimed at early recognition with prompt diagnosis and therapy so as to prevent irreversible loss of kidney function.

Clinical Findings

A. Symptoms and Signs

Nephritic syndrome can present with edema, oliguria, or uremic symptoms. Many patients have hypertension, which may even be malignant in some cases. Other physical examination findings depend on the underlying disorder. For example, malar rash and oral ulcers may be found in SLE, whereas palpable purpura is found in IgA vasculitis (formerly known as Henoch–Schönlein purpura) and cryoglobulinemia.

B. Laboratory Findings

1. Urinalysis—Patients often present with microscopic hematuria but may also present with macroscopic hematuria, which can have the appearance of tea- or cola-colored urine. Microscopic urine examination usually reveals RBCs. The RBCs are classically dysmorphic or misshapen as a result of the osmotic and chemical stress they incur as they

pass through the nephron. Urinary RBCs with membrane blebs or "bubble-like" projections (acanthocytes) are strong evidence of a glomerular cause of hematuria (Figure 24–3). RBC casts may also be observed. Urinary protein excretion

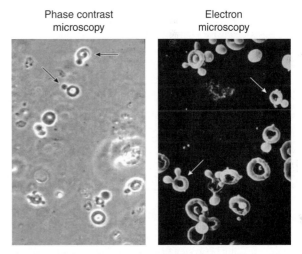

▲ **Figure 24–3.** Dysmorphic RBCs of glomerular hematuria. Phase contrast and Electron microscopy image demonstrating urinary red blood cells with acanthocytes (arrows). The presence of these membrane protrusions is consistent for glomerular hematuria. (From www.uptodate.com. Courtesy of Hans Kohler, MD.)

varies widely in nephritic syndromes, but it is generally less than 3 g of protein per day. Proteinuria can be quantified by either a 24-hour urine collection or can be estimated based on a single urine specimen by calculating the ratio of protein to creatinine.

2. Serum chemistries—A chemistry profile should be obtained to assess electrolyte status and to estimate the GFR in order to document the degree of renal dysfunction. A complete blood count (CBC) will often demonstrate anemia as well as possibly thrombocytopenia or leukopenia as seen in SLE. Additional useful tests depend on the patient's history and physical examination. These may include blood cultures if a fever or heart murmur is heard, streptozyme and antistreptolysin O (ASO) titers if a sore throat is or was recently present, or a hepatitis panel and cryoglobulins if a history of intravenous drug abuse (IVDA) is obtained or hepatomegaly palpated. Other helpful tests might include complement levels, anti-neutrophilic cytoplasmic antibodies (ANCAs), anti-GBM antibodies, and immune complex disease markers such as ANA and anti-dsDNA antibodies. It is important to note that up to 10% of patients with heavy proteinuria may have negative serologic findings at presentation due to loss of antibody in the urine or tissue deposition.

C. Imaging Studies

Chest X-ray may demonstrate pulmonary edema or findings suggestive of granulomatosis with polyangiitis or Goodpasture disease. An echocardiogram may identify a pericardial effusion or endocarditis. Renal ultrasound is frequently obtained when a decreased GFR is present in order to evaluate for kidney size. A kidney size of less than 9 cm suggests extensive kidney scarring with a low likelihood of reversibility.

D. Special Tests

Kidney biopsy is often used for definitive diagnosis and is helpful in distinguishing between primary and secondary causes of renal disease as well as subtypes in SLE. It can allow rapid diagnosis in cases of RPGNs where prompt diagnosis and treatment are essential in preserving renal function. Kidney biopsy can also yield information regarding the level of inflammation, extent of fibrosis, and overall prognosis.

▶ Differential Diagnosis

The differential diagnosis of nephritic syndromes requires distinguishing between a primary renal disease and one that occurs as a result of a systemic disease process. A useful clinical approach can be based on the results of serum complement levels, serologies, and immunofluorescence findings on kidney biopsy.

▶ Complications

Nephritic syndrome can lead to fluid retention with resulting edema and hypertension. Renal insufficiency also occurs and can require both short- and long-term renal replacement therapy. Anemia may occur as a result of resistance to erythropoietin or decreased production.

▶ Treatment

A. Underlying Renal or Systemic Disease

1. Corticosteroids—For many kidney diseases presenting as nephritic syndrome, high-dose corticosteroids (doses often in range of 1 mg/kg) are used as primary treatment (such as in IgA nephropathy) or in combination with other immunosuppressive agents.

2. Cytotoxic agents—Diseases such as anti-glomerular basement membrane disease (anti-GBM, formerly known as Goodpasture disease), granulomatous polyangiitis (GPA, formerly known as Wegener granulomatosis), and the more aggressive subtypes of lupus nephritis may require treatment with cytotoxic agents such as cyclophosphamide, mycophenolate mofetil, calcineurin inhibitors (cyclosporine or tacrolimus), and/or azathioprine. There have been a few studies suggesting that treating lupus nephritis with a combination of different immunosuppression agents may be beneficial.

3. Biological agents—Rituximab has been used in anti-GBM disease, GPA, and cryoglobulin-associated MPGN with good results. Rituximab has also been used in lupus nephritis but typically reserved for those who failed to respond to cytotoxic agents or used in conjunction with cytotoxic agents to limit corticosteroid exposure.

4. Plasmapheresis—Plasmapheresis is used to remove circulating pathogenic autoantibodies seen in diseases such as anti-GBM disease. Plasmapheresis is also used in pauci-immune crescentic glomerulonephritis and cryoglobulin-related MPGN in select individuals.

5. Others—Successful treatment of infections such as hepatitis B with lamivudine, hepatitis C with direct-acting antivirals agents, or HIV infection with HAART may lead to substantial improvement in renal dysfunction. Fish oil in doses of 6–12 g/day has been employed to prevent or slow the rate of loss of renal function in IgA nephropathy, though evidence for significant clinical benefit is lacking. On the other hand, treatment of postinfectious glomerulonephritis is only supportive, as the use of antimicrobial agents does not prevent or attenuate its course. However, antibiotics should be given if there is evidence of an ongoing infection.

B. Complications of Nephritic Syndrome

1. Edema—Though less frequently observed than in nephrotic syndrome, salt and water restriction in conjunction with diuretics is often beneficial.

2. HTN—Antihypertensive treatment is usually achieved with ACEI or ARB as these have the added anti-proteinuric benefits via reduction in the intraglomerular capillary hydrostatic pressure.

3. Renal insufficiency—If renal failure is severe or progressive, renal replacement therapy will often be necessary.

▶ Prognosis

Prognosis of the nephritic syndrome depends on the underlying etiology of the disease. In cases of postinfectious glomerulonephritis the prognosis is excellent with spontaneous recovery of renal function occurring in 70–85% of adults.

However, in diseases such as lupus nephritis, renal prognosis is mainly determined by severity of disease at presentation and response to treatment. Other diseases such as granulomatosis with polyangiitis and anti-GBM disease may be fatal if left untreated. However, with treatment, a dramatic recovery may be achieved.

KEY READINGS

Liu Z et al: Multitarget therapy for induction treatment of lupus nephritis: a randomized trial. Ann Intern Med 2015;162:18.

Ronco P, Debiec H: Anti-phospholipase A_2 receptor antibodies and the pathogenesis of membranous nephropathy. Nehron Clin Pract 2014;128:232.

Specks U et al: Efficacy of remission-induction regimens for ANCA-associated vasculitis. N Engl J Med 2013;369:427.

■ CHAPTER REVIEW QUESTIONS

1. A 19-year-old African–American man is seen in your clinic. He reports over the past 2 weeks progressive swelling of his feet to the point it is difficult to wear shoes. He now also noticed his eye lids are puffy in the morning. He denies shortness of breath, abdominal swelling, chest pain, arthralgia, rash, or gross hematuria. He has had no significant past medical history. He takes no medications and denies illicit drug use. He reports his father and paternal uncle both had a history of kidney disease and needed dialysis but denies family history of malignancy.

On physical examination, temperature is 37°C, blood pressure 142/85 mm Hg, pulse rate is 85 beats/min, and respiratory rate is 18 breaths/min. Cardiac and pulmonary examination is normal except for pitting edema to his knees. Abdominal examination is negative for hepatosplenomegaly and he has no flank tenderness.

Laboratory studies:
  CBC: within normal values

Renal function panel:

Sodium	140
Potassium	3.8
Chloride	107
Bicarbonate	23
BUN	15
Creatinine	1.0
Albumin	2.5
Calcium	8.0
Phos	3.5
Spot urine protein:	456 mg/dL
Spot urine creatinine:	99 mg/dL
Urinalysis:	3+ protein; no erythrocytes or leukocytes noted

Which of the following diagnostic tests is the most appropriate diagnostic test to perform?
A. Antinuclear antibody and anti-dsDNA antibody assay
B. Kidney biopsy
C. Anti-phospholipase A_2 receptor antibody assay
D. Serum protein electrophoresis (SPEP)

2. A 25-year-old woman comes to your office for evaluation of intermittent gross hematuria. She reports almost daily episodes of gross hematuria over the past month. She reports that she initially thought it was the start of her menstrual period, but it has not stopped when her normal menstrual period is only 5 days. She was diagnosed 2 years ago with SLE when she had joint pain, rash, and positive ANA. She has no prior history of lupus nephritis. She takes hydroxychloroquine for her lupus but no other medications. She denies worsening joint pain, dysuria, shortness of breath, chest pain, nausea, recent ingestion of beets, or lower extremity edema.

On physical examination, temperature is 37.5°C, blood pressure 115/71 mm Hg, pulse rate is 76 beats/min, and respiratory rate is 16 breaths/min. Cardiac and pulmonary examination is normal. Abdominal examination is normal, and she has no flank tenderness. Vaginal examination is normal without evidence of bleeding.

Laboratory studies:
　CBC:
　　Hemoglobin　　　9.6 g/dL
　　Leukocyte count　2.8 × 10⁹/L
　　Platelets　　　　223 × 10⁹/L

　Renal function panel:
　　Sodium　　　　138
　　Potassium　　　4.1
　　Chloride　　　104
　　Bicarbonate　　25
　　BUN　　　　　15
　　Creatinine　　1.1
　　Albumin　　　3.2
　　Calcium　　　8.9
　　Phos　　　　4.0
　　C3　　　　　10 (low)
　　C4　　　　　15 (low)
　ANA + 1:320
　dsDNA +
　Spot urine protein: 200 mg/dL
　Spot urine creatinine: 125 mg/dL
　Urinalysis: 2+ protein; 20–30 RBC/HPF, 0–5 WBC/HPF
　Kidney biopsy: moderately active class IV lupus nephritis

Which of the following treatment options would NOT be an appropriate first-line treatment option in this patient?
A. Mycophenolate mofetil and corticosteroids
B. Tacrolimus, mycophenolate mofetil, and corticosteroids
C. Cyclophosphamide plus corticosteroids
D. Plasmapheresis only

3. A 72-year-old man is seeing you for follow-up for his recent diagnosis of minimal change disease 3 weeks ago. At the time of his diagnosis, he was started on corticosteroids to treat the minimal change disease and diuretics with salt and water restriction for his edema. He reports feeling well today without any new complaints or concerns. He reports adhering to the medication regimen. He denies hematuria but still notes some bubbles in his urine. He denies over-the-counter medications, and his only medications include prednisone and furosemide.

On physical examination, temperature is 36.7°C, blood pressure 156/92 mm Hg, pulse rate is 71 beats/min, respiratory rate is 16 breaths/min, and BMI is 29. Cardiac and pulmonary examination is normal except for 2+ lower extremity edema. Abdominal examination is normal.

Laboratory studies:
　Serum creatinine is stable at 1.0
　Serum albumin improved to 3.1 (from 2.5–3 weeks ago)
　Spot urine protein: 680 mg/dL
　Spot urine creatinine: 180 mg/dL
　Urinalysis: 3+ protein; no erythrocytes or leukocytes noted

Which of the following treatment options is best to treat his proteinuria?
A. Start lisinopril
B. Increase furosemide dose
C. Start high-dose indomethacin
D. Start both valsartan and lisinopril

4. A 69-year-old white woman is seen in your clinic for routine follow-up. Her past medical history includes difficult to control diabetes mellitus type 2, hypertension, and hyperlipidemia. Her medications include glargine insulin, lisinopril, metformin, and atorvastatin. She reports feeling generally well. She states she attempts to adhere to her medication regimen but admits she does not adhere to a low-sodium, diabetic diet and occasionally forgets to take her medicines. She has no family history of kidney disease or malignancy.

On physical examination, temperature is 36.9°C, blood pressure 146/87 mm Hg, pulse rate is 86 beats/min, respiratory rate is 18 breaths/min, and BMI is 37. Funduscopic examination shows microaneurysms, dot and blot hemorrhages, and cotton wool spots consistent with moderate diabetic retinopathy. Cardiac and pulmonary examination is normal except for 1+ lower extremity edema. Abdominal examination is normal. Monofilament examination of lower extremities shows decrease sensation bilaterally.

Laboratory studies:
Serum creatinine: 1.1 mg/dL
Serum glucose: 250 mg/dL
Serum albumin: 3.4 mg/dl
Hemoglobin A$_{1C}$: 9.8%
Urinalysis: 3+ protein, 2+ glucose, 0–5 erythrocytes/HPF, and no leukocytes noted
Spot urine protein: 405 mg/dL
Spot urine creatinine: 80 mg/dL
ANA: Negative
C3 and C4: Normal
Hepatitis C antibody: Negative
HIV antibody: Negative

What is the most likely cause for her nephrotic syndrome?
A. Systemic lupus erythematosus
B. Hepatitis C–related MPGN
C. Primary Focal Segmental Glomerulosclerosis
D. Diabetic nephropathy

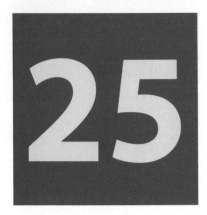

Minimal Change Disease

Elaine S. Kamil, MD

Minimal change disease (MCD) is a term used to describe the pathologic findings in a group of patients who present with heavy proteinuria, typically leading to nephrotic syndrome. On kidney biopsy the findings include apparently normal glomeruli on light microscopy, negative immunofluorescence, and diffuse podocyte foot process effacement on electron microscopy (Figure 25–1). While occasionally MCD may be secondary to another condition such as lymphoma, in the majority of cases MCD is one of the idiopathic renal diseases. Because MCD is most likely to be the diagnosis in children presenting with the nephrotic syndrome, the majority of children do not undergo a kidney biopsy, but receive empiric treatment without one. Seventy percent of children with MCD present before age 5 years, and 20–30% of adolescents who present with nephrotic syndrome have MCD. Nevertheless, MCD is the third most common finding in adults with nephrotic syndrome, after membranous nephropathy and focal, segmental glomerulosclerosis (FSGS). The typical patient with MCD responds to therapy but experiences recurrent relapses.

ESSENTIALS OF DIAGNOSIS

► Heavy proteinuria, typically leading to nephrotic syndrome.

► Renal biopsy with minimal changes on light microscopy, negative immunofluorescent microscopy, and podocyte foot process effacement on electron microscopy (see Figure 25–1).

► Usually there is no known etiology, although secondary MCD may be associated with neoplastic disease, toxic or allergic reactions to drugs, infections, autoimmune disorders, or other miscellaneous disorders.

General Considerations

MCD is the most common cause of nephrotic syndrome in children and the third most common cause of nephrotic syndrome in adults, affecting 10–15% of nephrotic adults. In children the incidence of nephrotic syndrome is 2–7 cases per 100,000 children and the prevalence is estimated at 16–100 cases per 100,000. In young children there is a male predominance of 2:1, but by adolescence the genders are equally affected. While most patients with MCD respond to therapy and have a good long-term prognosis, there are risks of developing serious complications such as infection and thrombosis, and the risks of complications from therapy. The treatment of the MCD patient who is resistant to or dependent on corticosteroid therapy remains a challenge, despite the several therapeutic options available.

Pathogenesis

Since first postulated by Shaloub in the 1970s, the pathogenesis of MCD has been associated with the presence of a circulating factor capable of inducing proteinuria. Presumably, the circulating factor is secreted by lymphoid cells and functions as a vascular permeability factor or directly affects the function of the podocyte. The induction of remission by immunosuppressive medications further strengthens the argument that the circulating factor is secreted by immune cells whose function is inhibited by these agents. Recent research has shown that T-cell regulation and function play a role in podocyte injury in MCD with an imbalance of T-cell subpopulations during relapse. In addition, patients who develop end-stage renal disease from MCD or FSGS are at risk for recurrent disease occurring rapidly after transplant. To date, the most promising candidate circulating factors include hemopexin; interleukin (IL)-4, IL5, IL9, IL10, and IL13; vascular endothelial growth factor (VEGF);

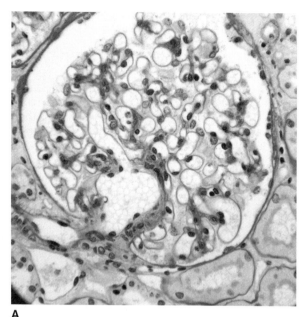
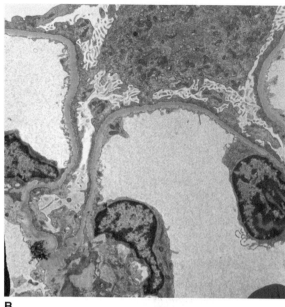

▲ **Figure 25–1. A:** Light microscopy (PAS stain) shows a completely normal looking glomerulus. **B:** Electron microscopy is normal except for the characteristic foot process effacement. (Photomicrographs courtesy of Arthur Cohen, MD.)

low-molecular-weight (<100 kDa) non-Ig permeability factors; and heparanase. The recently discovered clinical effectiveness of B-cell depletion from rituximab therapy has uncovered a role for B cells in the pathogenesis of MCD. It is likely that multiple factors are playing complex roles. The isolation and identification of the pathogenic circulating factors remain a "Holy Grail" in nephrotic syndrome research.

▶ Clinical Findings

A. Symptoms and Signs

The symptoms of MCD are related to the presence of nephrotic syndrome, including peripheral swelling, abdominal discomfort from ascites, occasional diarrhea from edema of the bowel wall, and, in extreme cases, pain from scrotal swelling and shortness of breath because of pleural effusions. Patients may experience oliguria, occasionally leading to acute kidney injury, especially in adults, because of renal hypoperfusion. There is an increased susceptibility to infection, especially from encapsulated bacteria, and patients may present with signs of peritonitis or septic shock. They are also at an increased risk for thromboembolic phenomena, which may present with signs of deep venous thrombosis, flank pain and hematuria from renal venous thrombosis (rare), or a central nervous system catastrophe from a sagittal sinus

thrombosis (also rare). MCD patients are at increased risk of developing clots in central lines. An occasional patient has only minimal swelling.

B. Laboratory Findings

Urinalysis in patients with MCD shows dipstick positive proteinuria (3+ to 4+); about 15% of patients with MCD also have microscopic hematuria at presentation that might clear during remission. The urinary protein-to-creatinine ratio (in milligrams/milligram) is 3.5 or greater in adults (or ≥2–3 in children) and can be obtained on a random sample, alleviating the need for a 24-hour urine collection. As a consequence of the heavy proteinuria, the patient develops hypoalbuminemia. The magnitude of proteinuria in MCD tends to be much greater than that seen in other glomerular diseases, leading to more profound hypoalbuminemia. Hypogammaglobulinemia may also be seen secondary to urinary losses of immunoglobulin G (IgG) or due to impaired IgG production and/or IgG catabolism in MCD. Children with MCD who have low IgG levels also have elevated immunoglobulin M (IgM) levels, changes in γ-globulins that may persist during periods of remission. Though not typically measured, there are elevated levels of circulating fibrinogen, factors V and VIII, and protein C and low levels of antithrombin III during relapses.

Renal function is typically normal, although there might be a minor increase in creatinine as a consequence of intravascular volume contraction. In severe cases, the hemoglobin and hematocrit will also be elevated from volume contraction, and platelets may also be elevated. Serum cholesterol and triglycerides are elevated and return to normal slowly after the induction of a remission. At presentation it is appropriate to draw C3 complement level and antinuclear antibody to rule out other causes of nephrotic syndrome; these will be normal in MCD.

C. Imaging Studies

Renal ultrasound is not necessarily indicated in nephrotic syndrome, but patients with MCD tend to have enlarged kidneys on ultrasound along with ascites fluid. A Doppler study will be helpful if there is suspicion of a renal venous thrombosis, which may be a complication of active nephrotic syndrome, especially in adults. Chest radiograph will be normal or may show pleural effusions.

D. Special Tests

Adults with nephrotic syndrome are diagnosed with MCD following a percutaneous kidney biopsy that is usually performed with ultrasound or computed tomography (CT) guidance. Since the vast majority of young children with nephrotic syndrome have MCD, they do not undergo a biopsy at presentation unless they have features suggesting a diagnosis other than MCD such as age less than 1 year, positive family history of nephrotic syndrome, extrarenal disease (eg, arthritis, rash, anemia), symptoms due to intravascular volume expansion, renal failure, or an active urine sediment. Children will undergo a renal biopsy, however, if they follow a steroid-resistant or steroid-dependent course. It is important to have the biopsy tissue studied by immunofluorescent and electron microscopy in addition to light microscopy. The presence of mesangial IgM on biopsy may portend a more therapy-resistant course.

Search for diseases leading to secondary MCD should be considered in adults with MCD (Table 25–1).

▶ Differential Diagnosis

The differential diagnosis of a patient with nephrotic syndrome and minimal to no hematuria includes MCD, FSGS, and membranous nephropathy. These lesions are differentiated on renal biopsy, although early FSGS may look like MCD since only some of the glomeruli show segments of sclerosis, and the sclerotic lesions, which tend to appear first in the deep, corticomedullary glomeruli, can be missed in a superficial biopsy.

▶ Complications

The complications of MCD are those seen with nephrotic syndrome, including infection, thromboembolic phenomenon,

Table 25–1. Selected secondary causes of minimal change disease.

Neoplasia: Hodgkin disease, non-Hodgkin lymphoma, leukemia, thymoma, renal cell carcinoma, mesothelioma, bronchogenic carcinoma, colon carcinoma, pancreatic carcinoma, urothelial cancer, prostate carcinoma, renal oncocytoma, multiple myeloma, eosinophilic lymphoid granuloma

Drugs: Gold, antimicrobials, nonsteroidal anti-inflammatory drugs (NSAIDs), trimethadione, paramethadione, lithium, interferon (α, γ), methimazole, tamoxifen, enalapril, penicillamine, provenecid, mercury, tioproin, immunizations

Infections: Syphilis, human immunodeficiency virus, mycoplasma, ehrlichiosis, echinococcus, schistosomiasis

Atopy: Pollen, cow's milk, house dust, cat fur, pork, bee stings, poison oak/ivy

Superimposed on another renal disease: IgA nephropathy, systemic lupus erythematosus, diabetes mellitus (type 1), autosomal dominant and recessive polycystic kidney disease, HIV-associated nephropathy

Miscellaneous: Sclerosing cholangitis, sclerosing mesenteric inflammation, vigorous exercise, acute decompression sickness, sarcoidosis, Graves' disease, thyroiditis, vasculitis, partial lipodystrophy, myasthenia gravis, renal artery stenosis, bisalbuminemia, Guillain–Barré syndrome, dermatitis herpetiformis

Adapted with permission from Glassock R: Secondary minimal change disease. *Nephrol Dial Transplant* 2003;18(Suppl 6):vi52.

and cardiovascular disease, in addition to the potential side effects of therapy. Increased susceptibility to infections, especially infections from encapsulated organisms, is multifactorial. Patients with MCD exhibit defective opsonization of bacteria secondary to low levels of factors B and I and experience low levels of total IgG and IgG subclass deficiencies. Treatment with immunosuppressive medications enhances the susceptibility to infections that can be life threatening. The most common infections include peritonitis (especially pneumococcal), cellulitis, and pneumonia. Patients with nephrotic syndrome should receive both pneumococcal vaccines (the 13 valent and 23 valent pneumococcal vaccines), preferably during remission and when they are off-immunosuppressive medications. Varicella immune status should be assessed in all patients with MCD, with prompt administration of varicella-zoster immune globulin or prophylactic acyclovir to nonimmune patients after exposure to an active case of varicella infection. Treatment with acyclovir may be lifesaving in an MCD patient on immunosuppressive medication who develops a varicella infection. Varicella vaccine is given during remission while off-steroid therapy appears to be safe and effective in children with MCD. Patients with MCD should also receive yearly influenza vaccine.

Children with MCD appear to be at a lower risk of thrombotic events than adults with MCD, but still they may experience life-threatening thrombosis such as sagittal sinus thrombosis, pulmonary artery thrombosis, or inferior vena caval thrombosis, while nephrotic adults are more prone to deep vein or renal venous thrombosis. The hypercoaguable state in nephrotic syndrome is due to several factors, including increased clotting factor synthesis (fibrinogen, II, V, VIII, IX, X, XIII, protein C), urinary losses of anticoagulants (antithrombin III), platelet abnormalities (thrombocytosis, increased aggregability), hyperviscosity, and hyperlipidemia. Thromboembolic risks are also associated with the presence of central lines and infections, with immobilization, and with thrombophilic genetic factors.

Most patients with MCD experience periods of remission during which their lipid profiles eventually return to normal. Thus, use of lipid lowering agents is not indicated solely on the basis of the MCD. However, adults with nephrotic syndrome have a higher incidence of coronary heart disease and children with therapy-resistant MCD or steroid dependency may well be at an increased risk of cardiovascular complications. Corticosteroid treatment and hypertension undoubtedly add to the cardiovascular risk.

Other complications include a risk of acute kidney injury secondary to renal hypoperfusion during relapse (more frequent in adults with MCD) iron deficiency anemia secondary to loss of iron-binding proteins during relapse, and vitamin D deficiency, also due to loss of vitamin D–binding proteins during relapse.

▶ **Treatment**

First-line therapy in MCD is corticosteroids. Children with MCD are highly likely (>95%) to experience a prompt (75% are in remission by 2 weeks), complete remission with steroid therapy while adults seem to be slower to respond. Once-a-day corticosteroid therapy is equally as effective as divided-dose therapy. Most pediatric protocols recommend 60 mg/m^2 of prednisone daily for 6 weeks followed by 40 mg/m^2 every other day for 6 weeks for a minimum duration of therapy of 12 weeks. Though it was felt that a taper after the 12-week induction period might be beneficial in reducing the subsequent incidence of frequently relapsing nephrotic syndrome, recent studies have questioned this practice. In children relapses are treated with a more abbreviated course of 60 mg/m^2 of prednisone daily until the urine dipstick is negative for protein for 3 days, followed by 40 mg/m^2 every other day for an additional 4 weeks.

Corticosteroid therapy remains first-line therapy in adults with MCD, but typically the adult patient requires a more prolonged course of steroids to achieve a complete remission. The current recommended induction therapy is 1 mg/kg of prednisone daily (maximum dose 80 mg) for 16 weeks. The course of daily prednisone may be abbreviated to 4 weeks if the patient goes into remission promptly. There is no consensus on a tapering regimen after remission is achieved, though tapering by 5–10 mg/week seems reasonable. Adults, however, are less likely than children to

experience relapses after a steroid-induced remission, but relapse rates in two recent studies were 42–73% and 27–41%.

The majority of steroid-sensitive children, and some adults, with MCD experience relapses that typically follow an infection, and remain responsive to treatment with steroids. Relapses are treated with shorter courses of prednisone; prolonged treatment of a relapse does not influence the subsequent frequency of relapses. However, most of these patients with frequent relapses will develop steroid-induced side effects such as hypertension, Cushingoid appearance, hyperactive behavior (in the younger children), mood changes, hyperglycemia, decreased bone density, and poor growth. Some patients will do well on a prolonged course of low-dose, alternate-day prednisone therapy.

Other therapies should be considered for MCD patients with frequent relapses, steroid dependency, and steroid toxicity. The goal of therapy for these patients is to avoid the complications of nephrotic syndrome by sustaining a remission while minimizing the side effects of the treatments. These therapies include alkylating agents, calcineurin inhibitors, mycophenolate, levamisole, and rituximab. A course of treatment with alklylating agents such as cyclophosphamide or chlorambucil has been shown to lead to a prolonged remission in children and adults who are frequent relapsers or are steroid dependent. Cyclophosphamide (2 mg/kg) for 12 weeks in children and 8 weeks in adults is more commonly used and may induce remission lasting several years. Patients must be monitored for bone marrow toxicity with weekly complete blood counts and prompt treatment with varicella-zoster immune globulin or acyclovir therapy on exposure to the varicella virus if they are not immune to varicella infection. Courses longer than 12 weeks may lead to gonadal toxicity. In practice, many patients begin cyclophosphamide therapy while on alternate-day steroids, which are weaned gradually over the course of 3–6 months.

Cyclosporine and tacrolimus have been shown to be useful therapy in the patient with frequent relapsing, steroid-dependent, and probably even steroid-resistant MCD. Because of their toxicity profiles, cyclosporine and tacrolimus should be prescribed only by physicians who are experienced in their use. Side effects of cyclosporine include hirsutism, gingival hyperplasia, hypertension, hypomagnesemia, and nephrotoxicity. The usual starting dose is 3–5 mg/kg/day divided in two doses with close monitoring of cyclosporine levels (target trough levels of 50–125 ng/mL), renal function, and magnesium levels. The typical course of therapy is 1–2 years, followed by a slow taper. Many patients experience relapses after discontinuation of cyclosporine; if continued therapy is needed, kidney biopsies should be performed to monitor for nephrotoxicity. Some patients also require alternate-day steroid therapy in conjunction with cyclosporine. Tacrolimus, also a calcineurin inhibitor, is dosed at 0.05–0.1 mg/kg/day in two divided doses and also requires close monitoring with target trough levels of 5–7. Tacrolimus may also be nephrotoxic and cause hypertension, but it does not have the cosmetic side effects of cyclosporine.

Other treatments include a 1- to 2-year course of mycophenolate, and most recently rituximab. Typically rituximab is administered intravenously at a dose of 375 mg/m^2 for two to four doses 1 week apart. A rituximab-induced remission may last indefinitely though many patients will relapse after 6–12 months. Mean time to relapse in one study was 18 months. While generally safe, rare serious side effects have been reported. Although not available in the United States, levamisole for 1–2 years has been shown to be helpful for many of these patients. Levamisole has been shown to reduce the incidence of relapses in children with frequent relapses but not in children with steroid dependence. If the patient has not yet had a kidney biopsy, many pediatric nephrologists will perform one prior to using another agent.

The majority of patients with steroid resistance are likely to have FSGS. Patients with secondary MCD may experience a remission after successful treatment of the disease inducing the MCD. Angiotensin-converting enzyme (ACE) inhibition or angiotensin receptor blockade is a useful adjunct for patients with steroid resistance even in the absence of hypertension. All patients with MCD should follow a no added salt diet during periods of relapse. Children with marked anasarca, pleural effusions, or signs of renal hypoperfusion should benefit from the cautious use of intravenous albumin (25%)—1 g/kg given over 2–4 hours followed by a 1 mg/kg dose of furosemide. The albumin infusion can be repeated up to every 12 hours to achieve a sustained diuresis. However, the patient's urine output must be closely monitored. A patient who has acute kidney injury as a complication of renal hypoperfusion may not respond to the albumin and furosemide infusions and is thus at risk for developing pulmonary edema. In addition, intravenous γ-globulin (IVIg) may be useful acutely in a nephrotic patient with hypogammaglobulinemia experiencing sepsis or once monthly in a chronically nephrotic patient with sustained hypogammaglobulinemia to reduce the incidence of sinus infections or bacteremia.

▶ Prognosis

The outcome in MCD is largely based on the patient's response to steroid therapy. In children, prompt remission within 7–9 days of therapy, absence of microhematuria, and age greater than 4 years at presentation predict fewer relapses. By 10 years from diagnosis, only 16% of children still experience relapses. Many children will "outgrow" their disease by or during puberty, although some continue to experience relapses into adulthood. During periods of relapse, patients remain vulnerable to life-threatening infections and thrombotic events. The long-term cardiovascular risk in children with MCD who have experienced long periods of steroid therapy and periods of hyperlipidemia and hypertension is largely unknown. Adults with MCD may have an increased risk of coronary artery disease. Patients with MCD who become resistant to steroids later in their course are likely to have FSGS with its high risk for end-stage renal disease.

KEY READINGS

Alpay H et al: Varicella vaccination in children with steroid-sensitive nephrotic syndrome. Pediatr Nephrol 2002;17:181.

Bagga A et al: Mycophenolate mofetil and prednisone in children with steroid-dependent nephrotic syndrome. Am J Kidney Dis 2003;42:1114.

Canetta PA et al: The evidence-based approach to adult-onset idiopathic nephrotic syndrome. Front Pediatr 2015;3:78.

Davin JC: The glomerular permeability factors in idiopathic nephrotic syndrome. Pediatr Nephrol 2016;31:207.

Glassock RJ: Secondary minimal change disease. Nephrol Dial Transplant 2003;18:vi52.

Hahn D et al: Corticosteroid therapy for nephrotic syndrome in children. Cochrane Database Syst Rev 2015;3:CD001533.

Kidney Disease Improving Global Outcomes Glomerulonephritis Workgroup: KDIGO clinical practice guidelines for glomerulonephritis. Kidney Int Suppl 2012;163:177.

Kyrieleis HA et al: Long-term outcome of biopsy-proven, frequently-relapsing minimal change nephrotic syndrome in children. Clin J Am Soc Nephrol 2009;4:1593.

Lombel RM et al: Treatment of steroid sensitive nephrotic syndrome: new guidelines from KIDGO. Pediatr Nephrol 2013;28:415.

Mathieson PW: Immune dysregulation in minimal change nephropathy. Nephrol Dial Transplant 2003;18:vi26.

Palmer SC et al: Interventions for minimal change disease in adults with nephrotic syndrome. Cochrane Database Sys Rev 2008;(1):CD001537.

Rüth EM et al: Children with steroid-sensitive nephrotic syndrome come of age: long-term outcome. J Pediatr 2005;147:202.

Vivarilli M et al: Minimal change disease. Clin J Am Soc Nephrol 2017;12:332.

■ CHAPTER REVIEW QUESTIONS

1. A 2-year-old boy is brought to his pediatrician's office because of progressive abdominal and periorbital swelling. He has had only two wet diapers in the past 24 hours, his appetite is less than his baseline, and he has had a runny nose for the past 1 week. He has had no fever or vomiting and remains playful. He has been a healthy boy with no previous illnesses except for otitis media at age 16 months. His pregnancy and delivery were uneventful. There is no family history of cardiac, liver, thromboembolic, or kidney disease.

On physical examination, his temperature is 37.4°C, his blood pressure is 93/47 mm Hg, and his heart rate is 96 beats/min. His examination is normal except for moderate periorbital edema, dullness on percussion of his lung bases, marked abdominal distension, and mild scrotal swelling. His urinalysis shows a pH of 6.0, specific gravity of 1.030, and negative dipstick except for 4+ protein. His H/H is 13.7/48, platelets are 434,000, and his white blood count (WBC) is 9.4 with a normal differential.

What additional testing is indicated at this time?
A. Blood culture, urine culture, and strep testing
B. Kidney biopsy
C. Urine total protein/creatinine ratio, serum cholesterol, C3 complement, antinuclear antibody (ANA), and blood chemistries—electrolytes, blood urea nitrogen (BUN), creatinine, serum albumin
D. Echocardiogram

2. A 38-year-old woman comes into your office with complaints of progressive ankle and leg swelling over the past 2–3 weeks. She has gained 15 lb, notices that her eyelids are swollen in the morning, and the waist of her pants is very tight. Her stools have been loose, and she has mild intermittent abdominal pain. Her knee and ankle joints feel tight. She denies any red or brown urine, preceding illness, sore throat, rashes, fever, shortness of breath, or other constitutional symptoms. She has a current history of allergic rhinitis and formerly had asthma as a child. Otherwise she has been healthy and works as an elementary school teacher. There is a family history of hypertension but no family history of heart disease, diabetes, kidney disease, liver disease, or arthritis.

On physical examination she is alert and comfortable with mild periorbital edema, clear lungs, mild abdominal fullness with no fluid wave, and 2+ foot, ankle, and pretibial edema up to her mid calf region. There are no rashes or joint inflammation. Her blood pressure was 118/65 mm Hg, and she was afebrile. Initial laboratory evaluation shows a urinalysis with a pH of 5, specific gravity of 1.030, dipstick with 4+ protein, 2+ blood, 5–10 RBCs, and 2 WBCs per high-power field on microscopic examination. Her H/H is 13.7/42, platelets are 380,000, and her WBC is 7.8 with a normal differential. Her chemistry panel showed a creatinine of 0.8, BUN 27, albumin 2.2, serum cholesterol 320, ANA negative, and C3 complement was normal. Urine total protein/creatinine ratio was 4.7.

What is the next appropriate step?
A. After checking a tuberculosis (TB) test, begin empiric therapy with daily prednisone 2 mg/kg daily.
B. Schedule a kidney biopsy.
C. Check serologies for hepatitis B and C.
D. Start therapy with a diuretic.

3. A 7-year-old boy has steroid dependent nephrotic syndrome that was diagnosed 4 years ago. He has always responded promptly to steroid therapy and does reasonably well on alternate-day prednisone, but you have been unable to wean the dose to less than 1 mg/kg every other morning without him relapsing, up to three times a year. His height was at the 75% at diagnosis, but over the years he has dropped down to the 50% and both his parents are tall. He has mild Cushingoid features, and his weight percentile has increased to the 95%. He developed mild hypertension, but that is well controlled with low-dose enalapril. His examination for cataracts was negative, and his renal function remained excellent. During relapses, he only shows nephrotic range proteinuria and has not had any microscopic hematuria. He has not developed any complications requiring hospitalization.

What is your next step?
A. Schedule a kidney biopsy.
B. Recheck a C3 complement and ANA.
C. Continue the alternate-day prednisone therapy and continue trying to wean the prednisone dose as tolerated.
D. Review second-line immunosuppressive therapics with his parents, including cyclophosphamide, mycophenolate, tacrolimus, levamisole, and rituximab.

4. A 3-year-old, recently diagnosed, previously healthy, nephrotic syndrome patient has been on daily steroids for 1 week when he presents to the emergency room with a fever of 104°F, tachycardia, and mild tachypnea. His blood pressure is 92/57 mm Hg. On examination he is ill-appearing and irritable. He has anasarca, clear lungs, and abdominal tenderness with rebound. He also has mild scrotal edema and no rashes though he has facial flushing. The emergency room team ordered a chest X-ray that showed a questionable infiltrate in the left lower lobe and small pleural effusions. His cardiac silhouette is not enlarged. The WBC is 22,000 with a left shift, H/H is 14.8/49, and his platelets are 920,000. Serum creatinine is 1, BUN 30, and serum albumin 1.8. He just urinated 10 cc, and his urine showed a specific gravity of 1.030, 4+ protein, and a negative microscopic examination.

What are your next steps?
A. Draw blood and urine cultures and perform a paracentesis for fluid culture, Gram stain, and WBC prior to starting antibiotics with coverage to include good coverage for pneumococcus.
B. Check a fractional excretion of sodium on his urine sample, and if the patient is conserving sodium, begin 25% albumin intravenously, 1 g/kg over 2–4 hours.
C. Place a good peripheral intravenous line and monitor the patient closely in the pediatric intensive care unit (PICU) for neurologic checks, vital signs, strict intake and output, and after a fluid bolus of normal saline, give intravenous fluids at insensible plus urine output replacement.
D. All of the above.

5. A 18-year-old patient with MCD and her parents want guidance about her long-term prognosis. She presented at age 4 and initially followed a steroid-dependent, frequently relapsing course. Because of some relative steroid resistance, she underwent a kidney biopsy at age 12 and it showed MCD. Over the years she received a course of cyclophosphamide that led to a 2-year remission, multiple courses of steroids for relapses, a 3-year course of tacrolimus, and she is currently on mycophenolate. She still has about one relapse per year despite maintenance mycophenolate for which she is treated with about 6–8 weeks of steroids. She experienced menarche at age 13, and her height and weight are at the 40% while her siblings are at the 75%. Her menstrual periods are regular. Her mild hypertension is well managed on enalapril, and her renal function remains excellent.

What do you tell her and her family about her future course?
A. The patient will likely develop end-stage kidney disease at some time and will need a kidney transplant.
B. It is likely that she will not experience any further relapses after age 21.
C. She is at risk for continuing relapses into adulthood with pregnancy being a trigger for relapse, but it is unlikely that she will develop end-stage kidney disease.
D. If she requires a kidney transplant, it is highly likely that she will get recurrent nephrotic syndrome after transplant.

Focal Segmental Glomerulosclerosis

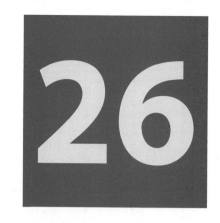

Howard Trachtman, MD
Debbie S. Gipson, MD, MSPH

ESSENTIALS OF DIAGNOSIS

▶ Focal segmental glomerulosclerosis (FSGS) can be primary or secondary.

▶ Diagnosis requires the presence of the characteristic histopathologic lesion.

▶ Genetic abnormalities in podocyte proteins may account for 25% of primary FSGS in high-risk populations.

▶ The presenting complaint is usually proteinuria or nephrotic syndrome.

▶ Nearly 50% of cases progress to end-stage renal disease (ESRD) over 5–10 years and disease recurs in up to 20% of those who receive a kidney transplant.

▶ Failure to respond to corticosteroid treatment is a poor prognostic sign and there is no proven therapy in these patients.

▶ General Considerations

A. Epidemiology

Focal segmental glomerulosclerosis (FSGS) is an important glomerulopathy because it has a high risk of progression to end-stage renal disease (ESRD). It is not a distinct disease but rather represents a pattern of response to injury that originates in or focuses on the podocyte. FSGS occurs in all ethnic groups, both sexes, and all geographic locales. Recent data indicate that the incidence of FSGS is rising, especially in black patients. This has been confirmed in reviews of kidney biopsy findings in the United States and Canada that demonstrate a two- to threefold increase in the incidence of FSGS over the period from 1984 to 2002. In addition, according to the North American Pediatric Renal Transplant Collaborative Study, FSGS is the most frequent form of acquired renal disease necessitating renal replacement therapy in pediatric patients in the United States. Similarly, it is the most common cause of idiopathic nephrotic syndrome in adults and is a major cause of ESRD.

B. Presenting Complaints

FSGS usually presents with asymptomatic proteinuria or overt nephrotic syndrome. In those patients who are diagnosed with isolated proteinuria, the abnormality is usually detected on a routine urinalysis. The clinical picture in those who present with nephrotic syndrome is almost indistinguishable from those with minimal change nephrotic syndrome (MCNS). Hematuria, evidence of tubular dysfunction such as glycosuria, hypertension, and mild azotemia, may be present in 15–30% of patients with new onset nephrotic syndrome and these features may increase the clinical suspicion that a patient has FSGS. However, the key feature that prompts further investigation to establish the diagnosis of FSGS is failure to respond to a standard course of corticosteroids. It is this clinical finding that triggers the performance of a diagnostic kidney biopsy; however, the utilization and timing of this procedure may differ among those who care for children or adults. Although the prognosis may be better in patients who present with subnephrotic-range proteinuria versus nephrotic syndrome, this difference has not been confirmed in patients of all ages.

C. Pathologic Findings

The diagnosis of FSGS requires histopathologic evidence of segmental glomerular sclerosis and hyalinosis. The lesion often manifests in juxtamedullary nephrons during the early stages of disease and it can be associated with periglomerular scarring, tubular atrophy, and interstitial fibrosis in the vicinity of the affected glomerulus (Figure 26–1). Generally, immunofluorescence studies are unrevealing. In a subgroup of patients, there are deposits of IgM and C3 in segmentally sclerosed lesions. Work by Thurman and colleagues suggests

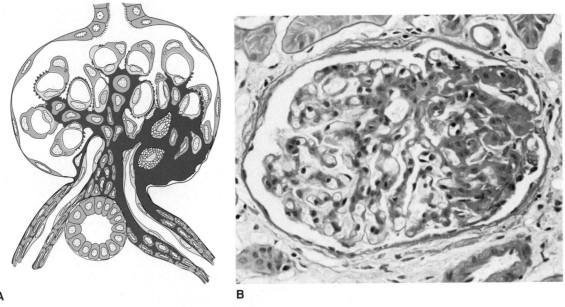

A

B

▲ **Figure 26–1.** **A.** Focal segmental glomerulosclerosis with a segmental scar shown from 4 to 6 o'clock. (Courtesy of J. C. Jennette, MD.) **B.** Human glomerulosclerosis with a segmental scar shown from 12 to 5 o'clock.

that these immunoreactants may activate innate immunity and contribute to glomerular injury. Electron microscopy demonstrates foot process effacement, the absence of immune deposits, and mesangial sclerosis.

In view of the widely divergent clinical course that patients with FSGS may follow, an attempt has been made to classify FSGS into distinct histologic subcategories. A scheme that has been proposed includes five variants: perihilar, tip, cellular, collapsing, and not otherwise specified. The collapsing variant has consistently been shown to have the poorest long-term prognosis among these five variants. Future work to define subtypes of FSGS based on the molecular mechanisms of disease may yield a more informative classification scheme than the current one based on histopathology.

▶ Pathogenesis

A. Primary Focal Segmental Glomerulosclerosis

This form has also been called idiopathic FSGS. Based on clinical evidence of variable response to immunosuppressive medications, the presumption has been that primary FSGS reflects a disturbance in the immune system. However, unlike MCNS, no consistent abnormality has been demonstrated except for altered synthesis and release of tumor necrosis factor (TNF) in peripheral blood leukocytes. In addition, various circulating factors, including hemopexin and immunoglobulin-like molecules, have been isolated

from the sera of patients with FSGS. Recent work suggests that soluble urokinase-type plasminogen activator receptor (suPAR) may be a molecule that mediates podocyte dysfunction in FSGS. However, the specificity of this circulating factor for FSGS requires further investigation. Removal of these circulating factors, using plasmapheresis or immunoadsorption columns, has been associated with disease remission and infusion into animals has resulted in glomerular proteinuria. Further work on the nature of these substances may help identify the cause of proteinuria in FSGS and define better treatments.

Exciting findings over the past 10 years underscore the pivotal role of the podocyte in maintaining the integrity of the glomerular permselective barrier. A number of proteins have been identified that are components of the cell membrane or actin cytoskeleton of the podocyte. These include nephrin, α-actinin-4, podocin, CD2AP, Wilms tumor suppressor (WT1), and TRPC6 (Figure 26–2). Mutations in the genes for these proteins, occurring in autosomal dominant and recessive patterns, have been associated with steroid-resistant nephrotic syndrome and biopsy-proven FSGS (Table 26–1). Mutations that affect mitochondrial function, nuclear transport, and lipid metabolism may also contribute to the pathogenesis of FSGS. Recent series suggest that up to 30% of familial and sporadic cases of steroid-resistant nephrotic syndrome in Europe are related to these genetic abnormalities. The role of genetic mutations is a subject of ongoing research as investigators improve filtering strategies

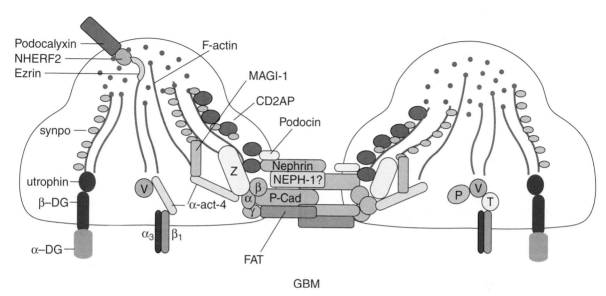

▲ **Figure 26–2.** Podocyte architecture. α-act-4, α-actinin-4; DG, dystroglycan; GBM, glomerular basement membrane; P, paxillin; P-Cad, P-cadherin; synpo, synaptopodin; T, talin; V, vinculin. (Reproduced with permission from Mundel P, Shankland SJ: Podocyte biology and response to injury. J Am Soc Nephrol 2002;13:3005.)

to distinguish disease-causing alterations from normal variations in both healthy and diseased subjects. The response to standard immunosuppressive medications and the risk of recurrent disease after transplantation may be markedly lower in patients with a genetic basis for FSGS. Clarification of these issues is imperative in designing an optimal approach to the evaluation and treatment of patients with FSGS.

B. Secondary Focal Segmental Glomerulosclerosis

The FSGS lesion represents a nonspecific response to podocyte injury and can arise in a variety of disease states. These include infections with viral agents including HIV and parvovirus B19. A variety of medications including lithium,

Table 26–1. Genetic mutations associated with focal segmental glomerulosclerosis.

Gene Product	Gene	Chromosome	Inheritance
Podocin	NPHS2	1q25–31	AR
α-Actinin-4	ACTN4	19q13	AD
CD2AP	CD2AP	6p12	AD
WT-1	WT-1	11p13	AD or AR
TRPC6	TRPC6	11q21–22	AD

AD, autosomal dominant; AR, autosomal recessive.

pamidronate, and illicit drugs such as heroin have been associated with FSGS. Reduced renal mass secondary to surgical ablation (e.g., surgery, trauma), reflux nephropathy, and low birth weight can lead to an adaptive response that results in FSGS. Finally, secondary FSGS can occur in patients with a normal renal mass but who have obesity, sickle cell anemia, or cyanotic congenital heart disease (Table 26–2). Identification of these causes and treatment of reversible conditions leads to regression of the FSGS lesions.

▶ Clinical Findings

A. Symptoms and Signs

The presentation of FSGS can be subtle with few or no presenting symptoms or may be apparent with the typical findings of nephrotic syndrome. Overtly nephrotic patients may manifest edema, ascites, and weight gain secondary to fluid retention. Edema is typically dependent in the lower extremities when upright and in the periorbital and presacral areas when supine. Edema of the scrotum and labia may also be present. Hypertension is found in approximately 60% of patients at presentation even among the nonedematous patients. Freshly voided urine may be foamy secondary to the effects of significant proteinuria.

B. Laboratory Findings

1. Urine—The urine contains from 1 to greater than 20 g of protein in a 24-hour collection. Determination of

Table 26–2. Secondary causes of focal segmental glomerulosclerosis.

Drugs
Adriamycin
Heroin
Interferon-α
Lithium
Pamidronate
Infections
HIV
Malarial nephropathy
Parvovirus B19
SV40 virus
Schistosomiasis
Malignancies
Hodgkin lymphoma
Non-Hodgkin lymphoma
Nephron loss
Reflux nephropathy
Surgical ablation
Genetic/familial
Alport syndrome
Branchiootorenal syndrome
Charcot–Marie–Tooth disease
Partial lecithin-cholesterol acyltransferase deficiency
Spondylometaphyseal dysplasia
Miscellaneous
Cyanotic congenital heart disease
Eclampsia
Residual from focal proliferative nephritis
Obesity
Sarcoidosis
Sickle cell nephropathy
Systemic sclerosis
Type I glycogen storage disease

proteinuria can be screened with a simple urinalysis but should be verified with a measurement of urine protein as either a single voided specimen (protein-to-creatinine ratio) or 24-hour timed urine collection for quantification of protein and creatinine. Proteinuria of 1 g/day/1.73 m^2 or a urine protein-to-creatinine ratio of 1 g/g or more is considered a level suggestive of a glomerular lesion. Microscopic hematuria is found in approximately 20%, but gross hematuria is rare. Glycosuria may also be documented in 10–20% of patients. Oval fat bodies and hyaline casts are commonly found when proteinuria is greater than 3 g/day/1.73 m^2.

2. Blood—Blood chemistries reveal the typical findings of hypoalbuminemia and dyslipidemia in patients with frank nephrotic syndrome. Serum albumin concentration may be less than 1.0 g/dL. Serum cholesterol, triglycerides, and very low-density lipoproteins are elevated in patients with severe hypoalbuminemia. Total serum calcium concentration is low because of the hypoalbuminemia; however, the ionized calcium is not usually reduced proportionately. However, with long-standing disease, there can be disturbances in vitamin D metabolism and modest reduction in the ionized calcium concentration and an elevated PTH level. Serum sodium may be low due to water retention. However, pseudohyponatremia secondary to hyperlipidemia is no longer a concern because automated serum chemistry analyzers use an ion selective electrode. At diagnosis FSGS patients may have an elevated serum creatinine concentration representing a loss of kidney function that may be acute or chronic. Acute kidney injury may occur secondary to severe intravascular volume contraction or renal interstitial edema leading to tubular obstruction.

Hematocrit may be elevated in patients with volume contraction or depressed in the patient with chronic loss of kidney function. Platelet counts may be significantly elevated as are coagulation factors V, VII, VIII, X, and fibrinogen. Antithrombin III and factors XI and XII may be decreased. These changes in clotting factors are related to the severity of the proteinuria and contribute to the risk of thrombosis in the grossly nephrotic patient.

The laboratory evaluation of a patient with FSGS may aid in the diagnosis of a primary or secondary lesion. Secondary forms of FSGS may be identified or confirmed by laboratory tests specific to the primary disease such as serology for HIV-associated FSGS. Although an unusual etiology, parvovirus B19 or SV40 can be confirmed by polymerase chain reaction (PCR).

C. Imaging Studies

Radiographic procedures such as renal ultrasound or computerized tomography may serve to exclude secondary or alternative conditions. For example, the patient with vesicoureteral reflux nephropathy may have evidence of hydronephrosis, hydroureter, or renal parenchymal scarring suggesting a urinary tract abnormality. Any patient with advanced glomerular sclerosis, whether from FSGS or from an alternative cause, may have small kidneys with a pattern of increased echogenicity in the kidney ultrasound.

D. Special Tests

The assessment of genetic markers of familial FSGS is not universally available. In 2006, the only gene test associated with FSGS available in commercial laboratories in the United States was the NPHS2 (podocin). Currently, a test battery including nearly 30 genes can be performed in a clinically certified laboratory and the results can be used to guide patient care. Research laboratories make other candidate gene testing available in a limited fashion but not for clinical use.

E. Special Examinations

The diagnosis of FSGS is based on the kidney biopsy finding of glomerular scaring in portions (segmental) of some (focal) of the glomeruli. Indeed, the finding of a single glomerulus with a segmental scar may be adequate to establish the diagnosis. Generally, if the kidney biopsy contains at least 10 glomeruli, then the likelihood of making the correct diagnosis of FSGS is high. Immunofluorescence staining is minimal and electron microscopy shows only foot process effacement. The pattern of scarring lesions has been used to classify FSGS into five subtypes. Using either the traditional classification or the newest classification scheme, the pattern of collapsing FSGS with glomerular capillary collapse and visceral epithelial cell hyperplasia has been associated with the worst prognosis among patients with primary FSGS. Collapsing FSGS has also been associated with HIV infection. All patients with FSGS should be evaluated for HIV as the treatment considerations differ according to etiology. The FSGS tip lesion has been considered the subtype most likely to respond to corticosteroid therapy with reduction or normalization of urine protein excretion and long-term kidney survival. However, all primary FSGS variants may respond to therapy or may progress to ESKD.

▶ Differential Diagnosis

Distinguishing primary from secondary FSGS has important therapeutic and prognostic implications. Primary FSGS is defined by confirmation by biopsy of the kidney pathology; the medical history, serology, and imaging studies confirm the absence of an alternative cause.

Disease entities such as Alport syndrome or immunoglobulin A (IgA) nephropathy may be associated with the finding of focal glomerulosclerosis on kidney biopsy. Recent studies indicate that up to 10% of patients given the diagnosis of FSGS have mutations in type IV collagen. Additional findings of glomerular basement membrane abnormalities on electron microscopy in Alport syndrome or IgA staining on immunofluorescence microscopy will identify the primary pathologic entity.

Although controversy exists, C1q nephropathy is considered a distinct pathologic entity wherein patients may present with nephrotic-range proteinuria, nephritis with cellular casts and proteinuria, or hematuria alone. Although kidney tissue from patients with C1q nephropathy may not have a focal sclerosing lesion, those with an FSGS lesion will also have C1q dominant staining on immunofluorescence microscopy, which ensures the distinct diagnosis of this secondary lesion. Other investigators do not distinguish primary FSGS based on the presence or absence of C1q deposits. Further study is required to clarify this issue.

Obesity-related glomerulopathy is an entity that causes glomerulomegaly in addition to focal sclerotic lesions. Patients with obesity-related glomerulopathy tend to have a nonedematous body mass index of 40 kg/m^2 or greater. These patients may demonstrate a resolution of proteinuria with significant weight loss and, even without an effective weight loss program, tend to have a better long-term prognosis compared to those with the primary FSGS lesion. Immunosuppression therapy is not warranted in this obesity-induced lesion.

▶ Complications

A. Infection

Bacterial infections causing spontaneous bacterial peritonitis, sepsis, and cellulitis may complicate nephrotic syndrome from FSGS. Episodes of peritonitis typically manifest with abdominal pain, rebound tenderness, guarding, and anorexia with or without fever. This is a medical emergency that requires urgent identification and treatment. The diagnosis can be confirmed by performing a paracentesis, which demonstrates leukocytosis of the peritoneal fluid with a predominance of neutrophils and a positive peritoneal fluid culture. The most common causes of peritonitis in patients with nephrotic syndrome are *Streptococcus pneumoniae*, *Escherichia coli*, and a variety of gram-negative rods. The exclusion of alternate abdominal pathology is critical as a ruptured appendix, for example, may also present with abdominal pain, rebound tenderness, and guarding.

B. Thrombosis

Venous and arterial thrombosis and thromboemboli occur in less than 2% of patients with significant proteinuria. The increased risk of formation of thrombus is thought to be secondary to the urinary loss of factors responsible for inhibition of coagulation such as antithrombin III, protein S, and protein C. Increased platelet activation and a reduction in plasmin-mediated fibrinolysis may also play a role. Additional risk factors may relate to decreased mobility in the grossly edematous patient. The risk of thrombosis is approximately one order of magnitude lower in children versus adults with FSGS.

C. Acute Kidney Injury

Acute renal injury may be present at diagnosis or with episodes of severe volume contraction. The restoration of circulating volume is the treatment of choice in these cases. Chronic kidney disease may be present at the time of diagnosis of FSGS. Kidney biopsy may assist in determining the likelihood for renal function recovery based on the severity of the glomerular and tubulointerstitial fibrosis.

▶ Treatment

A. Corticosteroids

The course of untreated FSGS is generally one of persistent proteinuria and progressive kidney failure. Less than 5% of patients experience a spontaneous remission. The therapy of FSGS remains controversial because there are few randomized trials to support an evidence-based practice. Use of corticosteroids as initial therapy in pediatric and adult aged patients is common for primary disease. The treatment course is typically between 6 weeks and 6 months with response rates of 25–40%. Regional and racial/ethnic differences have been reported in steroid responsiveness, which may relate to duration of corticosteroid administration or varying prevalence of underlying genetic or other etiologic factors.

Persistent proteinuria after a course of corticosteroids is observed in the majority of patients with FSGS. The selection of a second-line therapy may include immunosuppressive agents, agents to control symptoms alone such as diuretics, antifibrotic therapy, and plasmapheresis (Table 26–3).

B. Calcineurin Inhibitors

Cyclosporine is the standard second-line therapy for patients with steroid-resistant FSGS or for patients unable to tolerate corticosteroids. A 50% or greater reduction in urinary protein excretion with preservation of kidney function is expected in approximately 50–70% of patients treated with cyclosporine. The lower response rates have been documented in studies that include a high proportion of patients of African ancestry. The risk for relapse after discontinuation of the treatment may be related to the duration of therapy and the degree of control of the proteinuria. In the FSGS Clinical Trial, 46% of patients treated for 1 year with cyclosporine had a favorable response. However, the relapse rate within 6 months was substantial. The desire to continue therapy to maintain a remission is offset by the risk for calcineurin inhibitor-induced nephrotoxicity, which may be severe and depend on duration of drug exposure. In short-term studies, kidney function was better preserved in those

Table 26–3. Treatment options in patients with steroid-resistant focal segmental glomerulosclerosis.

Immunosuppressive agents
Calcineurin inhibitors
Cyclosporine
Tacrolimus
Cyclophosphamide
Mycophenolate mofetil
Conservative therapy
Diuretics
Antifibrotic therapy
Angiotensin-converting enzyme inhibitors
Angiotensin receptor blockers
Aldosterone antagonists
Lipid-lowering drugs
Antioxidants
Plasmapheresis

treated with cyclosporine. Generalization of this response to the other calcineurin inhibitor, tacrolimus, has theoretical merit and is commonly used in clinical practice despite the dearth of supporting evidence.

C. Cyclophosphamide

A nonrandomized study using combined high-dose corticosteroids and cyclophosphamide suggested improved control of proteinuria compared with historical controls. In a randomized trial of cyclophosphamide plus alternate day steroids versus alternate day steroids alone, cyclophosphamide was not found to improve renal survival or control proteinuria better than the steroid-only group.

D. Mycophenolate Mofetil

Anecdotal reports of mycophenolate mofetil have suggested that this agent may improve proteinuria and preserve renal function in steroid-dependent or steroid-resistant nephrotic syndrome. In the FSGS Clinical Trial, mycophenolate mofetil was given in combination with dexamethasone and resulted in a 33% partial proteinuria remission. There are few studies that examine use of this drug as a solitary agent. At present an ideal approach to immunomodulatory therapy for FSGS has not been identified.

E. Diet and Diuretics

Sodium-restricted diet is the mainstay of therapy to control edema in a patient with hypoalbuminemia and edema. Even with sodium restriction, additional therapy with diuretic agents may be required until proteinuria excretion is controlled. Amiloride may be a useful drug based on experimental data indicating activation of the epithelial sodium channel in patients with nephrotic syndrome.

F. Antihypertensive Agents

Angiotensin-converting enzyme inhibitors and angiotensin receptor blockade are part of the standard regimen in steroid-resistant FSGS patients. In isolation or combination, these agents have been shown to reduce proteinuria up to 50% from baseline and lower the risk for progression to kidney failure in diabetic and nondiabetic kidney disease. Monitoring should include assessment of serum potassium to allow early identification of a need for potassium restriction and measurement of serum creatinine to ensure preservation of the glomerular filtration rate. A small rise in serum creatinine concentration is expected on these agents. Changes up to 20% should be tolerated and are generally reversible if the agent(s) are discontinued. Despite a mild increase in serum creatinine concentration, the agents are to be continued with the goal of long-term preservation of kidney function. If therapy with angiotensin-converting enzyme inhibitors and angiotensin receptor blockade does not control hypertension, additional antihypertensive agents should be prescribed. Aldosterone antagonists may reduce proteinuria and prevent renal fibrosis, although this effect has not been evaluated specifically in patients with FSGS.

G. Lipid Control

Lipid-lowering agents are included in the nephrotic syndrome armamentarium to control hyperlipidemia. Hypercholesterolemia in animal models has been shown to cause glomerulosclerosis. Therapy with the 3-hydroxy-3-methylglutaryl coenzyme A (HMG-CoA) reductase inhibitors, statins, diminishes the effects of lipemia on the kidney even with persistent hypercholesterolemia in animal and human investigation. The role of PCSK9 has been studied in nephrotic syndrome and monoclonal antibodies to this target may become a useful agent to treat hyperlipidemia in patients with refractory FSGS.

H. Vitamin E

Vitamin E is also considered a means of controlling proteinuria and progressive kidney disease through the antioxidant mechanism. One open-label pilot study reported a 50% reduction in protein excretion in 11 children with FSGS, while others have found no beneficial effect. Controversy continues to exist regarding the efficacy of vitamin E.

I. Combination Therapy

In general, a combination therapy approach may be resorted to for corticosteroid-resistant FSGS patients. A calcineurin inhibitor, angiotensin-converting enzyme inhibitor, angiotensin receptor blockade, and statin combination are commonly used. For those who fail conventional therapy participation in clinical trials will help identify effective treatments for this disorder. Novel therapies that are under investigation include rituximab, ACTH, abatacept, and LDL lipopheresis.

J. Plasmapheresis

The patient with FSGS-induced rapid progression to kidney failure has a 30% risk of FSGS recurrence in the kidney transplant and an 18% risk of graft failure from recurrent disease. In an effort to diminish the risk for recurrent disease and to preserve the survival of the transplanted organ, plasmapheresis may be used in the peritransplant period as a preventive therapy or in response to rapid return of proteinuria. Combination therapy with plasmapheresis and rituximab has been used for early transplant recurrence. Caution must be used as this results in profound immunosuppression when added to standard transplant induction therapy and increases the risk for serious infections. The success of this approach is apparently better in children than adults. Occasionally, long-term plasmapheresis has been used to sustain a response.

▶ Prognosis

Nearly 50% of cases of FSGS progress to ESRD over 5–10 years. Those at greatest risk to progress to kidney failure include those who show resistance to therapy with continued proteinuria and those with collapsing variant FSGS. For patients with progression to kidney failure, dialysis, and transplant support are options for therapy. Unfortunately, those who receive a kidney transplant may have a recurrence of FSGS in the transplanted kidney. Patients with FSGS who present with azotemia or progress rapidly to ESRD are more susceptible to disease recurrence in a kidney transplant. The impact of age, ethnicity, and donor type is controversial. The presence of a genetic mutation has been associated with a diminished, but not absent, risk for FSGS recurrence in the kidney transplant recipient.

KEY READINGS

Buemi M et al: Statins in nephrotic syndrome: a new weapon against tissue injury. Med Res Rev 2005;25:587.

Cattran DC et al: Mycophenolate mofetil in the treatment of focal segmental glomerulosclerosis. Clin Nephrol 2004;62:405.

Chun MJ et al: Focal segmental glomerulosclerosis in nephrotic adults: presentation, prognosis, and response to therapy of the histologic variants. J Am Soc Nephrol 2004;15:2169.

Crook ED et al: Effects of steroids in focal segmental glomerulosclerosis in a predominantly African-American population. Am J Med Sci 2005;330:19.

Gadegbeku CA et al: Design of the Nephrotic Syndrome Study Network (NEPTUNE) to evaluate primary glomerular nephropathy by a multidisciplinary approach. Kidney Int 2013;83:749.

Gipson DS et al: Clinical trial of focal segmental glomerulosclerosis in children and young adults. Kidney Int 2011;80:868.

Gohh RY et al: Preemptive plasmapheresis and recurrence of FSGS in high-risk renal transplant recipients. Am J Transplant 2005;5:2907.

Haas ME et al: The Role of Proprotein Convertase Subtilisin/Kexin Type 9 in Nephrotic Syndrome-Associated Hypercholesterolemia. Circulation 2016;134:61.

Hodson EM et al: Corticosteroid therapy for nephrotic syndrome in children. Cochrane Database Syst Rev 2005;CD001533.

Huang K et al: The differential effect of race among pediatric kidney transplant recipients with focal segmental glomerulosclerosis. Am J Kidney Dis 2004;43:1082.

Kronbichler A et al: Soluble urokinase receptors in focal segmental glomerulosclerosis: a review on the scientific point of view. J Immunol Res 2016;2016:2068691.

Malone AF et al: Rare hereditary COL4A3/COL4A4 variants may be mistaken for familial focal segmental glomerulosclerosis. Kidney Int 2014;86:1253.

Pollak M: Genetics of familial FSGS. Semin Nephrol 2016;36:467.

Rodriguez MM et al: Comparative renal histomorphometry: a case study of oligonephropathy of prematurity. Pediatr Nephrol 2005;20:945.

Ruf RG et al: Patients with mutations in NPHS2 (podocin) do not respond to standard steroid treatment of nephrotic syndrome. J Am Soc Nephrol 2004;15:722.

Strassheim D et al: IgM contributes to glomerular injury in FSGS. J Am Soc Nephrol 2013;24:393.

Teoh CW, Robinson LA, Noone D: Perspectives on edema in childhood nephrotic syndrome. Am J Physiol Renal Physiol 2015;309:F575.

Troyanov S et al: Focal and segmental glomerulosclerosis: definition and relevance of a partial remission. J Am Soc Nephrol 2005;16:1061.

Valdivia P et al: Plasmapheresis for the prophylaxis and treatment of recurrent focal segmental glomerulosclerosis following renal transplant. Transplant Proc 2005;37:1473.

■ CHAPTER REVIEW QUESTIONS

1. A 30-year-old African–American man presents with edema, hypertension, urine protein 8 g/24 hours, serum albumin is 2.5 g/dL, and serum creatinine of 1.9 mg/dL. HIV, hepatitis B and C testing demonstrates no evidence for acute or chronic infection.

   What is the next test needed to identify the diagnosis in this patient?
   A. Echocardiogram
   B. Urine protein electrophoresis
   C. Ultrasound guided kidney biopsy
   D. CT scan of the kidneys and bladder

2. The kidney biopsy of 30-year-old African–American man presenting with nephrotic syndrome, serum creatinine of 1.9 mg/dL, and negative testing for HIV and hepatitis B and C revealed focal and segmental glomerulosclerosis (FSGS). He has no family history of nephrotic syndrome, FSGS, or kidney failure. He asks if he should have genetic testing to guide his therapy.

   What factors should be considered to guide the recommendation for genetic testing?
   A. Family history
   B. Evaluation for kidney transplant preparation
   C. Age of FSGS onset
   D. Patient interest in research
   E. All of the above

3. A 17-year-old woman with sickle cell disease presents with proteinuria of 1.5 g/24 hour, serum albumin 3.5 g/dL, serum creatinine of 0.7 mg/dL and blood pressure of 126/64. She has a history of previous episodes of pain crises but is currently asymptomatic. Infection evaluation for HIV and hepatitis B and C is negative.

   Kidney biopsy reveals focal and segmental glomerulosclerosis (FSGS) with mild podocyte foot process effacement.

   Which of the following is the most appropriate treatment option for this patient?
   A. Corticosteroids
   B. Angiotensin-converting enzyme Inhibitor
   C. Scheduled red blood cell transfusions
   D. Kidney transplant

4. A 6-week-old male infant presents with edema, urine protein-to-creatinine ratio 11 (mg:mg), serum albumin is 1.5 g/dL, and serum creatinine of 0.9 mg/dL. His HIV testing demonstrates no evidence for acute or chronic infection.

   What is the next test needed to identify the diagnosis in this patient?
   A. Genetic testing
   B. Kidney biopsy
   C. Hepatitis B and C testing
   D. Ultrasounds of both parents

5. A 13-year-old African–American boy with FSGS has steadily declining kidney function. He is referred for evaluation for kidney transplantation.

   Which of the following features is associated with an increased risk of recurrence disease in a potential kidney allograft?
   A. Hypertension
   B. APOL1 genotype
   C. Living kidney donation
   D. Rapid decline in GFR from onset of disease

Membranous Nephropathy

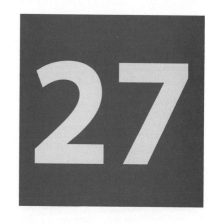

Talal A. Alfaadhel, MBBS, FRCP(C)

Fernando C. Fervenza, MD, PhD

Daniel C. Cattran, MD, FRCP(C)

ESSENTIALS OF DIAGNOSIS

▶ Nephrotic syndrome is the typical presenting feature.

▶ The glomerular basement membranes (GBMs) appear thickened on light microscopy.

▶ There is an absence of glomerular inflammation.

▶ Primary (PLA2R or THSD7A antigen related) membranous nephropathy (MN) is a leading cause of nephrotic syndrome in adults.

▶ Secondary MN forms can account for up to one-third of cases.

▶ Malignancy as a secondary cause increases with age.

▶ Conservative management should be the first step in management.

▶ Risk of progression of the disease needs to be considered because patients with a high risk of progression can benefit from immunosuppressive treatment.

▶ General Considerations

Seventy years ago, E.T. Bell coined the term membranous glomerulonephritis to describe the renal pathology in a group of patients with the clinical features of nephrotic syndrome in whom the kidney biopsy revealed marked glomerular basement membrane (GBM) thickening without significant inflammation. The terms extramembranous nephropathy and epimembranous glomerulonephritis were also used to describe the disease. The word glomerulonephritis is, however, misleading as one of the main features of the condition is the absence of glomerular inflammation; because of this the word nephropathy is now more often used. Idiopathic membranous nephropathy (MN) is a relatively common immune mediated glomerular disease and remains a leading cause of nephrotic syndrome in adults.

Until recently, the primary antigens were was unknown and the disorder was termed idiopathic, but now given the newly recognized two autoantibody systems (PLA2R and THSD7A) it more accurately should be designated primary MN. Secondary forms of MN may account for up to one-third of cases and are associated with autoimmune diseases (eg, systemic lupus erythematosus, SLE), infections (eg, hepatitis B and C viral infections), medications (eg, nonsteroidal anti-inflammatory drugs [NSAIDs], D-penicillamine, gold), and neoplasia (eg, colon kidney, prostate, and breast cancer) (Table 27–1). The presence of phospholipase A2 receptor (PLA2) antibodies or thrombospondin type 1 domain–containing 7A (THSD7A) antibodies (in the serum) or antigen localization on glomerular tissue staining helps in lowering the likelihood of secondary MN. However, since both primary and secondary forms have similar clinical presentations, the designation of primary requires appropriate ruling out of the secondary causes by a careful history, physical examination, and laboratory evaluation of the patient. This disease is rare in children, and when it occurs, is commonly associated with an immunologically mediated disorder such as SLE.

▶ Pathogenesis

For many years, the autoimmune nature of MN has been appreciated based on experimental models published by Heymann and colleagues in 1959. In these models, rats developed pathological disease resembling that seen in patients with MN with antibodies depositing in the subepithelial region of the GBM. The deposition of antibodies (mainly IgG) against antigens in the podocytes causes activation of the complement cascade, as evidenced by complement deposition in the biopsy. This complement activation causes direct injury to the podocytes, increased production of cytotoxic molecules that in turn lead to GBM damage. Complement activation can be determined by an increased urinary C5b-9, and its level may be a marker of disease

Table 27–1. Secondary membranous nephropathy.

Infections: Hepatitis B and C, syphilis (congenital and secondary), leprosy, filariasis, hydatid cyst disease, hepatosplenic schistosomiasis, echinococcus, post-streptococcal infection, malaria

Neoplasia: Carcinomas, leukemia, lymphoma, pheochromocytoma, carotid body tumor

Autoimmune: SLE,1 thyroiditis, rheumatoid arthritis, mixed connective tissue disease, sarcoidosis, angiolymphoid hyperplasia with eosinophilia (Kimura disease), primary biliary cirrhosis, Sjögren syndrome, ankylosing spondylitis, dermatitis herpetiformis

Drugs: NSAIDs (diclofenac), gold, D-penicillamine, mercury, captopril, formaldehyde, thiola, probenecid, bucillamine, tiopronin

Other: de novo renal transplant, sickle-cell disease, Gardner–Diamond syndrome, Guillain–Barré syndrome, graft-versus-host disease following bone marrow transplant, diabetes mellitus

NSAIDs, nonsteroidal anti-inflammatory drugs; SLE, systemic lupus erythematosus

activity. Ultimately, GBM damage leads to heavy proteinuria, which is the hallmark of the nephrotic syndrome seen in MN. Because the activation and deposition occurs on the urinary side of the basement membrane, the inflammatory response is typically blunted, thus explaining the usual lack of inflammation on pathology.

It was appreciated some time ago that the target antigen in rats was megalin a relatively large transmembrane protein found in podocytes. However, megalin expression is absent in humans, and similar target antigens in humans were only recently identified. The first antigen identified was neutral endopeptidase (NEP), the target of antibodies transferred from mothers deficient of this antigen, after sensitization from prior pregnancies, were their fetuses, producing a very rare form of antenatal membranous nephropathy. In 2009, the breakthrough in understanding primary MN came after Beck et al described antibodies to the M-type phospholipase A2 receptor (PLA2R) in 70% of patients with primary MN, but not in those with secondary MN or other glomerular diseases. The exact function of this receptor is not yet known. There is a wide variability in the prevalence of PLA2R antibodies in MN ranging from 45–75% in different populations and in different geographic regions. Consistent with prior description of MN, these antibodies were mainly of the IgG4 subclass. The development of the PLA2R ELISA assay, compared to the original detection by Western blot has made antibody testing more widely available. On occasions, PLA2R serum antibody levels can be negative, yet glomerular tissue PLA2R antigen staining is positive. This condition may occur early in the course of disease when the serum antibodies may not yet have saturated all the tissue PLA2 receptors. This highlights the importance of looking for enhanced expression of PLA2R in kidney tissue as well as looking for circulating anti-PLA2R antibodies to improve the sensitivity of the diagnosis of primary MN.

More recently, antibodies to thrombospondin type 1 domain-containing 7A (THSD7A) were reported in 10% of patients with PLA2R antibody-negative primary MN in cohorts from Europe and the United States. Like PLA2R antibodies, the predominant associated IgG subclass found was IgG4. Dual positivity of PLA2R and THSD7A antibodies has been described but is very rare in less than 1% of primary MN. When both antibodies are considered, they account for 70–80% of patients with primary MN. This still leaves a significant number of patients without an identified antigen target in MN. This is a focus of ongoing research.

▶ **Pathology**

Kidney biopsy classically makes the diagnosis of MN. In the very early stage of MN, the glomeruli can appear normal by light microscopy (hematoxylin and eosin), although abnormalities may be seen in silver preparations and by immunofluorescence and electron microscopy. Capillary loops are widely patent and the glomeruli show no increase in cellularity and there is no nuclear crowding. As the number and size of subepithelial immune complexes increase, the GBM develops a diffuse and uniform thickening on light microscopy. These changes affect all the glomeruli. Thin sections examined by silver stain may demonstrate the classical "spike" pattern on the epithelial side of the basement membrane reflecting increased synthesis and deposition of GBM-like material around the immune deposits (Figure 27–1). As the disease progresses, thickening of the capillary wall becomes

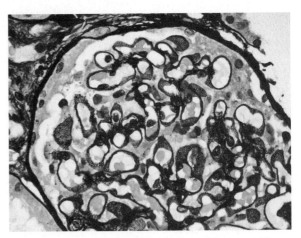

▲ **Figure 27–1.** Membranous nephropathy (stage II). Thicken the glomerular basement membrane with spikes and remodeling. Silver stain (×800). (Courtesy of Dr. Donna Lager, ProPath® Renal Pathology, Dallas, TX.)

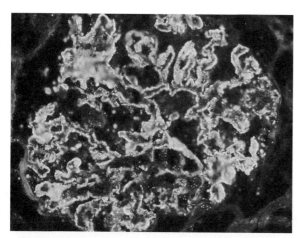

▲ **Figure 27–2.** Immunofluorescence staining showing intense diffuse finely granular IgG deposition along glomerular capillary walls (×600). (Courtesy of Dr. Donna Lager, ProPath® Renal Pathology, Dallas, TX.)

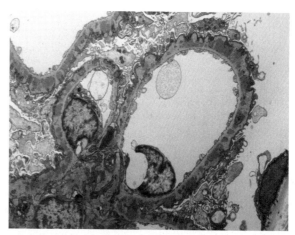

▲ **Figure 27–3.** Electron micrograph showing regularly distributed subepithelial deposits with well-developed glomerular basement membrane spikes and marked foot process effacement (×9600). (Courtesy of Dr. Donna Lager, ProPath® Renal Pathology, Dallas, TX.)

pronounced, the capillary lumen narrows, and eventually sclerosis and hyalinization of the glomerular tuft develop. Proximal tubules are remarkable for the lipid vacuoles in the cytoplasm and numerous proteinaceous casts in the lumen. In the initial stages, the interstitium is often normal, but with progression of the disease, fibrosis and lymphocyte infiltrates are seen.

Immunofluorescence microscopy shows a very characteristic and uniform deposition of IgG and C3 in a granular pattern along the epithelial side of the GBM (Figure 27–2). IgG (with IgG4 being the predominant IgG subclass) is present in 95% of cases, but C3 deposition can be seen less frequently (as low as 50%) in primary MN. It has been suggested that positive C3 staining represents active, ongoing immune deposit formation and complement activation at the time of biopsy whereas the absence of C3 reflects cessation of the immunopathologic process.

Electron microscopy demonstrates that the typical electron-dense deposits are localized in the subepithelial space associated with effacement of the foot processes (Figure 27–3). Deposits usually have a synchronous, homogeneous electron-dense appearance, but a heterogeneous pattern with dense deposits at various stages of formation can also be found.

A four-stage (I–IV; Table 27–2) classification system has been developed based on their specific localization. Unfortunately, the clinical and laboratory correlation with these stages is poor. Secondary forms of MN have histologic features that are like primary MN. However, the presence of deposits of immunoglobulins other than IgG (IgA and IgM), particularly in the mesangium, small subendothelial

deposits, tubular basement membrane deposits, and intense C1q deposition are more suggestive of membranous nephropathy secondary to SLE, hepatitis B, or drugs (gold, D-penicillamine). Positive glomerular tissue staining of PLA2R and/or THSD7A antigen in a pattern similar to the IgG staining along the GBM supports the diagnosis of primary MN, especially if secondary MN features are absent although caution should be taken in interpreting PLA2R IF

Table 27–2. Clinical features.[a]

Rare in children: <5% of total cases of NS
Common in adults: 15–50% of total cases of NS, depending on age; increasing frequency after age 40 years
Males > females in all adults groups
Whites > Asians > African–Americans > Hispanics
NS in 60–70%
Normal or mildly elevated BP at presentation
"Benign" urinary sediment
Nonselective proteinuria
Tendency to thromboembolic disease (DVT, RVT, PE)

BP, blood pressure; DVT, deep venous thrombosis; NS, nephrotic syndrome; PE, pulmonary embolism; RVT, renal vein thrombosis.
[a]Secondary causes are covered more extensively in Table 27–1.

staining, as this can be weakly positive in normal glomerular tissue and can also be seen in a proportion of secondary causes such as malignancy, infection, and autoimmune disorders. To be considered positive, the intensity of staining should be similar to the level of IgG IF staining. Negative staining does not rule out primary disease as the absence of anti-PLA2R and anti-THSD7A antibody staining in renal tissue may reflect an immunologically quiescent phase of the disease.

► Clinical Findings

The disease affects patients of all ages and races, but is more common in men than women by about a 2–3:1 ratio. Primary MN is most often diagnosed in middle age. Over the past two decades, the peak incidence age appears to have increased from the fourth and fifth decades to the fifth and sixth decade of life. It is relatively uncommon in patients less than 20 years. At presentation 60–70% of patients will have the nephrotic syndrome (NS) and its associated features: edema, hypoalbuminemia, and hyperlipidemia whereas the remaining 30–40% of patients are asymptomatic with subnephrotic proteinuria (<3.5 g/24 hours). The latter cohort is most commonly found at the time of routine examination performed for other indications. The presence of microscopic hematuria is common (30–40%), but macroscopic hematuria and red cell casts are rare and if present suggest a different histopathology. In patients with primary MN, serum C3 and C4 complement levels are always normal. At the time of diagnosis, most patients are normotensive. Renal function is also normal in most patients but a small fraction (10%) exhibits renal insufficiency at presentation (Table 27–3). This appears to be more common in older patients. Additional complications related to the disease include a variety of abnormalities in the lipid profile, potentially contributing to the increased cardiovascular risk seen in these patients, and a high prevalence of thromboembolic events including renal vein thrombosis and/or embolic events in 8–20% of patients.

► Differential Diagnosis

The differential diagnosis includes other causes of NS such as minimal change disease, focal segmental glomerulosclerosis, membranoproliferative glomerulonephritis, amyloidosis, light chain deposition disease, and diabetic nephropathy. It is also important to exclude secondary causes of MN, particularly, hepatitis B, SLE, malignancy, and drugs. Among those who are younger than 16 years old, secondary MN is most commonly due to viral infection or SLE, while in adults older than 60 years, secondary MN is more commonly due to malignancy or drugs (Table 27–4). In patients with MN, ruling out secondary causes, apart from a thorough history and physical examination, should involve appropriate laboratory evaluation including complement profile, hepatitis serology,

Table 27–3. The Ehrenreich and Churg "staging" of glomerular morphology in membranous nephropathy.[a]

Stage I or early stage: Light microscopy shows a normal glomeruli or slightly thickened capillary walls. There is no evidence of "spike-like" projections or only very scattered. Few and small, superficially placed, subepithelial electron-dense deposits on EM. Fusion of foot processes in the region of the deposits.

Stage II or fully developed lesion: Diffuse, uniform thickening of capillary walls on light microscopy. Prominent, "spike-like" projections along the GBM. Numerous, larger, and more confluent deposits cover the entire capillary loop on EM.

Stage III or advanced lesion: Highly irregular and thickened capillary walls ("moth-eaten" appearance). EM shows deposits (electron dense and lucent) have been encircled by the GBM ("domes") and become intramembranous.

Stage IV or late stage: Deposits become more lucent or absent, and fewer in numbers with numerous electron-lucent vacuolated areas seen within a markedly thickened GBM ("Swiss cheese"). Glomerular collapse and fibrosis are found on light microscopy.

EM, electron microscopy; GBM, glomerular basement membrane.
[a]The stages are based on the sequence of events observed primarily by electron microscopy. The extent to which individual patients will exhibit these sequential stages will vary according to the duration and the severity of the pathologic process.

antinuclear antibodies, a chest X-ray (CT scan for (ex) smokers), testing for occult blood in the stools or colonoscopy, a mammogram in women, and prostate-specific antigen testing in men. Finding a positive test for anti-PLA2R antibodies also helps to reduce the likelihood of secondary causes although after an initial high reported specificity of this antibody in primary MN, several studies have now reported anti-PLA2R antibody positivity in cases of malignancy, viral disease, sarcoidosis, and even in SLE. How such secondary causes can be mediated by anti PLA2R antibodies is unclear. This may represent two separate disease processes

Table 27–4. Secondary causes of membranous nephropathy according to age.

	Children <16 Years (%)	Adults >60 Years (%)
SLE[a]	27	1
Viral infection	53	2
Neoplasia	<1	54
Drugs	3	38
Other	17	5

[a]Systemic lupus erythematosus.

(eg, malignancy and primary MN) occurring simultaneously, or alternatively, similarity between the two autoantibody systems in these diseases. Antibody positivity should not deter investigating for possible secondary causes especially if there are any symptoms suggestive of autoimmune, viral or malignant disease present. In 345 MN patients tested prospectively for THSD7A, 2.6% tested positive. In their total cohort of over 1200 cases they found a higher percentage of these THSD7A positive cases associated with malignancy compared to the PLA2R + cohort, although the absolute numbers of cancer related cases were smaller given the much higher number in the PLA2R + cohort. Of the 40 patients THSD7A positive, 8 were found to have a malignancy within a median of 3 months from the time of diagnosis of MN. It is hypothesized that antigen(s) derived from the tumor are deposited in the glomeruli, where they trigger an antibody response and activation of the complement cascade, leading to disruption of the GBM integrity and podocyte injury. An alternative possible mechanism is the development of antibodies toward newly expressed tumor antigens and these antibodies cross react with similar antigens in the renal tissue. In some patients, proteinuria resolves with removal or adequate treatment of the tumor. There are, however, well-described cases in which no improvement or remission of the proteinuria occurred following removal of the tumor. True secondary MN is most commonly related to solid tumors of the lung, colon, prostate, breast, or kidney. The association with malignancy increases with age, reaching up to 20% in MN patients over the age of 60 years.

One of the other main differential diagnosis for MN especially in younger women is lupus nephritis. In a biopsy series from patients with SLE, MN histology accounts for 8–27% of cases of lupus nephritis. Patients with "pure" membranous lupus nephropathy often lack clinical symptoms that would suggest SLE and serologic markers of lupus activity, such as serum complement and anti-dsDNA levels, are frequently normal and do not correlate with disease activity. Hepatitis B–associated MN occurs most frequently in hepatitis B–prevalent areas of the world and affects both adults and children who are chronic carriers of hepatitis B virus (persistently positive hepatitis B surface antigen [HbsAg] or hepatitis B viral DNA) with or without a history of overt liver disease. In children with hepatitis B–associated MN the nephrotic syndrome usually has a benign course, but the development of progressive renal insufficiency in adulthood is common. The incidence of childhood hepatitis B–associated MN seems to be decreasing with the universal use of hepatitis B vaccination. In cases of MN secondary to drugs, discontinuation of the offending agent usually results in complete remission of the nephrotic syndrome. Although resolution of the proteinuria may occur quickly following discontinuation of the offending drug (eg, NSAIDs), drug-induced MN in the past, for example, gold or D-penicillamine may take years before remission of the proteinuria occurs (mean: 11 months).

A number of glomerular pathologies have been reported to occur in association with or superimposed upon MN. Such diseases include IgA nephropathy, focal and segmental glomerulosclerosis, crescentic glomerulonephritis (anti-GBM disease, ANCA-associated vasculitis), acute interstitial nephritis, and diabetic nephropathy. In some diabetic patients, MN may result as a consequence of the development of antiporcine insulin antibodies against porcine insulin that deposits along the GBM.

▶ Complications

The clinical course is characterized by great variability in the rate of disease progression. Even the natural course is difficult to assess, in part due to the different criteria used by local nephrologists in selecting patients for kidney biopsy. In a review of patients presenting with subnephrotic proteinuria followed for at least 1 year in the Toronto GN Registry, most patients (60%) progressed to nephrotic range proteinuria on follow up, with the others (40%) remaining subnephrotic throughout their average follow-up of 60 months. The rate of renal function decline was significantly faster in those who progressed to nephrotic range proteinuria and was comparable to those whose initial presentation was with a nephrotic picture. Based on a report from Spain in the era of renin–angiotensin system (RAS) blockers, spontaneous remission occurs in up to 30% of cases with nephrotic syndrome. However, in patients with proteinuria greater than 8 g/day, spontaneous remission was less frequent (24%) and the time to remission was slower (mean of 14 months) compared to those with lower levels of proteinuria. Historically, in untreated patients the 10-year kidney survival has varied from 50% to 70%, although many of these studies have included patients with proteinuria less than 3.5 g/day, thus producing a bias toward a more favorable prognosis, for example, a 72% renal survival was reported at 8 years for 100 untreated patients with MN. However, 37% of these patients were non-nephrotic (proteinuria <3.5 g/day) and in 56% of patients proteinuria was less than 5 g/day. Furthermore, the median follow-up was 39 months and deaths were excluded from the analysis. Even when these exceptions and the "benign" characteristics of the patients are taken into consideration, 25% still reached end-stage renal disease (ESRD) at the end of 8 years. In the most severely affected patients, progressive disease is more common, and up to 40–60% of patients eventually developing ESRD over a 15–20-year span. Despite the overall good short-term outcome, because of its high incidence rate compared to other types of GN, MN remains the second (in the United States) or third (in Europe) leading cause of ESRD among the primary types of glomerulonephritis.

Cardiovascular and thromboembolic events are increased in this population, especially in patients who remain nephrotic. When loss of renal function occurs more quickly than expected or there is an unexpected deterioration in renal function, a superimposed condition (eg, interstitial nephritis, anti-GBM disease, renal vein thrombosis) should be considered.

A. Predictors of Poor Outcome

An accurate early predictor of outcome of patients with primary MN would allow more specific targeting of immunosuppressive treatment to those who are at high risk of developing ESRD. Until recently, finding useful markers that predict this group has been difficult. Although age and gender influence outcome, with male sex and increasing age associated with a higher risk for renal failure, they do not predict rate of progression and cannot be altered by treatment. Similarly, the degree of glomerulosclerosis, tubulointerstitial fibrosis, and vascular disease seen on kidney biopsy has been associated with a poor prognosis but they commonly reflect preexisting injury rather than the severity of the MN disease process. The degree of renal impairment as measured by creatinine clearance at presentation also correlates with long-term renal survival. However, renal function at presentation is widely variable and can be independent of disease severity. A better and more sensitive predictor of long-term prognosis is the ongoing rate of renal function loss as measured by the decline of creatinine clearance over time but this is usually slow and may take years to establish a consistent rate of deterioration.

One of the better models for the identification of patients at risk was developed with data derived from the Toronto GN Registry and subsequently validated in two MN cohorts from Finland and Italy. This model takes into consideration the initial creatinine clearance, the slope of the creatinine clearance, and the lowest level of proteinuria during a 6-month observation period. This risk score assessment has good performance characteristics. In the validity data sets the sensitivity of the model varied from 60% to 89%, the specificity from 86% to 92%, and the overall accuracy from 79% to 87%. Based on data using this model, patients who present with a normal creatinine clearance, proteinuria less than 4 g/24 hours, and stable renal function over a 6-month observation period have an excellent long-term prognosis, and conservative treatment only is recommended. Since even in this group the worsening of proteinuria and renal function can occur, these patients need to have ongoing monitoring. In patients whose creatinine clearance remains unchanged during 6 months of observation, but continue to have proteinuria in the range of 4–8 g/24 hours, have a 55% probability of developing chronic renal insufficiency within 10 years. Patients with persistent proteinuria greater than 8 g/24 hours, independent of the degree of renal dysfunction, have a 66–80% probability of developing chronic renal insufficiency within 10 years (Table 27–5).

Table 27–5. Risk of progression categories.

Low risk	Normal serum creatinine and creatinine clearance, plus proteinuria <4 g/day over 6 months of observation
Medium risk	Normal or near normal creatinine clearance and persistent proteinuria ≥4 g/day to ≤8 g/day over 6 months despite maximum conservative treatment
High risk[a]	Deteriorating renal function and/or persistent proteinuria ≥8 g/day in <6 months of observation

[a]Presence of significant complications (thrombosis, severe hypoalbuminemia, dyslipidemia, refractory volume overload) from nephrotic syndrome should be considered as high risk.

B. Relapse After Complete or Partial Remission

About 30% of MN patients will relapse after a complete remission (CR). The majority who do, however, will relapse only to a subnephrotic range of proteinuria and usually have stable long-term function. In the two largest studies of patients with MN who achieved CR, only a few developed, over a long observation period, mild renal insufficiency and none progressed to ESRD. Based on data from the Toronto GN Registry, among 350 patients with nephrotic MN who were followed, the 10-year renal survival was 100% in the CR group, 90% in the partial remission (PR) group, compared to 45% in the no remission group. Thus, both CR and PR appear to be excellent predictors of long-term renal survival. This data has been reexamined recently and using a newer form of analysis (landmark analysis) indicated that regardless of age, baseline GFR, spontaneous or drug-induced remission, with every 3 month increase in duration of remission (CR or PR), there was an associated reduction in hard endpoints and prolonged kidney survival.

▶ Treatment

The international Kidney Disease Improving Global Outcomes (KDIGO) guidelines on the management of glomerulonephritis offer general principles on the management of primary MN as well as grading of the available evidence in regards to immunosuppressive treatment. Here we will emphasize the main practice points and highlight the related evidence as well as new data.

A. Nonimmunosuppressive Therapy

Conservative management should be directed at control of edema, treatment of high blood pressure and hyperlipidemia, dietary protein intake, and reduction of proteinuria through inhibition of the renin–angiotensin system.

1. Blood pressure—Blood pressure control is needed to protect against the cardiovascular risk of hypertension, to reduce proteinuria, and to slow the progression of the renal disease. The target blood pressure in patients with proteinuria remains a topic of debate. In general, a blood pressure of less than 130/80 mm Hg should be targeted. In the Modification of Diet in Renal Disease (MDRD) study, patients with proteinuria greater than 1 g/day had a significantly better outcome if their blood pressure was reduced to 125/75 mm Hg. Thus, in patients with proteinuric renal disease, including MN, a target blood pressure of 125/75 mm Hg may be preferable. Numerous studies have shown that angiotensin converting enzyme inhibitors (ACEI) and/or angiotensin II receptor blockers (ARBs) are renoprotective; they reduce proteinuria and slow progression of renal disease in both diabetic and nondiabetic chronic nephropathy patients. These classes of drugs reduce glomerular intracapillary pressure and protein ultrafiltration and improve glomerular barrier size selectivity.

Meta-analysis of some large renal protection trials with ACEI showed that the degree of protection is related to the degree of reduction of proteinuria; if proteinuria is not lowered, the benefit is substantially attenuated. Data from the RENAAL study (in patients with diabetic nephropathy) shows that the renal protective effect of angiotensin II blockade was nearly fully explained by its antiproteinuric effect. Previous studies have attempted to address this issue in patients with MN, but the numbers are small and follow up limited. In some, the use of ACEI has been associated with a significant improvement in the proteinuria, but in others the efficacy of ACEI appears to be modest at best (<30% reduction in proteinuria). Thus, improvement of proteinuria is unlikely to achieve a significant remission in patients with high-grade proteinuria (>8 g/24 hours). In those with a positive outcome, the antiproteinuric effect of these agents is almost always early (within 2 months of initiation of therapy). Patients at low risk for progression (proteinuria <4 g/24 hours) should be treated with RAS blockade since this may further reduce their proteinuria and offer additional renal protection with little risk of significant adverse effects.

Therefore, although these drugs should be tried first, achieving CR in patients with proteinuria greater than 5 g/24 hours using conservative treatment with ACEI and/or ARBs alone appears unlikely even when these are used at their highest recommended dosages. The use of combined ACEI and ARB treatment is not contraindicated. Data indicating increase complications from the combination from the ONTARGET trial do not apply to MN patients who are younger and do not have the CV comorbidities associated with patients with diabetes mellitus. However, it is rarely tolerated since MN patients are in general normotensive initially and not able to tolerate maximum approved ACE inhibition dosage let alone the addition of an ARB. If dual blockade is used, patients need frequent monitoring for hyperkalemia and further volume status since acute depletion states that can lead to acute kidney injury (AKI).

2. Diet modification—There is no strong evidence to make recommendations with regards to ideal protein intake in the setting of nephrotic syndrome. However, avoiding excessive protein, such as limiting intake to 0.8 g/kg ideal body weight per day of high-quality protein seems a judicious target. In the event of high-grade proteinuria, for instance greater than 15–20 g/day (can be as high as 50 g/day), replacement of urinary protein loss may be necessary. Although dietary protein restriction may reduce proteinuria (15–25%) and slow the progression of renal disease, it has never been shown to induce remission of the NS.

Dietary salt restriction to less than 100 mmol/day of sodium is highly recommended to improve both blood pressure control and reduce edema. Salt restriction is also necessary in order to allow ACEI and ARB treatment to exert their maximum antiproteinuric effects.

3. Dyslipidemia—Proteinuria is an independent risk factor for cardiovascular (CV) morbidity and mortality. Proteinuric patients have elevated cholesterol and triglycerides and markedly elevated CV risk, as illustrated by the almost six-fold increase in the incidence of myocardial infarction in this population. It is likely that the lipid abnormalities associated with proteinuria are important players in the high CV risk in these patients, and thus provide an important target for treatment. Statins are effective in improving the lipid profile and may reduce CV morbidity and mortality in hyperlipidemic and hypertensive patients and in patients with chronic kidney disease. These agents are also effective in reducing serum levels of total cholesterol and low-density lipoprotein (LDL) cholesterol in nephrotic patients and their use is appropriate in patients with hyperlipidemia (targeting LDL levels of <2 mmol/L). Although no study to date has been conducted to demonstrate that reducing cholesterol lowers the risk of CV events in nephrotic patients, the evidence derived from other studies strongly supports this concept. If the proteinuria persists at greater than 3 g/day even these agents may not completely normalize the lipid profile. The adverse risk profile with these agents in the nephrotic syndrome is like the normal population except for an increased incidence of rhabdomyolysis that may occur when used in conjunction with high-dose calcineurin inhibitor such as cyclosporine. Some studies have suggested a small synergistic antiproteinuric effect when statins are combined with ACEI. However, this effect is quite modest and is mainly seen in patients with subnephrotic proteinuria.

4. Thromboembolism—Patients with severe NS are at increased risk for thromboembolic complications. This risk is higher in patients with membranous nephropathy compared to other primary glomerular diseases. Prophylactic anticoagulation could potentially be of benefit in reducing fatal thromboembolic episodes in nephrotic patients with MN and high risk for thromboembolism (TE), for example, obese, bed ridden, previous history of DVT, factor V Leiden deficiency. Although no randomized trial has been done and there is no consensus as to whether prophylactic anticoagulation should be used in this disease, most physicians would consider using it for patients at high risk of a thromboembolic event. To help predict which patient belongs in this risk category that might benefit from prophylaxis, an assessment tool has been developed (gntools.com). This tool considers the risk of TE based mainly on the level of serum albumin relative to the bleeding risk; a score based on the patient's age, degree of anemia, and renal function as well as their comorbidities. This categorizes MN patients into categories of TE risk as well as risks of bleeding in order to assess who best to anticoagulate prophylactically versus where best to avoid. Traditionally, prophylactic agents included heparin, warfarin and in those with stable GFR low molecular weight heparin have been used. The new direct oral anticoagulants may also be appropriate medication for prophylaxis.

5. Severe nonremitting nephrotic syndrome—In patients with nonremitting severe nephrotic syndrome, who are not candidates for immunosuppressive treatment because of advanced kidney disease but are not yet on dialysis, complication from nephrosis can be severe. These complications include refractory volume overload that is difficult to control by diuretics. Drugs such ACEI and ARB can help reduce the proteinuria and ameliorate these complications but may fail to fully control the symptoms. Non-steroidal anti-inflammatory drugs (NSAIDs) have antiproteinuric effects, and can reduce proteinuria by 30–50% but caution should be taken, as these agents can lead to further renal complications (mainly AKI) and nonrenal complications (GI bleeding, and exacerbate cardiac disease) especially in those with significant renal impairment. Intentional renal artery thrombosis should be considered especially if the kidneys are small. Nephrectomy is a last resort for treatment of such uncontrolled nephrosis and should not be undertaken until all other options for treatment and the risks of surgery are considered.

B. Immunosuppressive Therapy

Several treatment strategies, including a variety of immunosuppressive agents and regimens, have been shown to reduce proteinuria in MN. However, questions to be asked when considering immunosuppressive treatment, should include

1. How long should you wait for spontaneous remission in patients on conservative therapy alone?

2. Which of the various therapeutic regimens should be considered first (taking into consideration specific patient characteristics, the regimens adverse event profile as well as effectiveness)?

3. How long should the drug be used before considering it a failure?

4. How long should the treatment be continued if it is successful?

Here we will briefly review the immunosuppressive treatments and the evidence behind each therapy. Table 27–6 summarizes therapies and doses of medications.

1. Corticosteroids—The early U.S. collaborative study of adult idiopathic nephrotic syndrome reported that a 2–3-month course of high-dose alternate-day prednisone (100–150 mg), when compared to placebo, resulted in a significant reduction in the progression to renal failure, although there was no effect on the degree of proteinuria. The short follow-up period and the worse than expected outcome of the control group raised major concerns, especially since subsequent data determined the close relationship between proteinuria reduction and outcome in MN. Subsequent controlled studies have shown no benefit from the use of corticosteroids on MN. The two largest randomized controlled trials, one by the British Medical Research Trial and the second by the Toronto Glomerulonephritis Study Group, found no significant benefit of corticosteroid treatment alone on either induction of remission or preservation of renal function. Currently, oral corticosteroids as monotherapy for the treatment of MN are not recommended in the Caucasian population.

2. Combined alkylating agents with corticosteroids—In patients with a moderate risk of progression, a significant benefit has been described when a cytotoxic agent alternating monthly with corticosteroids has been used. A number of randomized trials suggest that 6 months of this regimen (cyclophosphamide or chlorambucil as the cytotoxic agent) is four to five times more likely to induce a CR of the NS, and halt disease progression, compared to no therapy or corticosteroids alone. The largest studies with the longest observation time come from Ponticelli's group in Italy. The first study compared the effects of combined methylprednisolone (MTP) 1 g intravenously on the first 3 days of month 1, 3, and 5 followed by 27 days of oral methylprednisolone (0.4 mg/kg/day) or prednisone (0.5 mg/kg/day) alternating in months 2, 4, and 6 with chlorambucil at 0.2 mg/kg/day, versus conservative treatment in 67 patients with MN and nephrotic range proteinuria. The 32 patients who received the alkylating agent were followed for a mean of 31.4 ± 18.2 months. Complete remission was achieved in 38% and PR in 34% of the treated cases. Among the controls, CR was achieved in 7% and PR in 23% of the patients. The regimen was reported as safe with only two of the treated patients stopping therapy. After up to 10 years of follow-up, patients treated with combination therapy had a 92% probability of

Table 27–6. Common immunosuppressive regimens used for treatment of membranous nephropathy.

Treatment Class	Regimen	Special Considerations
Alkylating agents	Cyclophosphamide: *Ponticelli Based:* Methylprednisolone[a] 1 g IV for 3 days then prednisone 0.4 mg/kg daily for 27 days on months 1, 3, and 5 *alternating with* cyclophosphamide 2.5 mg/kg/day for 30 days on months 2,4, and 6 *Alternative (Dutch):* Methylprednisolone 1 g IV for 3 consecutive days then prednisone 0.5 mg/kg every other day for 6 months with subsequent tapering *plus* cyclophosphamide 1.5–2 mg/day for 1 y	Monitor WBC, serum creatinine, urine protein excretion every 2 wk for the first 2 mo then every month if stable on therapy Hold cyclophosphamide if WBC ≤3500/mm^3 until recovery to >4000/mm^3 then adjust the dose PJP prophylaxis should be considered. Gastric prophylaxis (eg, PPI) and bone protection (calcium and vitamin D ± bisphosphonate) for patients on prednisone
Calcineurin inhibitors	Cyclosporine: 3.5 mg/kg/day divided in 2 doses, 12 h apart, with or without prednisone (0.15 mg/kg/day) for 6 mo Tacrolimus: 0.05–0.075 mg/kg/day given in 2 equally divided doses 12 h apart, without prednisone for 6–12 mo	Target cyclosporine 12 h trough level of 125–175 ug/L Target tacrolimus 12 h trough level 4–8 ug/L Usually started at lower doses May need to extend the course for more than 1 y if only partial remission achieved
Rituximab	Most common: 375 mg/m^2 IV 4 weekly doses or 1 g IV 2 doses 15 days apart Alternative: Single dose 1 g IV with follow up of CD 19/20 lymphocyte count.	Caution of severe infusion reactions: Should be given in a monitored setting, especially the first dose. PJP prophylaxis should be instituted/maintained while CD20 count depleted. Monitoring of CD 19/20 lymphocyte count may be beneficial to determine further doses. Data on long-term side effects are still lacking.

[a]Monitor for signs of adrenal suppression on "off steroids" months. Eliminating high doses of methylprednisone IV may reduce overall steroid toxicity.

renal survival compared with 60% in the control group, and only 8% of treated patients versus 40% of untreated ones had reached ESRD. In addition, the slope of the reciprocal of serum creatinine remained significantly slower in the treated group than in the untreated controls for up to 90 months. In terms of proteinuria, only 42% of the treated group, versus 78% of the placebo group, spent time in a nephrotic state over the 10-year follow-up. Women and patients with mild glomerular lesions (stage I and II) were more likely to enter remission after combined therapy in this study, and no patients had significantly impaired renal function at entry.

A second study with 81 patients, compared 6 months of alternating monthly pulses of MTP (1 g), oral steroids, and chlorambucil as described above versus MTP pulses and steroids (0.4 mg/kg every other day) alone, found that at 3 years, 66% of the patients given steroids and chlorambucil versus 23% of the patients given steroids alone were in remission, the difference being significant. At 5 years, this difference remained statistically significant (73% in combined treatment versus 40% in control, $p = 0.026$). Combined therapy was also associated with a trend toward better preservation of renal function, as assessed by serum creatinine, although

the difference was not statistically significant. In a third study from the same group, patients were enrolled in a 6-month study comparing MTP/prednisone alternating with chlorambucil (same doses as the prior studies) to MTP alternating with oral cyclophosphamide (2.5 mg/kg/day). Among 87 nephrotic patients followed for at least 1 year, 82% of patients assigned to MTP and chlorambucil had complete or partial remission of the NS versus 93% of patients assigned to MTP and cyclophosphamide ($p = 0.116$, NS). The use of cyclophosphamide was associated with fewer side effects, but renal function was equally preserved in both groups for up to 3 years. However, a relapse rate in both treated groups of 25–30% was seen within 2 years. The incidence of CR 1 year following combined immunosuppressive treatment was approximately 28% in the first study, 20% in the second study, and 32% in the third study. All these studies excluded patients whose serum creatinine exceeded 1.7 mg/dL at entry. These observations have been confirmed by Jha et al, who reported the 10-year follow-up of a randomized, controlled trial on 93 patients of Asian origin allocated to either conservative therapy or to receive a 6-month course of alternating prednisolone and cyclophosphamide. Proteinuria was 5.9 ± 2.2 and 6.1 ± 2.5 g/24 hour in the conservative and immunosuppressive therapy group, respectively. Renal function was well preserved with estimated GFR rates above 80 mL/min in both groups. Of the 47 patients treated with immunosuppressive therapy, 34 achieved remission (15 CR and 19 PR), compared with 16 (5 CR and 11 PR) of 46 in the control group (p <0.0001). The 10-year dialysis-free survival was 89% and 65% (p = 0.016), and the likelihood of survival without death, dialysis, or doubling of serum creatinine was 79% in the treated versus 44% (p = 0.0006) in the control group. Both groups had a similar rate of infection.

Modified regimens of the Ponticelli course have been published with similar efficacy. These include daily oral cyclophosphamide (dose of 1.5–2 mg/kg/day) for 12 months combined with prednisone for 6 months (at a dose of 0.5 mg/kg every other day, with three consecutive doses of methylprednisolone 1 g IV at the beginning of the first, third, and fifth months). This regimen was used by the Dutch group who enrolled 65 patients with MN and significant renal impairment (serum creatinine >135 umol/L). Follow-up was 51 (5–132) months. Renal function improved or stabilized in all patients. Overall renal survival was 86% after 5 years and 74% after 7 years. A PR occurred in 56 patients followed by a CR in 17 patients. However, 11 patients had a relapse (28% relapse rate at 5 years), of whom nine were retreated because of deteriorating renal function. In contrast to the original Ponticelli regimens, treatment-related complications occurred in two-thirds of patients, mainly consisting of bone marrow suppression and infections. Not all patients received the IV doses of methylprednisone, and in routine practice, delivering such doses can be cumbersome (given the potential need for hospital admission). Moreover, administering the IV doses does increase the cumulative dose of steroids and their potential side effects.

Recently, a UK randomized controlled trial of immunosuppressive treatment in high risk of progression MN patients was published. This study included 108 patients (included patients with serum creatinine up to 300 umol/L, all with at least a 20% decline in GFR in the 2 years preceding enrollment). Patients were randomly assigned to chlorambucil and prednisone for 6 months (33 patients), cyclosporine for 12 months (37 patients), or supportive therapy (38 patients). Unconventionally, the primary end point was a further reduction in GFR by greater than 20% over the study period. The risk of further reduction of GFR was significantly lower in the combined chlorambucil and prednisone group (58%) versus the supportive therapy group (84%) and versus the cyclosporine group (81%). The frequency of side effects was high in all groups but significantly higher in the combined chlorambucil and prednisone group (56 events) compared to supportive group (24 events).

Thus, in several studies, both cyclophosphamide and chlorambucil in combination with corticosteroids appear to be effective in the treatment of patients with primary MN

and preserved renal function. The favorable effects are maintained well beyond the 6–12 months of treatment but relapse rates approached 35% at 2 years. This combination may also be effective in those with deteriorating renal function, but the supporting data are much less compelling, adverse effects are higher, and the likelihood of benefit is reduced in patients with severe renal failure (serum creatinine >3 mg/dL). The adverse effects of cyclophosphamide when used long term are the major drawbacks to the universal application of this form of therapy. These include increased susceptibility to infections, anemia, thrombocytopenia, nausea, vomiting, sterility, and in the long-term malignancy, in particular bladder cancer. In regard to chlorambucil, the additional major concern is the possibility of inducing acute leukemia or lymphoma. Even when chlorambucil was used in modified versions (lower doses) than in the original regimen, the rate of adverse effects was high.

3. Calcineurin inhibitors—cyclosporine—Early uncontrolled studies of cyclosporine suggested an initial benefit but a high relapse rate after cessation of treatment. In a single blind randomized controlled study by Cattran, 51 patients with steroid-resistant MN were treated with cyclosporine A (CSA) plus low-dose prednisone) compared to placebo plus prednisone. CsA was given at 3.5 mg/kg/day with a target whole-blood trough level of 125–175 ng/mL. All patients received prednisone at 0.15 mg/kg/day (up to a maximum of 15 mg/day). At the end of treatment at 26 weeks, 75% (21 of 28 patients) in the CsA group versus only 22% (5 of 23 patients) of controls had achieved a PR or CR (CR 2 in the CsA group versus 1 in the placebo group). CsA was well tolerated, and no one had to discontinue treatment because of adverse effects. Relapses occurred in approximately 40% of patients within 1 year of discontinuation of CsA treatment, not dissimilar to that found in controlled cytotoxic/corticosteroid regimens but at an earlier time point.

There has been one randomized controlled trial using CsA in patients with high-grade proteinuria and progressive renal failure, conducted by the Toronto group. In this study, 64 patients were placed on a restricted protein diet (0.9 g/kg) and followed for 12 months (phase 1). Seventeen patients with a loss in creatinine clearance of 8 mL/min/year (but with creatinine clearance >30 mL/min) and proteinuria greater than 3.5 g/ 24 hours were randomly assigned to either CsA treatment (3.5 mg/kg/day; nine patients) or placebo (eight patients) for 12 months (phase 2). After 12 months, there was a significant reduction in proteinuria and in the rate of loss of renal function in the CsA group compared with the group that received placebo. In the CsA group, the slope of creatinine clearance was reduced from 2.4 to 0.7 mL/min/month, whereas in the placebo group the change was insignificant, 2.2–2.1 mL/min/month (p = 0.02). This improvement was sustained in approximately 50% of the patients for up to 2 years after CsA was stopped.

Prolonging the treatment as reported by the German Cyclosporine in Nephrotic Syndrome Study Group results in a higher and more sustained rate of remission In this study, 41 high-risk patients with MN and proteinuria greater than 3.5 g/24 hours (mean 10.9 ± 5.7 g/24 hours) were treated with CsA (average dose = 3.3 ± 1.1 mg/kg/day) for a median of 353 days (159–586 days). Approximately 65% of the patients also received ACEI plus corticosteroid treatment (average 21 mg/day). Complete remission (proteinuria <0.5 g/24 hours) was achieved in 34% of the patients. The median treatment time to CR was 225 days (quartiles 120 days and 459 days). Similarly, Alexopoulos et al compared 12 months of low dose cyclosporine with prednisone to low-dose cyclosporine alone. The rates of CR and PR were comparable in the two groups. The renal function was unchanged in both groups. However, there were more relapses in the cyclosporine alone group than the combined group. A strong predictor of relapse was a low cyclosporine trough level (<100 ng/mL) in both groups. Taken together, these data would suggest that CsA induces a remission (CR or PR) of the NS in 50–60% of patients. It is important to emphasize that although reduction of proteinuria usually occurs within a few weeks, most CR occurred after more than 6 months of treatment. This would suggest that if urinary protein excretion is not significantly reduced within 3–4 months of initiating therapy it is unlikely that more prolonged therapy will result in a remission. This is an important observation and may explain why studies in which CsA was used for less than 6 months achieved low rates of CR, whereas studies using CsA for up to 1 year, albeit uncontrolled, reported complete remission rates close to 80%. However, significant adverse effects including hypertension, gingival hyperplasia, gastrointestinal complaints, muscle cramps, and more important nephrotoxicity can accompany prolonged CsA treatment. The latter is dose/duration dependent as well as age dependent. Patients at risk are those with initial impaired renal function, especially if accompanied by chronic vascular disease and tubulointerstitial damage on renal biopsy. On the other hand, there is little risk of nephrotoxicity with prolonged low-dose CsA (~1.5 mg/kg/day) and this approach could be considered for long-term maintenance of patients with preserved renal function who achieve a CR or PR, but then relapse.

Tacrolimus: Based on several studies including small RCTs and observational data, it appears that tacrolimus is as effective as cyclosporine in inducing remission of nephrotic syndrome in MN. A study by Praga et al evaluated tacrolimus monotherapy in MN. In this study 25 patients with normal renal function (mean proteinuria ~8 g/24 h), received tacrolimus (at a dose of 0.05 mg/kg/day) over 12 months with a 6-month taper, whereas 23 patients served as control. After 18 months, the probability of remission was 94% in the tacrolimus group but only 35% in the control group. Six patients in the control group and only one in the tacrolimus group reached the secondary end point of a 50% increase in their serum creatinine. Unfortunately, almost half of the patients relapsed after tacrolimus was withdrawn. Similarly, in a Chinese study by Yuan et al 42 patients with MN were treated with combined tacrolimus and prednisone for 6 months followed by either no treatment (20 patients) or long-term treatment with low-dose tacrolimus to 24 months (22 patients). Forty-five percent of the patients in the short-term treatment group relapsed after cessation of tacrolimus compared to none of the patients on the long-term tacrolimus therapy group. This suggests that similar to patients treated with CsA, maintenance of remission may require prolonged use of tacrolimus in low doses. It is important to recognize that based on this data calcineurin inhibitors work as monotherapy and there appears no additional benefit with the addition of corticosteroids.

4. Mycophenolate mofetil—Mycophenolate mofetil (MMF), a prodrug and its active ingredient mycophenolic acid (Myfortic) have been established as potent antirejection treatments. They are also commonly prescribed in the management of lupus nephritis as induction and maintenance therapy. Mycophenolic acid selectively inhibits T- and B-lymphocyte proliferation through inhibition of de novo purine synthesis and inactivation of inosine monophosphate dehydrogenase. It does not share azathioprine's profile in terms of myelotoxicity, hepatotoxicity, and mutagenesis. Unlike calcineurin inhibitors, these agents are not nephrotoxic. Recognized side effects are usually gastrointestinal (nausea, vomiting, diarrhea, abdominal pain) and less commonly myelosuppression (anemia and leukopenia). Some reports have indicated that gastrointestinal side effects are less common with Myfortic.

As with any immunosuppressive agent, patients on MMF are at a higher risk of infections. There has been a small number of studies using MMF in MN. Branten et al reported 32 patients with MN and renal insufficiency (serum creatinine 1.5 mg/dL) treated with MMF (1 g twice daily) for 12 months and compared to results obtained on 32 patients from a historic control group treated for the same duration with oral CYC (1.5 mg/kg/day). Both groups received high dose steroid treatment (methylprednisolone IV 1 g for 3 doses on months 1, 3, and 5 followed by oral prednisone 0.5 mg/kg every other day for 6 months, with subsequent tapering). Overall, 21 MMF-treated patients developed PR of proteinuria; in an additional six patients, proteinuria decreased by at least 50%, and no response was observed in five patients. Cumulative incidences of remission of proteinuria at 12 months were 66% in the MMF group versus 72% in the CYC group ($p = 0.3$). Side effects occurred at a similar rate between the two groups but relapses were much more common in the MMF treated group.

Following this, an open label randomized controlled trial from France compared MMF plus conservative therapy for 1 year to conservative therapy alone in patients with preserved GFR and medium risk proteinuria. The sample size was small with a total of 36 patients, 19 patients receiving MMF and 17 patients receiving conservative therapy only. The probability of CR or PR did not differ between the two groups after 12 months of treatment. Four patients who received MMF had serious adverse events (20%). Based on the available evidence, it does not appear that either MMF or mycophenolic acid are effective as monotherapy for MN. However, there may be a role for these agents as adjunctive therapy in patients who are unable to tolerate higher doses of CNI or who do not have an adequate response.

5. Rituximab—It has long been thought that rituximab would be a suitable therapy for primary MN, given its anti-CD 20 activity, which depletes B lymphocytes, the precursors for antibody synthesizing plasma cells. While this treatment was approved initially for treatment of lymphoma, over the past decade this agent has been gained widespread use (off-label) to treat primary MN. Initially, a pilot study in eight nephrotic MN were prospectively treated with a 4 weekly course of rituximab (375 mg/m^2) and followed for 1 year. All patients had complete depletion of circulating B cells for up to 1 year. Proteinuria significantly decreased from a mean of 8.6 g/24 hours at baseline to 4.3 ± 3.3 g (51%, p <0.005) at 3 months, 4.0 ± 3.1 g (53%, p <0.005) at 6 months, and to 3.0 ± 2.5 g (66%, p <0.005) at 12 months. At 12 months, proteinuria had decreased to less than 0.5 g/24 hours in two patients and less than 3.5 g/24 hours in three other patients. Proteinuria decreased in the remaining three patients by 74%, 44%, and 41%. Renal function remained stable in all patients. Adverse effects were reported as mild and included chills and fever in one patient and an anaphylactic reaction in another patient with drug infusion.

These findings were confirmed in a subsequent study by the same group, who treated 100 consecutive patients with persistent NS. After a mean follow up of 29 months, 65 patients achieved CR or PR. Notably, the median time to remission was 7.1 months. They reported no serious treatment related side effects. In the first randomized controlled trial, from France, after 6 months of conservative therapy, two doses of rituximab (375 mg/m^2 IV, on days 1 and 8) were given to 37 patients and compared to 38 patients who continued conservative antiproteinuric therapy for 6 more months. The median time of follow up was 17 months in both groups. After 6 months of treatment, 13 patients (35.1%) in the rituximab group achieved CR or PR, compared to eight patients (21.1%) in the conservative therapy group. This difference, the primary endpoint in the study, did not achieve statistical significance. However, anti-PLA2R titers were significantly reduced in the rituximab group (50%) compared to the conservative therapy (12%) at 6 months post-treatment (p = 0.004). During the follow-up observation period, remission of proteinuria was seen in 24 of 37 (64.9%) patients in the rituximab group compared to 13 of 38 (34.2%)

in the conservative treatment group (p <0.01). The mean time to remission was 7 months, comparable to the study by Ruggenenti et al. The authors concluded that the effects of rituximab on proteinuria continue to accrue beyond the 6 months period post-treatment, with patients demonstrating a reduction in PLA2R antibodies that appear to precede proteinuria remission. Safety and adverse events were similar in both groups. Currently a North American randomized controlled trial (MENTOR trial, NCT01180036) comparing rituximab to cyclosporine treatment is being conducted in MN patients with heavy proteinuria (>5 g/day).

6. ACTH—Adrenocorticotropic hormone (ACTH) derivatives have been used for treatment of nephrotic syndrome since the 1950s. The evidence for use of these agents specifically for treatment of primary MN is scarce, and based on small studies. Currently the drug is available in two forms. The first is a synthetic ACTH subcutaneous/intramuscular injection (Synacthen). A pilot study, compared synthetic ACTH (twice weekly IM injections) for 1 year to prednisone alternating with cytotoxic agent (using the Ponticelli protocol mentioned earlier) for 6 months. Each group had 16 patients with MN and nephrotic syndrome. Fourteen of 16 patients who received synthetic ACTH had CR or PR, compared to 15 of 16 patients on prednisone alternating with cytotoxic therapy. In both groups the median proteinuria decreased during follow-up. Two patients from each group developed significant side effects.

More recently, a prospective cohort of 20 high-risk patients with primary MN (defined as β_2-microglobulin excretion >500 ng/min) were selectively treated with intramuscular synthetic ACTH injections (maximum 1 mg twice weekly) for 18 weeks then tapered. Seventeen patients (85%) completed the treatment. The cumulative remission rate (four patients CR and seven patients with PR) was 55%. These were compared with historical controls treated with cyclophosphamide and steroids, who achieved 93% remission rate (13 patients with CR and 6 patients with PR out of total of 20 patients). There were significant different entry criteria and drug exposure in comparison to the original RCT making the two studies difficult to compare. The second form of the drug is natural product derived from processing porcine pituitary glands, ACTH gel (Acthar Gel) that has been studied in pilot trial of 20 patients randomized to receive either 40 or 80 IU twice weekly for 3 months. In a subset of patients who initially were on the 40 IU twice weekly dose, if there was no response, the dose was increased to 80 IU twice weekly for an additional 90 days. Patients were observed for changes in proteinuria, albumin, cholesterol, GFR, and anti-PLA2R antibody levels. The mean proteinuria was 9.1 ± 3.4 g/day, albumin 2.7 ± 0.8 g/dL and GFR 77 ± 30 mL/min. At 12 weeks of therapy, none of the nine patients who initially received 40 IU had a significant change in their proteinuria, but 5 out of 11 of the patients receiving the higher dose demonstrated at least 30% reduction in their urinary protein excretion. By 12 months of follow-up, there was a significant improvement in the proteinuria of the entire cohort, and a 50% reduction in proteinuria was observed in 65% with a trend of better outcomes in patients receiving a higher cumulative dose. The reduction in serum PLA2R antibody was noted in some but not all patients in parallel or prior to the reduction of proteinuria. Given the results of these studies, ACTH may have a role in the treatment of MN, especially in patients who have contraindications to CNI, cytotoxic, or rituximab therapy. To better understand the role of these agents, randomized controlled trials with greater number of patients are needed. There is also the issue of suppressing the hypothalamic-pituitary-adrenal axis with prolonged administration, which needs to be clarified in larger trials. In addition, its current high cost is an additional limitation to the widespread use of the drug.

▶ Prognosis

The prognosis of primary MN is closely associated with proteinuria. Based on previous studies, those who achieve CR or PR, whether with conservative therapy or with immunosuppressive treatment have a better long-term prognosis than those who remain nephrotic. Many studies have showed improved renal survival and a slower rate of decline of GFR in those achieving remission and that is directly related to its duration. In contrast to this improvement, there is good clinical evidence that higher sustained levels of proteinuria predict more rapid decline in renal function, more pronounced tubulointerstitial injury, and eventual kidney

failure. Moreover, the severity and duration of proteinuria are markers for thromboembolic and cardiovascular risk. Data from the Framingham study have showed that proteinuria predicts CV outcome. Other studies such as the LIFE and AASK trials have shown that CV risk increases incrementally with the increase in proteinuria, making the link between chronic renal disease and cardiac disease so strong that few patients develop chronic kidney disease without clinically apparent or occult cardiac disease.

Nephrotic patients are also at risk for thromboembolic events, with an incidence as high as 50% in patients with severe MN being reported. These events are associated with a mortality rate as high as 42% in high-risk patients. These data emphasize that these life-defining events, in addition to the potential of renal failure, are common in these patients. Therefore, even if the main benefit of immunosuppressive therapy is to speed up the induction of a remission that may eventually have occurred spontaneously, it still has long-term value. A treatment algorithm that combines the predictive factors and best evidence for immunosuppressive therapy is presented in Figure 27-4.

The KIDGO guidelines, recommend using cytotoxic/steroid or cyclosporine as the first line of therapy in the moderate or high-risk groups based on evidence from randomized trials. Recent controlled trials also support the addition of rituximab as first-line therapy. It is critical for the treating physician to consider the specific individual risks versus benefits as well as the patient's preference in deciding initial treatment. These immunosuppressive regimens are not mutually exclusive and if the first one chosen fails in reducing the proteinuria to the desired range and/or

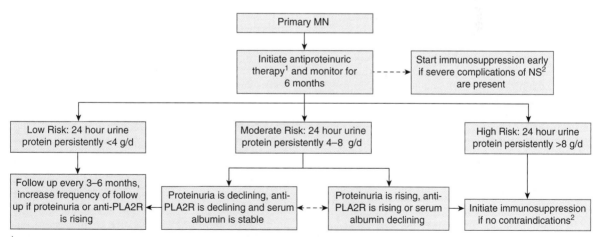

[1]Initiate low salt diet. Start ACEI/ARB, with target blood pressure <130/80 mm Hg
[2]Treat with an appropriate immunosuppressive agent (cyclophosphamide + prednisone, cyclosporine/tacrolimus, rituximab), must exclude infections, malignancy, severely reduced GFR (<30 mL/min) before initiating therapy

▲ **Figure 27-4.** MN treatment algorithm for membranous nephropathy. ACEI, angiotensin-converting enzyme inhibitor; ARB, angiotensin receptor blocker; BP, blood pressure.

adverse side effects make completion of a course of therapy untenable, a second or even third choice amongst these regimens may be effective (though the need for a drug holiday between such therapy should be considered). Patients who do not respond well or relapse after a first course of immunosuppression therapy may benefit from a second course of the same immunosuppression regimen if the first course was tolerated, and if the cumulative received dose of the immunosuppressant is acceptable (especially in the case of cyclophosphamide). Otherwise, if the first course has not been successful, a choice of another agent, with a different mechanism of action, should be considered. Patients with severe renal insufficiency (serum creatinine 3 mg/dL) are less likely to benefit to the same degree from any of the immunosuppression regimens and the risk of treatment is significantly higher. These patients should be considered for conservative therapy only and plans should be made for renal replacement therapy including transplantation in the future, assuming the immunologically active phase of the disease has resolved.

Prognostic value of anti-PLA2R antibody—Since the description of the pathologic role of PLA2R antibodies in primary MN, scientists have sought to determine how the levels of these antibodies correlate with disease activity. The populations studied have been somewhat heterogeneous in terms of from different geographic groups or varying severity of the disease, and in the timing of antibody testing in relation to disease onset and/or kidney biopsy, and in the treatment received. Earlier studies compared outcomes of patients with positive anti-PLA2R antibodies to those who were serologically negative. Hoxha et al reported in a multicenter prospective study, 133 patients with primary MN positive that were followed for changes in proteinuria and in antibody titer. The data indicated that patients who achieved remission at 1 year had lower anti-PLA2R levels at the time of study entry compared to a later remission rate in those with high anti-PLA2R antibody levels. In patients who received immunosuppression (CNI, rituximab or cytotoxic drug), antibody levels fell by 69–81% after 3 months of initiation of treatment, versus a reduction of proteinuria of only 38.8% at the same time point. In another study, 33 patients with non-nephrotic MN, were screened for anti-PLA2R antibodies and followed over a mean of 25 months. At study start, 16 patients (48%) tested positive for autoantibodies, of those 13 patients developed nephrotic proteinuria (81%). In the 17 patients who were antibody negative, only 5 developed nephrotic proteinuria (38.5%). Multivariate analysis showed that anti-PLA2R antibody levels were associated with an increased risk of development of nephrotic proteinuria (HR 3.66, CI 1.39–9.64, $p = 0.009$).

Beck et al tested anti-PLA2R antibodies in a retrospective cohort of 48 high-risk patients with progressive MN, from 1997 to 2005 whose initial median serum creatinine was 1.6 mg/dL. Twenty-two patients received MMF and 26 patients received cyclophosphamide, both in combination with steroids, for 12 months. Patients were followed up to 5 years from study entry. At baseline 34 patients (71%) were positive for PLA2R antibody. The response to immunosuppressive treatment was similar in patients who were antibody positive or negative. Anti PLA2R antibody levels did not predict the initial response to immunosuppressive therapy or the final outcomes (CR and PR). At the end of treatment, 24 of the 34 PLA2R antibody positive patients became negative and nine remained positive. None of those who remained PLA2R positive at the end of treatment (with three out of nine having partial remission) achieved a persistent remission over the follow-up. In a similar retrospective analysis among 132 patients with MN and persistent nephrotic syndrome treated with rituximab and screened for anti-PLA2R antibodies, 81 tested positive for the autoantibody. During follow-up, the outcomes of patients with and without antibodies were similar. However, in those who tested positive, lower antibody titers at baseline and antibody depletion at 6 months posttreatment better predicted remission. All the 25 patients who entered CR had preceding complete anti-PLA2R antibody depletion. It was noted that antibody depletion preceded proteinuria reduction by an average of 10 months.

In an additional study that addresses the prognostic value of the antibody titer, 73 patients with PLA2R-positive primary MN were divided into low (seronegative and tertile 1) and high (tertile 2, tertile 3) anti-PLA2R antibody levels were analyzed retrospectively. The samples were obtained at the time of renal biopsy. Patients were followed for a median period of 11.3 years. Patients with high PLA2R antibody levels had higher proteinuria compared to those with low antibody levels. The spontaneous remission rate was significantly higher in patients who were seronegative (88%) compared to those who were seropositive (43%). Spontaneous remission was also higher in those in the lowest antibody tertile (76%) compared to those in the highest (27%). During follow-up, 14 patients developed a relapse (five of whom were treated with immunosuppression); neither the tertile of PLA2R antibody level nor the severity of initial proteinuria was predictive of relapse. Thus, in patients who are positive for anti-PLA2R antibodies, the baseline level of antibody may not be as informative as the antibody response and the level of antibodies at the end of treatment. Monitoring the antibody levels may help predict remission, nonresponse or even relapse after remission and monitoring of patients positive for anti-PLA2R antibodies is informative, and should soon be integrated into primary MN patient care. A serology-based individualized approach to MN aiming to increase diagnostic and prognostic accuracy, limit unnecessary exposure to immunosuppression and optimize efficacy of treatment has been recently been proposed.

KEY READINGS

Alexopoulos E et al: Induction and long-term treatment with cyclosporine in membranous nephropathy with the nephrotic syndrome. Nephrol Dial Transplant 2006;21:3127.

Beck LH Jr et al: M-type phospholipase A2 receptor as target antigen in idiopathic membranous nephropathy. N Engl J Med 2009;361:11.

Beck LH Jr et al: Rituximab-induced depletion of anti-PLA2R autoantibodies predicts response in membranous nephropathy. J Am Soc Nephrol 2011;22:1543.

Branten AJ et al: Mycophenolate mofetil in idiopathic membranous nephropathy: a clinical trial with comparison to a historic control group treated with cyclophosphamide. Am J Kidney Dis 2007;50:248.

Branten AJ et al: Urinary excretion of beta 2-microglobulin and IgG predict prognosis in idiopathic membranous nephropathy: a validation study. J Am Soc Nephrol 2005; 16:169.

Cattran D: Management of membranous nephropathy: when and what for treatment. J Am Soc Nephrol 16:2005;1188.

Cattran DC et al: Cyclosporine in patients with steroid-resistant membranous nephropathy: a randomized trial for the North American Nephrotic Syndrome Study Group. Kidney Int 2001;59:1484.

Cravedi P et al: Titrating rituximab to circulating B cells to optimize lymphocytolytic therapy in idiopathic membranous nephropathy. Clin J Am Soc Nephrol 2007;2:932.

Dahan K et al: Rituximab for severe membranous nephropathy: a 6-month trial with extended follow-up. J Am Soc Nephrol 2017;28:348.

Debiec H et al: Antenatal membranous glomerulonephritis due to anti-neutral endopeptidase antibodies. N Engl J Med 2002;346:2053.

De Vriese AS et al: A proposal for a serology-based approach to membranous nephropathy. J Am Soc Nephrol 2017;28:421.

du Buf-Vereijken PW et al: Cytotoxic therapy for membranous nephropathy and renal insufficiency: improved renal survival but high relapse rate. Nephrol Dialysis Transplant 2004;19:1142.

du Buf-Vereijken PW, Wetzels JF: Efficacy of a second course of immunosuppressive therapy in patients with membranous nephropathy and persistent or relapsing disease activity. Nephrol Dialysis Transplant 2004;19:2036.

Fervenza FC et al: Rituximab therapy in idiopathic membranous nephropathy: a 2-year study. Clin J Am Soc Nephrol 2010;5:2188.

Hladunewich MA et al: A pilot study to determine the dose and effectiveness of adrenocorticotrophic hormone (H.P. Acthar® Gel) in nephrotic syndrome due to idiopathic membranous nephropathy. Nephrol Dial Transplant 2014;8:1570.

Hofstra JM et al: Treatment of idiopathic membranous nephropathy. Nat Rev Nephrol 2013;9:443.

Jha V et al: A randomized, controlled trial of steroids and cyclophosphamide in adults with nephrotic syndrome caused by idiopathic membranous nephropathy. J Am Soc Nephrol 2007;18:1899.

Kanigicherla D et al: Anti-PLA2R antibodies measured by ELISA predict long-term outcome in a prevalent population of patients with idiopathic membranous nephropathy. Kidney Int 2013;83:940.

Kidney Disease: Improving Global Outcomes (KDIGO) Glomerulonephritis Work Group. KDIGO Clinical Practice Guideline for Glomerulonephritis. Kidney Int Suppl 2012;2:139.

Perna A et al: Immunosuppressive treatment for idiopathic membranous nephropathy: a systematic review. Am J Kidney Dis 2004;44:385.

Ponticelli C et al: A randomized pilot trial comparing methylprednisolone plus a cytotoxic agent versus synthetic adrenocorticotropic hormone in idiopathic membranous nephropathy. Am J Kidney Dis 2006;47:233.

Ponticelli C, Glassock RJ: Glomerular diseases: membranous nephropathy—a modern view. Clin J Am Soc Nephrol 2014;3:609.

Praga M et al: Tacrolimus monotherapy in membranous nephropathy: a randomized controlled trial. Kidney Int 2007;71:924.

Ruggenenti P et al: Anti-phospholipase A2 receptor antibody titer predicts post-rituximab outcome of membranous nephropathy. J Am Soc Nephrol 2015;26:2545.

Ruggenenti P et al: Rituximab in idiopathic membranous nephropathy. J Am Soc Nephrol 2012;23:1416.

Seitz-Polski B et al: Epitope spreading of autoantibody response to PLA2R associates with poor prognosis in membranous nephropathy. J Am Soc Nephrol 2016;27:1517.

Thompson A et al: Complete and partial remission as surrogate end points in membranous nephropathy. J Am Soc Nephrol 2015;26:2930.

Timmermans SA et al: Anti-PLA2R antibodies as a prognostic factor in PLA2R-related membranous nephropathy. Am J Nephrol 2015;42:70.

Tomas NM et al: Thrombospondin type-1 domain-containing 7A in idiopathic membranous nephropathy. N Engl J Med 2014;371:2277.

Tomas NM et al: Autoantibodies against thrombospondin type 1 domain-containing 7A induce membranous nephropathy. J Clin Invest 2016;126:2519.

Troyanov S et al: Idiopathic membranous nephropathy: definition and relevance of a partial remission. Kidney Int 2004;66:1199.

Verhulst A et al: Inhibitors of HMG-CoA reductase reduce receptor mediated endocytosis in human kidney proximal tubular cells. J Am Soc Nephrol 2004;15:2249.

Vidt DG et al: Rosuvastatin-induced arrest in progression of renal disease. Cardiology 2004;102:52.

Yuan H et al: Effect of prolonged tacrolimus treatment in idiopathic membranous nephropathy with nephrotic syndrome. Pharmacology 2013;91:259.

■ CHAPTER REVIEW QUESTIONS

1. A 65-year-old man, with a past history of hypertension controlled on amlodipine, presented to the ER with bilateral lower limb swelling for the past 10 days. He has a 30-year history of smoking 1 pack per day but quit 5 years ago. On review he mentions increased frothiness in his urine. His physical examination reveals a blood pressure of 140/90 mm Hg, and a heart rate of 80 beats/min. He has bilateral lower limb swelling extending to the thighs. He weighs 80 kg compared to a baseline of 75 kg 3 months ago. Cardiovascular examination shows normal heart sounds. His chest is clear to auscultation. The rest of his examination is unremarkable. On laboratory investigations, his serum creatinine is 1.7 mg/dL, 24-hour urine protein is 10 g/day. Serum albumin is 11 g/L, hemoglobin 123 g/L. His kidney biopsy shows features of membranous nephropathy, with GBM thickening on light microscopy and by IF, IgG and C3 deposition in a granular fashion was seen and confirmed by subepithelial electron dense deposits on EM. His glomerular tissue staining for PLA2R is positive.

Which of the following steps in management should NOT be introduced at this time?
A. Add ramipril 5 mg once daily.
B. Start cyclosporine 125 mg twice daily.
C. Begin anticoagulation for venous thromboembolism prophylaxis.
D. Obtain CT chest to rule out lung cancer.

2. A 32-year-old woman, presents to the emergency department complaining of bilateral lower limb swelling for 1 week. Her past medical history and review of systems is unremarkable. On physical examination, she has bilateral lower limb swelling extending to the knees. Her blood pressure is 130/65 mm Hg, heart rate is 70 beats/min. Chest and cardiovascular examinations are unremarkable. Her laboratory investigations show, serum creatinine 0.7 mg/dL, serum albumin 10 g/L, Hb 121 g/L, platelets $202 \times 10(9)$/L, INR and APTT are normal. Urine PCR is 15,000 mg/g. Urinalysis shows positive protein and blood. On urine microscopy there are a few RBCs (4/Hpf) and no casts. Secondary workup including ANA, HIV, and hepatitis screening are negative. A kidney biopsy was performed and showed features of membranous nephropathy and she is started on conservative treatment. A week later she presents with left lower limb pain. Her Doppler ultrasound of the lower limbs show left femoral venous clot.

Which of the following is the next most appropriate step(s) in management?
A. Start anticoagulation and continue conservative management.
B. Start anticoagulation, continue conservative management, and start appropriate immunosuppression.
C. Screening to rule out malignancy.
D. Rule out hypercoagulable disease.

3. A 34-year-old woman was referred to the clinic with a 3-month history of intermittent bilateral lower limb edema and proteinuria. Her past medical history is unremarkable. She denies any skin rash and has no history of arthralgia. Her systemic review is unremarkable. On physical examination, she appears well but has trace bilateral edema. Her blood pressure is 120/60 mm Hg, and heart rate is 67 beats/min. Chest examination is clear to auscultation bilaterally. Cardiovascular examination is unremarkable. She has no skin rash and rheumatologic examination is unremarkable. On laboratory assessment, her serum creatinine is 0.6 mg/dL, albumin 30 g/L, and hemoglobin 119 g/L. INR and APTT are normal. ANA is positive, but anti-dsDNA is negative, C3 and C4 are normal. Twenty-four-hour urine protein is 4.5 g/day. A kidney biopsy is performed and this shows GBM thickening on light microscopy, with no increase in mesangial or endocapillary cells Immunofluorescence is positive for IgG (strong), IgA (strong), and IgM (weak) deposition, with C3 deposition (strong) and C1q (weak) in a granular fashion. EM shows subepithelial, and mesangial deposits. PLA2R glomerular tissue staining for antigen is negative.

Which of the following is true?
A. The lack of an inflammatory infiltrate makes lupus nephritis an unlikely diagnosis.
B. During the active phase of disease it is not uncommon for the PLA2R tissue antigen to be negative in primary MN.
C. A negative circulating anti-PLA2R antibody, test under these conditions assures the diagnosis is secondary MN.
D. Despite a negative test for double-stranded DNA and normal complement levels secondary MN (class V lupus nephropathy) is the likely diagnosis.

4. A 56-year-old man was diagnosed with primary membranous nephropathy a year ago with an initial 24-hour urine protein of 7 g/day, serum albumin of 30 g/L and normal serum creatinine. After 6 months of conservative therapy his 24-hour urine protein remains unchanged at 7 g/day. Immunosuppressive treatment options were reviewed with the patient and he chose to be treated with a calcineurin inhibitor, cyclosporine. After 6 months of treatment with appropriate trough levels his 24-hour urine protein was 3 g/day, his albumin was up to 34 g/L and his creatinine was unchanged. His latest 12-hour cyclosporine trough level was 143 ug/L. He has had no complaints related to his treatment.

Which of the following would be the next step in the management of this patient?

A. Cyclosporine should be discontinued as he has achieved a good response.

B. Cyclosporine should be discontinued and treatment with rituximab should be trialed as there is still residual disease.

C. A repeat renal biopsy should be considered to assess disease activity.

D. Cyclosporine should be continued since stopping this treatment at this stage is associated with a high risk of relapse.

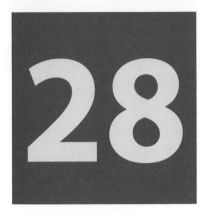

28

Immunoglobulin A Nephropathy and Henoch–Schönlein Purpura

Niti Madan, MD

Vicki J. Hwang, PhD

Jane Y. Yeun, MD

Robert H. Weiss, MD

IgA NEPHROPATHY

ESSENTIALS OF DIAGNOSIS

▶ IgA nephropathy is the most common form of glomerular disease in the world.

▶ IgA nephropathy is characterized by frequent bouts of microscopic and/or macroscopic hematuria, often following an upper respiratory infection (URI).

▶ The pathophysiology of IgA nephropathy is related to aberrant glycosylation of the IgA molecule.

▶ The pathogenesis of IgA nephropathy is considered to involve a "multi-hit" model.

▶ The diagnosis is established by kidney biopsy showing prominent globular deposits of IgA often accompanied by C3 and IgG in the mesangium.

▶ There is no specific treatment of IgA nephropathy and 10–20% of patients with the disease will progress to end-stage kidney disease within 10 years of diagnosis, and 25–40% within 20 years.

▶ General Considerations

IgA nephropathy (IgAN) is the most common form of glomerulonephritis in the developed world, yet despite this distinction, relatively little is known about noninvasive diagnostic as well as targeted treatment options. Patients may present at any age but the peak incidence is in second and third decade of life. The disease occurs with the greatest frequency in Asian and Caucasian races.

First described in 1968, IgAN continues to be a diagnostic as well as treatment dilemma even though there has been steady progress elucidating the molecular biology of its pathogenesis. The "classic" presentation of microscopic

hematuria and URI-induced macroscopic hematuria in an otherwise asymptomatic younger individual, after a negative urologic work-up, raises suspicion about the diagnosis. However, these are obviously nonspecific findings, thus with the current absence of serum or urine biomarkers, the only way to ensure a diagnosis is with an invasive kidney biopsy to include IgA immunofluorescence straining. Furthermore, there are as yet no targeted therapies which have been shown to be efficacious in this disease.

▶ Pathogenesis

A. Biology

The pathophysiology of IgAN is related to systemically decreased glycosylation of O-linked glycans in the hinge region of the IgA1 molecule, resulting in dysregulation and elevated serum levels of such galactose-deficient IgA1 (Gd-IgA1). Subsequently, these aberrant IgA1 molecules are deposited within the kidney mesangium leading to immune complex formation, promotion of cell growth, and production of proinflammatory cytokines, chemokines, and growth factors (Figure 28–1). Complement activation, stimulated by both polymeric IgA and Gd-IgA1, also plays a role in inflammation (although serum complement levels are generally not decreased). That IgAN is the manifestation of a systemic process is illustrated by the finding that this disease frequently recurs in kidney allografts in IgAN patients. However, the disease is cleared, from a pathological standpoint, in non-IgAN patients receiving IgAN kidneys.

The fact that some cases of IgAN are hereditary has been shown by the finding that 40–50% of first-degree relatives of IgAN patients have elevated serum levels of galactose-deficient IgA1 (see Genetic Considerations subsection). However, affected individuals do not have a parallel variation in serum IgA levels, suggesting that distinct mechanisms regulate the processes of IgA production and its

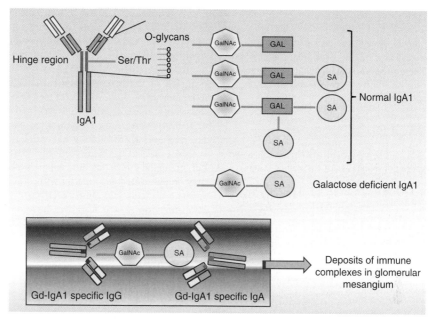

▲ **Figure 28–1.** IgA glycosylation changes and associated antibodies in IgAN. The hinge region of the IgA1 molecule encompasses the amino acids serine and threonine, which have hydroxyl functional groups that are O-glycosylated in the hinge region of the IgA1. The first glycan that is attached to these residues is GalNAc (N-acetylgalactosamine) . Following GalNAc, a galactose (GAL) molecule is added as the next step in the glycosylation of IgA1. A sialic acid (SA) molecule can be added in two different positions to the GAL or GalNAc. When the IgA1 lacks the GAL (as it happens in IgAN patients) SA binds to the GalNAc instead, which results in GAL deficient IgA1.

glycosylation; for this reason, the measurement of serum IgA is not a reasonable option for IgA diagnosis. In light of this, as well as the variability and nonspecificity of clinical presentation parameters, it is not surprising that there must be a large cohort of undiagnosed patients with IgA deposition in their mesangium. Conversely, IgA deposits may be seen incidentally in patients with no evidence of kidney disease. These issues call into question the true definition of IgAN, whether it is a pathological or clinical one.

Recent genome wide association studies (GWAS) have identified susceptibility variants responsible for only 6–8% of IgAN disease risk and have shown several potential pathways to be involved in pathogenesis, such as intestinal immunity and mucosal infections. In keeping with concepts most prevalent in the cancer field, IgAN has recently been described to be caused by distinct "hits" or pathogenic processes. Of the multiple hits thought to be important for IgAN pathogenesis, the initial (and most well-known) is the production of Gd-IgA1, but this is followed by the production of autoantibodies against this protein and their accumulation in the glomerular mesangium, with subsequent production of damaging inflammatory cytokines, chemokines, and extracellular matrix proteins within the kidney. Thus, the

levels of aberrantly glycosylated IgA1, although present in patients with IgAN, is not sufficient to cause disease and has not turned out to be a useful biomarker.

The finding that hematuria frequently accompanies pharyngitis suggests that defects in the response to mucosal immunity likely play some role in the pathogenesis of IgAN. Indeed, supporting this hypothesis, six new significant GWAS associations were found which were associated with either the risk of inflammatory bowel disease or maintenance of the intestinal epithelial barrier and response to mucosal pathogens.

B. Genetic Considerations

The majority of IgAN cases (90%) arise sporadically. Familial transmission occurs in the reminder of cases (10%) and is considered to be autosomal dominant with incomplete penetrance, although no specific genetic defect has been identified. Genetic factors have been shown to influence IgAN pathogenesis and transmission as 30–40% of first-degree relatives have serum Gd-IgA1 levels that are above the 90th percentile for healthy individuals. Risk alleles correlate well with disease epidemiology and specific loci have been identified within family cohorts, geographic locations, and ethnicities. East Asians carry the highest average number of risk alleles and have the highest prevalence of IgAN, whereas Africans have the lowest prevalence and carry the lowest burden of risk alleles. Some of these candidate genes and pathways include the antigen-processing and presentation pathway, the mucosal immunity pathway, and the alternative complement pathway.

KEY READINGS

Gharavi AG et al: Aberrant IgA1 glycosylation is inherited in familial and sporadic IgA nephropathy. J Am Soc Nephrol 2008;19:1008.

Kiryluk K et al: Discovery of new risk loci for IgA nephropathy implicates genes involved in immunity against intestinal pathogens. Nat Genet 2014;46:1187.

Lai KN, Leung JC, Tang SC: Recent advances in the understanding and management of IgA nephropathy. F1000Research 2016;5.

Moldoveanu Z et al: Patients with IgA nephropathy have increased serum galactose-deficient IgA1 levels. Kidney Int 2007;71:1148.

Suzuki H, Kiryluk K, Novak J, et al. The pathophysiology of IgA nephropathy. J Am Soc Nephrol 2011;22:1795.

▶ Clinical Findings

Patients with IgA nephropathy typically present in one of the three ways:

1. Approximately 40–50% present with one or recurrent episodes of visible hematuria, usually following 1–2 days of an upper respiratory infection or bacterial tonsillitis. This has been called "synpharyngitic hematuria." It is presumed, although not proven, that the first episode represents the onset of the disease. Patients may complain of acute flank pain which likely represents stretching of the kidney capsule. Most patients have only a few episodes of visible hematuria and episodes usually recur for a few years at most. The prevalence of hypertension in adult IgAN lies between 19% and 53% at the time of kidney biopsy. Patients can also present with malignant hypertension (7–15% of patients), which can result in rapid decline of kidney function if not promptly treated. Kidney biopsy in severely hypertensive patients might unmask patients who actually have malignant hypertension secondary to IgAN.

2. Another 30–49% patients have consistent microscopic hematuria and usually mild proteinuria, and are incidentally diagnosed in this manner on a routine examination. Gross hematuria will eventually occur in 20–25% of these patients.

3. Less than 10% present with either the nephrotic syndrome or rapidly progressive glomerulonephritis picture, characterized by edema, hypertension, and or kidney insufficiency as well as hematuria.

Rarely, patients develop acute kidney injury (AKI) with or without oliguria from crescentic IgA nephropathy or heavy glomerular hematuria, leading to tubular occlusion from red blood cell casts and subsequent acute tubular injury. This is usually a reversible phenomenon, although a significant proportion (25%) of IgAN patients with AKI do not recover to their baseline kidney function after the disappearance of macroscopic hematuria. Various risk factors like older age (>50 years), decreased baseline eGFR, longer duration of macroscopic hematuria (>10 days), and severity of acute tubular injury are associated with incomplete kidney recovery, which is consistent with other kidney diseases.

Most cases of IgAN are clinically restricted to the kidney but mesangial IgA deposition, which is often clinically silent, may be associated secondarily with other conditions, such as Henoch–Schönlein purpura, cirrhosis, celiac disease, and HIV infection. These disorders have a high frequency of glomerular IgA deposition, but most of these patients have little or no evidence of glomerular disease.

KEY READING

Gutierrez E et al: Factors that determine an incomplete recovery of renal function in macrohematuria-induced acute renal failure of IgA nephropathy. Clin J Am Soc Nephrol 2007;2:51.

▶ Laboratory Findings

A. Oxford Classification of IgA Nephropathy

A consensus on the pathologic classification of IgA nephropathy has been developed by the International IgA Nephropathy Network in collaboration with the Renal Pathology Society. As shown in Table 28–1, the following histologic variables correlate with kidney outcomes independent of the

Table 28–1. Histologic variables which correlated with kidney outcomes in IgAN.

Feature	Criteria	Classification
Mesangial hypercellularity (>3 cells/mesangial area)	Present in ≤50% of glomeruli	M0
	Present in >50% of glomeruli	M1
Segmental glomerulosclerosis	None	S0
	Any	S1
Endocapillary hypercellularity	None	E0
	Any	E1
Tubular atrophy/interstitial fibrosis	0–25% of cortical area	E0
	26–50% of cortical area	E1
	>50% of cortical area	E2

clinical features at baseline, the level of proteinuria, and the degree of blood pressure control. These variables may be less useful as prognostic markers in patients already treated with corticosteroids, and biopsies with fewer than eight glomeruli should be considered of uncertain value for prognosis. A major potential weakness of the above classification system is that it does not include crescents or necrotizing lesions as markers.

As previously mentioned, the gold standard for IgAN diagnosis is by kidney biopsy because there currently are no sufficiently sensitive and specific biofluid biomarkers. The pathognomonic finding is the presence of prominent globular deposits of IgA often accompanied by weaker staining for C3, IgG, and IgM in the mesangium on immunofluorescence microscopy, an absolute requirement in any kidney tissue sent to pathology to rule in IgAN. The deposited IgA is predominantly J chain, containing polymeric IgA1. Alternate complement pathway activation is generally seen in IgAN. The immunofluorescence findings in IgAN are the same as those in Henoch–Schönlein purpura (IgA vasculitis).

Light microscopic findings are variable and can reveal mesangial cell proliferation, mesangial expansion, focal or diffuse proliferative glomerulonephritis, crescentic glomerulonephritis, chronic sclerosing glomerulonephritis, and a membranoproliferative glomerulonephritis type I pattern, as well as endocapillary and extracapillary hypercellularity. Chronic stages of IgAN will show progression to focal or diffuse segmental and global glomerulosclerosis and interstitial fibrosis.

A subset of nephrotic patients with normal appearing glomeruli by light microscopy may have only prominent visceral epithelial cell foot process effacement on electron microscopy and appear indistinguishable from patients with minimal change disease. Electron microscopy confirms the presence of electron-dense deposits in the mesangium but may also occur in subendothelial and subepithelial spaces. The number and size of these deposits generally correlate well with the severity of changes seen on light microscopy.

Using biofluid biomarkers as an alternative to a kidney biopsy for diagnosis or to estimate disease progression in IgAN is highly desirable; however, no such markers have been validated for clinical use. Identifying such biomarkers is an active area of research. One potential candidate marker is Gd-IgA1 since aberrant synthesis of Gd-IgA1 is the initial pathogenic process in IgAN. However, current tests used to detect Gd-IgA1 are neither specific nor sensitive, and Gd-IgA1 levels do not predict progressive disease for most patients. Glycosylated IgA received some interest as a biomarker; however, some but not all IgAN patients have elevated levels of serum IgA (IgA1). Nevertheless, measurement of IgA levels has no diagnostic or prognostic value likely because increased levels of IgA alone are insufficient to cause disease, as remarked upon earlier.

Another biomarker candidate is an assay of autoantibodies, including those specific to Gd-IgA1: IgG anti-Gd-IgA1, since the formation of autoantibodies against Gd-IgA1 is the second pathogenic step in the development of IgAN. While the sensitivity of some studies to detect IgG anti-Gd-IgA1 is very low (<40%), other studies have been able to use IgG anti-Gd-IgA1 tests to diagnose IgAN with a sensitivity of 89% and a specificity of 92%.

MicroRNAs (miRNAs) are short, noncoding RNAs that regulate gene expression by degrading target mRNA or silencing translation. Specifically, miR-148b has been reported to be a prognostic biomarker as it targets the core 1, B1,3-galactosyltransferase 1 (C1GALT1) gene that controls IgA1 glycosylation. Indeed, upregulation of C1GALT1 in IgAN patients compared to healthy controls has been reported in several cohorts and transfection of miR-148b inhibitors in IgAN individuals led to a significant increase in C1GALT1 mRNA and normally glycosylated IgA1. Use of complement pathway biomarkers to monitor disease progression, specifically mannose binding lectin and C4d is promising; however, additional research needs to be accomplished in order to prove their usefulness.

The serum creatinine may be normal or elevated at presentation. Intermittent (generally following URI; see above section) or constant hematuria is nearly universal, and proteinuria is often present, but the nephrotic syndrome is uncommon (~10–15% of patients). Urine microscopy typically reveals dysmorphic red blood cells and red blood cell casts indicating bleeding of glomerular origin. Complement levels are generally normal.

Given the generally benign course of patients with IgA nephropathy who have isolated hematuria, a kidney biopsy is usually performed only if there are signs suggestive of more severe or progressive disease such as persistent protein excretion above 1000 mg/day or an elevated or rapidly rising serum creatinine concentration.

KEY READINGS

Cattran DC et al: The Oxford classification of IgA nephropathy: rationale, clinicopathological correlations, and classification. Kidney Int 2009;76:534.

Coppo R: Biomarkers and targeted new therapies for IgA nephropathy. Pediatr Nephrol 2017;32:725.

Hwang VJ et al: Biomarkers in IgA nephropathy. BiomarkMed 2014;8:1263.

Magistroni R et al: New developments in the genetics, pathogenesis, and therapy of IgA nephropathy. Kidney Int 2015;88:974.

Roberts IS: Pathology of IgA nephropathy. Nat Rev Nephrol 2014;10:445.

Roberts IS et al: The Oxford classification of IgA nephropathy: pathology definitions, correlations, and reproducibility. Kidney Int 2009;76:546.

Differential Diagnosis

The following diseases are often considered in the differential diagnosis of IgAN:

- Hematuria: nephrolithiasis, renal cancer
- Postinfectious glomerulonephritis, especially poststreptococcal
- Other glomerulonephritis, acute or chronic
- Alport syndrome and thin basement membrane nephropathy

Treatment

The optimal approach to treatment of IgAN is unclear, since the prognosis varies widely and the slowly progressive nature of the disease has hindered the design and execution of randomized controlled trials because of the required length of follow-up and/or number of patients. The few attempts at performing such trials resulted in low patient recruitment. As discussed above, an additional challenge lies in identifying early those patients who will progress before glomerulosclerosis and tubulointerstitial fibrosis is entrenched. The least controversial group consists of patients with minimal proteinuria (<500 mg/day), normal kidney function, and normal blood pressure at diagnosis and during follow-up, who require only close monitoring every 6 months or so as prognosis is excellent. Treatment of such patients with ramipril in a small (60 patients) randomized placebo controlled trial demonstrated no benefit. Current knowledge suggests that patients with abnormal kidney function (creatinine >1.25 mg/dL), significant proteinuria greater than 1 g/day, and hypertension may benefit from additional therapy, but not necessarily immunosuppression.

Treatment of IgAN can be divided broadly into two categories: "conservative" medical management and immunosuppression. Because hypertension and proteinuria are prominent risk factors associated with progressive decline in kidney function, much of conservative medical management revolves around controlling blood pressure and reducing proteinuria. Additional treatment considerations are anticoagulation, fish oil, and tonsillectomy. Immunosuppression ranges from use of corticosteroids to cytotoxic agents. Decision as to which route to pursue relies heavily on assessing the risk for progressive kidney function decline to determine if benefit from treatment outweighs treatment risk. This decision is made more difficult as most of the data on treatment is anecdotal and/or retrospective, and available randomized controlled trials are underpowered, of relatively short duration, and use reduction of proteinuria, rise in serum creatinine, or decline in estimated glomerular filtration rate as surrogate endpoints for ESKD.

A. Angiotensin Blockade

For patients at risk for progressive kidney injury, angiotensin converting enzyme inhibitors (ACEI) and angiotensin receptor blockers (ARB) are the first-line treatment. Two recent reviews conclude that ACEI and ARB are effective in reducing proteinuria and controlling blood pressure. Available studies were unable to demonstrate improved kidney outcomes convincingly because study quality were generally poor and used surrogate endpoints such as percentage change in creatinine clearance or serum creatinine. The data for combined use of ACEI and ARB in IgAN is anecdotal and demonstrates further reduction in proteinuria. In patients with persistent massive proteinuria despite treatment with ACEI or ARB, combined therapy may be considered provided the patient has relatively preserved kidney function and is at low risk for hyperkalemia. Whether patients with proteinuria between 0.5 and 1 g/day benefit from angiotensin blockade treatment is unclear.

B. Immunosuppression

Older randomized controlled trials report that addition of corticosteroids to supportive care reduced proteinuria in patients with IgAN, but had variable effects on preservation of kidney function. Based on these findings, the KDIGO (Kidney Disease: Improving Global Outcomes) guidelines published in 2012 recommended a 6-month course of corticosteroids for treating IgAN if proteinuria remained greater than 1 g/day despite 3–6 months of supportive therapy (blood pressure control and use of ACEI or ARB), provided eGFR is greater than 50 mL/min. However, in these studies, supportive care was not optimized since not all control patients received angiotensin II blockade and the degree of blood pressure control was variable.

Most studies evaluating mycophenolate mofetil, calcineurin inhibitors, or azathioprine in progressive IgAN did not find a benefit compared to control. The few that reported a benefit in either proteinuria reduction or slower decline of kidney function were retrospective, did not employ optimal supportive care, or treated patients with better preserved kidney function. Retrospective studies of corticosteroids and cyclophosphamide followed by azathioprine or mycophenolate mofetil maintenance therapy suggest a potential benefit, but only in patients with a serum creatinine less than 3 mg/dL.

The STOP-IGAN (Supportive versus Immunosuppressive Therapy for the Treatment of Progressive IgA Nephropathy) trial attempted to address some of the shortcomings of the previous studies. The trial employed a run-in period during which angiotensin II blockade was titrated upward to either maximal dose or maximal tolerated dose with additional antihypertensives as needed to lower the blood pressure to less than 130/80 mm Hg. One-third of the patients achieved a reduction of proteinuria to less than 0.75 g/day by the end of the run-in period and were ineligible for randomization. The remaining patients were randomized to continued maximal supportive care (control group) with or without immunosuppressive therapy (treatment group): corticosteroids in patients with eGFR greater than 60 mL/min, or corticosteroids and cyclophosphamide followed by azathioprine in those with eGFR of 30–59 mL/min. Immunosuppression reduced proteinuria at 12 months that was not sustained at 36 months but had no effect on the rate of decline of kidney function compared with maximal supportive care alone. Side effects were significant. The results of the STOP-IgAN study suggest that improved outcomes in the corticosteroid-treated groups in previous studies may be due to more use of angiotensin II blockade and better blood pressure control. However, limitations of the STOP-IgAN study include short follow-up (3 years), small number of patients in the two immunosuppression subgroups, inclusion of patients with eGFR down to 30 mL/min, and the lack of histologic data. Long-term follow-up studies of randomized controlled trials in IgAN suggest that kidney prognosis does not diverge until at least 2–3 years after treatment. These limitations may have reduced the power to detect a benefit with immunosuppression in this slowly progressive disease and included subjects with advanced disease and interstitial fibrosis that would not have responded to immunosuppression.

Taken together, a reasonable approach to treating patients with IgAN at increased risk of progression is

- Optimal supportive care for 3–6 months—control blood pressure to less than 130/80 mm Hg and proteinuria to less than 0.5–1 g/day using ACEI or ARB to maximal tolerated dose before titrating in other antihypertensives

- Persistent proteinuria greater than 1 g/day despite above—corticosteroids for 6 months if eGFR greater than 50 mL/min; continued optimal supportive care

- No role for corticosteroids if kidney function is impaired significantly or tubular dilation and interstitial fibrosis are prominent on histology

- No role for cytotoxic drugs except in special circumstances (see below)

Two corticosteroid regimens have been described in the literature, and either is acceptable:

- Methylprednisolone 1 g intravenously daily for 3 days at the beginning of months 1, 3, and 5; along with oral prednisolone 0.5 mg/kg daily on alternate days for 6 months

- Prednisone 0.8–1 mg/kg/day for 2 months, reduce by 0.2 mg/kg/day each month for the next 4 months

C. Special Circumstances

Corticosteroids are indicated as initial treatment in two special circumstances. First, patients with nephrotic syndrome and histologic findings of IgAN with diffuse foot process effacement typically achieve remission with corticosteroids, and behave like minimal change disease. Second, those with a rapidly progressive glomerulonephritis clinical presentation or with crescents and very active disease on histology may also benefit from corticosteroids in conjunction with cytotoxic agents.

Whether there is a role for corticosteroids and cytotoxic agents as initial treatment of patients with histologic evidence for active disease, eg, mesangial and endocapillary hypercellularity, remains to be determined. Future study designs should include the Oxford criteria to select patients who are more likely to respond to immunosuppression and have a longer follow-up period.

Pediatric IgAN may have a differing clinical course and prognosis and may benefit from combined dipyridamole and warfarin therapy, with or without concomitant immunosuppressive agents. Dipyridamole and warfarin have antiproliferative and antithrombotic effects, and dipyridamole inhibits mesangial proliferation in vitro. However, warfarin is associated with AKI from so-called warfarin or anticoagulant nephropathy and accelerated decline of eGFR.

For patients who progress to end-stage kidney disease (ESKD), kidney transplantation is a viable option. Histologic evidence of IgA deposition is reported in up to 60% of allografts by 10 years and 5–10% of affected allografts are lost to progressive disease. Earlier studies report that allograft survival in patients with IgAN is comparable to that of patients with other forms of kidney disease, but more recent studies suggest that risk for allograft loss after 15 years is increased compared with other kidney diseases, presumably due to recurrent IgAN. However, contemporary immunosuppression regimens with mycophenolate mofetil or three immunosuppressive agents may reduce the recurrence rate.

D. Other Possible Treatments

Fish oils rich in omega-3 fatty acids, eicosapentaenoic acid and docosahexaenoic acid, may protect the kidneys through reducing platelet aggregation and inflammation. Clinical trials assessing the benefit of fish oil have been inconclusive, with some demonstrating preservation of kidney function or reduction in proteinuria and others failing to do so. These conflicting results may be due to the short duration of the studies, the small number of patients enrolled, the lack of standardization of the type and dose of fish oil used, as well as patient selection and the severity of the IgAN at treatment. Given the lack of toxicity, high doses of fish oil (at least 3.3 g/day) can be added when patients have persistent proteinuria greater than 1 g/day despite 3–6 months of optimal therapy with ACEI or ARB.

Because the tonsils are a significant site of IgA1 production and may harbor pathogens, **tonsillectomy** has been proposed as a means to prevent disease progression. Most of the studies are retrospective, done in Asian populations, and compared tonsillectomy with corticosteroid to corticosteroid alone. Based on these data, a recent meta-analysis suggests that tonsillectomy, when added to corticosteroids, is more likely to induce remission of proteinuria and hematuria. Two recent randomized controlled trials in Asian populations confirmed these findings. Whether remission of proteinuria and/or hematuria translates into prevention of kidney failure is unclear, as these studies were underpowered to answer this question. Whether these findings may be generalized to other populations is also debated, as studies in non-Asian cohorts have not found a benefit to tonsillectomy. Given the inherent surgical risks and lack of definitive effect on kidney function, tonsillectomy is not recommended at present as primary therapy for IgAN, with the possible exception of patients with recurrent episodes of severe tonsillitis associated with gross hematuria.

E. Novel Treatments

Current therapies to treat IgAN, other than tight blood pressure control and use of ACEI or ARB, have yielded disappointing results with potentially serious adverse effects. With our improved understanding of its pathogenesis, clinical and animal studies are under way to determine if interference with B-cell maturation and mucosal IgA1 production will reduce disease activity and preserve kidney function. Budesonide delivered orally to the gastrointestinal mucosa has shown promise in a pilot study, and a larger multicenter, randomized controlled trial is in progress. Blisibimod and fostamatinib, which interfere with B-cell maturation and survival, and rituximab, which depletes B cells, are being studied to determine their efficacy and safety in IgAN treatment. Use of bacteria-derived IgA1 protease in a mouse model of IgAN appears to reduce hematuria, mesangial IgA deposits, and interstitial inflammation and fibrosis.

▶ Prognosis

The clinical course of IgAN is highly variable, due in part to variability in the timing of kidney biopsy, potential for geographic variability, as well as the effect of treatment. Variability in biopsy practices results in lead-time bias and/or inclusion of patients with milder disease. Whether genetic variability or geographic differences in diet and lifestyle practices can give rise to differences in prognosis remain unclear, but most studies suggest that the difference derives largely from timing of kidney biopsy and variations in risk factors for progression. In addition, the retrospective nature of many studies introduces confounding variables that may influence outcome independently, such as decisions to treat and the treatment itself. When prospective studies are conducted, conclusions are limited by the duration of follow-up because of the indolent nature of the disease. Aggregate data suggest that 10–20% of patients with IgAN will progress to ESKD within 10 years of diagnosis, and 25–40% within 20 years. The rate of progression varies from an annual decline in GFR of 1–4.4 mL/min, depending on the presence of risk factors.

Clinical risk factors for progression are hypertension, proteinuria, and reduced kidney function. More recent studies suggest that persistence of these risk factors appears to be as important, if not more important, than their presence at initial diagnosis, and that more stringent criteria for blood pressure control may be indicated:

- Blood pressure persistently greater than 130/80 mm Hg
- Time-averaged proteinuria greater than 1 g/day
- Serum creatinine greater than 1.25 mg/dL

Of these factors, persistence of proteinuria or development of proteinuria appears to be more important in predicting progressive decline in kidney function (Table 28-2). Compared with proteinuria less than 1 g/day, persistent proteinuria confers a higher hazard ratio for ESKD: 3.5 for

Table 28-2. Kidney survival by degree of time averaged (TA) proteinuria.

TA Proteinuria (g/day)	Rate of Decline of Kidney Function (mL/min per 1.73 m²/mo; Mean ± SD)	Risk for Kidney Failure [Hazard Ratio (95% CI)]
0 to 1	− 0.030 ± 0.46	Reference
1 to 2	− 0.326 ± 0.53	3.48 (1.8 to 6.7)
2 to 3	− 0.516 ± 0.66	5.17 (2.6 to 10.0)
>3	− 0.719 ± 0.61	9.89 (5.3 to 18.4)

As the degree of proteinuria increased, the slope or rate of deterioration in kidney function increased, accompanied by an increased risk for kidney failure.
Data from Reich HN et al: Remission of proteinuria improves prognosis in IgA nephropathy. *J Am Soc Nephrol* 2007;18:3177.

Table 28-3. Kidney survival correlates with remission of proteinuria.

Peak Proteinuria (g/d)	Rate of Decline of Kidney Function (mL/min per 1.73 m²/mo; Mean ± SD)	
	Partial Remission (<1 g/d)	No Remission (persistently >1 g/d)
1 to 2	− 0.20 ± 0.47	
2 to 3	− 0.14 ± 0.63	− 0.76 ± 0.59
>3	− 0.16 ± 0.37	

Patients achieving partial remission (<1 g/day) regardless of peak proteinuria, had similar rates of decline in kidney function, which compares favorably with the rate of decline (− 0.17 ± 0.47) observed in patients with no proteinuria (<0.3 g/day). In contrast, patients whose proteinuria does not remit with time have a much more rapid rate of decline in kidney function.
Data from Reich HN et al: Remission of proteinuria improves prognosis in IgA nephropathy. *J Am Soc Nephrol* 2007;18:3177.

1–2 g/day proteinuria, 5 for 2–3 g/day, and 10 for greater than 3 g/day. Reduction of proteinuria during 1–2 years of follow-up to less than 1 g/day conferred the same prognosis as those with minimal proteinuria throughout the course of the disease (Table 28–3). Whether proteinuria of less than 0.5 g/day offers additional kidney survival advantage is debated. Recent data suggest that albuminuria correlates higher with kidney prognosis and Oxford classification findings of glomerulosclerosis, adhesion, and extracapillary proliferation, than the degree of proteinuria.

Debate also persists as to whether reduced kidney function is a "legitimate" risk factor, as deterioration in kidney function is the endpoint of interest, and these patients are "self-selected" for worse prognosis. In the absence of an accepted risk model, impaired renal function remains an important clinical factor for assessing risk for progression to ESKD, precisely because these patients have "self-selected." Incidence for ESKD increases dramatically with higher serum creatinine concentrations (Cr): 2.5% for Cr less than or equal to 1.25 mg/dL, 26% for Cr 1.26–1.67 mg/dL, 68% for Cr 1.68–2.5 mg/dL, and 90% for Cr greater than 2.5 mg/dL.

Other clinical risk factors such as age, gender, degree of hematuria, hyperuricemia, and reduced serum protein are associated inconsistently with progressive kidney failure. These factors are less useful at the present time for risk stratification and assessing prognosis. The recently reported Oxford classification of kidney pathology is more reproducible, allows for standardization, and also impacts on prognosis.

Prognosis appears to differ in patients with AKI in the setting of gross hematuria or acute onset of nephrotic range proteinuria and/or nephrotic syndrome. Patients in the former category typically have crescents on kidney biopsy, and the latter have prominent foot process effacement. Whether these patients have clinical variants of IgA nephropathy or the presence of another glomerular disease such as crescentic glomerulonephritis or minimal change disease is unclear and may have significant impact on their differing prognosis.

In summary, prognosis and risk stratification is important in determining whether immunosuppression is indicated in treating what is otherwise an indolent disease. The side effect profile may be prohibitive in a patient at very low risk for developing ESKD, but acceptable in one who has progressive disease, culminating in the need for dialysis (assuming that treatment is effective). Various risk models have been proposed, but none have gained widespread acceptance, partly because of poor reproducibility of pathologic assessment, the indolent nature of the disease, the lack of agreement as to the importance of various proposed risk factors, and the inability of current risk models to predict response to treatment as the study populations include patients on treatment. The introduction of the Oxford classification and agreement on consistent risk factors may pave the way for a more widely acceptable risk model. One such risk model incorporating the Oxford classification has been proposed and appears to be highly discriminant in predicting risk for ESKD. However, because the presence of tubulointerstitial fibrosis and segmental glomerulosclerosis on histology play a prominent role in the prediction model, the model may be less effective in guiding therapy as such lesions are irreversible and unlikely to respond to immunosuppression. Additional research into novel biomarkers for activity and progression of disease may allow identification of patients at risk earlier in the disease and inform future risk models. For now, patients with less than 500 mg/day proteinuria, no hypertension, and normal kidney function are at very low risk for progressive kidney failure, with 10-year cumulative incidence of ESKD of near 0%. Patients with persistent proteinuria greater than 1 g/day, blood pressure greater than 130/80 mm Hg, and/or creatinine greater than 1.25 mg/dL are likely to develop progressive kidney failure and may benefit from more aggressive treatment earlier in the course of disease.

KEY READINGS

Barbour SJ, Reich HN: Risk stratification of patients with IgA nephropathy. Am J Kidney Dis 2012;59:865.

Berthoux F et al: Predicting the risk for dialysis or death in IgA nephropathy. J Am Soc Nephrol 2011;22:752.

Feehally J, Barratt J: Should immunosuppressive therapy be used in slowly progressive IgA nephropathy? Am J Kidney Dis 2016;68:184.

Floege J, Eitner F: Current therapy for IgA nephropathy. J Am Soc Nephrol 2011;22:1785.

Kamei K et al: For the Japanese Pediatric IgA Nephropathy Treatment Study Group. Long-term results of a randomized controlled trial in childhood IgA nephropathy. Clin J Am Soc Nephrol 2011;6:1301.

Kidney Disease: Improving Global Outcomes (KDIGO) Glomerulonephritis Work Group. KDIGO clinical practice guideline for glomerulonephritis. Kidney Int Suppl 2012;2:139.

Le WB et al: Long-term renal survival and related risk factors in patients with IgA nephropathy: results from a cohort of 1155 cases in a Chinese adult population. Nephrol Dial Transplant 2012;27:1479.

Li PK et al: Treatment of early Immunoglobulin A nephropathy by angiotensin-converting enzyme inhibitor. Am J Med 2013;126:162.

Lv J et al: For the TESTING Study Group: corticosteroid therapy in IgA nephropathy. J Am Soc Nephrol 2012;23:1108.

Moroni G et al: The long-term outcome of renal transplantation of IgA nephropathy and the impact of recurrence on graft survival. Nephrol Dial Transplant 2013;28:1305.

Rauen T et al: For the STOP-IgAN Investigators: intensive supportive care plus immunosuppression in IgA nephropathy. N Engl J Med 2015;373:2225.

Reid S et al: Non-immunosuppressive treatment for IgA nephropathy. Cochrane Database of Syst Rev 3:CD003962, 2011.

Tanaka S et al: Development and validation of a prediction rule using the Oxford classification in IgA nephropathy. Clin J Am Soc Nephrol 2013;8:2082.

Vecchio M et al: Immunosuppressive agents for treating IgA nephropathy. Cochrane Database Syst Rev 8:CD003965, 2015.

Yeo SC, Liew A, Barratt J: Emerging therapies in immunoglobulin A nephropathy. Nephrology 2015;20:788.

HENOCH–SCHÖNLEIN PURPURA

► General Considerations

Henoch–Schönlein purpura (HSP), also known as IgA vasculitis has many similarities in pathogenesis to IgAN, and hence it can be considered a systemic form of this disease. It is the most common vasculitis in children between the ages of 5 and 15 years, but can also affect adults. The circulating IgA1 in HSP has a similar defect in glycosylation to IgAN, and similarly results in formation of immune complexes, but in the case of HSP, such complexes cause small vessel and capillary damage.

► Pathogenesis

The pathologic findings in HSP are consistent with a leukocytoclastic vasculitis with IgA immune complexes in the affected organs. There have been numerous infectious agents linked to HSP, although causation has not been proven in these cases. As with IgAN, the damage that comes from the disease is related to the downstream effects of such immune complex deposition, including activation of complement and recruitment of cytokines and growth factors. However, why these pathological events in the case of HSP lead to systemic disease vasculitis and are not confined to the kidney as in IgAN is not well understood.

► Clinical Findings

HSP is self-limited in the vast majority of cases. The disease is characterized by a tetrad of clinical manifestations:

- Palpable purpura in patients with neither thrombocytopenia nor coagulopathy (present in most cases), which is histologically leukocytoclastic vasculitis with predominant immunoglobulin A (IgA) deposition. Symptoms and signs can occur in any order and at any time over a course of several days to weeks, and reflect the systemic leukocytoclastic vasculitis. The skin lesions usually appear as crops of palpable purpura on the lower limbs and buttocks (Figure 28–2). The rash is distributed symmetrically, and located primarily in gravity/pressure-dependent areas. Localized subcutaneous edema is a common feature that may be found in dependent and periorbital areas.

- Arthritis/arthralgia (75–80% of cases), is usually of acute onset. Joint involvement, consisting of arthralgias or

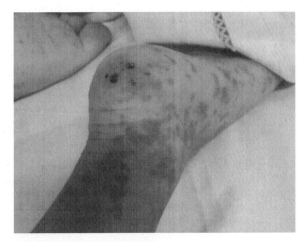

▲ **Figure 28–2.** Leukocytoclastic vasculitis as in a patient with HSP. (See Color Plate 1.)

frank arthritis, is typically oligoarticular (one to four joints), limited to the knees and ankles, and does not lead to permanent deformity. There is often periarticular swelling and tenderness, but usually without joint effusion, erythema, or warmth. Patients may have considerable pain and limitation of motion. The arthritis doesn't cause any chronic damage or sequelae. It may precede the appearance of purpura.

- Abdominal pain (50–75% of cases), usually diffuse and of acute onset. Gastrointestinal symptoms occur as mild (nausea, vomiting, abdominal pain, and transient paralytic ileus) to more significant findings (gastrointestinal hemorrhage, bowel ischemia and necrosis, intussusception, and bowel perforation). Gastrointestinal involvement is characterized by colicky abdominal pain sometimes associated with gastrointestinal bleeding (melena, hematochezia, or occult). Abdominal pain associated with HSP is caused by submucosal hemorrhage and edema. Purpuric lesions may be seen in endoscopy, commonly in the descending duodenum, stomach, and colon. The terminal ileum and jejunum may also be involved. Intussusception is the most common complication of HSP in children but rare in adults. It usually occurs in the small bowel as compared to idiopathic which is typically ileocolic.

- Kidney disease (20–54%), manifests usually as proteinuria and hematuria. Kidney manifestations may occur within days or up to several weeks after onset of the clinical presentation of HSP, but rarely precedes the other major components of the disease. Kidney findings include hematuria (microscopic or gross), none or mild proteinuria, and AKI, and are more prevalent in older children and adults. In adults risk of developing significant kidney involvement including end-stage kidney disease is much higher. The presence of microscopic papillary dermal edema and perivascular deposition of C3 on direct immunofluorescence of skin biopsy samples may be associated with development of kidney involvement. The findings on kidney biopsy are identical to those in IgAN.

Pulmonary, neurologic, genitourinary, and cardiac manifestations may also occur. Pulmonary manifestations can be impaired lung diffusion capacity, mild interstitial changes, and rarely pulmonary hemorrhage. Neurological involvement can be transient and manifest as headaches, seizures, encephalopathy, ataxia, and central and peripheral neuropathy.

Treatment

The majority of patients with or without kidney involvement require only supportive care, as the disease tends to remit spontaneously. However, because of the potential for recurrence, close follow-up to monitor both for systemic recurrence as well as kidney involvement is important. For those with severe symptoms, optimal treatment is debated, as most reports in the literature are anecdotal or retrospective. The few randomized studies available enrolled a small number of patients and were of short duration.

Corticosteroids may lead to faster resolution of arthritis and abdominal pain, but its role in treating Henoch–Schönlein purpura with nephritis (HSPN) is not clear. A recent Cochrane Database review concluded that there is no convincing data to support the use of corticosteroids, cytotoxic agents, dipyridamole, anticoagulants, plasma exchange, or immune globulin to treat HSP with kidney involvement. KDIGO guidelines suggest treating HSPN patients in the same manner as IgAN patients. Expert opinions disagree and instead recommends high dose corticosteroids for patients with severe kidney involvement (defined as marked proteinuria and/or AKI during an acute flare) supported by findings of crescents and inflammation with fibrinoid necrosis on kidney biopsy. Extrapolating from experience with other forms of kidney vasculitis, these experts argue that active and severe glomerular and interstitial inflammation can progress rapidly to glomerulosclerosis and tubulointerstitial fibrosis if treatment is delayed. Whether other immunosuppressive drugs such as cyclophosphamide or cyclosporine are of benefit is unclear. Prospective randomized controlled clinical trials are needed to evaluate the efficacy of these agents.

Kidney transplant is a viable treatment for patients who develop ESKD. Histologic recurrences of HSPN occur in up to 60% of kidney transplants within 24 months, with clinical recurrence of 2.5% at 5 years and 11.5% at 10 years, and graft loss due to recurrence of 2.5% at 5 years and 7.5% at 10 years. Compared with data from 1994 where 5-year clinical recurrence rate was 35% and graft loss rate 11%, prognosis of kidney allograft appears to have improved.

Prognosis

In the majority of patients, HSP resolves spontaneously, with complete recovery in 94% of children and 89% of adults at 19 and 22 months, respectively. However, one-third of patients will have one or more recurrences of symptoms. Transient hematuria and proteinuria typically resolve within several months. Spontaneous recovery may also occur in patients with severe kidney involvement although the risk for progressive kidney failure is higher.

The incidence of progressive kidney impairment varies among the different series in the literature, because of the retrospective nature of the studies, the small number of patients, and inclusion of patients with widely differing disease severity. The prognosis of HSPN in adults may be worse than that of children, with progressive CKD in up to one-third of adults at 15 years. Presence of nephrotic syndrome, persistent proteinuria, AKI at onset, greater than

50% crescents, and advanced tubulointerstitial disease on kidney biopsy are associated with a worse kidney prognosis. In contrast, only 5–15% of children have progressive kidney failure, although this is debated. Long-term follow-up studies (>20 years) of children with HSPN suggest that progressive CKD may be more common than suspected, even in those who appeared to have recovered fully, and kidney prognosis is comparable to that in adults if kidney involvement was severe at onset of disease.

KEY READINGS

Davin JC: Henoch–Schönlein purpura nephritis: pathophysiology, treatment, and future strategy. Clin J Am Soc Nephrol 2011;6:679.

Davin JC, Coppo R: Pitfalls in recommending evidence-based guidelines for a protean disease like Henoch–Schönlein purpura nephritis. Pediatr Nephrol 2013;28:1897.

Davin JC, Coppo R: Henoch–Schönlein purpura nephritis in children. Nat Rev Nephrol 2014;10:563.

Hahn D et al: Interventions for preventing and treating kidney disease in Henoch–Schönlein Purpura (HSP). Cochrane Database of Systematic Reviews. 8:CD005128, 2015.

Johnson EF et al: Henoch–Schönlein purpura and systemic disease in children: retrospective study of clinical findings, histopathology and direct immunofluorescence in 34 paediatric patients. Br J Dermatol 2015;172:1358.

Kanaan N et al: Recurrence and graft loss after kidney transplantation for Henoch–Schönlein purpura nephritis: A multicenter analysis. Clin J Am Soc Nephrol 2011;6:1768.

Thervet E et al: Histologic recurrence of Henoch–Schönlein purpura nephropathy after renal transplantation on routine allograft biopsy. Transplantation 2011;92:907.

■ CHAPTER REVIEW QUESTIONS

1. A 45-year-old Asian female is found on routine employment physical to have microscopic hematuria with normal serum creatinine and no casts in the urine. She denies ever seeing blood in her urine and is not menopausal but is currently not menstruating. Her blood pressure is 130/85 and she only takes birth control pills. She is an occasional smoker. She is an avid runner, and runs about 5 miles a day.

   How would you begin to work up the hematuria in this patient?
   A. Do an in and out urinary catheterization to see if the blood is coming from the urinary tract.
   B. Do a contrast CT of the urinary tract.
   C. Order a renal ultrasound.
   D. Do a renal biopsy.
   E. Do no further work-up.

2. A healthy 25-year-old white man developed gross hematuria one day after upper respiratory tract infection. He denies abdominal pain, rashes, or use of illicit drugs. Blood pressure is 160/95, pulse 80. Physical examination is remarkable only for pharyngeal injection without any discharge and nasal congestion. Urinalysis confirmed gross hematuria and also revealed occasional red blood cell cast, many dysmorphic red blood cells, and 2+ proteinuria. Serum creatinine is 2.5 mg/dL.

   What is the most appropriate next step in evaluating and treating this patient?
   A. Quantify the proteinuria
   B. Kidney biopsy
   C. High dose corticosteroid
   D. Serum IgA levels
   E. Serum anti-streptolysin O levels

3. A kidney biopsy was done for the patient described in Question 2 demonstrating IgA nephropathy with acute tubular necrosis. Patient was managed conservatively with blood pressure control. Kidney function recovered, but patient was left with persistent microscopic hematuria and 2 g of proteinuria. ACE inhibitor treatment was started once kidney function returned to baseline, with control of blood pressure to less than 130/80. He did well for 5 years with reduction of proteinuria to less than 500 mg/day, and then developed recurrent proteinuria to 2 g daily. He is interested in participating in a randomized controlled study for IgA nephropathy that offers the potential of definitively treating his disease.

   Which of the following study should he enroll in given his stated wish?
   A. Mycophenolate mofetil
   B. Tonsillectomy
   C. Fish oil
   D. IgA1 protease
   E. Anticoagulation therapy

4. An 18-year-old male patient presents with the abrupt onset of a lower extremity rash. He is otherwise entirely asymptomatic, except for complaints of intermittent episodes of mild abdominal pain. On physical examination, his blood pressure is 140/90 mm Hg, pulse is 78 beats/min, and respirations are 18 breaths/min. His head/eyes/ears/nose/throat exam is unremarkable. His pulmonary and cardiac examinations are negative. There is no abdominal tenderness. Extremities have no edema. There is a palpable purpuric lesion noted. Urinalysis reveals 12 dysmorphic red blood cells/high power field, 1+ protein, and 1 red blood cell cast. Laboratory studies reveal serum creatinine 1.0 mg/dL, serum C3 complement 125 mg/dL, and serum C4 complement 40 mg/dL. A renal biopsy revealed proliferative glomerulonephritis that is codominant for IgA and IgG.

Which one of the following is the MOST appropriate therapy?
A. Oral glucocorticoids
B. Mycophenolate mofetil
C. Oral glucocorticoids and azathioprine
D. An angiotensin-converting enzyme inhibitor
E. A diuretic

5. A 28-year-old man is found to have IgA nephropathy when a renal biopsy was performed for unexplained proteinuria, hematuria, and impaired renal function (serum creatinine 3.5 mg/dL). Extensive tubulointerstitial fibrosis and tubular atrophy were present and about 20% of the glomeruli revealed segmental fibrocellular crescents. Urine protein to creatinine ratio on first morning voided urine was 2 g protein/g creatinine. Blood pressure was 155/94 mm Hg.

Based on these findings, in addition to starting an angiotensin-converting enzyme inhibitor, which ONE of the following would be the BEST initial approach to treatment?
A. Start oral cyclophosphamide plus steroids.
B. Start oral mycophenolate plus steroids.
C. Start oral cyclosporine plus steroids.
D. Start intravenous methylprednisolone plus oral steroids.
E. No additional immunosuppressive therapy is indicated.

6. A 36-year-old Caucasian man with IgA nephropathy has persistence of proteinuria (2.8 g/day) despite 6 months of treatment with a combination of trandolapril and candesartan at maximal dosage. His BP is 122/76 mm Hg and his serum creatinine is now 1.3 mg/dL. The urinary protein excretion was 3.0 g/day and the serum creatinine 6 months ago was 1.2 mg/dL.

Which ONE of the following regimens would you recommend as treatment now?
A. A 6-months course of IV methylprednisolone, 1.0 g at the beginning of months 1, 3, and 5, plus oral prednisone, 0.5 mg/kg every other day.
B. Oral mycophenolate mofetil, 2.0 mg for 6 months.
C. Cyclosporin 4 mg/kg/day, plus oral steroids, 0.5 mg/kg every other day for 6 months.
D. Cyclophosphamide, 2.0 mg/kg/day for 3 months, followed by azathioprine, 2.0 mg for 1 year.
E. Fish oil, 12 g daily for 1 year.

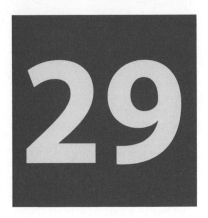

29

Membranoproliferative Glomerulonephritis

Howard Trachtman, MD

ESSENTIALS OF DIAGNOSIS

▸ Characterized by persistent hypocomplementemia.

▸ Disease is most often primary or idiopathic.

▸ Disease can occur secondary to immunoglobulin-mediated activation of the complement cascade or acquired or genetic abnormalities in the alternate pathway of complement.

▸ Fifty percent of patients progress to end-stage renal disease over 10–15 years.

▸ Prednisone is effective in pediatric patients but there is no proven treatment in adults.

▸ Disease recurs post-transplantation in approximately 25% of patients.

General Considerations

Membranoproliferative glomerulonephritis (MPGN) is the classic renal nomenclature monstrosity that spreads fear among house officers and practitioners. This disease was first described by Rene Habib in 1961 and was linked to decreased serum complement levels in 1965. Since then it has been a rare but well recognized cause of serious glomerular disease in pediatric and adult patients throughout the world and represents an important cause of end-stage kidney disease (ESKD). It is defined by a characteristic histopathologic appearance that consists of a lobulated shape to the glomerular tuft, glomerular hypercellularity, thickening of the capillary wall, and splitting of the glomerular basement membrane with a double contour ("tram tracking"). On ultrastructural examination of renal tissue, there are electron-dense deposits in the capillary wall and the distinctive localization of the deposits results in classification of MPGN into type I (subendothelial and mesangial), type II (intramembranous dense deposits), and type III (subendothelial, mesangial, and subepithelial).

In the last decade, the pivotal role of the alternate pathway of complement in this disorder has become increasingly evident. As a consequence, a new nomenclature, C3 glomerulopathy (C3G), has been introduced that overlaps with MPGN, types II and III. This is an evolving area and it is likely that terminology and definitions will become more standardized with time. MPGN is now classified into immune-complex (IC-GN) and complement C3G. For the purpose of this chapter, the new classification will be used namely, immunoglobulin (Ig) mediated MPGN I, C3 glomerulopathies, and Ig-mediated MPGN III.

Pathogenesis

The general mechanism of disease for the development of MPGN is dysregulated complement protein activation. Under normal circumstances complement activity, composed of various chemotactic factors and the membrane attack complex, is triggered either through the classical or alternative pathways. The third component of the cascade, C3, occupies a pivotal position in both pathways and is essential to the effector functions of the system. Therefore, a number of regulatory proteins are synthesized to modulate C3 convertase (C3bBb) activity and to prevent the deleterious consequences of uninterrupted complement activation. These include factors H and I, membrane cofactor protein (MCP), and decay accelerating factor.

MPGN is classified into primary and secondary forms. The pathogenesis of MPGN is linked to the underlying etiology of the glomerulopathy (Table 29–1). In the primary forms of MPGN, the mechanism of disease centers around abnormal activation of the complement cascade. In-depth studies of all components of the complement cascade suggest that there are three distinct patterns of complement activation in the three types of MPGN. Thus, in type I disease, the process

Table 29–1. Etiology of membranoproliferative glomerulonephritis.

Primary disease
  Type I
  Type II, dense deposit disease C3 nephritic factor
  Type III
Genetic forms
  Factor H defects
  C4 deficiency
Secondary
  Infections
    Lyme disease
    Hepatitis B
    Hepatitis C
    Bacterial endocarditis
    Hantavirus
    Malaria
    Schistosomiasis
  Chronic liver disease
  Collagen vascular disease
    Systemic lupus erythematosus
    Sjögren syndrome
  Other autoimmune disease
    Thyroiditis/type 1 diabetes mellitus
  Malignancy
    Chronic lymphocytic leukemia
    Non-Hodgkin lymphoma
    Monoclonal gammopathy
  Medications
    Granulocyte colony-stimulating factor
    Interferon-α therapy

is initiated by immune complex deposition within the glomerulus and involvement of the classical pathway. The source of the immune complexes is unknown in the idiopathic form of the disease. These patients have low levels of C3, C4, C6, C7, and/or C9. MPGN type I is sometimes associated with the presence of a circulating immunoglobulin (Ig)G or IgM autoantibody that stabilizes the C3 convertase (eg, C3 nephritic factor), thus engendering low C3 levels. A C4 nephritic factor has also been described. In the type II variant, the continuous overactivity of the complement cascade involves an amplification loop in the alternative pathway, characterized mainly by markedly depressed C3 levels. Abnormal complement activation in MPGN can also occur as a consequence of genetic mutations that result in reduced levels of endogenous inhibitors of the process, such as factor H, or because of the presence of C3 nephritic factor, the latter occurring in the majority of patients with C3 glomerulopathy (also called dense deposit disease or MPGN type II). Animal models in mice and pigs demonstrate the importance of factor H in regulating complement activation and the occurrence of MPGN when circulating levels of this protein are reduced. It is worth noting

that unlike hemolytic uremic syndrome, which can develop in patients who have heterozygous genetic defects in factor H, MPGN occurs only in patients who carry homozygous mutations. Other genetic causes of MPGN include isolated C4 deficiency. Finally, the pathogenesis of MPGN type III appears to have features in common with type I disease as well as evidence of activation of the terminal complement pathway with low C3, C5, and properdin levels. In adults, the type III form frequently occurs in association with systemic infection, inflammation, or neoplasm. The presence of MGPN type III in adults should stimulate a search for an underlying systemic process causing it.

Secondary forms of MPGN can occur as a result of various infections including hepatitis B and C, bacterial endocarditis, mixed cryoglobulinemia, malignancies, collagen vascular disease, and chronic liver disease (including specific entities such as α_1-antitrypsin deficiency). Indeed, most cases of MPGN, particularly in adults, are attributable to hepatitis C. The genetic forms of MPGN are rarely seen in adults. There are other entities that occur in rare association with MPGN such as Lyme disease and autoimmune thyroiditis. Moreover, the use of some newer medications has been linked to the occurrence of MPGN type I such as granulocyte colony-stimulating factor. Under these various circumstances, it is presumed that there is immune complex-mediated activation of the complement cascade. In animal models of cryoglobulinemia, overexpression of the membrane complement inhibitor, complement receptor 1-related gene/protein y (Crry), does not prevent the development of MPGN.

C3G is the term used to define glomerular disease that has an MPGN appearance in which C3 is the dominant immunoreactant (at least two scoring points higher than any other molecule) in the glomerulus. It overlaps with MPGN, types II and III and it has been introduced to highlight the key role of C3 activation in mediating glomerular injury. A recent consensus statement has been developed that clarifies the diagnosis of C3G and its relationship to MPGN. Figure 29–1 summarizes the linkage between the three major pathways of complement activation and the subtypes of MPGN.

▶ **Prevention**

MPGN is either idiopathic or secondary to an underlying condition. The former category of diseases cannot be prevented. Secondary causes can be avoided by minimizing exposure to the etiologic agent or by primary prevention of the underlying disease.

▶ **Clinical Findings**

A. Symptoms and Signs

The incidence of MPGN is low across the lifespan and accounts for 5–30% of patients with new-onset nephrotic

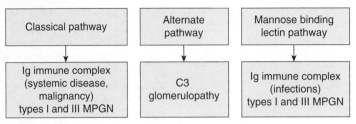

▲ **Figure 29–1.** This illustration summarizes the linkage between the three major pathways of complement activation and the subtypes of MPGN.

syndrome. It is lower in adults than in children. Several reports suggest that the incidence of MPGN has been declining over the past 10–20 years. Further epidemiologic studies are needed to clarify this issue. The disease is generally sporadic and familial cases are rare. Overall, the disease is equally prevalent in male and female patients but appears to be more common in white compared to black patients.

MPGN can present in a variety of fashions ranging from asymptomatic hematuria to a severe acute glomerulonephritis. In children, MPGN most often presents either as idiopathic nephrotic syndrome or an acute glomerulonephritis that closely resembles acute postinfectious nephritis. It accounts for approximately 5% of pediatric cases of new-onset nephrotic syndrome. The profile of MPGN is distinct from minimal change disease and focal segmental glomerulonephritis, which occurs more frequently in younger boys, because MPGN is more common in female patients over 8 years of age. The clinical suspicion of MPGN in a child with acute nephritis rises when the C3 levels fails to normalize during the standard 8–12 week observation period or the C4 level is decreased at the onset of disease because it is only rarely decreased in acute postinfectious glomerulonephritis. Cases such as these account for nearly 30% of all instances of MPGN and may have concomitant reduction in the glomerular filtration rate (GFR). Hypertension is present in 50–80% of cases of MPGN and can be severe. Because of concern that corticosteroid therapy may exacerbate the elevation in blood pressure and trigger malignant hypertension, it is advisable to rule out MPGN in a high-risk patient such as an older female child before initiation of daily treatment with steroids, in cases where steroids might otherwise be indicated.

Occasional patients with persistent glomerular hematuria lasting longer than 6 months and hypocomplementemia with MPGN detected on renal biopsy have been reported. Reports from Japan confirm early detection of MPGN in pediatric patients following findings of hematuria and/or proteinuria on routine annual screening urinalyses. Although this testing enables detection of disease prior to the onset of significant hypertension, proteinuria, and/or azotemia, the cost-effectiveness of this kind of program requires confirmation in other patient populations. In fact, there are even cases of typical MPGN in children being

diagnosed because of persistent hypocomplementemia in the complete absence of any urinary findings. In patients with asymptomatic urinary abnormalities, type III MPGN is more likely to be detected than type I or II disease.

In adult patients, the clinical presentation may be the consequence solely of the renal involvement with edema, hypertension, or gross hematuria. However, in those patients with secondary disease the symptoms and signs usually reflect the underlying cause. Thus, patients with cryoglobulinemia may have weakness, arthralgias involving the knees, hips, and shoulders, and palpable vasculitic lesions on the buttocks and lower extremities. These symptoms may fluctuate over time. The distribution of the purpura is reminiscent of Henoch–Schönlein purpura. Those patients with disease secondary to infection, malignancy, or collagen vascular disease will have manifestations associated with the underlying disease. Interestingly, MPGN may be the first manifestation of hepatitis C infection because affected patients often have no clinical evidence of hepatic disease.

B. Laboratory Findings

MPGN is characterized by hypocomplementemia, namely reduced C3 and CH50 levels, which is confirmed in 80–90% of patients. In patients with type I MPGN, approximately 40% of those with a low C3 level will also have a low serum C4 level. This is less common in patients with C3 glomerulopathy (type II) or type III MPGN. Although the different patterns of circulating complement component levels described above (see Pathogenesis) are useful in discriminating the types of MPGN, this comprehensive battery of tests is generally not performed in clinical chemistry laboratories and is available only in select research facilities. C3 nephritic factor activity is more common in type II disease, namely 60–70% of patients, compared to 20–25% of patients with type I or III disease. Interestingly, this autoantibody is also detectable in up to 50% of patients with secondary forms of MPGN. It is uncertain whether the presence of C3 nephritic factor indicates an increased risk of progression to ESKD. C3 nephritic factor can be measured in a hemolytic or a solid phase assay. In adults with cryoglobulinemia, testing should be performed for hepatitis B and C infection. Hepatitis serology should also be evaluated in pediatric patients with MPGN even in the absence of mixed cryoglobulinemia. Other laboratory abnormalities will be present depending upon the underlying disease.

C. Pathology

The characteristic pathology in MPGN is diffuse mesangial and endothelial cell proliferation, thickening of the capillary wall, and splitting of the glomerular basement membrane (Figure 29–2). Depending upon the severity of the disease, crescent formation may be noted in a substantial percentage of glomeruli. The hypercellularity is enhanced by leukocyte and monocyte infiltration of the glomerular tuft. Special stains such as silver methenamine may be required to visualize the splitting and broadening of the glomerular basement membrane and the trichrome stain to facilitate localization of deposits (Figure 29–3). This is important in classifying the three types of primary MPGN—type I with subendothelial and mesangial, type II with intramembranous, and type III with subendothelial, mesangial, and subepithelial deposits. The trichrome stain is also useful in assessing fibrosis. Special stains such as thioflavin T have been advocated to detect intramembranous dense deposits, especially in cases with focal distribution of the material. The extent of the basement membrane broadening, thought by some to be due to mesangial interposition into the basement membrane, may be a marker of disease severity, with those patients with diffuse changes having a more guarded prognosis compared to those with focal abnormalities. Thus, in type I MPGN focal changes may represent an early manifestation of the disease

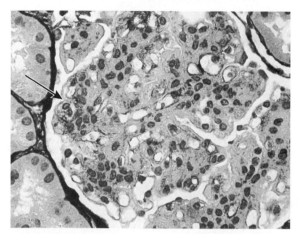

▲ **Figure 29–3.** Light micrograph of a silver-stained renal section illustrating classic splitting of the glomerular basement membrane and mesangial cell interposition (indicated by the black arrow) in a patient with membranoproliferative glomerulonephritis.

and explain the more favorable outcome in response to treatment. The histopathologic appearance of cryoglobulinemic MPGN, which is the most common secondary variant in children, closely resembles type I disease.

Immunofluorescence staining is usually positive for C3, IgG, and IgM in a capillary wall and mesangial distribution. Classical complement cascade components are seen in type I but not type II and III MPGN. When the new term C3G is applied to describe the renal histopathology in a patient with MPGN, it indicates that C3 staining on a 0–4+ scale is at least two levels higher than any other immunoreactant. Electron microscopy confirms the precise location of the deposits, namely subendothelial, mesangial, intramembranous, or subepithelial. The deposits can be numerous or sparse in number, are homogeneous in density, and have no defining ultrastructural appearance.

Figure 29–4 summarizes the role of a diagnostic kidney biopsy and select laboratory and genetic testing in the evaluation of patients who are being considered for the diagnosis of MPGN.

▶ Differential Diagnosis

Other entities that need to be considered in a patient who is being evaluated for MPGN depend upon the specific clinical circumstances. Patients with urinary findings alone may have a mild postinfectious nephritis, hereditary nephritis, or immunoglobulin A (IgA) nephropathy. In those with an overt nephritic syndrome, possibilities include postinfectious nephritis, lupus nephritis, Henoch–Schönlein purpura nephritis, and vasculitis. The likelihood of the last two

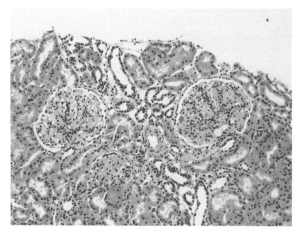

▲ **Figure 29–2.** Light micrograph of a hematoxylin and eosin-stained renal section illustrating the lobular appearance of the glomerulus, diffuse hypercellularity, and thickening of the capillary wall in a patient with membranoproliferative glomerulonephritis.

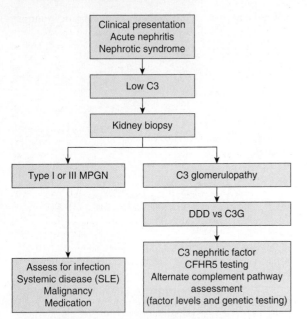

▲ **Figure 29–4.** This diagram summarizes the role of a diagnostic kidney biopsy and select laboratory and genetic testing in the evaluation of patients who are being considered for the diagnosis of MPGN.

diseases is increased in patients with a rash, arthralgias, or fever. There are patients who initially are considered to have postinfectious glomerulonephritis. However, because of persistent disease activity and laboratory abnormalities, ie, hypocomplementemia that last for more than 2–3 months, they are subsequently found to have evidence of activation of the alternate pathway of complement. They probably have MPGN or C3G that was triggered by the antecedent infection. In addition, patients with MPGN and monoclonal gammopathy have also been shown to have C3G resulting from the underlying plasma cell disorder.

In those patients who present with the nephrotic syndrome, depending upon the age, the differential diagnosis includes minimal change nephrotic syndrome, focal segmental glomerulosclerosis, and membranous nephropathy. Paraproteinemias (light chain nephropathy), thrombotic microangiopathies, and fibrillary glomerulonephritis can cause a histologic picture that resembles MPGN. Other than systemic lupus erythematosus (SLE) nephritis and atheroembolic renal disease, what distinguishes MPGN from all other diagnostic considerations is persistent hypocomplementemia.

▶ **Complications**

Patients with MPGN can develop sequelae related to the renal manifestations of the disease or the underlying illness.

Thus, patients with acute nephritis may experience severe hypertension or congestive heart failure. Those patients with nephrotic syndrome may develop local infections, peritonitis, or thromboembolic events.

Patients with dense deposit disease, which is more common in children than in adults, manifest partial lipodystrophy in nearly 25% of cases. This is characterized by a gradual loss of subcutaneous fat tissue in the face and upper body regions. In vitro studies demonstrate that addition of C3 nephritic factor to murine adipocytes results in cell lysis via a process that requires the presence of factor D and divalent cations. These findings may explain the linkage between MPGN and lipodystrophy. Leptin treatment of lipodystrophy in patients with MPGN for 4–36 months normalizes hyperfiltration and reduces proteinuria. The long-term consequences of this therapy on the progression of the renal disease have not been studied. Finally, there may be other associated findings in patients with MPGN such as mild visual fields and color defects. Retinal angiography demonstrates the presence of choroidal neovascularization.

Patients with MPGN in association with cryoglobulinemia may have ulcerative skin lesions, Raynaud's phenomenon, peripheral neuropathy, hepatomegaly, and signs of cirrhosis.

▶ **Treatment**

A. Pediatric Patients

Children with primary forms of MPGN who are clinically well and free of any symptoms, and who have only minor urinary abnormalities, generally do not require aggressive therapy. These patients may be treated with antihypertensive agents, specifically angiotensin-converting enzyme inhibitor (ACEI) or angiotensin receptor blocker (ARB), to reduce proteinuria and prevent progressive renal damage. However, after identification of the disease in 1965 and clarification of the ominous prognosis in the majority of patients, efforts were initiated to implement therapy to retard progression of MPGN. Initial studies performed by Clark West and colleagues at Cincinnati Children's Hospital indicated that prolonged alternate daily therapy with oral steroids favorably impacted on the disease course. The experience in 45 patients treated at that center was summarized in 1986. These patients were given prednisone 60 mg/m^2 or 2–2.5 mg/kg every other day for an average period of 6.5 years with an improved outcome compared to historic controls or patients treated at other centers. Hematuria resolved in 80%, renal function remained normal or improved in 73%, and 62% of those with nephrotic syndrome had normalization of serum albumin concentration. Hypocomplementemia resolves within 4–12 months of initiation of therapy in most patients. However, it may persist in some patients and does not necessarily indicate deteriorating renal histopathology. Repeat biopsies performed after 2 years of therapy indicated an increase in open capillary loops and a reduction in mesangial matrix expansion. However, it is important to note that there was an increase in glomerulosclerosis despite clinical improvement. This may reflect irreversible damage to nephrons prior to initiation of therapy. The efficacy of therapy was greater in patients who began treatment within 1 year of disease onset. In Japan where school urinary screening programs facilitate early detection of MPGN, treatment with prolonged alternate day steroids (4–12 years) after prednisolone pulse or cyclophosphamide therapy achieved remission and resulted in normalization of the urinalysis and stabilization of GFR in 15 patients and mild proteinuria in 4 others who were followed for 10–24 years.

The open-label treatment findings of the Cincinnati group have been confirmed in a randomized clinical trial performed by the International Study of Kidney Diseases in Children. Eighty children with MPGN (42 type I, 14 type II, 17 type III, and 7 nontypable) were assigned to prednisone 40 mg/m^2 every other day or placebo for an average of 41 months. All patients had significant proteinuria and a GFR greater than 70 mL/min/1.73 m^2. Treatment failure, defined as a 30% increase in the baseline serum creatinine or greater than 35 μmol/L increment, occurred in 55% of placebo versus 40% of prednisone-treated patients. Life table analysis indicated 61% renal survival at 130 months in prednisone-treated patients versus 12% in placebo-treated patients ($p = 0.07$). The response was comparable in type I and III MPGN. Although the outcome was less clear in patients with C3 glomerulopathy, a response to more prolonged alternate day steroids in this subtype has been documented.

Based on this experience, it is recommended that alternate steroid therapy be given to all pediatric patients for at least 2 years if the GFR is well preserved (>70 mL/min/1.73 m^2). The beneficial impact of treatment in patients with more advanced disease has not been established. The dose should be approximately 40–60 mg/m^2 every other day. Some investigators have reported good outcomes in a small series of patients given lower steroid doses; however, the minimum effective dose has not been systematically assessed. The need for prolonged therapy should be guided by the clinical response (serum complement level, degree of hematuria, urinary protein excretion, and calculated GFR) and repeat renal histopathologic assessment (after 2 years of steroid treatment, later in a course of therapy, or if there is evidence of recurrent disease).

There are recent reports suggesting that in patients with MPGN or C3 glomerulopathy who fail to respond to ACEI and corticosteroids, addition of mycophenolate mofetil may be beneficial. However, these open label observations require confirmation in randomized clinical trials.

B. Adult Patients

1. Steroid therapy—There is widespread concern about the risks of prolonged steroid therapy in adults. Therefore, the current evidence-based medicine recommendation is to prescribe steroids only for adults with nephrotic syndrome or impaired kidney function. Treatment is maintained for 6 months. The therapy may be extended until remission is achieved using the lowest possible dose of steroids. Patients with asymptomatic urinary findings and patients who fail to respond to steroids should be treated conservatively. ACEI have been demonstrated to be effective in reducing proteinuria in patients with MPGN.

2. Antiplatelet and anticoagulant therapy—It has been suggested that administration of the antiplatelet drug dipyridamole slowed deterioration in kidney function in patients with MPGN. However, a follow-up study failed to demonstrate efficacy of a combination of dipyridamole, cyclophosphamide, and warfarin. In a meta-analysis of five studies of antiplatelet therapy, no beneficial effect was discernible if the timing of the onset of treatment relative to the time of disease onset was accounted for. Thus, based on currently available evidence, these treatments are not recommended.

3. Cryoglobulinemic MPGN secondary to hepatitis C—In patients with hepatitis C infection and MPGN, interferon-α therapy for 6–12 months can achieve remission in 60% of patients. However, most will relapse within 3–6 months. Use of pegylated interferon and the addition of ribavirin to the regimen may improve the response. Current practice is to administer the combination of antiviral agents for 6 months and then switch to low dose every other day steroids. New anti-viral drugs that are highly active and effective in the treatment of hepatitis C may reduce the incidence of glomerular disease in association with this infection. Removal of cryoglobulins with cryofiltration is an experimental modality that may work by removing cryoglobulins from the circulation. Dosing regimens for both pegylated interferon and ribavirin are controversial in patients with diminished renal function. Serious side effects have been observed in patients treated with these agents whose renal function is impaired.

4. Other therapies—There have been isolated case reports claiming that plasmapheresis is a useful therapy in patients with severe idiopathic MPGN and acute renal failure or rapidly deteriorating disease. However, the response was not uniform. Moreover, this treatment modality is invasive and costly. Therefore, it should not be utilized routinely as a first-line treatment. Mycophenolate mofetil has been tried in patients with C3 glomerulopathy (type II MPGN) and cryoglobulinemic MPGN related to hepatitis B infection. Although treatment resulted in reduced proteinuria, viral replication was induced by the drug. Therefore, caution is advisable when considering this immunosuppressive agent for the treatment of MPGN. Plasmapheresis may be useful short term during the acute phase of treatment in patients with serious vasculitic flares from hepatitis C–associated cryoglobulinemia, although activation of the hepatitis is a concern. Finally, in C3 glomerulopathy (type II MPGN), there are small case series in which administration of eculizumab, a monoclonal antibody to C5, slowed the rate of progression of disease. Responses may be related to high serum levels of the soluble membrane attack complex (S5b-9). However, the efficacy of this therapy requires confirmation in a randomized clinical trial.

▶ Prognosis

A. Pediatric Patients

In general, the long-term outlook for untreated patients with MPGN is guarded. Although occasional children and adolescents have been described who achieve a spontaneous remission, nearly 50% of patients progress to end-stage renal disease over 10–15 years. An elevated serum creatinine concentration at the time of diagnosis, nephrotic-range proteinuria, severe hypertension, crescents in greater than 50% of glomeruli, diffuse interstitial fibrosis and tubular atrophy, and a reduced calculated GFR after 1 year of treatment are indicators of a poor outcome. The prognosis is worse in patients with primary versus secondary forms of MPGN. In addition, C3 glomerulopathy (type II MPGN) may have a more ominous long-term outlook compared to type I and III disease.

Recent reports confirm the poor prognosis of MPGN in pediatric patients. For example, in a series of 53 children, ranging in age from 13 months to 15 years, who were treated at two English centers over a 20-year period from January 1980 to December 1999, the mean renal survival time was 12.2 years. Interestingly, the histologic subtype, level of proteinuria below the nephrotic range, and specific therapy had no impact on the long-term outcome. However, the favorable experience in Japan, where MPGN is diagnosed as a result of school urinary screening programs, suggests that the prognosis may be improved following early detection and prompt implementation of corticosteroid therapy.

B. Adult Patients

Although there is an unstated concern that adults with MPGN do worse than children and adolescents, in general, the outcome of MPGN is comparable in adult versus pediatric patients. Thus, 50% of patients progress to ESKD within 5 years of the diagnostic renal biopsy and this percentage rises to 64% after 10 years of follow-up. The features associated with a poor prognosis are similar to those noted in pediatric patients, namely nephrotic syndrome at onset, more extensive tubulointerstitial lesions and interstitial fibrosis, and a reduced GFR. This is a compelling argument in favor of optimal control of blood pressure, preferably with an ACEI or ARB. Treatment for hepatitis C with antivirals before renal involvement occurs may alter the incidence and natural history of secondary MPGN as treatment becomes more commonly implemented. When analyzed from the perspective of the new diagnostic term, C3G, differences in disease presentation and response to treatment are similar to those reported for MPGN.

C. Recurrence Post-Transplantation

One of the more discouraging features about primary MPGN is that the disease recurs in 20–30% of patients who receive a kidney transplant. The risk approaches 90% in those with C3 glomerulopathy and dense deposit disease. Time after transplant, HLA B8DR3, and a living related donor may be risk factors for recurrent MPGN. Hepatitis C MPGN can also recur in transplants or develop *de novo*. It is important to distinguish recurrent MPGN from allograft nephropathy, which can have a similar histopathologic appearance. The presence of immune deposits points toward recurrent disease. Nearly 40% of patients with recurrent MPGN will experience irreversible loss of graft function. This compounds the problem immeasurably because the likelihood of recurrent MPGN increases with each subsequent transplant procedure. There is no therapy to reduce this risk and patients should be managed on a case by case basis.

KEY READINGS

Appel GB et al: Membranoproliferative glomerulonephritis type II (dense deposit disease: an update. J Am Soc Nephrol 2005;16:1392.

Bomback AS: Eculizumab in the treatment of membranoproliferative glomerulonephritis. Nephron Clin Pract 2014;128:270.

Cansick JC et al: Prognosis, treatment and outcome of childhood mesangiocapillary (membranoproliferative) glomerulonephritis. Nephrol Dial Transplant 2004;19:2769.

Cook HT, Pickering MC: Histopathology of MPGN and C3 glomerulopathies. Nat Rev Nephrol 2015;11:14.

Dimkovic N et al: Mycophenolate mofetil in high-risk patients with primary glomerulonephritis: results of a 1-year prospective study. Nephron Clin Pract 2009;111:c189.

Khalighi MA et al: Revisiting post-infectious glomerulonephritis in the emerging era of C3 glomerulopathy. Clin Kidney J 2016;9:397.

Medjeral-Thomas NR et al: C3 glomerulopathy: clinicopathologic features and predictors of outcome. Clin J Am Soc Nephrol 2014;9:46.

Pickering MC et al: Uncontrolled C3 activation causes membranoproliferative glomerulonephritis in mice deficient in complement factor H. Nature Genet 2002;31:424.

Pickering MC et al: C3 glomerulopathy: consensus report. Kidney Int 2013;84:1079.

Yanagihara T et al: Long-term follow-up of diffuse proliferative membranoproliferative glomerulonephritis type 1. Pediatr Nephrol 2005;20:585.

▶ Website

The website www.medicine.uiowa.edu/kidneeds/ is organized by Dr. Richard Smith at the University of Iowa and deals with MPGN type II. It is highly recommended by C. Fred Strife, MD, at the University of Cincinnati Children's Hospital.

■ CHAPTER REVIEW QUESTIONS

1. MPGN is associated with abnormal activation of in which of the following systems?
   A. Kallikrein system
   B. ACTH-adrenal axis
   C. Alternate pathway of complement
   D. Vasopressin-V2 receptor
   E. Th1 lymphocytes

2. A 62-year-old man is noted to have fatigue and impaired renal function. eGFR 46 mL/min/1.73 m². He has not traveled recently, He has nephrotic range proteinuria. He has no fever and his BP is 148/86. He has no jaundice and is breathing comfortably. The cardiac examination is normal. The ANA and ANCA titers are negative. A renal biopsy reveals type 1 MPGN. The most likely cause is

   A. Sarcoidosis
   B. Monoclonal gammopathy
   C. Malaria
   D. Hepatitis B
   E. Endocarditis

3. A 14-year-ol adolescent girl is noted to nephrotic syndrome. The eGFR is 101 ml/min/1.73 m² but the C3 is 36 mg/dl and the ANA titer is normal. Which of the following laboratory tests is most likely to establish the diagnosis?
   A. Serum amyloid protein
   B. Anti-neutrophil cytoplasmic antibody titer
   C. IgA level
   D. C3 nephritic factor
   E. Neutrophil gelatinase associated lipocalin

30

Anti-Glomerular Basement Membrane Disease (Goodpasture Disease)

Andrew J. Rees, MB, FRCP, FRSB, FMedSci

ESSENTIALS OF DIAGNOSIS

▸ Rapidly deteriorating renal function, with or without hemoptysis and pulmonary shadowing on chest radiograph characterizes this entity.

▸ Hematuria and proteinuria on urine dipstick and erythrocyte casts and/or dysmorphic erythrocytes are often seen on urine microscopy.

▸ Circulating antibodies directed against the glomerular basement membrane (GBM) are sometimes present.

▸ Kidney biopsy often demonstrates focal necrotizing glomerulonephritis with linear deposition of immunoglobulin.

▶ General Considerations

Anti-glomerular basement membrane (GBM) disease is a rare but uniquely well-defined form of glomerulonephritis characterized by pathogenic autoantibodies specific for a single component of the GBM—the NC1 domain of the α_3 chain of type IV collagen [α_3(IV)NC1]. The α_3 chain is only expressed in a small number of other basement membranes most notably those of pulmonary alveoli, which explains why the kidney and lung are the principal organs targeted in this disease. Typically these autoantibodies cause severe focal necrotizing glomerulonephritis with crescents resulting in rapidly progressing renal failure; while lung injury is characterized by alveolar hemorrhage. These are the features classic anti-GBM disease that is overwhelmingly the most common form. However, exceptional patients with linear deposition of IgG antibodies along the GBM have more chronic forms of glomerulonephritis. Standard assays for anti-GBM antibodies in these patients are usually negative in these patients who have been termed atypical anti-GBM disease (although the name is controversial).

The annual incidence of anti-GBM disease is between 1.5 and 2.5 cases per million population in the European caucasian, Japanese, and Chinese populations but it is exceptionally rare in those of African descent. Anti-GBM disease affects all age groups but is much less common in children and is more common in the third decade and the sixth or seventh decades. Lung hemorrhage is more common in younger patients, probably because of its close association with cigarette smoking. When this occurs, the condition has been known as Goodpasture disease but the 2012 Revised International Chapel Hill Consensus Conference Nomenclature of vasculitides, which includes anti-GBM disease as a small vessel vasculitis, recommends the term be discontinued.

KEY READINGS

Glassock RJ: Atypical anti-glomerular basement membrane disease: lessons learned. Clin Kidney J 2016;9:653.
Jennette JC et al: 2012 Revised International Chapel Hill Consensus Conference Nomenclature of Vasculitides. Arthritis Rheum 2013;65:1.

▶ Pathogenesis

The autoimmune response in anti-GBM disease is focused on the α_3(IV)NC1 domain of type IV collagen and the epitopes recognized by the patients' autoantibodies and auto-reactive T cells are known. Susceptibility to the disease is strongly influenced by the HLA complex: HLA types DR15 (and to a lesser extent DR4) predisposes to disease whilst HLADR1 and DR7 confer dominant protection which at least in the case of DR1 is mediated by inducing antigen specific regulatory T cells that suppress the autoimmune response. Much less is known about the environmental triggers that initiate the disease but three are commonly invoked: infection which is supported by the demonstration that anti-GBM occurs in geographical and temporal clusters, although specific organisms have not been identified; the release of GBM antigens into the circulation after physical damage such as extracorporeal shock wave lithotripsy or inflammatory injury that could explain the associations of anti-GBM disease with ANCA-associated vasculitis and membranous nephropathy; the therapeutic deletion T cells, most notably alemtuzumab in patients being treated for progressive multiple sclerosis, which might coincidentally remove regulatory T cells that suppress the anti-GBM response.

KEY READINGS

Canney M et al: Spatial and temporal clustering of anti-glomerular basement membrane disease. Clin J Am Soc Nephrol 2016; 11:1392.

Ooi JD et al: Dominant protection from HLA-linked autoimmunity by antigen-specific regulatory T cells. Nature 2017;545:243.

▶ Clinical Findings

A. Symptoms and Signs

1. Anti-GBM disease in native kidneys—Classically anti-GBM disease presents acutely with hemoptysis or symptoms of renal failure but these may be preceded by prodromal symptoms, principally malaise, arthralgia and weight loss. When these occur, they are invariably much less severe than the prodromal symptoms of ANCA-associated vasculitis (AAV), the other main cause of focal necrotizing glomerulonephritis. Anemia is also common and may be severe even in those with minimal hemoptysis.

In the past, pulmonary injury was extremely common in anti-GBM disease and hemoptysis provided an early warning of clinically silent glomerular disease. Nowadays pulmonary involvement is less common and occurs in 35–50% of cases that probably reflects the declining incidence of cigarette smoking that can trigger it. Lung injury varies considerably in severity from minor and transient hemoptysis in some to life-threatening pulmonary hemorrhage with respiratory failure in others. Typically, hemoptysis is intermittent at first and relatively mild before becoming more persistent and severe. As just mentioned, it is usually limited to current cigarette smokers or those exposed to unusual levels of inhaled toxins (such as gasoline fumes), which can also trigger it; it can also be provoked by intercurrent infection and fluid overload. The degree of hemoptysis correlates poorly with severity of pulmonary bleeding: chest radiographs and falls in hemoglobin concentration provide a better reflection, and it can be quantified by measurement of the lung diffusing capacity (D_{LCO}). Clinical signs include tachypnea, inspiratory crackles and bronchial breathing but cyanosis is rare because of concurrent anemia. Importantly, those that recover have no residual pulmonary symptoms or radiologic abnormalities although there may be minimal evidence of fibrosis on light microscopy.

Focal necrotizing glomerulonephritis is an invariable feature of classic anti-GBM disease and now occurs without pulmonary disease in well over half of patients. Renal inflammation itself rarely causes symptoms, although exceptional patients have macroscopic hematuria and loin pain. Accordingly, unless alerted by hemoptysis patients often present late with severe and largely irreversible renal failure. Glomerular inflammation is indicated by dipstick positive proteinuria (++ to +++) and hematuria (+++ to ++++) and an active urine sediment on microscopy with dysmorphic red blood cells and red blood cell casts. Hypertension is uncommon. Kidney disease may improve spontaneously in a small proportion of patients who present early but much more commonly injury progresses to end stage renal failure without the therapy to remove anti-GBM antibody concentrations. Indeed renal function can deteriorate very rapidly with progression from normal to established renal failure within 12 hours. Oliguria and anuria are signs of severe disease and a very poor prognosis.

Anti-GBM antibody synthesis is transient lasting for 12–18 months in those not given immunosuppressive drugs (such as anuric dialysis-dependent patients without lung involvement), and often less than 2 months in those treated with cytotoxic drugs and plasma exchange. Recurrence of anti-GBM disease is well recognized but rare and can be provoked by infection, inhaled toxins and occasionally by renal transplantation. Generally, recurrences are less severe than with the original presentation, possibly because of earlier diagnosis.

There is increasing recognition of a subgroup of patients with anti-GBM disease diagnosed on the basis of intense linear deposition of IgG along the GBM in whom standard clinical assays for anti-GBM antibodies are negative. Light microscopy of kidney biopsies from these patients demonstrate chronic endo-, mesangio-, or membranoproliferative glomerulonephritis rather than focal necrotizing glomerulonephritis and there are no immune deposits on electron microscopy. Pulmonary involvement was absent in all patients in the best characterized series but others have described individuals with recurrent and sometimes severe hemoptysis over many years. The paradox of linear staining and negative anti-GBM antibody assays is beginning to be understood: some of these patients have autoantibodies specific for an epitope distinct from $\alpha_3(IV)NC1$, the target in classic anti-GBM disease; in others the anti-GBM antibodies are restricted to IgG4 subclass; and in others to antibodies with a single λ or κ light chain but, with a single exception, without evidence of monoclonality. Thus atypical anti-GBM disease is heterogeneous both clinically and immunopathogenetically and those who present with it require expert specialist evaluation.

KEY READINGS

Alchi B et al: Predictors of renal and patient outcomes in anti-GBM disease: clinicopathologic analysis of a two-centre cohort. Nephrol Dial Transplant 2015;30:814.

Nasr SH et al: The clinicopathologic characteristics and outcome of atypical anti-glomerular basement membrane nephritis. Kidney Int 2016;89:897.

Rosales IA, Colvin RB: Glomerular disease with idiopathic linear immunoglobulin deposition: a rose by any other name would be atypical. Kidney Int 2016;89:750.

2. Anti-GBM disease in renal allografts—Anti-GBM disease recurs immediately in renal allografts of patients who still have circulating anti-GBM antibodies but is safe after the antibodies are undetectable. However, transplantation can reignite anti-GBM antibody synthesis in rare instances and so it is normally deferred for at least 6 months after the disappearance of circulating anti-GBM antibodies. Subsequently the recipients should be monitored closely thereafter with frequent examination of the urine sediment and anti-GBM assays.

De novo anti-GBM disease kidney transplantation develops in occasional patients with Alport syndrome, which is caused by mutations to genes encoding the α_3, α_4, and α_5 chains of type IV collagen. All three chains are absent from the GBM of Alport kidneys and their presence in allograft is a potential target an antibody-mediated alloimmunity. Fortunately, this is rarely severe enough to cause injury even though transient low concentrations of anti-GBM antibodies are quite common. However, between 3% and 5% develop a focal necrotizing glomerulonephritis with linear deposition of IgG and crescents in the allograft. The clinical course and morphologic appearances of alloimmune anti-GBM disease are indistinguishable from native anti-GBM disease and it usually destroys the graft despite aggressive treatment regimens. Recurrence in subsequent grafts is the norm and usually occurs within days of transplantation. Importantly, the anti-GBM alloantibodies in X-linked Alport are not directed against α_3(IV)NC1 and so are detected poorly, if at all, in standard anti-GBM antibody assays. Instead they are specific for conformational epitopes involving intact hexameric NC1 domains of the α_3, α_4, and α_5 chains. They can be detected by indirect immunofluorescence, which is insensitive or western blotting.

KEY READING

Mallett A et al: End-stage kidney disease due to Alport syndrome: outcomes in 296 consecutive Australia and New Zealand Dialysis and Transplant Registry cases. Nephrol Dial Transplant 2014;29:2277.

B. Laboratory Findings

The diagnosis of Goodpasture disease is dependent on the detection of anti-GBM antibodies either in the circulation or at renal biopsy. These antibodies are usually detected using an enzyme-linked immunosorbent assay (ELISA), and equivocal results can be confirmed by Western blotting. There is a clear correlation between the titer of anti-GBM antibodies and the severity of renal injury but the pattern of lung disease is independent of antibody titer. Circulating anti-GBM antibodies are not found in healthy individuals and highly specific for active disease and unlike anti-DNA antibodies and ANCA cannot be detected in archived sera from individuals who subsequently develop anti-GBM disease.

Hypochromic anemia is common and, as in other types of FNGN, may be associated with a mild microangiopathy on the blood film. Other laboratory findings reflect the presence of glomerulonephritis and the degree of renal failure.

C. Imaging Studies

The abnormalities in renal imaging are nonspecific and indistinguishable from other causes of acute renal failure. On chest radiographs, pulmonary hemorrhage causes widespread alveolar shadowing that typically spares the bases and upper lung fields that can be impossible to distinguish from infection or edema. However, hemorrhage itself is not associated with curly B-lines and is not limited by fissures. Typically the radiologic changes appear and resolve more quickly than is the case for infection.

D. Special Tests

A kidney biopsy is essential in the diagnosis and management of suspected anti-GBM disease. The early histologic changes include minor mesangial expansion and hypercellularity and are followed by the development of a focal and segmental glomerulonephritis, often with marked neutrophil infiltration. This progresses to a focal necrotizing glomerulonephritis with rupture of glomerular capillaries and leakage of blood into Bowman space (Figure 30–1). This initiates the formation of cellular crescents. Characteristically all the crescents are at the same stage of evolution, a feature that reflects the explosive nature of the disease and distinguishes it from pauci immune ANCA associated and other forms of focal necrotizing glomerulonephritis. Linear binding of antibody to GBM is found in all patients, regardless of the severity of the renal pathology (Figure 30–2). The antibodies are almost always IgG, which is accompanied by IgA or IgM in a third of cases; exceptional reports describe deposition of IgA or IgM alone. Linear C3 is seen in 60–70% of patients, and its presence does not influence the severity of the renal injury.

▶ Differential Diagnosis

Anti-GBM disease must be distinguished from other causes of combined acute renal and respiratory failure, the most important of which are listed in Table 30–1. The detection of circulating anti-GBM antibodies is unequivocal evidence of anti-GBM disease. However, the issue is more complicated with ANCA associated vasculitis because up to a third of

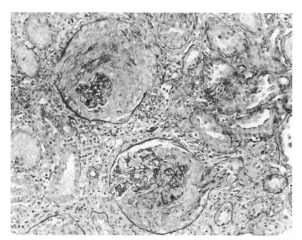

▲ **Figure 30–1.** Kidney biopsy from a patient with Goodpasture syndrome showing two glomeruli with segmental necrosis, leakage of blood into Bowman space, and crescent formation. Renal tubules contain red cell casts and there is perglomerular and interstitial inflammation. Stained with acid fuchsin orange G-stain (AFOG).

those with anti-GBM disease have positive ANCA, usually specific for myeloperoxidase, and signs of vasculitis beyond the glomerular and alveolar capillaries. The titer of anti-GBM antibodies is usually lower than in those patients with anti-GBM antibodies alone and more easily suppressed. These issues apply equally to anti-GBM disease in the absence of pulmonary hemorrhage. The prognosis for renal outcome is similar regardless of whether ANCA are present or not.

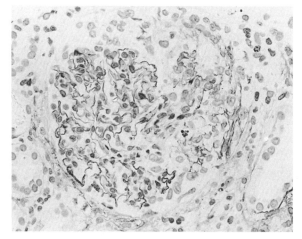

▲ **Figure 30–2.** Glomeruli from a patient with Goodpasture disease showing linear deposition of IgG along the glomerular basement membrane detected by the immunoperoxidase method.

Table 30–1. Differential diagnosis of acute renal and respiratory failure.

Autoimmune mediated
Anti-glomerular basement membrane disease
ANCA-associated vasculitis—microscopic polyangiitis, granulomatous polyangiitis (Wegeners), eosinophilic granulomatosis with polyangiitis (Churg–Strauss)
Systemic lupus erythematosus
Other vasculitides—rheumatoid vasculitis, Behçet disease, cryoglobulinemia

Infections
Severe pneumonia (especially *Legionella*) associated with acute tubular necrosis human immunodeficiency virus

Acute renal failure
Pulmonary edema secondary to acute renal failure of any etiology
Severe cardiac failure with renal hypoperfusion and pulmonary edema

Toxins
Paraquat poisoning

Others
Renal vein thrombosis with pulmonary emboli
Thrombotic microangiopathy (hemolytic uremic syndrome) with acute lung syndrome

Similarly, the demonstration of anti-GBM antibodies distinguishes anti-GBM disease from other types of FNGN that do not have linear IgG deposition in the GBM. One exception is that early fibrillary deposits in fibrillary glomerulonephritis, a rare cause of FNGN, can mimic linear deposition. However, assays for circulating anti-GBM antibodies are negative and the correct diagnosis can be made by electron microscopy.

KEY READING

Thomas JA et al: A case of mistaken identity: fibrillary glomerulonephritis masquerading as crescentic anti-glomerular basement membrane disease. Clin Nephrol 2016;85:114.

▶ **Treatment**

The prognosis for classical anti-GBM disease was dismal before treatment regimens that rapidly removed the pathogenic from the circulation became available: without them almost all patients develop irreversible renal failure or die from pulmonary hemorrhage. There is a severe risk of developing devastating renal injury as long as circulating anti-GBM antibodies persist, even those with relatively a normal serum creatinine concentration and few crescents on the kidney biopsy. This emphasizes the critical importance of early diagnosis and prompt treatment because severity of renal destruction before anti-GBM antibody concentrations are reduced is major determinant of renal prognosis. Those

Table 30–2. KDIGO guideline for the treatment of acute anti-GBM disease.

Methylprednisolone 500–1000 mg/day IV for 3 days followed by prednisolone 1 mg/kg/day orally for 2 wk (max 80 mg/day); then 0.6 mg/kg/day for weeks 2–4; 0.4 mg/kg/day for weeks 4–8; 30 mg/day for weeks 8–10; 25 mg/day for weeks 10–11; 20 mg/day for weeks 11–12; and then weekly reductions of 2.5 mg/day until 10 mg/day is reached at week 15.
Cyclophosphamide 2 mg/kg/day by mouth.
Daily exchange of 4 L of plasma for 5% human albumin for 14 days or until the circulating antibody is suppressed; in the presence of pulmonary hemorrhage, or when there is concern about bleeding, 300–400 mL of fresh frozen plasma should be given at the end of each treatment.

Note: Others have established that regimens that omit methyl prednisolone and have a more rapid early tapering of the dose of oral prednisolone. Specifically, prednisolone 1 mg/kg/day orally for 1 week (max. 80 mg/day); then reduce at weekly intervals to 45, 30, 25, 20, 15, 10, and 5 mg/day.

who are oligoanuric or have dialysis-dependent renal failure almost never regain renal function.

The KDIGO Clinical Practice Guideline for Glomerulo-nephritis recommends a treatment regimen that combines cyclophosphamide, prednisolone, and plasma exchange (Table 30–2). This recommendation is based on consensus rather than evidence from prospective randomized control trials (RCT) because the rarity of anti-GBM disease and its severity preclude suitably empowered studies. The single RCT performing immunosuppression with or without plasma exchange showed the plasma exchange group had significantly faster reduction in anti-GBM antibody concentrations and lower serum creatinine values but was flawed as it was too small, the protocol prescribed three plasma exchanges weekly rather than the 6 or 7 needed to reliably reduce anti-GBM antibody concentrations. Although the groups were clinically well matched at enrollment subsequent analysis of the renal biopsies showed the plasma exchange group had significantly fewer crescents. More compelling evidence comes from large single center cohorts from Europe, United States, China, and Japan that uniformly show much better prognosis for patients treated with plasma exchange combined with alkylating agents and corticosteroids than for those not receiving plasma exchange; and secondly the individual patient correlations between reducing autoantibody concentrations after plasma exchange and improving renal function. Analysis of these data provided the basis for the four KDIGO recommendations (Table 30-2).

1. Initiate immunosuppression with cyclophosphamide and corticosteroids plus plasmapheresis in all patients with anti-GBM glomerulonephritis except those who are dialysis-dependent at presentation and have 100% crescents in an adequate biopsy sample, and do not have pulmonary hemorrhage. (1B)

2. Start treatment for anti-GBM glomerulonephritis without delay once the diagnosis is confirmed. If the diagnosis is highly suspected, it would be appropriate to begin high-dose corticosteroids and plasmapheresis while waiting for confirmation. (Not graded)

3. Prescribe no maintenance immunosuppressive therapy for anti-GBM glomerulonephritis. (1D)

4. Defer kidney transplantation after anti-GBM glomerulonephritis until anti-GBM antibodies have been undetectable for a minimum of 6 months. (Not graded)

The KDIGO recommendations remain the basis for treating anti-GBM disease. Effective removal of anti-GBM antibodies is central to the regimen and daily treatments of one plasma volume remain the standard. Removing equivalent amounts of IgG with more recently developed methods, such as double filtration plasmapheresis or immunoabsorption, appears equally effective. There is early evidence that more intensive IgG removal made feasible by immunoabsorption reduces anti-GBM antibody concentrations more rapidly and may be more effective at rescuing severely damaged kidneys but more data are needed. Recent reports suggest that anti-B-cell therapy with rituximab may also be effective in controlling anti-GBM antibody synthesis in the longer term, but the delayed effect on antibody concentrations and the practical difficulties of combining therapeutic monoclonal antibodies with plasma exchange argue against its use in the acute stage.

Patients on treatment need close monitoring both to ensure effective control of anti-GBM antibody concentration and tissue injury, and to anticipate potential complications. Renal injury is most simply monitored by serum creatinine and lung injury by arterial po_2 concentration, chest radiographs and when necessary supplemented by measurement of the diffusing capacity of the lung (D_{LCO}) that increases with fresh pulmonary hemorrhage. Infection is a constant risk and the toxicity of immunosuppressive drugs should be monitored equally assiduously especially in the presence of severe renal failure. Careful monitoring of the complete blood count is essential, and cyclophosphamide should be discontinued if the white cell count falls below 3.5×10^9/L. Patients should also be assessed for fluid overload that can trigger renewed pulmonary hemorrhage and is a particular concern during the early stages because some replacement fluid used for plasma exchange have a high sodium concentration which can result in sodium overload.

KEY READINGS

Biesenbach P et al: Long-term outcome of anti-glomerular basement membrane antibody disease treated with immunoadsorption. PlosOne 2014;9:e103568.

Kidney Disease: Improving Global Outcomes (KDIGO) Glomerulonephritis Work Group. KDIGO Clinical Practice Guideline for Glomerulonephritis. Kidney Int 2012; Suppl 2:139.

Zhao C et al: Anti-glomerular basement membrane disease: outcomes of different therapeutic regimens in a large single-center Chinese cohort study. Medicine 2011;90:303.

Prognosis

Control of pulmonary injury is straightforward in most patients with anti-GBM disease and prognosis is dependent on the kidney. This is critically dependent on the degree of renal injury when treatment is instituted and most probably on the early introduction of plasma exchange. Reported renal survival at one year has ranged from 15% to 58% in large series with survival of concomitant patient between 67% and 94%. The most impressive results have come from the group that introduced the intensive plasma exchange regimen and have perhaps applied it most aggressively. Results in consecutive patients managed over a 25-year period and separated into three groups depending on the initial serum creatinine (creatinine <5.7mg/dL; >5.7 mg/dL but not requiring dialysis; and dialysis dependent with serum creatinine >5.7 mg/dL) were as follows: after 1 year, patient survival in the three groups was 100%, 82%, and 65%, respectively; and renal survival was 95% (and 74% at last follow-up), 82% (and 69% at last follow up), and 8% (5% at last follow-up). These results demonstrate both the need for early diagnosis and treatment, and the possibility of maintaining long-term independent renal function after aggressive treatment.

When to Refer

All patients with confirmed or suspected anti-GBM disease need urgent referral to a specialized unit able to perform intensive plasma exchange.

■ CHAPTER REVIEW QUESTIONS

1. A 54-year-old Caucasian woman is admitted with severe hypoxemia and a serum creatinine of 3.9 mg/dL (6 weeks previously it had been 1.9 mg/dL). She had a fever of 38°C and there were small patches of palpable purpura on both arms. There were no signs of fluid overload, her BP was 140/85 mm Hg but she had widespread crackles in both lungs. Urine was dipstick positive for protein (++) and blood (+++) and contained an active urinary sediment with red blood cell casts.

   Which one of the following tests is MOST likely to be positive?
   A. Urinary antigen test or PCR for *Legionella* spp
   B. Immunoassay for circulating anti-GBM antibodies
   C. Blood cultures for *Streptococcus pneumoniae*
   D. ANCA
   E. Toxicological screen for paraquat

2. A 48-year-old Caucasian woman was referred because of incidentally discovered dipstick positive proteinuria (+++) and hematuria (++). She was hypertensive (150/95) but otherwise the physical examination was normal. Serum creatinine was 1.8 mg/dL and proteinuria 4.8 g/24 hours. Kidney biopsy revealed membranoproliferative glomerulonephritis on light microscopy and intense linear deposition of IgG along the GBM was seen on immunofluorescence; no immune deposits were visible on electron microscopy. An immunoassay for circulating anti-GBM antibodies was negative.

   Which one of the following reasons for glomerular IgG deposition in this case is correct?

   A. Accentuation of the normal background GBM staining for IgG induced by the increased glomerular permeability
   B. Atypical anti-GBM antibodies with affinity for antigens other than $\alpha_3(IV)NC1$—the classic Goodpasture antigen.
   C. Fibrillary IgG deposits in early fibrillary glomerulonephritis mimicking linear staining by anti-GBM antibodies.
   D. Anti-GBM antibodies specific for $\alpha_3(IV)NC1$ of predominantly IgG4 subclass.

3. A 28-year-old man with renal failure due to X-linked Alport syndrome caused by a missense mutation of the α_5 chain of type IV collagen received a kidney allograft. Four weeks later his serum creatinine increases and his physicians are anxious that he has developed anti-GBM disease in the graft.

   Which one of the following statements is correct in this patient?
   A. The diagnosis is more likely because he has a missense mutation.
   B. A negative immunoassay for anti-GBM antibodies excludes the diagnosis.
   C. *De novo* anti-GBM disease occurs in less than 5% of allografts.
   D. Linear staining of the GBM is sufficient to make the diagnosis.

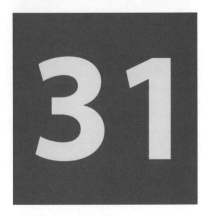

31

Bacterial Infection-Associated Glomerulonephritis

Samar M. Said, MD

Samih H. Nasr, MD

In the past, the majority of cases of bacterial infection-associated glomerulonephritis occurred in children following streptococcal upper respiratory tract or skin infections. Over the past four decades, there has been a shift in epidemiology, bacteriology, and outcome of this disease. A significant percentage of cases now target adults, particularly the elderly or immunocompromised. Streptococcus-associated glomerulonephritis generally begins after the pharyngeal (more common) or skin infection has either resolved spontaneously or has been effectively treated and therefore the term poststreptococcal glomerulonephritis is appropriate. In contrast, most of the other causes of bacterial infection-associated glomerulonephritis, including that due to staphylococcus infection, occur when the infection is still present and hence the term staphylococcus-associated glomerulonephritis is more appropriate. Streptococcus and staphylococcus are by far the most common bacteria responsible for bacterial infection-associated glomerulonephritis, although a large variety of other bacteria, such as Escherichia, Yersinia, Salmonella, and pseudomonas, can rarely cause the disease. We will limit our considerations to four specific disease entities: (1) acute poststreptococcal glomerulonephritis, (2) staphylococcus-associated glomerulonephritis, (3) infective endocarditis-associated glomerulonephritis, and (4) glomerulonephritis associated with infected atrioventricular shunts (shunt nephritis).

ESSENTIALS OF DIAGNOSIS

- Acute nephritic syndrome (hematuria, edema, hypertension, ± oliguria), occasionally nephrotic syndrome, and rarely rapidly progressive azotemia
- Recent bacterial infection (serology or culture)
- Reduced serum complement (CH50 and C3)
- Renal biopsy confirmation required in adults

- Exudative glomerulonephritis associated with streptococcus, crescentic glomerulonephritis with infectious endocarditis, and membranoproliferative glomerulonephritis with shunt nephritis
- Frequently IgA dominant glomerular staining on immunofluorescence in staphylococcus-associated glomerulonephritis

ACUTE POSTSTREPTOCOCCAL GLOMERULONEPHRITIS

General Considerations

The incidence of acute poststreptococcal glomerulonephritis (APSGN) has decreased dramatically in most industrialized countries. The association with alcoholism in adult patients has been noticed in central Europe. Nevertheless, in other countries, such as Singapore, Trinidad, and Venezuela, a poststreptococcal etiology is the causative factor in more than 70% of children admitted to the hospital with glomerulonephritis. The reason for these geographic variations in epidemiology may relate to the accessibility of early medical care and antibiotic treatment resulting from improvements in living standards. APSGN presents as sporadic cases, clusters of cases, or epidemics that follow streptococcal infections of the throat or the skin. The vast majority of epidemics and sporadic cases were due to group A streptococci, but several outbreaks caused by group C streptococci, group G streptococci, or milk-borne *Streptococcus zooepidemicus* have been reported.

Streptococci of M types 47, 49, 55, and 57 are frequently the etiologic agents of pyodermitis-associated nephritis while types 1, 2, 4, and 12 correspond to upper respiratory streptococcal infections causing nephritis. There is a wide variability in the incidence of nephritis following a nephritogenic streptococcal infection, but the incidence among siblings is close to 40%, which indicates a familial predisposition to the disease; however, a genetic marker of susceptibility for APSGN has not been found.

▶ Clinical Findings

APSGN is usually, but not exclusively, a disease of children and adolescents. The highest incidence occurs in patients between the ages of 4 and 15 years. Less than 5% of the patients are younger than 2 years and about 10% in most large series are older than 40 years. APSGN induces long-term protective immunity as demonstrated by the fact that repeated attacks of the disease are extremely rare.

A. Symptoms and Signs

The diagnosis of APSGN requires demonstration of antecedent streptococcal infection in a patient who presents with acute glomerulonephritis. Nephritis may follow approximately 7–15 days after streptococcal tonsillitis and 4–6 weeks after impetigo. It is not unusual for the active pyodermitis to have subsided at the time of APSGN but telltale skin scars and decoloration are present. Impetigo frequently complicates scabies and a clue to this association may be obtained by examination of the patient's siblings.

The acute nephritic syndrome, characterized by edema, gross or microscopic hematuria, hypertension, and frequently oliguria, is the usual clinical presentation of this glomerular disease. Hematuria, gross or microscopic, is almost universally present. Edema occurs in 80–90% of the patients, is usually the primary complaint, and varies in severity from swollen eyelids to anasarca, but in contrast with nephrotic syndrome, ascites is rarely present. Hypertension is found in 80% of patients and its severity is correlated with the degree of fluid retention. Pulmonary edema and hyperkalemia may sometimes be present if there is severe oliguria and excessive fluid intake. In contrast to the benign clinical picture in children, 40% of elderly patients with APSGN present with hypervolemia and congestive heart failure. Rarely, APSGN is complicated by hypertensive encephalopathy or a rapidly progressive course of kidney function loss due to the presence of a crescentic glomerulonephritis phenotype. The clinical manifestations of acute nephritic syndrome usually last less than 2 weeks.

Asymptomatic cases, manifested by microscopic hematuria, reduction of complement levels, and sometimes hypertension after a recent streptococcal infection, are in prospective studies four or five times more frequent than clinically apparent disease.

The clinical manifestations of APSGN in adults are different from those in children patients. Massive proteinuria and azotemia may occur in as many as 20% and 80%, respectively, of adults with this disease. Adults also frequently have a more protracted course, higher incidence of complications, and a poorer prognosis.

B. Laboratory Findings

The percentage of positive cultures in cases of APSGN has significant variability: 10–70% of the cases during epidemics and about 25% in sporadic cases. Most frequently, the poststreptococcal etiology is established by increasing titers of antistreptolysin O (ASO) (reported in 33–80% of the cases of APSGN that follow throat infections), anti-DNase B (increased in 73% of the post-impetigo cases), and the streptozyme test that measures antibodies to five antigens: (1) DNase B, (2) ASO, (3) hyaluronidase, (4) streptokinase, and (5) nicotinamide-adenine dinucleotidase (positive in >95% of patients with pharyngitis and in 80% of patients with skin infections). Anti-nephritis-associated plasmin receptor (NAPlr), anti-streptococcal cationic exotoxin B (SPE B), and anti-zymogen (SPE B precursor) antibody titers are positive in close to 90% of the APSGN patients, but their determination is not generally available.

The complement system is preferentially, but not exclusively, activated by the alternative pathway. C4 levels are usually normal, and CH50 and C3 are depressed in more than 90% of the cases and return to normal in less than 1 month. Normal serum complement in the acute phase as well as hypocomplementemia lasting longer than 1 month should raise suspicion of a diagnosis different than APSGN, such as IgA nephropathy, C3 glomerulonephritis (C3GN), or dense deposit disease. Serum IgG and IgM are usually elevated and IgA is normal. Cryoglobulins are present in one-third of the patients.

Urine sediment examination shows red blood cell casts and dysmorphic erythrocytes, characteristic of glomerular hematuria. The fractional excretion of sodium is frequently less than 0.5 and increases with the reestablishment of diuresis.

C. Kidney Biopsy

Kidney biopsy is generally not needed to confirm the diagnosis of epidemic APSGN and childhood APSGN unless there are characteristics that make the diagnosis doubtful or have prognostic significance and therapeutic implications. In contrast, kidney biopsy is generally required to establish the diagnosis of sporadic adulthood APSGN as the differential diagnosis is wide (see Differential Diagnosis below).

The classic light microscopic appearance of APSGN is diffuse endocapillary proliferative glomerulonephritis with abundant intracapillary neutrophils (Figure 31–1A). A diffuse crescentic pattern can rarely occur and manifests clinically as rapidly progressive glomerulonephritis.

Immunofluorescence shows C3-dominant glomerular immune staining. The majority of cases show coarsely granular glomerular wall and mesangial staining (so-called "starry sky pattern,") (Figure 31–1B). The remaining minority show mostly glomerular capillary wall staining ("garland pattern") or predominantly mesangial staining ("mesangial pattern"). The garland pattern, which corresponds to

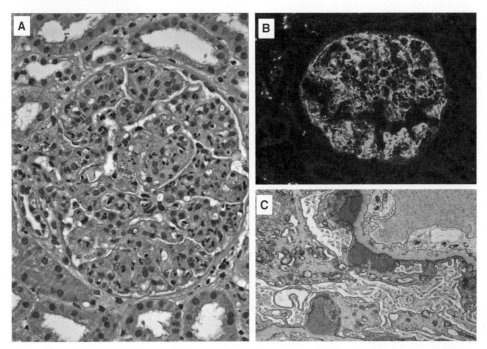

▲ **Figure 31–1.** Pathology of APSGN: **A.** The depicted glomerulus shows global occlusion of the peripheral capillaries by marked endocapillary hypercellularity including numerous intracapillary infiltrating neutrophils. **B.** Immunofluorescence shows coarsely granular mesangial and glomerular capillary wall staining for C3 ("starry sky pattern"). **C.** This electron microscopic image shows four large subepithelial hump-shaped electron dense deposits. (See Color Plate 2.)

numerous confluent subepithelial deposits, is associated with heavy proteinuria. Codeposition of IgG is less intense than C3 staining and not always present. IgM deposition is less common and less intense than IgG whereas IgA and C1q are typically absent.

The most characteristic finding on electron microscopy is scattered large subepithelial electron-dense deposits, which exhibit a "hump-shaped" appearance (Figure 31–1C). Humps are more frequent and abundant in APSGN than other forms of bacterial infection-associated glomerulonephritis. In the resolving phase of disease, humps are preferentially located where the glomerular basement membrane reflects over the mesangium (hinge region) and frequently exhibit a variegated texture as they begin to undergo reabsorption.

▶ Differential Diagnosis

The initial approach to the patient with acute nephritic syndrome should indicate if a systemic disease is associated with the acute glomerulonephritis or if the clinical picture results from a primary renal disease. Lack of fever, gastrointestinal and pulmonary manifestations, arthralgias, or vasculitic skin lesions suggests a primary renal disease. Serum complement

levels are helpful as a first-line laboratory test because fewer than 10% of the patients with APSGN have normal levels and such a finding should raise the possibility of other diseases such as IgA nephropathy, vasculitis, hemolytic uremic syndrome, or antiglomerular basement membrane disease. In addition, serum complement levels return to normal in less than a month in APSGN and a persistently low C3 should make the clinician consider C3 glomerulopathy (which encompass C3GN and dense deposit disease) or lupus nephritis. Circulating antineutrophil cytoplasmic antibodies (ANCA) are associated with higher serum creatinine concentrations and crescent formation in APSGN; therefore, ANCA testing is recommended when crescentic APSGN is present to rule out concurrent ANCA glomerulonephritis.

Episodic IgA nephropathy is often triggered by an upper respiratory infection, similar to the presentation of patients with APSGN. In contrast to APSGN, gross hematuria typically develops at time of infection (so-called "synpharyngitic nephritis") and there is a history of prior episodes of gross hematuria with IgA nephropathy.

Histologically, APSGN can be difficult to distinguish from C3GN. Most cases of C3GN demonstrate an MPGN pattern of injury, which is exceedingly rare in APSGN. However, some cases of C3GN lack the MPGN pattern and show subepithelial humps, mimicking APSGN. Glomerular positivity for C3 only (ie, without positivity for IgG, IgM, IgA, or C1q) is a prerequisite for C3GN, but is also common in APSGN, especially in the resolving phase. In patients with sole glomerular positivity for C3, the following clinico-pathologic findings favor C3GN over APSGN: (1) absence of clinical or laboratory evidence of preceding infection; (2) continuous depression of C3 or active glomerulonephritis for longer than several months despite clearance of infection; (3) MPGN pattern on light microscopy; or (4) large subendothelial, intramembranous, or mesangial electron dense deposits ultrastructurally. When this distinction is not possible, testing for defects in the regulation of the alternative pathway of complement is advised.

Treatment

Symptomatic therapy is recommended for APSGN. The management of acute nephritic syndrome requires hospital admission in the adult or elderly patient and in most children with APSGN. Some children without severe edema or hypertension and normal serum creatinine concentration may be followed closely at home, particularly in the first few days when the clinical picture may worsen. All patients should be instructed to restrict sodium and fluid intake; most will benefit from the administration of loop diuretics (such as furosemide) in the first 24–48 hours of the disease. Hypertension usually subsides after diuresis is established. Oral nifedipine is generally sufficient to control hypertension. If hypertensive encephalopathy develops, treatment with oral nifedipine, parenteral nicardipine, or nitroprusside is warranted. Pulmonary edema is treated with loop diuretics and oxygen. Hyperkalemia and uremia may require dialysis in severe cases.

There is no conclusive evidence that treatment with antibiotics after the onset of APSGN alters the course of disease, although penicillin therapy can control the spread of outbreaks of epidemic APSGN. Therefore penicillin prophylaxis should be given to family members during infectious epidemics. APSGN patients with recurrent streptococcal infection should be treated with a course of penicillin (oral or intramuscular) or with erythromycin if the patient is allergic.

Steroids and immunosuppressive agents are not generally recommended for treatment of APSGN, although patients with the crescentic phenotype who have persistent disease despite resolution of the preceding streptococcal infection can be treated with a short course of methylprednisolone to reduce glomerular inflammation.

Prognosis

Prognosis of the acute phase is excellent in children but in elderly patients the mortality in some series is as high as 20% because of associated cardiovascular complications. Mild proteinuria and hematuria may persist for several months after the acute attack. Long-term prognosis of APSGN has

been debated. Approximately 50% of the biopsies obtained up to 15 years after the acute attack show variable degrees of interstitial infiltration and glomerular sclerosis. The incidence of kidney function abnormalities in the reported studies has significant variability. For instance, most studies indicate that proteinuria is found in 4–13% of patients, but the range extends from 1.4% to 46%. Similarly, the reported frequency of hypertension ranges noted in the general population to as much as 46% of the patients. These discrepancies result, at least in part, from studying populations of different ethnic background, different age groups, and sporadic or epidemic cases. Nevertheless, the incidence of end-stage renal disease from collected studies with 15 years of follow-up is less than 1%. There is general agreement that long-term prognosis is worse in adult patients, in those with massive proteinuria, and in those with predisposing conditions such as diabetes or alcoholism. A disturbingly high incidence of impaired kidney function has been reported in an outbreak of APSGN occurring as a result of the ingestion of cheese contaminated with *Streptococcus zooepidemicus*. In this study, which included predominantly adult patients, 30% of the patients had impaired kidney function 2 years after the acute attack.

Pathogenesis

The pathogenesis of APSGN, which is an immune complex-mediated disease, has been studied extensively. Humoral and cellular immune mechanisms are involved. Immune complexes formed in the circulation or *in situ* induce local activation of the complement (preferentially by an alternative pathway) and coagulation systems (platelet consumption and activation) and the recruitment of inflammatory cells. Infiltration of helper T lymphocytes is an early feature and increased levels of interleukin (IL)-6, tumor necrosis factor-α (TNF-α), and platelet-derived growth factor (PDGF) have been demonstrated. In addition, there is evidence of autoimmune reactivity attributed in part to neuraminidase-induced desialization of normal components. ANCA, cryoglobulins, serum rheumatoid factor titers, C3eNef, and anti-immunoglobulin (Ig) G renal deposits have all been demonstrated. These manifestations of autoimmune reactivity have undefined clinical significance except for the demonstration of ANCA that is more frequent in cases of greater severity.

The nature of the nephritogenic streptococcal antigen is still controversial. Two candidate antigens identified are streptococcal plasmin receptor [NAPlr or glyceraldehyde-3-phosphate dehydrogenase (GAPDH)] and streptococcal cationic exotoxin B and zymogen precursor (SPE B). Serum antibody response to these antigens has been found in 70–90% of the patients and both GAPDH and SPE B have been detected in kidney biopsies obtained early in the course of the disease. Multicentric studies show that the anti-zymogen antibody titer is the best marker of nephritogenic streptococcal infection. Evidence of colocalization of NAPlr and glomerular plasmin-like activity has been found, suggesting that the ability to bind to plasmin plays a critical pathogenetic role in APSGN. Other potentially nephritogenic streptococcal antigens proposed to be important in the pathogenesis of APSGN are endostreptosin, streptokinase, and preabsorbing antigen. However, the specificity and pathogenetic role of NAPlr and the other above mentioned proposed nephritogenic streptococcal antigens remain questionable.

The finding of low serum CH50 and C3 with normal C4, the presence of sole C3 deposition in glomeruli (ie, C3 without immunoglobulins or C1q) in a significant proportion of cases, the detection of C3eNef and mutations in complement regulating proteins, and the histological similarities to C3GN suggest that bacterial infection-associated glomerulonephritis (including APSGN) in some patients could be due to mild defects in complement alterative pathway regulating proteins which trigger transient uncontrolled activation of the alternative pathway of complement and glomerulonephritis. This theory could explain why a large variety of bacterial organisms can cause glomerulonephritis and the fact that no reliable nephritogenic bacterial antigen has been identified so far despite extensive search.

KEY READINGS

Balter S et al: Epidemic nephritis in Nova Serrana, Brazil. Lancet 2000;20;355(9217):1776.

Nasr SH et al: Acute postinfectious glomerulonephritis in the modern era: experience with 86 adults and review of the literature. Medicine (Baltimore). 2008;87:21.

Oda T et al: Glomerular plasmin-like activity in relation to nephritis-associated plasmin receptor in acute poststreptococcal glomerulonephritis. J Am Soc Nephrol 2005;16:247.

Rodriguez-Iturbe B, Musser JM: The current state of poststreptococcal glomerulonephritis. J Am Soc Nephrol 2008;19:1855.

Yoshizawa N et al: Nephritis-associated plasmin receptor and acute poststreptococcal glomerulonephritis: characterization of the antigen and associated immune response. J Am Soc Nephrol 2004;15:1785.

STAPHYLOCOCCUS-ASSOCIATED GLOMERULONEPHRITIS

▶ General Considerations

Staphylococcus-associated glomerulonephritis (SAGN) is infrequent and primarily affects middle-aged and elderly patients. In the elderly, glomerulonephritis due to bacterial infection is more often due to staphylococcus than streptococcus. The site of staphylococcal infection is variable, including skin (38%), lung/pleura (22%), heart (10%), deep-seated abscesses (6%), or urinary tract infection (6%). Unlike APSGN, upper respiratory tract infection is generally not a cause of SAGN. Most cases are due to *Staphylococcus (S) aureus* with methicillin-resistant *S. aureus* being more frequent than methicillin-sensitive *S. aureus*. Less commonly, coagulase-negative staphylococcus such as *S. epidermidis* and *S. hemolyticus* can cause the disease. *S. epidermidis* is the most frequent causative bacterium in shunt nephritis. Many affected adults have a predisposition to staphylococcal infection particularly patients with diabetes, which is due to a higher incidence of staphylococcal colonization and infection of skin. Other predisposing conditions to SAGN are alcoholism, malignancy, and intravenous drug addiction.

▶ Clinical Findings

A. Symptoms and Signs

Patients with SAGN present clinically with a concurrent infection, hematuria, proteinuria, and a rising serum creatinine concentration. Peripheral edema is present in approximately half of patients and new onset hypertension in up to 29% of patients. New onset or exacerbated heart failure occurs in a third of elderly patients, owing to the higher prevalence of underlying cardiovascular disease and the reduced ability to handle the salt and water retention associated with glomerulonephritis. Purpuric skin rash occurs in up to 20% of patients, mimicking Henoch–Schönlein purpura or ANCA-associated vasculitis.

B. Laboratory Findings

Unlike APSGN, there are no serologic tests to detect staphylococcal infection and therefore a causative staphylococcal infection can only be identified from a positive culture. The urine sediment reveals hematuria in over 95% of patients with or without red blood cell casts. Leukocyturia is present in two-thirds of patients. The mean 24-hour urine protein is 3 g/day and one-third of patients have nephrotic syndrome. The mean serum creatinine concentration at the time of kidney biopsy is 5.1 mg/dL. Hypocomplementemia is not as frequent as in APSGN, reported in 48–78% of patients (most commonly low C3 with normal C4 but occasionally low C3 and C4). Positive ANCA serology has been reported in 8–22% of patients with SAGN, most commonly in the setting of infectious endocarditis (IE), and their presence is frequently associated with rapidly progressive glomerulonephritis due to crescentic phenotype.

C. Kidney Biopsy

Kidney biopsy is required to confirm the diagnosis of SAGN and exclude other forms of acute glomerulonephritides such as C3GN, lupus nephritis, ANCA glomerulonephritis, and IgA nephropathy (including IgA vasculitis) that may require prompt aggressive immunosuppressive therapy.

Most cases of SAGN exhibit exudative and endocapillary proliferative glomerulonephritis similar to APSGN, although focal endocapillary proliferative or pure mesangial proliferative patterns of injury can be seen in the resolving phase of disease. A crescentic phenotype can occur, particularly in the setting of IE, and manifests clinically as rapidly progressive glomerulonephritis. As a significant percentage of adults with SAGN have diabetes, changes of underlying diabetic glomerulosclerosis are common on biopsy.

Immunofluorescence typically shows C3 dominant glomerular staining. C3 can be the only immunoreactant detected by immunofluorescence (in 27% of patients), or there could be codeposition of one or more immunoglobulins, most commonly IgA (Figure 31–2). The vast majority of cases of IgA-dominant bacterial infection-associated glomerulonephritis (ie, glomerular staining for IgA stronger than IgG and IgM) are due to staphylococcal infection, and when present should prompt thorough search for underlying staphylococcal infection. This morphologic variant of bacterial infection-associated glomerulonephritis which is called "IgA-dominant staphylococcus-associated glomerulonephritis" can be confused histologically with IgA nephropathy (see Differential Diagnosis below).

Electron microscopy typically shows large, hump-shaped subepithelial electron dense deposits. Subepithelial humps are less abundant in SAGN than APSGN and examination of multiple glomeruli might be needed to identify them. Most cases also show small subendothelial, mesangial, and/or intramembranous electron dense deposits.

▶ Differential Diagnosis

Patients with suspected SAGN should have serologic testing to evaluate for other potential causes of acute

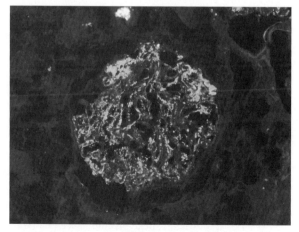

▲ **Figure 31–2.** Pathology of SAGN: The glomerulus in this case of IgA-dominant staphylococcus-associated glomerulonephritis shows bright granular global mesangial and segmental glomerular capillary wall staining for IgA. (See Color Plate 3.)

glomerulonephritis, including testing for ANA, ANCA, cryoglobulins, and hepatitis B and C. Whereas most patients with SAGN have low C3 and normal C4, some have depression of both C3 and C4, raising the differential diagnosis of lupus nephritis. Furthermore, some patients with SAGN, particularly in the setting of shunt nephritis, have positive ANA. The presence of C3 dominant staining on immunofluorescence (as opposed to "full-house" pattern) and subepithelial humps distinguishes SAGN from lupus nephritis.

SAGN can be difficult to distinguish from C3GN both clinically and histologically as depressed serum C3 with normal C4, C3 dominant glomerular staining, and subepithelial humps are characteristic of both conditions. Testing to exclude defects in the alternative pathway of complement is recommended in patients with glomerular staining for C3 only who have persistently low serum C3 levels or active glomerulonephritis despite eradication of infection.

Histologically, IgA-dominant SAGN can be difficult to distinguish from IgA nephropathy that is triggered or reactivated by infection. Features that favor IgA-dominant SAGN over IgA nephropathy include initial presentation at an older age or in a patient with diabetes, presence of hypocomplementemia, presence of exudative glomerulonephritis pattern of injury, stronger glomerular staining for C3 than IgA, and presence of subepithelial hump-shaped deposits.

▶ Treatment

The treatment of SAGN includes eradication of staphylococcal infection with appropriate antibiotics (and if needed with surgery) and management of complications of nephritis. Elderly patients who are vulnerable to complications such as congestive heart failure may require hospital admission for closer observation and therapy. Antihypertensive drugs, diuretics (preferably loop diuretics) and dietary salt restriction are often necessary in the acute setting to control hypertension and edema. In patients with persistent heavy proteinuria, renin-angiotensin system inhibitors can be given to slow disease progression.

The role of immunosuppressive therapy in the treatment of SAGN has not been investigated in randomized prospective studies. Retrospective studies found no beneficial effects for steroids on the outcome of bacterial infection-associated glomerulonephritis (including SAGN) in adults. In addition, in patients with an active staphylococcal infection, which is often the case in SAGN, high-dose glucocorticoid exposure can lead to worsening of the infectious condition or death.

▶ Prognosis

In young adults who do not have comorbidities, successful eradication of the staphylococcal infection results in resolution of the glomerulonephritis with stabilization of the serum creatinine, disappearance of hematuria, and normalization of complement levels, a process that may take months. In contrast, renal prognosis in elderly patients is guarded with

32% of patients have persistent renal dysfunction and 44% progress to ESRD. A dismal prognosis has been reported in SAGN superimposed on diabetic glomerulosclerosis in whom 64% of patients progress to ESRD.

Pathogenesis

While the pathogenesis of APSGN has been studied extensively, few studies have investigated the pathogenesis of SAGN and the etiology is largely unknown. SAGN is an immune-complex mediated disease. The antigen component of the immune complex is derived from the infective agent, similar to APSGN. Potential nephritogenic staphylococcal antigens include staphylococcal neutral phosphatase, a 70-kDa protein (p70), and staphylokinase. *In situ* immune complex formation may occur due to cationic staphylococcal antigens planted in the glomeruli. On the other hand, glomerular deposition of preformed circulating immune complexes might be more important in SAGN then APSGN. In patients with staphylococcal infection, the circulating antigens and the antibodies directed against these antigens coexist in the circulation for prolonged periods of time, predisposing to formation of immune complexes in the circulation, which then deposit in glomeruli causing glomerulonephritis and, rarely, in the extrarenal small vessels leading to cutaneous vasculitis. In contrast to APSGN, SAGN requires continued antigen production, and therefore continued active infection, to sustain the glomerular inflammation. If the staphylococcal infection is effectively treated, the activity of glomerulonephritis should eventually diminish.

A role for "superantigens" has been suggested for glomerulonephritis induced by methicillin-resistant *S. aureus* in which staphylococcal enterotoxins may act as superantigens, activating T cells which results in polyclonal B-cell activation and production of polyclonal IgA, IgG, and IgM. Some of these antibodies, often IgA, react with staphylococcal antigens. This may explain why glomerular immune deposits in patients with SAGN commonly show IgA dominant or codominant staining.

KEY READINGS

Koyama A et al: Glomerulonephritis associated with MRSA infection: a possible role of bacterial superantigen. Kidney Int 1995;47:207.

Nasr SH et al: Bacterial infection-related glomerulonephritis in adults. Kidney Int 2013;83:792.

Nasr SH et al: IgA-dominant acute poststaphylococcal glomerulonephritis complicating diabetic nephropathy. Hum Pathol 2003;34:1235.

Nasr SH et al: Postinfectious glomerulonephritis in the elderly. J Am Soc Nephrol 2011;22:95.

Satoskar AA et al: Staphylococcus infection-associated GN-spectrum of IgA staining and prevalence of ANCA in a single-center cohort. Clin J Am Soc Nephrol 2017;12:39.

INFECTIOUS ENDOCARDITIS-ASSOCIATED GLOMERULONEPHRITIS

General Considerations

In the United States, 10,000–15,000 cases of infective endocarditis are diagnosed every year. Male:female ratios range from 2:1 to 9:1 and the disease is increasingly frequent in elderly individuals and in patients with no underlying heart disease. Intravenous drug use, prosthetic heart valves, and structural heart disease are risk factors. Nosocomial endocarditis complicating bacteremia induced by invasive procedures or prosthetic devices may account for almost 10% of the cases of IE in some areas. Other less common predisposing conditions are HIV infection, immunosuppression, hemodialysis arteriovenous fistulas, central venous catheters, and ulcerative colitis (*Streptococcus bovis* endocarditis).

The average age of patients with endocarditis has increased to a current median age of 58 years. This change can be attributed to the decreasing prevalence of rheumatic heart disease, the increasing prevalence of underlying degenerative valve disease, and the increment of procedures and practices predisposing older patients to bacteremia. Isolated mitral or aortic valve is most common site of infection. *Streptococcus viridans* was the most common organism in the preantibiotic era and glomerulonephritis occurred in 50–80% of cases. With the use of prophylactic antibiotics in patients with valvular heart disease and the mounting frequency of intravenous drug abuse, *S. aureus* has replaced *S. viridans* as the leading cause of IE. The incidence of glomerulonephritis associated with *S. aureus* endocarditis ranges from 22% to 78%, with the higher figure consisting predominantly of intravenous drug users. Renal complications include infarcts, abscesses, and glomerulonephritis (all of which may coexist). In a study of 62 out of 354 patients with IE in whom kidney tissue was available for pathologic analysis (mostly autopsy tissue), localized infarcts were seen in 31%, half of which were septic; focal or diffuse glomerulonephritis in 26% of cases, of which many cases had vascular inflammation; interstitial nephritis, mostly attributable to antibiotics, in 10%; and cortical necrosis in 10%.

Clinical Findings

Recent series on IE-associated glomerulonephritis indicated a change in bacteriology, clinical features, and pathology of this disease compared to those described historically. It is now more common in older adults with a mean age at diagnosis of 48 years and about third of patients are elderly (≥60 years of age). There is male predominance (3.5:1). IE can be unrecognized at the time of nephrology consult (in up to 20% of patients). Predisposing conditions to endocarditis include intravenous drug use (29%), prosthetic valves (18%), and prior valvular disease (12%), although over half of patients do not have a known prior cardiac disease.

The cardiac valve infected in patients with IE-associated glomerulonephritis is tricuspid in 43%, mitral in 33%, and aortic in 29% of patients. IE-associated glomerulonephritis is twice as likely to be due to staphylococcus (53%, typically *S. aureus*) than Streptococcus (23%). Less common culprit pathogens include *Bartonella henselae, Coxiella burnetii, Cardiobacterium hominis, and Gemella.* Staphylococcal infection is by far the most common cause in association with intravenous drug abuse (77%), with the tricuspid valve affected in 83%.

A. Symptoms and Signs

The diagnosis of IE is usually suggested by the presentation of multiple clinical findings. A previous history of IE is obtained in 2–9% of the patients. The most common signs and symptoms in patients with IE-associated glomerulonephritis are fever and septic pulmonary emboli. Petechiae, splinter hemorrhages, intracranial hemorrhage, Osler's nodes, and conjunctival hemorrhage were seen in only a small minority of patients in recent series.

B. Laboratory Findings

Different from the other forms of bacterial infection-associated glomerulonephritis in which the most common presentation is nephritic syndrome, most (79%) patients with IE-associated glomerulonephritis present with rapidly progressive glomerulonephritis. The median serum creatinine concentration at diagnosis is 3.8 mg/dL. Almost all patients have hematuria. Proteinuria is common (median 1.8 g/day) but full nephrotic syndrome is exceptional. One-third of patients with IE-associated glomerulonephritis develop azotemia and the risk increases with age, previous history of hypertension, thrombocytopenia, and prosthetic valve infection.

The positive yield of blood cultures depends on the number of cultures taken from separate venipuncture sites (three cultures give 98%), the volume of blood (>5 mL of blood gives 92%), and the organism involved. The probability of endocarditis in patients with *S. aureus* bacteremia is particularly high. Other laboratory tests that are frequently positive in endocarditis are elevated erythrocyte sedimentation rate, normocytic normochromic anemia, and, especially in staphylococcal endocarditis, elevated white cell count.

Hypocomplementemia develops in 56% of patients (low C3 only in 37% of patients, low C3 and C4 in 16%, and low C4 only in 3%). ANA is positive in 15% of patients. ANCA seropositivity (P-ANCA or C-ANCA with equal frequency) has been reported in 28% of patients with IE-associated glomerulonephritis. High titers of rheumatoid factor, circulating immune complexes, and mixed cryoglobulins may also be present.

C. Kidney Biopsy

The most common pattern of glomerular injury in IE-associated glomerulonephritis is diffuse or focal crescentic

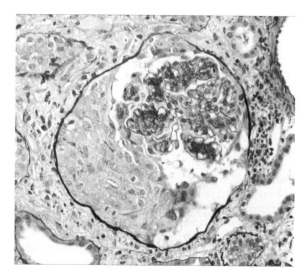

▲ **Figure 31–3.** Pathology of IE-associated glomerulonephritis: This case of IE-associated glomerulonephritis showed diffuse crescentic pattern on injury. The glomerulus shows a large cellular crescent. The underlying glomerular tuft exhibits mild mesangial and endocapillary hypercellularity (silver stain). (See Color Plate 4.)

glomerulonephritis (Figure 31–3) without associated endocapillary hypercellularity (53%). Diffuse endocapillary proliferative glomerulonephritis, with or without crescents, is present in 33% of patients and pure mesangial proliferative glomerulonephritis in 10% of patients. Active glomerulonephritis, particularly the crescentic variant, is usually associated with acute tubular injury, red blood cell casts and interstitial inflammation. Microabscesses and cortical necrosis are very rarely seen on renal biopsy nowadays.

On immunofluorescence, 94% of patients show dominant glomerular staining for C3, whereas glomerular positivity for IgG (27%), IgM (37%), and IgA (29%) is less common. In 37% of patients, isolated C3 glomerular staining is seen.

On electron microscopy, glomerular electron dense deposits are seen in 90% of patients, most commonly seen in the mesangium and the subendothelial space. Subepithelial humps are less common.

▶ Differential Diagnosis

IE-associated glomerulonephritis commonly exhibits a crescentic phenotype (occasionally with paucity of immune deposits) and about a quarter of cases are associated with ANCA seropositivity. Therefore, a major differential diagnosis in these cases is ANCA-associated pauci-immune crescentic glomerulonephritis. IE should be ruled out in patients presumed to have ANCA crescentic glomerulonephritis because of the attendant risks associated with immunosuppression. It remains unknown if positive ANCA serology in patients with IE are pathogenic or rather a secondary phenomenon triggered by the bacterial infection.

▶ Treatment

Antibiotic prophylaxis before dental procedures is recommended in patients at high risk for IE, including those with prosthetic heart valves, previous history of IE, or certain congenital heart defects (eg, cyanotic congenital heart disease that has not been fully repaired). Treatment of IE depends on the causative organisms and susceptibility results. Common to all therapies is the need to give antibiotic treatment for 4–6 weeks, which, when the antibiotic is appropriate, usually results in complete eradication of endocarditis with correction of serologic abnormalities. Preferred antibiotic selection is beyond the scope of the present work and requires determining bacterial resistance, but, in general, *S. viridans, bovis,* and other streptococcal species may be reliably treated with penicillin or ceftriaxone in allergic patients. Enterococci may be more successfully treated with a combination of antibiotics: penicillin or vancomycin (if there is a high level of penicillin resistance) in association with gentamycin. Native valve endocarditis due to *S. aureus* is best treated with nefcillin or oxacillin with perhaps the addition of gentamycin in the first few days of therapy. Standard treatment for methicillin-resistant staphylococci is vancomycin. For acutely ill patients with signs and symptoms strongly suggestive of IE, empiric therapy with vancomycin may be necessary after at least two sets of blood cultures have been obtained.

Immunosuppressive therapy should be avoided in most cases of IE-associated glomerulonephritis as it may worsen the infection. In patients with IE-associated glomerulonephritis with diffuse crescents/fibrinoid necrosis and positive ANCA serology in whom the infection is adequately treated but kidney function has not improved, a course of pulse steroids may be considered.

▶ Prognosis

The prognosis of IE depends on the severity and extent of the valvular damage and the infecting organism. Despite optimal care, 1 year mortality approaches 30%. Abnormal kidney findings, which include microscopic hematuria, proteinuria, and elevation of serum creatinine concentration, may persist for months after eradication of the infection. Normalization of C3 during the therapy correlates with a good outcome.

Immediate prognosis is generally good and is related to the prompt eradication of infection. In contrast, long-term prognosis is unknown. A recent study of IE-associated glomerulonephritis (38 patients followed for a mean of 25 months) reported that 32% of patients had complete kidney function recovery, 37% had persistent renal dysfunction, 10% progressed to ESRD, and 21% died. Patients with

a rapidly progressive course and severe crescentic phenotype have the worst prognosis.

▶ Pathogenesis

An immune complex mechanism is likely responsible for the production of this form of glomerulonephritis, particularly in cases characterized by glomerular deposition of immunoglobulins (IgG, IgA, and/or IgG) and C3. Support for this pathogenesis includes the demonstration of specific antibody in kidney eluates and detection of bacterial antigen in the deposits. Both *S. aureus* and hemolytic streptococcus antigens have been identified. Glomerular immune complex formation could result from passive trapping of immune complexes from the circulation or *in situ* formation following prior localization of exogenous cationic bacterial antigens.

However, in a significant percentage of cases of IE-associated glomerulonephritis, there is a paucity of immunoglobulin deposition, suggesting that glomerular immune complex formation may not be the principal pathogenic event in these cases. SPE B and other bacterial antigens independent of antibodies could activate the plasmin system or directly activate the alternative complement pathway through the mannose-lectin pathway (producing C3-dominant nephritis). In addition, *S. aureus* expresses "superantigens" that can also activate T cells directly.

KEY READINGS

Boils CL et al: Update on endocarditis-associated glomerulonephritis. Kidney Int 2015;87:1241.
Fernandez Guerrero ML et al: Infective endocarditis at autopsy: a review of pathologic manifestations and clinical correlates. Medicine (Baltimore) 2012;91:152.
Majumdar A et al: Renal pathological findings in infective endocarditis. Nephrol Dial Transplant 2000;15:1782.

SHUNT NEPHRITIS

▶ General Considerations

Shunt nephritis refers to an immune complex-mediated glomerulonephritis that develops as a complication of chronically infected ventriculoatrial or ventriculojugular shunts inserted for the treatment of hydrocephalus. The renal outcome of shunt nephritis is good if early diagnosis and treatment are provided. Ventriculovascular (VV) shunts may become infected in about 30% of cases. Glomerulonephritis may develop in 0.7–2% of the infected VV shunts in an interval of time ranging from 2 months to many years after insertion. *S. epidermidis* is the causative bacterium in about 70% of cases of shunt nephritis. Less common infective organisms include *Propionibacterium acne, S. aureus. Pseudomonas,* and *Serratia* spp. In contrast to VV shunts, ventriculoperitoneal shunts are rarely complicated with glomerulonephritis. Due to the wide clinical spectrum and indolent courses of shunt infections, the diagnosis is often delayed.

Clinical Findings

A. Symptoms and Signs

The clinical course typically consists of recurrent fever, weight loss, arthralgias, and frequently hepatosplenomegaly, in association with evidence of increased intracranial pressure. Hypertension is often present. However, signs of infection can be absent, resulting in a delay in diagnosis.

B. Laboratory Findings

Laboratory abnormalities indicative of kidney disease include hematuria (microscopic or gross), proteinuria (nephrotic syndrome in 30% of patients), and elevated serum creatinine concentration. Anemia, usually normochromic normocytic unless iron deficiency is also present, and elevated sedimentation rate and C-reactive protein levels are often present. Elevated titers of rheumatoid factor, cryoglobulinemia, hypocomplementemia (C3, C4, and CH50), and the presence of circulating immune complexes have all been demonstrated. Positive titers of ANCA specific for proteinase 3 have been reported in these patients.

C. Kidney Biopsy

Glomeruli typically exhibit membranoproliferative glomerulonephritis, but a mesangial proliferative pattern may occasionally be present. By immunofluorescence, granular mesangial and glomerular capillary wall positivity for IgG, IgM, and C3 is seen. On electron microscopy, mesangial and subendothelial electron dense deposits are present in most cases.

Treatment

Antibiotic therapy and prompt removal of the infected device usually lead to remission of the glomerulonephritis. However, cases of progressive chronic renal failure have been reported. Delay in the diagnosis and in the removal of the shunt worsens the prognosis of the renal lesion.

Pathogenesis

The presence of persistent antigenemia derived from an infectious agent likely stimulates immune complex formation which induces activation of the classical pathway of complement, which in turn mediates glomerular injury and local inflammation.

KEY READING

Haffner D et al: The clinical spectrum of shunt nephritis. Nephrol Dial Transplant 1997;12:1143.

■ CHAPTER REVIEW QUESTIONS

1. A 68-year-old male was admitted for management of pneumonia and septicemia. While in the hospital he developed acute kidney injury, hematuria, and subnephrotic proteinuria. He had depressed serum C3 and normal C4. ANA, ANCA, and hepatitis serologies were negative. Kidney biopsy performed showed endocapillary proliferative and exudative glomerulonephritis on light microscopy. Based on the immunofluorescence findings shown, blood cultures will likely grow one of the following pathogens:

(See Color Plate 5.)
A. *Chlamydia pneumoniae*
B. *Staphylococcus aureus*
C. *Legionella*
D. *Streptococcus pneumoniae*
E. *Mycoplasma pneumonia*

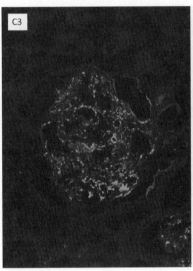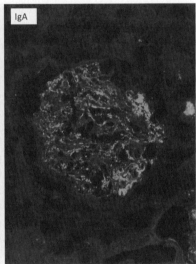

2. Which one of the following features favors IgA-dominant staphylococcus-associated glomerulonephritis over primary IgA nephropathy?
   A. Normal serum complement
   B. Concurrent respiratory tract infection
   C. Bright glomerular staining for C3 and IgA on immunofluorescence
   D. Subepithelial hump-shaped electron dense deposits on electron microscopy
   E. Mesangial proliferative glomerulonephritis on light microscopy

3. The depicted pattern of glomerular injury is more likely to be associated with one of the following types of bacterial infection:

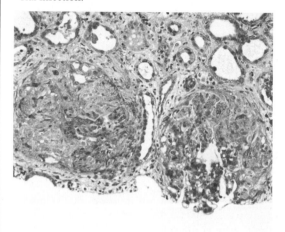

(See Color Plate 6.)
A. Upper respiratory tract infection
B. Cellulitis
C. Urinary tract infection
D. Shunt nephritis
E. Infectious endocarditis

4. One of the following statements is true with regards to bacterial infection-associated glomerulonephritis caused by streptococcus:
A. It typically occurs when the infection is still present
B. On immunofluorescence, there is almost always glomerular staining for C3 and IgG
C. The incidence of this disease is increasing worldwide
D. Renal biopsy confirmation is needed to establish the diagnosis in adults
E. Streptococcus is responsible for most cases of bacterial infection-associated glomerulonephritis in the elderly

5. One of the following statements is correct in shunt nephritis:
A. S. epidermidis is the causative bacterium in most patients
B. It is more commonly associated with ventriculo-peritoneal than ventriculovascular shunts
C. Most patients present with rapidly progressive glomerulonephritis
D. Renal biopsy typically shows endocapillary proliferative and exudative glomerulonephritis with glomerular positivity of C3, IgG, and IgM
E. Subepithelial hump-shaped deposits are seen on electron microscopy in most cases

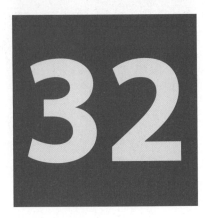

Vasculitides

Renu Regunathan-Shenk, MD

Jai Radhakrishnan, MD, MS

ESSENTIALS OF DIAGNOSIS

▸ Vasculitides affecting the kidneys are typically associated with hematuria and proteinuria, frequently presenting as a rapidly progressive glomerulonephritis.

▸ Glomerular injury occurs in the setting of the small vessel vasculitides, associated with antineutrophil cytoplasmic autoantibodies (ANCA), antiglomerular basement membrane antibodies (anti-GBM), or the presence of immune complex formation such as with Henoch–Schönlein purpura (HSP), cryoglobulinemic vasculitis, and systemic lupus erythematosus (SLE).

▸ They may affect the kidneys alone, but are more frequently part of a multiorgan disease that may affect the skin, upper and lower respiratory tracts, and the musculoskeletal, gastrointestinal, and nervous systems.

GENERAL CONSIDERATIONS

Vasculitides are inflammatory diseases of the blood vessels, which are typically classified by their size (Figure 32–1 and Table 32–1). The following sections will provide an overview of the various kinds of vasculitides. The remainder of this chapter will focus on small vessel vasculitis (SVV) because of its association with glomerulonephritis. The International Chapel Hill Consensus Conference (CHCC) has developed one of the most widely used nomenclature systems which specifies the names and definitions for most forms of vasculitis.

▶ Large Vessel Vasculitis

Large vessel vasculitis affects the aorta and its major branches. The acute phase of disease is characterized pathologically by granulomatous inflammation that often contains giant cells in the inflammatory infiltrates. Biopsy during the chronic phase demonstrates extensive vascular sclerosis with little or no active inflammation. Inflammatory and sclerotic thickening of the arteries causes narrowing of lumina, which in turn leads to ischemia and the resultant symptoms of claudication. Involvement of the renal artery may cause renovascular hypertension.

The two major large vessel vasculitides are Takayasu arteritis and giant cell arteritis. Takayasu arteritis most often involves the aorta and its major branches, although the pulmonary arteries may also be affected. Clinical manifestations include diminished pulses, vascular bruits, claudication, and renovascular hypertension. It is most commonly diagnosed on angiogram. An estimated 80–90% patients with the disease are female, and the disease is much more common in children and young adults, rarely occurring in patients over the age of 40. It is more prevalent in patients of Asian descent. The main treatment is steroids as well as other immunosuppressive medications; for large vessel damage, endovascular or surgical repair may be necessary.

Giant cell arteritis also affects the aorta and its major branches; however, it has a much greater predilection for the extracranial branches of the carotid artery. Common symptoms include headache, jaw claudication, blindness, deafness, tongue dysfunction, extremity claudication, and reduced peripheral pulses. Pathologic involvement of the renal artery is common in giant cell arteritis, but symptomatic renovascular hypertension is rare. Polymyalgia rheumatica occurs in 40–60% of patients with giant cell arteritis. The presence of polymyalgia rheumatica may be useful for diagnosis, but symptoms may occur before, simultaneously, or after the onset of giant cell arteritis. In contrast to Takayasu arteritis, giant cell arteritis rarely occurs in patients younger than 50 years and is most common in patients of northern European ethnicity. Treatment consists chiefly of steroid therapy.

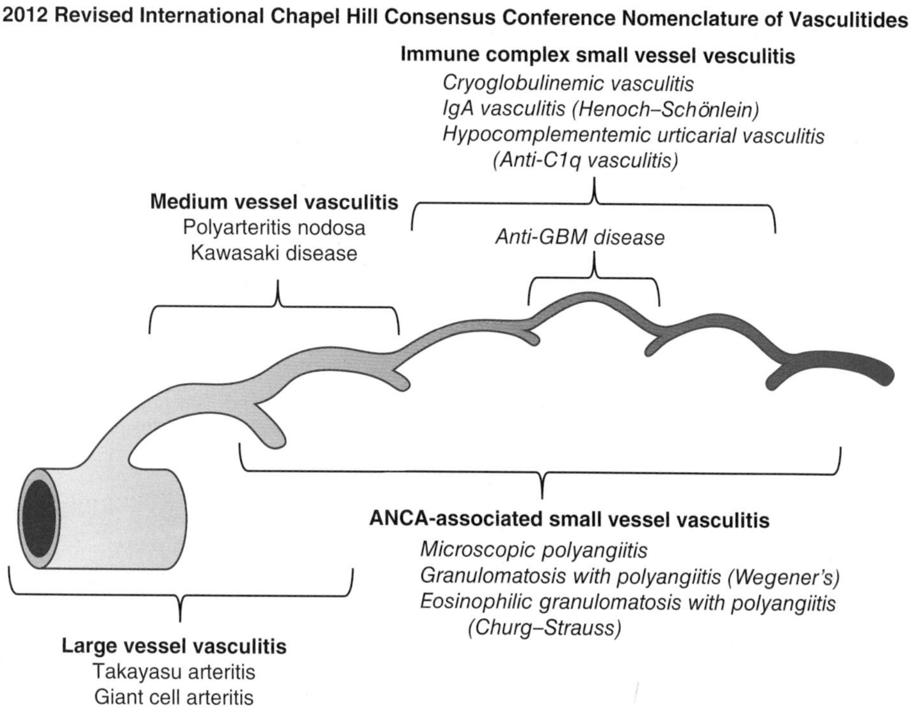

2012 Revised International Chapel Hill Consensus Conference Nomenclature of Vasculitides

Immune complex small vessel vesculitis
Cryoglobulinemic vasculitis
IgA vasculitis (Henoch–Schönlein)
Hypocomplementemic urticarial vasculitis
(Anti-C1q vasculitis)

Medium vessel vasculitis
Polyarteritis nodosa
Kawasaki disease

Anti-GBM disease

ANCA-associated small vessel vasculitis
Microscopic polyangiitis
Granulomatosis with polyangiitis (Wegener's)
Eosinophilic granulomatosis with polyangiitis
(Churg–Strauss)

Large vessel vasculitis
Takayasu arteritis
Giant cell arteritis

▲ **Figure 32–1.** Distribution of vessel involvement by large vessel vasculitis, medium vessel vasculitis, and SVV. Note that there is substantial overlap with respect to arterial involvement, and an important concept is that all three major categories of vasculitis can affect any size artery. Large vessel vasculitis affects large arteries more often than other vasculitides. Medium vessel vasculitis predominantly affects medium arteries. SVV predominantly affects small vessels, but medium arteries and veins may be affected, although immune complex SVV rarely affects arteries. Not shown is variable vessel vasculitis, which can affect any type of vessel, from aorta to veins. The diagram depicts (from left to right) aorta, large artery, medium artery, small artery/arteriole, capillary, venule, and vein. ANCA, antineutrophil cytoplasmic antibody; Anti-GBM, antiglomerular basement membrane. (Reproduced with permission from Jennette JC et al: 2012 revised International Chapel Hill Consensus Conference Nomenclature of Vasculitides. Arthritis Rheum 2013;65:1.)

▶ Medium-Sized Vessel Vasculitis

The medium-sized vessel vasculitides have a predilection for arteries that lead to major viscera and their initial branches. In the kidneys, the major targets are the interlobar and arcuate arteries, with less frequent involvement of the main renal artery and interlobular arteries. The two most common medium-sized vessel vasculitides are **polyarteritis nodosa (PAN)** and **Kawasaki disease**. Histologically, both are characterized in the acute phase by necrotizing arteritis with transmural inflammation that can lead to the formation of pseudoaneurysms. In just a few days, the lesions evolve from an acute neutrophil-rich inflammation to a "chronic" inflammation with mononuclear leukocyte predominance. Secondary complications of the arteritis include thrombosis,

infarction, and hemorrhage. Sites of thrombosis and necrosis also develop progressive scarring. Although medium sized vessel vasculitides do not cause glomerulonephritis by definition, they can cause hematuria, proteinuria (usually less than 2 g in 24 hours), and renal insufficiency as a result of renal infarction. Pseudoaneurysms near the renal surface may rupture and cause severe, even fatal, retroperitoneal and intraperitoneal hemorrhage.

Although the diagnostic term "polyarteritis nodosa" previously included all patients with any pattern of necrotizing arteritis, current classification distinguishes it from vasculitides that predominantly affect small arterioles, capillaries, and venules (such as microscopic polyangiitis). By this approach, the presence of glomerulonephritis or pulmonary alveolar capillaritis with pulmonary hemorrhage rules out a

Table 32–1. Names and definitions of vasculitis adopted by the Chapel Hill Consensus Conference on the nomenclature of systemic vasculitis.

Large vessel vasculitis[1]	
Giant cell arteritis	Granulomatous arteritis of the aorta and its major branches, with a predilection for the extracranial branches of the carotid artery. Often involves the *temporal artery*. Usually occurs in patients older than 50 years and often is associated with *polymyalgia rheumatica*.
Takayasu arteritis	Granulomatous inflammation of the aorta and its major branches. Usually occurs in patients younger than 50 years.
Medium-sized vessel vasculitis[1]	
Polyarteritis nodosa	Necrotizing inflammation of medium-sized or small arteries without glomerulonephritis or vasculitis in arterioles, capillaries, or venules.
Kawasaki disease	Arteritis involving large, medium-sized, and small arteries, and associated with mucocutaneous lymph node syndrome. *Coronary arteries are often involved*. Aorta and veins may be involved. Usually occurs in children.
Small vessel vasculitis[1]	
Granulomatosis with polyangiitis[2]	Granulomatous inflammation involving the respiratory tract, and necrotizing vasculitis affecting small to medium-sized vessels, eg, capillaries, venules, arterioles, and arteries. Necrotizing glomerulonephritis is common.
Eosinophilic granulomatosis with polyangiitis[2]	Eosinophil-rich and granulomatous inflammation involving the respiratory tract and necrotizing vasculitis affecting small to medium-sized vessels, and associated with *asthma and blood eosinophilia*.
Microscopic polyangiitis[2]	Necrotizing vasculitis with few or no immune deposits affecting small vessels, eg, capillaries, venules, or arterioles. Necrotizing arteritis involving small and medium-sized arteries may be present. Necrotizing glomerulonephritis is very common. Pulmonary capillaritis often occurs.
Henoch–Schönlein purpura	Vasculitis with IgA-dominant immune deposits affecting small vessels, eg, capillaries, venules, or arterioles. Typically involves skin, gut, and glomeruli and is associated with *arthralgias or arthritis*.
Cryoglobulinemic vasculitis	Vasculitis with cryoglobulin immune deposits affecting small vessels, eg, capillaries, venules, or arterioles, and associated with cryoglobulins in serum. *Skin and glomeruli are often involved*.
Cutaneous leukocytoclastic angiitis	Isolated cutaneous leukocytoclastic angiitis without systemic vasculitis or glomerulonephritis.

[1]"Large artery" refers to the aorta and the largest branches directed toward major body regions (eg, to the extremities and the head and neck); "medium-sized artery" refers to the main visceral arteries (eg, renal, hepatic, coronary, and mesenteric arteries); and "small artery" refers to the distal arterial radicals that connect with arterioles. Note that, large and medium-sized vessel vasculitides do not involve vessels other than arteries.
[2]Strongly associated with ANCA.
Reproduced with permission from Jennette JC et al: Nomenclature of systemic vasculitides. Proposal of an international consensus conference. Arthritis Rheum 1994;37(2):187.

diagnosis of PAN and indicates the presence of some type of SVV. Testing for ANCA is typically negative in PAN. About 30% of patients with PAN will test positive for chronic hepatitis B.

Kawasaki disease is an acute febrile illness of childhood that is characterized by mucocutaneous lymph node syndrome, which includes nonsuppurative lymphadenopathy, polymorphous erythematous rash, erythema of the oropharyngeal mucosa, erythema of the palms and soles, conjunctivitis, and indurative edema and desquamation of the extremities. The necrotizing arteritis of Kawasaki disease is pathologically indistinguishable from PAN. A major cause for morbidity and mortality in patients with Kawasaki disease is the development of a necrotizing arteritis with a predilection for coronary arteries. Symptomatic renal involvement is rare in this disease.

Because Kawasaki disease and PAN are treated differently, differentiation between the two arteritides is very important. The presence or absence of the mucocutaneous lymph node syndrome is an effective diagnostic discriminator. Kawasaki disease usually is treated with aspirin and intravenous γ-globulin therapy, with the goal to prevent coronary arteritis. Timely treatment with intravenous immunoglobulin (IVIG) and aspirin has been shown to reduce the incidence of cardiac lesions from 20–40% to <5%. Aspirin alone has not been shown to reduce cardiac sequelae but combined therapy with IVIG appears to have an additive anti-inflammatory effect. If the patient fails initial treatment, repeated doses of IVIG, pulse methylprednisolone, cyclophosphamide, methotrexate, cyclosporine, and plasmapheresis have been used. Recent data suggest that infliximab may be an alternative therapy for patients with refractory disease.

Idiopathic PAN is usually treated with high-dose corticosteroids and cyclophosphamide. This form of therapy has been shown to be beneficial, especially in those who have adverse prognostic factors. The optimal length of treatment is unknown, but a recent study has suggested that 6 months of therapy may be less effective than that of 12 months. For patients with hepatitis B virus-associated PAN, therapy with antiviral agents improves outcomes.

▶ Small Vessel Vasculitis

Small vessel vasculitides (SVV) are characterized by necrotizing inflammation primarily targeting venules and capillaries, although arteries, arterioles, and veins may also be involved. Unlike vasculitides of larger vascular beds, small vessel vasculitides frequently cause glomerulonephritis (Table 32–1).

The two major categories of SVV include the "pauci-immune small vessel vasculitides" and the "immune complex small vessel vasculitides" (Table 32–2). Immune complex vasculitides, such as **Henoch–Schönlein Purpura (HSP)**, **cryoglobulinemic vasculitis, lupus vasculitis**, and **anti-glomerular basement membrane (anti-GBM) vasculitis**, have

Table 32–2. Small vessel vasculitides.

Pauci-immune small vessel vasculitis (usually ANCA[1] positive)
Microscopic polyangiitis
Granulomatosis with Polyangiitis (formerly known as Wegener's Granulomatosis)
Eosinophilic Granulomatosis with Polyangiitis (formerly known as Churg–Strauss syndrome)
Drug-induced ANCA vasculitis
Immune complex small vessel vasculitis
Henoch–Schönlein purpura
Cryoglobulinemic vasculitis
Lupus vasculitis
Rheumatoid vasculitis
Goodpasture's syndrome
Serum sickness vasculitis
Hypocomplementemic urticarial vasculitis
Drug-induced immune complex vasculitis
Infection-induced immune complex vasculitis
Behçet's disease
Paraneoplastic small vessel vasculitis
Lymphoproliferative neoplasm-induced vasculitis
Carcinoma-induced vasculitis
Myeloproliferative neoplasm-induced vasculitis
Inflammatory bowel disease vasculitis

[1]ANCA, antineutrophil cytoplasmic autoantibodies.

extensive localization of immunoglobulin (Ig) and complement in vessel walls due to the deposition of circulating immune complexes or *in situ* immune complex formation between circulating antibodies and planted or constitutive antigens. In contrast, pauci-immune necrotizing small vessel vasculitides have little or no vascular wall localization of immunoglobulins. They often present with a necrotizing and crescentic glomerulonephritis, either alone or as a component of a systemic disease. Pauci-immune crescentic glomerulonephritis is the most common type of crescentic glomerulonephritis (Table 32–2).

The three major systemic pauci-immune small vessel vasculitides, known as Anti-Neutrophil Cytoplasmic Antibody (ANCA) associated vasculitis, are **microscopic polyangiitis (MPA), granulomatosis with polyangiitis (GPA)**, and **eosinophilic granulomatosis with polyangiitis (EGPA)**. MPA is a necrotizing angiitis involving capillaries, venules, and arterioles of the kidneys, lungs, skin, spleen, liver, heart, and muscle. Organ inflammation can occur simultaneously or individually. GPA, formerly known as Wegener granulomatosis, causes necrotizing granulomatous inflammation in the upper or lower respiratory tract and may occur without overt vasculitis. EGPA, formerly known as Churg–Strauss syndrome, occurs in patients with a history of asthma and eosinophilia, and causes an eosinophil-rich granulomatous inflammation of the vascular bed. The necrotizing glomerulonephritis and vasculitis found in all three diseases can be pathologically identical, characterized by segmental fibrinoid necrosis, crescent formation, and the absence of immunofluorescence staining. Given the heterogeneity of presentation of these diseases, many clinicians prefer to classify them by their serologic testing (discussed later in this chapter).

ANCA SVV predominantly affects older adults; in fact, a retrospective study of renal biopsy in the very elderly (over 80 years old) found that pauci-immune GN was the most common pathologic diagnosis, affecting nearly 20% of biopsied patients. It is more common in whites than in African–Americans, with a ratio of 7–8:1. Females and males are equally affected.

KEY READINGS

Burns JC et al: Infliximab treatment for refractory Kawasaki syndrome. J Pediatr 2005;146:662.

Guillevin L et al: Short-term corticosteroids then lamivudine and plasma exchanges to treat hepatitis B virus-related polyarteritis nodosa. Arthritis Rheum 2004;51:482.

Guillevin L et al: Treatment of polyarteritis nodosa and microscopic polyangiitis with poor prognosis factors: a prospective trial comparing glucocorticoids and six or twelve cyclophosphamide pulses in sixty-five patients. Arthritis Rheum 2003;49:93.

Jennette JC et al: 2012 revised International Chapel Hill Consensus Conference Nomenclature of Vasculitides. Arthritis Rheum 2013;65:1.

Moutzouris D-A et al: Renal biopsy in the very elderly. CJASN 2009;4:6.

Royle J et al: The diagnosis and management of Kawasaki disease. J Paediatr Child Health 2005;41:87.

PATHOGENESIS

Conceptually, vasculitides may be organized on the basis of three different mechanisms of injury: (1) Immune complex-mediated vasculitis, (2) direct antibody-mediated attack, or (3) pauci-immune necrotizing vasculitides. Immune complex vasculitis includes HSP, cryoglobulinemic vasculitis, rheumatoid vasculitis, and lupus vasculitis, and will be described in detail in other chapters. Direct antibody attack-mediated diseases include anti-GBM-mediated glomerulonephritis, Goodpasture syndrome, and Kawasaki disease. The pauci-immune small vessel vasculitides associated with ANCA will be the focus of this chapter.

CLINICAL FINDINGS

▶ Symptoms and Signs

Renal manifestations of ANCA SVV include microscopic hematuria (with dysmorphic RBCs and casts), proteinuria, and elevated creatinine. Proteinuria is usually moderate (2–3 g/day) but may be as much as 20 g/day. ANCA-associated glomerulonephritis frequently presents as a rapidly progressive glomerulonephritis, although the syndromes of asymptomatic hematuria with minimal amounts of proteinuria or acute nephritis are possible.

At least 50% of patients with ANCA associated glomerulonephritis have pulmonary disease spanning from fleeting alveolar infiltrates to severe life-threatening pulmonary hemorrhage. Massive pulmonary hemorrhage affects about 10% of patients with ANCA glomerulonephritis, and is associated with higher mortality. The evaluation of pulmonary disease in the setting of a glomerulonephritis must exclude the possibility of infection, especially when pulmonary infiltrates develop in the setting of prior or ongoing immunosuppressive treatment. Recurrent vasculitis must be differentiated from infectious etiologies, with special attention to opportunistic pathogens such as *Pneumocystis carinii*, *Mycobacterium tuberculosis*, and fungi. Bronchoscopy and bronchial alveolar lavage help differentiate infection from alveolar hemorrhage. Similarly, infections of the upper respiratory tract may mimic vasculitic lesions in the nose, sinus, and ear. Fiberoptic transillumination of the upper airways with biopsy may allow differentiation of vascular inflammation from infection.

Common dermatologic findings include palpable purpura (usually in the lower extremities), petechia, ulcers, nodules, urticaria, ecchymoses, and bullae. The typical neurologic manifestations of ANCA SVV are peripheral neuropathies (such as mononeuritis multiplex), while central nervous system involvement, specifically granulomatosis meningeal inflammation, is uncommon. Several other organ systems may also be involved. Gastrointestinal disease, which affects one-third of patients with ANCA SVV, may present with vasculitic ulcers of the small and large intestine causing bleeding or perforation. Iritis, uveitis, and episcleritis result in red, painful eyes. These lesions frequently present in a "subclinical" fashion and require slit-lamp ophthalmologic evaluation. Almost all patients have a prodrome of a "flu-like illness" with malaise, myalgias, and arthralgias that may last weeks to months prior to the development of more overt findings.

▶ Laboratory Findings

Testing for ANCA is useful in diagnosing pauci-immune SVV or renal-limited pauci-immune glomerulonephritis. ANCA reacts with constituents of neutrophils and monocytes. By indirect immunofluorescence microscopy on alcohol-fixed neutrophils, two patterns of staining can be distinguished: a cytoplasmic pattern (C-ANCA) and a perinuclear pattern (P-ANCA). The majority of C-ANCAs react with the lysosomal enzyme proteinase 3 (PR3). In necrotizing SVV, P-ANCA reacts with myeloperoxidase (MPO). Approximately 90% of patients with SVV will test positive for either MPO or PR3. PR3 has a high specificity and sensitivity for granulomatosis with polyangiitis, but as many as 20% of patients with disease may have MPO. MPO is more commonly found in patients with microscopic polyangiitis and eosinophilic granulomatosis with polyangiitis, but has been reported in other conditions such as lupus, rheumatoid arthritis, and inflammatory bowel disease. Thus, despite a predominance of antigenic specificity for each of the diseases, neither ANCA subtype completely differentiates between the three phenotypes of necrotizing vasculitis. Other tests that are elevated in settings of disease activity include the erythrocyte sedimentation rate (ESR) and the C-reactive protein (CRP).

▶ Special Tests

A. Monitoring Disease Activity

Physicians should evaluate disease activity clinically as well as through serologic markers. Clinical assessment tools used in research trials include the Birmingham Vasculitis Activity Score (BVAS), the Vasculitis Damage Index (VDI), and the SF-36 patient questionnaire, which monitors patient physical and mental function. These instruments may be helpful for clinicians to monitor patient symptoms (both renal and extrarenal) and response to therapy.

Serologic monitoring of ANCA titers has become common practice in the management of ANCA vasculitis, but should be exercised with caution, as the correlation between laboratory values and disease activity can be poor for some individuals. Clinical remission may occur in the setting of a persistently elevated ANCA titer, and conversely, clinical relapses occur in the setting of a persistently negative or low ANCA titer. Furthermore, what constitutes a clinically significant change in ANCA titer has been defined differently in various studies and remains to be determined for each of the various ANCA tests.

In a cohort study of patients with ANCA positive SVV with or without renal manifestations, rises in the ANCA titer correlated strongly with relapse in patients with renal involvement, but was less reliable in non-renal SVV. Two small retrospective studies suggest that patients with persistently elevated ANCA titers are more likely to suffer a relapse than patients with negative or declining titers. In a prospective study of patients with GPA, 0 of 9 patients preemptively treated with cyclophosphamide for 9 months after a more than or equal to 4-fold increase in titer suffered a relapse [versus 6 of 11 (55%) nontreated patients]. Of note, it is unclear when a relapse will occur in relation to a change in antibody titer; some relapses occurred more than a year after the rise in titer.

Given the risks of toxicity from treatment of ANCA disease, the decision to start treatment based on ANCA titer should be weighed carefully. A combination of clinical findings, urine and blood studies, and antibody titers should all be taken into account when considering a repeat course of immunosuppressive therapy.

B. Role of the Kidney Biopsy

Whether a renal biopsy is essential for the management of ANCA glomerulonephritis rests on the accuracy of the ANCA methodology, the risks associated with therapy, and the "pretest probability" based on the features of the patient's clinical syndrome. Based on a study of 1000 patients with proliferative and/or necrotizing glomerulonephritis, the sensitivity and specificity of ANCA for pauci-immune glomerulonephritis was 80% and 89% respectively, corresponding to a positive predictive value of 86%, a false-positive rate of 14%, and a false-negative rate of 16%. These results preclude the use of ANCA testing alone as the determinant for treatment. Conversely, if the pretest probability of ANCA vasculitis is high based on the presence of characteristic clinical findings, a positive ANCA test may be sufficient to establish a diagnosis of pauci-immune necrotizing glomerulonephritis. In the setting of a rapidly progressive glomerulonephritis, or a pulmonary-renal vasculitic syndrome, initiation of pulse methylprednisolone and consideration of plasmapheresis should not be delayed until a biopsy result is obtained, as prompt initiation of treatment is an essential determinant of outcome. Renal biopsy should nevertheless be pursued, if possible, to assess disease activity and confirm diagnosis.

KEY READINGS

Han WK et al: Serial ANCA titers: useful tool for prevention of relapses in ANCA-associated vasculitis. Kidney Int 2003;63:1079.

Kemna MJ et al: ANCA as a predictor of relapse: useful in patients with renal involvement but not in patients with nonrenal disease. J Am Soc Nephrol 2015;26:537.

Langford CA: Antineutrophil cytoplasmic antibodies should not be used to guide treatment in Wegener's granulomatosis. Clin Exp Rheumatol 2004;22:S3.

Slot MC et al: Positive classic antineutrophil cytoplasmic antibody (C-ANCA) titer at switch to azathioprine therapy associated with relapse in proteinase 3-related vasculitis. Arthritis Rheum 2004;51:269.

DIFFERENTIAL DIAGNOSIS

The differential diagnosis of ANCA-associated pauci-immune SVV also includes direct antibody-mediated and immune complex SVV. Despite a great deal of overlap in organ system involvement among different types of small vessel vasculitides, certain clinical serologic, and histologic features—described in Tables 32–3 and 32–4—differentiate among MPA, GPA, EGPA, cryoglobulinemic vasculitis, and HSP. Testing for ANCA, anti-GBM, cryoglobulins, hepatitis C or B, ANA, and complement component levels helps focus the potential etiologies. Direct immunofluorescence microscopy of vessels in biopsy specimens, such as glomerular capillaries or dermal venules, demonstrates IgA-dominant vascular Ig deposits in HSP, IgG, and IgM deposits in cryoglobulinemic vasculitis, and little or no Ig in pauci-immune SVV.

The differential diagnosis of rapidly progressing glomerulonephritis includes lupus nephritis, anti-GBM disease, IgA nephropathy, HSP, and ANCA SVV. Patients with thrombotic microangiopathies may present with a picture that mimics necrotizing glomerulonephritis. However, these patients do not demonstrate MPO- or PR3-ANCA positivity and have biopsy features typical of a microangiopathic hemolytic disease. About 20% of patients with anti-GBM disease may concomitantly express ANCA.

Drug induced vasculitis should be considered in patients on hydralazine, methimazole, propylthiouracil, and in cocaine users. Many patients with drug induced ANCA SVV will demonstrate dual positivity for MPO and PR3 as well as other positive serologic testing (such as positive ANA).

COMPLICATIONS

The very nature of systemic SVV exposes patients to a number of potential complications as a result of the disease itself or its therapy. Patients may suffer from end stage renal disease (ESRD), chronic pulmonary dysfunction, hearing loss, destructive sinus disease, proptosis, motor or sensory neurologic deficits, and blindness.

Table 32–3. Comparison of approximate frequency of manifestations of microscopic polyangiitis with other forms of small vessel vasculitis.

	Pauci-Immune			Immune Complex	
	Microscopic Polyangiitis (%)	GPA (%)	EGPA Syndrome (%)	Henoch–Schönlein Purpura (%)	Cryoglobulinemic Vasculitis (%)
Cutaneous	40	40	60	90	90
Renal	90	80	45	50	55
Pulmonary	50	90	70	<5	<5
Ear, nose, and throat	35	90	50	<5	<5
Musculoskeletal	60	60	50	75	70
Neurologic	30	50	70	10	40
Gastrointestinal	50	50	50	60	30

Adapted from Jennette JC, Falk RJ: Small vessel vasculitis. N Engl J Med 1997;337:1512.

ANCA vasculitis can present with acute life-threatening manifestations. Diffuse pulmonary hemorrhage causes gross hemoptysis and respiratory failure requiring mechanical ventilation. It is associated with a 50% mortality rate without the use of plasmapheresis (in addition to immunosuppressive therapy). Patients with granulomatosis with polyangiitis may also present with acute critical subglottic stenosis causing stridor and respiratory failure, and often require emergency tracheostomy. Unfortunately, surgical interventions on the trachea in this disease are characterized by poor healing and scarring, requiring repeat interventions. For this reason, early detection of subglottic involvement and the prompt institution of intralesional as well as systemic corticosteroids and immunosuppressant therapy are essential to avoid surgery or tracheostomy.

ESRD may be the result of the acute injury or from progressive scarring. In a cohort of 350 patients with ANCA vasculitis, 22% of patients presented with or reached ESRD

Table 32–4. Differentiation among various small vessel vasculitides.

	Immune Complex		Pauci-Immune		
	Henoch–Schönlein Purpura	Cryoglobulinemic Vasculitis	Microscopic Polyangiitis	GPA (Wegener Granulomatosis)	EGPA (Churg–Strauss Syndrome)
Small vessel vasculitis signs and symptoms[1]	+	+	+	+	+
IgA-dominant immune deposits	+	–	–	–	–
Cryoglobulins in blood and vessels	–	+	–	–	–
ANCA in blood	–	–	+	+	+
Necrotizing granulomas	–	–	–	+	+
Asthma and eosinophilia	–	–	–	–	–

[1]All of these small vessel vasculitides can manifest any or all of the shared features of small vessel vasculitides, such as purpura, nephritis, abdominal pain, peripheral neuropathy, myalgias, and arthralgias. Each is distinguished by the presence and just as importantly the absence of certain specific features.
ANCA, antineutrophil cytoplasmic autoantibodies.
Adapted from Jennette JC, Falk R: Small vessel vasculitis. N Engl J Med 1997;337:1512.

within 2 months of presentation. In addition, 10% of patients who responded to initial therapy later progressed to ESRD in a median of 106 months without clinical evidence of disease relapse. Of note, many patients with ANCA related renal disease may require dialysis at presentation; however, nearly all who recover will do so within the first 3 months of treatment.

Perhaps less recognized is the increased risk of venous thrombotic disease among patients with GPA. This was illustrated in a recent large clinical trial that detected an incidence of venous thrombosis of 7 per 100 patient-years, with 75% of the events occurring at the time of, or shortly preceding, clinically active vasculitis.

The complications met during the course of vasculitis are often iatrogenic. Common to all forms of immunosuppression is the risk of serious infections including bacterial, viral, and fungal opportunistic organisms. The risk of serious infection is compounded by treatment-related neutropenia, which may occur in up to 55% of patients treated with cyclophosphamide or azathioprine. Monthly pulse cyclophosphamide substantially lowers the risk of neutropenia and associated infections compared with daily oral regimens.

Treatment with cyclophosphamide is also associated with long-term risks of infertility, in both men and women, and malignancies, especially cutaneous, hematologic, and urothelial cancers. These risks are commensurate with the cumulative dose of cyclophosphamide and other cytotoxic or antimetabolite therapies received during the course of treatment. Glucocorticoid use is associated with multiple short- and long-term complications including weight gain, diabetes mellitus, osteoporosis, avascular necrosis of bone, myopathy, and cataracts. Rituximab is generally well tolerated, but has been associated with reactivation of hepatitis B and tuberculosis.

KEY READINGS

Gluth MB et al: Subglottic stenosis associated with Wegener's granulomatosis. Laryngoscope 2003;113:1304.

Hoffman GS et al: Treatment of subglottic stenosis, due to Wegener's granulomatosis, with intralesional corticosteroids and dilation. J Rheumatol 2003;30:1017.

Jayne D et al: A randomized trial of maintenance therapy for vasculitis associated with antineutrophil cytoplasmic autoantibodies. N Engl J Med 2003;349:36.

Klemmer PJ et al: Plasmapheresis therapy for diffuse alveolar hemorrhage in patients with small-vessel vasculitis. Am J Kidney Dis 2003;42:1149.

Knight A et al: Urinary bladder cancer in Wegener's granulomatosis: risks and relation to cyclophosphamide. Ann Rheum Dis 2004;63:1307.

Merkel PA et al: Brief communication: high incidence of venous thrombotic events among patients with Wegener granulomatosis: the Wegener's Clinical Occurrence of Thrombosis (WeCLOT) Study. Ann Intern Med 2005;142:620.

TREATMENT

▶ Induction Therapy

The current KDIGO guidelines recommend a combination of corticosteroids and cyclophosphamide as first line therapy for ANCA vasculitis, with rituximab as an alternative in patients without severe disease (or for whom cyclophosphamide is contraindicated). Treatment studies in moderate ANCA disease have demonstrated that rituximab is non-inferior to cyclophosphamide for induction therapy. Plasmapheresis is recommended for patients with rapidly rising creatinine (or requiring dialysis), diffuse pulmonary hemorrhage, and concomitant anti-GBM disease.

Steroid therapy has a rapid anti-inflammatory effect and may reduce the amount of antibody producing plasma cells. Recommended initial steroid therapy includes a 3-day course of intravenous methylprednisolone (500 mg) daily, then oral prednisone (1 mg/kg/day) for 1 month, not to exceed 60 mg daily. After at least 2 months of treatment, it is recommended to taper the dose with the goal to terminate steroids after 6 months.

Several studies have shown that plasmapheresis effectively treats diffuse alveolar hemorrhage and limits pulmonary toxicity. In addition, the MEPEX trial examined the utility of plasma exchange in newly diagnosed patients with ANCA associated glomerulonephritis and a serum creatinine above 5.8 mg/dL (>500 µmol/L). Patients were randomized to initial therapy with pulse IV methylprednisolone or seven rounds of plasma exchange; both groups subsequently received oral cyclophosphamide and prednisone. At 3 months, 69% of patients who received plasmapheresis were alive and dialysis independent, compared with 49% of patients randomized to steroids ($p < 0.02$) and plasma exchange was associated with a reduction in risk of progression to ESRD (from 43% to 19%) at 1 year. However, over a median follow-up period of 3.95 years, the group receiving plasma exchange was similar in terms of the primary outcome of ESRD or death compared to IV methylprednisolone; hazard ratio 0.81 (95% confidence interval 0.53–1.23).

Cyclophosphamide is administered either by monthly intravenous pulses (0.5–1 g/m^2) or orally (1–2 mg/kg/day). Patients treated with either intravenous or oral cyclophosphamide have a long-term remission rate of 60–85%. In general, the intravenous regimen allows for 2–3 times smaller total dose of cyclophosphamide than the oral regimen with equal effectiveness in inducing disease remission. In prospective and retrospective analyses, intravenous therapy was associated with a significant decrease in the rate of clinically significant neutropenia and other complications. All forms of cyclophosphamide dosage should be titrated to keep the nadir leukocyte count more than 3000 cells/mm^2. In a meta-analysis of three randomized controlled trials comparing pulse versus oral continuous cyclophosphamide, intravenous cyclophosphamide also resulted in a statistically higher rate of remission (odds ratio for failure to achieve remission 0.29; 95% CI 0.12–0.73) and lower rates of leukopenia (odds ratio 0.36; 95% CI 0.17–0.78) and infections (odds ratio 0.45; 95% CI 0.23–0.89). The final outcomes of patients (death or ESRD) were no different in the two groups despite a (statistically not significant) lower rate of relapse in the oral cyclophosphamide group.

The optimum length of therapy with cyclophosphamide has not been determined and is the subject of ongoing controversy. In patients achieving complete remission within 6 months of therapy, treatment can be stopped with the institution of close patient follow-up. In those individuals with persistently active disease at 6 months, it is reasonable to continue cyclophosphamide therapy for a full 12 months. An alternative regimen consists of switching cyclophosphamide to oral azathioprine at the end of 3 months if the patient is in remission. Azathioprine is then continued for 18 months. This regimen offers the advantage of a limited use of cyclophosphamide and results in rates of remission and relapse similar to the cyclophosphamide-only-based therapies.

Two large randomized controlled trials demonstrated that rituximab therapy was non-inferior to cyclophosphamide for initial treatment of mild to moderate ANCA disease. The RAVE trial included 197 patients who were randomized to either rituxmab or oral cyclophosphamide. Of note, the mean creatinine clearance of the participants was 62 mL/min, indicating moderate renal disease. Patients achieved similar rates of remission, as well as similar rates of serious adverse events and deaths. The RITUXIVAS trial compared a combination of rituximab and intravenous cyclophosphamide with intravenous cyclophosphamide alone in a smaller group of patients with a median eGFR of 18 mL/min/1.73m^2. Remission, adverse events, and death rates were also similar amongst the study and control groups.

Maintenance Treatment Strategies

Expert consensus recommends at least 18 months of maintenance therapy for patients who achieve remission and against further therapy in patients who progress to ESRD (without extrarenal manifestations of disease). The goal of maintenance therapy is to reduce the incidence and severity of potential relapse. Patients who suffer recurrence are at risk for progression to ESRD as well as serious pulmonary complications. While some studies sustained patients on low-dose prednisone (such as 7.5 mg daily) for over 1 year, there are several preferred non-steroidal therapies described in this section.

The KDIGO preferred maintenance agent is azathioprine, dosed at 1–2 mg/kg/day. In a study comparing it to oral cyclophosphamide, it was equally effective in preventing relapse. Patients who are unable to tolerate azathioprine can alternatively use mycophenolate mofetil 1 g twice daily. It should be noted that in a large trial comparing long-term

therapy with azathioprine or mycophenolate mofetil, there was a higher relapse rate in the mycophenolate group, thus the drug should be reserved for patients unable to take azathioprine. For patients intolerant to both antimetabolites, methotrexate is another option, but should be used with caution in patients with estimated GFR below 60 due to the risk of renal toxicity. In a large randomized control trial comparing methotrexate to azathioprine, there was no difference in the rate of relapse; however, there was a higher rate of adverse events in the methotrexate group. In patients with upper respiratory tract disease, additional therapy with sulfamethoxazole-trimethoprim should be considered as it has been shown to decrease the rate of recurrent pulmonary disease. When used as a single agent, sulfamethoxazole-trimethoprim has not been shown to successfully prevent disease recurrence outside of the respiratory tract.

Rituximab is emerging as a potentially more effective maintenance therapy over azathioprine. In a study of 115 patients with GPA, MPA, and renal limited ANCA disease who achieved remission with a combination of glucocorticoids and cyclophosphamide, patients randomized to rituximab infusions were less likely to relapse than patients randomized to azathioprine (hazard ratio 6.61, $p = 0.002$). Rates of serious adverse events were similar between the two groups. Further studies are planned to investigate the use of rituximab for maintenance therapy.

Transplantation

As many patients with ANCA SVV will progress to ESRD, the option of renal transplantation should also be carefully considered. Expert consensus suggests that transplantation be delayed until a patient has achieved a complete remission for 1 year, although controversy exists as to the optimal timing for transplant. The presence of circulating ANCA at the time of transplant does not increase the risk of recurrent disease, thus transplantation should not be delayed until a negative ANCA serology is attained.

Recurrence of ANCA vasculitis after renal transplantation occurs in about 10% of patients. Time to recurrence varies widely, from a few days to several years post-transplantation. Patients with PR3 related disease appear more likely to relapse than patients with MPO related disease. In the majority of reported cases, recurrent disease after transplantation responded well to treatment with cyclophosphamide and pulse corticosteroids. Patient and graft survival rates are similar to other non-diabetic kidney disease, with a 5-year survival of 92% and 88% respectively, and a 10-year survival of 68% and 67%, respectively.

Supportive Therapy

As corticosteroids and cyclophosphamide remain the cornerstone of therapy of ANCA SVV, special effort must be exercised to minimize the short- and long-term complications of treatment. Whenever corticosteroids are used, the development of osteoporosis can be minimized with the early institution of calcium and vitamin D supplementation, and in patients with established osteoporosis, calcitonin or bisphosphonates (if not contraindicated by renal failure or esophagitis). Rigorous control of blood pressure with sodium restriction and antihypertensive therapy is essential to minimize the additive effect of hypertension in loss of renal function following active nephritis. Hormonal manipulation during cytotoxic therapy may allow the preservation of gonadal function. The prevention of cyclophosphamide-induced infertility was reported with the use of testosterone in men and leuprolide in women.

KEY READINGS

Booth A et al: Prospective study of TNF alpha blockade with infliximab in anti-neutrophil cytoplasmic antibody-associated systemic vasculitis. J Am Soc Nephrol 2004;15:717.

de Groot K et al: Randomized trial of cyclophosphamide versus methotrexate for induction of remission in early systemic anti-neutrophil cytoplasmic antibody-associated vasculitis. Arthritis Rheum 2005;52:2461.

Guillevin L et al: Rituximab versus azathioprine for maintenance in ANCA-associated vasculitis. N Engl J Med 2014; 371:1771.

Jayne D et al: Randomized trial of plasma exchange or high dose methylprednisolone as adjunctive therapy for severe renal vasculitis. J Am Soc Nephrol 2007;18:2180.

Jones RB et al: Rituximab versus cyclophosphamide in ANCA-associated renal vasculitis. N Engl J Med 2010;363:211.

Langford CA et al: Mycophenolate mofetil for remission maintenance in the treatment of Wegener's granulomatosis. Arthritis Rheum 2004;51:278.

Metzler C et al: Maintenance of remission with leflunomide in Wegener's granulomatosis. Rheumatology (Oxford) 2004;43:315.

Moran S, Little MA. Renal transplantation in antineutrophil cytoplasmic antibody-associated vasculitis. Curr Opin Rheum 2014;26:37.

Specks U: Methotrexate for Wegener's granulomatosis: what is the evidence? Arthritis Rheum 2005;52:2237.

Stone JH et al: Rituximab versus cyclophosphamide for ANCA-associated vasculitis. N Engl J Med 2010;363:221.

PROGNOSIS

Untreated, systemic vasculitis is associated with an 80% mortality at 1 year. The introduction of steroids, azathioprine, cyclophosphamide, and rituximab have led to a marked improvement in survival; however, patients with SVV still have a significantly higher mortality rate than the general population (estimated 24–44% at 4–10 years). Predictors of death include increasing age and creatinine at presentation, disease extent and severity at diagnosis, pulmonary hemorrhage, progression to ESRD, and treatment-related infection. Presence of relapse has not been shown to increase mortality. Common causes of death include infection, pulmonary failure, renal failure, and cardiovascular disease.

Response to Treatment

The terms "remission" and "relapse" are defined in Table 32–5. Patients treated with either intravenous or oral cyclophosphamide have a long-term remission rate of between 70% and 92%. Based on a large observational cohort of 350 patients with ANCA vasculitis, female gender, black race, and potentially older age were associated with a higher likelihood of treatment resistance. Whether socioeconomic factors and access to health care account for these differences in response to treatment is unknown.

Relapse

The risk of relapse after an initial response to treatment is of the order of 40%, but reports vary between 11% and 57%. The risk of relapse is not uniform among all patients with ANCA vasculitis. An increased risk of relapse has been associated with a diagnosis of GPA (as opposed to MPA). Based on a multivariate analysis of 258 patients, the presence of PR3-ANCA and lung and upper respiratory tract involvement were independent risk factors for relapse. Among patients presenting with none of the three risk factors, 26% relapsed in a median of 62 months (the median among those who relapsed was 20 months). In contrast, 47% of the patients presenting with a single risk factor experienced

Table 32–5. Criteria for treatment response.

Remission: Stabilization or improvement of the renal function (as measured by serum creatinine), resolution of hematuria, and resolution of extrarenal manifestations of systemic vasculitis. Persistence of proteinuria was not considered indicative of persistence of disease activity.

Remission on therapy: The achievement of remission while still receiving immunosuppressive medication or corticosteroids given at a dose greater than 7.5 mg/day of prednisone or its equivalent.

Treatment resistance: (1) Progressive decline in renal function with the persistence of an active urine sediment, or (2) persistence or new appearance of any extrarenal manifestation of vasculitis despite immunosuppressive therapy.

Relapse: Occurrence of at least one of the following: (1) rapid rise in serum creatinine accompanied by an active urine sediment; (2) a renal biopsy demonstrating active necrosis or crescent formation; (3) hemoptysis, pulmonary hemorrhage, or new or expanding nodules without evidence for infection; (4) active vasculitis of the respiratory or gastrointestinal tracts as demonstrated by endoscopy with biopsy; (5) iritis or uveitis; (6) new mononeuritis multiplex; (7) necrotizing vasculitis identified by biopsy in any tissue.

Data from Nachman PH et al: Treatment response and relapse in antineutrophil cytoplasmic autoantibody-associated microscopic polyangiitis and glomerulonephritis. J Am Soc Nephrol 1996;7:33.

a relapse in a median of 39 months (corresponding to a 2-fold increased risk for relapse; 95% CI: 1.1, 3.9, $p = 0.038$). Among patients presenting with all three risk factors, 73% relapsed in a median of 17 months (median time to relapse among those who relapsed was 15 months), corresponding to a 3.7 times increased risk of relapse (95% CI: 1.4, 9.7, $p = 0.007$) compared to those with no risk factor.

Relapse typically occurs in the same organ system initially affected by the disease, although new organ system involvement can also develop. Relapses in the kidney are heralded by the recurrence of microscopic hematuria, red blood cell casts, and worsening renal function. Fluctuations in the amount of proteinuria are not good indicators of active disease as they may be related to glomerulosclerosis rather than active disease.

Fortunately, a similar rate of response is achieved in the treatment of relapse and initial disease. Full vasculitic relapse should be treated with a repeat course of induction therapy, with steroids, consideration of plasmapheresis, and either cyclophosphamide or rituximab. Rituximab is emerging as a better treatment for recurrent disease over cyclophosphamide, as a subgroup analysis of the RAVE study showed that rituximab was more effective in treating relapsed disease than cyclophosphamide. How to best treat milder relapses is a matter of substantial investigation. In an effort to limit the exposure of relapsing patients to repetitive cycles of cytotoxic drugs and their associated risks, alternative or adjunctive, less toxic therapies are being evaluated.

▶ **Prognostic Factors**

Several studies have examined the question of prognostic factors in ANCA SVV. The presence of pulmonary hemorrhage is the most important determinant of patient survival, whereas other pulmonary findings (eg, infiltrates, nodules, or cavities) did not increase the risk of death. The risk of ESRD is largely determined by the degree of renal dysfunction at the time of diagnosis. Serum creatinine is the single most important prognostic marker for long-term renal outcome as exemplified by a 1.24-fold increased risk for ESRD for each 1 mg/dL increase in serum creatinine at baseline. Nevertheless, there is no threshold of initial renal dysfunction below which treatment is futile, as remission occurs in 57% of individuals with an estimated GFR less than 10 mL/min. Histopathologic measures of chronic renal scarring (glomerulosclerosis, interstitial fibrosis, and tubular atrophy) have consistently been associated with poor renal outcomes. The impact of renal damage as a predictor of resistance emphasizes the importance of early diagnosis and prompt institution of therapy.

KEY READINGS

Booth AD et al: Outcome of ANCA-associated renal vasculitis: a 5-year retrospective study. Am J Kidney Dis 2003;41:776.

Booth AD et al: Renal vasculitis—an update in 2004. Nephrol Dial Transplant 2004;19:1964.

Hogan SL et al: Predictors of relapse and treatment resistance in antineutrophil cytoplasmic antibody-associated small-vessel vasculitis. Ann Intern Med 2005;8:1709.

Sanders JS et al: Risk factors for relapse in anti-neutrophil cytoplasmic antibody (ANCA)-associated vasculitis: tools for treatment decisions? Clin Exp Rheumatol 2004;22:S94.

Stone JH et al: Rituximab versus cyclophosphamide for ANCA-associated vasculitis. N Engl J Med 2010;363:221.

■ CHAPTER REVIEW QUESTIONS

1. A 40-year-old previously healthy woman presents to her primary care physician with night sweats, weight loss, joint pain, and fatigue for 4–5 weeks. On examination she is normotensive and afebrile. Her physical examination is normal. Laboratory testing shows 1+ protein and 30–40 RBC/HPF in the urine, serum creatinine 1.8 mg/dL, ESR 80 mm/hour, urine cultures negative. She is referred to a nephrologist who notes that only a PR3 ANCA is positive at 40 U/mL (negative <0.4 U/mL), with negative antiglomerular basement antibody, negative lupus profile, negative workup for monoclonal gammopathy, and normal complements.

The kidney biopsy is likely to show which of the following immune staining patterns in this patient?
A. Negative immune staining
B. Linear glomerular basement staining
C. Granular staining for IgG, IgA, IgM, C3, and C1q along the capillary wall
D. Staining with IgG and only kappa light chain along the basement membrane

2. A 55-year-old man, with past medical history of coronary artery disease requiring percutaneous intervention is admitted with low-grade fevers and arthralgia for 2 weeks prior to admission. His admission vital signs show normal BP, temperature of 99°F, and physical examination is notable for few petechiae over his lower extremities. His laboratory tests show mild normocytic anemia with hemoglobin 9 g/dL, serum creatinine 2.5 mg/dL, urinalysis with 2+ proteinuria and 10–15 RBC. His serological tests show negative antiglomerular basement membrane antibody, positive myeloperoxidase ANCA, normal complements, and negative lupus serologies. Electrocardiogram shows an old inferior wall infarct. A kidney biopsy is performed and results are pending. After 72 hours of admission, he develops frank hemoptysis and develops respiratory distress requiring intubation. He is noted to have frank blood from his endotracheal tube. His chest X-ray shows diffuse bilateral opacities. His echocardiogram shows wall motion abnormalities in the inferior wall and troponin levels are normal.

What is your next step in management for this patient?
A. Perform a bronchoscopy
B. Start pulse steroids and plasmapheresis
C. Left and right heart catheterization
D. Await results of kidney biopsy

3. A 70-year-old man is being treated with monthly intravenous cyclophosphamide and corticosteroids for a relapse of PR3-ANCA-associated vasculitis. This is his 3rd relapse over 5 years and manifested mainly with joint pain, myalgias, and worsening hematuria and proteinuria in the setting of rising PR3-ANCA titers. Three months into his treatment, he noted shortness of breath with low-grade fevers and sweats. The dyspnea now occurs at rest and he is admitted for workup. On examination his breathing is labored, his vital show a temperature of 100°F and oxygen saturation on room air is 88%. His physical examination reveals bilateral crackles on lung examination, but is otherwise normal. His laboratory tests show elevated WBC count 15×10^9/L, Hb 8.8 g/dL and normal platelets. His PR3-ANCA titers are positive but 50% lower than at the time of relapse. His urinalysis is normal and creatinine is at baseline. His chest X-ray shows reticulonodular opacities bilaterally.

What is your next step in management for this patient?
A. Pulse steroids
B. Plasmapheresis
C. Bronchoscopy
D. Lung biopsy

4. A 50-year-old woman with past medical history of hypertension, asthma, and non-ischemic cardiomyopathy was admitted with worsening kidney function. One month prior to admission, she developed a sore throat with myalgias, low-grade fevers and chest congestion that persisted until the time of admission. Her home medications include carvedilol, hydralazine, losartan, albuterol, spironolactone, montelukast, trazodone, atorvastatin, and famotidine.

Her physical examination was notable for BP 150/90 and bilateral mild pedal edema but was otherwise normal. Serum creatinine was 1.5 mg/dL (increased from her baseline of 1.07 mg/dL. UPr/Cr is 4.9 g/g, serum albumin 3.1 g/dL and hemogram showed total WBC count 5×10^9/L, hemoglobin 7.9 g/dL, and platelets 176 $\times 10^9$/L. Her serological tests were notable for elevated MPO ANCA, positive ANA, positive anti-histone IgG, positive SSA, and positive SSB, and borderline elevated anti-dsDNA antibody. Her antiglomerular basement antibody, HIV antibody, serum-free light chains ratio, complements C3 and C4, anti-streptolysin-O, anti-PR3 ANCA, hepatitis panel, urine culture, and blood culture were all normal or negative. Her chest X-ray shows cardiomegaly and normal lung fields. A kidney biopsy showed diffuse crescentic necrotizing glomerulonephritis without any antibody staining ("pauci immune").

What is the most likely underlying reason for this patient's clinical syndrome?
A. Cardiomyopathy (cardiorenal syndrome)
B. Sarcoidosis
C. Hydralazine
D. Upper respiratory infection

5. A 60-year-old woman with PR3-ANCA associated vasculitis is being seen for follow-up. She presented 4 months ago with rapidly progressive renal failure (peak serum creatinine 4.5 mg/dL, vasculitic skin lesions, and hemoptysis. She was treated with pulse steroids, plasma exchange and intravenous cyclophosphamide. At the present time she has no symptoms. She is taking prednisone 5 mg daily and she received her fourth dose of intravenous cyclophosphamide 2 weeks ago. Her physical examination is normal. Laboratory tests are notable for normal hemogram, serum creatinine 1.8 mg/dL, normal urinalysis, normal sedimentation rate and negative ANCA titers.

What is your next step in the management of this patient?
A. Stop all medications
B. Switch to azathioprine
C. Reduce cyclophosphamide to 3-monthly infusions
D. Switch to etanercept

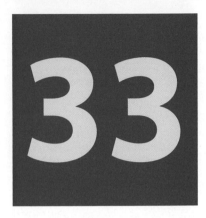

Lupus Nephritis

James E. Balow, MD

▶ Systemic lupus erythematosus (SLE): this diagnosis is based on presence of at least four clinical and laboratory features: rash, photosensitivity, mucosal ulcers, arthritis, serositis or renal, neurologic, hematologic, immuno-logic disorder, or antinuclear antibody; while not formal criteria, complement components, C3 and/or C4, are commonly depressed.

▶ Lupus nephritis (LN): this diagnosis often represents an exception to the usual basal requirement for a formal diagnosis SLE based on systemic disease cri-teria; diagnosis of LN is made on the basis of urinary findings (hematuria, cellular casts, and/or proteinuria), autoantibodies (antinuclear and/or anti-DNA), and kidney biopsy showing immune complex mediated glomerulonephritis.

▶ LN spans a spectrum of pathology and cases are assigned to one of six major classes, along with semi-quantitative scores to reflect degrees of activity and chronicity.

▶ Deposition of nephritogenic immune complexes that characteristically starts in the mesangium may extend into the subendothelial space in the case of prolifera-tive LN, or presumptively qualitatively different types of immune complexes may form in the subepithelial space in the case of membranous nephropathy, along tubular basement membranes in the case of interstitial nephri-tis, or in vascular bed in the case of lupus vasculopathy.

▶ General Considerations

Lupus nephritis (LN) develops in the majority of patients with systemic lupus erythematosus (SLE). The clinical spectrum ranges from mild and indolent to severe and progressive glomerulonephritis. Autoantibodies to a range of constitutive nuclear antigens contribute to the diagnosis of SLE. Anti-DNA antibodies appear to be the most nephri-togenic, although other autoantibodies are clearly involved in many cases of LN.

The main determinants of the occurrence, form, and severity of LN derive from the quantity and affinity of circulating immune complexes for glomerular structures. Immune complexes initially accumulate in the mesangial interstices. Deposits may be limited to the mesangium in mild LN (Classes I and II, Mesangial Lupus Nephritis). Complexes may spill over into the subendothelial space where they evoke inflammatory processes and endocap-illary hypercellularity (Classes III, Focal, and Class IV, Diffuse Proliferative Lupus Nephritis). The pathogenesis of Class V, Membranous Lupus Nephropathy, is less well understood. The leading hypothesis for formation of the characteristic subepithelial immune complex deposits is that autoantibodies react with either constitutive or planted anti-gens expressed on podocyte membranes. Mononuclear cells (macrophages and lymphocytes) are typically present in the tubulointerstitial compartment. Thus, there is inference that imprecisely defined cell-mediated immune mechanisms may contribute to the pathogenesis of LN.

Understanding of the complex mechanisms leading to LN continues to evolve. Current models are based on a multitude of factors which include the following: genetic susceptibility, epigenetic modifiers, loss of self-tolerance to nuclear antigens, overactive and dysregulated lymphoid cells, overproduction of stimulatory cytokines and circulat-ing growth factors, hyperglobulinemia and autoantibody production, ready availability of nuclear antigens from high rates of apoptotic cell death, overproduction and impaired clearance of immune complexes, complement activation, inflammation, coagulation, repair and fibrosis. Extrapolat-ing from the complexity of this paradigm, it is easy to under-stand the rationale for the ever-expanding armamentarium of interventional strategies being tested as methods to interdict the pathologic consequences of SLE.

Clinical Findings

The clinical manifestations of SLE are extremely protean. In the context of clinical practice, diagnosis of SLE should be suspected when there is evidence of multisystemic disease along with autoantibodies to nuclear antigens. Ideally, the diagnosis of SLE should be based on the presence of four or more criteria defined by the American College of Rheumatology, but it should be emphasized that these criteria are intended to standardize eligibility criteria for inclusion of subjects in SLE research studies and are less rigorously used to establish the diagnosis of SLE in clinical practice.

A. Symptoms and Signs

Glomerulonephritis is uncommonly the sentinel manifestation of SLE. An exception to this principle is Class V, Membranous Lupus Nephropathy, wherein up to 25% of patients present with no extrarenal manifestations and diagnosis of SLE may emerge only during extended follow-up.

The key challenge for diagnosticians is to detect clinically significant LN prior to overt symptoms. Patients with a likely or proven diagnosis of SLE should be carefully queried for what they may ordinarily consider to be trivial changes in urine color, nocturia, and foam-producing urination, each of which may mark the onset of occult LN.

B. Laboratory Findings

Evidence of hematuria, proteinuria, or pathologic urine sediment (dysmorphic RBCs, RBC casts, etc.) on screening urinalysis usually confirms the presence of LN. However, the astute clinician should be mindful that false-negative urinalyses, particularly urine sediment abnormalities, are relatively common in high-throughput clinical laboratories. It is judicious to "flag" urinalyses from patients with SLE for special scrutiny by laboratory personnel.

Proteinuria is traditionally quantified by 24-hour urine collection. However, spot urine protein/creatinine ratio (the value of which approximates the number of grams per day of proteinuria) is becoming widely accepted as the more convenient alternative for patients, particularly for monitoring changes in proteinuria over time.

Serologic testing includes antinuclear, anti-DNA, and antiphospholipid antibodies, which are useful for the diagnosis of SLE and its complications. The clotting diathesis conferred by the antiphospholipid syndrome may compound the thromboembolic risk of persistent nephrotic syndrome. Elevated anti-DNA titers and depressed levels of C3 and C4 complement levels correlate with active proliferative LN; changes in levels of these serologies tend to be more useful than their absolute levels for monitoring activity of nephritis during follow-up.

C. Special Tests

Kidney biopsy is primarily valuable for staging the type and severity of LN. The current classification scheme (Table 33–1) has evolved from multiple revisions over the past several decades. Discordances among clinicopathologic findings are common over time and repeat renal biopsy may be needed to stage (or potentially reclassify) the kidney disease. Figures 33–1, 33–2, and 33–3 are provided to illustrate the spectrum of the pathology of LN.

In the past few years, a relatively rare and previously unrecognized entity called lupus podocytopathy has received increasing attention. Lupus podocytopathy has been used to describe patients, whose biopsies are conventionally categorized as Class I or Class II LN, who present unexpectedly with heavy, nephrotic range proteinuria. Ultrastructural studies of biopsies from these patients show extensive podocyte foot process effacement reminiscent of minimal change disease or focal segmental glomerulosclerosis. Lupus podocytopathy often responds to a limited course of corticosteroids with relapses characteristic of minimal change disease. However, it is not definitively proven where such patients have two coincidental glomerular diseases or whether lupus podocytopathy is a previously unrecognized form of LN.

Table 33–1. Classification of lupus nephritis (LN).

Class I*
- **Minimal mesangial LN:** Normal light microscopy; mesangial immune deposits

Class II*
- **Mesangial proliferative LN:** Mesangial hypercellularity, matrix expansion and deposits

Class III
- **Focal Proliferative LN:** Fewer than 50% of glomeruli display active or inactive segmental (<50% of the tuft) or global (>50% of the tuft) endocapillary or extracapillary glomerulonephritis; subendothelial deposits are usually present but a pauci-immune process akin to ANCA vasculitis may be operant in some cases

Class IV
- **Diffuse Proliferative LN:** More than 50% of glomeruli have endocapillary or extracapillary glomerulonephritis typically with subendothelial deposits; segmental (IV-S) and global (IV-G) diffuse LN are defined by >50% of affected glomeruli having segmental and global lesions, respectively

Class V
- **Membranous LN:** Capillary loop thickening in association with subepithelial immune deposits by immunofluorescence and electron microscopy

Class VI
- Advanced **sclerosis LN:** >90% of glomeruli are globally sclerosed

*May include a unique subset called lupus podocytopathy (described in text).

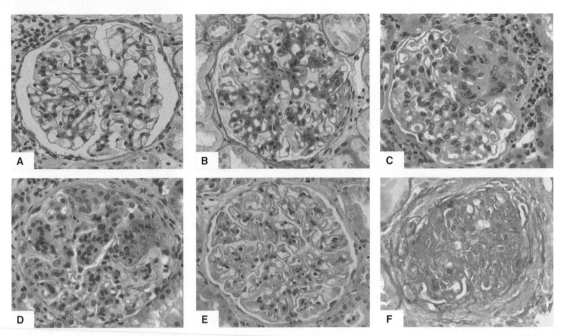

▲ **Figure 33–1.** Classes of lupus nephritis (LN). **A.** Class I. Minimal abnormality: essentially normal glomerular cellularity and capillary loop patency (PAS stain). **B.** Class II. Mesangial LN: increased mesangial cellularity and expanded mesangial matrix (PAS stain). **C.** Class III. Focal proliferative LN: segmental endocapillary proliferation with loss of capillary loop patency in right upper quadrant of this glomerulus (H&E stain). **D.** Class IV. Diffuse proliferative LN: nearly global endo-capillary proliferative changes which characteristically vary from segment to segment; nuclear karyorrhexis is evident in the solidified segment on the right (H&E stain). **E.** Class V. Membranous LN. Global thickening of capillary loops with modest mesangial matrix expansion (H&E stain). **F.** Class VI. Sclerosing LN. Glomerular tuft has collapsed with expanded mesangial matrix, fibrosis and loss of capillary circulation (PAS stain). (See Color Plate 7.)

Knowledge of the findings of kidney biopsy pathology strongly influences therapeutic decisions in LN. Institution of intensive therapy, particularly cytotoxic drugs, has been shown to occur earlier when clinicians have the benefit of renal pathology data.

▶ Differential Diagnosis

Several systemic diseases, particularly the systemic vasculitides, have features that commonly overlap those of SLE and LN. Antineutrophil cytoplasmic antibodies (ANCA) usually allow discrimination between LN and renal vasculitis, but it is prudent to be mindful that a small subset of patients with a definitive diagnosis of SLE have concurrent ANCA auto-antibodies, though their role in pathogenesis is uncertain.

Patients with rheumatoid arthritis may have hematuria in association with mild mesangial nephritis or proteinuria in association with membranous nephropathy. Mixed connective tissue disease has been infrequently associated with glomerulonephritis, which, however, may be indistinguishable from the various classes of LN.

Thrombotic microangiopathy is known to occur as a superimposed process in some patients with SLE and LN. The potential role of anticardiolipin or antiphospholipid antibodies as a cause of lupus kidney disease is unresolved, but it seems to account for some cases of extraglomerular vasculopathy in patients with SLE.

▶ Complications

The complications of LN result from the pathophysiology intrinsic to the glomerular disease, including hypertension, nephritic and nephrotic syndromes, and renal failure, as well as from side effects of treatment. While clinicians treating patients with LN have traditionally focused on therapeutic interventions to reduce the risks of renal failure, there is emerging appreciation that treatment may be required to interdict the cardiovascular and thromboembolic complications engendered by protracted nephrotic syndrome. Indeed, evidence of the benefit of achieving even partial remission of proteinuria (to the subnephrotic level) has a salutary effect on patient and renal survival. Beyond

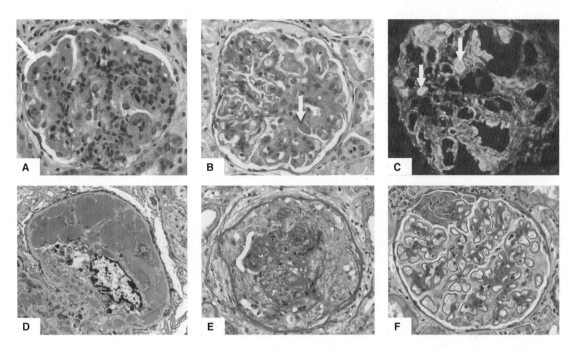

▲ **Figure 33–2.** Spectrum of pathology within classes IV and V lupus nephritis (LN). **A.** Class IV LN with classic "wire loop" lesions (white arrow) along with severe endocapillary proliferation in a near global pattern (H&E stain). **B.** Class IV LN with hyaline thrombi (white arrow) representing massive immune complex deposits across a continuum from wire loops to capillary loop occlusion (PAS stain). **C.** Class IV LN. Immunostaining for IgG deposits in same case as B; heavy capillary wall deposits and luminal thrombi (white arrows) (Immunofluorescence microscopy). **D.** Class IV LN. Ultrastructure of immune complex deposits in same case as B; note the extensive subendothelial deposits which continue to accumulate as massive luminal deposits that compromise capillary circulation (Electron microscopy). **E.** Class IV LN. The tuft of this glomerulus is severely compressed by a circumferential cellular crescent (PAS stain). **F.** Class V + Class III LN. This glomerulus exhibits nearly uniform capillary loop thickening and a superimposed segmental proliferative lesion near the top of this figure (PAS stain). (See Color Plate 8.)

standard immunosuppressive therapies, the full armamentarium of renal protection strategies, particularly angiotensin antagonists and lipid-lowering statin drugs, is warranted in management of LN.

▶ **Treatment**

Optimal care of patients with LN usually requires integrated expertise of nephrologists and rheumatologists. Most SLE patients will require some dosage of corticosteroids, antimalarials, and nonsteroidal anti-inflammatory drugs for control of their commonly debilitating extrarenal disease, which are best evaluated and managed by rheumatologists. Conversely, delineation of the more arcane aspects of renal disease and integration of the results of kidney biopsy are best evaluated and managed by nephrologists. Conjointly staffed clinics offer the best environment for effective communication and comprehensive care of patients with SLE and LN.

Immunosuppressive drug options for management of patients with LN are summarized in Table 33–2. Evidence-based clinical recommendations derived from completed controlled clinical trials are limited and consensus in developing clinical practice guidelines has not been achieved. Results of ongoing multicentered clinical trials are necessary to assist in prioritizing the multiplicity of therapeutic options for treatment of the various forms of LN.

A. Corticosteroids

Patients with new onset Class III, IV, or V LN warrant a limited therapeutic trial of high-dose corticosteroids, though several European investigators continue to explore the benefit/risk profile of steroid-free regimens. Currently, it is recommended that patients failing to achieve full remission of nephritis within 6–8 weeks of high-dose corticosteroids should be treated with adjunctive cytotoxic drug

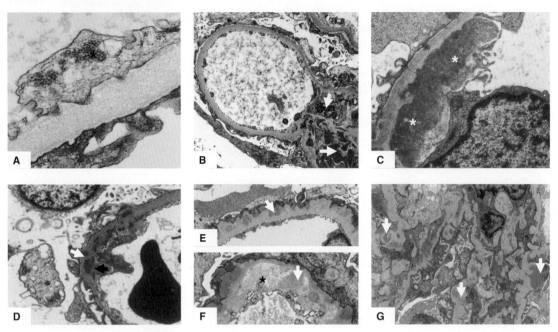

▲ **Figure 33–3.** Characteristic ultrastructural lesions in lupus nephritis (LN). **A.** Tubuloreticular inclusion (black asterisk) in the cytoplasm of a glomerular endothelial cell; these structures putatively reflect condensation of cytoplasmic organelles caused by interferon. **B.** Earliest evidence of immune complex deposition; dark electron-dense deposits appear first in the mesangial stalk (white arrows). **C.** Subendothelial deposits (white asterisks) characteristic of Class III and IV LN. **D.** Class IV LN with predominant subendothelial deposits (black arrow) is often accompanied by scattered subepithelial deposits (white arrow); when the subepithelial deposits are more extensive and regularly distributed along the capillary wall, it is best described as mixed membranous and proliferative LN. **E.** Class V LN. Stage 2 membranous nephropathy; regularly distributed subepithelial electron dense deposits are evident (white arrow); projections of glomerular basement membrane outwardly between the subepithelial deposits tend to produce a spiked appearance to the capillary loops. **F.** Class V LN. Stage 3–4 membranous nephropathy; electron-dense deposits have become incorporated with the capillary wall (white arrow) and have begun to disintegrate (black asterisk). **G.** Glomerular sclerosis. This appearance of collapsed, wrinkled glomerular basement membranes is seen across all classes of LN but predominantly in Class VI; residual electron-dense deposits (white arrows) are interspersed in the sclerosing process. (See Color Plate 9.)

(cyclophosphamide or mycophenolate mofetil) or calcineurin inhibitor. Based on current evidence, those patients with substantial fibrinoid necrosis or cellular crescents on kidney biopsy should be directly initiated on therapy with combined pulse methylprednisolone and pulse cyclophosphamide for a period of 6 months or more.

B. Cyclophosphamide

Results of early treatment of murine LN and meta-analyses of human trials indicate that cyclophosphamide is among the most effective immunosuppressive drugs for LN. Adverse effects of daily cyclophosphamide are formidable, particularly beyond 3 months, and for this reason, prescription of daily therapy has become limited. The therapeutic index of cyclophosphamide is improved by administration of intermittent pulse therapy, which has become widely

accepted as the standard approach to administration of cyclophosphamide therapy.

The emergence of pulse cyclophosphamide as the interim therapeutic standard for proliferative LN arose from observations in several long-term clinical trials reported from the National Institutes of Health. The composite of evidence indicated that pulse cyclophosphamide achieved the most sustained rates of renal remission, the lowest rates of cumulative damage on kidney biopsy, and ultimately the lowest rate of progression to end-stage renal disease (ESRD). Relapse occurs in approximately 20% of patients, depending on the effectiveness of maintenance therapies such as mycophenolate and/or azathioprine. The substantive risk of gonadal toxicity incurred with extended courses of pulse cyclophosphamide has been the major impetus to continue the search for shorter treatment cycles and alternative drug therapies in LN.

Table 33–2. Immunosuppressive drug options and guidelines for administration in lupus nephritis.

Corticosteroids
- **Prednisone:** Start with 1 mg/kg/day for approximately 6–8 weeks; taper to approximately 0.25 mg/kg/day over the next 6–8 weeks; strive for low-dose alternate-day maintenance therapy; patients with membranous LN are often initiated on treatment with comparable doses of alternate-day prednisone.
- **Pulse methylprednisolone:** Start with three daily intravenous pulses, 1 g each; continue with single monthly pulses for 6 or more months in patients with severe LN (usually in conjunction with pulse cyclophosphamide).

Cyclophosphamide
- **Pulse cyclophosphamide:** If the estimated glomerular filtration rate (GFR) is >30 mL/min, start single monthly doses of 0.75 g/m^2 body surface area (BSA) administered intravenously over 1 hour; if the GFR is <30 mL/min, the starting dose is 0.5 g/m^2 BSA; adjust the subsequent doses to a maximum of 1.0 g/m^2 BSA according to the white blood cell (WBC) nadir count (should not be <1500) at days 10 and 14 after treatment. All cyclophosphamide pulse treatments should include bladder protection by administration of oral or intravenous mesna, forced fluids to achieve a diuresis of >150 mL/hour, and frequent voiding for 24 hours; consider preemptive antiemetic treatment with dexamethasone 10 mg single dose plus ondansetron or granisetron prior to cyclophosphamide infusions; pulse regimens usually continue monthly for 3–6 months with conversion to quarterly pulse cyclophosphamide or to alternative maintenance therapies with mycophenolate or azathioprine.
- **Daily oral cyclophosphamide:** Start with 2 mg/kg/day (as single morning dose); taper the dose as necessary to keep WBC >4000; the duration of therapy is usually <3 months; after 3 months, consider a transition to maintenance therapy with azathioprine or mycophenolate.

Azathioprine
- Start at 2 mg/kg/day as maintenance therapy.

Mycophenolate mofetil
- Start at 0.5 g twice daily, escalating weekly to a target of 1.5 g twice daily or 1.0 g three times daily according to gastrointestinal tolerance.

Cyclosporine
- Start at 5 mg/kg/day adjusting the dose downward according to side effects, particularly azotemia, hyperkalemia, or hirsutism.

C. Mycophenolate Mofetil

Mycophenolic acid was initially tested and shortly abandoned for treatment of rheumatic diseases in the 1960s. It was reformulated and initially compared to azathioprine in renal allograft recipients. Mycophenolate was licensed on the basis of its advantage over azathioprine in achieving a reduced frequency of acute rejection episodes. Doubts have been raised about the superior cost effectiveness of mycophenolate because of its high cost and its lack of proven benefit in extending allograft survival.

Several uncontrolled trials of mycophenolate in LN suggested that this therapy may be useful in patients failing to achieve satisfactory responses to cyclophosphamide. Over the past several years, multiple controlled trials comparing induction therapy with mycophenolate mofetil versus cyclophosphamide have indicated comparable rates of renal remission and short- to intermediate-term kidney survival. Mycophenolate initially appeared to have an advantage over cyclophosphamide in terms of adverse effect profile; however, the current perspective is that mycophenolate and cyclophosphamide-based regimens confer substantively similar frequencies of major adverse effects, though each conveying somewhat different types of infection diathesis, teratogenic potential, and malignancy diathesis.

Because historical studies have shown that several treatments, including azathioprine, cyclophosphamide, a combination of azathioprine and cyclophosphamide, and even prednisone alone, achieve comparable short- and intermediate-term renal survival rates, many have argued that the definitive choice among the newer immunosuppressive drugs must await ascertainment of long-term renal outcomes after 5 or more years of observation.

D. Azathioprine

Azathioprine is a relatively weak immunosuppressive drug in studies of both murine and human LN. It has mostly been relegated to use as a steroid-sparing agent and as a less costly and well-tolerated maintenance after cyclophosphamide or mycophenolate induction therapies.

E. Plasma Exchange Therapy

Plasma exchange has been of historical interest in LN based on the evidence that preformed circulating immune complexes are the key nephritogenic mechanism for LN. Large numbers of anecdotal reports have been published claiming a salutary effect, but prospective controlled trials have shown that plasma exchange (without adjunctive chemical immunosuppressive drug therapy) is ineffective in LN.

F. Experimental Therapies

Several studies involving novel therapeutic agents for LN are underway. The agents being evaluated in these studies are summarized in Table 33–3. The website ***www.clinicaltrials.gov*** leads to a potentially useful resource in searching for

Table 33–3. Selected experimental therapies for SLE and lupus nephritis*

Calcineurin inhibitors
- Tacrolimus
- Sirolimus

Monoclonal antibodies (targets)
- Rituximab (CD20, B cells)
- Obinutuzumab (CD20, B cells)
- Anifrolumab (interferon-α)
- Belimumab (BLyS cytokine)
- Tocilizumab (interleukin-6 receptor)
- Infliximab (tumor necrosis factor)
- Eculizumab (complement C5)

Costimulation inhibitors
- CTLA4-Ig, Abatacept, Belatacept (CD80/86)

Tyrosine kinase inhibitors
- Tofacitinib (JAK/STAT)

Proteasome inhibitors
- Bortezomib (Plasma cells)
- Ixazomib (Plasma cells)

Tolerogens
- Abetimus, LJP-394 (anti-DNA)

Autologous stem cell transplants

*Search website address for latest updates: www.clinicaltrials.gov.

studies that may be recruiting patients, along with information about eligibility and exclusion criteria.

G. Membranous Lupus Nephropathy

Patients with Class V Membranous LN with normal kidney function and subnephrotic proteinuria may not warrant aggressive immunosuppressive therapy and are usually managed with diuretics, antiproteinuric angiotensin antagonists and lipid-lowering statins.

Patients with Class V disease and high-grade nephrotic-range proteinuria, particularly if protracted and unimproved by angiotensin antagonists, are usually treated with moderate dose corticosteroids plus cyclophosphamide or mycophenolate. If kidney function is well preserved, cyclosporine is also an effective alternative in patients with membranous LN. The optimal duration of treatment is undefined, but relapse of proteinuria is particularly likely after cessation of cyclosporine. This has prompted a very protracted slow tapering of cyclosporine before discontinuation (unless there is clinical suspicion or pathologic evidence of significant cyclosporine nephrotoxicity).

Experimental studies currently underway using rituximab monotherapy or combination rituximab and calcineurin inhibitor therapy for primary, idiopathic membranous nephropathy may yield evidence that could be relevant to Class V Lupus Membranous Nephritis.

▶ Prognosis

The prognosis of Classes III and IV proliferative LN has improved from a 5-year renal survival of less than 20% during the period 1960–1980 to more than 80% during the period 1980–2000. This improvement in prognosis has been ascribed mostly to increasing use of cyclophosphamide. While preliminary data based on achievement of renal remission suggest that mycophenolate may have comparable benefits, it remains to be established if mycophenolate will achieve comparable long-term renal survival.

In patients progressing to ESRD due to LN, there is considerable controversy about the prevalence of active SLE during maintenance dialysis and the risk of recurrent LN in renal allografts. In general, patients should be clinically and serologically inactive for approximately 1 year before kidney transplantation. Recent reports suggest that recurrence of low-grade LN is common, but fortunately clinically significant nephritis and allograft loss are rare.

KEY READINGS

Anders H-J et al: A pathophysiology-based approach to the diagnosis and treatment of lupus nephritis. Kidney Int 2016;90:493.

Dall'Era M: Treatment of lupus nephritis: current paradigms and emerging strategies. Curr Opin Rheumatol 2017;29:241.

Hanaoka H et al: Comparison of renal response to four different induction therapies in Japanese patients with lupus nephritis class III or IV: a single-centre retrospective study. PLOS One 2017;12:e0175152.

Paramalingam S et al: Recurrent podocytopathy in a patient with systemic lupus erythematosus. SAGE Open Med Case Rep 2017;5:2050313X17695997.

Parikh SV et al: The kidney biopsy in lupus nephritis: past, present and future. Semin Nephrol 2015; 35:465.

Parikh SV et al: Current and emerging therapies for lupus nephritis. J Am Soc Nephrol 2016;27:2929.

Tamirou F et al: A proteinuria cut-off level of 0.7 g/day after 12 months of treatment best predicts long-term renal outcome in lupus nephritis: data from the MAINTAIN Nephritis Trial. Lupus Sci Med 2015;2:e000123.

■ CHAPTER REVIEW QUESTIONS

1. A 23-year-old woman with a 3-year history of SLE and biopsy-proven Class IV Diffuse Proliferative LN (high-activity index, low-chronicity index) received induction therapy with pulse cyclophosphamide monthly for 6 months and then switched to mycophenolate mofetil 1 g twice daily and low dose prednisone as maintenance therapy. Extrarenal disease remitted and lupus serologies and kidney function had normalized by the 1 year follow-up visit. Despite excellent compliance with the treatment regimen, between months 12 and 16 proteinuria steadily rose from a nadir, partial-remission value of 0.6–5.6 g/day and creatinine increased from a nadir value of 1.3–2.4 mg/dL. Urinalysis showed minimal hematuria along with granular, broad and waxy casts. Anti-DNA and complement that had normalized during induction therapy remained unchanged.

   Which of the following would represent the best approach to the escalating proteinuria and deteriorating renal function?
   A. Consider that the latest clinical scenario represents a flare of Class IV LN and reinstitute the previously successful induction regimen
   B. Consider that the new clinical scenario might represent a change in class of LN and proceed to a repeat kidney biopsy to gather evidence that will determine the need for possible change in therapies
   C. Consider that the patient has failed the best available therapies and prepare the patient for the inevitable need for end-stage renal failure therapies
   D. Switch to a completely different therapeutic approach to the flare using a combination of calcineurin inhibitor and rituximab

2. A 25-year-old woman with inactive SLE seeks your counsel about the implications of starting a family. She had a 3-year history, starting at age 21, of active SLE, including Class IV Diffuse Proliferative LN. Induction therapy comprised of pulse methylprednisolone, prednisone, and 3 g/day of mycophenolate was very effective. She achieved complete clinical remission which has been sustained for the past year. Her maintenance treatment includes low-dose prednisone and 1.5 g/day of mycophenolate, along with lisinopril and birth control pills. Serum creatinine concentration is 1.4 mg/dL, C3, and C4 are normal; anti-DNA has improved during induction but has persisted at low titers.

   Which of the following approaches would represent sound advice to this patient?
   A. Success of pregnancy and risks of complications to mother and fetus should be minimal if stable remission can be maintained by the current treatment regimen
   B. The persistently abnormal levels of anti-DNA predict high-risk of pregnancy complications, despite the presence of other criteria for complete remission
   C. Attempting pregnancy is acceptable, but lisinopril must be continued because of its superior efficacy for hypertension management and for renoprotection
   D. Attempting pregnancy is acceptable, but only after a period of time to ensure that azathioprine is tolerated as a substitute for mycophenolate

3. A 19-year-old woman with a several month history of apparent chronic fatigue syndrome was given a clinical diagnosis of SLE; ANA and IgM antiphospholipid antibodies were positive, but anti-DNA was negative and complement levels were normal. There was no evidence of kidney disease by urinalysis. Initial treatment included hydroxychloroquine and naproxen which led to improvement of constitutional symptoms. Approximately 6 months later, the patient had an uncomplicated first trimester spontaneous abortion. At 9 months, she developed rapid weight gain and was documented to have nephrotic syndrome. Blood pressure and kidney function remained normal. Urinalysis showed hyaline and granular casts with a urine protein/creatinine ratio of 8.7 (>90% albumin). Lupus serology profile was unchanged from the time of diagnosis of SLE.

   Which of the following is the most likely cause of the rapid onset of kidney disease?
   A. Renal vasculopathy related to antiphospholipid syndrome
   B. Coincidental post-infectious glomerulonephritis
   C. Lupus podocytopathy
   D. Acute interstitial nephritis due to NSAIDs

4. Which of the following is correct regarding the pathology of LN?
   A. Membranoproliferative glomerulonephritis is a simple way to describe the findings of mixed membranous and proliferative LN
   B. The class of renal pathology for a given case of LN tends to remain static over time
   C. A high Chronicity Index is a better predictor of renal prognosis than the Activity Index for LN
   D. At the light microscopy level, the pathologic manifestations of the glomerular capillary deposition of subendothelial immune complexes is best described as thrombotic microangiopathy
   E. Negative urinalysis findings reported by high-throughput clinical pathology laboratories is a reliable method to rule out LN

5. Which of the following is correct regarding the efficacy and adverse effects for various treatments for LN?
   A. Rates of Complete or Partial Remission are valid surrogates for hard renal outcomes in LN and are reliable measures of the relative efficacies of various therapies for LN

B. The natural history, prognosis, and response to various therapies are quite heterogeneous among various racial, ethnic, and socioeconomically-defined populations with LN
C. Complete normalization or seronegativity of immunologic tests for SLE occurs in the majority of patients achieving Complete Remission of LN
D. Malignancy diathesis associated with cyclophosphamide therapy is substantially higher that that associated with mycophenolate or azathioprine therapy
E. All contemporary immunosuppressive drug regiments for LN share similar risks of JC virus reactivation and progressive multifocal leukoencephalopathy (PML)

Plasma Cell Dyscrasias

Nelson Leung, MD

Samih H. Nasr, MD

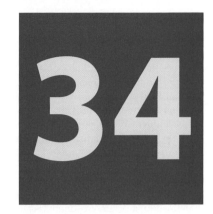

ESSENTIALS OF DIAGNOSIS

▶ Immune deposits are considered monotypic if they display light chain restriction.

▶ Heavy chain restriction without light chain restriction is not considered monotypic as several polyclonal diseases can have heavy chain isotype restriction.

▶ C3 glomerulonephritis and thrombotic microangiopathy do not have immunoglobulin deposits but can be due to monoclonal gammopathy.

▶ Immunofluorescence (IF) on paraffin tissue after protease digestion should be performed on all cases of C3 glomerulonephritis with monoclonal gammopathy to look for masked immunoglobulin deposits.

▶ All amyloidosis cases should undergo tissue typing prior to initiation of chemotherapy.

PLASMA CELL DYSCRASIAS

General Considerations

Plasma cell dyscrasias are diseases or conditions secondary to clonal proliferation of plasma cells. These conditions are typically characterized by the overproduction of a monoclonal protein causing a monoclonal gammopathy. Plasma cell dyscrasias are categorized by their clonal burden and end organ damage. Classically, the categories are monoclonal gammopathy of undetermined significance (MGUS), smoldering multiple myeloma (SMM), and symptomatic multiple myeloma (MM). Patients with MGUS have less than 10% bone marrow clonal plasma cells and less than 3 g/dL of monoclonal (M) protein in the serum. By definition, no end organ damage can be present as a result of the plasma cell dyscrasia. SMM is characterized by more than 10% bone marrow clonal plasma cells or more than

3 g/dL of M-protein also without end organ damage. MM is defined by the presence of end organ damage in someone who meets the criteria for SMM. End organ damage has been represented by the mnemonic CRAB (hyperCalcemia, Renal impairment, Anemia, and Bone lesions). Recently, three additional diagnostic criteria were added to the definition of MM. They are an involved to uninvolved free light chain (FLC) ratio more than 100 with the involved FLC having a level of more than 10 mg/dL, bone marrow plasma cells more than 60% and more than 1 focal boney lesion on MRI. However, it has been increasingly appreciated that the kidney can be injured without meeting the criteria for MM. Since treatment is currently only recommended for patients with MM, a conflict is created by these patients. To resolve the conflict, the term monoclonal gammopathy of renal significance (MGRS) was created. MGRS encompasses all B-cell/plasma cell proliferative disorders that do not meet criteria for MM or malignant lymphoma but are associated with a kidney disease. These clones usually have lower proliferative rates and behave more like MGUS than MM. However, they produce a nephrotoxic M-protein which differentiates them from MGUS. Kidney diseases associated with plasma cell dyscrasias are the focus of this discussion. It is important to note that these diseases are not exclusive to plasma cell clones. Kidney diseases can arise from any clone producing a nephrotoxic M-protein.

KEY READINGS

Kyle RA et al: Monoclonal gammopathy of undetermined significance (MGUS) and smoldering (asymptomatic) multiple myeloma: IMWG consensus perspectives risk factors for progression and guidelines for monitoring and management. Leukemia 2010;24:1121.

Leung N et al: Monoclonal gammopathy of renal significance: when MGUS is no longer undetermined or insignificant. Blood 2012;120:4292.

Rajkumar SV et al: International Myeloma Working Group updated criteria for the diagnosis of multiple myeloma. Lancet Oncol 2014;15:e538.

LIGHT CHAIN CAST NEPHROPATHY

Light chain cast nephropathy (CN) is the most common kidney disease in patients with MM; it is also called myeloma CN. It is the result of tubular obstruction by casts formed from the binding and precipitation of monoclonal immunoglobulin light chains to Tamm–Horsfall protein. The casts are quite immunogenic and cause a secondary tubular injury by recruitment of inflammatory infiltrates. Recently, CN has been made a myeloma-defining event by the International Myeloma Working Group. This is because CN always occurs in high-tumor burden condition. The incidence of CN is unknown since its diagnosis can only be confirmed by a renal biopsy. The incidence of acute renal impairment as defined by a serum creatinine (Scr) of more than 2 mg/dL is about 20% in patients with newly diagnosed MM. This incidence increases as the stage of disease advances. In autopsy series, CN is found in 32–62% of patients who died from MM.

Hematologic Characteristics

Nearly all patients with CN also meet the definition of SMM or MM. Two risk factors have been identified for the development of CN. First, CN is extremely rare in patients with less than 50 mg/dL of serum FLC. Once above this cutoff, the incidence of CN increases with the level of the serum FLC. Patients with renal impairment with less than 50 mg/dL of serum FLC should therefore undergo evaluation for alternative explanation for their kidney failure, which may include a kidney biopsy. Another prerequisite for development of CN is urinary excretion of FLC or Bence Jones proteinuria. Less than 2% of patients without Bence Jones proteinuria develop kidney failure but the incidence increases to 50% when urinary FLC excretion is above 12 g/g of creatinine. CN has been called a high-risk feature in MM as patients in whom the myeloma defining event is CN have poorer outcomes than those who develop MM via other criteria. Studies have found that reversal of the kidney failure can improve the prognosis.

Clinical Manifestations

CN can be the first manifestation of MM or it may occur for the first time during relapsed disease. It usually presents as rapidly progressive acute kidney injury (AKI) resulting in an acute rise in Scr over a period of days. Renal impairment is variable and ranges from moderate to severe requiring dialysis. Several precipitating factors have been identified. These include the use of non-steroidal anti-inflammatory drugs (NSAIDs), angiotensin converting enzyme (ACE) inhibitors, and intravenous contrast. Unfortunately, NSAIDs are often taken or prescribed as a result of back pain due to compression fractures. An incidence of 1.25% was reported for AKI after the use of intravenous contrast in patients with MM in comparison to the 0.15% in the general population. Even higher rates have been reported in smaller studies but the role of intravenous contrast has been challenged recently as the severity of illness requiring the use of contrast has been associated with the developed AKI. Dehydration via vomiting and diarrhea and severe infections can also precipitate CN. These patients should have a serum FLC above 50 mg/dL. Median proteinuria is 2.0 g/day, which should be predominately from FLC rather than albuminuria.

Pathologic Findings

On light microscopy, periodic acid–Schiff (PAS) negative intraluminal casts are seen in the distal tubular lumina while glomeruli are spared. The casts can have a waxy to crystalline appearance. The number of casts can vary and may have prognostic significance. Fracturing of the casts during the slide preparation is quite characteristic of light chain casts. Another characteristic feature is the macrophage derived giant cell reaction surrounding the casts. Tubular rupture may occur as a result of the tubular obstruction, which can induce an intense inflammatory infiltrate resembling interstitial nephritis. On IF study, only a single light chain corresponding to the circulating monoclonal immunoglobulin should stain in the casts. On electron microscopy (EM), the casts show highly electron dense granular material or crystalline-like structures.

Treatment

The most important goal in the treatment of CN is the rapid reduction of the serum FLC. Studies have found a minimum reduction of 60% is needed for recovery of kidney function. However, this is time dependent as prolonged exposure to the light chain casts can invoke secondary inflammatory injuries. It has been shown that the 60% reduction of serum FLC should be accomplished within 14 days to ensure recovery of kidney function while 80% reduction is required at 21 days to attain the same goal. Anti-myeloma chemotherapy is the main method of reducing serum FLC production. In the past, patients with AKI were less responsive to alkylator-based therapy resulting in early deaths and a significantly inferior long-term prognosis. More recently, in a randomized trial, bortezomib (a proteasome inhibitor) based therapy has been shown to be capable of overcoming the effects of kidney failure on the long-term survival. However, a significant number of early deaths still occurred. Immunomodulatory drugs (IMiDs) have also been studied. Thalidomide and pomalidomide are not metabolized by the kidney and can be used without dosage adjustment but pomalidomide is not approved for front line use currently. Lenalidomide, which is approved for front line therapy, is cleared by the kidney and requires dosage adjustment. Trial data showed that lenalidomide is effective in patients with renal failure but the incidence of adverse events was increased. The results from alkylator particularly melphalan have been discouraging. On the other hand, cyclophosphamide is much better tolerated and can be used in combination with bortezomib. Other alkylators such as bendamustine are not extensively metabolized by the kidney and can be used without significant dosage adjustment.

In addition to chemotherapy, extracorporeal removal of the FLC has been studied extensively. This was initially done with plasma exchange (PLEX). The first report of a successful use of PLEX was in 1976 in a young man with MM and AKI. Since then, three randomized trials have been performed. The first one with 29 patients with severe renal dysfunction randomized patients to PLEX and hemodialysis versus peritoneal dialysis. Eleven of 13 patients who required dialysis became dialysis independent in the PLEX group and only one patient died during follow-up. In comparison, two patients in the peritoneal dialysis group recovered kidney function and five patients died during follow-up. While this was a positive trial, it was criticized for the use of peritoneal dialysis in the non-PLEX arm. The higher earlier mortality rate may have also influenced the kidney recovery rate. A second trial with 21 patients with severe renal impairment was performed. This time, both groups received hemodialysis if renal replacement therapy was needed. In this study, five of 10 patients without PLEX and seven of 11 patients with PLEX had improvement in their kidney function. Of those who were dialysis dependent, none of the patients treated with hemodialysis alone improved while three of seven patients treated with hemodialysis and PLEX became dialysis independent. The difference was not statistically significant ($p = 0.09$) given the small number of patients. A third trial was conducted where 104 patients were randomized. A composite score that included: death, dialysis dependence, and an estimated glomerular filtration rate (eGFR) of less than 30 mL/min/1.73 m^2 at 6 months was used to evaluate these patients. The results showed no statistical difference between groups. The composite outcome was met by 69.2% of the control group versus 57.9% of the PLEX group. No significant differences in the secondary outcomes, which included: death (33.3% versus 32.8%), dialysis dependence (26.9% versus 12.8%), discontinuation of dialysis excluding death (36.8% versus 41.6%), starting dialysis (20.0% versus 20.9%) were noted between the control and PLEX group respectively. However, serum FLC was not used for guidance and few kidney biopsies were performed to confirm the diagnosis in this study.

The use of high cutoff (HCO) dialyzer showed promising results in a preliminary study of patients with CN. The HCO dialyzer chosen had a surface area of 1.1 m^2 and molecular cutoff of 45 kilodaltons (kD). This allows for easy removal of FLCs, which has the molecular weight of 25 kD for kappa and 50 kD for lambda (dimer). Fourteen of the 19 dialysis dependent patients recovered kidney function after HCO dialyzer treatment. However, while all patients

who had continuous chemotherapy became dialysis independent, only one of six patients whose chemotherapy was interrupted became dialysis independent. Given the promising results, two randomized trials: (1) The European Trial of Free Light Chain Removal by Extended Haemodialysis in Cast Nephropathy (EuLITE) and (2) Studies in Patients with Multiple Myeloma and Renal Failure Due to Myeloma Cast Nephropathy (MYRE) were undertaken and have finished accruing patients. The results of these trials were reported in abstract form in 2016. Eulite showed no differences in renal recovery at 3 months between HCO dialyzer and control treated patients while renal recovery was improved by HCO hemodialysis in MYRE at 6 month. It is important to keep in mind that the two trials had many design differences which may explain the differences in response rates. Formal comparison will need to be performed once these trials are reported in manuscript format.

KEY READINGS

Dimopoulos MA et al: Significant improvement in the survival of patients with multiple myeloma presenting with severe renal impairment after the introduction of novel agents. Ann Oncol 2014;25:195.

Drayson M et al: Effects of paraprotein heavy and light chain types and free light chain load on survival in myeloma: an analysis of patients receiving conventional-dose chemotherapy in Medical Research Council UK multiple myeloma trials. Blood 2006;108:2013.

Hutchison CA et al: Early reduction of serum-free light chains associates with renal recovery in myeloma kidney. J Am Soc Nephrol 2011;22:1129.

Leung N et al: Urinary albumin excretion patterns of patients with cast nephropathy and other monoclonal gammopathy-related kidney diseases. Clin J Am Soc Nephrol 2012;7:1964.

Nasr SH et al: Clinicopathologic correlations in multiple myeloma: a case series of 190 patients with kidney biopsies. Am J Kidney Dis 2012;59:786.

Yadav P, Cook M, Cockwell P: Current trends of renal impairment in multiple myeloma. Kidney Dis (Basel) 2016;1:241.

Yadav P et al: The use of immunoglobulin light chain assays in the diagnosis of paraprotein-related kidney disease. Kidney Int 2015;87:692.

AIg AMYLOIDOSIS

While CN is the most common kidney disease in MM, immunoglobulin-related (AIg) amyloidosis is most common form of glomerular disease. AIg amyloidosis is a group of diseases that consists of three subtypes: immunoglobulin light chain (AL), heavy and light chain (AHL), and the rarest of all immunoglobulin heavy chain (AH) amyloidosis. AL amyloidosis represents the majority of cases of AIg amyloidosis and the discussion will focus on AL amyloidosis since nearly all of the data come from patients with AL amyloidosis.

Hematologic Characteristics

AL amyloidosis can be seen as a complication of MM but actually majority of cases are due to MGRS. Up to 40% of patients with AL amyloidosis may have 10% or more bone marrow plasma cells but only ~15% meet the definition of MM. One study of over 1000 patients with MM found only 1% was diagnosed with AL amyloidosis prior, 3% within 30 days of diagnosis of MM, and 2% were diagnosed afterwards. Patients with both diagnoses have the worst prognosis compared to either one alone. This has not changed despite modern therapies. It is also important to remember that AL amyloidosis is not exclusive to MM, it can also be the result of Waldenström macroglobulinemia, CLL, and other B-cell lymphomas. Lambda light chains are more likely to form amyloid (60–70%) than kappa light chains.

Pathologic Findings

Amyloid deposits appear as eosinophilic material that stain PAS-negative or weak and silver-negative (Figure 34–1). Deposits can be found in all kidney compartments but most cases exhibit glomerular and vascular involvement. In the glomeruli, the deposits first appear in the mesangium causing acellular mesangial expansion and later extend into the peripheral capillary wall. Amyloid spicules, resulting from parallel alignment of amyloid fibrils in the subepithelial zone perpendicular to the glomerular basement membrane, are frequently seen on silver stain and by EM. The amount of deposit ranges from minimal to massive and may not correlate with the degree of proteinuria. This explains why AL amyloidosis is sometimes misdiagnosed as minimal change disease. Proteinuria is dependent on the site of deposition. Patients with amyloid deposits limited to the vascular/interstitial compartment have little (<1 g/day) to no proteinuria and mainly present with progressive renal insufficiency. This can be seen in about 5% of cases.

All amyloid display anomalous colors (yellow/orange/green) under polarized light after staining with Congo red. Solid fibers ranging from 7 to 12 nm in diameter are seen on EM in a randomly arranged fashion (Figure 34–1). However, the diagnostic process is not complete until the amyloid is typed. IF staining is the initial step in renal amyloid typing. Positive IF staining to one light chain should be demonstrated in AL (Figure 34–1), to one heavy and one light chain in AHL and to one heavy chain with negative staining for both light chains in AH. IgG subtyping ensure the heavy

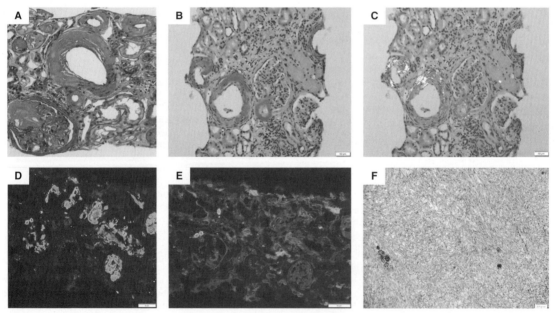

▲ **Figure 34–1.** Pathologic findings in a case of AL-lambda amyloidosis. **A.** Acellular, PAS-weak amyloid deposits involving a glomerulus, an interlobular artery and two arterioles. **B.** Amyloid deposits are strongly Congo red positive. **C.** Under polarized light, they exhibit anomalous colors (yellow/orange/green) (so-called "apple-green birefringence). **D.** On immunofluorescence, glomerular, and vascular amyloid deposits show strong smudgy staining for lambda. **E.** Amyloid deposits are negative for kappa. **F.** On electron microscopy, amyloid deposits are composed of solid randomly oriented fibrils with a mean thickness of 9 nm (range 7–12)(×200 for A–C, ×100 for D&E, ×46,000 for **F**). (See Color Plate 10.)

chain is monotypic. IF is quite useful in diagnosing AL amyloidosis since it is readily available, but sensitivity and specificity can be a problem particularly for the diagnosis of AHL and AH. The gold standard for amyloid typing currently is laser microdissection assisted liquid chromatography-tandem mass spectrometry (LMD/MS-MS). Unfortunately, expertise is required for interpretation and limited availability makes it less useful.

Clinical Presentation

AL amyloidosis is a systemic disease capable of affecting any visceral organ. The kidney and the heart are the most commonly involved organs. The median age of these patients is in the mid 60s. It is rare to affect patients younger than 30 years of age. Approximately 70% of patients present with proteinuria (often in the nephrotic range) and renal insufficiency. Unlike myeloma CN, the proteinuria in AL amyloidosis is predominately albuminuria. Renal insufficiency is often mild at presentation but is progressive. Rare manifestations such as Fanconi syndrome with renal tubular acidosis and nephrogenic diabetes insipidus have been reported with amyloid deposition in the proximal tubule and collecting duct respectively. Renal impairment is seen in 50% patients with a median serum creatinine (Scr) of 1.2 mg/dL at diagnosis. Twenty to 26% of patients have Scr more than 2.0 mg/dL. In a large combined Italian German study, end stage renal disease (ESRD) was present in 4–5% of patients at diagnosis. ESRD was reported in 15% of the Italian patients and 31% of the German patients after treatment. ESRD occurs predominately in patients who presented with renal involvement. Over a median follow-up of 11 years, 42% of patients with renal involvement versus 5% without renal involvement at presentation developed ESRD. Hypoalbuminemia was found to be a significant risk factor for progression to ESRD. The prognosis of patients with ESRD is poor but had improved significantly over the past few years. The median survival was 11 months after starting dialysis in patients between 1994 and 1997, but improved to 39 months in more recent studies.

The most important organ that determines overall survival in AL amyloidosis is the heart. Patients with advance cardiac involvement have a median survival of 6 months, which has not been changed by modern chemotherapy. These patients present with progressive congestive heart failure. Syncopal or near syncopal episodes can occur especially if autonomic nerve dysfunction is present. Peripheral neuropathy can occur with or without autonomic neuropathy. A change in bowel habits suggests gastrointestinal involvement. Diarrhea may be severe and can be due to bacterial overgrowth. Liver involvement is often silent presenting with elevated alkaline phosphatase and hepatomegaly.

Laboratory Testing

In AL amyloidosis, evaluation should include monoclonal protein tests, kidney function tests, liver function tests as well as cardiac biomarkers. Organ involvement and clonal burden all contribute to prognosis. Since the clonal burden is generally less than that of MM, the sensitivity of the diagnostic tests is also lower. Compared to MM, the sensitivity of serum protein electrophoresis is 66% in AL amyloidosis versus 88% in MM. Inclusion of serum immunofixation improves the sensitivity to 74% while the addition of serum FLC assay increases sensitivity to over 97%. Serum FLCs are not only important diagnostically and prognostically, but they are also a key biomarker for assessment of response to therapy. Although urine protein electrophoresis does not improve the monoclonal protein detection rate, it is used to measure renal response.

Treatment

Significant breakthrough began with the use of autologous stem cell transplant (ASCT) in patients with AL amyloidosis. Prior to that, median survival was around 18 months with various chemotherapeutic regimens. With ASCT, median survival as high as 6.3 years has now been achieved. However, patients with advance cardiac involvement are at high risk for treatment related mortality (TRM) and alternative treatment should be sought. The development of AKI has also been associated with poor outcomes during ASCT. Recently, hypoalbuminemia (<2.5 g/dL) and low eGFR (<40 mL/min/1.73 m^2) have been found to be risk factors for development of AKI and TRM during ASCT independent of cardiac biomarkers. Interestingly, the risk returns to baseline if a patient is on stable hemodialysis prior to the ASCT. Melphalan and dexamethasone is an effective treatment that has been shown in a randomized trial to have a significantly lower TRM than ASCT for patients with advanced heart involvement, but its slower time to response still leaves the sickest patients without a good alternative. Melphalan is also not preferred if there is significant renal impairment. Small studies have shown promising results with bortezomib-based therapies which have a more rapid response time. It does not require renal dosing adjustment and is not considered nephrotoxic. Larger trials are needed to evaluate the true efficacy of bortezomib based therapies.

Regardless of therapy, achievement of a very good partial response (VGPR) as defined by the difference between the involved and uninvolved free light chain (dFLC) of less than 4 mg/dL or more than 90% reduction of the dFLC has been shown to increase the likelihood of a renal response (Table 34–1). Renal response has been classically defined as 50% reduction in proteinuria without significant (>25%) loss in kidney function. The main issue with this definition is that 50% reduction in proteinuria can take up to 12 months to achieve. In addition, some have questioned whether 50% is sufficient.

Table 34–1. AL amyloidosis hematologic response criteria.

Response	Definition
CR	Negative serum and urine IFE and normal serum FLC ratio
VGPR	dFLC <4 mg/dL (or >90% reduction in dFLC)
PR	>50% reduction in dFLC
NR	<50% reduction in dFLC

CR, complete response; dFLC, difference of involved to uninvolved FLC; FLC, free light chain; IFE, immunofixation; NR, no response; PR, partial response; VGPR, very good partial response.

A new response criteria introduced proposes the use of 30% proteinuria reduction at 6 months with less than 25% reduction in kidney function. Achievement of renal response by the new criteria has been shown to significantly reduce the incidence of end stage renal disease in these patients. Achieving a renal response is an independent marker of treatment success.

Kidney transplantation has been successfully performed in patients with AL amyloidosis. Patients without significant cardiac involvement and severe hypotension may be suitable candidates. Adequate disease control is a must. The achievement of a complete response (CR) should eliminate the risk of recurrence. CR is defined by a negative serum and urine immunofixation and normal serum FLC ratio. This can be achieved before or after the kidney transplantation but may be best to do so prior to avoid injury to the renal allograft during treatment or recurrence.

KEY READINGS

Cibeira MT et al: Outcome of AL amyloidosis after high-dose melphalan and autologous stem cell transplantation: long-term results in a series of 421 patients. Blood 2011;118:4346.

Glavey SV et al: Long-term outcome of patients with multiple myeloma-related advanced renal failure following auto-SCT. Bone Marrow Transplant 2013;48:1543.

Jaccard A et al: High-dose melphalan versus melphalan plus dexamethasone for AL amyloidosis. N Engl J Med 2007;357:1083.

Kyle RA, Gertz MA: Primary systemic amyloidosis: clinical and laboratory features in 474 cases. Semin Hematol 1995;32:45.

Palladini G et al: A staging system for renal outcome and early markers of renal response to chemotherapy in AL amyloidosis. Blood 2014;124:2325.

Pinney JH et al: Outcome in renal AL amyloidosis after chemotherapy. J Clin Oncol 2011;29:674.

Said SM et al: Renal amyloidosis: origin and clinicopathologic correlations of 474 recent cases. Clin J Am Soc Nephrol 2013;8:1515.

Venner CP et al: Cyclophosphamide, bortezomib, and dexamethasone therapy in AL amyloidosis is associated with high clonal response rates and prolonged progression-free survival. Blood 2012;119:4387.

MONOCLONAL IMMUNOGLOBULIN DEPOSITION DISEASE

Monoclonal immunoglobulin deposition disease (MIDD), like AL amyloidosis, is a group of diseases resulting from deposition of monoclonal Ig. In this case, the deposits are neither fibrillar nor congophilic. This group is also represented by three entities: light chain deposition disease (LCDD), the most common variant, light- and heavy-chain deposition disease (LHCDD), and heavy-chain deposition disease (HCDD). Also like AL amyloidosis, MIDD is a multisystemic disease capable of affecting multiple organs. Despite the similarity, there are important clinical differences that help differentiate MIDD from AL amyloidosis.

▶ Hematologic Characteristics

MIDD is usually the result of a plasma cell dyscrasia. A small number of cases have also been reported in patients with CLL, Waldenström macroglobulinemia, and other B-cell lymphomas. An older study found 65% of patients with LCDD had MM and 3% had CLL. However, the percentage of patients with MM decreases dramatically when myeloma-defining events are used in the definition. A recent study from France and one from the Mayo Clinic, both reported a rate of 20% for MM at the time of diagnosis. Waldenström macroglobulinemia accounted for 2% and the rest had MGRS. In one study the MGRS patients were further broken down to MGUS (42%) and SMM (36%). Kappa is the preferred immunoglobulin light chain accounting for ~80% of the clones in MIDD. As with AL amyloidosis, patients with concomitant MM have significantly poorer prognosis from the renal and overall survival standpoint.

▶ Laboratory Testing

Serum protein electrophoresis and serum immunofixation are not very sensitive in MIDD. The sensitivity rate ranges from 43% to 73%. One study suggests sensitivity is much higher in patients with LHCDD than LCDD and HCDD. Urine protein electrophoresis and immunofixation actually outperform serum studies in MIDD. Fortunately, serum FLC assay is 99–100% sensitive in MIDD making it the test of choice. Serum FLC assay is abnormal even in HCDD since the abnormal heavy chain is unable to bind the immunoglobulin light chain resulting in excess circulating FLC.

▶ Clinical Manifestations

MIDD is a systemic disease with Ig deposition in various organs. The median age at diagnosis is in the mid 50s, about 10 years earlier than AL amyloidosis. Kidney involvement is the dominant presentation in these patients. Kidney injury is present in over 90% of patients and proteinuria is nephrotic in 50%. Hematuria and hypertension are also common.

Median proteinuria ranges from 2 to 4 g/day but patients with HCDD can have massive proteinuria (>10 g/day). Liver and cardiac involvement is seen in one-fourth of patients but most are asymptomatic. Hepatomegaly with mild abnormalities in liver function tests is the most common manifestations of liver involvement. Diastolic dysfunction similar to cardiac amyloidosis may be seen with cardiomegaly and heart failure. Deposits may also be seen in nerve fibers, bone marrow, and lymph nodes. Extrarenal involvement is less common in HCDD.

Pathologic Findings

The diagnosis of MIDD can only be made by a kidney biopsy. Glomeruli characteristically show nodular mesangial matrix expansion by PAS positive material resembling diabetic glomerulosclerosis (Figure 34–2). There may be mild mesangial hypercellularity. Crescents may be seen especially with alpha

type HCDD. PAS positive material can also be seen along the tubular basement membrane, vessels, and interstitium. The diagnostic finding on IF is diffuse linear staining of glomerular, tubular, and vascular basement membranes for the pathogenic immunoglobulin light chain and/or heavy chain (Figure 34–2). Complement activation with C1q deposition may be seen in some cases especially with HCDD involving the γ1 or γ3 chains. The deposits have a finely granular powdery appearance on EM and can be seen along the outer aspect of tubular basement membranes and inner aspect of lamina densa of the glomerular basement membranes (Figure 34–2).

Treatment

The recent advances in the treatment of MM have also benefitted patients with MIDD. The use of novel agents has substantially improved the outcomes of patients especially

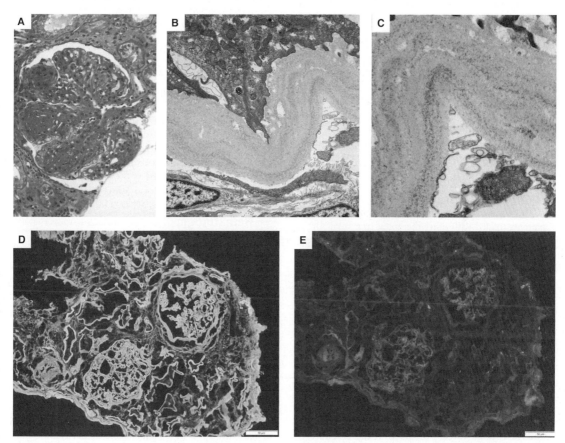

▲ **Figure 34–2.** Pathologic findings in a case of kappa-LCDD: **A.** The glomerulus shows nodular mesangial expansion by PAS positive immune deposits. There is also mild mesangial hypercellularity. On electron microscopy, punctate, powdery electron dense deposits are seen along the tubular basement membranes. **(B&C)** On immunofluorescence, there is bright diffuse linear staining of glomerular and tubular basement membranes for kappa **D.** with negative staining for lambda **(E)** (×200 for A, ×11,000 for B, ×23,000 for C, ×100 for D&E). (See Color Plate 11.)

those with MGRS who were previously suboptimally managed. One study reported kidney survival rate of 67% and 37% at 1 year and 5 year respectively with melphalan and prednisone. Patient survival was 89% and 70% at 1 year and 5 year respectively. In comparison, a study of patients treated with novel agents (thalidomide, lenalidomide, bortezomib, and alkylator) and ASCT from the United Kingdom showed a median renal survival of 5.4 years and a median patient survival of 14 years. In this study, 11.3% of patients had more than 10% bone marrow plasma cells. Kidney survival in this study was significantly shorter for patients presenting with CKD stage IV and V than II and III (2.7 years versus 9 years respectively, $p = 0.004$). CR was achieved in 88.9% of patients treated with bortezomib as front line agent versus 27.3% of those treated with thalidomide. Hematologic response was improved with ASCT where 13 of 16 patients achieved a CR, two patients had partial response (PR) and one patient died of complications during ASCT. Achievement of VGPR with first line therapy was significantly associated with better renal survival (83.7% versus 36.4% respectively, $p = 0.005$). In a French study with 49 patients, 20% of whom had MM, 70.4% achieved a VGPR or better after treatment with bortezomib based therapy. In this study, ASCT did not improve hematologic response. Renal response was again found closely associated with achievement of VGPR or better. In this study, 71% of patients with VGPR or better also achieved renal response versus 22% of those who did not ($p < 0.001$). Another study from the Mayo Clinic with 88 patients confirmed the finding of superior renal survival with the achievement of VGPR or better. Renal response was noted in 57% of patients who achieved a VGPR or better versus 17% of these with less than VGPR. VGPR and CR were achieved by 77% of patients who underwent ASCT versus 56% of patients using proteasome inhibitors versus 6% of patients treated with other therapies. In a small Greek study of 18 patients treated with bortezomib-based therapy, four patients of whom also received ASCT, CR was achieved in 45.5% and VGPR in 9% of patients. No patient with VGPR or better developed ESRD while 25% of those who achieved PR or less developed ESRD. Improvement in eGFR was also better in patients who had VGPR or better (7.7 mL/min/17.3 m^2 versus 0.8 mL/min/17.3 m^2). Unfortunately, due the small study, neither of these findings was statistically significant.

Kidney transplant in MIDD is risky if hematologic response is not achieved prior to transplant. In a single center study, 71.4% of patients had recurrence of disease at a median of 33 months. A review of seven cases in the literature found a recurrence rate of 85.7%. Graft lost was common after discovery of recurrence. In the United Kingdom study above, all three patients who did not receive chemotherapy prior to kidney transplant lost their graft to recurrence. In comparison, four patients who were treated with ASCT and achieved a CR all had preserved kidney function without signs of recurrence. In the French study, three patients underwent kidney transplant after bortezomib

treatment. One lost the graft at 3 years without evidence of recurrence on biopsy while the other two had stable graft function without signs of recurrence at 1 and 2 years posttransplant. Two of the patients had achieved a CR and one VGPR prior to kidney transplant.

KEY READINGS

Cohen C et al: Bortezomib produces high hematological response rates with prolonged renal survival in monoclonal immunoglobulin deposition disease. Kidney Int 2015;88:1135.

Kourelis TV et al: Outcomes of patients with renal monoclonal immunoglobulin deposition disease. Am J Hematol 2016;91:1123.

Nasr SH et al: Renal monoclonal immunoglobulin deposition disease: a report of 64 patients from a single institution. Clin J Am Soc Nephrol 2012;7:231.

Pozzi C et al: Light chain deposition disease with renal involvement: clinical characteristics and prognostic factors. Am J Kidney Dis 2003;42:1154.

Sayed RH et al: Natural history and outcome of light chain deposition disease. Blood 2015;126:2805.

LIGHT CHAIN PROXIMAL TUBULOPATHY

Light chain proximal tubulopathy (LCPT) is a rare complication of plasma cell dyscrasia and other B-cell lymphoproliferative disorders. LCPT is often accompanied by multiple electrolytes wasting, glycosuria, and aminoaciduria known as acquired Fanconi syndrome. However, patients with LCPT can present with full Fanconi syndrome, partial or none. This is further complicated by the fact that electrolytes wasting become less apparent with diminishing renal function.

▶ Hematologic Characteristics

Like many of the other lesions described above, LCPT is more commonly associated with MGRS. Two recent large series showed MM accounted for 20–33% of the hematologic diagnosis. In these series, MGRS was present in 60–80% of patients. Other hematologic conditions including CLL, Waldenström macroglobulinemia, and non-Hodgkin lymphoma accounted for 6–8% of cases. Monoclonal protein was detected in the serum in 71% and urine in 94% of patients. Serum FLC was abnormal in 91–100% of patients. In this disease, 95% of the light chains are kappa.

▶ Clinical Manifestations

The median age of these patients is between 58 and 60 years of age. Two-thirds of the patients are men. Renal insufficiency (<60 mL/min/1.73 m^2) is present in 83–95%. Median eGFR at presentation was 33–38 mL/min/1.73 m^2. Proteinuria is usually subnephrotic ranging between 2–3 g/day at presentation. Fanconi syndrome is reported in 40% in one series. This is manifested by type 2 renal tubular acidosis, aminoaciduria, hypophosphatemia, hypouricemia, and glycosuria. Patients with phosphaturia, aminoaciduria but without glycosuria are considered to have partial Fanconi syndrome. It is important to realize that hypophosphatemia and hypouricemia pseudonormalize as kidney function declines. However, aminoaciduria, abnormal fractional excretion of uric acid and phosphate, and glycosuria can still be found in 70–100% of patients at any kidney function. Recently, two studies have found that Fanconi syndrome is associated with the presence of crystalline light chain deposition in the proximal tubule cells. Patients without crystalline inclusions do not have Fanconi syndrome. Interestingly, the light chains in the crystals are nearly always kappa while lambda restricted monoclonal light chains often do not form crystals. Thus, Fanconi syndrome is mainly seen in patients with monoclonal kappa light chain. In addition to the renal manifestations, osteodystrophy can occur as a result of the Fanconi syndrome. In one series, 40% of the patients had suffered stress fractures either before, at the time of diagnosis or afterward. These are often atraumatic or minimally traumatic.

▶ Pathologic Findings

In majority of cases, the crystalline deposits in the proximal tubular cells dominate the pathologic features of LCPT. The crystals stain strongly eosinophilic, weakly PAS-positive, and trichrome-red. Some crystal may appear clear with all stains. Crystals can show various shapes ranging from rhomboid, hexagonal, pentagonal, triangular, to rod or needle shaped, which are best appreciated on EM (Figure 34–3). Signs of acute tubular injury are often present, but in contrast to myeloma CN secondary interstitial inflammation is infrequent. Intracytoplasmic vacuoles and proximal tubular cell distension can be present with or without crystal inclusions. Tubular atrophy and interstitial nephritis with mononuclear interstitial infiltrate can be mild to moderate. Due to their extensive crystallization and intracellular localization, the crystals in LCPT are frequently negative for kappa and lambda by standard IF on frozen tissue. However, in most of these cases, IF on protease-digested, paraffin-embedded tissue will demonstrate that the proximal tubular crystals stain for kappa with negative staining for lambda.

▶ Treatment

Up until recently, treatment of LCPT without MM was not recommended. The use of alkylator based therapies produced inadequate renal response. More important, it resulted in several mortalities due to complication from myelodysplastic syndrome. The risk of myelodysplasia has certainly changed with the novel agents but renal outcomes remains less certain. Renal outcomes were mixed in one study of 46 patients where every patient treated with chemotherapy and ASCT has either improved or stable renal function. In comparison, 67% of the patients treated with chemotherapy alone and 71.4% of patients treated

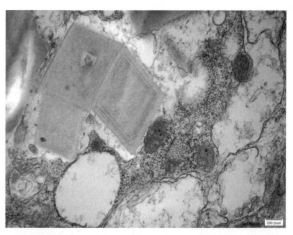

▲ **Figure 34–3.** Pathology of light chain proximal tubulopathy. Rhomboid shaped crystals composed of immunoglobulin kappa light chain are seen within a proximal tubular cell. Mitochondria and cytoplasmic vacuoles are present adjacent to the crystals (×46,000).

conservatively had improved or stable renal function. The percentage of patients with improved kidney function was 40% with chemotherapy and ASCT, 25% with chemotherapy alone, and 14% with conservative therapy. However, 33% of patients treated with chemotherapy alone and 37.5% of patients treated with conservative therapy died. In another study of 49 patients, eGFR improved by 14% in patients who achieved a VGPR or better while those that achieved a PR had a loss of 19% of eGFR. Kidney function improved or stabilized in 93%, 91%, 100%, and 67% of patients treated with ASCT, bortezomib based chemotherapy, immunomodulatory agents, and alkylating agents. Recurrence has been reported after kidney transplant often rapidly so hematologic response should be achieved prior to kidney transplant.

KEY READINGS

El Hamel C et al: Crystal-storing histiocytosis with renal Fanconi syndrome: pathological and molecular characteristics compared with classical myeloma-associated Fanconi syndrome. Nephrol Dial Transplant 2010;25:2982.

Ma CX et al: Acquired Fanconi syndrome is an indolent disorder in the absence of overt multiple myeloma. Blood 2004;104:40.

Messiaen T et al: Adult Fanconi syndrome secondary to light chain gammopathy. Clinicopathologic heterogeneity and unusual features in 11 patients. Medicine (Baltimore) 2000;79:135.

Stokes MB et al: Light chain proximal tubulopathy: clinical and pathologic characteristics in the modern treatment era. J Am Soc Nephrol 2016;27:1555.

Vignon M et al: Current anti-myeloma therapies in renal manifestations of monoclonal light chain-associated Fanconi syndrome: a retrospective series of 49 patients. Leukemia 2017;31:123.

MEMBRANOPROLIFERATIVE GLOMERULONEPHRITIS ASSOCIATED WITH MONOCLONAL GAMMOPATHY

Membranoproliferative glomerulonephritis (MPGN) is a heterogeneous group of kidney diseases, which shares the same histologic features on light microscopy. This group of diseases was previously categorized by their EM features. However, this classification is unable to differentiate the etiology. A new classification system has been proposed using IF characteristics. With the IF based classification, MPGNs can now be separated by the nature of the deposits: Ig (monoclonal versus polyclonal), complement or no deposits (thrombotic microangiopathy). Three rare entities make up the monoclonal Ig associated MPGN. These are proliferative glomerulonephritis with monoclonal immunoglobulin deposits (PMGMID), MPGN with masked Ig deposits, and C3 glomerulopathy with monoclonal gammopathy.

▶ PGNMID

PGNMID is a recently described glomerulonephritis characterized by non-organized monoclonal Ig deposits. The most common histological feature is MPGN but other patterns such as endocapillary proliferative glomerulonephritis and membranous glomerulonephritis can also be seen. Crescents either cellular or fibrous can be found in nearly a-third of cases. On IF, deposits are limited to the glomeruli and are seen along the glomerular capillary walls and mesangium. The Ig deposits should show restriction to a single light chain isotype and a single heavy chain isotype (and subtype in the case of IgG). In PGNMID, 50% of cases are due to a monoclonal IgG3 kappa and another 15% are due to IgG3 lambda. Other Ig heavy chains (IgA and IgM) and light chains alone (without heavy chains) have also been noted to cause this lesion. Most cases display C3 and C1q deposits in the same distribution as the monoclonal Ig. On EM, the deposits are mainly seen in the mesangium and subendothelial zone but can be present in a subepithelial location. By definition, the majority of deposits in PGNMID should appear granular (ie, without substructure). Rarely, a minority of otherwise granular deposits exhibits lattice-like arrays or ill-defined fibrils.

Patients with PGNMID usually present with high-grade proteinuria (median 5.7 g/day) and severe renal impairment (serum creatinine 2.8 mg/dL). The average age at diagnosis is 54 years but ranges from 20 to 81. PGNMID is a very low tumor burden disease. In a large series, only 4% of patients were noted to have MM. In fact, monoclonal protein was detectable in less than 30% of patients. A pathologic clone was identifiable in 100% of cases when both the serum immunofixation and serum FLC ratio were abnormal. Clone detection rate drops to 75% when only the serum immunofixation was positive and 17% when only the serum FLC ratio was abnormal. A pathologic clone could not be identified when both immunofixation and serum FLC ratio were normal. Patients with non IgG deposits were more likely to have a clone identified. Patients with IgG3 deposits are less likely to have a nephropathic clone identified compared with those with IgG1 or IgG2 deposits. As a consequence, deciding the chemotherapy and monitoring response to therapy can be challenging when no monoclonal protein exists. In these patients, response assessment is made via renal response. Patients with PGNMID have a high-recurrence rate after kidney transplant often resulting in allograft dysfunction within months of transplantation. More sensitive methods of monoclonal protein detection are desperately needed for PGNMID.

▶ C3 Glomerulopathy with Monoclonal Gammopathy

C3 glomerulopathy is a rare group of kidney diseases characterized by principally C3 deposits with little to no immunoglobulin deposition. Two diseases are represented by C3 glomerulopathy: C3 glomerulonephritis (C3GN) and dense deposit disease (DDD). On light microscopy C3GN may exhibit MPGN, endocapillary proliferative GN, or mesangial proliferative GN patterns of injury. Neutrophilic infiltrates in the glomerular tufts are not uncommon. IF shows diffuse and bright granular staining for C3 in the mesangium and capillary walls with negative or trivial immunoglobulin and C1q staining. On EM the deposits in C3GN are typically mesangial and subendothelial but subepithelial deposits including subepithelial hump are not uncommon. The pathologic hallmark of DDD is segmental transformation of the lamina densa of the glomerular basement membrane by highly electron dense deposits. Severe proteinuria often in the nephrotic range and severe renal impairment are common for these patients. Low C3 but normal C4 is present in half of the patients consistent with activation of the alternative pathway of complement. In fact, in children and young adults, complement dysregulation secondary to mutations of the complement regulatory peptides or cascade is one of the most common etiologies. Infection prior to development of C3 glomerulonephritis is also commonly reported in these patients.

The association between monoclonal gammopathy and C3 glomerulopathy was recently reported. This was first reported in a series of six patients in France. All but one patient were older than 50 years of age. A study from the Mayo Clinic found 31% of patients with C3GN also had a monoclonal gammopathy. MGUS was reported in 90% of these patients and CLL in the other 10%. The age of the patients with MG was significantly higher than the patients without (54 years versus 31 years respectively). The same institution also reported the presence of a monoclonal gammopathy in 71.4% of patients with DDD over the age of 49 years. All had MGUS at the time of diagnosis but one progressed to MM after follow-up of 120 months. These results are similar to a report from the University of Utah which found monoclonal gammopathy in 83% of patients with C3GN patients that are 49 years or older. In this cohort, MM or SMM were found in 40%, MGRS in 40%, and 10% had polyclonal plasmacytosis.

The pathogenesis of C3 glomerulopathy by monoclonal gammopathy remains poorly understood. By definition, there can be no significant monoclonal immunoglobulin deposition in the kidney biopsy. This has been confirmed by LMD/MS-MS. It has been suggested that the monoclonal Ig can act as a C3 nephritic factor (C3nef), but in large series, C3nef has been found in less than 20% of patients. No disease causing mutations have been found in these patients but a few (10–20%) carry the risk allele H402 (and rarely Y402) for factor H. The high rate of monoclonal gammopathy makes this unlikely to be a mere coincidence. Recurrence after kidney transplantation has been reported.

▶ MPGN with Masked Immunoglobulin Deposits

As above, C3GN is characterized by an MPGN pattern with C3-predominant deposits. In true C3GN, no significant immunoglobulin deposit is found even with LMD/MS-MS. However, a recent study from Arkana Laboratories and Mayo Clinic found that one-third of patients with monoclonal gammopathy and C3GN diagnosed based on standard IF on frozen tissue in fact have masked monoclonal deposits in glomeruli that required performing IF on paraffin tissue after antigen retrieval by proteinase K or pronase for detection. The majority of these patients are older than 50 years of age. Low C3 and normal C4 are detected in some of the patients just like in C3 glomerulopathy with monoclonal gammopathy. Hematologically, most of these patients have MGRS but some carry the diagnosis of MM, Waldenström macroglobulinemia, or CLL. It is of interest that none of these patients had humps on EM. While more patients are needed to verify the results, these data suggest that the diagnosis of C3GN with monoclonal gammopathy should only be made after exclusion of masked monoclonal deposits by protease IF. Interestingly, in the above noted study, no case of DDD with monoclonal gammopathy showed masked monoclonal deposits by protease IF; hence, protease IF is not warranted in patients with DDD with monoclonal gammopathy.

KEY READINGS

Nasr SH et al: Proliferative glomerulonephritis with monoclonal IgG deposits. J Am Soc Nephrol 2009;20:2055-64.

Zand L et al: C3 glomerulonephritis associated with monoclonal gammopathy: a case series. Am J Kidney Dis 2013;62:506-14.

Chauvet S et al: Treatment of B-cell disorder improves renal outcome of patients with monoclonal gammopathy-associated C3 glomerulopathy. Blood 2017;129:1437-1447.

Larsen CP et: Membranoproliferative glomerulonephritis with masked monotypic immunoglobulin deposits. Kidney Int 2015;88:867-73.

■ CHAPTER REVIEW QUESTIONS

1. What are the most important risk factors in the development of cast nephropathy?
   A. More than 60% bone marrow plasma cells and more than one focal bone lesion on MRI
   B. Anemia and hypercalcemia
   C. Lytic bone lesions
   D. Serum free light chain level more than 50 mg/dL and a high-urinary free light chain excretion
   E. The use of non-steroidal anti-inflammatory drugs and intravenous contrast agent

2. Which of these is the most helpful in predicting the recovery of renal function after cast nephropathy?
   A. The isotype of the immunoglobulin light chain
   B. The baseline free light chain ratio
   C. The percent reduction of the serum-free light chain
   D. The cytogenetic FISH results of the multiple myeloma
   E. The serum M-spike

3. What is the minimum level of hematologic response required to increase the chances of a renal response in AL amyloidosis?
   A. A complete response: the absence of a monoclonal protein by serum and urine immunofixation and a normal free-light chain ratio
   B. A very good partial response: dFLC less than 4 mg/dL or more than 90% reduction of the dFLC
   C. A partial response: 50% reduction of the dFLC
   D. Absent of clonal plasma cells in the bone marrow
   E. Normal serum-free light chains

4. What percentage of patients with monoclonal immu-noglobulin deposition disease also have symptomatic multiple myeloma?
   A. 10%
   B. 20%
   C. 30%
   D. 40%
   E. 50%

5. A monoclonal protein is found in less than 30% of patients with PGNMID. What laboratory value helps predict the identification of a pathologic clone in these patients?
   A. A positive serum immunofixation
   B. An abnormal serum-free light chain ratio
   C. The presence of IgG3 on the kidney biopsy
   D. A and B
   E. None of the above

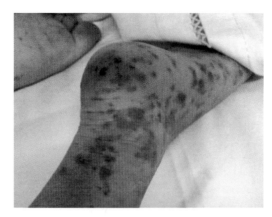

▲ **Plate 1.** Leukocytoclastic vasculitis as in a patient with HSP. (See Figure 28-2.)

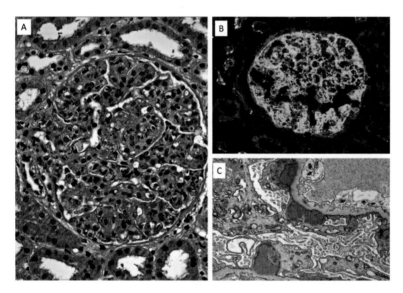

▲ **Plate 2.** Pathology of APSGN: **A.** The depicted glomerulus shows global occlusion of the peripheral capillaries by marked endocapillary hypercellularity including numerous intracapillary infiltrating neutrophils. **B.** Immunofluorescence shows coarsely granular mesangial and glomerular capillary wall staining for C3 ("starry sky pattern"). **C.** This electron microscopic image shows four large subepithelial hump-shaped electron dense deposits. (See Figure 31-1.)

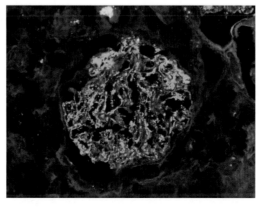

▲ **Plate 3.** Pathology of SAGN: The glomerulus in this case of IgA-dominant staphylococcus-associated glomerulonephritis shows bright granular global mesangial and segmental glomerular capillary wall staining for IgA. (See Figure 31-2.)

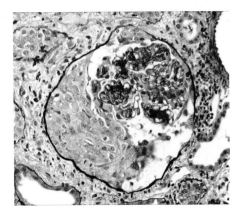

▲ **Plate 4.** Pathology of IE-associated glomerulonephritis: This case of IE-associated glomerulonephritis showed diffuse crescentic pattern on injury. The glomerulus shows a large cellular crescent. The underlying glomerular tuft exhibits mild mesangial and endocapillary hypercellularity (silver stain). (See Figure 31-3.)

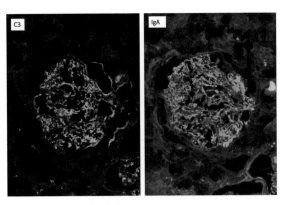

▲ **Plate 5.** (See Chapter Review Question 31-2.)

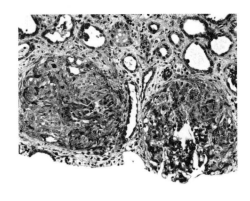

▲ **Plate 6.** (See Chapter Review Question 31-3.)

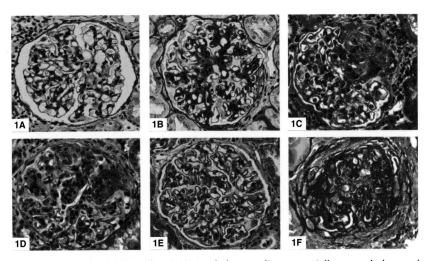

▲ **Plate 7.** Classes of lupus nephritis (LN). **A.** Class I. Minimal abnormality: essentially normal glomerular cellularity and capillary loop patency (PAS stain). **B.** Class II. Mesangial LN: increased mesangial cellularity and expanded mesangial matrix (PAS stain). **C.** Class III. Focal proliferative LN: segmental endocapillary proliferation with loss of capillary loop patency in right upper quadrant of this glomerulus (H&E stain). **D.** Class IV. Diffuse proliferative LN: nearly global endocapillary proliferative changes which characteristically vary from segment to segment; nuclear karyorrhexis is evident in the solidified segment on the right (H&E stain). **E.** Class V. Membranous LN. Global thickening of capillary loops with modest mesangial matrix expansion (H&E stain). **F.** Class VI. Sclerosing LN. Glomerular tuft has collapsed with expanded mesangial matrix, fibrosis and loss of capillary circulation (PAS stain). (See Figure 33-1.)

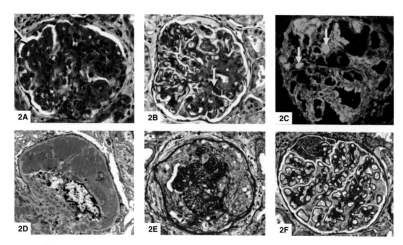

▲ **Plate 8.** Spectrum of pathology within classes IV and V lupus nephritis (LN). **A.** Class IV LN with classic "wire loop" lesions (yellow arrow) along with severe endocapillary proliferation in a near global pattern (H&E stain). **B.** Class IV LN with hyaline thrombi (yellow arrow) representing massive immune complex deposits across a continuum from wire loops to capillary loop occlusion (PAS stain). **C.** Class IV LN. Immunostaining for IgG deposits in same case as B; heavy capillary wall deposits and luminal thrombi (yellow arrows) (Immunofluorescence microscopy). **D.** Class IV LN. Ultrastructure of immune complex deposits in same case as B; note the extensive subendothelial deposits which continue to accumulate as massive luminal deposits that compromise capillary circulation (Electron microscopy). **E.** Class IV LN. The tuft of this glomerulus is severely compressed by a circumferential cellular crescent (PAS stain). **F.** Class V + Class III LN. This glomerulus exhibits nearly uniform capillary loop thickening and a superimposed segmental proliferative lesion near the top of this figure (PAS stain). (See Figure 33-2.)

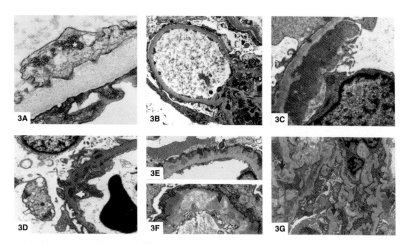

▲ **Plate 9.** Characteristic ultrastructural lesions in lupus nephritis (LN). **A.** Tubuloreticular inclusion (yellow asterisk) in the cytoplasm of a glomerular endothelial cell; these structures putatively reflect condensation of cytoplasmic organelles caused by interferon. **B.** Earliest evidence of immune complex deposition; dark electron-dense deposits appear first in the mesangial stalk (pink arrows). **C.** Subendothelial deposits (pink asterisks) characteristic of Class III and IV LN. **D.** Class IV LN with predominant subendothelial deposits (yellow arrow) is often accompanied by scattered subepithelial deposits (pink arrow); when the subepithelial deposits are more extensive and regularly distributed along the capillary wall, it is best described as mixed membranous and proliferative LN. **E.** Class V LN. Stage 2 membranous nephropathy; regularly distributed subepithelial electron dense deposits are evident (pink arrow); projections of glomerular basement membrane outwardly between the subepithelial deposits tend to produce a spiked appearance to the capillary loops. **F.** Class V LN. Stage 3–4 membranous nephropathy; electron-dense deposits have become incorporated with the capillary wall (pink arrow) and have begun to disintegrate (yellow asterisk). **G.** Glomerular sclerosis. This appearance of collapsed, wrinkled glomerular basement membranes is seen across all classes of LN but predominantly in Class VI; residual electron-dense deposits (pink arrows) are interspersed in the sclerosing process. (See Figure 33-3.)

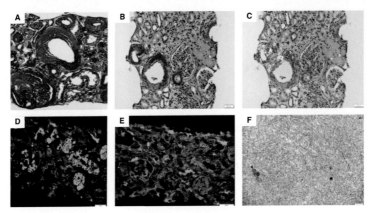

▲ **Plate 10.** Pathologic findings in a case of AL-lambda amyloidosis. **A.** Acellular, PAS-weak amyloid deposits involving a glomerulus, an interlobular artery and two arterioles. **B.** Amyloid deposits are strongly Congo red positive. **C.** Under polarized light, they exhibit anomalous colors (yellow/orange/green) (so-called "apple-green birefringence). **D.** On immunofluorescence, glomerular, and vascular amyloid deposits show strong smudgy staining for lambda . **E.** Amyloid deposits are negative for kappa. **F.** On electron microscopy, amyloid deposits are composed of solid randomly oriented fibrils with a mean thickness of 9 nm (range 7–12)(×200 for A–C, ×100 for D&E, ×46,000 for F). (See Figure 34-1.)

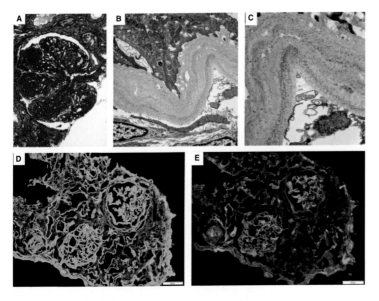

▲ **Plate 11.** Pathologic findings in a case of kappa-LCDD: **A.** The glomerulus shows nodular mesangial expansion by PAS positive immune deposits. There is also mild mesangial hypercellularity. On electron microscopy, punctate, powdery electron dense deposits are seen along the tubular basement membranes. (**B&C**) On immunofluorescence, there is bright diffuse linear staining of glomerular and tubular basement membranes for kappa **D.** with negative staining for lambda (**E**) (×200 for A, ×11,000 for B, ×23,000 for C, ×100 for D&E). (See Figure 34-2.)

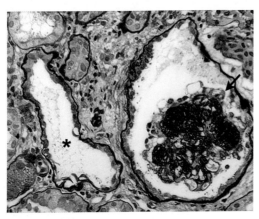

▲ **Plate 12.** Typical histopathologic findings in HIVAN. Periodic acid–Schiff staining demonstrates focal glomerulosclerosis with collapse of the glomerular tuft and overlying podocyte proliferation (arrow), microcystic tubular dilation (asterisk), interstitial inflammation, and interstitial fibrosis. Magnification, ×200. (See Figure 36-2.)

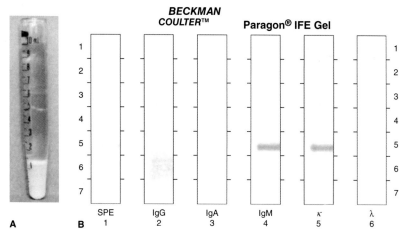

▲ **Plate 13. A.** Whitish cryoprecipitates forming in Wintrobe tube after standing at 4°C for 72 hours followed by centrifugation at 400 × g for 10 minutes. The cryocrit is approximately 30%. **B.** Immunofixation of the washed, dissolved cryoprecipitate detected a monoclonal IgMκ with polyclonal IgG. By definition, these are type II cryoglobulins. (Courtesy of Dr Janette S.Y. Kwok, Department of Pathology and Clinical Biochemistry, Queen Mary Hospital, Hong Kong, China.) (See Figure 36-5.)

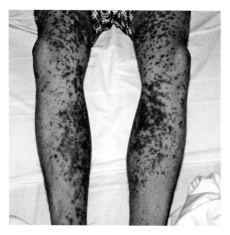

▲ **Plate 14.** Palpable purpuric skin lesions in the lower limbs of a patient with cryoglobulinemia. Such lesions are characteristic of any causes of small vessel vasculitis, but not pathognomonic of the rashes in cryoglobulinemia. (Courtesy of Dr. Chi-keung Yeung, Department of Medicine, Queen Mary Hospital, Hong Kong, China.) (See Figure 36-6.)

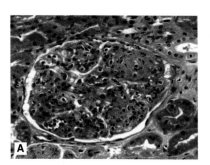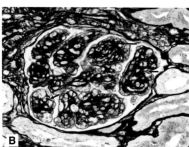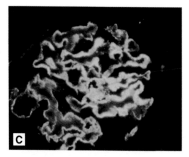

▲ **Plate 15.** Pathology of membranoproliferative glomerulonephritis type I associated with cryoglobulinemia. **A.** Glomerulus exhibits a diffuse increase in mesangial cellularity and matrix with accentuation of lobulation of tuft architecture, obliteration of capillary lumens, and leukocytic infiltrate (×200, H&E). **B.** Periodic acid–Schiff and methenamine silver staining reveals prominent double contours or tram-tracking (arrows) of the glomerular basement membrane (GBM) (×400). **C.** Immunofluorescence reveals granular deposits of C3 (shown here) and IgG in the mesangium and in peripheral capillary loops (×200). (Courtesy of Dr. Kwok-wah Chan, Department of Pathology, Queen Mary Hospital, Hong Kong, China.) (See Figure 36-8A-C.)

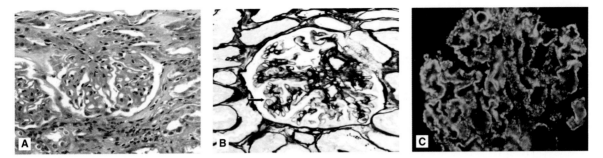

▲ **Plate 16.** Pathology of hepatitis B virus (HBV)-associated membranous nephropathy (MN). **A.** On light microscopy, the characteristic glomerular lesion is a diffuse thickening of glomerular capillary walls to form thick "membranes" (H&E, ×200). **B.** Periodic acid–Schiff and methenamine silver staining highlights the characteristic epimembranous "spike" formation (arrow), projections of glomerular basement membrane (GBM) material between immune complexes that lead to a saw tooth-like appearance of the GBM (×400). **C.** Immunofluorescence reveals granular deposits of IgG (shown here) together with C3. IgM, IgA, and C1q may be present. (Courtesy of Dr. Kwok-wah Chan, Department of Pathology, Queen Mary Hospital (A–C), and Dr. Yun-hoi Lui and Dr. Chung-ying Leung, Department of Pathology, United Christian Hospital (D), Hong Kong, China.) **(See Figure 36-9A-C.)**

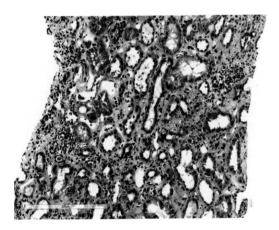

▲ **Plate 17.** Renal histology findings in drug-induced ATIN showing lymphoplasmacytic tubulointerstitial infiltrate and tubulitis. The patient had lung adenocarcinoma on anti-PD1 therapy (Lambrolizumab) and presented with rising creatinine and adrenalitis. The patient was also on a proton pump inhibitor for years prior to starting anti-PD1 therapy. Urine sediment had numerous white blood cells. (See Figure 37-2.)

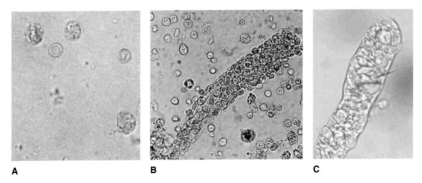

A   B   C

▲ **Plate 18.** **A.** White blood cell and red blood cell in urine of a patient with CTIN. **B.** White blood cell cast with surrounding white blood cells and renal tubular epithelial cells in urine of patient with CTIN. **C.** Waxy, non-cellular hyaline cast in patient with diabetic nephropathy with significant chronic tubulointerstitial changes. (See Figure 38-2.)

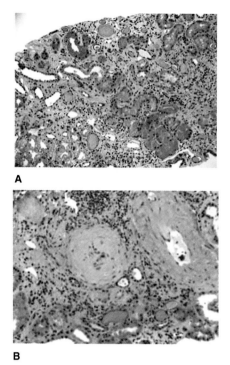

A

B

▲ **Plate 19.** **A.** Tubulointerstitial disease from a patient with CTIN. Tubulules show dilatation and atrophy. Proteinacious hyaline casts can be seen in some tubules. Interstitium has a cellular infiltrate with diffuse fibrosis. **B.** Sclerotic glomerulus in patient with CTIN. Note the periglomerular infiltration. Thickened vessel suggestive of long standing hypertension. (See Figure 38-3.)

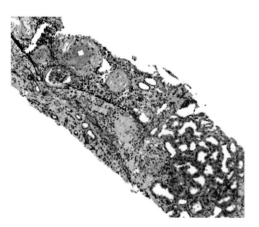

▲ **Plate 20.** CTIN from a patient with longstanding tacrolimus use in the setting of a previous liver transplant. Noted are areas of intense infiltrate and fibrosis juxtaposed to areas of tubular injury without interstitial infiltrate or fibrosis. This represents the so-called "stripped-fibrosis" pattern seen with CNI nephrotoxicity. (See Figure 38-4.)

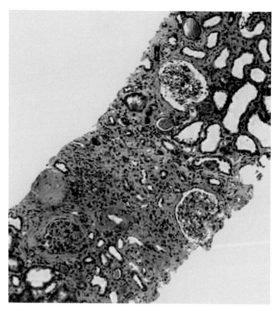

▲ **Plate 21** CTIN from a patient with treated PR3 vasculitis. Note the areas of continued interstitial inflammation and marked fibrosis. Tubules demonstrate dilatation and atrophy. Patient has undetectable PR3 titers and remained on maintenance rituximab for 1 year at time of biopsy. (See Figure 38-5.)

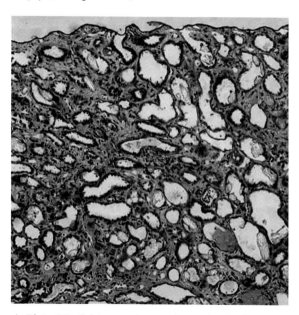

▲ **Plate 22.** Calcium oxalate nephropathy. Birefringent crystals in the lumen of many tubules. Tubules demonstrate marked dilatation and atrophy. Interstitium has cellular infiltration and fibrosis. (See Figure 38-6.)

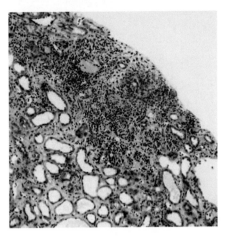

▲ **Plate 23.** CTIN from a patient with IgG4 related disease. Tubules show dilatation and atrophy with intervening interstitial fibrosis. Dense area of infiltration rich in eosinophils. (See Figure 38-7.)

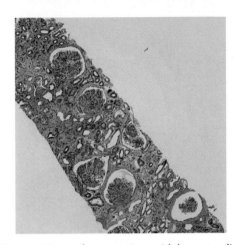

▲ **Plate 24.** Biopsy from a patient with long standing diabetic nephropathy. Glomerular show classical basement membrane thickening with nodules. Tubules show dilation and atrophy. Interstitium shows infiltrate and fibrosis. (See Figure 38-8.)

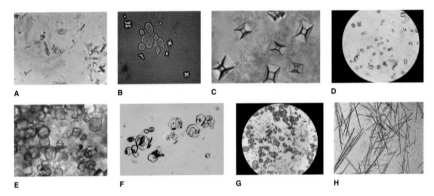

▲ **Plate 25.** Types of crystals which may be seen in urine. **A.** Calcium oxalate monohydrate. **B.** Calcium oxalate dehydrate. **C.** Struvite crystals. **D.** Uric acid crystals. **E.** Uric acid crystals under a polarized light. **F.** Cystine crystals. **G.** Sulfadiazine crystals. **H.** Acyclovir crystals. (See Figure 39-2.)

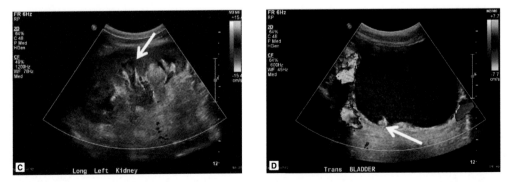

▲ **Plate 26.** Imaging study findings in a sickle cell disease patient presenting with hematuria. **C.** Renal US shows dilated renal pelvis and calyces with echogenic material consistent with blood. **D.** The urinary bladder is distended with echogenic material consistent with blood, with a small clot seen dependently. (Courtesy of Dr. Matilda Jude, UCLA-Olive View Medical Center, Sylmar, California.) (See Figure 48-1C & D.)

Thrombotic Microangiopathies

Joshua M. Thurman, MD
Ashley Frazer-Abel, PhD

ESSENTIALS OF DIAGNOSIS

- ▶ Thrombotic microangiopathy is caused by thrombosis within the microvasculature of various organs.
- ▶ Patients typically present with thrombocytopenia, hemolytic anemia, and dysfunction of affected organs (most commonly the kidneys and brain).
- ▶ ADAMTS13 activity and the presence of Shiga-like toxin in stool should be evaluated in all patients with suspected TMA. Specific tests for other causes of TMA are based upon the clinical scenario.

▶ General Considerations

The thrombotic microangiopathies (TMAs) are a group of diseases caused by thrombosis in the microvasculature of tissue beds throughout the body. Patients present with microangiopathic hemolytic anemia, thrombocytopenia, and injury of affected organs. TMA can develop in patients exposed to a wide range of different diseases or stressors, including infections, cancers, drugs, autoimmune diseases, and pregnancy. There are also two primary forms of TMA: thrombotic thrombocytopenic purpura (TTP) and hemolytic uremic syndrome (HUS).

HUS and TTP are caused by distinct pathologic processes that cause similar clinical presentations. The treatment of these diseases is different, so the proper diagnosis is important. For the secondary causes of TMA, the approach is to treat or remove the triggering event. Episodes of HUS and TTP can be triggered by illness, medications, or pregnancy, however, so in practice the distinction of the primary and secondary forms of TMA can be difficult.

THROMBOTIC THROMBOCYTOPENIC PURPURA

ESSENTIALS OF DIAGNOSIS

- ▶ TTP has traditionally been described as presenting with thrombocytopenia, hemolytic anemia, neurologic symptoms, renal insufficiency, and fever. However, patients do not usually present with all five of these findings.
- ▶ Low activity (<10% activity) of ADAMTS13 [a protease that cleaves von Willebrand factor (vWF)] is considered diagnostic of TTP.
- ▶ Plasma exchange is the treatment of choice for patients with TTP, and immunosuppression with corticosteroids and rituximab may be beneficial in some patients.

▶ General Considerations

TTP is associated with decreased function of the zinc metalloprotease ADAMTS13 (A Disintegrin And Metalloprotease with ThromboSpondin-1-domains, type 13). The incidence of TTP is estimated to be less than 2 cases per million people and it is more common in women than in men. TTP typically presents in patients between 20 and 50 years old, although patients with congenital deficiency of ADAMTS13 usually present in childhood.

▶ Pathogenesis

Endothelial cells produce large multimers of vWF that are normally cleaved by ADAMTS13. Decreased ADAMTS13 activity permits the persistence of unusually large vWF multimers that can bind to extracellular matrix and platelets, inducing platelet aggregation, thrombocytopenia, thrombosis, and ischemia of affected organs. Some patients have congenital deficiency of ADAMTS13, a condition termed Upshaw–Shulman syndrome. In most adult patients with TTP, however, ADAMTS13 activity is reduced due to an inhibitory autoantibody to the protein.

▶ Clinical Findings

A. Symptoms and Signs

TTP is traditionally described as manifesting with microangiopathic hemolytic anemia, thrombocytopenia, fever, neurologic symptoms, and renal failure, but only a small percentage of patients have all five of these findings. Patients frequently feel fatigue due to anemia, and thrombocytopenia can cause bleeding and purpura. Any organ system can be involved, and patients commonly present with mild neurologic symptoms and gastrointestinal symptoms, including abdominal pain and bloody diarrhea (which should raise concerns for mesenteric ischemia). Patients can have cardiovascular symptoms, including those of myocardial ischemia and congestive heart failure. The clinical presentation of TTP is very similar to that of HUS. In general, platelet count tends to be lower in TTP, whereas renal function tends to be more severely affected in with HUS. Patients with congenital TTP may develop disease shortly after birth, but the disease may not present until adulthood. Pregnancy can trigger a first episode of TTP in women with congenital ADAMTS13 deficiency.

B. Laboratory Findings

Patients with TTP usually have laboratory evidence of microangiopathic hemolytic anemia (low hemoglobin, elevated lactate dehydrogenase and direct bilirubin, low haptoglobin, and presence of schistocytes). The platelet count is usually very low, and can be less than $10 \times 10^3/\mu L$. Coagulation times are usually normal, and the direct antiglobulin test (DAT, or Coombs test) is negative.

ADAMTS13 functional activity should be promptly measured in all patients with suspected TMA so that TTP can be diagnosed and treated as quickly as possible (Figure 35–1). ADAMTS13 activity less than 10% is diagnostic of TTP (Figure 35–1). Many laboratorys also test for the presence of an ADAMTS13 inhibitor, but the presence or absence of an inhibitor does not change the approach to treatment. Plasma infusion or plasma exchange alters ADAMTS13 activity, so it is critical that the activity level is measured in a sample obtained prior to the administration of plasma. Renal failure is usually mild in TTP. A platelet count of less than $30 \times 10^3/\mu L$, a serum creatinine (Cr) less than 2.3 mg/dL, and a positive antinuclear antibody are predictive of low ADAMTS13 activity.

C. Biopsy Findings

Light microscopic examination of renal biopsies often reveals fibrin and platelet thrombi in the glomerular capillaries (Figure 35–2). Thrombi can also be seen in arterioles and small arteries. Schistocytes can sometimes be seen within the vessel walls. Microthrombi in TTP may be more platelet rich compared to HUS, and the heart and pancreas are more frequently affected in TTP. By electron microscopy the endothelial cells can appear swollen and fibrin can be seen. Chronically the disease causes double contour formation within the capillary wall, and glomeruli develop a membranoproliferative pattern. However, immunofluorescence microscopy typically does not reveal IgG or C3 deposits. In approximately 3% of patients the diagnosis of TMA is made by kidney biopsy, and the clinical features of TMA may be absent in these patients.

▶ Differential Diagnosis

All of the causes of TMA should be considered in patients suspected of having TTP (Table 35–1). Disseminated intravascular coagulation causes many of the same findings as TTP, but is associated with abnormal coagulation tests. Immune-mediated thrombocytopenia (ITP) should also be considered in patients presenting with very low platelet counts, but ITP is not associated with hemolytic anemia or with the other systemic findings seen in TTP. Systemic lupus erythematosus (SLE) is associated with antiphospholipid antibody syndrome (APS) and can cause clinical findings similar to those seen in TTP. Detection of lupus-related autoantibodies may indicate a diagnosis of SLE. If ADAMTS13 activity is low, however, patients should be treated with plasma exchange for presumptive TTP.

1. Pregnancy-associated TTP—Pregnancy can provoke the first presentation of disease in patients with congenital defects in ADAMTS13 activity, and it is associated with flares of the disease in patients with acquired TTP. Absence of an inhibitory antibody suggests a genetic deficiency in this setting, and genetic testing can confirm this diagnosis.

Diagnosis of TTP in pregnant patients can be particularly challenging. Anemia and thrombocytopenia are seen with normal pregnancy and the diagnosis of TMA can be missed. Several different forms of TMA can complicate pregnancy, and there is overlap in the presentations of TTP, pre-eclampsia, and HELLP syndrome (hemolysis, elevated liver enzymes, low platelets). TTP typically occurs in the second or third trimester, and usually does not improve after delivery, whereas pre-eclampsia and HELLP syndrome do. Although ADAMTS13 activity falls during normal pregnancy, an activity level less than 10% distinguishes pregnancy-associated TTP from other causes of TMA. In pregnant patients with severe TMA (eg, a platelet count <50,000/μL, hemolytic anemia, neurologic symptoms, and

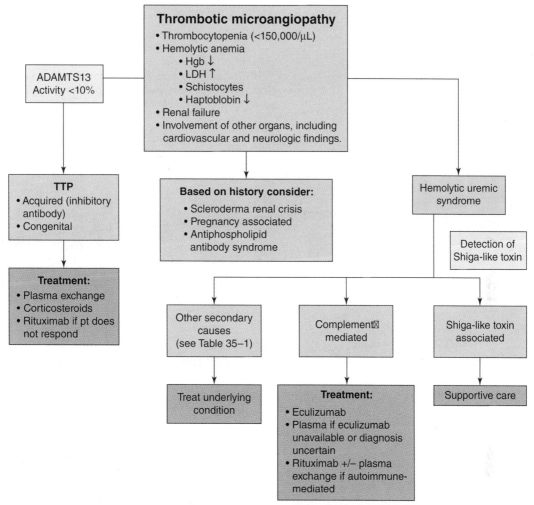

▲ **Figure 35–1.** Approach to patients with thrombotic microangiopathy. Thrombotic microangiopathy is a clinical diagnosis based on the detection of thrombocytopenia and hemolytic anemia. Ischemia of target tissues can also lead to organ ischemia, and commonly affected tissues include the kidney and central nervous system. ADAMTS13 activity and detection of Shiga-like toxin should be performed in all patients suspected of having thrombotic microangiopathy. Depending on the clinical history and examination findings, specific tests should be performed for other causes of thrombotic microangiopathy. All patients suspected of having thrombocytopenic thrombotic purpura should be treated with plasma exchange while awaiting the results of ADAMTS13 activity. Patients suspected of having hemolytic uremic syndrome should be treated with eculizumab, a complement inhibitory drug.

renal impairment) plasma exchange can be started even before ADAMTS13 activity results are obtained.

2. TTP in patients with infections—Various bacterial, fungal, and viral infections have been documented in patients with TMA, including cytomegalovirus (CMV) and human immunodeficiency virus (HIV). Infections may trigger TTP in susceptible patients, but a large number of different systemic infections can directly cause TMA in patients with normal ADAMTS13 activity (Table 35–1). Clinical presentation of infection-induced TMA in patients with normal or non-diagnostic ADAMTS13 activity can be indistinguishable from TTP. In these patients the underlying infection should be treated and plasma exchange should not be performed. Patients with ADAMTS13 activity less than 10%, on the other hand, should be treated for TTP.

Complications

TTP can affect any organ system through the body. Kidney involvement is typically milder than in HUS, but TTP can lead to irreversible kidney injury and in some cases end stage renal disease (ESRD). Neurologic manifestations are also usually mild and/or transient, but seizures and cerebrovascular accidents can occur.

Treatment

Plasma exchange is the cornerstone of treatment for TTP. Diagnosis of TTP requires documentation of low ADAMTS13 activity, but plasma exchange should be started right away in patients suspected of having the disease. Prompt plasma treatment is been associated with a better prognosis, and treatment should not be delayed while awaiting confirmation

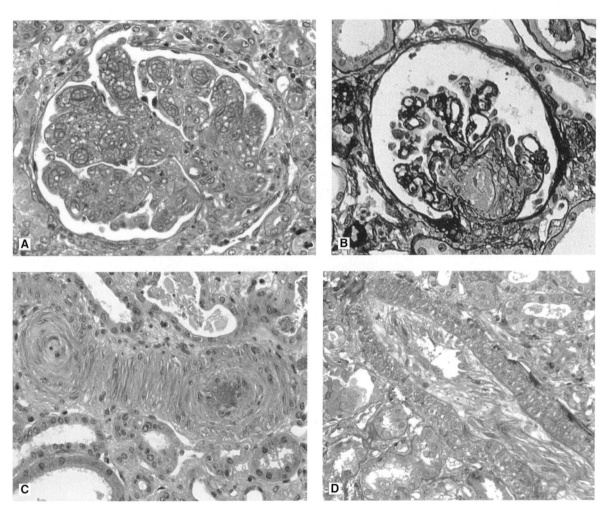

▲ **Figure 35–2.** Renal findings in thrombotic microangiopathy. **A.** Glomerulus with a lobular configuration, mesangiolysis, and thrombosed capillary lumina (×400). **B.** thrombosis of intraglomerular arteriole. The glomerulus is ischemic with wrinkled and partially collapsed capillary walls (×400). **C.** Arteriole showing muscular hypertrophy with an "onion skin" appearance, absent lumen, and focal thrombosis (×200). **D.** Artery with mucoid intimal thickening and swollen endothelial cells (×200). **E.** Immunofluorescence of an artery demonstrating fibrin throughout the thickened vascular intima. **F.** Electron micrograph of a glomerular capillary wall showing a markedly expanded subendothelial zone containing flocculent granular material (altered fibrin) with narrowing of the lumen. (Figure reproduced from Nast CC, Adler SG: Thrombotic microangiopathies. In: *Current Diagnosis & Treatment: Nephrology & Hypertension.* Lerma EV, Berns JS, Nissenson AR (eds). McGraw-Hill, New York, 2009.)

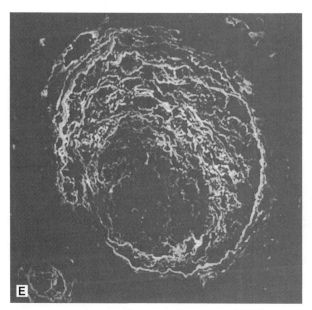

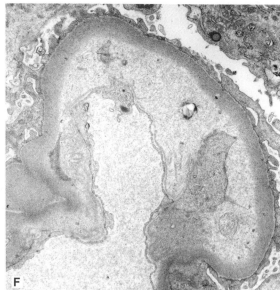

▲ **Figure 35–2.** (*Continued*)

of the diagnosis. Plasma exchange should be used in pregnant patients and infected patients if the ADAMTS13 activity is very low or if alternative diagnoses are not found.

When available, plasma exchange is preferable to plasma infusion because larger volumes of plasma can be administered without causing volume overload. Plasma exchange may also have the benefit of removing circulating ADAMTS13 inhibitors as well as ultralarge vWF multimers. Treatments should replace 1–1.5 plasma volumes with fresh frozen plasma. Alternative (non-plasma) replacement fluids should not be used, as fresh frozen plasma has the benefit of restoring ADAMTS13 activity.

Blood counts and LDH should initially be measured daily in order to assess the response to treatment, and plasma exchange should be repeated daily until the platelet count is more than 150,000/µL for two successive days. Patients with severe disease, such as those with neurologic manifestations, can be treated with twice daily plasma exchange until they show signs of improvement.

Steroids may reduce the production of ADAMTS13 inhibitors, and patients should be empirically started on corticosteroids (prednisone 1 mg/kg/day), unless there is evidence of an underlying infection. This dose can be continued until the blood counts improve and can then be tapered over several weeks. Although the optimal dose of steroids is uncertain, there may be a benefit to treating patients with high-dose intravenous methylprednisolone followed by oral steroids. Rituximab may be beneficial in patients with severe or refractory disease. Patients can be transfused with platelets if they have bleeding complications or in anticipation of invasive procedures. On the other hand, TTP patients may be at increased risk of venous thrombosis, particularly after their platelet counts improve. Ambulation and intermittent compression systems can be used to lower the risk of thrombosis.

1. Refractory or relapsing disease—Patients who do not respond to plasma therapy after 4–7 days or who show signs of clinical deterioration after the initiation of treatment are considered to have refractory disease. Plasma exchange and corticosteroids should be continued in these patients, and rituximab is probably also beneficial. Patients with early relapse of the disease after initially responding to treatment should be retreated with plasma exchange, corticosteroids, and rituximab. Because plasma exchange removes rituximab, some investigators recommend waiting 48 hours after rituximab dosing before the next plasma exchange treatment. Based on each patient's course physicians must weigh the risks of withholding plasma exchanges for this period versus delaying the administration of rituximab. Most relapses occur within the first year after disease onset, but relapses can occur after years of remission.

▶ **Prognosis**

Untreated, TTP is fatal in more than 90% of patients, but with plasma therapy survival rates are higher than 80%. Patients who respond to plasma therapy usually have complete hematologic recovery between episodes of the disease.

Table 35–1. Causes of thrombotic microangiopathy.

Disease	Clinical Characteristics	Diagnostic Tests
Thrombotic thrombocytopenic purpura (TTP) • Genetic (Upshaw–Shulman syndrome) • Acquired (ADAMTS13 inhibitor) • Infection associated • Pregnancy associated	• Very low platelet count (often $<30 \times 10^3/\mu L$) • Mild kidney injury (creatinine usually <2.3 mg/dL)	In all patients: • ADAMTS13 activity <10% • ADAMTS13 inhibitor In appropriate clinical setting: • Genetic testing for ADAMTS13 mutation
Hemolytic uremic syndrome • Shiga-toxin associated • Complement mediated • Pregnancy associated • Infection associated • Neuraminidase producing *Streptococcus pneumoniae* • Cobalamin deficiency (homozygous deficiency) • Diacylglycerol kinase ε (*DGKE*) mutation (homozygous or compound heterozygous)	• Platelet count usually $>30 \times 10^3/\mu L$ • Moderate to severe kidney injury	In all patients: • Shiga toxin in stool • Complement tests In appropriate clinical setting: • Complement protein levels and genetic screen (see text) • Polysaccharide *Streptococcal* antigen detection • High homocysteine, low methionine levels • Genetic analysis of *DGKE* gene
Drug-associated thrombotic microangiopathy	• Kidney injury is common • Can present as sudden onset disease with systemic symptoms • Can present as slowly progressive disease	• Onset correlates with use of drug associated with TMA (see Table 35–2) • Improvement with discontinuation of drug
Cancer associated and hematopoietic stem cell-associated thrombotic microangiopathy	• Cancer-associated usually presents with pulmonary involvement • SCT-associated usually presents with renal involvement	Diagnosis of exclusion. Consider also: • Drug associated • Graft versus host disease • Infectious
Scleroderma renal crisis	• Sudden onset hypertension	In appropriate clinical setting: • Anti-RNA polymerase III • Anti-Th/To RNP • Anti-topoisomerase III (Scl-70)
Antiphospholipid antibody syndrome	• Frequently associated with autoimmune disease	In appropriate clinical setting: • Anticardiolipin • Anti-β2 glycoprotein I • Lupus anticoagulant tests
Malignant hypertension	• Severe hypertension • Platelet count usually $>60 \times 10^3/\mu L$	Improvement after treatment with antihypertensive drugs

Infections:
  Bacteria
  • *Acinetobacter baumannii*
  • *Bacteroides fragilis*
  • *Campylobacter jejuni*
  • *Clostridium difficile*
  • *Enterococcus faecalis*
  • *Enterobacter aerogenes/cloacae*
  • *Legionella pneumophila*
  • *Mycobacterium tuberculosis*
  • *Mycoplasma pneumonia*
  • *Pseudomonas aeruginosa*
  • *Rickettsia rickettsia*
  • *Salmonella typhi*
  • *Staphylococcus aureus/epidermidis*
  • *Streptococcus pyogenes/pneumoniae/viridans*
	Viruses
	• CMV
	• Hepatitis A
	• Human immunodeficiency virus (HIV)
	
	Fungi
	• *Aspergillus fumigatus*
	• *Blastomyces dermatiditis*
	• *Candida albicans*
	• *Cryptococcus neoformans*
		Test for infections in appropriate settings.

Patients who develop acute kidney injury during acute episodes of TTP usually have residual renal dysfunction. Ischemia of other tissues can also lead to permanent organ damage, and patients may develop hypertension, cardiovascular disease, or cognitive deficits as a result of disease flares.

Persistently low ADAMTS13 activity or detectable circulating inhibitors are associated with an increased risk of relapse. The activity may vary over time, however, and preemptive treatment based on low ADAMTS13 activity is not generally performed.

▶ When to Refer/When to Admit

Ideally, all patients with suspected TTP should be admitted to a hospital capable of performing plasma exchange. When plasma exchange is not available, patients should be admitted for plasma infusions. Improving or stable patients can be treated on an outpatient basis.

KEY READINGS

Balduini CL et al: High versus standard dose methylprednisolone in the acute phase of idiopathic thrombotic thrombocytopenic purpura: a randomized study. Ann Hematol 2010;89:591.

Coppo P et al: Predictive features of severe acquired ADAMTS13 deficiency in idiopathic thrombotic microangiopathies: the French TMA reference center experience. PloS One 2010;5:e10208.

George JN, Clinical practice: Thrombotic thrombocytopenic purpura. N Engl J Med 2006;354:1927.

George JN et al: Lessons learned from the Oklahoma thrombotic thrombocytopenic purpura-hemolytic uremic syndrome registry. J Clin Apher 2008;23:129.

Lim W, Vesely SK, George JN. The role of rituximab in the management of patients with acquired thrombotic thrombocytopenic purpura. Blood 2015;125:1526.

HEMOLYTIC UREMIC SYNDROME

ESSENTIALS OF DIAGNOSIS

▶ HUS classically presents with the clinical triad of thrombocytopenia, hemolytic anemia, and renal failure.

▶ Most cases of HUS occur in patients with enteric infections caused by bacteria that produce Shiga-like toxin (Stx).

▶ "Atypical HUS" is a term used for patients with HUS not caused by Stx-producing bacteria. Most patients with atypical HUS have underlying abnormalities in their ability to control activation of the alternative pathway of complement, such as mutations in complement regulatory proteins.

▶ General Considerations

The discovery that TTP is associated with abnormal ADAMTS13 activity strengthened the classification of TTP and HUS as distinct diseases. Stx is a causative factor in most cases of HUS, and Stx-associated HUS is usually caused by infections with *Escherichia coli* O157:H7. Non-Stx HUS is referred to as atypical HUS. Historically, HUS was classified as diarrhea associated (D+) or non-diarrheal (D−). Atypical HUS flares can be triggered by diarrheal illness; however, the presence or absence of diarrhea is not diagnostically helpful. Stool of patients with HUS should be tested for Stx, and these results can be used to classify patients as having Stx-HUS or atypical HUS. Most patients with atypical HUS have defective regulation of the complement cascade.

▶ Pathogenesis

HUS is caused by damage to the endothelium of the microvasculature, followed by thrombosis and inflammation. Platelet count falls because of consumption in thrombi, and erythrocytes are mechanically hemolyzed as they pass through the thrombi. Thrombi cause ischemia of affected organs, leading to tissue damage. In Stx-HUS, Stx binds to the globotriasylceramide Gb3 receptor, primarily on the renal endothelium. This causes impaired protein synthesis and production of proinflammatory cytokines. In patients with atypical HUS, endothelial injury triggers complement activation, and this process is not adequately controlled due to impaired function of complement regulatory proteins (factor H, factor I, membrane cofactor protein, and thrombomodulin). In approximately 10% of childhood atypical HUS cases, dysregulation of the complement system is caused by autoantibodies to the complement regulator factor H that inhibit its function.

▶ Prevention

Proper hygiene and food preparation can prevent the spread of infections by Stx-producing bacteria. Complement inhibition with eculizumab may prevent disease flares in patients with complement-mediated atypical HUS, but patients with underlying mutations in the genes for the complement regulatory genes are at life-long risk of recurrence. Given that eculizumab can only be administered intravenously, it increases patients' risk of infection, and is very expensive; the role of complement inhibition to prevent flares is unclear.

▶ Clinical Findings

A. Symptoms and Signs

Patients with HUS often present with oliguric renal failure. In both Stx and atypical HUS the disease may follow an infection, most frequently diarrheal illness. Pneumococcal pneumonia is also associated with the development of HUS, primarily in children. Patients may experience complications from renal failure, including volume overload, hypertension, and edema.

In addition to the kidneys, other organ systems throughout the body can be affected. Atypical HUS may affect the cardiovascular system in up to 10% of affected patients. Patients can develop cardiomyopathies, and microangiopathy has been detected within the hearts of affected patients. Neurologic involvement may affect up to 20% of patients with Stx-HUS, but is less common in patients with atypical HUS. Patients can present with altered mentation, seizures, pyramidal symptoms, and extrapyramidal symptoms. Patients can develop hypertensive encephalopathy, and posterior reversible encephalopathy syndrome (PRES) has been reported.

B. Laboratory Findings

Classic laboratory findings in patients with HUS are similar to those of TTP, including a low platelet count, hemolytic anemia, and renal failure. As with other forms of hemolysis, the lactate dehydrogenase (LDH) is usually elevated, and the haptoglobin is decreased. These laboratory data are usually the basis for the clinical suspicion of the disease, but there have been cases where the diagnosis was made only after tissue biopsy and not all of the classic laboratory abnormalities were present (eg, platelet count was normal). Most patients have microscopic hematuria and some degree of proteinuria. DAT is negative, and coagulation times (PT and PTT) are close to normal.

1. Complement testing in patients with atypical HUS— Unfortunately there is no specific test to accurately identify patients with complement-mediated HUS. Altered levels of circulating complement proteins or mutations in the genes for complement proteins are suggestive of complement-mediated disease, but are neither required for nor specific for this diagnosis. Measurement of total C3 is widely available, but the levels are decreased in only approximately 50% of patients with complement-mediated disease. The terminal complement complex (TCC or sC5b-9) is generated during complement activation and may be a more sensitive indicator of complement activation than low C3 levels. Levels of sC5b-9 are often elevated in Stx-HUS, however, limiting the utility of this test for differentiating HUS types. Total complement activity (CH50) and sC5b-9 are useful for monitoring the effectiveness of eculizumab treatment. If the complement system is sufficiently inhibited during treatment, the CH50 levels should be well below normal and sC5b-9 levels should be normal or low.

Mutations in the genes for several different complement proteins have been identified in patients with atypical HUS, including the genes for factor H, factor I, membrane cofactor proteins (MCP, or CD46), C3, and thrombomodulin. Mutations are found in only around 60% of atypical HUS patients,

however, and the presence or absence of complement mutations is not sufficient to determine whether a patient has complement-mediated disease. Factor H autoantibodies can account for around 10% of the pediatric cases. Detection of these antibodies informs treatment strategy, and the assay should be performed in pediatric patients with suspected HUS.

C. Biopsy Findings

Biopsy findings in Stx and atypical HUS are similar to those of TTP, although fibrin deposits may be more prominent in the thrombi in HUS than in TTP.

▶ Differential Diagnosis

As discussed elsewhere in this chapter, a large number of infections, drugs, stressors, and systemic diseases can trigger TMA. Historically, many of these cases have been described as having secondary HUS. Diagnosis can be difficult because some of these conditions directly cause TMA and some trigger TMA in susceptible patients, such as those with genetic complement defects. Specific laboratory tests can help distinguish HUS from the other causes of TMA (Table 35–1), but HUS should be considered in patients who do not improve even after the putative cause has been removed or treated.

HUS can also present similarly to acute glomerulonephritis. Hematologic abnormalities often indicate that that the underlying process is a TMA, but anemia and thrombocytopenia are also hallmarks of diseases such as SLE. A kidney biopsy is sometimes necessary to determine whether a patient has TMA or glomerulonephritis.

1. Pregnancy-associated HUS—Diagnosis of HUS in pregnant and postpartum patients can be particularly challenging. Pregnancy is a common trigger of HUS in patients with underlying complement defects, but several other causes of TMA are also seen during pregnancy. The different causes of TMA can sometimes be distinguished by the clinical presentation. For example, pregnancy-associated HUS usually develops in the postpartum period. TTP, in contrast, usually develops during the second or third trimester of pregnancy and is associated with low ADAMTS13 activity levels. Pre-eclampsia and HELLP syndrome usually improve after delivery, whereas HUS usually does not. HUS should therefore be considered in patients with suspected pre-eclampsia or HELLP if they do not improve after delivery.

2. TMA caused by malignant hypertension—Malignant hypertension can cause TMA, and the clinical and laboratory presentation of these patients is similar to that of HUS. Patients typically present with acute kidney injury, and their platelet counts are on average approximately 60,000/μL. The primary treatment of hypertension-induced TMA is to control the blood pressure. Other causes of TMA can cause hypertension; however, making it difficult to determine whether hypertension is the primary cause of disease in these patients.

Complications

Kidney involvement in Stx- and atypical-HUS is typically more severe than it is in TTP. Any organ system can be involved in both diseases.

Treatment

1. Stx-HUS—There is currently no specific treatment for Stx-HUS, and care is primarily supportive. Antibiotics may increase the risk of developing HUS in patients infected with Stx-producing bacteria, and are only recommended in patients with bacteremia. There is no proven benefit to treatment with plasma exchange, anticoagulation, or corticosteroids. Angiotensin-converting enzyme inhibitors may be beneficial for reducing renal complications after the acute episode has resolved. Kidney transplant is safe in patients who reach ESRD.

2. Complement-mediated HUS—Eculizumab is a monoclonal antibody to complement C5 that prevents generation of C5a and C5b-9. Several clinical trials have now shown that eculizumab is effective for treating atypical HUS. It has been approved by the Food and Drug Administration, and is currently the treatment of choice for this disease. The main adverse effect of eculizumab is an increased risk of meningococcal infections. All patients treated with eculizumab should receive meningococcal vaccination and/or treated with prophylactic antibiotics. There is not evidence, at this point, to support the use of eculizumab in other forms of TMA, although there are some reports of its efficacy in Stx-HUS, HELLP, and APS. Eculizumab may be indicated in pregnancy-associated HUS, particularly if renal failure develops postpartum. A large percentage of these patients may have underlying defects in complement regulation, and there are several reports of postpartum patients in whom eculizumab was effective.

Patients with atypical HUS have long been treated with plasma infusion or plasma exchange, and plasma exchange should be performed if eculizumab is not available. Factor H and factor I are plasma proteins, and plasma infusion is effective in some patients in whom the function of these proteins is impaired. Plasma exchange also removes autoantibodies to factor H. Plasma exchange and immunosuppression (corticosteroids, mycophenolate mofetil, and rituximab) may be beneficial in patients with autoimmune disease, but further studies are needed to determine the optimal approach in these cases.

Prognosis

In spite of supportive care, approximately 1–5% of patients with Stx-HUS die of the disease, and another 5% of patients develop ESRD or stroke. Nearly half of the patients with Stx-HUS have residual renal abnormalities, such as hypertension, proteinuria, or chronic kidney disease (CKD). Permanent impairment of other affected organs can also occur. Atypical HUS can lead to rapid, irreversible renal failure. Prior to the introduction of eculizumab, the majority of patients with atypical HUS either died or progressed to ESRD. More than half of the patients treated with eculizumab show clear clinical improvement, but more patients need to be treated before the overall effect on prognosis can be assessed.

When to Refer/When to Admit

HUS can cause multi-organ failure and lead to rapid clinical deterioration. Patients with HUS should be admitted to the hospital and treated by experienced specialists. Improving or stable patients can be treated on an outpatient basis.

KEY READINGS

Greenbaum LA et al: Eculizumab is a safe and effective treatment in pediatric patients with atypical hemolytic uremic syndrome. Kidney Int 2016;89:701.
Loirat C et al: An international consensus approach to the management of atypical hemolytic uremic syndrome in children. Pediatr Nephrol 2016;31:15.
Spinale JM et al: Long-term outcomes of Shiga toxin hemolytic uremic syndrome. Pediatr Nephrol 2013;28:2097.

DRUG-INDUCED THROMBOTIC MICROANGIOPATHY

ESSENTIALS OF DIAGNOSIS

▶ Multiple different drugs have been associated with the development of TMA.

▶ Drug-induced TMA should be suspected in patients who are being treated with drugs previously associated with the development in TMA, or in patients whose disease onset is temporally related to treatment with the drug.

▶ The offending drug should be discontinued in patients suspected of having drug-induced TMA.

General Considerations

Many different drugs have been associated with the development of TMA (Table 35–2). Historically, cases of drug-induced TMA have been referred to as "secondary" TTP or HUS, but there is evidence that some drugs directly cause TMA through unique mechanisms. Many of the drugs associated with TMA are used to treat cancers, infections, and

Table 35–2. Drugs associated with thrombotic microangiopathy.

High likelihood of association:	
• Bevacizumab	• Penicillin
• Bortezomib	• Pentostatin
• Cafilzomib	• Quetiapine
• Clopidogrel	• Quinine
• Cocaine	• Sirolimus
• Cyclosporine	• Sulfisoxazole
• Docetaxel	• Sunitinib
• Everolimus	• Tacrolimus
• Gemcitabine	• Ticlopidine (lower
• Interferon alpha/beta/polycarboxylate	evidence)
• Mitomycin	• Trielina
• Muromonab-CD3	• Vancomycin
• Oxaliplatin	• Vincristine
Possible association:	
• Adalimumab	
• Alendronate	• Mefloquine
• Carmustine	• Metronidazole
• Ciprofloxacin	• Oxymorphone (intrave-nous injection of Extended release formulations)
• Cytarabine	
• Ecstasy (MDMA; 3.4-methylenedioxy-N-methylamphetamine)	• Taxotere
	• Trimethoprim-sulfamethoxazole

kidney diseases, so it can be difficult to determine whether TMA is caused by a drug or the underlying disease. Cyclosporine and tacrolimus, for example, are calcineurin inhibitors (CNIs) that are part of the standard treatment patients with kidney transplants, autoimmune diseases, or graft versus host disease (GVHD). In some patients it may be preferable to discontinue the CNI to reduce the toxicity of the drug, whereas in other patients it may be better to increase the dose of CNI in order to better treat the underlying condition.

Pathogenesis

Drug-induced TMA can be caused by two general mechanisms. Some drugs cause an immune-related process in which patients form antibodies that bind to cells in the presence of the drug. Quinine causes TMA by this mechanism and is the most common cause of drug-induced TMA. In patients with autoimmune TMA, re-exposure to even low doses of the drug can cause disease recurrence. Other drugs cause TMA through a toxic effect on target cells. In these cases, the duration and magnitude of the exposure affect disease severity. In some patients with toxicity-mediated disease, TMA may resolve at lower doses of the drug.

Prevention

Culprit drugs should be avoided when possible, particularly in those with a history of immunologic drug-induced TMA.

Quinine carries a Black Box warning for TMA and its use as a prescription medication is limited. Since quinine is present in beverages and in herbal supplements, care must also be taken to avoid exposure from these non-pharmacologic sources. CNIs have been implicated in the development of *de novo* TMA in transplant recipients. In retrospective analyses, however, they do not seem to increase the risk of TMA or HUS recurrence after solid organ or hematopoietic stem cell transplantation (SCT), and they should not be avoided in transplant recipients.

Clinical Findings

Laboratory abnormalities in patients with drug-induced TMA are similar to those in HUS and TTP, and the same laboratory workup should be undertaken as in these diseases. Patients with immune-mediated drug-induced TMA usually have acute onset of disease and systemic involvement. Patients often have fevers, gastrointestinal symptoms, neurologic symptoms, and liver involvement. Renal failure is more common and more severe in drug-induced TMA than it is in TTP, and it is particularly common in quinine-induced disease. Some patients with quinine-induced disease may have a positive direct antibody test (DAT).

Drug-induced TMA caused by the toxicity of the drug is usually more slowly progressive. In some cases of drug-induced toxicity-mediated TMA the standard TMA laboratories (hematocrit, platelet count, LDH, serum creatinine) do not point to the diagnosis, or they are confounded by other underlying medical problems. In these cases the diagnosis may only be made after a tissue biopsy.

Differential Diagnosis

Drug-induced TMA can be particularly difficult to diagnose because many affected patients are taking multiple drugs or have underlying medical problems that are associated with TMA, such as cancer or organ transplantation. Furthermore, many drugs can cause isolated thrombocytopenia, anemia, or kidney injury. Drug-induced TMA is usually not associated with decreased ADAMTS13 levels, and patients with low ADAMTS13 levels should be treated for TTP with plasma exchange.

Renal failure is common in patients with drug-induced TMA, and clinically these patients are similar to those with HUS. Complement-mediated HUS should be considered in patients with severe renal failure, particularly those who require hemodialysis. Mutations in complement regulatory genes have been identified in some patients suspected of having drug-induced TMA. Unfortunately, there are no reliable tests for rapidly distinguishing these diseases. Treatment with eculizumab should therefore be considered when there is uncertainty about the role of medications in the disease and in patients who do not improve after cessation of the suspected drugs.

Complications

A majority of patients develop severe renal failure, and in some series more than 50% of patients have required hemodialysis.

Treatment

The offending drug should be stopped when drug-induced TMA is suspected. Plasma exchange is not beneficial in cases caused by drug toxicity, although it may be beneficial in patients with immune-mediated disease such as that caused by quinine exposure. There are reports of patients with drug-induced disease who improved after treatment with eculizumab, but more data is needed before this approach can be recommended.

In transplant patients who develop *de novo* TMA, many clinicians reduce the dose of CNIs or switch from one type of CNI to another. There is little data to guide the treatment of these patients, however, and the proper approach is further complicated by the difficulty of distinguishing TMA from vascular rejection and transplant glomerulopathy.

Prognosis

Although TMA usually resolves after discontinuation of the offending medication, most patients who develop drug-induced TMA and kidney injury have residual CKD.

When to Refer/When to Admit

Patients with drug-induced TMA can develop slowly progressive disease or fulminant disease with systemic symptoms. Those with worsening or critical labs should be admitted to the hospital, and alternative diagnoses should be considered. All patients should be monitored carefully after discontinuation of the offending medication to confirm improvement.

KEY READINGS

Al-Nouri ZL et al: Drug-induced thrombotic microangiopathy: a systematic review of published reports. Blood 2015;125:616.
Reese JA et al: Drug-induced thrombotic microangiopathy: Experience of the Oklahoma Registry and the Blood Center of Wisconsin. Am J Hematol 2015;90:406.

CANCER AND HEMATOPOIETIC STEM CELL TRANSPLANT (SCT)-ASSOCIATED THROMBOTIC MICROANGIOPATHY

ESSENTIALS OF DIAGNOSIS

- Cancer-associated TMA can occur in patients with a wide range of different malignancies, and can occur in patients whose cancer has not yet been diagnosed.
- Patients are at particularly high risk for TMA after SCT.
- Patients who develop SCT-associated TMA may benefit from early plasma exchange, and some patients may benefit from complement inhibition.

General Considerations

Cancer and SCT are both associated with the development of TMA. Cancers probably directly cause TMA in some patients. SCT patients are at a particularly high risk for developing TMA. TMA may occur in more than 60% of patients, although estimates vary widely depending on the diagnostic criteria. In both of these clinical settings a diagnosis of TMA may be obscured by numerous other causes of thrombocytopenia, anemia, and kidney failure. It can be difficult to distinguish the relative contribution of the underlying cancer, treatments (chemotherapy and radiation therapy), GVHD, and infections to the development of the disease.

Pathogenesis

Cancer-associated TMA is caused by cancer emboli that lodge in small blood vessels, primarily in the lungs. SCT-associated TMA is probably due to endothelial damage caused by multiple factors, including the underlying cancer, medications, radiation therapy, and GVHD. There is evidence that dysregulated complement activation contributes to injury in some SCT patients.

Prevention

Although multiple risk factors for developing SCT-associated TMA have been identified, these usually cannot be avoided. TMA is more common after allogeneic than autologous bone marrow transplantation, although it does occur in both settings. Risk factors for TMA include high-dose chemotherapy, radiation therapy, infection, an unrelated donor, a male donor to female recipient, and GVHD. Sirolimus, an immunosuppressive drug that also inhibits vascular endothelial growth factor, is also a risk for TMA in SCT recipients.

Clinical Findings

Patients with cancer-associated TMA may present with weight loss, progressive weakness, pain, and respiratory symptoms. Low ADAMTS13 activity has been reported in patients with cancer-associated TMA.

SCT-associated TMA usually occurs within the first 100 days after transplantation. Postmortem histologic analysis indicates that the kidneys are almost always involved, and extrarenal involvement is seen in fewer than 50% of patients. SCT-associated TMA has the same histologic appearance in the kidneys as HUS. Although some autopsy series have reported that all patients with a clinical diagnosis of TMA also had histologic disease, other series have found a poor correlation between the clinical and histologic findings. ADAMTS13 activity is usually not decreased in patients with SCT-associated TMA. Antibodies to factor H have been identified in patients with SCT-associated TMA, suggesting that complement dysregulation sometimes contributes to TMA in this setting.

Differential Diagnosis

Diagnosis of TMA in patients with cancer or who have undergone SCT is particularly difficult. These patients are at risk for many other conditions that can cause the hallmarks of TMA. Cancer, infections, medications, delayed bone marrow engraftment, and disseminated intravascular coagulation can cause a complex clinical picture, and it is common to see varying degrees of anemia, thrombocytopenia, elevated LDH, renal failure in these patients.

Complications

Cancer associated TMA primarily affects the lungs. SCT-associated TMA primarily affects the kidneys and causes renal failure. TMA in both settings is associated with a high mortality, and the cause of death in these patients is usually infection.

Treatment

Treatment of cancer-associated TMA involves treatment of underlying cancer while therapy for SCT-associated TMA is primarily supportive. Contributing medications such as CNIs and sirolimus should be reduced or discontinued if possible. These medications may be important for the treatment of GVHD, however. Rituximab or daclizumab may be beneficial as alternative drugs for treating GVHD while minimizing drug-induced injury of the vasculature, and eculizumab has been used in some patients. Although most studies do not support the use of plasma exchange in SCT patients, one small study did find that early plasma exchange is beneficial.

Prognosis

SCT-associated TMA has been associated with mortality as high as 100% in some series, although the most common cause of death in these patients is infection. CKD is common in patients who survive.

When to Refer/When to Admit

Both cancer-associated and SCT-associated TMA are severe conditions that carry a poor prognosis. Patients suspected of TMA in these settings should be admitted to the hospital and cared for by clinicians with experience treating these conditions.

KEY READINGS

Changsirikulchai S et al: Renal thrombotic microangiopathy after hematopoietic cell transplant: role of GVHD in pathogenesis. Clin J Am Soc Nephrol 2009;4:345.
Jodele S et al: Abnormalities in the alternative pathway of complement in children with hematopoietic stem cell transplant-associated thrombotic microangiopathy. Blood 2013;122:2003.

SCLERODERMA RENAL CRISIS

ESSENTIALS OF DIAGNOSIS

▶ Scleroderma renal crisis is characterized by an abrupt onset of severe hypertension decreased kidney function.

▶ Renal crisis is more common in patients with diffuse systemic sclerosis than in those with limited disease.

▶ Primary treatment of scleroderma renal crisis is angiotensin converting enzyme (ACE) inhibition.

General Considerations

Scleroderma renal crisis is a life-threatening complication of scleroderma that presents with severe hypertension and renal failure. It affects up to 20% of patients with scleroderma, and is more common in patients with diffuse cutaneous scleroderma. In contrast, it is rare in patients with localized systemic sclerosis or CREST (calcinosis, Raynaud's phenomenon, esophagitis, sclerodactyly, telangiectasias) syndrome.

Pathogenesis

Scleroderma causes vascular injury and medial hypertrophy resulting in narrowing of small blood vessels. Scleroderma renal crisis is an acute event, and may develop in response to endothelial injury. Structural changes in the arteries and acute injury may reduce renal perfusion, which causes activation of the renin-angiotensin system.

Prevention

Scleroderma renal crisis may be more common in patients treated with glucocorticoids or CNIs, and minimizing the exposure of patients to glucocorticoids may reduce the risk of developing renal crisis. ACE inhibitors are the primary treatment for scleroderma renal crisis, although there is no evidence that therapy with these drugs prevents this complication.

Clinical Findings

A. Symptoms and Signs

Patients with scleroderma renal crisis usually present with acute kidney injury and severe hypertension. In a subset of patients the hypertension is within the normal range, but this is often in patients who previously had low blood pressures. Patients may develop complications of the acute, severe hypertension, including headache and heart failure. Patients can also have arrhythmias, and seizures can occur. On physical examination patients sometimes display hypertensive retinopathy and papilledema.

B. Laboratory Findings

Patients with scleroderma renal crisis can present with the usual hallmarks of microangiopathic hemolytic anemia. Anemia is found in approximately half of the patients with renal crisis. Thrombocytopenia is also common, but platelet counts are rarely less than 50,000/μL. Autoantibodies reactive to RNA polymerase III are more common in scleroderma patients who develop renal crisis than in those who do not. Patients with renal crisis are also more likely to have anti-Th/To RNP antibodies and anti-topoisomerase III (Scl-70).

C. Biopsy Findings

The pathologic hallmarks of TMA can also seen in the kidneys of patients with scleroderma renal crisis, including double contours in the capillary walls and fibrin thrombi. Interlobular and arcuate renal arteries have mucoid thickening of the intima. Proliferation in this layer causes an "onion-skin" appearance and the lumen is often narrowed.

Differential Diagnosis

Acute kidney injury (AKI) in patients with scleroderma can be precipitated by other manifestations of the disease, such as pulmonary hypertension or medications. Patients with scleroderma can also rarely develop antineutrophil cytoplasmic antibody (ANCA)-associated small vessel vasculitis. Antibodies are usually reactive with myeloperoxidase (MPO) and patients develop a necrotizing glomerulonephritis.

Complications

Severe hypertension in patients with scleroderma renal crisis can cause neurologic symptoms and hypertensive encephalopathy. The abrupt increase in blood pressure can also cause other complications such as acute cardiac events and congestive heart failure.

Treatment

Blood pressure control with ACE inhibitors is the treatment of choice for patients with scleroderma renal crisis, even for those who are normotensive. Captopril has been used in many of the studies, and its short half-life allows rapid titration of the drug. The blood pressure should be treated promptly with the goal of bringing it into the normal range over 2–3 days. Serum creatinine may increase as the blood pressure is controlled since vascular hypertrophy may reduce renal perfusion at a lower blood pressure, but ACE inhibition should be continued in this setting. Treatment should also be continued for patients who require hemodialysis, as patients can show a delayed recovery of renal function.

Prognosis

In some series more than 50% of patients require hemodialysis during a renal crisis. Of these patients, many recover sufficient renal function to discontinue dialysis and recovery of renal function can be seen up to 18 months after the acute episode. Even with treatment, mortality may be as high as 30% in patients with renal crisis.

When to Refer/When to Admit

Renal crisis is a medical emergency. Patient suspected of having this condition should be admitted to the hospital and cared for by specialists to ensure proper treatment and monitoring.

KEY READINGS

Penn H et al: Scleroderma renal crisis: patient characteristics and long-term outcomes. QJM 2007;100:485.
Teixeira L et al: Mortality and risk factors of scleroderma renal crisis: a French retrospective study of 50 patients. Ann Rheum Dis 2008;67:110.

ANTI-PHOSPHOLIPID ANTIBODY SYNDROME

ESSENTIALS OF DIAGNOSIS

▸ The diagnosis of anti-phospholipid syndrome (APS) involves detection of anti-phospholipid antibodies (aPLs) in patients who have also had a thromboembolic event or an unexplained pregnancy loss after 10 weeks of gestation.

▸ APS can cause thrombosis in renal arteries and veins. Involvement of the glomeruli causes TMA.

▸ Treatment for APS is anticoagulation.

General Considerations

APS is an autoimmune syndrome characterized by venous, arterial, or microvascular thrombosis, or recurrent pregnancy loss. It can occur as a primary disease and is also commonly associated with systemic autoimmune diseases, particularly SLE. Thrombosis is caused by antibodies that bind phospholipids or to β_2-glycoprotein I, a phospholipid binding protein. Approximately 9% of patients with APS have kidney involvement, but the incidence may be higher in patients with lupus and APS.

Pathogenesis

aPLs bind to phospholipids or phospholipid binding proteins on the vascular endothelium. The antibodies can disrupt the anticoagulant function of endothelial cells, and they can also activate the complement cascade on the endothelial surface.

Prevention

For patients with aPLs but who have not had a documented thrombotic event, treatments that reduce cardiovascular risk, such as blood pressure control and statins, may be beneficial. Aspirin reduces the risk of thrombosis in patients with lupus and aPLs, and hydroxychloroquine may also be protective.

Clinical Findings

The diagnosis of APS requires detection of aPLs and at least one thrombotic event. The thrombotic event can be venous, arterial, or within the small capillaries. It can also manifest as recurrent miscarriages or unexplained fetal loss after 10 weeks of gestation. The main clinical finding of APS involving the kidneys is often hypertension, and about half of the patients have an elevated serum creatinine. Migraine and neurologic findings are common in patients with APS, and patients frequently develop livedo reticularis as part of the disease. Laboratory assays detect aPLs that bind to cardiolipin and β_2-glycoprotein I. The lupus anticoagulant assay is a functional test that measures the effects of aPL in patient serum with a phospholipid-dependent clotting assay. To make a diagnosis of APS at least one of these tests must be positive on two separate occasions at least 12 weeks apart.

Patients with APS present with hypertension, renal failure, and proteinuria. The thrombocytopenia and anemia in APS are usually milder than in TTP and HUS. Catastrophic APS (CAPS) is a term used to describe patients with at least three involved organs. Patients with CAPS usually have renal involvement and present with severe hypertension.

Differential Diagnosis

Patients with APS present with many of the findings of acute glomerulonephritis. A kidney biopsy is often necessary to make a definitive diagnosis of APS, particularly in patients with lupus. Detection of the aPLs can help distinguish APS from the other causes of TMA.

Complications

The presence of aPLs may be a risk factor for glomerulosclerosis and CKD in patients with lupus. APS may also be a risk factor for bleeding after kidney biopsy in patients with lupus nephritis. Patients with APS can develop sterile cardiac vegetations (Libman–Sacks endocarditis) and valvular disease of the heart. Patients with CAPS can develop rapid multi-organ failure.

Treatment

The primary treatment for APS is anticoagulation. Warfarin is usually used to maintain the international normalized ratio (INR) within the 2–3 range. Unfractionated heparin or low molecular weight heparin can be used until the INR is in the target range. Low molecular weight heparin should also be used in pregnant patients. Newer anticoagulants, such as direct thrombin inhibitors, have not been specifically tested in APS and should not be used. Immunosuppression may be beneficial in APS, but there is not sufficient data to recommend it at this time.

Patients with CAPS should be treated with immunosuppressive drugs. Corticosteroids and cytotoxic agents have been used, particularly in patients who also have autoimmune disease. Intravenous immunoglobulin may also be beneficial. Plasma exchange should be used to rapidly remove the aPLs in patients with CAPS, and the plasma can be replaced with non-plasma fluids. Rituximab and eculizumab have been used in selected patients. Data supporting the use of these drugs are limited, but it is reasonable to try these drugs in patients who are deteriorating or are resistant to therapy.

Prognosis

APS is associated with increased mortality, primarily because of thromboembolic complications. Patients with lupus nephritis who also have aPLs have a worse prognosis than those who do not, and aPLs are associated with an increased likelihood of developing CKD. For patients with CAPS the mortality may be higher than 50%. The survival for CAPS patients who survive the initial episode is generally good, but they are usually continued on long-term anticoagulation.

When to Refer/When to Admit

Patients with APS should be treated by experienced clinicians. Patients with acute thrombotic events should be hospitalized. CAPS is a medical emergency and patients should be admitted to hospitals that can provide appropriate care, such as plasma exchange.

KEY READINGS

Cervera R, Rodriguez-Pinto I, Espinoza G on behalf of the Task Force on Catastrophic Antiphospholipid Syndrome. Catastrophic antiphospholipid syndrome: task force report summary. Lupus 2014;23:1283.

Shapira I et al: Brief report: induction of sustained remission in recurrent catastrophic antiphospholipid syndrome via inhibition of terminal complement with eculizumab. Arthritis Rheum 2012;64:2719.

Tektonidou MG et al: Antiphospholipid syndrome nephropathy in patients with systemic lupus erythematosus and antiphospholipid antibodies: prevalence, clinical associations, and long-term outcome. Arthritis Rheum 2004;50:2569.

■ CHAPTER REVIEW QUESTIONS

1. A 47-year-old woman is admitted with weakness and fevers. Laboratory testing reveals a hemoglobin level of 7.4 g/dL and a platelet count of 20,000/μL. Further testing reveals a serum creatinine of 1.5 mg/dL and proteinuria (1+ by dipstick testing). Her medical history is otherwise unremarkable and she is not on any medications. Blood and urine cultures are sent.

   Which ONE of the following should be done next?
   A. Transfusion of packed red blood cells and platelets while awaiting blood culture results.
   B. Treatment with corticosteroids and rituximab.
   C. ADAMTS13 activity should be measured, and the patient should be empirically treated with plasma exchange while awaiting the results.
   D. The patient should be started on captopril, and the dose should be titrated to achieve a blood pressure of less than 140/80 mm Hg.
   E. Computed tomography and bone marrow biopsy should be performed to look for an occult tumor.

2. A 15-year-old girl is admitted with a 1-day history of anuria and anasarca. Her serum creatinine is 5.4 mg/dL, her hemoglobin level is 8 g/dL, and the platelet count is 50,000/μL. Testing for Shiga-like toxin is negative and ADAMTS13 activity is 30%. A presumptive diagnosis is atypical hemolytic uremic syndrome is made, and treatment with the complement inhibitor eculizumab is planned.

   Which ONE of the following should be done next?
   A. A renal biopsy should be performed to confirm the diagnosis.
   B. The patient should empirically be treated with corticosteroids and plasma exchange.
   C. The patient should be tested for systemic lupus erythematosus, and corticosteroids should be empirically started while awaiting the results.
   D. The patient should be empirically treated with ciprofloxacin for a possible asymptomatic enteric infection.
   E. The patient should be immunized for meningococcus and empirically treated to cover meningococcal infection for 2 weeks.

3. A 57-year-old woman is admitted with fevers, chills, and bruising. Laboratory testing reveals a hemoglobin level of 6.4 mg/dL and a platelet count of 15,000/μL. ADAMTS13 activity has been tested, but the results are still pending. The patient is a Jehovah's Witness and refuses transfusion of any blood products. Her past medical history is unremarkable except for occasional headaches and leg cramps. Within the past several weeks she has taken ibuprofen once and has taken pills for leg cramps that she got from her neighbor.

   Which of the following is the best approach?
   A. The patient may have quinine-induced thrombotic microangiopathy. Plasmapheresis may remove pathogenic antibodies in this condition, but replacement with donor plasma is not necessary.
   B. The patient should be treated with plasma exchange. Although this is against her medical wishes, she has a life-threatening condition and her refusal of treatment is evidence that she is not competent to make medical decisions.
   C. If the patient's plasma C3 level is low she should be treated with eculizumab, a therapeutic complement inhibitor.
   D. The patient should be started on lisinopril and pravastatin to reduce endothelial dysfunction.
   E. Antiplatelet agents should be used to prevent thrombosis in the microvasculature.

4. A 12-year-old boy develops hemolytic uremic syndrome during an outbreak of Shiga-toxin producing *Escherichia coli*. He requires hemodialysis, and his kidney function does not recover after the illness resolves.

Which ONE of the following is true regarding renal transplantation in this patient?
A. Calcineurin inhibitors should not be used in this patient because they increase the risk of disease relapse.
B. He should receive eculizumab for 6 months after transplantation.
C. He should not receive a kidney from a related donor.
D. He is unlikely to develop recurrent hemolytic uremic syndrome.
E. Nephrectomy of the patient's native kidneys will reduce the risk of recurrent hemolytic uremic syndrome.

5. A 60-year-old woman with a history of mixed connective tissue disease presents with several days of weakness. Her hemoglobin level is 9 g/dL and her platelet count is 65,000/μL. Her serum creatinine is 2.4 mg/dL and her blood pressure is 170/90 mm Hg. Testing reveals a low C3 level and autoantibodies reactive against RNA polymerase III and topoisomerase III (Scl-70).

The most appropriate treatment is:
A. Treatment with captopril for possible scleroderma renal crisis.
B. Treatment with the complement inhibitor eculizumab because it is effective in both atypical hemolytic syndrome and antibody-mediated autoimmune disease.
C. Empiric anticoagulation for presumed catastrophic antiphospholipid antibody syndrome.
D. ADAMTS13 activity should be measured, and the patient should be empirically treated with plasma exchange and corticosteroids while awaiting the results.
E. High dose corticosteroids should be administered for possible immune-mediated thrombotic microangiopathy.

Glomerular Disorders Due to Infections

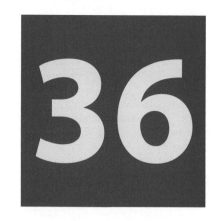

Jeremy S. Leventhal, MD
Michael J. Ross, MD
Kar Neng Lai, MD, DSc
Sydney C. W. Tang, MD, PhD

▼ HIV-RELATED KIDNEY DISEASE

Jeremy S. Leventhal, MD and Michael J. Ross, MD

ESSENTIALS OF DIAGNOSIS

▸ HIV-associated Nephropathy (HIVAN) is a distinct pathological entity characterized by the combination of collapsing FSGS, microcystic dilation of renal tubules, and interstitial inflammation found in HIV infected individuals

▸ HIVAN is caused by expression of HIV-1 genes in renal epithelial cells and is highly associated with APOL1 risk alleles:

• Combination antiretroviral therapy (cART) is the most effective treatment to retard progression of glomerular filtration decline and proteinuria:

○ Though cART protects against HIVAN, some individual agents are associated with a spectrum of renal manifestations from benign spurious changes in serum creatinine to fulminant acute kidney injury (AKI)

• Small studies suggest a beneficial effect of angiotensin converting enzyme inhibitors and steroids in selected patients

▸ HIV-positive patients are predisposed to AKI

▸ HIV-associated immune complex kidney (HIVICK) disease includes a heterogeneous spectrum of glomerular diseases occurring in HIV-infected patients characterized by glomerular immune complex deposition

▸ Thrombotic microangiopathy is an HIV-related complication most commonly found in patients with untreated/advanced HIV disease

▸ HIV infection increases the risk of diabetic kidney disease progression, and may also promote progression of other common forms of chronic kidney disease (CKD).

▸ General Considerations

At the onset of the HIV epidemic, little was known concerning the ability of the virus to cause end-organ damage. As treatment options evolved, so too, did the spectrum of kidney diseases caused by the virus. Initially, the lack of therapeutic options permitted the most severe of renal phenotypes, HIV-associated nephropathy (HIVAN), a clinical syndrome of nephrotic proteinuria and rapid renal function deterioration, to appear. The advent of combined antiretroviral therapy (cART) decreased the prevalence of fulminant HIVAN; however, its efficacy in treating other HIV-associated kidney complications including immune complex related disease, thrombotic microangiopathy (TMA), acute kidney injury (AKI), and synergy with other forms of glomerular disease are poorly defined. Though cART has markedly improved patient outcomes and reduced the incidence of end-stage renal disease (ESRD) due to HIVAN, several agents used in cART, can have nephrotoxic effects. In this chapter, we discuss the presentation, pathogenesis, and treatment of HIVAN, the prototypical HIV-induced kidney disease, as well as the spectrum of HIV-associated kidney diseases.

KEY READING

Razzak Chaudhary S et al: Trends in the outcomes of end-stage renal disease secondary to human immunodeficiency virus-associated nephropathy. Nephrol Dial Transplant 2015;30:1734.

▸ Pathogenesis

In the United States, HIVAN occurs almost exclusively in persons of African descent. International studies evaluating HIV-infected patients with proteinuria corroborate the U.S. data. In fact, HIVAN has the strongest racial predisposition of any form of acquired renal disease leading to ESRD.

Recently, discoveries explain the genetic predisposition to HIVAN amongst persons of African descent. Polymorphisms in the gene for *Apolipoprotein L1* (*APOL1*) explain the majority of excess race-attributed risk in blacks for nondiabetic ESRD. Patients with two copies of risk-associated APOL1 alleles, which provide protection against endemic trypanosomal illness have a 10-fold greater risk of non-HIV related FSGS. Remarkably those with the renal risk genotype have a 29-fold increased risk of developing HIVAN. Plasma APOL1 levels are not associated with CKD in HIV infected patients whereas survival of transplanted kidneys from African–Americans is associated with donor APOL1 genotype. Studies to date suggest that APOL1 promotes nephropathy via local expression by renal parenchymal cells but the mechanisms remain unclear.

The mechanisms through which infection with HIV-1 results in the HIVAN phenotype are not completely known. However, research has elucidated important aspects of disease pathogenesis.

The HIV-1 genome encodes nine genes, including three structural genes (*env*, *gag*, and *pol*) two regulatory genes (*tat* and *rev*) and four accessory genes (*vif*, *vpr*, *vpu*, and *nef*) (Figure 36–1). Studies have demonstrated that HIV infection of renal epithelial cells and expression of viral genes is a critical determinant of HIVAN pathogenesis. Interestingly, active viral replication is not necessary to produce the HIVAN phenotype and renal expression of *nef*, *vpr*, and possibly *tat* are sufficient to produce the HIVAN phenotype in genetically susceptible hosts. Renal expression of these genes induces cellular injury, cell cycle dysregulation and inflammation. It is not yet known how polymorphisms in APOL1 promote the ability of HIV to induce renal injury. It is also important to note that the kidney can serve as a reservoir for the HIV virus and efforts to cure HIV will therefore need to also eradicate the virus from the kidney.

KEY READINGS

Abbott KC et al: Human immunodeficiency virus/acquired immunodeficiency syndrome-associated nephropathy at end-stage renal disease in the United States: patient characteristics and survival in the pre highly active antiretroviral therapy era. J Nephrol 2001;14:377.

Blasi M et al: Renal epithelial cells produce and spread HIV-1 via T-cell contact. AIDS 2014;28:2345.

Bruggeman LA et al: Nephropathy in human immunodeficiency virus-1 transgenic mice is due to renal transgene expression. J Clin Invest 1997;100:84.

Bruggeman LA et al: Plasma apolipoprotein L1 levels do not correlate with CKD. J Am Soc Nephrol 2014;25:634.

Freedman BI et al: Apolipoprotein L1 gene variants in deceased organ donors are associated with renal allograft failure. Am J Transplant 2015;15:1615.

Genovese G et al: Association of trypanolytic ApoL1 variants with kidney disease in African Americans. Science 2010;329:841.

Husain M et al: HIV-1 Nef induces dedifferentiation of podocytes in vivo: a characteristic feature of HIVAN. AIDS 2005;19:1975.

Kopp JB et al: APOL1 genetic variants in focal segmental glomerulosclerosis and HIV-associated nephropathy. J Am Soc Nephrol 2011;22:2129.

System USRD. USRDS 1999 annual data report. 1999.

Zuo Y et al: HIV-1 genes vpr and nef synergistically damage podocytes, leading to glomerulosclerosis. J Am Soc Nephrol 2006;17:2832.

▶ Clinical Findings

A. Symptoms and Signs (in the absence of cART)

- Low CD4+ Count—Most but not all patients with HIVAN have advanced HIV disease, with CD4+ count less than 200 cells/mm³.

- Severe Proteinuria—HIVAN is characterized by proteinuria that can frequently be in the nephrotic range.

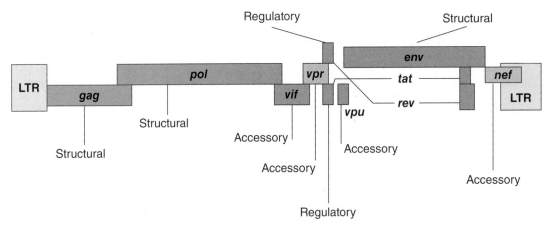

▲ **Figure 36–1.** A schematic representation of the HIV genome flanked by its LTR promoter regions. *Vpr* and *nef* are most important HIV genes contributing to HIVAN pathogenesis and are colored lighter blue.

One series of 57 patients with biopsy proven HIVAN had an average 24 hours protein excretion of 4.1 g.

- Rapid Deterioration of Renal Function.

  Prior to the availability of cART, the clinical course of HIVAN was characterized by a rapid decline of renal function resulting in the need for renal replacement therapy within weeks to months after diagnosis. Patients with biopsy-proven HIVAN most often present with obvious signs of kidney disease. Severe proteinuria and impaired glomerular infiltration rates are common indications for biopsy in patients with renal disease. However, as demonstrated by Han et al., even the presence of microalbuminuria may herald the presence of the HIVAN. While the incidence of "classic HIVAN" leading to rapid progression to ESRD has decreased since the advent of cART, HIV may promote more indolent phenotype in genetically susceptible patients treated with cART.

B. Imaging Studies

- Renal Ultrasound—Patients with HIVAN have echogenic, enlarged kidneys.

C. Special Studies

- Renal Biopsy

The most common pathologic finding in biopsy specimens from patients with HIVAN is collapsing focal segmental glomerulosclerosis (FSGS) (Figure 36–2). HIVAN

is also notable for the presence of proliferating glomerular epithelial cells in Bowman space, which can sometimes appear similar to crescentic glomerulonephritis. However, the absence of glomerular hematuria indicates the absence of glomerulonephritis and these "pseudocresents" are similar to those found in the cellular variant of FSGS. Prominent tubulointerstitial disease is present in HIVAN, and includes interstitial inflammation and fibrosis and tubular abnormalities include flattening and atrophy of tubular epithelial cells and "microcytstic" dilation of the tubules which can involve all segments of the nephron. On electron microscopy, there is prominent effacement of podocyte foot processes and the visceral epithelial cytoplasm can have large, electron dense resorption droplets. The endothelium may have large tubuloreticular inclusions (also found in other kidney diseases characterized by high interferon levels including lupus nephritis) although their absence does not preclude the diagnosis, especially since they are less common in more recent series, likely due to lower serum interferon levels in patients treated with cART.

KEY READINGS

Atta MG et al: Nephrotic range proteinuria and CD4 count as noninvasive indicators of HIV-associated nephropathy. Am J Med 2005;118:1288.

Bigé N et al: Presentation of HIV-associated nephropathy and outcome in HAART-treated patients. Nephrol Dial Transplant 2012;27:1114.

Choi AI et al: The impact of HIV on chronic kidney disease outcomes. Kidney Int 2007;72:1380.

D'Agati V, Appel GB: Renal pathology of human immunodeficiency virus infection. Semin Nephrol 1998;18:406.

D'Agati V et al: Pathology of HIV-associated nephropathy: a detailed morphologic and comparative study. Kidney Int 1989;35:1358.

Han TM et al: A cross-sectional study of HIV-seropositive patients with varying degrees of proteinuria in South Africa. Kidney Int 2006;69:2243.

Razzak Chaudhary S et al: Trends in the outcomes of end-stage renal disease secondary to human immunodeficiency virus-associated nephropathy. Nephrol Dial Transplant 2015;30: 1734.

Ross MJ et al: Microcyst formation and HIV-1 gene expression occur in multiple nephron segments in HIV-associated nephropathy. J Am Soc Nephrol 2001;12:2645.

Wyatt CM, Klotman PE, D'Agati VD: HIV-associated nephropathy: clinical presentation, pathology, and epidemiology in the era of antiretroviral therapy. Semin Nephrol 2008;28:513.

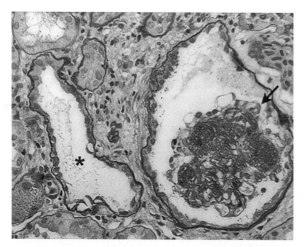

▲ **Figure 36–2.** Typical histopathologic findings in HIVAN. Periodic acid–Schiff staining demonstrates focal glomerulosclerosis with collapse of the glomerular tuft and overlying podocyte proliferation (arrow), microcystic tubular dilation (asterisk), interstitial inflammation, and interstitial fibrosis. Magnification, ×200. (See Color Plate 12.)

▶ **Differential Diagnosis**

- Primary FSGS
- Drug-Induced FSGS
- Membranous Nephropathy (MN)
- HIV-associated Immune Complex Kidney Disease

- Diabetic Nephropathy
- Minimal Change Disease

▶ Treatment

Strategies for the prevention and/or treatment of HIVAN have never been evaluated in prospective randomized controlled studies and most studies on the treatment of HIVAN have been retrospective and/or lack proper controls. The types of medical therapy for HIVAN that have been studied in humans include antiretroviral therapy, corticosteroids, and angiotensin converting enzyme inhibitors. Below, we briefly discuss the evidence supporting use of these agents for treating patients with HIVAN.

A. Antiretroviral Therapy

Studies demonstrating that HIV infection of kidney parenchymal cells is necessary for the development of HIVAN suggest that antiretroviral medications should be beneficial for treating and/or preventing HIVAN. Though the efficacy of cART for the prevention and treatment of HIVAN has never been tested in a randomized trial, a wealth of epidemiologic data strongly support the conclusion that cART is effective in this setting. However, it remains possible that in some patients, cART may not fully prevent/cure HIVAN and may instead alter the phenotype to more indolent disease that is less likely to be evaluated by diagnostic renal biopsy.

B. Angiotensin Converting Enzyme Inhibitors, Receptor Blockers, and Steroids

Blockade of renin-angiotensin system (RAS) has been shown to attenuate proteinuria in various glomerular diseases. Similarly, evidence suggests that use of RAS blockers in patients with HIVAN is associated with both stabilization of serum creatinine and reduction of proteinuria. Although randomized trials were never performed in patients with HIVAN, use of RAS blockers in HIV-positive patients with proteinuric kidney disease should be considered as in HIV-negative patients.

C. Corticosteroids

Tubulointerstitial inflammation is one of the most prominent histopathologic findings in HIVAN and the inflammatory response of renal parenchymal cells to HIV infection is an important component of HIVAN pathogenesis. It is therefore plausible that anti-inflammatory agents may be useful in the treatment of HIVAN. Several case series and small case control studies from the pre-cART era suggested that prednisone may be efficacious in HIVAN. However, since most patients with HIVAN have advanced HIV disease/AIDS, and already have suppressed immune systems, use of immunosuppressive medications may expose these patients to excess risk of infection and/or malignancy. We believe that steroids should be reserved for short-term use while other more effective agents (ie, ACE inhibitors and cART) are initiated or in cases where they have failed.

KEY READINGS

Atta MG et al: Antiretroviral therapy in the treatment of HIV-associated nephropathy. Nephrol Dial Transplant 2006;21:2809.

Bruggeman LA et al: Nephropathy in human immunodeficiency virus-1 transgenic mice is due to renal transgene expression. J Clin Invest 1997;100:84.

Burns GC et al: Effect of angiotensin-converting enzyme inhibition in HIV-associated nephropathy. J Am Soc Nephrol 1997;8:1140.

Lucas GM et al: Highly active antiretroviral therapy and the incidence of HIV-1-associated nephropathy: a 12-year cohort study. AIDS 2004;18:541.

Ross MJ et al: HIV-1 infection initiates an inflammatory cascade in human renal tubular epithelial cells. J Acquir Immune Defic Syndr 2006;42:1.

Smith MC et al: Prednisone improves renal function and proteinuria in human immunodeficiency virus-associated nephropathy. Am J Med 1996;101:41.

▶ Prognosis

Early in the epidemic, patients with HIVAN progressed to ESRD with a dismal prognosis; most died after approximately 1 year on dialysis. Since cART became widely available, the renal outcomes of HIV-infected patients with HIVAN have improved but remain poor. Amongst 57 patients presenting with HIVAN, 30 progressed to ESRD despite initiating cART. Similarly, despite overall decreased excess mortality in patients with HIVAN who progress to ESRD, these patients continue to experience an almost threefold greater mortality than patients with non-HIVAN causes of ESRD. Unfortunately, despite the improvements in the efficacy of medical treatment, the prevalence of both HIV/AIDS and ESRD in African–Americans, the group at highest risk of developing HIVAN, has continued to increase, highlighting the need for novel eradicative therapies (Figure 36–3).

KEY READINGS

Bigé N et al: Presentation of HIV-associated nephropathy and outcome in HAART-treated patients. Nephrol Dial Transplant 2012;27:1114.

Carbone L et al: Course and prognosis of human immunodeficiency virus-associated nephropathy. Am J Med 1989;87:389.

Centers for Disease Control and Prevention. HIV/AIDS Surveillance Report. 2015;11.

Ortiz C et al: Outcome of patients with human immunodeficiency virus on maintenance hemodialysis. Kidney Int 1988;34:248.

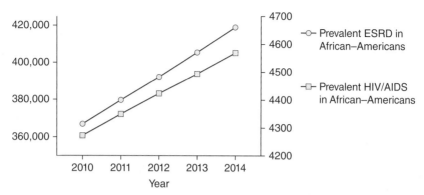

▲ **Figure 36–3.** The prevalence of African–American patient with ESRD (cases/million population) continues to increase in parallel with the prevalence of HIV/AIDS in African–Americans, the group at highest risk of developing HIVAN. Data adapted from 2016 USRDS annual report and the 2015 CDC HIV/AIDS Surveillance Report. Notice: The data here have been supplied by the USRDS. The interpretation and reporting of these data are the responsibility of the author(s) and in no way should be seen as an official policy or interpretation of the US Government.

Razzak Chaudhary S et al: Trends in the outcomes of end-stage renal disease secondary to human immunodeficiency virus-associated nephropathy. Nephrol Dial Transplant 2015;30:1734. System USRD. USRDS 2016 Annual Report. 2016.

HIV-ASSOCIATED IMMUNE COMPLEX DISEASE

While HIVAN was the initial dominant manifestation of HIV-associated renal disease, also noted in biopsy studies is a group of HIV-associated immune complex kidney diseases (HIVICD). In contrast to the defined features of HIVAN, HIVICD encompasses a pleomorphic set of glomerular pathology that includes, amongst others, membranoproliferative glomerulonephritis (MPGN), mesangioproliferative glomerulonephritis, and IgA nephropathy. A 2009 study of HIV-infected patients found glomerulonephritis as the third most common renal abnormality on autopsy, even in the absence of overt CKD. HIVICD was also present in more than 30% of biopsies from HIV-infected patients in a John Hopkins study.

The variable manifestations of HIVICD suggest a varied pathogenesis. A case report documented IgA against HIV protein-specific IgM detected in the plasma and eluted from the kidney of a patient with IgA nephropathy, suggesting disease produced by HIV-reactive immune complex deposition. Alternatively, HIVICD could arise from infected renal parenchyma or planted viral antigens that locally generate an immune response. A lack of animal models has limited our understanding of HIVICD pathogenesis. Unlike HIVAN, it is less clear whether ART affects disease trajectory. One biopsy series found ART use, associated with decreased ESRD in patients with biopsy diagnosed HIVAN, but not in those with HIVICD.

▶ Renal Toxicities of cART Agents

Despite their efficacy in prolonging life and retarding or reversing HIVAN, a growing experience with cART has defined a spectrum of nephrotoxic effects associated with use of these agents (Table 36–1).

1. Tenofovir—Tenofovir is the most commonly prescribed cART agent. Use of tenofovir, a nucleotide reverse transcriptase inhibitor, is associated with a variety of renal toxicities which include AKI, tubular dysfunction (ie, RTA, hyperphosphaturia), non-nephrotic proteinuria, and CKD.

Table 36–1. Potential renal complications of cART agents.

cART Agent	Renal Manifestation	Reversibility
Tenofovir	• AKI • Proximal tubular dysfunction • CKD • Proteinuria	• Most features resolve with cessation of drug: AKI may involve fibrosis and not fully resolve
Atazanavir/ Indinavir	• Nephrolithiasis/ Crystalluria • CKD	• Reversible after cessation
Ritonavir-boosted Lopinavir	• CKD • Increased Tenofovir toxicity	• Unclear if reversible
Cobicistat, Dolutegravir, and Ritonavir	• Increase in serum creatinine	• Change is due to altered tubular creatinine secretion not parenchymal damage

Despite these associations, the absolute risk AKI tenofovir use may be as low as 0.15% per year, so other causes of AKI should also be sought. Due to concerns about renal toxicity and higher tenofovir levels in patients with impaired GFR, tenofovir is should not be initiated in patients with eGFR less than 60 mL/min or in patients whose regimen includes a ritonavir-boosted protease inhibitor. Tenofovir should also be discontinued in patients with declining renal function without other obvious reversible causes. The recent approval of tenofovir alafenamide, a new formulation of tenofovir allowing for lower serum levels of tenofovir might further mitigate renal toxicity associated with tenofovir.

2. Protease Inhibitors—

- Atazanavir/Indinavir—Both agents are associated with an increased risk crystalluria and nephrolithiasis. Indinavir is now rarely used, but atazanavir use is common and has been associated with higher progression to CKD (eGFR <60 mL/min) than tenofovir. GFR reductions appear reversible in patients who discontinue atazanavir.

- Ritonavir-boosted Lopinavir—Use of this agent is associated with increased risk of CKD and increased risk of tenofovir associated toxicity.

3. cART agents that block tubular creatinine secretion— Cobicistat is a component of some cART regimens and does not possess anti-HIV activity but is used to prolong the half-life of protease inhibitors. Cobicistat can cause a rapid but modest increase in serum creatinine by inhibiting tubular creatinine secretion. Cobicistat can therefore mimic mild AKI similar to that seen with cimetidine or trimethoprim. Importantly, other cART medications including dolutegravir, rilpivirine, and ritonavir can also inhibit tubular secretion of creatinine. Clinicians therefore need to be aware that creatinine changes after initiation of cART do not always reflect renal injury. The most important clinical clue to separate true toxicity from blocking tubular creatinine secretion is that in the latter case, creatinine will rise by a small amount and then stabilize whereas ongoing injury will be associated with continued rise in creatinine.

ACUTE KIDNEY INJURY

HIV-infected patients are at higher risk for developing AKI in both the inpatient and ambulatory settings. Factors most likely associated with AKI include low CD4+ count, exposure to nephrotoxins (eg, cART), and pre-existing CKD.

HIV-ASSOCIATED THROMBOTIC MICROANGIOPATHY

TMA and associated conditions are a complication of advanced HIV infection noted since early in the epidemic. The pathogenesis of this condition is not known and can occur independent of ADAMTS13 levels in contrast to the traditional pathogenesis of TMA from thrombotic thrombocytopenic purpura (TTP). While direct endothelial infection is unlikely, cytotoxic HIV proteins can circulate, and thus may form the initiating event/injury. This suggests that TMA related to HIV infection is due to uncontrolled disease/active viral replication. Consistent with this idea, a review of TMA in cohorts of HIV-infected patients found a TMA rate of 1.4% prior to, and 0% after the introduction of cART. Moreover, TMA associated with traditional pathophysiology (ie, ADAMTS13 depletion) conveyed a better prognosis in HIV-infected patients than when it occurred independent of ADAMTS13 levels. This suggests that uncontrolled HIV infection predisposes to a TMA occurring through different mechanism than ADAMTS13 abundance and may therefore confer greater risk. Because cART has decreased the incidence of TMA in HIV-infected patients its initiation should be part of the treatment in addition to the traditional treatments that are independent of HIV infection.

DIABETIC RENAL DISEASE AND HIV RENAL DISEASE

Recent evidence suggests that HIV infection and diabetes mellitus can interact to promote progressive CKD. In a study comparing risk of progressive CKD in US Veterans with diabetes, HIV, diabetes and HIV, or neither, patients with HIV and diabetes had significantly higher risk for progressive CKD compared to those with HIV or diabetes alone, after controlling for known risk factor. These findings were later replicated in an murine model where HIV transgenic mice developed worsened diabetic kidney injury. Physicians should be therefore be aware that patients with both HIV and diabetes are at increased risk CKD.

KEY READINGS

Boccia RV et al: A hemolytic-uremic syndrome with the acquired immunodeficiency syndrome. Ann Intern Med 1984;101:716.

Couser WG, Johnson RJ: The etiology of glomerulonephritis: roles of infection and autoimmunity. Kidney Int 2014;86:905.

Foy MC et al: Comparison of risk factors and outcomes in HIV immune complex kidney disease and HIV-associated nephropathy. Clin J Am Soc Nephrol 2013;8:1524.

Franceschini N et al: Incidence and etiology of acute renal failure among ambulatory HIV-infected patients. Kidney Int 2005;67:1526.

Gervasoni C et al: Thrombotic microangiopathy in patients with acquired immunodeficiency syndrome before and during the era of introduction of highly active antiretroviral therapy. Clin Infect Dis 2002;35:1534.

Kimmel PL et al: Brief report: idiotypic IgA nephropathy in patients with human immunodeficiency virus infection. N Engl J Med 1992;327:702.

Lepist EI et al: Contribution of the organic anion transporter OAT2 to the renal active tubular secretion of creatinine and mechanism for serum creatinine elevations caused by cobicistat. Kidney Int 2014;86:350.

Lucas GM et al: Clinical practice guideline for the management of chronic kidney disease in patients infected with HIV: 2014 update by the HIV Medicine Association of the Infectious Diseases Society of America. Clin Infect Dis 2014;59:e96.

Malak S et al: Human immunodeficiency virus-associated thrombotic microangiopathies: clinical characteristics and outcome according to ADAMTS13 activity. Scand J Immunol 2008;68:337.

Mallipattu SK et al: Expression of HIV transgene aggravates kidney injury in diabetic mice. Kidney Int 2013;83:626.

Medapalli RK et al: Comorbid diabetes and the risk of progressive chronic kidney disease in HIV-infected adults: data from the Veterans Aging Cohort Study. J Acquir Immune Defic Syndr 2012;60:393.

Mocroft A et al: Estimated glomerular filtration rate, chronic kidney disease and antiretroviral drug use in HIV-positive patients. AIDS 2010;24:1667.

Nobakht E et al: HIV-associated immune complex kidney disease. Nat Rev Nephrol 2016;12:291.

Wyatt CM et al: Acute renal failure in hospitalized patients with HIV: risk factors and impact on in-hospital mortality. AIDS 2006;20:561.

Wyatt CM et al: The spectrum of kidney disease in patients with AIDS in the era of antiretroviral therapy. Kidney Int 2009;75:428.

HEPATITIS-ASSOCIATED GLOMERULONEPHRITIS

Kar Neng Lai, MBBS, MD and Sydney C. W. Tang, MD, PhD

HEPATITIS C VIRUS-ASSOCIATED RENAL DISEASES

ESSENTIALS OF DIAGNOSIS

- The presence of circulating hepatitis C viral RNA and antibody.

- Type I membranoproliferative glomerulonephritis.

- Circulating type II mixed cryoglobulins (polyclonal immunoglobulin [Ig]G and monoclonal IgMκ rheumatoid factor).

- Strong association with hepatitis C virus (HCV) infection chronicity.

- Very low serum C4, C1q, and CH50, but normal C3 levels.

- Direct acting antivirals are highly effective in attaining sustained viral remission in HCV-infected subjects.

▶ General Considerations

A. Historic Perspective

The clinical manifestations associated with "mixed" cryoglobulinemia (MC) were first described in 1966. They included a constellation of clinical features that consisted of the triad of palpable purpura, arthralgias, and weakness plus variable degrees of glomerulonephritis, lymphadenopathy, and hepatosplenomegaly in some patients. Cryoglobulinemia in these patients had a "mixed" composition of IgG and IgM rheumatoid factor (RF). The cause of this disease was unknown in those days, and its association with hepatitis C virus (HCV) infection became increasingly apparent only after its discovery in 1989. It is now apparent that the classic clinical triad occurs in a minority of patients and that the main characteristic of the disease is the markedly heterogeneous manifestations of a systemic vasculitis, with purpuric skin lesions that show leukocytoclastic vasculitis on biopsy being an almost constant and predominant feature.

B. Hepatitis C Virus Virology

Since its discovery 27 years ago, the structure and life cycle of the HCV has been further elucidated which have been key to the recent development of new antiviral therapies. HCV is an enveloped, single-strand, positive-sense, RNA virus that undergoes proteolytic cleavage. The resultant components include two structural envelope glycoproteins (E1 and E2) and the core protein (C). The remaining components are non-structural proteins (NS2, NS3, NS4A, NS4B, NS5A, and NS5B) that are necessary for viral propagation. NS2/3 and NS3/4A comprise proteases responsible for cleaving the HCV polyprotein. NS5B is an RNA dependent RNA polymerase required for viral replication. NS5A is involved in assembly of the cytoplasmic membrane-bound replication complex (Figure 36–4). The evolution of HCV has been characterized by the emergence of six major genotypes based on sequence homology, and more than 50 subtypes.

C. Epidemiology

Globally, around 130–150 million individuals are estimated by the World Health Organization to have chronic HCV infection, which is 18% lower than a decade ago. A significant number of those who are chronically infected will develop liver cirrhosis or cancer, and approximately 700,000 people die each year from HCV-related liver diseases. Its prevalence varies widely among countries, being highest in several African and Eastern Mediterranean countries. Most studies report findings of genotypes 1–3, though a large number of patients worldwide have genotypes 4–6. HCV genotype 6 is mostly found in South-East Asia, ranging from 18% in Thailand, 23.6% in Hong Kong, and 49% in Myanmar. It is the second most common genotype in southern China after genotype 1. HCV genotype 1 patients are largely infected through blood transfusion, while HCV genotype 6 is commonly found in intravenous drug users.

Although HCV infection appears to be primarily a disease that is almost exclusively confined to the liver, a wide variety of extrahepatic disease manifestations have been

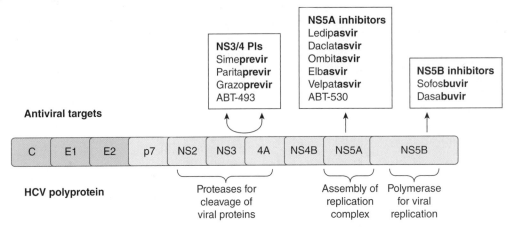

▲ **Figure 36–4.** HCV polyprotein and targets of direct acting antiviral agents. Structural proteins are shown in dark blue and non-structural proteins in light blue. PIs, protease inhibitors.

reported to be associated with HCV infection. The prevalence of extrahepatic diseases is not known with certainty, but it suggests that HCV is involved in nonhepatic pathologic processes.

D. Extrahepatic Manifestation

Up to 40–74% of patients with HCV infection develop at least one extrahepatic manifestation (EHM) during their lifetime. Occasionally, EHMs might be the leading clinical manifestation of HCV infection and can determine the overall prognosis of the disease.

The disorder with the strongest link to HCV infection is MC, defined by the presence of circulating cryoglobulins, which are immunoglobulins that precipitate at reduced temperatures (Figure 36–5A). Therefore, blood samples obtained from patients for detection of cryoglobulins must be stored and transported at 37°C. Overall, cryoglobulins can be found in 19–55% of HCV-infected individuals. There are three different types of cryoglobulinemia. In type I, immunoglobulins are of monoclonal origin. This variant is mainly found in B-cell malignancies, such as multiple myeloma, Waldenström macroglobulinemia, or idiopathic monoclonal gammopathy. HCV infection is associated in 60–96% of cases with type II and III cryoglobulinemia which both contain at least one polyclonal "mixed" component in the precipitating immunoglobulins. Therefore they are called MCs. In type II a polyclonal IgG and a monoclonal IgMκ element with rheumatoid factor activity can be found whereas in type III all cryoglobulins are of polyclonal origin (Table 36–2).

Up to 30% of patients with detectable cryoglobulins develop MC-related symptoms collectively called MC syndrome. Patients with MC syndrome may develop systemic vasculitis. Other common symptoms are peripheral polyneuropathy, Raynaud syndrome and Sicca-like symptoms. Around 10% of patients develop a B-cell lymphoma at some stage. Clinically, the most relevant manifestation of MC is a MPGN, which appears in 30–36% of cases and is associated with significantly increased morbidity and mortality.

In addition, HCV is associated with insulin resistance, type 2 diabetes, and involvement of the central nervous system giving rise to chronic fatigue, depression or general cognitive impairment.

The most frequent form of renal involvement in HCV infection is MPGN, described mainly in the United States and Japan. The real prevalence of MPGN without detectable cryoglobulinemia is difficult to assess. Such cases might represent a subclinical form of cryoglobulinemia because of failure to detect circulating cryoglobulins by standard laboratory techniques or inadequate methods. In addition, the production of IgM antibodies with anti-IgG activity might induce immune complexes without cryoprecipitable properties. Finally, these patients may develop detectable circulating cryoglobulinemia only later in the course of the disease.

▶ Pathogenesis

Two immunologic features of HCV may predispose to chronic infection. First, HCV is known to evade immune elimination, and leads to chronic infection and accumulation of circulating immune complexes. MPGN associated with HCV infection may be the result of this phenomenon. The second feature is the ability of HCV to induce production of monoclonal rheumatoid factors (mRF). The pathogenesis of cryoglobulinemic GN associated with HCV infection is related to the deposition of immune complexes containing HCV proteins, anti-HCV antibodies and rheumatoid factor IgM with activity anti-IgG.

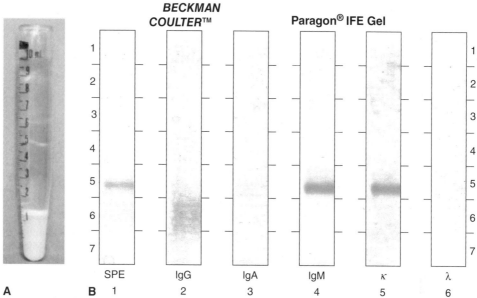

▲ **Figure 36–5.** **A.** Whitish cryoprecipitates forming in Wintrobe tube after standing at 4°C for 72 hours followed by centrifugation at 400 × g for 10 minutes. The cryocrit is approximately 30%. **B.** Immunofixation of the washed, dissolved cryoprecipitate detected a monoclonal IgMκ with polyclonal IgG. By definition, these are type II cryoglobulins. (Courtesy of Dr Janette S.Y. Kwok, Department of Pathology and Clinical Biochemistry, Queen Mary Hospital, Hong Kong, China.) (See Color Plate 13.)

Cryoglobulins are deposited in the mesangium during their macromolecular trafficking in the glomerulus. They can be seen ultrastructurally as finger print-like mesangial and subendothelial dense deposits or filamentous or microtubular structures. This can also lead to intense IgM immunofluorescent staining along capillary walls. Their nephrotoxicity may be partly related to special affinity of the IgMκ-RF for fibronectin in the mesangial matrix.

Immune complex formation is another mechanism for kidney injury induced by HCV. Viral RNA amplified from nephrons obtained by laser capture microdissection has been observed. The findings of IgM, IgG, IgA, and complement components at the site of glomerular and tubular locations coinciding with HCV strongly support this connotation, with the virus being the target for circulating immunoglobulins and possibly complement activation and production of proinflammatory proteins.

Table 36–2. Classification of cryoglobulins.

Type	Immunoglobulin Composition	RF Activity	Most Common Disease Association	Other Disease Associations
I	Single monoclonal IgG, IgA, or IgM	No	Multiple myeloma	Waldenström macroglobulinemia Idiopathic monoclonal gammopathy Chronic lymphocytic leukemia
II[1]	Polyclonal IgG and monoclonal IgM	Yes	HCV infection	Chronic lymphocytic leukemia Lymphoproliferative disease Essential[2]
III[1]	Polyclonal IgG and polyclonal IgM	Yes	Connective tissue disease, particularly RA	Lymphoproliferative disease Chronic liver disease Essential[2]

[1]Also known as mixed cryoglobulinemia due to the presence of more than one Ig type.
[2]When no definite disease association is found, these are known as essential mixed cryoglobulinemias.
HCV, hepatitis C virus; Ig, immunoglobulin; RA, rheumatoid arthritis; RF, rheumatoid factor.

▶ Clinical Findings

A. Symptoms and Signs

1. Hepatitis C virus-related cryoglobulinemia—Full-blown symptomatic cryoglobulinemia occurs infrequently, and the typical symptoms are fatigue and palpable purpura, which histologically consists of a leukocytoclastic vasculitis (with complexes of anti-HCV antibody and HCV in injured tissue). These lesions are usually found on the lower limbs (Figure 36–6), although they can occur anywhere, and represent small vessel vasculitis. A smaller proportion of patients have fever, arthritis, Raynaud phenomenon, and neuropathy. Peripheral neuropathy is usually characterized by paresthesias and variable degrees of motor deficits. Abdominal pain arises from mesenteric vasculitis, and may mimic an acute abdomen during disease flare. Hepatosplenomegaly is due to chronic liver disease as a result of HCV. Cryoglobulinemia is more common in women than men and typically occurs after a prolonged period, often years or decades, of HCV infection. Although the course of illness tends to wax and wane, occasionally the systemic illness can be severe or

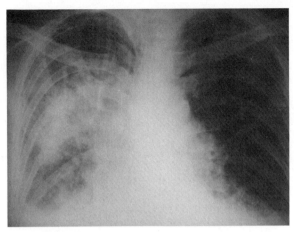

▲ **Figure 36–7.** Nodular pulmonary infiltrates in a patient with cryoglobulinemia. Note also a right internal jugular venous catheter *in situ* for plasmapheresis and hemodialysis.

even fulminant. For instance, nodular pulmonary infiltrates from deposition of cryoglobulins leading to respiratory failure (Figure 36–7) and non-Hodgkin B cell and splenic lymphomas have been reported to arise in the setting of cryoglobulinemia.

2. Cryoglobulinemic glomerulonephritis—The clinical signs and symptoms of HCV-related MC can precede the onset of kidney involvement for years. The principal renal manifestation of HCV infection is MPGN type I, usually in the context of cryoglobulinemia. Type II MPGN (eg, dense deposit disease) has not been described in association with HCV infection. From studies in Italy, the United States, and Japan, MPGN associated with type II cryoglobulinemia is the predominant type of glomerulonephritis clinically associated with HCV infection. The prevalence of MPGN in HCV type II cryoglobulinemia is approximately 30%. On the other hand, the prevalence of anti-HCV antibody among patients with MPGN is much lower in Chinese people. MPGN is also occasionally observed in patients with hepatitis C in the absence of cryoglobulinemia.

Renal disease is rare in children and the typical age of disease onset is in the fifth or sixth decade of life after longstanding infection, often in association with mild subclinical liver disease. Clinically, patients may have other symptoms of cryoglobulinemia, such as palpable purpura and arthralgias. Renal manifestations include nephrotic (20%) or nonnephrotic proteinuria and microscopic hematuria. Acute nephritic syndrome is the presenting feature in about 25% of cases. More than 50% of patients have

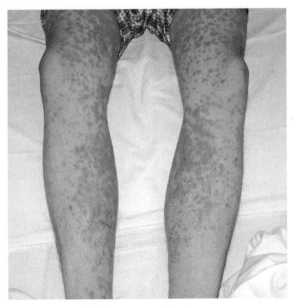

▲ **Figure 36–6.** Palpable purpuric skin lesions in the lower limbs of a patient with cryoglobulinemia. Such lesions are characteristic of any causes of small vessel vasculitis, but not pathognomonic of the rashes in cryoglobulinemia. (Courtesy of Dr. Chi-keung Yeung, Department of Medicine, Queen Mary Hospital, Hong Kong, China.) (See Color Plate 14.)

refractory hypertension. Progression to uremia is associated with male gender and old age. Renal insufficiency, frequently mild, occurs in about 50% of patients. Over 80% of patients have refractory hypertension upon presentation, which may be responsible for a considerable number of cardiovascular deaths.

The natural history of HCV-related cryoglobulinemia remains poorly defined. The clinical course can vary dramatically. The renal disease tends to have an indolent course and does not progress to uremia despite the persistence of urine abnormalities in the majority of patients. Around 15% of patients eventually require dialysis according to an Italian series.

B. Laboratory Findings

Laboratory testing coupled with renal biopsy establishes the diagnosis of HCV-related MPGN. Most patients will have anti-HCV antibody, as well as HCV RNA, in serum. Serum transaminase levels are elevated in 70% of patients. Cryoglobulins are detected in 50–70% of patients. Serum electrophoresis and immunofixation reveal type II mixed cryoglobulins (Figure 36–5B), in which the mRF, almost invariably an IgMκ, is a distinguishing feature of cryoglobulinemic glomerulonephritis. Their amount, usually measured as a cryocrit, varies from one patient to another,

and varies from time to time in a given patient (ranging between 2% and 70%). Urine κ light chains are also commonly present. The serum complement pattern, which does not change much with clinical activity, is also discriminative. Characteristically, the early complement components (C4 and C1q) and CH50 are at very low, or even undetectable, levels, while the C3 level tends to remain normal or only slightly depressed.

Renal histologic evaluation typically shows evidence of immune complex deposition in glomeruli and changes of MPGN. MPGN refers to a pattern of glomerular injury characterized by diffuse mesangial proliferation and thickening of the capillary wall, hence the synonym of mesangiocapillary glomerulonephritis (Table 36–3). In cryoglobulinemic MPGN, light microscopy reveals an increased number of mesangial cells, expansion of the mesangial matrix, and diffuse accentuation of glomerular tufts, which gives a lobular appearance to the glomeruli (Figure 36–8A). Glomerular capillary walls appear thickened because of the interposition of the mesangial matrix between the glomerular basement membrane (GBM) and the endothelium. Staining of the GBM with periodic acid–Schiff or silver stain shows splitting ("double contour") or "tram-tracking" due to insertion of the mesangial matrix (Figure 36–8B). Immunofluorescence reveals granular deposits of C3 and IgG in the mesangium

Table 36–3. Comparison of glomerulonephritis related to chronic hepatitis virus infection.

	HBV Membranous/Mesangiocapillary GN	HCV Mesangiocapillary GN
Route of infection	Vertical or horizontal in children, intravenous or sexual in adult	Intravenous
Occurrence	Children and adult	Adult (fifth and sixth decade)
Male:female	3:1	2:3
History of liver disease	Absent in endemic areas	Yes
Abnormal liver function	Occasional	Yes
Renal presentation	Nephrotic syndrome/proteinuria	Microscopic hematuria/proteinuria, nephrotic syndrome <20%
Hypertension	25–40%	80%
Renal insufficiency	Occasional, 29% in 5 years	15% in 10 years
10-year probability of survival without dialysis	75–90%	49% mainly due to extrarenal complications
Extrarenal complications	Uncommon	40%—CVA, hematologic malignancy, infection, liver failure

CVA, cerebrovascular accident; GN, glomerulonephropathy; HBV, hepatitis B virus; HCV, hepatitis C virus.

and in peripheral capillary loops (Figure 36–8C). A similar morphologic appearance may be seen with infective endocarditis and infected ventriculoatrial shunts (shunt nephritis). In addition, glomerular capillaries may have marked inflammatory cell infiltrates with both mononuclear cells and polymorphonuclear leukocytes (Figure 36–8A), a distinguishing feature from noncryoglobulinemic MPGN. Intracapillary globular accumulations of eosinophilic material representing precipitated immune complexes or cryoglobulins may also be present. Viral HCV-containing antigens had previously been detected in glomerular structures using a three-stage

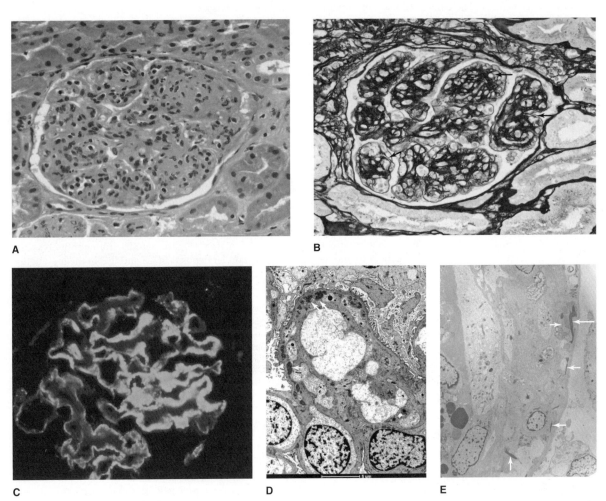

▲ **Figure 36–8.** Pathology of membranoproliferative glomerulonephritis type I associated with cryoglobulinemia. **A.** Glomerulus exhibits a diffuse increase in mesangial cellularity and matrix with accentuation of lobulation of tuft architecture, obliteration of capillary lumens, and leukocytic infiltrate (×200, H&E). **B.** Periodic acid–Schiff and methenamine silver staining reveals prominent double contours or tram-tracking (arrows) of the glomerular basement membrane (GBM) (×400). **C.** Immunofluorescence reveals granular deposits of C3 (shown here) and IgG in the mesangium and in peripheral capillary loops (×200). **D.** Electron microscopy shows markedly increased glomerular cellularity and subendothelial deposits (arrowheads), indicative of cryoglobulin deposition. **E.** Several tactoids are also seen. These are highly electron-dense deposits (arrows) that are most likely crystalline immune complexes as they are surrounded by accompanying nonstructured, less electron-dense materials (arrowhead) (×7,800). (Courtesy of Dr. Kwok-wah Chan, Department of Pathology, Queen Mary Hospital, Hong Kong, China.) **(For Parts A-C, see Color Plate 15.)**

indirect immunohistochemical monoclonal antibody technique but this has not been confirmed by subsequent studies. Electron microscopy shows subendothelial deposits (Figure 36–8D) that may have a tactoid pattern, size, and distribution (Figure 36–8E), suggestive of cryoglobulin deposition. These tend to be of 15–30 μm in size, distinguishing them from the smaller fibrillary deposits (12–25 μm). The presence of immunotactoid glomerulonephritis in a viral disease confirms the association of immunotactoid glomerulonephritis with a systemic disorder, while fibrillary glomerulonephritis is more frequently a "primary" condition. Fibrillogenesis may be favored by circulating paraproteins interacting with matrix proteins in the glomerulus, such as fibronectin. The animal model of MPGN derived from induction of MC strongly suggests a pathogenetic role of cryoglobulins rather than a direct etiologic role of HCV infection. Of interest, however, and again in animal models, both rheumatoid factor and cryoglobulinemic properties may be necessary for the development of skin vasculitis, but cryoglobulin activity alone is sufficient to induce glomerular lesions.

Other forms of glomerular injury have been associated with HCV infection in individual case reports and small series, including membranous glomerulonephritis, IgA nephropathy, focal and segmental glomerulosclerosis, fibrillary glomerulonephritis, immunotactoid glomerulopathy, rapidly progressive glomerulonephritis, exudative–proliferative glomerulonephritis, and lupus nephritis. MN in HCV carriers is characterized by the absence of cryoglobulins and male predominance.

▶ Treatment

The treatment of HCV infection has progressed markedly over the last 3 years. As with any glomerulopathy with proteuinuria and hypertension, renoprotection with antihypertensives and antiproteinuric agents, in particular renin-angiotensin-aldosterone system blockade, should be used judiciously. The HCV life cycle comprising early steps, polyprotein synthesis, maturation of viral proteins, replication, and finally late steps of viral particle formation, offers a large number of potential targets of intervention for the development of specific antiviral drugs, including direct-acting antiviral drugs and host-targeted agents.

In general, therapy can be directed at two levels: (1) removal of cryoglobulins by plasmapheresis and (2) reducing the generation of immune complexes through either attenuation of the immune responses (using corticosteroid, cytotoxic agents or biologic) or suppression of viral replication (using interferon and ribavirin in the past decade or direct acting antivirals [DAAs], as a more promising approach).

Before the association between HCV and cryoglobulinemic MPGN was unraveled, corticosteroid and cyclophosphamide were the mainstay of treatment. High-dose pulse methylprednisolone (1 g/day for three consecutive days), followed by oral steroids, was used to control the systemic illness. Plasmapheresis may be applied to remove circulating cryoglobulins, thus preventing their deposition in glomeruli and blood vessel walls. Cyclophosphamide ameliorates the vasculitic injury and inhibits the production of mRFs by B-lymphocytes.

Our current understanding of the association between MC and HCV infection has resulted in a more rational approach. For the past decade the standard of care for patients with chronic HCV infection has been pegylated interferon (peg-IFN) alfa in combination with ribavirin (RBV). In patients with moderate proteinuria, stable kidney function and mild-to-moderate histologic lesions at kidney biopsy, anti-HCV therapy with peg-IFN, and ribavirin are recommended by the KDIGO. In a meta-analysis, antiviral therapy was found to be more efficacious at lowering proteinuria compared with immunosuppressive therapy (corticosteroids and cyclophosphamide); however, both treatment regimens failed to show any significant improvement in serum creatinine.

Rituximab is a human-mouse chimeric monoclonal antibody against the B-cell surface antigen CD20 that interferes with the synthesis of cryoglobulins and IgMκ-RF by B-cells. It has been used in treatment of HCV-MPGN with or without cryoglobulinemia with significant decreases in proteinuria. In patients with HCV-related mixed cryoglobulinemic vasculitis, addition of rituximab to peg-IFN and ribavirin therapy has been shown to improve elimination of cryoglobulins.

In severe acute flares of cryoglobulinemia with glomerulonephritis or vasculitis and nephritic range proteinuria, an appropriate approach is to include high-dose corticosteroids and cyclophosphamide to control severe cryoglobulinemic symptoms in addition to combination antiviral therapy. In the most severe cases, plasmapheresis (three to four times weekly exchanges of 3 L of plasma for 2–3 weeks) might be used in association with rituximab to remove circulating cryoglobulins. Rituximab may rarely form a complex with IgMκ-RF and lead to increased cryoprecipitation and, hence, should be administered after plasma exchange in patients with high-baseline cryoglobulin levels.

With the approval by the Food and Drug Administration in 2014 of three oral regimens of DAAs which possess potent and rapid virological efficacy, it is likely that current guidelines will be updated to recommend IFN-free anti-HCV treatment regimens using DAAs for patients with cryoglobulinemic vasculitis and HCV-related MPGN. Treatment with DAAs should be proposed to any patient with renal impairment in order to reduce renal and extrarenal complications. Multiple DAAs directed against different targets of the HCV genome are now available (Figure 36–4). To date, the best regimen for patients with renal impairment is unknown. The combination of grazoprevir (protease inhibitor) and elbasvir (NS5A inhibitor), which does not require dose adjustment to eGFR, led to 99% SVR in per protocol analysis in a randomized controlled study in genotype 1–infected patients with CKD stage 4–5. It must be borne in mind that DAAs as of today are highly costly, being priced at US$ 83,320–150,000 for a typical 3-month course in the United States.

KEY READINGS

Chevaliez S et al: Virology of hepatitis C virus infection. Best Pract Res Clin Gastroenterol 2012;26:381.

Gupta A et al: Glomerular diseases associated with hepatitis B and C. Adv Chronic Kidney Dis 2015;22:343.

Ladino M et al: Hepatitis C virus infection in chronic kidney disease. J Am Soc Nephrol 2016;27:2238.

Roth D et al: Grazoprevir plus elbasvir in treatment-naïve and treatment-experienced patients with hepatitis C virus genotype 1 infection and stage 4–5 chronic kidney disease. (the C-SURFER Study): a combination phase 3 study. Lancet 2015;386:1537.

HEPATITIS B VIRUS-ASSOCIATED RENAL DISEASES

ESSENTIALS OF DIAGNOSIS

▸ Membranous nephropathy is the most frequent association.

▸ The presence of circulating hepatitis B virus (HBV) DNA.

▸ The presence of HBV-specific antigen(s) or viral genome in the glomerulus.

▸ Serum C3 and C4 levels may be low in 20–50%.

▸ General Considerations

A. Historic Perspective

Following the landmark discovery in 1965 of the Australian antigen, subsequently renamed the hepatitis B surface antigen (HBsAg), the occurrence of MN due to glomerular deposition of Australian antigen-containing immune complexes was described in a 53-year-old man in 1971. Different histologic types of glomerular lesions have since been described in association with HBV carriage; however, the most striking is still MN.

B. Hepatitis B Virus Virology

HBV is a hepatotropic, double-stranded DNA virus belonging to the family Hepadnaviridae. The 42 nm infectious virion has an internal capsid (core particle) of 27 nm to shield a partially double stranded DNA genome of unusual structure. The DNA genome contains only four genes that encode viral proteins. These include the surface (S) gene, which encodes the three forms of HBsAg, the precore/core (PC/C) gene, which encodes the core protein and hepatitis B e antigen (HBeAg), the X gene, which encodes the X protein, and the polymerase (P) gene, which encodes the viral DNA polymerase. HBV is itself not cytopathic; hepatitis develops as a result of the host's immune reaction toward infected hepatocytes. HBV utilizes a replication strategy closely related to retroviruses, in that transcription of RNA into DNA is a critical step. Unlike retroviruses, HBV DNA is not integrated into host cell DNA during replication. After an HBV particle binds to and enters a hepatocyte, HBV DNA enters the cell nucleus where the relaxed circular DNA (rcDNA) is released and converted into covalently closed circular DNA (cccDNA), which is highly stable acting as the intermediate template for transcription of RNA copies. This pregenomic mRNA is transported to the cytoplasm and has the dual functions of acting as a template for synthesis of new HBV DNA and carrying genetic information to direct the synthesis of viral proteins.

C. Epidemiology

An estimated 240 million people worldwide are now chronically infected with HBV. The reported prevalence of HBV-associated nephropathy, particularly MN, closely parallels the geographic patterns of prevalence of HBV. HBV infection occurs throughout the world and is endemic in sub-Saharan Africa, East Asia, the Amazon basin of South America, and the southern parts of eastern and central Europe, where between 5% and 10% of the adult population is infected. In the Middle East and the Indian subcontinent, an estimated 2–5% of the population is infected. Less than 1% of the population of Western Europe and North America are infected.

In endemic areas, transmission is usually vertical from infected mother to child. Horizontal transmission occurs via direct contact with blood (as in blood transfusions) or mucous membranes (as in sexual contacts), or via the percutaneous route upon contact with blood or body fluids (as in illicit intravenous drug use and needle-sharing practices). As such, HBV is an important occupational hazard for healthcare workers.

▸ Pathogenesis

It is generally believed that host immune response directed toward the surface, core, and extracellular antigens leads to the formation of pathogenic immune complexes to deposit in the mesangium, subepithelial and subendothelial spaces. In addition, HBV can directly infect glomerular cells. Finally, host HLA-related risk alleles and viral genotypes have been implicated to play a role. Yet, the only definitive means to prove that a particular glomerulopathy is etiologically associated with HBV infection is to fulfill the following criteria:

1. The presence of circulating HBV antigen or DNA and HBV-specific antigen(s) or the viral genome in the glomerulus or viral particles identified on ultrastructural examination.

2. The absence of other causes of renal disease.

3. Regression of the pathologic lesion with viral eradication.

4. Reproducibility of the pathology in animal models infected with the virus.

▶ Clinical Findings

A. Symptoms and Signs

Pediatric and adult patients tend to have slightly different clinical manifestations of HBV-related MN. In children, the mean age of presentation is 6 year and there is a strong male preponderance. The most frequent presentation is nephrotic syndrome together with microscopic hematuria and normal or mildly impaired renal function. Pediatric chronic HBV carriers often do not have overt liver disease, and transaminase levels are usually normal. Hypertension occurs in less than 25% of patients. In adults, proteinuria and the nephrotic syndrome are the most common manifestations, though male predominance is less obvious than that observed in children. In addition, adults are more likely than children to have hypertension, renal dysfunction, and clinical evidence of liver disease.

The prognosis of HBV-associated MN in children is favorable with stable renal function and high rates of spontaneous remission reported in several high-prevalence areas, including Hong Kong, South Africa, and Turkey. On the other hand, adults with HBV-associated MN typically develop progressive disease. In Hong Kong, up to 29% of patients had progressive renal failure, and another 10% developed ESRD over 5 years. The prognosis is even worse in patients with nephrotic-range proteinuria and overt hepatitis at presentation, with over 50% of patients requiring renal replacement therapy over 3 years.

B. Laboratory Findings

Laboratory tests to be followed for diagnostic purposes and also to assess response to treatment include standard liver biochemistries (serum alanine aminotransferase, γ-glutamyltransferase, and bilirubin levels) and HBV serologies (HBsAg, HBeAg, anti-HBe, and anti-HBc antibodies). HBeAg is present in 80% of patients, who may also have high titers of anti-HBc. Subjects with biochemical hepatitis should also be tested for circulating HBV DNA levels and should undergo liver biopsy. In addition, α-fetoprotein assay could be an important adjunct. Serum C3 and C4 levels may be low in 20–50% of patients.

More recently, antibodies against phospholipase A2 receptor (anti-PLA2R) can help differentiate idiopathic MN from HBV-MN. In the original study, reactivity to this 185-kDa glycoprotein eluted from glomeruli was present in 70% of subjects with idiopathic MN, but none in secondary MN patients. In a subsequent study in the Chinese population, 82% of patients with idiopathic MN were positive for anti-PLA2R, compared with only 1 in 16 in HBV-MN patients. The subclass of IgG also differs between idiopathic MN which features IgG4 from HBV-MN and other secondary forms of MN in which IgG1 tends to be the predominant IgG subclass. Hence, among HBV carriers with MN, the presence of IgG1 in the glomeruli favors the diagnosis of HBV-MN.

Light microscopic findings are similar to that of idiopathic MN, with some differentiating features. The characteristic glomerular lesion is a diffuse thickening of the glomerular capillary walls to form thick "membranes" (Figure 36–9A). It is now firmly established that this alteration is caused by immune complexes that accumulate subepithelially on the outer aspect of the GBM, which assumes a "membranous" morphology in a stepwise manner. Other pertinent light microscopic findings are reflected in the reactive structural changes of the GBM induced by immune complexes. Therefore special stains highlighting the GBM, such as methenamine silver and periodic acid–Schiff (PASM or silver stain) are more useful (Figure 36–9B). The earliest change on silver staining is a mottled appearance best seen on tangential sections and represents slight indentations of the GBM by immune complexes adhering to its surface. The most specific change of the GBM is the so-called "spike" formation (Figure 36–9B). These are projections of GBM material between immune complexes that lead to a saw tooth-like appearance of the GBM. This pattern is pathognomonic of full-blown membranous glomerulonephropathy. Disease progression results in a diffuse thickening of the GBM. The major constituents of the immune complexes are IgG together with C3 (Figure 36–9C and D). IgM, IgA, and C1q may be present. Ultrastructural findings typically consist of both subepithelial and occasional subendothelial deposits. The presence of subendothelial deposits favors a secondary case of MN such as HBV associated rather than idiopathic MN. The presence of mesangial proliferation on light microscopy is helpful in distinguishing this form of secondary MN from idiopathic MN.

Apart from MN, other renal pathologies have also been associated with HBV infection. These include MPGN with or without cryoglobulinemia, mesangial proliferative glomerulonephritis, and IgA nephropathy. Polyarteritis nodosa

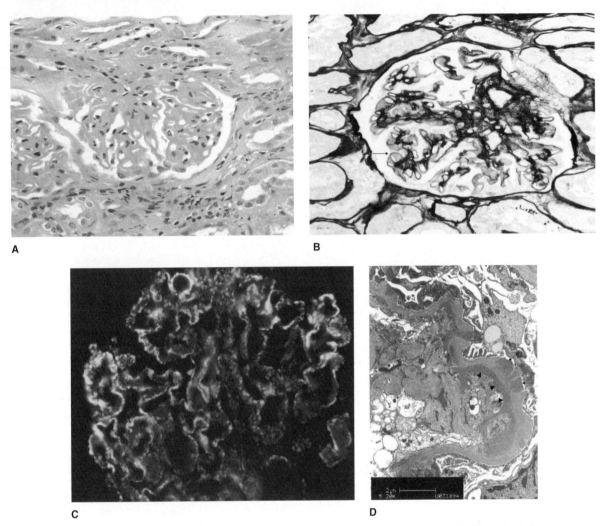

▲ **Figure 36–9.** Pathology of hepatitis B virus (HBV)-associated membranous nephropathy (MN). **A.** On light micros-copy, the characteristic glomerular lesion is a diffuse thickening of glomerular capillary walls to form thick "membranes" (H&E, ×200). **B.** Periodic acid–Schiff and methenamine silver staining highlights the characteristic epimembranous "spike" formation (arrow), projections of glomerular basement membrane (GBM) material between immune complexes that lead to a saw tooth-like appearance of the GBM (×400). **C.** Immunofluorescence reveals granular deposits of IgG (shown here) together with C3. IgM, IgA, and C1q may be present. **D.** Ultrastructural findings typically consist of both subepithelial (arrows) and occasional subendothelial (arrowheads) deposits. The presence of subendothelial deposits favors a secondary case of MN, such as HBV-related rather than idiopathic MN. (Courtesy of Dr. Kwok-wah Chan, Department of Pathology, Queen Mary Hospital (A–C), and Dr. Yun-hoi Lui and Dr. Chung-ying Leung, Department of Pathology, United Christian Hospital (D), Hong Kong, China.) **(For Parts A–C, see Color Plate 16.)**

has also been reported in some patients with HBV and may respond to corticosteroids and interferon-α therapy. Occasionally, overlapping of these pathologic forms leading to double glomerulopathies may be seen. For instance, MN and IgAN have been reported to coexist in an HBV carrier.

Regardless of the pathologic finding, it is important to localize HBV-specific antigens in the biopsy. To document an etiologic association between HBV and MN or other forms of glomerular lesion, the demonstration of HBVspecific antigens by immunofluorescence is indispensable. The three major antigens are: (1) HBsAg, (2) HBeAg, and (3) hepatitis B core antigen (HBcAg). Monoclonal antibodies recognize a single antigenic epitope and are in general less sensitive than polyclonal antibodies that bind to more than one epitope. Commercial polyclonal anti-HBc preparations cross-react with both anti-HBc and anti-HBe, as HBeAg is an integral component of HBcAg. HBsAg is characteristically localized in the mesangium while HBeAg is found in the capillary loop. Furthermore, HBV DNA and mRNA have been detected in the glomerulus and tubular epithelia by polymerase chain reaction and *in situ* hybridization with specific HBV RNA probes.

▶ Treatment

Unlike childhood disease in which there is a high rate of spontaneous remission, adults with HBV-associated MN typically develop progressive disease. Various strategies have been tried, although an ideal agent has yet to be found. Treatment for HBV-associated renal disease should ideally achieve the following objectives:

1. Amelioration of nephrotic syndrome and its complications, such as hyperlipidemia, edema, infection, and venous thrombosis.

2. Preservation of renal function.

3. Normalization of liver function and prevention of hepatic complications of HBV.

4. Permanent eradication of HBV.

In view of the immune complex nature of the disease, immunosuppressive therapy, similar to that applied in the idiopathic form of the disease, was once fashionable. Although it has previously been reported that corticosteroids achieve symptomatic relief in isolated cases, the contemporary view is that steroids and cytotoxic agents may cause deleterious hepatic flares or even fatal decompensation by enhancing viral replication upon treatment withdrawal.

Another approach is treatment with an antiviral agent. Interferon-α is a naturally occurring cytokine produced by B-lymphocytes, null lymphocytes, and macrophages, and possesses antiviral, antiproliferative, and immunomodulatory effects. While reported to be useful in children, interferon-α has produced mixed results in adults with HBV-associated MN.

Nucleos(t)ide analogues have become the standard of care in patients with chronic HBV hepatitis. Following the introduction of lamivudine in the late 1990s, we now have adefovir, entecavir, tenofovir, and telbivudine in the armamentarium. In children and adults with HBV-associated MN, lamivudine has been anecdotally reported to induce remission of nephrotic syndrome and suppress viral replication. In an analysis of 10 adult nephrotic patients with HBV-related MN who received lamivudine treatment versus 12 matched historic control subjects who presented in the prelamivudine era, lamivudine treatment significantly improved proteinuria, ALT levels, and renal outcome over a 3-year period (Figure 36–10). A potential limitation of prolonged treatment with lamivudine is the emergence of drug-resistant strains due to the induction and selection of HBV variants with mutations at the YMDD motif of DNA polymerase. These could be overcome by switching to another more effective antiviral agent. Dose adjustments are needed in patients with impaired renal function.

A meta-analysis indicated that combining steroids with antiviral drugs led to a marked improvement in proteinuria and kidney function without significantly worsening liver function. There is a paucity of clinical trials to define the optimal treatment of HBV-MN. Current KDIGO guidelines recommend that patients with HBV-GN receive treatment with IFN or with nucleoside analogues following standard clinical practice guidelines for HBV infection in general. It is apparent that such guideline requires updating.

Although nucleos(t)ide analogues are effective in suppressing viral replication, it is unable to completely eradicate the virus from the host. In the absence of an ideal agent for treatment of HBV-associated glomerulopathy, active immunization remains the most effective measure of immunoprophylaxis. Vaccination for all

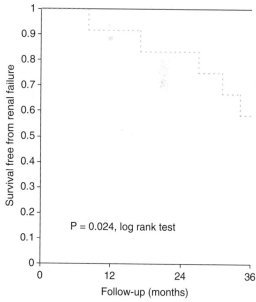

▲ **Figure 36–10.** Renal survival in 10 patients who received lamivudine treatment for hepatitis B virus-associated membranous nephropathy (MN) (solid line) versus 12 matched patients from the prelamivudine era (dotted line).

newborns in some endemic areas such as Hong Kong has dramatically reduced the incidence of chronic HBV infection and its associated complications in children and adolescents. In Taiwan, the introduction of active immunization to all newborns since 1984 has led to a dramatic (10-fold) decline in the incidence of neonatal HBV infection and its subsequent sequelae. In the United States, universal vaccination of infants began in 1991, and a 67% reduction in HBV infection was recorded 10 years later. The introduction of nationwide HBV vaccination in China in 1992 led to significant decreases in childhood glomerular disease. In 2003, the World Health Organization recommended that all countries provide universal HBV immunization programs for infants and adolescents.

KEY READINGS

Infection-related glomerulonephritis. The Kidney Disease: Improving Global Outcomes Clinical Practice Guidelines. Kidney Int 2012;2:200.

Lai KN et al: Membranous nephropathy related to hepatitis B virus in adults. N Engl J Med 1991;27:225.

Qin W et al: Anti-phospholipase A2 receptor antibody in membranous nephropathy. J Am Soc Nephrol 2011;22:1137.

Sun L et al: Effect of hepatitis B vaccine immunization on HBV associated nephritis in children. Zhonghua Er Ke Za Zhi 2003;41:666.

Tang S et al: Lamivudine in hepatitis B-associated membranous nephropathy. Kidney Int 2005;68:1750.

Zheng XY et al: Meta-analysis of combined therapy for adult hepatitis B virus-associated glomerulonephritis. World J Gastroenterol 2012;18:821.

■ CHAPTER REVIEW QUESTIONS

HIV Associated Renal Disease

1. A 34-year-old African–American man who was first diagnosed as HIV positive 10 years ago but has refused antiretroviral therapy presents to an emergency room with nausea and vomiting. The symptoms started over the last few days and have worsened. Prior to the onset of nausea and vomiting, he noted a metallic taste in his mouth and anorexia. He has a previous history of injection drug use but quit 5 years ago. He takes no medications and has no allergies. His most recent serum creatinine was 1.2 mg/dL 1 year ago.

Vital Signs:
Temp—37.2
Blood Pressure—133/86
Pulse—95

Physical Examination:
Young man in apparent distress, occasional retching. Head and neck examination remarkable for oral thrush. Chest is clear to auscultation, Heart rate is normal, normal rhythm, abdominal examination is without tenderness or distension. Pulses are 2+ bilaterally in both extremities. Both lower extremities with trace edema.

Lab Results:
Sodium—141
Potassium—6.1
Chloride—105
CO_2—16
BUN—101 mg/dL
Creatinine—7.9 mg/dL

Urinalysis:
Protein—4+
BLD—NEG
LE—NEG
NITRITE—NEG

Renal Ultrasound—Bilaterally enlarged echogenic kidneys without obstruction or stones.

Which therapy is most likely to be effective in improving the patient's renal function?
A. Prednisone 60 mg daily for 6 months
B. Maximum dose ACE-inhibitor
C. Rituximab
D. Combination antiretroviral therapy

2. A 59-year-old woman diagnosed with HIV 11 years ago presents to her infectious disease specialist's office for follow-up of lab results. The patient has been on a tenofovir-based cART regimen (tenofovir, emtricitabine, and raltegravir for the past 3 years and has had undetectable HIV plasma RNA. Her serum creatinine has been stable at 0.7 mg/dL over the last 3 years. Recently, to decrease her pill burden, she was prescribed a fixed-dose combination therapy with Stribild (elvitegravir, cobicistat, emtricitabine, and tenofovir).

Lab Results:
HIV Viral Load—Undetectable
Sodium—139
Potassium—4.2
Chloride—105
CO_2—28
BUN—25 mg/dL
Creatinine—1.0 mg/dL

Urinalysis:
Protein—None
Blood—None
RBC—0/hpf
WBC—0/hpf

What is the next appropriate step in response to the increase in serum creatinine?

A. Conservative management with continued periodic monitoring of serum creatinine and urinalysis
B. Maximum dose ACE-inhibitor
C. Change to a non-tenofovir based cART regimen
D. Renal biopsy

3. A 42-year-old man presents to his infectious disease specialist's office complaining of weakness. He tested positive for HIV-1 approximately 1 year ago. His initial CD4 count was 25 and he was started on combined antiretroviral therapy with emtricitabine, tenofovir, and lopinavir-ritonavir. The patient responded well and most recent CD4 count is 438 with an undetectable viral load. Approximately 2 months ago, the patient noted onset of myalgias and weakness that have steadily progressed.

Medications:
1. Emtricitabine
2. Tenofovir
3. Lopinavir-Ritonavir
4. Atorvastatin
5. Hydrochlorothiazide
6. Lisinopril

Physical Exam:
Temp—36.5
Blood Pressure—122/78
Pulse—95
O_2 Saturation—100% on room air

Phosphorus—1.0 mg/dL
CPK—899 U/L
Total protein—11 g/dL
Albumin—3.9 g/dL
SPEP—no monoclonal band noted

Lab Values:
Sodium—137 meq/L
Potassium—3.3 meq/L
Chloride—115 meq/L
CO_2—15 meq/L
BUN—25 mg/dL
Creatinine—1.2 mg/dL
  (1.0 two months ago)

Urinalysis:
Protein—None
Blood—None
RBC—0/hpf
WBC—0/hpf

The patient was hospitalized and aggressive electrolyte repletion was initiated.

Which of the following is the most appropriate management?

A. Bone marrow biopsy
B. Replace Hydrochlorothiazide with a potassium sparing diuretic

C. Discontinue Lipitor
D. Change to a non-tenofovir containing cART regimen

4. A 58-year-old woman presents to an emergency room with complaints of flank pain and gross hematuria for 1 day. The flank pain preceded the hematuria and was accompanied by nausea and vomiting. The patient has a history of chronic hepatitis C with cirrhotic liver changes, hypertension, congestive heart failure and HIV infection. His HIV is treated with a combination of lamivudine, tenofovir, ritonavir, and atazanavir.

Vital Signs and Physical Examination:
Temp—36.9
Blood Pressure—159/88
Pulse—95
O_2 Saturation—100% on room air
General—Patient writhing in pain on gurney
Abdominal—Diffuse abdominal tenderness; no rebound, no guarding

Medications:
1. Amlodipine
2. Metoprolol
3. Furosemide
4. Atorvastatin
cART: lamivudine, tenofovir, ritonavir, and atazanavir

Lab Values:
Sodium—137 meq/L
Potassium—4.7 meq/L
Chloride—103 meq/L
CO_2—30 meq/L
BUN—25 mg/dL
Creatinine—1.3 mg/dL
Calcium—9 mg/dL
Phosphorus—2.5 mg/dL
Uric Acid—5 mg /dL

Urinalysis:
pH—6.5
Protein—1+
Blood—4+
RBC—50+/hpf
WBC—3–5/hpf
Casts—none
Crystals—+needle-shaped

Renal Ultrasound—Left kidney with 6 mm stone in the lower pole

Which of the following is the most appropriate treatment?

A. Discontinue atazanavir
B. Begin potassium citrate therapy
C. Discontinue tenofovir
D. Proceed to renal biopsy

5. A 67-year-old Caucasian patient presents to a nephrologist consultant's office for evaluation of proteinuria. Patient noticed the onset of lower extremity edema 2 months ago. Twenty-four hours urine collection resulted in 4.2 g of protein detected. The patient has a history of HIV diagnosed 19 years ago treated with elvitegravir, cobicistat, emtricitabine, and tenofovir resulting in undetectable serum viral load. Patient has additional history of hypertension and diabetes mellitus, diagnosed at the age of 50.

Vital Signs and Physical Examination:
Temp—37.3
Blood Pressure—138/74
Pulse—62
O_2 Saturation—100% on room air
Lower Extremities—4+ pitting edema bilaterally extending to the thigh

Lab Values:
Sodium—137 meq/L
Potassium—4.9 meq/L
Chloride—101 meq/L
CO_2—28 meq/L
BUN—27 mg/dL
Creatinine—1.5 mg/dL
Albumin—2.6 g/dL
SPEP—no monoclonal protein

Urinalysis:
pH—5
Protein—4+
Blood—NONE
RBC—0 /hpf
WBC—0/hpf
Casts—none

Which of the following is the most likely diagnosis?
A. HIVAN
B. Membranous nephropathy
C. HIV-associated immune complex kidney disease
D. Diabetic nephropathy

Hepatitis-Associated Glomerulonephritis

1. A 53-year-old woman is evaluated for a 3-month history of swelling of the face, hands, and feet. She has untreated hepatitis C virus infection. She takes metformin for diabetes mellitus. She has no additional symptoms. On physical examination, temperature is normal, blood pressure is 131/86 mm Hg, pulse rate is 71/min, and respiration rate is 18/min. Bilateral periorbital edema and swelling of the hands and legs are noted. The remainder of the examination is unremarkable.

Laboratory Studies:

Hemoglobin	10.7 g/dL
Platelet	48,000/μL (48 × 10⁹/L)
Sodium	141 meq/L (141 mmol/L)
Potassium	4.6 meq/L (4.6 mmol/L)
Albumin	16 g/L
Serum creatinine	1.5 mg/dL (133 μmol/L)
Rheumatoid factor	Negative
Hepatitis B surface antigen	Negative
Hepatitis C virus antibodies	Positive with high RNA titer
HIV antibodies	Negative
Urinalysis	4+ protein; 4–7 erythrocytes/hpf; 4–7 leukocytes/hpf
Urine albumin–creatinine ratio	8.7 mg/mg

Ultrasound shows normal-sized kidneys.

What of the following diagnostic studies is the most appropriate next step in this patient's management?
A. Twenty-four-hour urine protein
B. Cryoglobulins
C. Cystoscopy
D. Kidney biopsy

2. A 61-year-old ex-intravenous drug addict man presents with bilateral purpuric skin rashes in his lower extremities. He complains of increasing fatigue and notices swelling in his feet. Physical examination reveals palpable purpuric skin lesions in both lower limbs, and bilateral pitting ankle edema. Temperature is normal, blood pressure is 142/85 mm Hg, pulse rate is 74/min. Abdominal examination is unremarkable. There was also loss of sensation in the glove-and-stocking distribution. The remainder of the examination is unremarkable. You order laboratory work on the patient and it shows the following:

Blood picture	Normal
Sodium	141 meq/L (141 mmol/L)
Potassium	4.6 meq/L (4.6 mmol/L)
Albumin	26 g/L
Serum creatinine	1.9 mg/dL (168 μmol/L)
Serum ALT	123 U/L
Immunofixation	Monoclonal IgMκ with polyclonal IgG
Hepatitis B surface antigen	Negative
Hepatitis C virus antibodies	Positive
HIV antibodies	Negative
Urinalysis	3+ protein; 4–7 erythrocytes/hpf
Urine albumin–creatinine ratio	2.7 mg/mg

Kidney biopsy reveals glomerulomegaly with accentuated lobulations, presence of C3 and IgG immunostaining, and subendothelial electron dense deposits.

What of the following is the best next step in management?

A. Perform a skin biopsy and bone marrow biopsy and refer to a hematologist
B. Check HCV RNA titer and refer to a hepatologist for antiviral treatment
C. Check HCV RNA titer and perform a liver biopsy
D. Check C3 and other immune markers, then start corticosteroid and rituximab
E. Check C3 and other immune markers, then start pegylated interferon-alpha and ribavirin

3. A 40-year-old businessman was detected to be seropositive for HBsAg 2 years ago during an insurance medical examination. He has promiscuity especially when he was travelling overseas. Laboratory tests at the same medical examination revealed that he was seronegative for HBeAg with detectable serum level of HBeAb. The liver enzymes were raised by twofold with normal liver echotexture by Fibroscan. Anti-HCV and HIV screening were negative. He was advised to undergo repeated liver enzymes at 6-monthly interval. Two months ago, he noticed frothy urine. Spot urine examination revealed proteinuria of 580 mg/L with no microscopic hematuria. The serum creatinine and albumin were within normal limits. The patient requested antiviral therapy for hepatitis B infection.

Which of the following is the most appropriate step in his management?

A. Start antiviral treatment (eg, Entecavir) immediately
B. Perform a kidney biopsy
C. A therapeutic trial of corticosteroid to reduce the proteinuria
D. Serum HBV DNA to determine the viral load
E. Administration of a full course of HBV vaccination

Acute Tubulointerstitial Nephritis

Dennis G. Moledina, MD

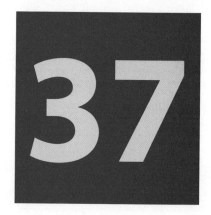

ESSENTIALS OF DIAGNOSIS

▶ Clinical suspicion of tubulointerstitial nephritis is raised by acute to subacute rise in serum creatinine, presence of sterile pyuria, and exposure to offending medications.

▶ Diagnosis of tubulointerstitial nephritis requires a kidney biopsy.

▶ On histology, tubulointerstitial nephritis is characterized by presence of lymphocytes in the interstitium, presence of lymphocytes infiltrating into the tubular space ("tubulitis"), and varying degree of interstitial eosinophils. The glomeruli are usually spared except in nonsteroidal anti-inflammatory drug-induced tubulointerstitial nephritis, which may show global foot process effacement.

▶ Medications are the most common cause of tubulointerstitial nephritis in the United States; autoimmune diseases are an uncommon etiology of tubulointerstitial nephritis in the elderly, but may be seen in the young.

▶ Antibiotics, proton pump inhibitors and nonsteroidal anti-inflammatory drugs are the most common causes of tubulointerstitial nephritis in the United States. Immune checkpoint inhibitors are the newest class of drugs implicated in the tubulointerstitial nephritis.

General Considerations

Acute tubulointerstitial nephritis (ATIN) is a common histological diagnosis characterized by presence of inflammatory cells in the renal interstitial space, varying degree of interstitial eosinophils, and infiltration of these inflammatory cells into the tubular space ("*tubulitis*"). ATIN suspicion is raised clinically by an acute or subacute decrease in glomerular filtration rate (GFR) indicated by a rise in serum creatinine, or by an abnormal urinalysis and urinary sediment examination in a patient with clinical scenario suspicious for ATIN. This is usually followed by a kidney biopsy to establish the diagnosis as there is as yet no reliable noninvasive test for ATIN. Most biopsy series report that 2–3% of all kidney biopsies carry a diagnosis of ATIN. In patients with acute kidney injury (AKI), however, the reported proportion of this diagnosis increases to 13–20%. Thus, ATIN is a relatively common cause of AKI cases that require a biopsy. ATIN incidence is also on the rise, particularly in the elderly population.

▶ Etiology

A number of causes of ATIN have been described (Table 37–1). The following describes those that are most common and of highest interest for clinicians.

1. Medications: Drug-induced interstitial nephritis is responsible for over 70% causes of ATIN. While over 120 medications have reportedly been associated with ATIN, the most frequently implicated drug classes are antibiotics, proton pump inhibitors (PPIs), and nonsteroidal anti-inflammatory drugs (NSAIDs). Among the antibiotics, beta-lactams, fluoroquinolones, vancomycin, sulfonamides and rifampin are the most common culprits. Due to their easy availability without a prescription in the United States, perceived safety and widespread use, PPIs have become a common ATIN cause. Multiple recent studies have demonstrated higher ATIN, AKI, chronic kidney disease (CKD), and end stage renal disease (ESRD) risk in individuals taking PPIs. Recently, ATIN has also been described in association with immune checkpoint inhibitors (or "immunotherapy") including cytotoxic T-cell antigen-4 (CTLA-4) inhibitors such as ipilimumab and PD1/PDL-1 inhibitors such as pembrolizumab and nivolumab. These drugs act by restoring T-cell activity against tumor cells. These drugs have revolutionized therapy of melanoma, non-small cell

Table 37–1. Typical features and therapy of various forms of acute tubulointerstitial nephritis.

Etiology of ATIN	Clinical and Laboratory Features	Typical Histopathologic Features	Therapy
Drug-induced	Most common etiology (over 70% in developed countries)	Lymphocytic infiltrate with eosinophils	Discontinue offending agent; Consider trial of glucocorticoids
Proton pump inhibitors	Long latent period; few typical clinical features.		
Nonsteroidal anti-inflammatory drugs	ATIN is often associated with massive proteinuria; long latent period; rarely present with typical allergic manifestations.	Interstitial eosinophilia may be absent. Glomerular lesions are sometimes present.	Questionable benefit of corticosteroids.
Antibiotics	More likely to present with systemic allergic manifestations of rash, eosinophilia, and fever (particularly with methicillin and penicillin). Short latent period.	Interstitial eosinophilia is common. Granuloma sometimes present.	
Immune-mediated diseases	More common in younger individuals.	Mononuclear cell infiltration. Granuloma seen with certain diseases.	Therapy directed at the specific etiology. Immunosuppressive agents often used.
SLE nephritis	Systemic features of lupus. Positive lupus serologies, evidence of complement activation.	Usually seen in association with focal or diffuse proliferative glomerulonephritis with "full house" immunofluorescence staining.	
Sarcoidosis	Many other renal manifestations such as hypercalcemia, hypercalciuria, and nephrolithiasis.	Focal lymphocytic infiltrate and interstitial noncaseating granulomas composed of giant cells, histiocytes, and lymphocytes.	Excellent response to corticosteroid therapy.
Sjögren syndrome	Characterized by dry eyes and dry mouths. Serologies often positive.	Lymphoplasmacytic infiltrate.	Immunosuppressive therapy in the form of corticosteroids, azathioprine, cyclophosphamide, and mycophenolic acid.
IgG4-related	Systemic disorder with elevated serum IgG4 level. Other organ involvement: salivary glands, pancreas, retroperitoneum and kidneys.	Lymphoplasmacytic interstitial infiltrate with IgG4-positive plasma cells and interstitial fibrosis in a "storiform" pattern.	Long-term corticosteroid treatment; steroid-sparing agents.
Tubulointerstitial nephritis and uveitis syndrome	Uveitis: painful red eyes, photophobia; renal failure; common in younger individuals. Uveitis can occur months after nephritis.	Mixed inflammatory infiltrate with granuloma formation.	3–6 months of prednisone with slow taper. Both ocular and renal manifestations improve dramatically upon initiation of corticosteroids.

ATIN, acute tubulointerstitial nephritis; SLE, systemic lupus erythematosus.

lung cancer and renal cell carcinoma, and are actively being investigated in many other cancers. However, these drugs have been associated with various immune phenomena due to increased T-cell activity, including ATIN.

2. Systemic autoimmune disorders are the second most common causes of ATIN in the developed world. Autoimmune ATIN is more common in the young, but uncommon in the elderly. ATIN is found in association with **sarcoidosis,** where it is one of many other renal manifestations such as hypercalcemia, normocalcemic hypercalciuria, nephrocalcinosis, nephrolithiasis, and various glomerular lesions. **Sjögren syndrome** involves the kidney in 15–67% cases in the form of ATIN. Systemic lupus erythematosus- and ANCA vasculitis-associated renal disease can show isolated ATIN; however, it is more commonly associated with glomerulonephritis. ATIN is also seen as part of **tubulointerstitial nephritis and uveitis syndrome (TINU),** which involves the eyes and kidneys. **IgG4-related kidney disease** is part of a group of disorders characterized by elevated serum levels of IgG4 subclass antibodies, tissue deposition of IgG4, and involvement of various organ systems including salivary glands, pancreas, retroperitoneum, and kidneys.

3. Infections are an uncommon cause of ATIN in the developed world and account for less than 5% of cases. ATIN has been described in association with tuberculosis, Hantavirus, leptospirosis, legionellosis, histoplasmosis, cytomegalovirus, and Epstein–Barr virus. Bacterial pyelonephritis should be suspected when the interstitial infiltrate consists predominantly of neutrophils.

Pathogenesis

Since the majority of ATIN is caused by medications, we will focus on the pathogenesis of drug-induced ATIN. The kidneys are particularly sensitive to drug hypersensitivity and kidneys are often affected in the absence of systemic manifestations. ATIN is a rare consequence of drug exposure as immune responses in the kidneys seem to be self-regulatory. Immune checkpoint inhibitors, which cause loss of this immune tolerance, lead to ATIN. In reported cases of immune checkpoint inhibitor-associated ATIN, patients were tolerant to drugs known to cause this lesion for months (such as PPIs), subsequently becoming intolerant after initiating immune checkpoint inhibitor therapy.

The typical histological ATIN findings are predominantly in the renal tubulointerstitium. In ATIN, the renal tubular epithelial cells acquire the ability to present antigens to CD4+ T-helper cells by expressing the HLA-DR molecules. Drug-specific CD4+ T-cells have also been isolated from the blood and renal interstitium in antibiotic-induced ATIN. The interstitial infiltrate in ATIN consists primarily of CD4 and CD8 T-cells. As the interstitial infiltrate consists predominantly of T-cells, immunosuppressive therapies aimed at suppressing this inflammation are often employed as therapy. Eosinophils in the interstitium are often present in drug-associated ATIN; however, their absence doesn't exclude the diagnosis, particularly in cases of PPI- or NSAID-associated ATIN, which rarely show eosinophils. Ongoing and unchecked interstitial inflammation can rapidly progress to interstitial fibrosis, which is irreversible and leads to CKD. Thus, early recognition is key in ATIN management.

Clinical Presentation, Risk Factors, and Diagnostic Testing

Most patients with drug-associated ATIN are asymptomatic. History may reveal the presence of medication triggered allergic reaction. Manifestations of an allergic reaction such as hives, fever, or rash may be present, particularly with antibiotics, but characteristically absent in PPI- or NSAID-associated ATIN. The classic clinical "triad" of fever, rash, and eosinophilia is observed in less than 10% of patients with drug-induced ATIN, almost always seen in association with antibiotic-associated ATIN. Patients with systemic diseases associated with ATIN (sarcoidosis, SLE, Sjögren syndrome, IgG4, etc.) often have known history of these diseases. In TINU, uveitis manifests with painful red eyes and photophobia, and may come to clinical attention months after the renal diagnosis. Thus, younger individuals without known etiology of ATIN should be monitored for development of uveitis. The clinical features and therapies of the various forms of ATIN are noted in Tables 37–1 and 37–2.

The period from drug initiation to ATIN diagnosis varies based on the drug involved and prior exposure. Time from drug initiation to diagnosis is usually a few days for antibiotics as compared to weeks to months for PPIs and NSAIDs. This may represent either a long latent period or failure to recognize the disease early due to its indolent nature (due to lack of symptoms/signs), or a combination of both. Thus, ATIN need not occur due to a new exposure, and should be on the differential diagnosis list even if no new medication has been recently added.

Table 37–2. Clinical and laboratory manifestation of acute tubulointerstitial nephritis.

Clinical features	Manifestations of allergic reaction: Fever, rash, eosinophilia ("Triad" <10%)
	History of drug-intake
	Latent period varies by drug-class: few days for antibiotics, days to weeks for NSAIDs, weeks to months for PPIs
	More common in elderly and those with underlying chronic kidney disease
Serum tests	Subacute (typical) or acute (uncommon) decrease in glomerular filtration rate (indicated by rise in serum creatinine)
	Eosinophilia (non-specific, but suggestive)
Urine tests	Sterile pyuria, white blood cell casts, granular casts
	Low-grade proteinuria ("tubular range"); except NSAID-associated ATIN, which may have nephrotic range proteinuria
	"Normal sediment" in ~20%
	Urine eosinophil testing is not recommended
Imaging	Ultrasound and CT scan: needed to rule out other causes of renal disease.
Kidney biopsy	"Gold Standard"; typical findings include interstitial inflammatory cell infiltrate, "tubulitis," interstitial eosinophils

CT, computed tomography; NSAID, nonsteroidal anti-inflammatory drugs; PPIs, proton pump inhibitors.

The elderly seem to be at higher risk of drug-associated ATIN. One study noted a steep rise in proportion of ATIN present on biopsies in the elderly in recent years. Medications account for a larger proportion of ATIN cases in the elderly (>65 years) as compared with the young (<65 years) (87% versus 64%), while autoimmune diseases as a cause of ATIN is fairly uncommon in the elderly as compared to the young (7% versus 27%). IgG4-related kidney disease typically affects middle-aged men. CKD is also a known risk factor for ATIN, and a significant proportion of patients diagnosed with this lesion have underlying CKD. Thus, ATIN should be suspected in any patient with unusually rapid progression of CKD, particularly in the setting of an offending agent.

The first clinical clue for the clinician is often a slow decline in kidney function indicated by an elevation in serum creatinine concentration. Due to slower decline in kidney function, up to 50% patients with biopsy-proven ATIN do not meet the KDIGO AKI criteria (defined as rise in serum creatinine of 50% from baseline within 7 days), but have a much slower decline (over months) that is indistinguishable from progressive CKD. This often leads to a delay in ATIN recognition and treatment.

Due to the nature of tubulointerstitial kidney injury with ATIN, some urinary abnormality is often present. Pyuria or presence of WBC casts in urine is highly suggestive of ATIN (Figure 37–1); however, these casts may also be seen with inflammatory glomerulonephritides. ATIN can also present with low-grade ("tubular") proteinuria. NSAID-associated ATIN is an exception, however, and can present with nephrotic-range proteinuria (and associated glomerular disease). *Urine* eosinophil testing is inaccurate for diagnosing ATIN, and is often misleading. This lack of accuracy of a test, once considered reliable for ATIN diagnosis, is due to the significant change in the etiology of this renal lesion since the original studies in urine eosinophil testing were conducted. Finally, up to 20% of ATIN patients can present with "normal" urinary sediment and ATIN cannot be excluded as a diagnosis purely based on the presence of normal urinary sediment. While significant *serum* eosinophilia may point toward ATIN, the diagnosis cannot be made based on this test alone. In ATIN, ultrasound and computed tomography imaging studies serve to rule out other causes of kidney injury, but don't help in recognizing ATIN. IgG4-related kidney disease may demonstrate obstructive renal disease due to retroperitoneal fibrosis.

One small study that found elevation in novel markers of tubular dysfunction such as Monocyte Chemoattractant Protein-1 (MCP-1), Neutrophil Gelatinase-associated Lipocalin (NGAL), α1-microglobulin, and *N*-acetyl-beta-D-glucosaminidase (NAG) in ATIN as compared to healthy individuals. However, the clinical applicability of these results is limited due to the fact that the control group in these biomarker studies was normal, healthy volunteers, rather than individuals with kidney disease.

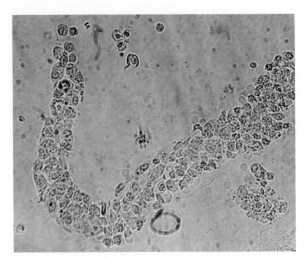

▲ **Figure 37–1.** White blood cell cast observed in spun urine sediment of patient with ATIN.

Thus, noninvasive ATIN diagnosis is quite challenging as there is no typical clinical feature, the kidney function decline is slowly progressive, and there is no definitive non-invasive test. Thus, it is necessary to maintain a high index of suspicion. Cases of non-resolving or progressive AKI should be carefully evaluated to assess the need for an early kidney biopsy. ATIN often occurs in those with CKD, and cases of atypical renal function decline in previously stable CKD should also prompt consideration of this kidney disease.

▶ Pathology

The "gold standard" of ATIN diagnosis remains histological examination of kidney tissue sample via percutaneous kidney biopsy.

A. Tubulointerstitium

The typical findings of ATIN are predominantly in the tubulointerstitium. ATIN is characterized by infiltration of the renal interstitium with lymphocytes (Figure 37–2). These lymphocytes often cross the renal tubular basement membrane and enter the renal tubules, a phenomenon termed "tubulitis." Tubulitis is often best seen on periodic acid–Schiff (PAS) stain and presence of tubulitis leads the renal pathologist to suspect ATIN. These cells in the tubular space are excreted in the urine leading to the clinical finding of pyuria and WBC casts in the urine. Tubulitis also leads to significant degree of renal tubular injury, likely contributing significantly to AKI. Thus, it is not uncommon to find renal tubular epithelial cells and casts in the urine of ATIN patients. Eosinophils are often seen in the interstitium in ATIN; however, their absence doesn't exclude drug-induced ATIN. This is particularly true in cases of ATIN associated

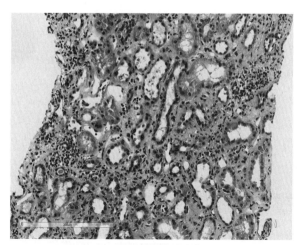

▲ **Figure 37–2.** Renal histology findings in drug-induced ATIN showing lymphoplasmacytic tubulointerstitial infiltrate and tubulitis. The patient had lung adenocarcinoma on anti-PD1 therapy (Lambrolizumab) and presented with rising creatinine and adrenalitis. The patient was also on a proton pump inhibitor for years prior to starting anti-PD1 therapy. Urine sediment had numerous white blood cells. (See Color Plate 17.)

with PPIs and NSAIDs. Scattered eosinophils are also seen in the infiltrates of inflammatory glomerulonephritides. Thus, the finding of urine eosinophils is neither sensitive nor specific for ATIN diagnosis. The presence of a significant number of neutrophils should raise the possibility of pyelonephritis or other infectious agent. Pathologically, ATIN can be characterized into acute (developing over days to weeks) or chronic (developing over months to years) based on degree of interstitial fibrosis and the type of cells involved.

Diagnosis of ATIN is challenging in patients with renal transplantation, where an interstitial infiltrate is most commonly due to transplant rejection, which is characterized by interstitial infiltrate by lymphocytes, and other cells. It has been suggested that more than 20 eosinophils/high power field may indicate ATIN. This kidney lesion can also present with a granulomatous interstitial nephritis characterized by non-caseating granulomas comprised of macrophages and multinucleated giant cells. This is particularly seen in sarcoidosis. Granulomatous interstitial nephritis with eosinophils is very suspicious for drug-induced ATIN. IgG4-related tubulointerstitial nephritis is characterized by presence of numerous plasma cells and characteristic "storiform" (cartwheel) fibrosis.

Glomeruli and blood vessels are typically spared in this kidney disease. In NSAID-induced ATIN, glomerular lesions such as minimal change disease or membranous nephropathy may be present correlating with the significant proteinuria noted clinically. Changes related to underlying CKD such

as diabetic nephropathy and hypertension may be seen with ATIN superimposed on these findings. Late biopsy in ATIN will reveal significant interstitial fibrosis and tubular atrophy.

Immunofluorescence is typically unremarkable in ATIN. Very rarely, linear tubular basement membrane staining with C3 and immunoglobulin G (anti-TBM antibodies) has been reported with drugs such as methicillin. Immunofluorescence is primarily used to rule out other causes of interstitial nephritis. For example, systemic lupus erythematosus nephritis can present with isolated interstitial lesions. In such cases, presence of mesangial full house staining is indicative of lupus nephritis. IgG4 positivity is noted within the plasma cells in IgG4-related kidney disease.

▶ Differential Diagnosis

The differential diagnosis of acute to subacute rise in serum creatinine includes a myriad of kidney diseases including known causes of AKI such as acute tubular injury from various causes, various glomerulonephritides, and obstructive kidney disease, and causes of progressive CKD such as diabetic kidney disease and hypertensive kidney disease. The differential diagnosis of interstitial inflammation and tubulitis includes ANCA-associated vasculitis and lupus nephritis, and acute rejection in the transplant setting.

▶ Prevention

Given that ATIN is most commonly caused by medications, preventive strategies are aimed at reducing exposure to medications associated with this lesion. This is particularly important in high-risk groups such as the elderly and those with CKD. Such patients should be specifically questioned about their over-the-counter drug use as PPIs and NSAIDs, both of which are available without a prescription and are taken by 10–15% of US adults. PPI-use is associated with various adverse effects and its use should be avoided outside of clear indications. NSAIDs also have myriad of renal toxic effects are their use should be minimized in those with advanced CKD, if possible.

▶ Treatment

A. Identification and Discontinuation of Offending Agent

The mainstay of ATIN management is identification of the offending agent and prompt discontinuation. When a diagnosis of ATIN is confirmed or suspected, culprit drugs should be substituted with alternative agents where possible. Drug-associated ATIN is often a class effect and switching to another agent in the same class is generally not recommended. Some clues can help identify an offending drug. For example, temporal association of initiation with worsening of laboratory parameters may point to the new drug as an offender. In addition, the presence of hypersensitivity features (eosinophilia, fever, rash) may suggest beta-lactams or sulfonamides, and the coexistence of glomerular lesions such as minimal change disease may point toward NSAIDs.

B. Immunosuppressive Therapy

Given the underlying immune mechanism in ATIN and extensive inflammatory infiltrate observed on kidney biopsy, immunosuppressive therapy is an attractive treatment option in ATIN. There are, however, no randomized controlled trials in ATIN, and the existing evidence is derived from retrospective studies. The decision to use steroids in these studies was determined by treating clinician based on clinical severity, and hence these studies are highly susceptible to bias. Moreover, these are all small studies and clearly underpowered to detect any potential benefit of steroids, if one existed. One study evaluated 187 patients with ATIN, of whom 158 were treated with steroids and found higher eGFR in steroid treated group despite comparable baseline characteristics including baseline eGFR and interstitial fibrosis. Two other smaller studies also showed lower serum creatinine at follow-up in those treated with steroids. On the other hand, one study found lower eGFR at follow-up in steroid treated ATIN patients. However, in this study steroid treated patients had lower eGFR at the start of the study. Another study of 133 patients found no improvement in eGFR in steroid treated patients. In view of the conflicting results of these retrospective studies and given the underlying immune pathogenesis in ATIN, the current evidence suggests careful consideration of a short course (<4 weeks) of glucocorticoid therapy in those that have potential for renal recovery (indicated by low-interstitial fibrosis) and without significant contraindication to glucocorticoid therapy. Those responding to therapy may be continued for 4–6 weeks, whereas in the absence of response within 3–4 week, this therapy should be promptly tapered off. A reasonable approach is to start therapy with either 3 days of intravenous pulse steroids (250–500 mg) or with prednisone at 1 mg/kg. An exception to this is NSAID-induced ATIN, where the underlying mechanism makes this form of ATIN unlikely to respond to immunosuppressive therapy.

There is also some evidence to suggest that the timing of glucocorticoid initiation may be important in ATIN. One study found that patients with complete recovery to baseline serum creatinine concentration had a shorter duration between diagnosis and steroid administration as compared to those without complete recovery, and there was a positive correlation between delay in steroid initiation and final serum creatinine. Another study found a correlation between delay from onset of AKI or biopsy to initiation of steroids and recovery. Thus, if glucocorticoid therapy is being considered, it should be initiated early. As mentioned before, these recommendations are based on retrospective studies representing low-quality evidence, and therapy must be individualized in each case.

Treatment of other forms of secondary ATIN is described in respective chapters throughout this textbook.

▶ Prognosis

ATIN is considered reversible upon early recognition and withdrawal of the offending agent. However, delay in diagnosis, longer exposure to offending drugs, and delay in initiation of steroids are associated with incomplete recovery. Other markers of poor prognosis include presence of granulomas on kidney biopsy, and degree of tubular atrophy and interstitial fibrosis.

▶ When to Refer/Admit

ATIN should be diagnosed and managed by a nephrologist. A patient with acute to subacute rise in serum creatinine concentration should be referred to a nephrologist as soon as possible. The offending agent should be discontinued or substituted, if possible. Evaluation and management can be conducted in the outpatient setting, if a biopsy can be performed and evaluated in a timely manner.

KEY READINGS

Arora P, Gupta A, Golzy M, et al: Proton pump inhibitors are associated with increased risk of development of chronic kidney disease. BMC Nephrol 2016;17:112.

Bhaumik SK et al: Evaluation of clinical and histological prognostic markers in drug-induced acute interstitial nephritis. Ren Fail 1996;18:97.

Brewster UC, Perazella MA: Acute kidney injury following proton pump inhibitor therapy. Kidney Int 2007;71:589.

Clarkson MR et al: Acute interstitial nephritis: clinical features and response to corticosteroid therapy. Nephrol Dial Transplant 2004;19:2778.

Cortazar FB et al: Clinicopathological features of acute kidney injury associated with immune checkpoint inhibitors. Kidney Int 2016;90:638.

D'Agati VD et al: Interstitial nephritis related to nonsteroidal anti-inflammatory agents and beta-lactam antibiotics: a comparative study of the interstitial infiltrates using monoclonal antibodies. Mod Pathol 1989;2:390.

Davison AM, Jones CH: Acute interstitial nephritis in the elderly: a report from the UK MRC Glomerulonephritis Register and a review of the literature. Nephrol Dial Transplant 1998;13:12.

Goicoechea M, Rivera F, Lopez-Gomez JM: Increased prevalence of acute tubulointerstitial nephritis. Nephrol Dial Transplant 2013;28:112.

Gonzalez E et al: Early steroid treatment improves the recovery of renal function in patients with drug-induced acute interstitial nephritis. Kidney Int 2008;73:940.

Ivanyi B, Hamilton-Dutoit SJ, Hansen HE, Olsen S. Acute tubulointerstitial nephritis: phenotype of infiltrating cells and prognostic impact of tubulitis. Virchows Arch 1996;428:5.

Izzedine H: Tubulointerstitial nephritis and uveitis syndrome (TINU): a step forward to understanding an elusive oculorenal syndrome. Nephrol Dial Transplant 2008;23:1095.

Izzedine H et al: Kidney injuries related to ipilimumab. Invest New Drugs 2014;32:769.

Lazarus B et al: Proton pump inhibitor use and the risk of chronic kidney disease. JAMA Intern Med 2016;176:238.

Mahevas M et al: Renal sarcoidosis: clinical, laboratory, and histologic presentation and outcome in 47 patients. Medicine (Baltimore) 2009;88:98.

Maripuri S et al: Renal involvement in primary Sjögren's syndrome: a clinicopathologic study. Clin J Am Soc Nephrol 2009;4:1423.

Moledina DG, Perazella MA: PPIs and kidney disease: from AIN to CKD. J Nephrol 2016;29:611.

Muriithi AK et al: Biopsy-Proven Acute Interstitial Nephritis, 1993–2011: A Case Series. Am J Kidney Dis 2014;64:558.

Muriithi AK et al: Clinical characteristics, causes and outcomes of acute interstitial nephritis in the elderly. Kidney Int 2015;87:458.

Muriithi AK, Nasr SH, Leung N: Utility of urine eosinophils in the diagnosis of acute interstitial nephritis. Clin J Am Soc Nephrol 2013;8:1857.

Peng YC et al: Association Between the Use of Proton Pump Inhibitors and the Risk of ESRD in Renal Diseases: A Population-Based, Case-Control Study. Medicine (Baltimore) 2016;95:e3363.

Perazella MA: Diagnosing drug-induced AIN in the hospitalized patient: a challenge for the clinician. Clin Nephrol 2014;81:381.

Perazella MA, Markowitz GS: Drug-induced acute interstitial nephritis. Nat Rev Nephrol 2010;6:461.

Prendecki M, Tanna A, Salama AD, et al: Long-term outcome in biopsy-proven acute interstitial nephritis treated with steroids. Clin Kidney J 2017;10:233.

Raissian Y et al: Diagnosis of IgG4-related tubulointerstitial nephritis. J Am Soc Nephrol 2011;22:1343.

Raza MN et al: Acute tubulointerstitial nephritis, treatment with steroid and impact on renal outcomes. Nephrology 2012;17:748.

Ren H et al: Renal involvement and followup of 130 patients with primary Sjögren's syndrome. J Rheumatol 2008;35:278.

Shirali AC, Perazella MA, Gettinger S: Association of Acute Interstitial Nephritis With Programmed Cell Death 1 Inhibitor Therapy in Lung Cancer Patients. Am J Kidney Dis 2016;68:287.

Valluri A et al: Acute tubulointerstitial nephritis in Scotland. QMJ 2015;108:527.

Wu Y et al: Pathological significance of a panel of urinary biomarkers in patients with drug-induced tubulointerstitial nephritis. Clin J Am Soc Nephrol 2010;5:1954.

Xie Y, Bowe B, Li T, Xian H, Balasubramanian S, Al-Aly Z. Proton pump inhibitors and risk of incident CKD and progression to ESRD. J Am Soc Nephrol 2016;27:3153.

■ CHAPTER REVIEW QUESTIONS

1. A 50-year-old Caucasian woman with a 30-year history of type 1 diabetes presents to the nephrology office for routine follow-up of proteinuria. She works as a marketing executive at a beauty product firm. She is asymptomatic. She is on an insulin pump for diabetes, on losartan for proteinuria and has started omeprazole 6 months ago for endoscopically diagnosed reflux esophagitis. On her last ophthalmological examination, she had mild nonproliferative diabetic retinopathy. Her vital signs show a blood pressure of 130/80. Her physical examination is unremarkable. On laboratory examination, her creatinine has increased from 1 to 1.4 mg/dL and her eGFR has dropped from 66 to 40 mL/min/1.73 m^2 over the past year. On review of her past records, her creatinine had increased from 0.7 to 1 mg/dL over 10 years. Hemoglobin A$_{1c}$ is 6.5%. Urinalysis shows 1+ protein and 0–5 white blood cells/HPF. Rest of her serum tests are normal. What is the best next step in management of this patient?

   A. Follow-up in 1 year
   B. Urine eosinophil testing
   C. Refer to endocrinology for better control of diabetes
   D. Refer to ophthalmology for follow-up of diabetic retinopathy
   E. Discuss renal biopsy to rule out drug-induced tubulointerstitial nephritis

2. A 75-year-old African–American man is admitted to the hospital for fever and elevated white blood cell count with diagnosis of cellulitis of left foot. His past medical history is significant for extensive atherosclerotic vascular disease including coronary artery disease requiring a drug-eluting stent to his left anterior descending artery and peripheral vascular disease. He is treated with ampicillin-sulbactam leading to improvement in cellulitis. On day 3 of his hospitalization he has a new rash and his serum creatinine increases from baseline of 1–1.5 mg/dL. Nephrology is consulted and a kidney biopsy is performed. Review of light microscopy shows presence of extensive lymphocytes in the renal interstitium with 1–5 lymphocytes crossing the tubular basement membrane into the tubular space. There are also 5–10 eosinophils per HPF. Trichrome stain demonstrates 50% fibrosis in the interstitium. Which of the following is the best determinant of long-term renal prognosis after an episode of drug-induced tubulointerstitial nephritis?

   A. Number of eosinophils in the interstitium
   B. Degree of tubulointerstitial fibrosis
   C. Presence of extra-renal manifestations such as rash
   D. Type of drug responsible for tubulointerstitial nephritis

3. You are reviewing a kidney biopsy with the renal pathologist. The biopsy is from a 57-year-old man who was biopsied for unexplained, slow rise in creatinine and proteinuria. His eGFR had decreased from 85 mL/min/1.73 m^2 to 50 mL/min/1.73 m^2 over the past 3 months. The biopsy demonstrates 35 glomeruli, of which two are globally sclerotic. The other glomeruli look unremarkable. The tubulointerstitium demonstrates an extensive lymphocytic infiltrate, lymphocytes infiltrating into the tubular space, but no eosinophils. There is 20% interstitial fibrosis on trichrome stain. Immunofluorescence shows absence of any immune deposits. Electron microscopy demonstrates global foot process effacement. You and the renal pathologist conclude that this may non-steroidal anti-inflammatory drug (NSAID)-induced tubulointerstitial nephritis and you decide to call the patient to obtain over-the-counter medication history. Which of the following statements is true regarding NSAID-induced tubulointerstitial nephritis?
   A. Absence of eosinophils on the kidney biopsy rules out drug-induced tubulointerstitial nephritis
   B. NSAID-induced tubulointerstitial nephritis may present with glomerular changes of global foot process effacement and clinical finding of nephrotic-range proteinuria
   C. Tubulointerstitial nephritis is never associated with NSAID use
   D. Renal biopsy is unnecessary in most cases of clinically suspected NSAID-induced tubulointerstitial nephritis

4. A 80-year-old woman presents to you for evaluation of new onset rise in serum creatinine. Her past medical history includes hypertension for which she has been taking hydrochlorothiazide for the past 20 years. She volunteers at the local hospital and is independent in her daily activities including driving, cooking, and finances. Her annual PPD test was positive this year after she cared for a patient with tuberculosis. After a chest radiograph demonstrated absence of active tuberculosis she was started on rifampin prophylaxis. One month later, her creatinine increased from 0.7 to 1.2 mg/dL. You recommend a kidney biopsy to rule out tubulointerstitial nephritis. All of the following statements are true in tubulointerstitial nephritis except:

A. Degree of interstitial fibrosis is the best determinant of long-term prognosis
B. Medications are the most common cause of tubulointerstitial nephritis in the United States
C. Medications are not a common cause of tubulointerstitial nephritis in the elderly
D. Tubulointerstitial nephritis does not meet the KDIGO acute kidney injury definition in over half the cases

5. A 59-year-old man who works for a brokerage firm comes to you for evaluation of new onset rise in creatinine. He has significant past medical history of hypertension for over 10 years for which he takes amlodipine. He is also on atorvastatin for elevated cardiovascular risk from high cholesterol. He does not take any supplements or any other prescription medications. He takes over-the-counter omeprazole twice a day for heart burn, which he has been taking regularly for over 20 years. On review of laboratory tests, he has low grade proteinuria (0.6 mg/mg) and a rise in serum creatinine from 1 mg/dL (5 years ago) to 1.6 mg/dL. His hepatitis serologies are unremarkable. He does not have HIV. He has normal hemoglobin A1c. You inform him that while the differential diagnosis of rise in creatinine is broad, you suspect that he might have proton pump inhibitor (PPI)-induced interstitial nephritis and you recommend a kidney biopsy for further evaluation. All of the following statements are true regarding PPI-induced tubulointerstitial nephritis except:
   A. Healthy individuals taking PPI are at increased risk of chronic kidney disease
   B. PPI-related tubulointerstitial nephritis is a class effect and switching to another PPI is generally not recommended if tubulointerstitial nephritis is suspected
   C. PPI-related tubulointerstitial nephritis can occur months after starting therapy
   D. PPI-related tubulointerstitial nephritis is characterized by fever, rash and eosinophilia in over 25% of affected patients
   E. PPI-use has been associated with increased risk of hypomagesemia

Chronic Tubulointerstitial Nephritis

38

Dominique Dorsainvil, MD

Randy L. Luciano, MD, PhD

INTRODUCTION

Chronic tubulointerstitial nephritis (CTIN) is an inflammatory process that involves the peritubular space or interstitium of the kidneys resulting in interstitial scarring with fibrosis, a lymphomonocytic infiltrate, tubular dilation, and atrophy. These forms of injury are very similar regardless of the inciting cause. Usually asymptomatic, it presents as a slowly progressive impairment in renal function leading to chronic kidney disease (CKD). Any structural damage, either glomerular, tubular, or a direct injury to the interstitium from an acute nephritis that has not appropriately resolved can amount to CTIN.

The most common etiologies are medication-induced lesions and infections. However, a wide variety of other diseases can lead to CTIN, including heavy metal toxicities or exposures, chronic obstructive nephropathy, reflux disease, nephrolithiasis, immunologic disease, metabolic disorders, genetic disease, neoplasia, and chronic renovascular, ischemia (Table 38–1). The following will provide an overview of select causes of CTIN.

ESSENTIALS OF DIAGNOSIS

Analgesic Nephropathy

▶ Most common cause of drug induced CTIN

▶ Seen with phenacetin, acetaminophen, aspirin, and NSAIDs

▶ Presents with CTIN, papillary necrosis, hypertension

▶ Despite association with nephropathy, number of patients is relatively low given the total amount of non-narcotic analgesics prescribed or available without prescription

Lithium-Induced Renal Disease

▶ Approximately 15–20% of patients treated with lithium will develop kidney disease

▶ Latent period to development of ESRD is approximately 20 years

▶ Renal manifestations include: FSGS, MCD, distal RTA, diabetes insipidus, and CTIN

▶ Stopping lithium may delay progression, but progression to ESRD tends to occur if serum creatinine >2.5 mg/dL

Aristolochic Acid Nephropathy

▶ Exposure through herbal supplements containing ingredients from Aristolochia species

▶ Rapid progression to ESRD of approximately 2 years

▶ Biopsy reveals hypocellular infiltrate with severe fibrosis

▶ 40–45% prevalence of urothelial carcinomas

▶ Treatment with glucocorticoids may delay progression to ESRD

▶ Balkan endemic nephropathy is a prolonged variant of AAN with progression to ESRD occurring over decades

Renal Sarcoidosis

▶ Immune mediated disease affecting several organs including lungs and kidney

▶ Renal involvement can be in the form of hypercalcemia with AKI to CTIN with granulomatous lesions

▶ Glucocorticoids remains first line of therapy

TINU

▶ Anterior uveitis usually occurs after nephritis

▶ CTIN is usually mild with low grade proteinuria

▶ β_2-microglobulin can be used as a non-specific marker of disease activity

▶ Nephritis can resolve spontaneously; however, glucocorticoids can be used for relenting disease

IgG4 Related Disease

- Associated with autoimmune infiltration of various organs
- Kidney biopsy will show a dense lymphoplasmacytic infiltrate that stains positive for IgG4 antibody
- Serum IgG4 levels >135 mg/dL are supportive but not specific nor sensitive
- Prolonged glucocorticoid therapy can lead to remission

OVERVIEW OF DIAGNOSIS AND TREATMENT

Clinical manifestations are usually non-specific. Renal insufficiency as manifested as a decreased estimated glomerular filtration rate (eGFR) and a rising serum creatinine is common; however, depending on the degree of interstitial involvement, the chronicity, and underlying comorbid conditions, serum creatinine, and eGFR may appear normal. Patients may also have mild proteinuria (in the range of 1 g of protein/day); however, nephrotic range proteinuria (proteinuria >3.5 g/day) may be present especially in advanced CKD or in patients with other comorbid renal disease that can cause glomerular injury. Proteinuria is best screened with a urinalysis, which detects urinary albumin excretion only. Normally some degree of protein is filtered at the glomerulus; however, the low molecular weight proteins are usually reabsorbed in the proximal tubules leading to minimal urinary protein excretion (<0.2 g/day). However, with CTIN, tubular damage and interstitial fibrosis can significantly alter the ability of the proximal tubule to reabsorb filtered protein, thereby leading to increased urinary protein excretion (Figure 38–1). The presence of protein on a urinalysis should always be quantified with both albumin and total protein to creatinine urinary ratios. Measurements of urinary β_2-microglobulin, a low molecular weight protein, can also be useful in diagnosing CTIN. β_2-microglobulin would normally be low, but can be dramatically elevated in the urine of a patient with CTIN. In addition to impaired tubular protein reabsorption, other functional abnormalities of renal tubules may be seen with CTIN, including renal tubular acidosis, potassium disorders (hypokalemia or hyperkalemia), hyperuricemia, hypercalcemia, impaired urine concentration defects, normoglycemic glycosuria, phosphaturia, and renal sodium wasting (Table 38–2).

Urine sediment analysis may also be useful in diagnosing CTIN. As CTIN is a chronic inflammatory disease of the interstitium and tubules, the presence of urinary white blood cells (WBCs) and renal tubular epithelial (RTE) cells, may suggest tubulointerstitial disease (Figure 38–2A). In addition, cells may be incorporated into casts with the presence of WBC casts, RTE cell casts or mixed cell casts (Figure 38–2B).

Table 38–1. Causes of chronic tubulointerstitial disease.

Medications
Analgesics: Phenacetin, Acetaminophen, Aspirin
NSAIDs
Lithium
Chemotherapeutic agents: Platinum based agents, Ifosfamide, Carmustine
Calcineurin inhibitors: Tacrolimus, Cyclosporine
Aristolochic acid herbal medications
Phosphate preparations

Immunologic disease
Sarcoidosis
Sjögren syndrome
Tubulointerstitial nephritis with uveitis
Vasculitis
Systemic lupus erythematosus
Cryoglobulinemia
Amyloidosis
IgA nephropathy/vasculitis
IgG4 related disease
Idiopathic hypocomplementemic interstitial nephritis

Neoplastic/Hematopoietic disease
Lymphoma/Leukemia
Multiple myeloma
Sickle cell disease
Light chain disease
Lymphoproliferative disorders

Occupational and environmental exposures
Heavy metal: Lead, Cadmium, Mercury
Mycotoxins

Metabolic disorders
Hypercalcemia
Hypokalemia
Oxalosis
Hyperuricemia
Cystinosis

Infections
Bacterial pyelonephritis
Xanthogranulomatous pyelonephritis
Malacoplakia
Viral mediated nephritis: BK, Epstein–Barr virus

Hereditary disorders
Medullary cystic disease
Polycystic kidney disease
Karyomegalic interstitial nephritis

Miscellaneous
Diabetic nephropathy
Hypertensive nephrosclerosis
Obstructive uropathy
Radiation nephritis
Mesoamerican nephropathy
Sri-Lanka chronic kidney disease

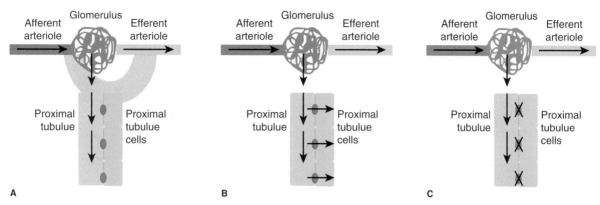

▲ **Figure 38–1. A.** Small molecular weight proteins are freely filtered in the glomerulus. This does not reflect glomerular dysfunction. **B.** Approximately 99.9% of filtered low molecular weight proteins are reabsorbed proximally. **C.** In the setting of tubular dysfunction from CTIN, reabsorption is impaired leading to increased proteinuria.

Although less common, the sediment may show red blood cells, usually a byproduct of interstitial inflammation and less so from glomerular injury. More often, CTIN will often present with a bland sediment or minimally cellular urine sediment with possible hyaline or waxy casts (Figure 38–2C).

Imaging studies are helpful to establish chronicity. Renal ultrasound may show altered corticomedullary differentiation and increased echogenicity of the cortex. It is also possible that with chronicity, the kidneys may appear small in size (typically <7 cm in length depending on patient gender and height).

The gold standard for diagnosing CTIN is through kidney biopsy. Depending on the chronic disease and the rate of progressive CKD, a biopsy may not be necessary. However, if the patient has nephrotic range proteinuria, hematuria with dysmorphic red blood cells suggestive of glomerular disease, or a rapidly rising creatinine, a biopsy should be performed. Biopsy will show a lymphocytic infiltrate, interstitial fibrosis, and tubular atrophy (Figure 38–3A). In certain diseases chronic glomerular lesions can also be seen including segmental sclerosis of the glomerulus and periglomerular fibrosis (Figure 38–3B).

The first step in treatment of CTIN is discontinuation of any offending agent or exposure that may be contributing to disease. However, if CTIN is thought secondary to a disease such as diabetes mellitus, hypertension, or an autoimmune disease, then treatment would focus on controlling the underlying disease process. Since damage associated is often irreversible, treatment should also include avoiding medications or exposures that can contribute to future renal injury. This includes avoiding medications that have a moderate to high risk of leading to CKD in selected patients, including non-steroidal anti-inflammatory drugs (NSAIDs), proton pump inhibitors (PPIs) and various herbal medications that may have NSAID-like properties. In addition to preventing progression of disease, treatment should also focus on management of CKD complications, including hypertension, proteinuria, anemia, metabolic acidosis, electrolyte abnormalities, renal osteodystrophy, and hypervolemia.

Table 38–2. Clinical features of chronic tubulointerstitial nephritis.

Proximal tubular defects
Proximal renal tubular acidosis
Fanconi syndrome
Proteinuria (<1 g/day)

Distal tubular defects
Distal renal tubular acidosis
Concentrating defects
Salt wasting nephropathy
Nephrogenic diabetes insipidus

Nephrolithiasis
Calcium oxalate stones
Calcium phosphate stones
Uric acid stones

Papillary necrosis
Analgesic nephropathy
Pyelonephritis
Sickle cell nephropathy

▼ INFECTIOUS CHRONIC TUBULOINTERSTITIAL NEPHRITIS

EPSTEIN–BARR VIRUS

Epstein–Barr virus (EBV) has been proposed as a possible etiology of a primary CTIN. In biopsy specimens from patients diagnosed with idiopathic CTIN, EBV was detected

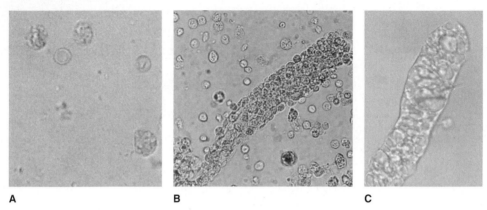

▲ **Figure 38–2. A.** White blood cell and red blood cell in urine of a patient with CTIN. **B.** White blood cell cast with surrounding white blood cells and renal tubular epithelial cells in urine of patient with CTIN. **C.** Waxy, non-cellular hyaline cast in patient with diabetic nephropathy with significant chronic tubulointerstitial changes. (See Color Plate 18.)

by polymerase chain reaction primarily in the proximal tubule cells. This was not seen in patients with glomerular and vascular diseases or other iatrogenic causes. The literature regarding the potential role of EBV either as a causative or consequent process remains inconclusive.

BK VIRUS

BK virus is ubiquitous to the general population. BK nephropathy (BKN) is more common in renal transplant patients compared to other solid organ or hematologic transplants. A high index of suspicion is required for diagnosis. Reactivated in immunosuppressed states, it is a recognized cause of CTIN in transplanted kidney. Involvement of native kidneys in the setting of other solid organ transplant or immunosuppressed conditions is an emerging entity.

The primary infection is believed to occur in childhood, usually as an upper respiratory tract infection. Acute infection is usually subclinical. Rare reports of urinary tract involvement during the acute infection have been described. The virus has a tropism for renal tubular and transitional urothelial cells where it remains dormant. Intracellular virion (in transitional cells) called decoy cells can be seen in urine microscopy. Presence of viremia or viruria does not consistently correlate with impaired renal function or histopathological evidence of BK nephropathy. Risk factors for BKN are the degree of immunosuppression, induction with rabbit anti-thymoglobulin, the use of tacrolimus and mycophenolate, age, and male gender.

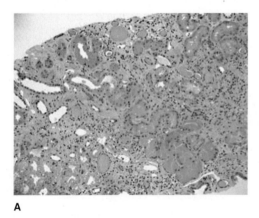
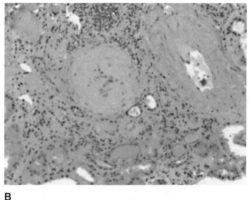

▲ **Figure 38–3. A.** Tubulointerstitial disease from a patient with CTIN. Tubulues show dilatation and atrophy. Proteinacious hyaline casts can be seen in some tubules. Interstitium has a cellular infiltrate with diffuse fibrosis. **B.** Sclerotic glomerulus in patient with CTIN. Note the periglomerular infiltration. Thickened vessel suggestive of long standing hypertension. (See Color Plate 19.)

Clinical Manifestations

With declining renal function in an allograft, BKN must be considered. It has a very similar clinical presentation to acute renal allograft rejection with ureteral stenosis, bacterial urinary tract infection, and hematuria suggesting BKN. Hemorrhagic cystitis however is more frequently reported in hematologic transplants with BKN.

Kidney biopsy remains the gold standard for diagnosis with tubulointerstitial nephritis, tubulitis, and some degree of tubular injury with varying degrees of fibrosis depending on the chronicity seen. Tissue from specimens positive for BKN will characteristically stain positive for SV40 (immunochemistry assay).

Treatment

Progression to end stage renal disease (ESRD) in the setting of BKN in either native kidneys or transplanted renal patients remains a significant risk, and therefore, treatment should be aggressive. Preemptive reduction of immunosuppression or periodic monitoring of BK viremia or viruria is possible preventive measure in high-risk patients.

Once BKN is present, the mainstay of management is reduction of immunosuppressive therapy or substitution of mycophenolate mofetil with an mTOR (mechanistic target of rapamycin) inhibitor (everolimus or sirolimus) or switching from the calcineurin inhibitor tacrolimus to cyclosporine. Several drugs may be useful in treating BKN, including the fluoroquinolone class of antibiotics, cidofovir, brincidofovir, leflunomide, and intravenous immunoglobulin (IVIg). However, used either alone or in combination, the outcome with these medications still remains poor with a high rate of allograft dysfunction and progression to ESRD.

PYELONEPHRITIS

Clinical Manifestations

Acute pyelonephritis is a complicated urinary tract infection involving the upper urinary tract. Flank pain or discomfort with costovertebral angle tenderness on physical examination is a common presentation. This can be associated with fever and rigors, dysuria, urinary urgency and frequency, nausea, and vomiting. Urine microscopy shows pyuria, bacteria, WBCs, RTE cells, RBCs, and WBC casts, and seldom bacterial casts. If isolated, acute pyelonephritis will rarely progress to chronic renal dysfunction secondary to CTIN and fibrosis. However, chronic pyelonephritis can occur from repetitive urinary tract infections, vesicoureteral reflux, or obstructive uropathy. Fever, chills, flank pain, dysuria, and hypertension are common clinical manifestations. Some patients may have urine concentrating defects with hyperkalemia, salt wasting reflecting a distal tubular dysfunction. Urinary sediment is similar to that seen in acute pyelonephritis.

Biopsy will reveal significant lymphocytic and monocytic interstitial infiltration, while edema and tubular atrophy are seen in the interstitium along with intratubular WBCs. Fibrosis will vary based on chronicity. Glomeruli are sometimes involved with periglomerular inflammation. Tubular thyroidization, although not specific of CTIN, has been described.

Treatment:

Appropriate antibiotic coverage, tailored to the organism identified on culture, is the hallmark of treatment. Recurrent infections, non-compliance to prescribed therapy, or failure to respond to antibiotic therapy are the main causes of chronic pyelonephritis.

XANTHOGRANULOMATOUS PYELONEPHRITIS

Xanthogranulomatous pyelonephritis is used to define persistent localized chronic pyelonephritis. It is characterized by granulomatous inflammation in the renal interstitium. The mechanism is unknown. It leads to progressive destruction of the renal parenchyma with accumulation of lipid laden macrophages called "foam cells".

Most often seen in middle aged women, it is associated with chronic urinary tract infection from *Escherichia coli*, *Proteus mirabilis*, and *Klebsiella spp*, chronic urinary tract obstruction from vesicoureteral reflux, obstructive calculi (most frequently staghorn calculus) and other causes of obstruction.

Clinical Manifestations

Presentation in xanthogranulomatous pyelonephritis is similar to that seen with chronic pyelonephritis (discussed previously). In most cases, at the time of diagnosis, there may be little to no function in the affected kidney. Renal ultrasound can show obstructing renal calculi, hydronephrosis, dilated calices, and multiple fluid-filled hypoechoic intraparenchymal collections (abscesses). In some incidences, a parenchymal mass that is difficult to differentiate from a renal cell carcinoma is noted. CT or MRI is helpful to better define a mass, but depending on renal function, contrast studies can be problematic.

On kidney biopsy, the characteristic findings are xanthomatous histiocytes with an abundant foamy and lipid-laden cytoplasm. The inflammatory infiltrate is pleomorphic (lymphocytes, neutrophils, plasma cells, and histiocytes) with the presence of cholesterol clefts. If present, necrotic lesions are surrounded by a granulomatous response. Fibrosis is usually quite profound.

Treatment

Current treatment recommendations consist of broad-spectrum intravenous antibiotics narrowed down once the responsible pathogen is identified. Relief of obstruction and/or stone removal may be required. Total or partial nephrectomy is curative and may be necessary in refractory or resistant cases.

DRUG AND TOXIN RELATED NEPHROPATHY

Drug-induced kidney injury is the most common type of tubulointerstitial injury. CTIN can occur even at therapeutic doses. Acute manifestations of the tubulointerstitial injury are not always evident and therefore may go unnoticed for some time. Drugs can cause insidious tubulointerstitial damage with prolonged use, eventually leading to chronic and irreversible changes. Certain drugs are well known for toxic effects, including NSAIDs, PPIs, and chemotherapeutic agents.

ANALGESIC NEPHROPATHY

Analgesics are the most common etiology, class of drugs causing CTIN. It was first believed that only phenacetin containing analgesics caused CKD and was removed from the market. However, CKD has been associated with other non-narcotic analgesics, including aspirin, acetaminophen, and NSAIDs.

Analgesic nephropathy was first described in the setting of prolonged use of over-the-counter analgesics in certain European countries. It was presumed to be related to elevated drug concentrations leading to toxic levels in the kidney. The most common medications implicated in analgesic nephropathy are NSAIDs. Current preparations available in the United States are not associated with classic analgesic nephropathy when used in moderate doses. Risks for developing CTIN with NSAID use include older age, existing comorbidities (eg, cirrhosis, congestive heart failure, diabetes mellitus, dehydration), CKD, or concurrent use with other medications (such as angiotensin converting enzyme inhibitors) known to impair glomerular hemodynamics. Both selective and non-selective NSAIDs are associated with CTIN. However, it should be noted that the number of patients developing CTIN from NSAID use is still relatively small compared with the total number of doses prescribed or purchased.

▶ Pathogenesis

The main site of injury in analgesic nephropathy is the renal medulla, primarily because of its inherent low oxygen tension. Toxic metabolites of various analgesic compounds may accumulate due to the countercurrent mechanism, thereby exacerbating injury. The mechanism of injury is not well known, but thought to be due to the impairment of renal prostaglandin production, leading to a proinflammatory leukotriene dominant state. Vasoconstrictive effects from prostaglandin inhibition can also leads to ischemic injury and eventually interstitial fibrosis.

▶ Clinical Manifestations

Analgesic nephropathy is commonly seen in elderly females over 60 years of age who have chronic pain syndromes. Clinical renal syndromes include progressive CKD, nephrotic range proteinuria or nephrotic syndrome, hematuria, sodium and water retention with possible edema, hyperkalemia, hyponatremia, hypertension, and acute kidney injury (AKI). Renal mechanisms of NSAID injury are secondary to dysregulation of renal prostaglandins and subsequent kidney function.

CTIN is most often seen in patients who have been using NSAIDs for a prolonged period of time reflecting dose and duration dependency. This is in contrast to patients who demonstrate and acute rise in serum creatinine after starting NSAIDs, as this process is related to reduced glomerular filtration. Laboratory findings associated with NSAID-induced CTIN often include a slowly progressive decline in eGFR and the possible presence of nephrotic range proteinuria. The latter is due to the effect of prostaglandins on maintaining podocyte integrity. Urinalysis is often bland, but may show sterile pyuria, microscopic or macroscopic hematuria with WBC or RTE cell casts. Imaging is usually uninformative, but decreased kidney size may indicate chronicity, and CT scan may demonstrate small kidneys, papillary calcifications, and irregular renal contours.

▶ Treatment

Management is supportive. Stopping these agents may slow the progression of CKD. As mentioned above, complications of CKD need to be treated.

LITHIUM-INDUCED RENAL DISEASE

Lithium is used in the management of refractory depression and bipolar disorder. Chronic lithium use causes several forms of kidney disease, including, focal segmental glomerulosclerosis (FSGS), minimal change disease (MCD), distal renal tubular acidosis (RTA)ly, diabetes insipidus, and CTIN.

Approximately 15–20% of patients treated with lithium will develop mild CKD from CTIN; however, if the medication is not discontinued, CKD can progress to ESRD. The average latent period to progression to ESRD is about 20 years. Major risk factors are long-standing lithium treatment (usually more than one to two decades), advanced age, and cumulative dose of lithium.

▶ Clinical Manifestations

CTIN manifests generally as mild renal insufficiency, which may include polyuria, polydipsia, hypovolemia, hypernatremia, incomplete distal renal tubular acidosis, and hypercalcemia. Urinalysis is usually bland and may yield low-grade proteinuria. Nephrotic range proteinuria has also been reported, but is usually seen in association with glomerular involvement. Renal ultrasound may show multiple small cortical and medullary cystic lesions.

Treatment

In patients with mild renal insufficiency, stopping the drug can slow down or alter the progression of tubulointerstitial damage and delay CKD progression. However, patients with serum creatinine concentrations greater than 2.5 mg/dL at the time of presentation tend to progress to ESRD despite discontinuation of lithium.

Amiloride, a potassium-sparing diuretic that blocks the collecting tubule epithelial sodium channel (ENaC), has been shown to reduce polyuria by preventing lithium entry into tubular cells via this channel. Thiazides can be used to reduce polyuria; however, they should be used cautiously as they can induce volume depletion and complicate univalent and divalent abnormalities if present.

CALCINEURIN INHIBITOR NEPHROPATHY

Calcineurin inhibitors (CNI) (cyclosporine and tacrolimus) are currently the leading immunosuppressive agents used in both solid and hematopoietic organ transplants. Nephrotoxicity, either acute or chronic renal insufficiency, is a major side effect of CNI use. The development and progression of CKD in native kidneys or the kidney allograft are frequent complications of chronic CNI therapy, which can ultimately lead to ESRD. The nephrotoxic effects of both tacrolimus and cyclosporine are equivalent. CNI nephropathy is not common in hematopoietic stem cell transplants mainly due to the shorter duration and lower dosing of the CNI.

Acutely, CNIs cause afferent arteriole vasoconstriction, thereby leading to decreased GFR. If detected early enough, these changes can be reversed by cessation or dose reduction. However, chronic use may lead to ischemia and structural damage with the development of tubulointerstitial fibrosis. This usually occurs after several years of treatment with a CNI, but may be accelerated in states of hypovolemia, CKD from other causes, or the use of additional medications that may lead to afferent arteriolar vasoconstriction (eg, NSAIDs).

Clinical Manifestations

Other than increased serum creatinine, CNI nephrotoxicity can present with hyperkalemia, a non-anion gap metabolic acidosis, hypomagnesemia, hypophosphatemia, and hyperuricemia, all suggestive of a combination of reduced GFR and tubulointerstitial injury.

Kidney biopsy in a patient with chronic CNI toxicity will demonstrate a very characteristic appearance of striped interstitial fibrosis. Striped fibrosis is a "band-like" interstitial fibrosis found in both the cortex and medulla (Figure 38–4). Apart from striped interstitial fibrosis, other lesions often seen include tubular atrophy, glomerulosclerosis, arteriolar hyalinosis, and less commonly, thrombotic microangiopathy (TMA).

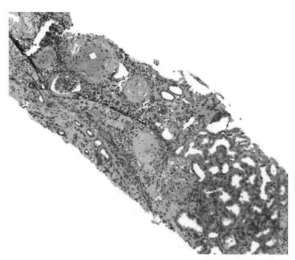

▲ **Figure 38–4.** CTIN from a patient with longstanding tacrolimus use in the setting of a previous liver transplant. Noted are areas of intense infiltrate and fibrosis juxtaposed to areas of tubular injury without interstitial infiltrate or fibrosis. This represents the so-called "stripped-fibrosis" pattern seen with CNI nephrotoxicity. (See Color Plate 20.)

Treatment

The mainstay of management is either stopping or reducing the dose of the medication. This often results in an improvement in renal function, but is concerning as it can increase the risk of rejection. Therefore, when the CNI must be stopped, other maintenance immunosuppressive agents may be used.

ARISTOLOCHIC ACID NEPHROPATHY

CKD resulting from exposure to Chinese herbs was first identified in the 1990s. It is a complication from the toxic effects of an active ingredient, aristolochic acid, found in a Chinese herbal weight loss pill. Aristolochic acid exposure has been associated with an increased risk of both nephropathy (termed aristolochic acid nephropathy, AAN) and urothelial cancer. Fairly rapid progression to ESRD has been reported; median time from exposure of approximately 2 years.

Clinical Manifestations

Acute nephrotoxicity manifests as acute tubular necrosis with renal failure, tubular dysfunction resulting in renal tubular acidosis and Fanconi syndrome. Proteinuria can be present. Chronically, progressive renal failure is observed. Severe interstitial fibrosis with a pleomorphic hypocellular infiltration is the main pathological finding. In addition to the severe kidney disease, AAN is associated with a 40–45% prevalence of urothelial carcinomas.

▶ Treatment

As with other forms of CTIN, the mainstay of therapy is stopping the herbal preparation containing aristolochic acid. In certain cases, glucocorticoids have been shown to delay progression to ESRD. There has been no consensus on treatment duration and stopping steroids at 6 months, if there is no response to therapy is advisable.

Given the high prevalence of urothelial carcinoma, close cancer surveillance is warranted. Prophylactic bilateral nephroureterectomy should be done prior to renal transplantation given the high incidence of urothelial cancer and the potential for progression of cancer development in transplanted patients on immunosuppressive agents.

▼ BALKAN ENDEMIC NEPHROPATHY

Balkan endemic nephropathys is a form of CTIN characterized by a slow onset and progressive renal function deterioration. Endemic to the countries in the Southeast European peninsula, also known as the Balkan states, the specific etiology of this disease was elusive until recently. Genetic and immune-related factors have been identified but that show a relationship to AAN. The theory is that Balkan endemic nephropathy is a more gradual and slowly progressive form of AAN that is the result of a decreased amount yet more chronic exposure to Aristolochia seeds.

The clinical presentation is very similar to that of AAN. Biopsy findings are similar with a hypocellular interstitial infiltrate yet with a more moderate amount of fibrosis. As with AAN, there is a high prevalence of urothelial cancer with Balkan endemic nephropathy (40–60% of those affected). Treatment is mainly supportive.

Aside from the Balkan territories, CTIN accounts for as much as 28% of all CKD in India. Aristolochia species are a large part of traditional Indian herbal remedies and medicines. It is thought that an AAN-like disease is an underrepresented cause of CKD in India.

CHEMOTHERAPY INDUCED NEPHROPATHY

A wide variety of chemotherapeutic agents are associated with acute and chronic tubulointerstitial injury. One class of agents that can cause both an acute and chronic forms of injury are the platinum based chemotherapy agents, cisplatin and to a lesser degree carboplatin and oxalaplatin. Acutely these agents can cause acute tubular injury with profound acute tubular necrosis. This renal injury is usually reversible and often will result in a delay if not a change to the chemotherapeutic agent.

Chronic manifestations of platinum based chemotherapeutic agents can occur months to years after treatment. CTIN often presents with hypomagnesemia, Fanconi-like syndrome, anemia and less commonly salt wasting nephropathy.

Histologic findings consist of interstitial lymphomonocytic infiltration, tubular atrophy, and interstitial fibrosis, suggestive of chronic inflammatory process. Other agents that behave similarly to platinum based chemotherapy agents include ifosfamide and carmustine.

PHOSPHATE NEPHROPATHY

Phosphate nephropathy is associated with the use of oral laxatives, bowel enemas, or bowel cleansing preparations for colonoscopies that contain sodium phosphate. Its incidence along with the exact mechanism of acute tubular injury is not well known. The renal injury is related to a severe increase in serum phosphate with subsequent calcium phosphate crystal deposition occurring within the renal parenchyma. The risk factors associated with phosphate nephropathy are phosphate dosing, advanced age, female gender, volume depletion, underlying CKD, concomitant use of ACEi's or angiontensin receptor blockers (ARBs), NSAIDs, or diuretics.

▶ Clinical Findings

Patients often present with an elevated serum creatinine, low-grade proteinuria, and significant hyperphosphatemia. Urine microscopy may show calcium phosphate crystals, but this is an uncommon finding. Both acute and chronic histopathological findings can be seen on biopsy. Acute tubular injury and interstitial edema are initial findings, which progress to tubular atrophy and tubulointerstitial fibrosis. Calcium phosphate crystals found in the distal and collecting tubules are the hallmark of this entity, and in some cases interstitial crystal deposits can be seen. Calcium phosphate crystals are not birefringent when polarized and they characteristically stain positive for the von Kossa stain, allowing for differentiation from the more common calcium oxalate crystals. CKD is a noted complication.

▶ Treatment

Management of phosphate nephropathy includes hydration to flush the crystals out of the tubules and general supportive measures including avoiding other nephrotoxic medications. However, once chronic changes are seen on biopsy, the goal is to prevent progression by avoiding further medications that can contribute to nephrotoxicity.

▼ HEAVY METALS

CADMIUM

Prolonged occupational (industrial battery plants, shipyards, industrial paints, fertilizers, metal industry) and environmental exposure (food, air, plastics, cigarettes, fashion jewelry) to cadmium (Cd) have been associated with CKD. The association of low-level environmental exposure is however controversial.

Clinical studies have shown that elevated plasma levels of cadmium positively correlated with CKD after adjustment for other confounders such as hypertension or diabetes mellitus. In addition, low-level environmental exposure to cadmium has been associated with CKD in the general population in those with hypertension and diabetes mellitus. This can slowly progress to ESRD.

In humans, 50% of the body cadmium accumulates in the renal cortex, mainly in the proximal tubule. Clinical manifestations include proximal tubular dysfunction with Fanconi syndrome. Treatment of cadmium-associated nephrotoxicity is supportive.

LEAD TOXICITY

Exposure to lead can come from a variety of places, but is most often associated with occupational exposures with plumbers, lead miners, smelters, and refiners, automobile technicians, construction workers, and battery manufacturers. In addition, lead can be found in older homes, mainly in paints or plumbing. Moonshine made in homemade lead contaminated stills is another source of lead intoxication.

These various exposures and elevated blood levels are associated with CKD. Approximately 90% of the body lead concentration is within bone. In the kidney, lead can accumulate in the proximal tubule. In acute exposure the serum level will be elevated; however, prolonged exposure and accumulation in the kidneys will eventually amount to chronic interstitial changes with tubular atrophy and diffuse fibrosis. Serum lead levels often do not correlate with the degree of renal dysfunction.

▶ Clinical Manifestations

Lead toxicity can lead to multisystem impairment including neurological (ataxia, hyperirritability, mental developmental delays, convulsions, coma), hematologic (hypochromic anemia, hemolysis), gastrointestinal (anorexia, vomiting, constipation, abdominal pain), and cardiovascular (hypertension) sequelae. Renal involvement is consistent with proximal tubule dysfunction leading to glycosuria with normal serum glucose, aminoaciduria, hyperuricemia, and hyperphosphaturia.

The diagnosis of lead nephropathy is established by increased urinary excretion of chelated lead, after administration of ethylenediaminetetraacetic acid (EDTA). Cumulative body stores of lead are estimated by the EDTA mobilization test or by X-ray fluorescence, which determines bone lead content. In the EDTA mobilization test, 2 g of EDTA is administered either by the intravenous or intramuscular route, with subsequent measurement of 24-hour urine lead excretion. Urinary lead more than 0.6 g/day is considered abnormal. One major limitation of the EDTA mobilization test is that it cannot mobilize lead deposits in bone. Reduced levels of erythrocyte aminolevulinate

dehydrase (ALAD) compared to levels of ALAD "restored" by the addition of dithiothreitol may be even more efficient in detecting increased body lead burden in CKD patients.

▶ Treatment

The treatment of lead toxicity is chelation therapy with EDTA or oral succimer until improvement of the symptoms. This has been shown to prevent CKD and slow its progression if present. However, response depends on the degree of tubulointerstitial fibrosis present.

MERCURY

Like lead and cadmium, mercury is another heavy metal that can lead to nephrotoxicity at high levels. But chronic low-level exposure from either occupational or environmental sources like contaminated water, food, air, dental amalgam (less common nowadays), and seafood, may result in chronic renal insufficiency. Mercury accumulates in the body with a predominance in the kidneys.

▶ Clinical Manifestations

Mercury toxicity can manifest with symptoms of the gastrointestinal (abdominal pain, diarrhea, hematemesis, perforated viscus), pulmonary (cough, dyspnea), neurological (headache, tremors, encephalopathy, ataxia), and dermatologic (pruritic maculopapular rashes) systems. Mercury accumulates in the proximal tubules leading to a proximal tubulopathy just as cadmium and lead. Histologic renal lesions are consistent with tubulointerstitial disease, mainly cellular infiltration and tubular atrophy with fibrosis.

▶ Treatment

Chelation is the mainstay of treatment with dimercaprol or D-penicillamine. Newer agents, DMSA (meso-2,3-dimercaptosuccinic acid) and DMPS (2,3-dimercaptopropane-1-sulfonate) have been shown to be the two most efficacious chelating agents, effectively reducing the burden of mercury from the kidneys and brain.

▼ IMMUNE MEDIATED NEPHROPATHY

SARCOIDOSIS

Sarcoidosis is a systemic non-caseating granulomatous disease that usually involves the lungs and mediastinum. Other organ systems can be involved to various degrees. Renal involvement is common in sarcoidosis, and may even be the initial presentation. Renal sarcoidosis can consist of several different forms. Renal involvement is most often from increased production of 1,25-dihydroxyvitamin D_3 by activated macrophages leading to abnormal metabolism of calcium resulting in hypercalcemia. Hypercalcemia has a vasoconstrictive effect on the afferent arteriole, leading to decreased GFR and possible tubular ischemia. In addition, hypercalcemia can lead to hypercalciuria that can result in nephrolithiasis. Other complications, like nephrogenic diabetes insipidus, can stem from the chronic hypercalcemic state. Glomerular lesions such as membranous glomerulonephritis, rarely amyloidosis and exceptionally IgA nephropathy have been described.

Clinical Manifestations

Renal sarcoidosis rarely manifests as severe AKI. Findings like distal renal tubular acidosis, hypokalemia, urine concentrating defect, non-nephrotic range proteinuria, and sterile pyuria are often present. Kidney biopsy frequently reveals tubulointerstitial nephritis marked by interstitial cellular infiltrate, edema, tubular atrophy, and possible granulomatous lesions. Non-caseating granulomas on biopsy are highly suggestive of sarcoidosis and should initiate a workup for this disease process.

Treatment

Steroids remain the first line treatment. Renal function, hypercalcemia and extra renal symptoms improve rapidly with institution of steroids especially if started early in the course, prior to fibrosis. The prognosis is usually excellent with early diagnosis; however, incomplete resolution with CKD can be seen in late diagnosis or delayed treatment.

SJÖGREN SYNDROME

Sjögren syndrome related CTIN clinically manifests as a distal (Type 1) renal tubular acidosis with hypokalemia, normal anion gap metabolic acidosis; mild proteinuria can also be seen. The proposed mechanism is the presence of autoantibodies against carbonic anhydrase II. Although not common, proximal tubule involvement has been described in case reports resulting in a Fanconi-like syndrome. Kidney biopsy findings reveal a lymphomonocytic infiltrate, tubular atrophy, and varying degrees of fibrosis.

Treatment

Treatment has been successful with high dose steroids leading to improvement of renal function. Other drugs, such as antiproliferatives (mycophenolate mofetil), calcineurin inhibitors (tacrolimus, cyclosporine), and cyclophosphamide have been used in cases of steroid resistance with variable degrees of success.

TUBULOINTERSTITIAL NEPHRITIS WITH UVEITIS SYNDROME

Tubulointerstitial nephritis with uveitis (TINU) is characterized by bilateral non-granulomatous anterior uveitis with tubulointerstitial nephritis. TINU is usually seen in adolescents and young female adults with a 3:1 female to male ratio. TINU has been associated with preexisting systemic disease, autoimmune disease, infections or previous use of medications such as antibiotics and NSAIDs. Significant genetic associations exist with HLA-DQA1*01, HLA-DRB1*01, and HLA-DQB1*05 which are believed to confer a risk of development of the disease.

Clinical Manifestations

Patients with TINU present with signs and symptoms of anterior uveitis manifested as painful eye movements, red eye, eyelid edema, blurry vision, and photophobia. Uveitis can occur well after the systemic symptoms have resolved and may develop after nephritis. However, this is not absolute and uveitis may precede nephritis by weeks to months.

Renal manifestations include mild renal insufficiency, mild proteinuria, or sterile pyuria. Markers of tubular protein reabsorption such as β_2-microblobulin can serve as non-specific markers of disease activity. Renal histopathology reveals an interstitial inflammatory interstitial infiltrate with predominantly CD4+ T lymphocytes, plasma cells, and histiocytes. Macrophages and monocytes and non-caseating granulomas have also been reported. Delayed diagnosis, chronic disease or refractory disease can result in a chronic tubulointerstitial pattern with marked tubular atrophy and interstitial fibrosis.

Treatment

Nephritis frequently resolves spontaneously but evolution to CKD has been reported. In cases of progressive renal failure, oral prednisone (at a dose of 1 mg/kg/day) usually results in improvement. Length of therapy depends on the response but typically requires 3–6 months as recurrence rates are high. The uveitis component often has a relapsing course that my need more aggressive therapy.

VASCULITIDES

Large to small vessel vasculitis can present with kidney involvement. Glomerular involvement is the most common renal injury seen on biopsy, with a necrotizing glomerulonephritis, with or without crescents, being the most frequent pattern observed in pauci immune vasculitis. However, tubulointerstitial lesions often associated with glomerular and vascular lesions.

Clinical Manifestations

Clinical findings include renal failure that may progress fairly rapidly, variable degrees of proteinuria (usually non-nephrotic range), an active urine sediment, and hypertension. Systemic (fever, fatigue, weight loss, arthralgia, skin lesions), and extrarenal manifestations (pulmonary, central nervous system, upper respiratory) may also be present.

Tubulointerstitial lesions can appear initially as active tubulointerstitial nephritis with lymphocytic, plasmocytic, and sometimes eosinophilic infiltrates. There may also be small to medium vessel fibrinoid necrosis and transmural vasculitis. Perivascular and peritubular granulomas may also be present, but are rare. If the vasculitis is refractory to treatment or there has been a delay in diagnosis, chronic lesions of tubular atrophy and interstitial fibrosis will be apparent.

▶ Treatment

Management of the underlying disease with a combination of plasmapheresis, induction and maintenance immunosuppressive agents, and supportive therapy including blood pressure control are the cornerstones of therapy. However, despite these therapies, re-biopsy studies in patients with "treated" vasculitis have shown significant CTIN with severe fibrosis and tubular atrophy that can impact long-term renal prognosis (Figure 38–5).

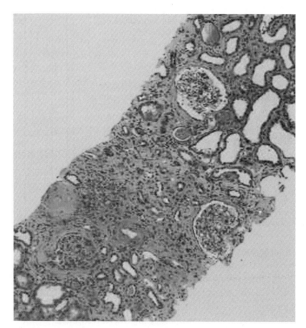

▲ **Figure 38–5.** CTIN from a patient with treated PR3 vasculitis. Note the areas of continued interstitial inflammation and marked fibrosis. Tubules demonstrate dilatation and atrophy. Patient has undetectable PR3 titers and remained on maintenance rituximab for 1 year at time of biopsy. (See Color Plate 21.)

IDIOPATHIC HYPOCOMPLEMENTEMIC INTERSTITIAL NEPHRITIS

Idiopathic hypocomplementemic interstitial nephritis is a rare entity that is usually seen in elderly men. It is characterized by idiopathic hypocomplementemia (C3 or C4) and is associated with tubulointerstitial nephritis with lymphocytic infiltrate and tubular basement membrane IgG and complement deposition. The classical pathway is predominantly affected. Presentation is non-specific with renal insufficiency with mild proteinuria and bland urine. This appears to be a diagnosis of exclusion after thoroughly excluding other autoimmune diseases. Treatment with glucocorticoids or other immunosuppressive agents has variable rates of success depending on the degree of tubulointerstitial fibrosis.

▼ METABOLIC CAUSES

OXALATE NEPHROPATHY

Hyperoxaluria can be the result of genetic disease or secondary to increased oxalate intake or absorption. While the former is an autosomal recessive disorder the latter is due to the excessive ingestion of food high in oxalate (star fruit, certain mushrooms, peanuts, chocolate, strawberries, rhubarb, spinach, beets, tea), increased enteric absorption (diarrhea, gastric bypass, small bowel resection, inflammatory bowel disease), medications (ascorbic acid, orlistat), or toxic ingestions (ethylene glycol or inhalation of methoxyflurane).

Oxalate derives from both endogenous and dietary sources. In its ionic form, oxalic acid or oxalate, it is highly soluble in water. When coupled with calcium it forms insoluble salts of calcium oxalate, which crystalize rapidly. Common complications of hyperoxaluria are nephrolithiasis and oxalate nephropathy.

▶ Clinical Manifestations

Renal insufficiency stems from a combination of ATN and tubulointerstitial inflammatory process. Hypokalemia, distal RTA, hyperoxaluria, hypercalcemia, and hypocitraturia can also be seen. Urine microscopy can be bland but may show calcium oxalate crystals, RTE cell or granular casts, and microscopic hematuria. Kidney biopsy may show calcium oxalate crystal deposition in the tubular lumens and interstitium causing tubulointerstitial nephritis. Gray white birefringent crystals can be seen on polarized light microscopy of with peritubular and interstitial infiltrate, edema and fibrosis (Figure 38–6).

▶ Treatment

Prevention of nephrolithiasis includes increases increasing daily fluid intake to 3 L/day and increasing dietary citrate (increase the urinary solubility of calcium oxalate crystals)

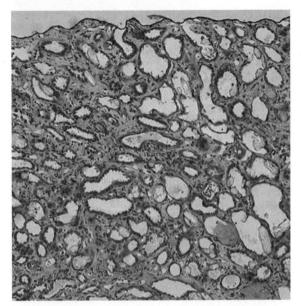

▲ **Figure 38–6.** Calcium oxalate nephropathy. Birefringent crystals in the lumen of many tubules. Tubules demonstrate marked dilatation and atrophy. Interstitium has cellular infiltration and fibrosis. (See Color Plate 22.)

and calcium (calcium will bind enteric oxalate thus preventing reabsorption and urinary excretion thus increasing urinary oxalate levels). If dietary means fail, potassium citrate supplements can be prescribed.

When oxalate nephropathy is diagnosed or suspected, aggressive hydration with intravenous fluids in attempt to flush the crystals from renal tubules may help. Steroids to reduce tubulointerstitial inflammation may help, but needs further study. Treatment is largely supportive and CKD may develop if exposure is significant or chronic. More than 30% of patients will not fully recover despite traditional treatment and develop progressive CKD that may eventually lead to ESRD.

CHRONIC URIC ACID NEPHROPATHY

Uric acid (UA) is a degradation product of purine that is excreted by the kidneys but is also highly insoluble in the urine. Elevated serum UA levels appear to be associated with CKD. A recent meta-analysis based on observational cohort studies showed that hyperuricemia was an independent predictor of new onset CKD development. A previous epidemiologic study of healthy subjects followed over 7 years showed a linear relationship with increased UA levels and new onset CKD, approximately 6–7 mg/dL in women and 7–8 mg/dL in men. Above these levels the associated risk increases rapidly, as high as a threefold increase in its incidence.

Several mechanisms have been proposed to explain the role of UA on renal function: (1) UA is believed to have a role in the activation of RAAS (renin angiotensin aldosterone system and cyclooxygenase-2 pathway leading to vasoconstrictive effect on the arterioles; (2) hyperuricemia induced arteriolopathy of preglomerular vessels impairing the autoregulatory response of afferent arterioles resulting in glomerular hypertension and vascular wall thickening producing severe renal hypoperfusion; and (3) direct entry of UA into both endothelial and vascular smooth muscle cells resulting in inhibition of endothelial nitric oxide (NO) levels, upregulation of reactive oxidative species, activation of TNF-α that can lead to the stimulation of vascular smooth muscle cell proliferation, and stimulation of vasoactive and inflammatory mediators leading to tubulointerstitial fibrosis. In addition, an acute rise in serum UA levels as seen in tumor lysis syndrome can result in hyperuricosuria. This may lead to deposition of UA crystals in the interstitium leading to tubular atrophy with interstitial inflammation and eventual fibrosis. Finally, hyperuricemia can be complicated by UA nephrolithiasis. Approximately 20% of patients with elevated serum level of UA will develop kidney stones. Kidney stones are also associated with an increased risk of CKD.

▶ Treatment

Several studies have looked at treatment of asymptomatic hyperuricemia, with either allopurinol or febuxostat, and improvement of CKD parameters. Outcomes have been inconclusive. There are no current recommendations on treating hyperuricemia to delay the progression of CKD.

CHRONIC HYPOKALEMIA

Chronic hypokalemia reportedly enhances interstitial scarring and progression of CKD. However, the association of hypokalemia with the progression to ESRD remains unclear. In the CKD population the most common causes of hypokalemia are chronic diuretic use, poor nutritional status, and resistance to RAAS blockade.

Mechanisms by which hypokalemia contribute to CTIN include the stimulation of RAAS despite direct suppression of aldosterone synthesis leading to salt sensitive hypertension, intrarenal vasoconstriction and ischemia and the increase in inflammatory mediators leading to enhanced oxidative stress and impaired angiogenesis. Prolonged hypokalemia has been accompanied by the development of multiple renal medullary cysts, tubular degeneration, marked interstitial fibrosis and macrophage infiltration.

Currently, the only treatment is the adequate supplementation of potassium to normal levels with caution to overcorrection in CKD patients with moderate to substantial reductions in GFR.

▼ MISCELLANOUS

RADIATION NEPHROPATHY

Radiation therapy to the kidneys or in the vicinity of the kidneys can lead to CTIN. In a dose dependent manner, the total exposed kidney volume (>30% of bilateral kidneys needed) is an important factor to consider in the incidence of radiation nephropathy. More than 1500 to 2000 rads, equivalent to more than 20 Gray, has been established as the threshold dose required for kidney injury.

▶ Clinical Manifestations

Radiation nephritis has both an acute and chronic phase. Acute nephritis usually manifests itself 6–12 months after exposure to radiation with renal failure, hypertension (malignant hypertension occasionally), edema, non-nephrotic range proteinuria, and normocytic anemia (sometimes microangiopathic hemolytic anemia). Chronic radiation nephritis occurs after more than 18 months. Clinical findings are similar to those of the acute onset with progression of CKD to ESRD. This can be further classified into primary or secondary nephritis. Primary chronic nephritis refers to an initial presentation within 2 years of radiation therapy whereas secondary chronic radiation nephritis occurs after an episode of acute nephritis that never resolved and progressed to CKD.

Proposed pathogenesis is direct tubular epithelial injury, endothelial cell injury and edema leading to vascular occlusion and ultimately to chronic ischemic injury. Concomitant chemotherapy may enhance the injurious effects of radiation therapy.

▶ Treatment

Damage sustained from radiation nephritis is generally irreversible. Prevention of radiation nephropathy includes shielding the kidneys during radiation therapy or limiting the dose or fractioning the total doses over several sessions. Treatment is limited to CKD management. Hypertension should preferably be managed with an ACEi, as suppression of the RAAS has been shown to be beneficial in animal models.

IgG4 RELATED DISEASE

Immunoglobulin G4-related disease is a fibroinflammatory disease of unknown etiology characterized by a dense lymphoplasmacytic infiltrate that positively stains for IgG4 antibody. IgG4 is the least common of the four IgG subclasses, representing less than 5% of the total IgG concentration.

IgG4-related disease is associated with autoimmune pancreatitis (AIP) and other autoimmune diseases infiltrating multiple organs, hence the initial proposition of an autoimmune etiology. In 2011 a Japanese group proposed that the various diseases linked with IgG4 fall under the new entity of IgG4-related diseases: AIP, autoimmune thyroiditis, retroperitoneal fibrosis, inflammatory aortic aneurysm (aneurysmal aortitis), interstitial pneumonitis, Mikulicz disease (chronic swelling of both lacrimal and salivary glands), hypophysitis and tubulointerstitial nephritis.

The diagnosis can most often be based on biopsy findings of any involved organ that show lymphoplasmacytic infiltration of the affected organ with IgG4 positive plasma cells and lymphocytes with fibrosis with storiform features. Serum IgG4 ≥135 mg/dL, although supportive are neither specific nor sensitive for IgG4 related disease. CT or PET scans may show focal organ infiltration (mass-like lesions) and encasement by inflammatory and fibrotic tissue.

▶ Clinical Manifestations

Clinical manifestations are non-specific ranging from normal to mild renal insufficiency and non-nephrotic range proteinuria. Urine microscopy is usually bland. CT abdomen/pelvis with contrast may show enlarged kidneys with or without intraparenchymal low-attenuated lesions, diffuse wall thickening of the renal pelvis with a smooth intraluminal surface, or retroperitoneal disease with hydronephrosis.

Pathognomonic findings on kidney biopsy include a dense lymphoplasmacytic infiltrate organized in "storiform" pattern with positive immunostaining of plasma cells for anti-IgG4. An obliterative phlebitis and mild to moderate eosinophil infiltrate can be seen (Figure 38–7). Lymphocytic infiltration consists of both T cell diffusely spread and B cells. The latter tend to aggregate in a germinal layer.

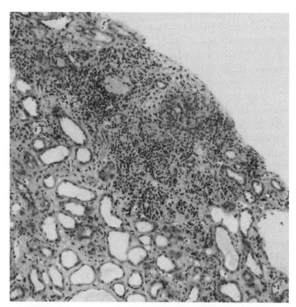

▲ **Figure 38–7.** CTIN from a patient with IgG4 related disease. Tubules show dilatation and atrophy with intervening interstitial fibrosis. Dense area of infiltration rich in eosinophils. (See Color Plate 23.)

Membranous glomerular lesions have also been reported with IgG4-related disease.

Treatment

Glucocorticoids are the mainstay of the treatment with prednisone (0.6 mg/kg) for 2–4 weeks followed by progressive tapering, usually over months to years. If remission is achieved, the glucocorticoids can be stopped, but about 20% of patients will relapse. In cases of failure or resistance to glucocorticoid therapy, various immunosuppressive agents have been used including rituximab, azathioprine, or mycophenolate mofetil.

SICKLE CELL NEPHROPATHY

Sickle cell disease is an inherited autosomal recessive hemoglobinopathy that affects the gene that encodes β globin leading to the formation of hemoglobin S, which polymerizes with deoxygenation. Erythrocytes lose their deformability (sickle cell) and obstruct the lumen of small vessels. This clinically manifests as vaso-occlusive crisis. Renal involvement develops early in homozygotes, usually in the third decade of life while it occurs later in heterozygotes, fifth to sixth decades. The prevalence of ESRD in sickle cell disease is not well known. It is in an independent risk factor for mortality in sickle cell patients. Long-term survival on hemodialysis and with renal transplantation is poor.

Several mechanisms are thought to be involved in the pathogenesis of sickle cell nephropathy. Early hyperfiltration is believed to be the main mechanism involved in the glomerular lesions of sickle cell nephropathy, which may persist until early adulthood. It is the result of compensatory secretion of vasodilatory prostaglandins in response to obstructed small vessels.

Apoptosis of tubular cells by ischemia-reperfusion can induce tubulointerstitial lesions. Ischemia induces NO release leading to hyperperfusion and ultimately hyperfiltration. NO stimulates the reactive oxygen species (ROS) pathway that can promote fibrosis by augmenting apoptosis when unregulated.

Clinical Manifestations

Renal involvement in sickle cell disease includes hypertension, proteinuria (non-nephrotic to nephrotic range), chronic microscopic hematuria, macroscopic hematuria, severe anemia, incomplete renal tubular acidosis, and urine concentrating defects with polyuria.

Early in the disease, prominent enlarged glomeruli and minimal tubulointerstitial fibrosis are present. This progressively evolves to FSGS, usually the perihilar variant. Tubulointerstitial nephritis is sometimes seen in the medulla with a neutrophilic infiltrate, edema, and occasionally necrosis. Papillary necrosis may also be seen.

Treatment

Treatment is supportive. Hydration is imperative to prevent the vaso-occlusive crises especially in polyuric patients. Sodium bicarbonate is used for metabolic acidosis and to reduce intra-renal sickling. Hypertension should be managed preferably with an ACRE-I or ARB especially if proteinuria is present.

MESOAMERICAN NEPHROPATHY

Epidemic on the pacific coast of Central America, Mesoamerican nephropathy (MeN), first described in 2002, is characterized by an asymptomatic CKD. Histopathological changes demonstrate primarily CTIN, with chronic glomerular lesions sometime present. Of unknown etiology, MeN was initially identified in male sugarcane field workers, but now been observed in other male field workers (cotton, beans, corn), fishermen, miners, construction, and transportation workers.

MeN is thought to be related to strenuous physical activities under extremely hot conditions. These conditions predispose to recurrent dehydration causing repetitive renal injury from a prerenal picture leading to ATN. An animal model of dehydration showed that mice exposed for 5 weeks to the same working conditions as the farmers developed renal insufficiency and tubulointerstitial fibrosis.

An emerging theory is that hyperuricosuria may lead to the chronic tubulointerstitial changes. Urine UA levels more than 100 mg/dL/day were detected in sugarcane field workers, similar to that seen in patients with AKI complicating tumor lysis syndrome. Hyperuricemia develops in the setting of hyperosmolar plasma, a consequence of water and salt loss from dehydration. This activates an enzymatic system present in the proximal tubule, aldolase reductase-sorbitol dehydrogenase-fructokinase that converts glucose to fructose, which in turn is metabolized into UA. Hyperuricosuria predisposes to tubular injury and crystalluria with possible UA crystals deposition, especially in the setting of dehydration and acidic urine. Subclinical rhabdomyolysis, which can occur with intense exercising under heat stress, may also develop in these workers, further increasing UA production.

Clinical Manifestations

Generally asymptomatic, patients often present late with uremia; however, mild proteinuria, microscopic hematuria, sterile pyuria, "sandy urine," and dysuria (from passing crystals) are common. Hypertension is not frequent.

Management

Adequate hydration while working, especially during the hottest time of the day, and allopurinol prophylaxis are suggested as preventive measures.

SRI-LANKAN CHRONIC KIDNEY DISEASE

Sri Lanka is another country with hot climate where endemic CKD of unknown etiology is predominant ($\geq$70%) in middle-aged male farmers (30–60 year old), specifically paddy rice farmers. Prevalent in the agricultural North Central region of the country, occupational exposure is speculated to be the cause of CKD (pesticides, agricultural chemicals, contaminated water/soil). This is challenged by several reports of women and non-farmers that have also CKD of an unknown etiology in the region.

At the time of diagnosis the majority of patients had stage 3 and 4 CKD with inconsistent proteinuria. Sterile pyuria and erythrocytes can be present. Histopathological findings are typical of CTIN with the interstitial infiltrate chiefly composed of lymphocytes, monocytes, with prominent interstitial fibrosis and tubular atrophy. Glomerular sclerosis may also be observed.

▶ Treatment

Extensive kidney disease was found on histopathology despite mild elevations in serum creatinine. Therefore, in the presence of mild renal insufficiency with mild proteinuria in middle-aged men should prompt a CKD workup. However, management thus far remains supportive.

DIABETIC NEPHROPATHY

Diabetic nephropathy (DN) is the leading cause of ESRD in developed countries. Prevalent in about 40% of the ESRD population, the incidence of DN in diabetes mellitus type 2 is increasing, possibly due to the increased rates of obesity and metabolic syndrome in the general population. Progression to ESRD occurs over one to two decades from initial diagnosis. This can be accelerated in those who develop early nephrotic range proteinuria.

▶ Clinical Manifestations

The first clinical manifestation of DN is albuminuria. At different stages of the disease, proteinuria ranges from microalbuminuria to macroalbuminuria and possibly nephrotic range proteinuria in cases of uncontrolled diabetes. A decrease in GFR or renal function is seen later, usually within 5–15 years of diagnosis.

Histopathological lesions are present early, usually within 2 years of the onset of diabetes. Glomerular and tubular hypertrophy, as well as glomerular and tubular basement membrane thickening, are seen. As the disease progresses, the pathognomonic lesion of nodular mesangial expansion and sclerosis known as Kimmelstiel–Wilson nodules is seen. Apart from the glomerular lesions, extensive tubulointerstitial lesions with interstitial fibrosis and tubular atrophy are also seen (Figure 38–8). The degree of interstitial fibrosis has been shown to be an important independent predictor of renal failure in diabetic patients.

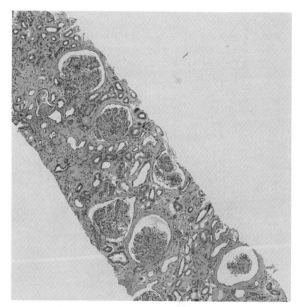

▲ **Figure 38–8.** Biopsy from a patient with long standing diabetic nephropathy. Glomerular show classical basement membrane thickening with nodules. Tubules show dilation and atrophy. Interstitium shows infiltrate and fibrosis. (See Color Plate 24.)

▶ Treatment

Management of CTIN aims at preventing or slowing the rate of progression of DN. Appropriate glucose control (target hemoglobin A1C 7%), blood pressure control (preferably with a RAAS inhibitor even in the absence of proteinuria), and weight loss (improved insulin sensitivity hence better glucose control) have all proven to reduce the progression of diabetes nephropathy. The SGLT2 inhibitors have shown promise in slowing progression of diabetic kidney disease.

KEY READINGS

Aguilar MC, Lonngi M, de-la-Torre A: Tubulointerstitial nephritis and uveitis syndrome: case report and review of the literature. Ocul Immuno Inflamm 2016;24:415.

Akiyama M et al: Acute kidney injury due to renal sarcoidosis during etanercept therapy: a case report and literature review. Intern Med 2015;54:1131.

Beck LH, Salant DJ: Glomerular and tubulointerstitial diseases. Prim Care 2008;35:265.

Bensefa-Colas L, Andujar P, Descatha A: Mercury poisoning. Rev Med Interne 2011;32:416.

Cartery C et al: Oxalate nephropathy associated with chronic pancreatitis. Clin J Am Soc Nephrol 2011;6:1895.

Chang YK et al: Increased risk of end-stage renal disease (ESRD) requiring chronic dialysis is associated with use of nonsteroidal anti-inflammatory drugs (NSAIDs): nationwide case-crossover study. Medicine (Baltimore) 2015;94:e1362.

Edeani A et al: Radiation Nephropathy. ASN Chapter 10. Onco-Nephrology Curriculum. http://www.asn-online.org/education/distancelearning/curricula/onco/. January 6, 2017.

Fioretto P et al: Tacrolimus and cyclosporine nephrotoxicity in native kidneys of pancreas transplant recipients. Clin J Am Soc Nephrol 2011;6:101.

Fogo AB et al: Pauci-immune necrotizing crescentic glomerulonephritis. Am J Kidney Dis 2016;68:e31.

Glew RH et al: Nephropathy in dietary hyperoxaluria: a potentially preventable acute or chronic kidney disease. World J Nephrol 2014;3:122.

Hou J, Herlitz LC: Renal infections. Surg Pathol Clin 2014;7:389.

Jalal DI: Hyperuricemia, the kidneys, and the spectrum of associated disease: a narrative review. Curr Med Res Opin 2016;32:1863.

Jayasumana C et al: Chronic interstitial nephritis in agricultural communities: a worldwide epidemic with social, occupational and environmental determinants. Nephrol Dial Transplant 2016 Oct 13.

John R, Herzenberg AM: Renal toxicity of therapeutic drugs. J Clin Pathol 2009;62:505.

Jung JH et al: Nonsteroidal anti-inflammatory drug induced acute granulomatous interstitial nephritis. BMC Res Notes 2015;8:793.

Kang DH et al: A role for uric acid in the progression of renal disease. J Am Soc Nephrol 2002;13:2888.

Kim NH et al: Environmental heavy metal exposure and chronic kidney disease in the general population. J Korean Med Sci 2015;30:272.

Kovic SV et al: Prevention of renal complications induced by non-steroidal anti-inflammatory drugs. Curr Med Chem 2016;23:1953.

Krejci K et al: Calcineurin inhibitor-induced renal allograft nephrotoxicity. Biomed Pap Med Fac Univ Palacky Olomouc Czech Repub 2010;154:297.

Kubo K, Yamamoto K: IgG4-related disease. Int J Rheum Dis 2016;19:747.

Le Roy V, Delmas Y, Verdoux H: Chronic renal complications induced by lithium. Encephale 2009;35:605. French.

Luciano RL et al: Aristolochic acid nephropathy: epidemiology, clinical presentation, and treatment. Drug Saf 2015;38:55.

Mahfoudhi M et al: Systemic sarcoidosis complicated of acute renal failure: about 12 cases. Pan Afr Med J 2015;22:75.

Meola M, Samoni S, Petrucci I: Clinical scenarios in chronic kidney disease: chronic tubulointerstitial diseases. Contrib Nephrol 2016;188:108.

Mikhalkova D et al: Epstein-Barr virus-associated nephrotic syndrome. Clin Kidney J 2012;5:50.

Muji A et al: Oxalate nephropathy: a new entity of acute kidney injury in diabetic patients? Rev Med Suisse 2015;11:493, 496. French.

Nava F et al: Everolimus, cyclosporine, and thrombotic microangiopathy: clinical role and preventive tools in renal transplantation. Transplant Proc 2014;46:2263.

Obermayr RP et al: Elevated uric acid increases the risk for kidney disease. J Am Soc Nephrol 2008;19:2407.

Okada H et al: An atypical pattern of Epstein-Barr virus infection in a case with idiopathic tubulointerstitial nephritis. Nephron 2002;92:440.

Pan Y et al: Status of non-steroidal anti-inflammatory drugs use and its association with chronic kidney disease: a cross-sectional survey in China. Nephrology (Carlton) 2014;19:655.

Rahman S, Malcoun A: Nonsteroidal anti-inflammatory drugs, cyclooxygenase-2, and the kidneys. Prim Care 2014;41:803.

Remy P, Audard V, Galacteros F: Kidney and hemoglobinopathy. Nephrol Ther 2016;12:117. French.

Roncal-Jimenez CA et al: Heat stress nephropathy from exercise-induced uric acid crystalluria: a perspective on mesoamerican nephropathy. Am J Kidney Dis 2016;67;20.

Roncal-Jimenez CA et al: Mesoamerican nephropathy or global warming nephropathy? Blood Purif 2016;41:135.

Said SM, Nasr SH: Silent diabetic nephropathy. Kidney Int 2016;90:24.

Selvarajah M et al: Clinicopathological correlates of chronic kidney disease of unknown etiology in Sri Lanka. Indian J Nephrol 2016;26:357.

Shankar S et al: Renal involvement in ANCA associated vasculitis. Indian J Rheum 2013;8:73.

Stone JH et al: IgG4-related disease. N Engl J Med 2012;366:539.

Sutariya HC, Pandya VK: Renal papillary necrosis: role of radiology. J Clin Diagn Res 2016;10:TD10.

Umehara H et al: Comprehensive diagnostic criteria for IgG4-related disease (IgG4-RD), 2011. Mod Rheumatol 2012;22:21.

Vigil D et al: BK nephropathy in the native kidneys of patients with organ transplants: clinical spectrum of BK infection. World J Transplant 2016;6:472. Review.

Wang HH et al: Hypokalemia, its contributing factors and renal outcomes in patients with chronic kidney disease. PLoS One 2013;8:e67140.

Wang SM et al: Increased risk of urinary tract cancer in ESRD patients associated with usage of Chinese herbal products suspected of containing aristolochic acid. PLoS One 2014;9:e105218.

Yaxley J, Lifting T: Non-steroidal anti-inflammatories and the development of analgesic nephropathy: a systematic review. Ren Fail 2016;38:1328.

■ CHAPTER REVIEW QUESTIONS

1. A 39-year-old man is referred to you for the evaluation of glucosuria. The patient is not a diabetic and has had a recent hemoglobin A1c of 5.5%. Additional lab works reveal a serum glucose of 78 mg/dL, a creatinine of 1.7 mg/dL, a serum bicarbonate of 19 mmol/L, and a serum phosphate of 1.8 mg/dL. His urinalysis demonstrates 3+ glucose, 1+ protein, and trace leukocyte esterase. A protein to creatinine ratio shows 1.1 gm/gm creatinine. His urine sediment is bland with no cellular elements, casts, or crystals. His history is unremarkable and his father only has well-controlled hypertension. He works restoring older homes. How can you explain his laboratory findings?
   A. Diabetic nephropathy (early stages)
   B. Urinary tract infection
   C. Chronic tubulointerstitial nephritis
   D. Isolated glucosuria due to mutation in glucose transporter

2. You are evaluating a 42-year-old man in the emergency room with AKI. Two weeks ago the patient had a presumed rotator cuff tear secondary to a sports related injury. Other than mild hypertension for which he is taking lisinopril 10 mg daily, the patient has no significant medical history. For the last 2 weeks he has been using ibuprofen 800 mg three times daily. Three days ago he developed nausea and diarrhea with a low-grade fever. The symptoms have since resolved but routine lab work for a shoulder MRI on the day of presentation demonstrated a creatinine of 4.2 mg/dL (prior baseline 1.6 mg/dL 3 months ago). Urinalysis shows 2–3 RBC/hpf and 1–2 WBC/hpf. There is 3+ protein. What is the most likely cause of the kidney injury in this patient?
   A. Interstitial nephritis from NSAID use
   B. Post-infectious glomerulonephritis from his recent infection
   C. IgA nephropathy given his recent infection
   D. Acute tubular necrosis

3. A 52-year-old woman is being seen in your office to establish care. She has had a gradual rise in creatinine over the last 2 years from a baseline creatinine of 1.5 mg/dL to now 2.5 mg/dL. She has HTN and is currently on hydrochlorothiazide 25 mg daily. In addition she had Roux-en-Y bypass surgery 5 years ago and has had a dramatic 150 pound weight loss since then. She takes occasional ibuprofen (200 mg every 2 weeks for headaches) and denies any herbal medications. Her history is only remarkable for an episode of pyelonephritis in her early thirties and a kidney stone when she was pregnant with her daughter 25 years ago. Examination is unremarkable and urine sediment evaluation shows 5–10 WBC/hpf, 3–5 RBC/hpf, and 2–3 envelope shaped birefringent crystals/hpf. What is the most likely cause of the elevated creatinine in this patient?
   A. Uric acid nephropathy
   B. Calcium oxalate nephropathy
   C. Obstructive uropathy secondary to kidney stones
   D. Chronic interstitial nephritis secondary to ibuprofen use

4. You are evaluating a 42-year-old woman ESRD patient in transplant clinic. The patient developed ESRD after using a weight loss supplement that contained Aristolochia. The patient has been on dialysis for 3 years and is compliant with all treatments and medications. She no longer uses herbal medications. How should you proceed with transplant workup at this time?
   A. The patient should be immediately listed for transplant without any further workup at this time.
   B. The patient will need a bilateral nephrectomy in order to be listed for transplant.
   C. The patient will need a bilateral nephroureterectomy in order to be listed for transplant.
   D. The patient is not a transplant candidate given the strong association of Aristolochia with the development of urothelial carcinomas.

5. You are seeing a 62-year-old woman with newly diagnosed pancreatitis and a progressive AKI. The patient has a history of diabetes mellitus, currently on insulin glargine in the morning and insulin lispro at meals, coronary artery disease with stent placement 3 years ago, and nephrolithiasis, with her last kidney stone 12 years ago. Her creatinine has increased from a baseline of 1.4 mg/dL to 2.2 mg/dL over the last 3 months. A kidney biopsy is performed and shows a dense lymphoplasmacytic infiltrate organized in "storiform" pattern. Given the biopsy finding you make the diagnosis of IgG4 related kidney disease. How would you proceed with treatment?
   A. Start the patient on glucocorticoid treatment
   B. Start the patient on mycophenolate mofetil given her diabetes mellitus
   C. Start the patient on Rituximab
   D. No treatment necessary as there is a high spontaneous remission rate.

39

Nephrolithiasis

David Geller, MD, PhD

Neera K. Dahl, MD, PhD

ESSENTIALS OF DIAGNOSIS

▶ Renal colic is classically described as a waxing and waning pain, which starts in the flank and may radiate to the groin. It may be accompanied by hematuria.

▶ An ultrasound is an appropriate first test to diagnose a kidney stone, a helical non-contrast CT scan—either low dose or standard dose may also be considered.

▶ Chemical analysis of the stone is very helpful in determining further treatment.

▶ Individuals with multiple stones, very early age of onset of stones, or multiple risk factors should undergo further metabolic workup to determine appropriate treatment for stones.

General Considerations

Kidney stones are becoming more common and are associated with significant morbidity. The overall prevalence of kidney stones has increased from 3.8% of the population in 1976–1980 to 8.8% of the population in 2007–2010 based on NHANES data. Non-Hispanic white men have the highest prevalence of stones, followed by Hispanic men, non-Hispanic white women, and Hispanic women. Non-Hispanic black men and women have the lowest prevalence of stones at 4.8% and 4.2% respectively.

Risk Factors

Nutritional factors also play a role in the development of kidney stones. Diets rich in magnesium, potassium and calcium with good fluid intake decrease the risk of kidney stones while diets high in fructose, sucrose, or sodium with low fluid intake increase risk of kidney stones. Being overweight or obese increases the risk for a kidney stone in both

men and women. Lower household income also increased risk of developing a kidney stone. Stones are more common in warmer climates.

An initial evaluation of a kidney stone patient should include a detailed medical history. Bowel disease leading to chronic diarrhea and malabsorption increases risk of kidney stones. Bariatric surgery (Roux-en-Y gastric bypass), small bowel resection, and ileostomy will increase risk. Systemic diseases which increase urine or serum calcium will also increase risk and include primary hyperparathyroidism and sarcoidosis. Certain medications, such as topiramate and carbonic anhydrase inhibitors will increase risk. Diabetes, gout, and hyperthyroidism will increase risk of kidney stones.

Certain occupations may also increase risk of kidney stones (Table 39–1). For example, taxi cab drivers, who have infrequent access to restrooms, are at higher risk, as are those who work in hot environments or with infrequent access to fluids.

Pathogenesis of Kidney Stone Formation

The urine of most individuals is supersaturated at least sometimes with respect to calcium and oxalate, meaning that the potential for stone formation exists in most people. Nevertheless, clinical nephrolithiasis occurs in only a small subset of the population. Much work has gone into understanding how stones form in the urine. At high concentrations of calcium and oxalate, homogeneous crystal formation may occur spontaneously, but these levels are not commonly observed. However, at the calcium and oxalate concentrations more typically observed, spontaneous crystal formation is less likely, and thus, stone formation may not occur even in the presence of urine supersaturated with respect to calcium and oxalate. The key step, therefore, in the formation of a stone is the formation of the initial crystal nidus. Many years ago, Randall hypothesized that areas of

Table 39–1. Specific concerns for stone formers which increase risk for recurrent stones.

	Metabolic Risk	Stone Type
Inflammatory bowel disease or chronic diarrhea	hyperoxaluria	Calcium oxalate
Intestinal surgery, including ileostomy or colectomy	Volume depletion, bicarbonate loss	Calcium oxalate or uric acid
Roux-en-Y, gastric bypass	hyperoxaluria	Calcium oxalate
Sarcoidosis, primary hyperparathyroidism, immobilization, hyperthyroidism	Hypercalciuria	Calcium phosphate and calcium oxalate stones
Distal renal tubular acidosis	Low urine citrate but high urine pH	Calcium phosphate stones
Gout	High serum uric acid	Uric acid stones
Metabolic syndrome, obesity, diabetes mellitus	Low urine citrate, low urine pH	Uric acid stones, calcium oxalate stones
Renal anomaly	Urine Stasis	Multiple stone types
Recurrent UTI with a urea-splitting organism	High urine pH	Struvite stones
Medications: Topiramate Sulfa-containing drugs Anti-retroviral therapy	Low urine citrate, high urine pH Crystallization in urine Crystallization in urine	Calcium phosphate stones Sulfa (medication)stone Anti-retroviral stone (Indinavir)
Nephrocalcinosis (medullary calcification without medullary sponge kidney) seen on imaging	Hyperparathyroidism, distal RTA, chronic loop diuretic use	Calcium phosphate or calcium oxalate
Medullary calcification with ductal ectasia (medullary sponge kidney)	Urine stasis	Calcium oxalate or calcium phosphate

Source: Adapted from Worcester EM, Coe FL: Clinical practice. Calcium kidney stones. *N Engl J Med* 2010;363:954.

apatite plaque in the renal tubule serve as a base for stone formation and development, serving as an initial nidus where stones can attach and grow. Once a nidus has formed, the potential exists for stone growth in situations where the free concentrations of oxalate and calcium exceed the solubility of calcium oxalate (Figure 39–1). Thus, conditions in which increased oxalate or calcium reside in the urine increase the likelihood of stone formation. Other factors, however, affect stone formation as well. Promoters of stone formation include low urine volume (thus concentrating other substituents such as calcium and oxalate), sodium, low urine pH, and urate. In contrast, other urinary components, including inorganic compounds like citrate and magnesium, or organic compounds, such as osteopontin, urinary prothrombin fragment 1, and glycosaminoglycans, serve as inhibitors to stone formation. The organic compounds are thought to adsorb to the surface of the crystal, directly inhibiting further crystal growth. It should be noted that while Randall's plaques are thought to be critical in the formation of calcium oxalate stones, in recent years it has been learned that other groups of stone formers have been identified in whom alternate histologies exist. In addition, small amounts

of other inorganic compounds composing the elementome may be important in stone formation.

Clinical Findings

A. Signs and Symptoms of an Obstructing Kidney Stone

Many patients may have an incidental finding of a kidney stone found on abdominal imaging. Only kidney stones that cause obstruction of urine flow and stretching of the renal capsule are thought to cause renal colic. Thus, a patient may have one or more stones, including a staghorn calculus, and not have symptoms. An obstructing stone will typically cause hydronephrosis or hydroureter, which should be apparent by imaging. Renal colic typically presents as severe, acute flank pain which waxes and wanes over time. The patient may also have hematuria, dysuria, or urinary urgency. Renal colic, with an obstructing stone on imaging, coupled with a fever or high white blood cell (WBC) count should raise concern for an associated urinary tract infection and is a surgical emergency. An obstructing stone in a solitary kidney or with associated AKI should also be treated promptly.

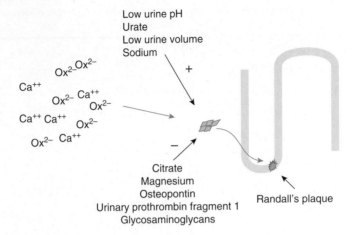

▲ **Figure 39–1.** Schematic of calcium oxalate stone formation. At high levels of calcium oxalate supersaturation, calcium oxalate crystals form and deposit in the basement membrane of Randall's plaque, which is classically found in the thin limb of the loop of Henle. Once a crystal nidus has been generated, crystal growth occurs until a stone forms.

B. Imaging Studies

Imaging plays an important role in the evaluation of kidney stones. A KUB will show larger, calcium-containing stones, but may miss small calcium-containing stones, or uric acid or cystine stones. Calcium-containing stones are more radiopaque, while cystine and uric acid are radiolucent, which are difficult to visualize on KUB.

Non-contrast, helical, computed tomography (CT) is considered the imaging modality of choice for the evaluation of nephrolithiasis. CT has several advantages. The size of a stone can be accurately determined. Small stones and/or ureteral stones are easily visualized (Figure 39–2). The Hounsfield units (HU) of the stone may also be measured by CT. In general, a HU less than 500 is consistent with

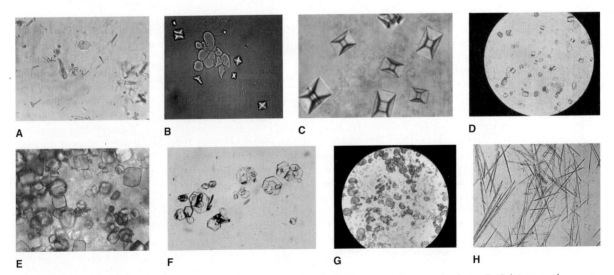

▲ **Figure 39–2.** Types of crystals which may be seen in urine. **A.** Calcium oxalate monohydrate. **B.** Calcium oxalate dehydrate. **C.** Struvite crystals. **D.** Uric acid crystals. **E.** Uric acid crystals under a polarized light. **F.** Cystine crystals. **G.** Sulfadiazine crystals. **H.** Acyclovir crystals. (See Color Plate 25.)

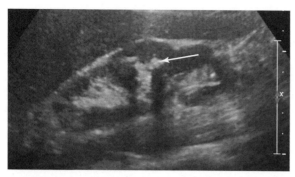

▲ **Figure 39–3.** Ultrasound of the right kidney showing two non-obstructing kidney stones. Both stones cause shadowing which helps identify stones.

a uric acid stone, which may be amenable to medical dissolution therapy regardless of size. Ultrasound is also helpful for the diagnosis of nephrolithiasis (Figure 39–3). Cost and radiation concerns make ultrasound a reasonable and preferable imaging modality especially in younger patients. Patients with an initial negative ultrasound who still have signs and symptoms of renal colic may benefit from CT scanning (Figure 39–4). Low-dose, non-contrast CT scans are a nice option, when available, for minimizing radiation exposure.

Patients with multiple stones are at high risk of recurrence, and should be counseled to undergo a more thorough evaluation to identify stone risk factors. Similarly, patients with only a solitary kidney and stones should also undergo further evaluation and close follow-up. Finally, evidence of nephrocalcinosis might suggest distal renal tubular acidosis (dRTA), primary hyperparathyroidism or medullary sponge kidney, for which further evaluation is necessary.

C. Treatment of an Obstructing Kidney Stone

In the absence of fever or sepsis, initial treatment of an obstructing kidney stone consists of hydration to maintain urine flow, and pain management. Stones smaller than 6 mm may pass spontaneously with aggressive hydration while larger stones may require surgical intervention. Patients who do not require immediate surgical intervention should be sent home with a strainer and instructions to strain their urine to capture the stone, which will allow subsequent stone analysis. Patients may also benefit from medical expulsive therapy, or the use of a medication to help promote stone passage. The most common medication used for medical expulsive therapy is tamsulosin, a selective alpha blocker which promotes ureteral relaxation.

Patients with large (>6 mm) obstructing stones will benefit from surgery. The timing and type of surgery depends on a variety of factors including location and size of the stone. Ureteroscopy with basket stone extraction and/or laser lithotripsy, shock wave lithotripsy (SWL), ureteral stenting, percutaneous nephrolithotomy, open lithotomy or laparoscopy may be considered.

D. Decreasing Risk of Additional Stone Formation

All stone formers should receive appropriate dietary counseling. Recurrent stone formers should undergo an evaluation including a medical and dietary history, serum chemistries, urinalysis and urine microscopy, and a 24-hour urine. Stone formers who are found to have specific metabolic risks may benefit from further pharmacologic therapy.

E. Determining the Risk of a Second Stone

The overall risk of a second kidney stone is about 10% per year, and about 50% in 5 years. However, some individuals are much more likely to develop a second stone. Factors associated

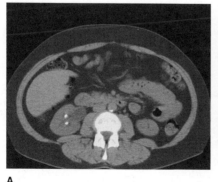
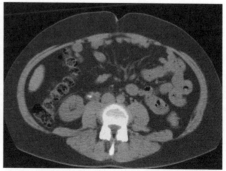

A   B

▲ **Figure 39–4.** Abdominal CT Scan without IV Contrast showing two non-obstructing kidney stones and hydronephrosis (Panel A) in the right kidney, and an obstructing stone in the right ureter (Panel B).

with an increased likelihood of a second stone include first stone at a young age, Caucasian race, male, or with a family history of kidney stones. Uric acid stones are most likely to recur. A stone at the renal pelvis or lower pole is associated with a higher risk of recurrence than a stone at the ureterovesicular junction. Any other incidentally noted stones will increase risk of a second stone. These factors form the basis of the ROKS (recurrence of kidney stone) nomogram for predicting stone recurrence (Table 39–2).

F. Laboratory Findings Important in Medical Management of Kidney Stones

1. Stone Analysis—The chemical composition of a stone can help guide therapy as dietary guidelines and pharmacologic therapy are specific for each stone type. Therefore, it is important to send at least one stone for analysis of chemical composition. Stone composition can vary by time of year, and by the age and sex of the patient. Young women tend to submit more calcium phosphate and struvite stones, while men tend to submit more calcium oxalate and uric acid stones. Uric acid stones are more common after the age of 55, and calcium oxalate and uric acid are more common in the summer. The initial stone analysis may be the first time a rare stone such as drug-containing stone, struvite, or cystine stone is diagnosed. Any patient who has recurrent stones while on appropriate therapy should have a repeat chemical analysis to determine if the stone type has changed.

2. Urinalysis/Urine Microscopy—It may provide important diagnostic information. Uric acid stones tend to form in acidic urine. A high urine pH is associated with calcium phosphate or struvite stones. Examination of the urine sediment may also be helpful. Crystals may be seen in the urine, which

Table 39–2. AUA guidelines for evaluation of risk of kidney stones.

A clinician should perform a screening evaluation consisting of a detailed medical and dietary history, serum chemistries, and urinalysis on a patient with newly diagnosed kidney or ureteral stones
When a stone is available, clinicians should obtain a stone analysis at least once
Clinicians should review available imaging to quantify stone burden
Clinicians should perform additional metabolic testing in high-risk or interested first-time stone formers and recurrent stone formers
Metabolic testing should consist of one or two 24-hour urine collections obtained on a random diet and analyzed at a minimum for total volume, pH, calcium, oxalate, uric acid, citrate, sodium, potassium, and creatinine

Source: Perle MS et al: Medical Management of Kidney Stones: AUA guideline. *J Urol.* 2014;192:316.

may help determine the type of stone present (Figure 39–2). Both calcium oxalate and struvite crystals have distinctive shapes which can be easily recognized, calcium oxalate dehydrate presenting with envelope shaped crystals and struvite presenting with a pyramidal shape (Figures 39–2A-C). Uric acid stones are distinguished by their polychromatic appearance under polarized light (Figures 39–2D, E), and cystine stones form pathognomic hexagonal crystals (Figure 39–2F). Certain drugs form characteristic crystals in the urine, including the "shocks of wheat" sulfadiazine crystals (Figure 39–2G) and the birefringent needle-shaped crystals of acyclovir (Figure 39–2H). Finally, urine specific gravity is a helpful marker of hydration status. Ideally, a kidney stone patient drinking appropriate amounts of fluid is making dilute urine with a low specific gravity (SG <1.015).

3. Chemistries—A basic metabolic panel may provide useful clues to the cause of kidney stones. A high serum calcium could reflect primary hyperparathyroidism, or inappropriately high levels of 1,25-OH vitamin D which may be seen with sarcoid or other granulomatous diseases. Low serum bicarbonate and low potassium concentrations may reflect a distal RTA. A high BUN to creatinine ratio may reflect underlying volume depletion.

4. 24-Hour Urine Measurement—Recurrent stone formers should undergo an evaluation that includes a medical and dietary history, serum chemistries, UA, and a 24-hour urine that measures volume, pH, calcium, oxalate, uric acid, pH, citrate, sodium, potassium, and creatinine. Measurement of 24-hour urine should be performed when the patient is eating and drinking typically, as it provides only a single snapshot of that day's intake. One or two initial measurements should be performed.

It is important to remember that all 24-hour measurements are continuous variables. Thus, a patient with a "normal" urinary calcium who forms calcium-containing stones may still benefit from treatment to reduce urinary calcium. In pediatrics, a spot urinary calcium/creatinine ratio is also used for monitoring urinary calcium because of ease of collection.

Many commercial laboratories will also provide measurements of supersaturation for common stone types including calcium oxalate, calcium phosphate, uric acid, and struvite (Table 39–3). A urine supersaturation above the reference range indicates that the patient is at risk for forming that type of stone in the urine. A urine supersaturation below the reference range is the goal of treatment.

▶ Treatment

A. Calcium Stones

Patients with uric acid, struvite, or cystine stones typically require therapy specific to their stone type. The management of calcium stones, however, is often more nuanced. The risk

Table 39–3. Components of a 24-hour urine measurement for metabolic analysis.

Component in Urine	Unit	Goal of Therapy for Stone Formers
Volume	Liter/day	>2–3 L/Day
pH		Depends on Stone type. Treatment for CaOx, UA, and cystine stones includes increasing urine pH. CaP stones are more likely to form >6.3
Calcium	mg/day	<250 (men), <200 (women) for calcium-containing stones
Oxalate	mg/day	<40 for calcium oxalate stone formers
Citrate	mg/day	>450 (men), >550 (women) for uric acid, calcium oxalate, and dRTA stone formers
Uric Acid	mg/day	<800 (men), <750 (women)
Phosphate	mg/day	about 1000
Magnesium	mg/day	>80 for calcium-containing stones
Sulfate	mmol/day	<30 if low urine pH is a risk factor
Ammonium	mmol/day	Range is 15–60. Helps determine treatment
Sodium	mmol/day	<100 for calcium-containing stones
Potassium	mmol/day	>50 for calcium or uric acid stones
Creatinine	mg/day	Men produce 18–24 mg/kg/day, women 15–20 mg/kg/day
Protein Catabolic Rate (PCR)	g/kg/day	<1 for uric acid and calcium containing stones
Supersaturation		Lowest achievable for stone type

CaOx, calcium oxalate; CaPhos, calcium phosphate (also called brushite or apatite); UA, uric acid.

of stone recurrence is roughly 50% over 10 years, and that risk can be lowered further by simple dietary measures and maintaining high fluid intake. An educated patient may reasonably choose to forego taking medicine every day for the next 10 years to avoid a 50% risk of a frequently painful, but typically benign, recurrence of nephrolithiasis. As such, the first question that must be answered in any calcium stone former is to determine which patients are deserving of a full evaluation. Certainly, any child with stones should be fully evaluated, as the stone is often an indicator of an underlying metabolic abnormality.

B. Conditions Deserving of Further Evaluation in a First Time Adult Stone Former

1. Distal renal tubular acidosis—This is a rare condition in which the kidney is unable to appropriately acidify the urine. A low serum bicarbonate is a clue to the diagnosis, particularly in the setting of an alkaline urine (pH >6.5). The resultant systemic acidosis leads to increased calcium liberation from the bone and hypercalciuria. Hypocitraturia and hypokalemia are typical and the confluence of all of these abnormalities predisposes to nephrolithiasis. Calcium

phosphate stones are the typical outcome in the setting of alkaline urine. Genetic etiologies predominate in children. In adults, the most common etiology is Sjögren syndrome, but it can also occur secondary to certain collagen vascular diseases and hyperglobulinemic conditions. Acidemia is straightforward to manage—provision of alkali, usually in the form of potassium citrate, is typically sufficient to reverse the hypercalciuria and will serve to correct the hypokalemia and hypocitraturia as well.

2. Primary hyperparathyroidism—Hyperparathyroidism is suggested by the presence of hypercalcemia and hypercalciuria and has been associated with an increased risk of calcium nephrolithiasis. Hypophosphatemia is often seen as well. The finding of a non-suppressed PTH is suggestive of the diagnosis, as long as the patient is not lithium, which can trigger abnormal PTH secretion. Surgical excision of the parathyroid is recommended. Although calcimimetics have been used in patients in whom surgical options are not available, their general use is not recommended due to their cost.

3. Sarcoid—Sarcoidosis and other granulomatous disorders such as lymphoma and tuberculosis can also be associated with hypercalcemia and hypercalciuria. Sarcoidosis is associated with an approximate 20-fold increased incidence of nephrolithiasis, and renal stones are the presenting manifestation of sarcoid in 6% of patients. The mechanism is increased conversion of 25-OH vitamin D to 1-25-OH vitamin D by activated monocytes, which leads to increased gut calcium absorption as well as increased renal reabsorption of calcium. Treatment is directed at the underlying disease, typically steroids for sarcoidosis.

4. Intestinal disease—A variety of intestinal disorders are contributory to stone disease, and any patient with a new stone should be questioned for telltale signs of bowel disease, particularly a history of diarrhea. Intestinal disorders predispose to calcium nephrolithiasis in a variety of ways. First of all, volume loss from frequent diarrhea results in decreased urine volume and thus a more concentrated urine. Similarly, the systemic acidemia that results from stool bicarbonate losses leads to hypocitraturia, an important risk factor for calcium stones, as well as liberation of bone calcium, leading to an increase in urine calcium.

Enteric hyperoxaluria is a complication of a number of intestinal disorders, and it deserves special mention as it is increasingly problematic. Hyperoxaluria is commonly observed in fat malabsorption disorders such as Crohn's disease, short bowel syndrome, in intestinal bypass procedures done for obesity, and obesity drugs such as orlistat (induces fat malabsorption). Calcium normally serves to bind oxalate in the gut and prevent its absorption. It is believed that malabsorbed fat adsorbs calcium in the gut. The reduction in free calcium caused by fat malabsorption in these disorders leads to a significant increase in oxalate absorption. Avoidance of a high fat, high oxalate diet is recommended. In addition, calcium supplements are recommended with meals and cholestyramine has been recommended to bind excess fatty acids as well. Given that the hyperoxaluria in these disorders has been associated not just with nephrolithiasis, but also acute and chronic oxalate nephropathy and occasionally end-stage renal disease (ESRD), therapy directed at hyperoxaluria must be aggressive in these circumstances.

C. Patients with Recurrent Calcium-Containing Stones with Abnormal 24-hour Urine Results

Patients with signs or symptoms consistent with any of the above conditions should be further evaluated to ensure that any underlying disorder predisposing to stones is identified. Here, we will review abnormalities that may appear on 24-hour urine.

1. Low urine volume—Studies have consistently found that low urine volume, less than 2 L/day, predisposes to nephrolithiasis and that increasing urine volume to greater than 2 L (or ideally 3 liters) significantly lowers the stone recurrence risk. While this would seem to be straightforward to manage,

there are a number of circumstances that limit the ability or interest in increasing fluid intake. Patients in certain occupations, such as truck drivers, and (typically) older individuals may wish to limit fluid intake to avoid the need for frequent urination. Patients who live or work in a hot and humid climate may lose significant fluid via perspiration and may find it challenging to remain appropriately hydrated throughout the day. Patients with intestinal illnesses may find it challenging to maintain fluid volume in the face of ongoing stool losses. Efforts should be made to help such patients find a hydration regiment that works within their lifestyle.

2. Hypercalciuria—Hypercalciuria (>200 mg/24 hours in women, or >250 mg/24 hours in men) is a common finding in patients with calcium nephrolithiasis. In most cases, conditions associated with calcium wasting, such as hyperparathyroidism, sarcoidosis, vitamin D excess, malignancy, immobilization, and excessive calcium intake are absent, and thus, this is termed idiopathic hypercalciuria. The mechanisms underlying hypercalciuria are typically unknown, although there does seem to be a clear genetic component. What has become increasingly clear, however, is that most patients with idiopathic hypercalciuria have net negative calcium balance—urine losses exceed GI absorption. As such, patients with idiopathic hypercalciuria are at long-term risk for bone demineralization. Thiazide diuretics coupled with a sodium restricted diet have been shown to be quite useful in reducing stone propensity in such individuals via their effect on reducing urine calcium excretion, with the added benefit that they may limit net bone loss as well. However, they may predispose to potassium losses, which can lead to hypocitraturia, and thus potassium supplementation with potassium citrate is recommended. If urine pH rises above 6.2, potassium chloride can be substituted, as an overly basic urine can predispose to calcium phosphate stones.

Dietary measures are also useful to limit hypercalciuria. Both high sodium and high protein intake predispose to renal calcium wasting, and thus, hypercalciuric stone formers should be counseled to maintain a low sodium diet (<2 g daily) and avoid excessive protein intake. Conversely, a low calcium diet has been shown to be harmful, presumably due to its effects on gut oxalate absorption, and likely increases the risk of further bone demineralization. Calcium gluttony as well as calcium supplementation should be avoided, but the patient should be cautioned that avoidance of calcium containing foods will paradoxically increase their risk of calcium stone recurrence.

3. Hypocitraturia—Hypocitraturia, often defined as less than 550 mg/day (women), less than 450 mg/day (men), is a common risk factor for calcium stones. Citrate complexes calcium in the urine, thereby lowering calcium's availability to participate in stone formation. Urine citrate is reduced in individuals with an underlying metabolic acidosis, such as is seen in patients with distal renal tubular acidosis or a chronic diarrheal illness, but is also reduced in individuals with high sodium or animal protein intake as well as in individuals with hypokalemia, or metabolic syndrome. Hypocitraturia is typically treated with potassium citrate, about 50–60 mEq daily. Trials of potassium citrate for the prevention of recurrence of nephrolithiasis have generally suggested a reduction in stone recurrence comparable to that seen in patients prescribed a thiazide. Sodium citrate has never been formally assessed in trials, due to the theoretical concerns of sodium intake increasing both blood pressure and renal calcium excretion. However, patient with underlying CKD and hyperkalemia may not tolerate potassium citrate and require sodium citrate.

4. Hyperuricosuria—Hyperuricosuria (>800 mg/24 hours in men, >750 mg/24 hours in women) is a common finding in calcium stone formers, occurring in up to one third of such patients. Uric acid has been proposed as a nidus for calcium stone nucleation, thereby lowering the chemical threshold for stone initiation, but others have proposed that uric acid may trigger a "salting-out" mechanism whereby the threshold for calcium stone formation is lowered by the presence of uric acid. One small clinical trial showed that allopurinol induced a reduction in calcium stone recurrence in patients with hyperuricosuria and normocalciuria. While allopurinol would not be considered a first-line therapy for patients with nephrolithiasis, its use could be considered in challenging patients with hyperuricosuria.

5. Dietary hyperoxaluria—As noted above, certain intestinal conditions are associated with hyperoxaluria. Hyperoxaluria can also occur as a byproduct of excessive dietary intake, although this is usually not the primary cause of oxalate containing stones. Although oxalate is found in a variety of foods of plant origin such as nuts, cocoa, and dark leafy greens, the most common sources of oxalate in an American diet tend to be spinach and potatoes. Low calcium intake is typically associated with dietary oxaluria, as the absence of intestinal calcium favors oxalate absorption from the gut over oxalate precipitation and excretion from the gut. Avoidance of oxalate rich foods and a normal (800–1000 mg daily) calcium intake are recommended.

Table 39–4 provides a summary of the available treatments for calcium-containing stones based on the underlying metabolic defect detected.

D. Uric Acid Stones

Uric acid stones are most often radiolucent by plain film. They are readily identifiable by CT, as generally the HU are less than 500. Uric acid stones, even those that are quite large, may respond to medical dissolution therapy that consists of increasing the urine pH, generally with potassium citrate. Uric acid is insoluble and will precipitate leading to stone

Table 39–4. Summary of treatment for calcium-containing stones.

Metabolic Defect	Treatment
All calcium stone formers	Dietary counseling: low salt (<100 mEq), high fluid (2.5 L), 3–5 servings of fruits/vegetables daily, and 1000 mg of dietary calcium daily. A low salt DASH diet is appropriate
Hyperoxaluria	Modest restriction of high oxalate foods. https://regepi.bwh.harvard.edu/health/Oxalate/files/Oxalate%20Content%20of%20Foods.xls contains an accurate list of the oxalate content of food
Hypocitraturia	Consider potassium citrate, typically 20–60 mEq daily
Idiopathic hypercalciuria	Consider treatment with a long acting thiazide diuretic (chlorthalidone or indapamide, or BID hydrochlorothiazide). Aim for the lowest dose which achieves an effective decrease in urinary calcium
Hyperuricosuria and normal urine calcium	Consider treatment with allopurinol or febuxostat
Recurrent stone formers with no metabolic defect	Consider empiric therapy with either potassium citrate or a long-acting thiazide
Mixed calcium-oxalate and calcium-phosphate stones or predominantly calcium phosphate stones	Cautious use of potassium citrate therapy may be warranted. If the starting urine pH is low (<6.2) then the goal should be to raise the pH to about 6. If the starting urine pH is high (>6.2), then the goal should be to increase urinary citrate to correct hypocitraturia. Since a high-urine pH promotes calcium phosphate stones, overall risks and benefits of therapy must be individualized.

formation or growth at an acid pH. The solubility increases with increasing pH. The goal is a pH above 6.0, which generally requires about 20 mEq thrice daily of potassium citrate. Repeat imaging after several months of dissolution therapy will help determine if treatment has been successful, or if surgical intervention is needed. Since uric acid stones have an increased tendency to recur, life-long prophylactic therapy may be considered. The dose of potassium citrate should be adjusted to the lowest possible to maintain a urine pH of 6. All patients should be counseled on following an alkali-rich (or fruit and vegetable rich) diet with good fluid intake. Drugs such as allopurinol or febuxostat are considered second line therapy as the primary risk for most patients is a low urine pH rather than hyperuricosuria.

E. Struvite Stones

Struvite stones are composed of magnesium ammonium phosphate. A typical UA from a struvite stone former will have a high urine pH and classic "coffin lid" shaped crystals. Patients with recurrent upper tract infections with a urea-splitting bacterium such as *Proteus* or *Klebsiella* are at high risk of struvite stones. Women, patients with a neurogenic bladder or with a urinary diversion are at higher risk. Since stone fragments remaining in the kidneys may form a nidus for recurrent infection, the goal of surgical therapy is to completely remove all stones. For patients whom effective surgical treatment is not possible, acetohydroxamic acid, a urease inhibitor, or antibiotic suppressive therapy may be considered. Since struvite stones can occur in combination with other stone types, particularly calcium phosphate, full metabolic evaluation is still important to minimize other risk factors.

F. Cystine Stones

Patients with an autosomal disorder resulting in a defect in proximal tubular uptake of cysteine, ornithine, lysine, and arginine (COLA), are at risk of forming cystine stones. Patients with autosomal recessive disease have defects in SLC3A1, while patients with autosomal dominant disease have defects in SLC7A9. A typical presentation for a cystine stone former would be the presence of unilateral or bilateral staghorn calculi, often at a young age. Urinalysis with microscopy may show classic hexagonal crystals. A cyanide-nitroprusside test will be positive.

Cystine is the oxidized dimer form of the amino acid cysteine. Cystine is relatively insoluble in urine, particularly at low pH. The goals of therapy for cystine stones include alkalinizing the urine to increase cystine solubility, reducing the concentration of cystine in the urine below the threshold for precipitation (generally about 243 mg/L or 1 mmol/L) by increasing fluid intake, and maintaining cysteine in a monomeric state.

The goal for cystine stones is a urine pH >7.0. This is usually achieved with potassium citrate at a dose of 20–30 mEq twice daily. The urinary excretion of cystine should be measured in a 24-hour urine, and an individualized fluid prescription should be determined to maintain the urine concentration of cystine below 243 mg/L. For example, a patient who excretes 1000 mg of cystine in a 24-hour collection should be instructed to drink at least 4 L of fluid a day.

If urinary alkalinization and increased fluid intake are not sufficient to limit further cystine stone formation then treatment with thiol-containing drugs should be considered. Thiol-containing drugs reduce cystine to more soluble cysteine-containing compounds. D-penicillamine or tiopronin are typically used. Both drugs have significant adverse effects such as diarrhea, dysgeusia, skin rash, proteinuria, thrombocytopenia, leukopenia, and nausea, which may limit use.

Since cystine stones are caused by a genetic defect in cysteine transport, life-long adherence to therapy is required.

Otherwise recurrent stones can increase risk of renal insufficiency and ESRD.

G. Medication-induced Stones

Some medications may indirectly lead to an increased risk of kidney stones while others precipitate within the kidney and directly cause kidney stones. Zonisamide, and topiramate have carbonic anhydrase activity leading to hypocitraturia and a high urine pH, which favors calcium phosphate stones. Furosemide (and other loop diuretics) leads to increased urinary calcium excretion and increased calcium oxalate and calcium phosphate stones. Other medications are renally cleared, with high concentrations in the urine favoring crystallization. Common drugs in this class include indinavir, triamterene, sulfadiazine, and allopurinol. Finally, stones may be caused by contaminants in food such as silica in milk or melamine in infant formula.

▶ Future Directions

A. The Gut Microbiome

In recent years, there has been substantial interest in the contribution of the gut microbiome toward stone formation. *Oxalobacter formigenes* (OF) is a species of bacteria that reside in the colon of vertebrates including humans. It relies exclusively on metabolism of oxalate for their energy, breaking it down into formate and carbon dioxide. Interest in oxalobacter spiked with the finding that recurrent calcium oxalate stone formers are significantly less likely to be colonized with OF than controls, leading to the hypothesis that the absence of intestinal oxalobacter might predispose to oxalate absorption and stone formation. It is not clear, however, whether provision of oxalate metabolizing bacteria to the gut yields any clinical benefit at the present time. More recently, however, Stern and colleagues in a small study demonstrated a distinctive gut microbiome in kidney stone formers, in whom there was an increased finding of *Bacteroides* (OR = 3.26) and an inverse association with *Prevotella* (OR = 0.37). Furthermore, they demonstrated trends toward a correlation of *Eubacterium* with oxalate levels and *Escherichia* with citrate levels. Results of this study will need to be confirmed in larger studies, but they raise the question of whether adjustment of the gut microbiome may play a role in the management of calcium oxalate nephrolithiasis in the future.

B. Genetics

One area that has received increased interest in recent years is the role of genetics in kidney stone formation. It has long been known that the prevalence of stone formers is higher among relatives of stone-forming patients than among relatives of healthy individuals. A number of rare monogenic disorders have been linked to nephrolithiasis, and these should certainly be considered in a child presenting with renal stones, but these account for only a small fraction of the heritability of nephrolithiasis. Family and twin studies have calculated that the heritability of calcium nephrolithiasis is about 50%, making this trait more heritable than diseases such as hypertension and type 2 diabetes. However, the genetic signals underlying this predisposition have remained for the most part elusive.

In recent years, however, there has been progress in this direction that may herald a new understanding in our understanding of stone formation. Oddsson and colleagues performed a genome wide association study (GWAS) on 28.3 million sequence variants in 2636 Icelanders with a history of stone formation. Interestingly, they found significant associations with sequence variants in the ALPL locus, a tissue specific alkaline phosphatase, the Claudin 14 locus, which is involved in renal calcium and magnesium reabsorption, and a suggestive locus at CASR, the calcium sensing receptor. The ALPL locus is intriguing as loss of function mutations in ALPL have previously been shown to affect urine levels of pyrophosphate, a known inhibitor of stone formation. They furthermore identified rare missense coding sequence variants in SLC34A1, the principal site for renal phosphate reabsorption, and in TRPV5, the principal site of regulated renal calcium reabsorption. While further work is no doubt necessary, it is certainly intriguing that this work has identified significant associations in genes intimately involved in calcium homeostasis. These findings suggest a day when personalized genomic medicine may aid in the management of stones.

C. Association of Nephrolithiasis with Chronic Kidney Disease and Coronary Artery Disease

Nephrolithiasis is associated with a twofold increase risk of chronic kidney disease (CKD) and ESRD independent of other known CKD risk factors. Similarly, a large cohort study demonstrated that patients with nephrolithiasis have an approximately 18% increased risk of coronary artery disease (CAD) compared to non-stone formers. The causes of these associations have not been fully elucidated, but a number of mechanisms have been posited. Some of the explanation is likely patient-specific. For example, patients with the metabolic syndrome are predisposed to nephrolithiasis as well as CAD and CKD. Patients with anatomic urinary tract abnormalities that predispose to stone formation may also be predisposed to renal disease, and those with infection stones may develop renal scarring due to chronic infection. Furthermore, patients with CKD are known to be at increased risk of cardiovascular disease. Whether there are other mechanisms underlying these associations, including lifestyle, genetics, or diet for example, remains to be discovered. As such, the precise meaning of these associations is not clear at this time, but it will be interesting to see if new insights into the physiology of stone formation and its interaction with renal disease can be determined.

KEY READINGS

Borghi L et al: Urinary volume, water and recurrences in idiopathic calcium nephrolithiasis: a 5-year randomized prospective study. J Urol 1996;155:839.

Buckalew VM Jr.: Nephrolithiasis in renal tubular acidosis. J Urol 1989;141:731.

Daudon M, Jungers P: Drug-induced renal calculi: epidemiology, prevention and management. Drugs 2004;64:245.

Ettinger B et al: Randomized trial of allopurinol in the prevention of calcium oxalate calculi. N Engl J Med 1986;315:1386.

Ferraro PM, D'Addessi A, Gambaro G: When to suspect a genetic disorder in a patient with renal stones, and why. Nephrol Dial Transplant 2013;28:811.

Ferraro PM et al: History of kidney stones and the risk of coronary heart disease. JAMA 2013;310:408.

Ingimarsson JP, Krambeck AE, Pais VM Jr: Diagnosis and management of nephrolithiasis. Surg Clin North Am 2016;96:517.

Keddis MT, Rule AD: Nephrolithiasis and loss of kidney function. Curr Opin Nephrol Hypertens 2013;22:390.

Lieske JC et al: Stone composition as a function of age and sex. Clin J Am Soc Nephrol 2014;9:2141.

Matlaga BR et al: The role of Randall's plaques in the pathogenesis of calcium stones. J Urol 2007;177:31.

Moore CL et al: Ureteral stones: implementation of a reduced-dose CT protocol in patients in the emergency department with moderate to high likelihood of calculi on the basis of STONE score. Radiology 2016;280:743.

Oddsson A et al: Common and rare variants associated with kidney stones and biochemical traits. Nat Commun 2015;6:7975.

Parks J, Coe F, Favus M: Hyperparathyroidism in nephrolithiasis. Arch Intern Med 1980;140:1479.

Pearle MS et al: Medical management of kidney stones: AUA guideline. J Urol 2014;192:316.

Prywer J, Torzewska A, Płociński T: Unique surface and internal structure of struvite crystals formed by Proteus mirabilis. Urological Research 2012;40:699.

Ramaswamy K et al: The elementome of calcium-based urinary stones and its role in urolithiasis. Nat Rev Urol 2015;12:543.

Rizzato G, Fraioli P, Montemurro L: Nephrolithiasis as a presenting feature of chronic sarcoidosis. Thorax 1995;50:555.

Rule AD et al: The ROKS nomogram for predicting a second symptomatic stone episode. J Am Soc Nephrol 2014;25:2878.

Scales CD Jr. et al: Prevalence of kidney stones in the United States. Eur Urol 2012;62:160.

Siva S et al: A critical analysis of the role of gut Oxalobacter formigenes in oxalate stone disease. BJU Int 2009;103:18.

Smith-Bindman R et al: Ultrasonography versus computed tomography for suspected nephrolithiasis. N Engl J Med 2014;371:1100.

Stern JM et al: Evidence for a distinct gut microbiome in kidney stone formers compared to non-stone formers. Urolithiasis 2016;44:399.

Taylor EN, Curhan GC: Oxalate intake and the risk for nephrolithiasis. J Am Soc Nephrol 2007;18:2198.

Taylor EN, Fung TT, Curhan GC: DASH-style diet associates with reduced risk for kidney stones. J Am Soc Nephrol 2009;20:2253.

Teichman JM: Clinical practice. Acute renal colic from ureteral calculus. N Engl J Med 2004;350:684.

Worcester EM, Coe FL: Clinical practice. Calcium kidney stones. N Engl J Med 2010;363:954.

Zuckerman JM, Assimos DG: Hypocitraturia: pathophysiology and medical management. Rev Urol 2009;11:134.

■ CHAPTER REVIEW QUESTIONS

1. A 45-year-old woman comes to renal clinic for medical management of kidney stones. She had a stone at the age of 35, diagnosed during her first pregnancy. An ultrasound shows she has small bilateral non-obstructing stones. She is on no medications except a multivitamin. On examination she is an obese woman in NAD. VSS. UA: SG 1.020, pH 6.5, trace ketones. Which of the following is not a risk factor for kidney stones?
   A. Low fluid intake which correlates with the high urine SG of 1.020
   B. Exercising (Zumba class) 3×/week
   C. Her young age at initial diagnosis
   D. Multiple bilateral kidney stones
   E. Her obesity

2. A 60-year-old man presents to the ED with acute, left renal colic. He is found to have a 9 mm obstructing stone causing mild hydronephrosis. The stone has an HU of 352. After his pain is managed, he appears well with no fever and stable vital signs. Appropriate initial therapy includes
   A. Treatment with allopurinol for a uric acid stone
   B. Treatment with potassium citrate therapy for a uric acid stone
   C. Treatment with tamsulosin (medical expulsive therapy)
   D. Treatment with a long-acting thiazide for a calcium-containing stone

3. A 24-year-old woman has a history of recurrent calcium-containing stones. She was well until 1 year ago. However, she has passed 3 stones over the last 12 months. Each stone has been a mixture of calcium oxalate and calcium phosphate. Her initial laboratories are notable for a calcium of 10.5 mg/dL, and a urinary calcium of 500 mg/day. Her urinary citrate is normal. Which of the following is the most likely cause of her recurrent kidney stones?
   A. Primary hyperparathyroidism
   B. A hereditary distal RTA
   C. Dent disease
   D. Surreptitious abuse of a thiazide diuretic for weight loss
   E. Surreptitious abuse of a loop diuretic for weight loss.

4. A 35-year-old woman patient had an abdominal ultrasound to evaluate for abdominal pain. She was found to have bilateral nephrocalcinosis without nephrolithiasis. Her past medical history is notable for a diagnosis of toxic multinodular goiter. She underwent a complete thyroidectomy 3 months ago. Her TSH is now within normal limits on thyroid hormone replacement therapy. Appropriate further workup for the nephrocalcinosis includes
   A. Testing for primary hyperparathyroidism
   B. Testing for a distal RTA
   C. Testing for medullary sponge kidney
   D. No further workup is needed
   E. Genetic testing for this hereditary condition

5. Appropriate dietary advice for a patient with recurrent calcium oxalate stones and hypercalciuria includes
   A. A low salt, low calcium (<400 mg/daily), high fluid intake diet
   B. A low salt, high calcium (1000 mg/daily), high fluid intake diet
   C. A high protein, high fiber diet such as the South Beach diet
   D. Dietary oxalate restriction, with high fluid intake
   E. Dietary oxalate restriction with high calcium (1000 mg/daily) intake

Primary (Essential) Hypertension

Hala Yamout, MD
George L. Bakris, MD

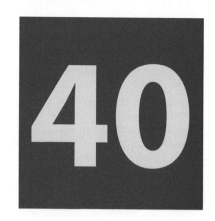

40

ESSENTIALS OF DIAGNOSIS

- Primary hypertension in adults aged 18 years and older is defined as blood pressure of 140/90 mm Hg or more, based on an average of two or more properly measured seated blood pressure (BP) readings at each of two or more clinic visits.

- Normal BP is a systolic BP (SBP) <120 mm Hg and diastolic BP (DBP) <80 mm Hg.

- Prehypertension is defined as an SBP of 120–139 mm Hg or DBP of 80–89 mm Hg.

- Stage 1 hypertension is defined by an elevation in either SBP 140–159 mm Hg or diastolic BP of 90–99 mm Hg.

- Stage 2 hypertension is defined by an elevation in either SBP of ≥160 mm Hg or DBP of ≥100 mm Hg.

- The BP should be measured properly (see text) and on at least two separate occasions before confirming the diagnosis. It should also interpreted in the context of the overall cardiovascular risk of the patient, which is most easily estimated by evaluating other concomitant disorders and target-organ damage (TOD) and using the lifetime risk equation (http://clincalc.com/cardiology/ascvd/pooledcohort.aspx or http://professional.heart.org/professional/GuidelinesStatements/Prevention-Guidelines/UCM_457698_Prevention-Guidelines.jsp)

▶ General Considerations

Hypertension affects 29% of all adult Americans and its prevalence increases with age. Indeed, data from the Framingham health study suggest that people with a normal BP (<120/80 mm Hg) at 55 years of age have a 90% lifetime risk of developing hypertension. Additionally, it is now

well established that a linear relationship exists between BP and risk of cardiovascular events, thus the more elevated the BP the greater the likelihood of myocardial infarction, congestive heart failure, kidney failure, or stroke.

Despite the increased prevalence of hypertension and its associated morbidity and mortality, current control rates are inadequate. Despite the availability of multiple treatments only 53% of people with hypertension have their BP controlled to a goal of less than 140/90 mm Hg. Key factors for the inadequate BP control include failure of physicians to prescribe: (1) lifestyle modifications, (2) adequate doses of antihypertensive medications, and (3) appropriate drug combinations and increased occurrence of pure systolic hypertension in the elderly, which is considerably more difficult to treat.

▶ Risk Factors

The American Heart Association recommends that specific public health interventions such as eating a diet high in vegetables and fruits, reducing sodium intake, and increasing physical activity be strongly encouraged. This strategy can achieve a downward shift in the distribution of a population's BP and thus potentially decrease the lifetime risk of morbidity and mortality from hypertension in an individual.

▶ Clinical Evaluation

A. Measurement of Blood Pressure

Accurate measurement and interpretation of BP is crucial for the diagnosis and treatment of hypertension. The recommendations outlined below will help standardize the technique and improve the accuracy of BP readings (see Essentials of Diagnosis):

- Patients should abstain from drinking caffeine or alcohol-containing beverages or using tobacco within 30 minutes prior to a BP measurement.

- The cuff size appropriate for the patient's arm circumference should be used (the cuff bladder should encircle at least 80% of the arm).

- The cuff bladder should be centered over the brachial artery, with its lower edge within 2.5 cm of the antecubital fossa.

- Listen over the brachial artery using the bell of the stethoscope with minimal pressure exerted on the skin. Inflate the cuff 20 mm Hg higher than the pressure at which the palpable pulse at the radial artery disappears. Use a properly calibrated sphygmomanometer.

- The deflation rate of the column of mercury should be 2–3 mm Hg/second.

- Multiple measurements should be made on different occasions in the sitting position with the back supported for 5 minutes and the arm supported at heart level.

- At least two readings should be taken on each visit separated by as much time as possible.

- Attempt to avoid "terminal digit preference" (>20% of measurements ending with a specific even digit).

- Measure BP in both arms initially, and in the arm with the higher BP thereafter if the difference is greater than 10/5 mm Hg.

1. Home blood pressure measurements—Home BP measurements are indicated for (1) evaluating white-coat hypertension, (2) assessing target-organ damage (TOD) in response to antihypertensive drug therapy, and (3) improving patients' adherence to therapy. Use of home readings are associated with better blood pressure control and are better predictors of cardiovascular risk than office readings alone. Additionally, they are associated with better patient adherence.

2. Ambulatory blood pressure monitoring—Ambulatory BP readings provide BP data during daily activities and sleep and correlate better than office readings with cardiovascular event rates. They are indicated for the evaluation of white-coat hypertension in the absence of TOD, episodic hypertension, apparent drug-resistant hypertension, drug-induced hypotensive symptoms, and autonomic dysfunction. As in home BP readings patients are considered to have hypertension if their mean BP during the day is more than 135/85 mm Hg or more than 125/75 mm Hg during sleep. Outcome studies have demonstrated increased cardiovascular risk associated with abnormal ambulatory blood pressure monitoring (ABPM) profiles (eg, "nondipping" of BP at night). It is also important in the diagnosis of masked hypertension, where home readings are higher than clinic readings.

ABPM important and use in the context of office and home BP is summarized in Table 40–1. Note that if properly done home BP has been validated against daytime ABPM and is strongly correlated; both are better than office BP.

Table 40–1. Indications and validity of ambulatory and home blood pressure.

	Ambulatory Blood Pressure (ABPM)	Home Blood Pressure
Indications	White coat hypertension; masked hypertension	White coat hypertension
Information obtainable	(a) Dietary sodium intake presence of salt sensitive hypertension; (b) detects white coat hypertension; (c) detects masked hypertension; (d) detects presence of nocturnal dipping and correlates with sleep disorders	(a) white coat hypertension; (b) shown to improve medication adherence if done routinely;* (c) masked hypertension*

*If patient is properly instructed how to take blood pressure and when to take it at home (early morning when first awaken before meds) results are validated against daytime ABPM).

WHITE-COAT HYPERTENSION—**Up to 20%** of those with hypertension have BP readings that are considerably higher in the doctor's office or hospital than those measured at home, at work, or by ABPM. This occurs more commonly among the elderly. The clinical consequences of this diagnosis are higher risk for cardiovascular events and related mortality as compared to normotensive, non-white-coat hypertension patients, but with a lower risk than those with primary hypertension. Twenty-four-hour ambulatory monitoring is needed along with a normal physical examination to confirm the diagnosis. It has been suggested that such stimuli raise BP only transiently and reversibly while others think that these patients will all eventually become sustained hypertensives. Currently, lifestyle modifications with frequent BP monitoring are recommended.

MASKED HYPERTENSION—With an estimated prevalence of 10–25%, this is when home readings are higher than clinic readings. This can be from higher nocturnal or daytime pressures, especially in patients with high stress jobs. Ambulatory readings of more than 135/85 mm Hg with normal clinic readings will confirm the diagnosis. These patients appear to have higher cardiovascular risk than those without hypertension and at higher risk of developing hypertension in the future. Treatment includes lifestyle modifications with use of short-acting antihypertensive agents during the time of elevated readings.

B. Laboratory Findings

Patients with essential hypertension should undergo a limited work-up because extensive laboratory testing may be unrewarding.

1. Cardiac evaluation—Left ventricular hypertrophy (LVH) is an objective measure of both the severity and duration of hypertension and has been associated with higher cardiovascular morbidity and mortality. It should be routinely evaluated in all patients with an electrocardiogram although an echocardiogram appears to be a better predictor of future cardiovascular events. Other initial laboratory tests include a 9–12 hour fasting lipid profile that includes high-density lipoprotein (HDL), low-density lipoprotein (LDL), and triglycerides, hematocrit, and glucose to assess other risk factors for heart disease.

2. Kidney function tests—Current recommendations for evaluation of kidney function include a serum blood urea nitrogen and creatinine, estimated glomerular filtration rate (GFR), electrolytes, and spot urinalysis to detect red blood cells, white blood cells, casts, or proteinuria. Optional tests include measurement of urine albumin excretion or albumin/creatinine ratio and microalbuminuria (protein excretion between 30 and 300 mg/day). Note: All patients with even trace positive protein on routine dipstick should have a spot urine albumin: creatinine checked.

These tests should to assess if work-up for secondary causes of hypertension is warranted.

C. Special Examinations

The initial clinic evaluation of a person with elevated BP readings should include the following objectives:

- Determine an accurate diagnosis of hypertension.
- Define the presence or absence of TOD related to hypertension (see Essentials of Diagnosis).
- Screen for other cardiovascular (CV) risk factors or comorbidity that often accompany hypertension (Table 40–2).
- Stratify the risk for cardiovascular disease.
- Assess the likelihood of secondary hypertension and initiate further diagnostic testing to confirm or exclude the diagnosis.
- Obtain data that may be helpful in the choice of therapy and prognosis.

The most important aspects of the history include the natural history of the hypertension, aggravating factors, the extent of TOD, and the presence of other risk factors. Clinical clues suggestive of the possible presence of secondary hypertension must be recognized. The main goals of the physical examination are to evaluate for features of TOD and for evidence of secondary hypertension. Key areas include verification of the BP in the contralateral arm, fundoscopy, body mass index, waist circumference, auscultation for carotid, abdominal, and femoral bruits, and detection of lower extremity edema.

Table 40–2. Cardiovascular risk factors and target-organ damage associated with hypertension.

Major risk factors
Cigarette smoking
Obesity (body mass index ≥30)
Physical inactivity
Dyslipidemia
Diabetes mellitus
Microalbuminuria or chronic kidney disease
Age (men >55 years or women >65 years)
Family history of premature cardiovascular disease (men >55 years or women >65 years)
Target-organ damage
Left ventricular hypertrophy
Angina pectoris or prior myocardial infarction
Prior coronary revascularization
Congestive heart failure
Chronic kidney disease
Stroke or transient ischemic attack
Peripheral artery disease
Retinopathy

▶ Complications

Hypertension is associated with major cardiovascular risks such as cardiovascular disease, congestive heart failure, LVH, stroke, chronic kidney disease (CKD), and end-stage renal disease.

▶ Treatment

The primary goal of antihypertensive therapy is to reduce cardiovascular and renal morbidity and mortality using the least intrusive means possible. Indeed, in clinical trials adequate BP control has been associated with mean reductions of more than 50% in the incidence of congestive heart failure, more than 20% in myocardial infarction, and more than 35% in stroke.

The Expert Panel Report released management guidelines in 2014 that recommended target blood pressure goals for different subgroups of the population as determined by evidence from randomized controlled trials. All adults regardless of the presence of DM or CKD should have a goal blood pressure of less than 140/90 mm Hg. Since those guidelines came out, the SPRINT trial (A Randomized Trial of Intensive versus Standard Blood-Pressure Control) demonstrated, in those at high cardiovascular risk but without DM, aiming for a systolic blood pressure of 120 mm Hg as compared to 140 mm Hg reduced cardiovascular events and death. Note that the way BP was measured in this trial is different than almost all office measurement and translates into a 5–10 mm Hg higher systolic pressure in office. Hence, the 120 goal is closer to 125–130 mm Hg as measured by most practices.

Additionally, the HOPE 3 trial demonstrates that reduce BP in people who are already normotensive does NOT provide additional cardiovascular benefit. Thus, both the long-term follow-up of the ACCORD trial and the SPRINT demonstrate reduction in cardiovascular events when BP is reduced well below a currently recommended goal of less than 140/90 mm Hg. In the updated ADA BP consensus report the evidence further demonstrates that those who can achieve a lower systolic BP in the range of 125–130 mm Hg will have further risk reduction. Note that measurement of office BP in both SPRINT and ACCORD is very different than routine office practice and can yield a systolic BP 7–10 mm Hg higher than seen in these trials.

Appropriate lifestyle modifications are strongly recommended for all patients with either prehypertension or hypertension. Antihypertensive medications should be started if the BP is not at goal despite an adequate trial of nonpharmacologic treatment. The initiation of two drugs should be strongly considered in all patients with a baseline BP of more than 20/10 mm Hg above goal or stage 2 hypertension. This strategy will increase the likelihood of achieving goal BP within a reasonable time but should be used cautiously in patients with diabetes and the elderly who are at a higher risk of developing orthostatic hypotension.

A. Life-Style Modification

The American Heart Association recommends weight loss for overweight or obese patients with hypertension, limitation of dietary sodium intake to less than 100 mEq/L/day (ie, 2.4 g of sodium or 6 g of sodium chloride) as part of the Dietary Approaches to Stop Hypertension (DASH) eating plan, and moderate alcohol intake of no more than two drinks per day. Increased physical activity such as brisk walking for at least 30 minutes for about 5 days/week is also advised (Table 40–3).

Assessment of adherence with a low-sodium diet requires use of a 24-hour urinary sodium as well as total creatinine to ensure adequate collection. As an estimate roughly 15 mg/kg creatinine reflects an adequate collection within about 10%. Spot urine sodium estimates are inaccurate and at best only correlate 65–70% with a 24-hour Sample.

Additionally, smoking cessation is also recommended to improve cardiovascular health. The benefits of these interventions include lowering BP, enhancement of antihypertensive efficacy, and reduction of cardiovascular risks.

Table 40–3. Lifestyle modifications to manage essential hypertension.[1]

Modification	Recommendation	Approximate Reduction in Systolic Blood Pressure[2]
Weight reduction	Maintain normal body weight (body mass index 18.5–24.9 kg/m^2	5–20 mm Hg/10 kg
Adopt DASH eating plan	Consume a diet rich in fruits, vegetables, and low-fat dairy products with a reduced content of saturated and total fat	8–14 mm Hg
Dietary sodium reduction	Reduce dietary sodium intake to no more than 100 mmol/day (2.4 g sodium or 6 g sodium chloride)	2–8 mm Hg
Physical activity	Engage in regular aerobic physical activity such as brisk walking (at least 30 minutes/day, most days of the week)	4–9 mm Hg
Moderation of alcohol consumption	Limit consumption to no more than two drinks (eg, 24 oz beer, 10 oz wine, or 3 oz 80-proof whiskey) per day in most men and to no more than one drink per day in women and in lighter-weight persons	2–4 mm Hg

[1]For overall cardiovascular risk reduction, stop smoking.
[2]The effects of implementing these modifications are dose and time dependent and could be greater for some individuals. DASH, dietary approaches to stop hypertension.

B. Pharmacologic Treatment

Multiple clinical trials have convincingly shown that reduction of BP by most antihypertensive agents will reduce the cardiovascular and renal morbidity and mortality associated with hypertension. The JNC 8 recommends using any of several first line agents or their combination in the treatment of hypertension. In the general nonblack population, thiazide-type diuretics, calcium channel blockers (CCBs), renin-angiotensin system (RAS) blockers, such as ACE inhibitors and ARBs, can be used. In the general the African–American population is recommended to have first line agents as CCBs and thiazide- type diuretics (chlorthalidone or indapamide). Most patients will need two or more antihypertensive agents to achieve the recommended BP goal. Treatment can be started with one medication with up titration of its dose as needed, or a combination of two agents can be used especially if the initial blood pressure is more than 20/10 mm Hg above goal. Other antihypertensive agents can be added sequentially or substituted at monthly intervals until the BP goal is reached (Figure 40–1). If combination therapy is needed, use of CCBs and RAS blockers have been found to improve cardiovascular outcomes in high-risk patients. After the BP goal, has been achieved and remains stable, patients can be followed up at 3- to 6-month intervals.

C. Treatment of Specific Clinical Conditions

The general recommendations for initial therapy should be adapted for clinical conditions in which specific antihypertensive agents have been shown to be beneficial by outcome data from clinical trials. These include the demonstration that renin–angiotensin–aldosterone blockers such as ACE inhibitors or ARBs improve outcome in high-cardiovascular risk settings such as patients with diabetes mellitus, congestive heart failure, myocardial infarction, stroke, CKD, or albuminuria and that β-blockers improve survival in patients with systolic heart failure and prior myocardial infarction.

1. Diabetes and hypertension—The combination of hypertension and diabetes significantly increases the risk of cardiovascular events and end-stage renal disease compared to either risk factor alone. Recent clinical outcome trials and

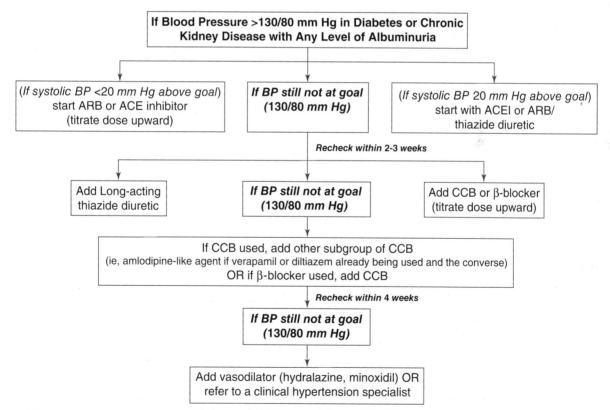

▲ **Figure 40–1.** Algorithm for the management of essential hypertension in kidney disease. ACE, angiotensin-converting enzyme; ACEI, ACE inhibitors; ARB, angiotensin receptor blockers; BP, blood pressure; CCB, calcium channel blockers.

guidelines have solidified the role of RAS blockers in delaying the progression of diabetic nephropathy among those with pre-existing diabetic nephropathy, that is, more than 300 mg/day albuminuria and eGFR less than 60 mL/min/1.73 m². In the absence of nephropathy RAS blockers are an option to control blood pressure along with calcium antagonists and thiazide type diuretics. Combinations of two or more antihypertensive drugs are usually needed to achieve the recommended goal BP of less than 140/90 mm Hg and for those with nephropathy less than 130/80 mm Hg. If the BP goal is not achieved other drugs such as CCBs, diuretics, and vasodilating β-blockers are added until goal BP is attained. Two agents blocking the RAS system should not be used together.

2. Congestive heart failure (CHF)—Hypertension is a major risk factor for the development of both systolic and diastolic heart failure. For many patients, LVH is an important intermediate step, resulting in "hypertensive heart disease" with impaired LV filling and increased ventricular stiffness. The BP goal for most patients with CHF is less than 140/90 mm Hg. Asymptomatic patients with "reduced LV function" [left ventricular ejection fraction (LVEF) <40%] improve both their BP and long-term prognosis with an ACEI and β-blocker while patients with symptomatic systolic heart failure will require additional agents such as ARBs, aldosterone antagonists, and loop diuretics. The use of a new agent class of angiotensin receptor-neprilysin inhibitors can also be used in those with reduced LV function and symptomatic heart failure instead of ACEI and ARBs. Treatment of hypertension in CHF patients with preserved LV function has not been as well studied. In general, β-blockers, ACEI/ARBs, diuretics, or nondihydropyridine (DHP)-CCBs are recommended for treatment however major trials are lacking.

3. Coronary artery disease (CAD)—The coexistence of CAD and hypertension is an indication for therapy with multiple antihypertensive drugs to achieve a goal BP of less than 140/90 mm Hg. In patients with hypertension and stable angina, β-blockers are strongly recommended but long-acting CCBs are suitable and effective alternatives based on the results of outcome trials such as the International Verapamil/Trandolapril Study in which more than 22,000 patients with hypertension and coronary disease were randomized to either atenolol or verapamil. Patients with acute coronary syndromes or post-myocardial infarction should be initially treated with ACE inhibitors, β-blockers, and aldosterone antagonists. Additional recommendations include intensive treatment of dyslipidemia (to achieve or exceed an LDL-cholesterol target of <100 mg/dL) and anti-platelet therapy with aspirin.

4. Left ventricular hypertrophy (LVH)—LVH is a well-recognized independent risk factor for cardiovascular events and premature death. It is common in the elderly and is often associated with diastolic dysfunction. Intensive BP management with agents that induce regression of LVH and reduce BP to a goal of less than 140/90 mm Hg is recommended. Medical treatment includes use of ACEI/ARBs and CCBs were better at reducing LV mass than beta-blockers.

5. Stroke—In acute ischemic stroke, the optimal level of BP is controversial. Acute lowering of the BP may lead to a reduction in blood flow to "watershed" areas of the brain with worsening of the neurologic function. In this setting, control of BP to is recommended at less than 220/120 mm Hg, unless fibrinolytic therapy needed then target less than 180/105 mm Hg. In stable patients, ACE inhibitors and thiazide diuretics are recommended to reduce recurrence of stroke. Target blood pressure should be less than 140/90 mm Hg; however, there may be some benefit in reducing recurrence of stroke with blood pressure of less than 130/80 mm Hg.

6. Chronic kidney disease—Most patients with CKD have hypertension and the therapeutic goals are to slow the progression of renal disease and to prevent cardiovascular disease. Optimal BP control to a goal of less than 140/90 mm Hg is recommended by guidelines. Among those with less than 300 mg of albuminuria less than 130/80 mm Hg is recommended. ACE inhibitors and ARBs are recommended for initial therapy because they have been shown to retard the progression of both diabetic and nondiabetic renal disease. An increase of the serum creatinine level by as much as 35% over baseline after initiation of these drugs should not lead to discontinuation because of the long-term benefits of these agents. For increases of serum creatinine larger than 35%, an assessment for concomitant nonsteroidal anti-inflammatory drug (NSAID) use, volume depletion, and/or renovascular hypertension is appropriate. Most patients will require three or more BP drugs to achieve the goal BP and thiazide diuretics are substituted with loop diuretics when the estimated GFR is less than 30 mL/min/1.73 m².

7. Albuminuria/proteinuria—In all patients with hypertension, albuminuria or proteinuria is an established risk marker for progression of renal disease and has also emerged as an independent marker of cardiovascular risk. Recent pharmacologic interventions with agents that lower BP and reduce albuminuria have resulted in a significant delay and even an arrest in the progression of microalbuminuria to CKD. Moreover, a reduction in proteinuria of more than 50% from baseline following 6 months of treatment reduces the risk of end-stage renal disease by 72% at 5 years. Current guidelines recommend that patients with hypertension and albuminuria should be started on agents that block the RAS system, such as ACE inhibitors or ARBs. Although it has also been shown that maximal dose combinations of ACE inhibitors and ARBs agents further reduce albuminuria by an additional 30–35% over either agent alone, this has not been shown to improve renal outcome and increased risk of adverse effects such as hyperkalemia. Nondihydropyridine CCBs such as verapamil or diltiazem also reduce proteinuria in patients with hypertension with proteinuric kidney disease, and have additive effects when combined with ACE inhibitors.

KEY READINGS

Agarwal R: Implications of blood pressure measurement technique for implementation of Systolic Blood Pressure Intervention Trial (SPRINT). J Am Heart Assoc 2017;6. pii: e004536.

Ando K: Increased salt sensitivity in obese hypertension: role of the sympathetic nervous system. Curr Hypertens Rev 2014;9:264.

Ando K, Fujita T: Pathophysiology of salt sensitivity hypertension. Ann Med 2012;44:S119.

Bakris GL et al: Differential effects of calcium antagonist subclasses on markers of nephropathy progression. Kidney Int 2004;65:1991.

Bakris GL: The Implications of blood pressure measurement methods on treatment targets for blood pressure. Circulation 2016;134:904.

Bakris GL, Weir MR: Angiotensin-converting enzyme inhibitor-associated elevations in serum creatinine: is this a cause for concern? Arch Intern Med 2000;160:685.

Benavente OR et al: Blood-pressure targets in patients with recent lacunar stroke: the SPS3 randomised trial. Lancet 2013;382:507.

Booth JN 3rd, et al: Evaluation of Criteria to Detect Masked Hypertension. J Clin Hypertens (Greenwich) 2016;18:1086.

Brostrom A et al: Sex-Specific Associations Between Self-reported Sleep Duration, Cardiovascular Disease, Hypertension, and Mortality in an Elderly Population. J Cardiovasc Nurs 2017; online.

Chobanian AV et al: The Seventh Report of the Joint National Committee on the Detection, Evaluation, and Treatment of High Blood Pressure (JNC 7). JAMA 2003;289:2560.

de Zeeuw D et al: Proteinuria, a target for renoprotection in patients with type 2 diabetic nephropathy: lessons from RENAAL. Kidney Int 2004;65:2309.

Eckel RH et al: 2013 AHA/ACC guideline on lifestyle management to reduce cardiovascular risk: a report of the American College of Cardiology/American Heart Association Task Force on Practice Guidelines. Circulation 2014;129:S76.

Erdem F et al: A new diagnostic tool for masked hypertension: impaired sleep quality. Arch Med Sci 2016;12:1207.

Fihn SD et al: 2012 ACCF/AHA/ACP/AATS/PCNA/SCAI/STS guideline for the diagnosis and management of patients with stable ischemic heart disease: a report of the American College of Cardiology Foundation/American Heart Association task force on practice guidelines, and the American College of Physicians, American Association for Thoracic Surgery, Preventive Cardiovascular Nurses Association, Society for Cardiovascular Angiography and Interventions, and Society of Thoracic Surgeons. Circulation 2012;126:e354.

Fried LF et al: Combined angiotensin inhibition for the treatment of diabetic nephropathy. N Engl J Med 2013;369:1892.

Gradman AH et al. American Society of Hypertension Writing G: Combination therapy in hypertension. J Clin Hypertens (Greenwich) 2011;13:146.

Guo X et al: Epidemiological evidence for the link between sleep duration and high blood pressure: a systematic review and meta-analysis. Sleep Med 2013;14:324.

Hirsch S et al: Tolerating increases in the serum creatinine following aggressive treatment of chronic kidney disease, hypertension and proteinuria: pre-renal success. Am J Nephrol 2012;36:430.

Jamerson K et al: Benazepril plus amlodipine or hydrochlorothiazide for hypertension in high-risk patients. N Engl J Med 2008;359:2417.

James PA et al: 2014 evidence-based guideline for the management of high blood pressure in adults: report from the panel members appointed to the Eighth Joint National Committee (JNC 8). JAMA 2014;311:507.

Jauch EC et al: Guidelines for the early management of patients with acute ischemic stroke: a guideline for healthcare professionals from the American Heart Association/American Stroke Association. Stroke 2013;44:870.

Klingbeil AU et al: A meta-analysis of the effects of treatment on left ventricular mass in essential hypertension. Am J Med 2003;115:41.

Lewington S et al: Age-specific relevance of usual blood pressure to vascular mortality: a meta-analysis of individual data for one million adults in 61 prospective studies. Lancet 2002;360:1903.

Lima NK, Moriguti JC, Ferriolli E: Uncontrolled hypertension in older patients: Markers and associated factors to masked and white-coat effect. J Geriatr Cardiol 2016;13:672.

Margolis KL et al: Outcomes of combined cardiovascular risk factor management strategies in type 2 diabetes: the ACCORD randomized trial. Diabetes Care 2014;37:1721.

Niiranen TJ et al: Home-measured blood pressure is a stronger predictor of cardiovascular risk than office blood pressure: the Finn-Home study. Hypertension 2010;55:1346.

Pepine CJ et al: A calcium antagonist vs a non-calcium antagonist hypertension treatment strategy for patients with coronary artery disease. The International Verapamil-Trandolapril Study (INVEST): a randomized controlled trial. JAMA 2003;290:2805.

Pickering TG, Shimbo D, Haas D: Ambulatory blood-pressure monitoring. N Engl J Med 2006;354:2368.

Ruggenenti P, Remuzzi G: Dealing with renin-angiotensin inhibitors, don't mind serum creatinine. Am J Nephrol 2012;36:427.

Standards of Medical Care in Diabetes-2017: Summary of Revisions. Diabetes Care 2017;40:S4.

Sternlicht H, Bakris GL: Hypertension and chronic kidney disease. IN: Bakris GL, Sorrentino M (eds). *Hypertension-Companion to Braunwald's The Heart*, 3rd ed. Elsevier, Philadelphia, 2018, pp. 311-320.

Sternlicht H, Bakris GL: The kidney in hypertension. Med Clin North Am 2017;101:207.

Stewart DL et al: Stress and salt sensitivity in primary hypertension. Curr Hypertens Rep 2015;17:2.

Thomas SJ, Calhoun D: Sleep, insomnia, and hypertension: current findings and future directions. J Am Soc Hypertens 2017;11:122.

Vakili BA, Okin PM, Devereux RB: Prognostic implications of left ventricular hypertrophy. Am Heart J 2001;141:334.

Uhlig K et al: Self-measured blood pressure monitoring in the management of hypertension: a systematic review and meta-analysis. Ann Intern Med 2013;159:185.

Uzu T et al: High sodium intake is associated with masked hypertension in Japanese patients with type 2 diabetes and treated hypertension. Am J Hypertens 2012;25:1170.

Wright JT Jr et al: A Randomized Trial of Intensive versus Standard Blood-Pressure Control. N Engl J Med 2015;373:2103.

Yano Y, Bakris GL: Recognition and management of masked hypertension: a review and novel approach. J Am Soc Hypertens 2013;7:244.

Yancy CW et al: 2016 ACC/AHA/HFSA Focused Update on New Pharmacological Therapy for Heart Failure: An Update of the 2013 ACCF/AHA Guideline for the Management of Heart Failure: A Report of the American College of Cardiology/American

Heart Association Task Force on Clinical Practice Guidelines and the Heart Failure Society of America. Circulation 2016;134:e282.

Yoon SS, Carroll MD, Fryar CD: Hypertension Prevalence and Control Among Adults: United States, 2011–2014. NCHS Data Brief 2015;1.

Yusuf S et al: Blood-pressure and cholesterol lowering in Persons without cardiovascular disease. N Engl J Med 2016;374:2032.

Ziegler MG, Milic M: Sympathetic nerves and hypertension in stress, sleep apnea, and caregiving. Curr Opin Nephrol Hypertens 2017;26:26.

■ CHAPTER REVIEW QUESTIONS

1. A 67-year-old man with home BP—170/95 mm Hg, heart rate—56 and serum creatinine of 2.2 (eGFR = 38), presents for better management. He states the he is aware of low-sodium diet which he follows and sleeps well. Denies other lifestyle issues that could affect his BP. Other medical problems include hypercholesterolemia which is well controlled with rosuvastatin 10 mg daily. He denies sleep apnea with a negative sleep study and is not obese. His current BP meds include clonidine 0.2 mg twice daily, metoprolol tartrate 50 mg twice daily and HCTZ 12.5 mg daily. You switch the metoprolol tartrate to metoprolol succinate 100 mg daily and start to taper the clonidine as well as increase HCTZ to 25 mg daily. Additionally, you start amlodipine 10 mg daily. The patient returns in 2 weeks off clonidine with a BP 148/88 mm Hg and heart rate of 64 and repeat eGFR-35 mL/min. Which of the following is an appropriate way to achieve BP goal in this patient?
   A. Switch to chlorthalidone 25 mg daily from HCTZ
   B. Increase the metoprolol to 200 mg daily
   C. Add a RAS blocker to the regimen
   D. Add spironolactone
   E. Switch to furosemide 40 mg daily

2. A 62-year-old, black woman presents with a BP of 154/90 mm Hg but was previously well controlled in the range of 125–130 mm Hg for many years with amlodipine 5 mg and ramipril 5 mg daily. She has gained 30 lbs in the last 2 years and is not exercising anymore due to a recent leg sprain. Additionally, she has been eating out more due to her job. Her examination is remarkable for pedal edema 1+ but no new findings. Which of the following could be contributing to her elevated BP?
   A. Increased job stress
   B. Increased weight
   C. Increased weight and salt intake
   D. Decreased exercise
   E. She is getting older and hence BP goes higher

3. A 58-year-old African–American man presents with a long history of poor blood pressure control and nonadherence to medications. Now states he is concerned because he was told he has kidney disease. Past history positive for 30 pack year (py) smoking history but stopped 6 years ago and hypercholesterolemia but was taking atorvastatin 10 mg daily. Physical examination-BP 168/100 mm Hg, pulse 84 and regular, BMI-31, remaining examination positive for pedal edema 1+ and 2/6 systolic murmur at apex. Labs-eGFR 50 mL/min/1.73 m^2 serum creatinine 1.4 mg/dL, K=3.8 mEq/L, all other labs are normal. Renal ultrasound shows no evidence of renal artery stenosis. Medicines: Amlodipine 5 mg, lisinopril 40 mg/day and HCTZ 25 mg daily (patient admits to only taking all these medicines over last week). You decide to make the following changes: Increase amlodipine to 10 mg daily, change lisinopril to olmesartan 40 mg daily, change HCTZ to chlorthalidone 25 mg daily and add spironolactone 25 mg daily. Patient instructed to check BP at home. He returns in one month with BP 134/82 mm Hg and heart rate 76 and regular and no orthostasis. Repeat labs: K = 4.4 mEq/L, serum creatinine 1.7 mg/dL, eGFR = 40 mL/min.

   Which of the following is the next appropriate step in the care of this patient?
   A. Stop the olmesartan because renal function got worse
   B. Stop spironolactone because over volume depleted
   C. Continue present therapy as BP controlled and creatinine did not rise by 30%
   D. Stop olmesartan and start a beta blocker because heart is still elevated
   E. Call for a nephrology consult

4. A 76-year-old woman has been having trouble sleeping for the past few months, comes in because she is concerned about her blood pressure being high and fluctuating during the day. She denies other issues including snoring and had a sleep apnea study a year earlier that was negative. She says she feels fine other than being tired and wanting sleep in the afternoon. PMH unremarkable except for arthritis and hypertension × 26 years. Her physical examination is unremarkable except for BP 172/84 mm Hg, heart rate 92 otherwise unremarkable BMI-27. Current meds include: amlodipine 10 mg daily, losartan 100 mg daily and HCTZ 25 mg daily. Her labs are normal including K = 4.3 mEq/L and eGFR = 62 mL/min/1.73m^2.

Which of the following would be the best approach to reduce blood pressure variability in this patient?

A. Dose medications at night
B. Start spironolactone
C. Change HCTZ to chlorthalidone and dose losartan twice daily
D. Given sleep medication such as trazadone or zolpidem to improve sleep
E. Refer for another sleep apnea study

5. A 72-year-old Caucasian woman presents with a complaint of BP always being elevated at night around 7–10 pm. She states it gets as high as 170–180 mm Hg while in the morning when awakening it is 130–140 mm Hg. She has checked it through the day and finds it is fine until after dinner. She denies any other problem and states her lifestyle is stable but she has been going out more with her husband for dinner over the last month but always watches how much food she eats to avoid gaining weight. There have been no change in medications and all labs are stable and normal. There have also been no significant new findings on physical examination.

Which of the following most likely accounts for this lady's elevated pressure in evening?

A. She is having major disagreements with her spouse
B. She has gained weight although since she does not weigh herself has not noted it
C. She is eating much more sodium than she appreciates and has masked hypertension
D. She is wearing new support stockings that are elevating her pressure
E. She becomes more anxious about going out but has not told her spouse

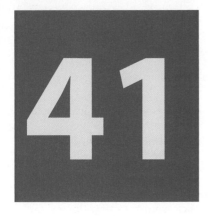

Secondary Hypertension

Debbie L. Cohen, MD

Muriel Ghosn, MD

Jonathan Suarez, MD

Raymond R. Townsend, MD

▼ INTRODUCTION

Secondary hypertension accounts for about 5–10% of all cases of hypertension with most hypertension being attributed to essential hypertension. It is important to identify patients early with secondary hypertension as timely diagnosis of secondary hypertension can result in potential cure or significant improvement in hypertension with improved quality of life and lower cardiovascular morbidity. Secondary hypertension should be suspected in the following patients (Table 41–1): initial presentation of hypertension at the extremes of age (<30 or >70 years of age), spontaneous hypokalemia, drug resistant hypertension (use of at least three medications at maximal tolerated dose with at least one medication being a diuretic), negative family history of hypertension, recent exacerbation of hypertension that has previously been well controlled, labile hypertension, symptoms of palpitations, sweating and headaches and differential BP in arms and legs. Patients with an identifiable secondary cause of hypertension typically present with a relatively abrupt onset of symptoms (BP ≥160/100 mm Hg) and with considerable target-organ damage (TOD). They typically do not respond as well to lowering BP and to antihypertensive drug therapy as do patients with primary hypertension. The BP-lowering response to specific antihypertensive drugs may offer important clues to the presence and type of secondary hypertension; for example, patients with early renovascular hypertension (RVHT) often have an impressive BP-lowering response to an angiotensin-converting enzyme (ACE) inhibitor or angiotension receptor blocker (ARB) and those with bilateral adrenal hyperplasia as a cause of primary aldosteronism respond well to spironolactone, but not vice versa. The initial evaluation for secondary hypertension is shown in Table 41–2 and will be discussed in detail in the chapter. The choice of tests and the order in which they are obtained depend not only on the pretest probability of the disease, but also on safety, availability, local expertise with the test, and its cost.

▼ RENOVASCULAR HYPERTENSION

Jonathan Suarez, MD

▶ General Considerations

A. Clinical Clues

Recognition of important clinical clues for RVHT is paramount in the clinical diagnosis of this condition. RVHT probably occurs in less than 1% of unscreened patients with mild hypertension; however, 10–30% of white patients with severe or refractory hypertension may have renal artery disease. One study found that among patients with resistant hypertension 24% had at least 50% stenosis by renal angiography. Pertinent clinical clues for RVHT are summarized in Table 41–3.

B. Epidemiology

Of the 5–10% of hypertensive patients with secondary hypertension, RVHT accounts for 0.2–3%. However, at autopsy the prevalence of anatomic RAS attributable to atherosclerosis in the elderly is quite common. In addition, studies have shown that patients with atherosclerosis have a significantly increased risk of death compared to patients without atherosclerosis. Clinically, atherosclerosis increases with age and may coexist in 20–25% of patients undergoing cardiac catheterization for coronary artery disease (CAD). Similarly, approximately 6–11% of patients with end-stage renal disease (ESRD) have a concomitant diagnosis of atherosclerotic renal artery stenosis (ARAS) and studies have shown that ARAS is associated with increased mortality compared to all other causes of ESRD, except diabetes mellitus. However, it is unclear whether

Table 41–1. Who to work up for secondary hypertension.

New onset hypertension at young age (<30 years old; >70 years old)

Negative family history of hypertension

Acute exacerbation of previously well controlled hypertension

Resistant hypertension (three drugs prescribed at optimal doses with one drug being a diuretic)

Spontaneous hypokalemia

Headaches, sweating, and palpitations

Epigastric bruit

Differential BP in arms and legs

Hypertension and an adrenal mass

Table 41–3. Clinical clues to renovascular hypertension.

Severe or refractory hypertension

Age of onset younger than 30 years or older than 55 years

Abrupt acceleration of stable hypertension

Severe hypertension in the setting of generalized atherosclerosis

Systolic–diastolic bruit in the epigastrium

Flash pulmonary edema

Unexplained azotemia ACE inhibitor- or ARB-induced renal dysfunction

ACE, angiotensin-converting enzyme; ARB, angiotensin receptor blocker.

the occlusive RAS was etiologic in the development of end-stage kidney failure.

C. Etiology

The etiology of renal artery stenosis (RAS) is usually attributable to atherosclerosis or fibromuscular disease (FMD). As can be seen in Table 41–4, atherosclerosis accounts for over 80% of RAS. It is generally seen in an older hypertensive population with concomitant diffuse atherosclerosis in other vascular beds (eg, coronary, carotids, and peripheral circulation). The RAS lesion due to atherosclerosis occurs at the ostium or in the proximal 2 cm of the renal artery. In contrast, FMD accounts for 10–20% of RAS and is typically seen in young to middle aged female hypertensive patients. FMD affects not only the renal arteries, but also medium sized arteries like the carotid arteries and the lesion is typically located in the mid and distal portion of the artery. FMD appears like a "string of beads" on angiography.

▶ Pathogenesis

The pathophysiology of RVHT is best explained by the sentinel animal experiments by Goldblatt. These animal models consist of occluding one or both renal arteries with

constricting clips. The two-kidney one-clip (2K-1C) model represents unilateral RAS whereas the two-kidney two-clip (2K-2C) model represents bilateral RAS. The mechanism of development of hypertension is mediated via the renin–angiotensin–aldosterone system (RAAS) with salt and water retention. In unilateral RAS (2K-1C model), renal perfusion pressure is decreased in the kidney distal to the stenosis, which leads to increased renin production, which in turn forms angiotensin II (AT II). AT II causes vasoconstriction directly and also stimulates aldosterone production, which causes salt and water retention. The normal contralateral kidney undergoes a pressure natriuresis, which maintains volume status. Due to the constantly elevated levels of renin in the 2K-1C model, this form of RAS is referred to as renin-mediated.

On the other hand, in the 2K-2C or 1K-1C models representing bilateral RAS or RAS to a solitary kidney,

Table 41–2. Initial evaluation for secondary hypertension.

Plasma renin and serum aldosterone levels

Plasma or urine metanephrine levels

Sleep study

Renal Doppler

CT angiogram/MR angiogram

TSH

24 urine cortisol (if indicated)

Table 41–4. Etiology of renovascular hypertension.

Cause	Prevalence (%)	Clues/Characteristics
Atherosclerosis (ASO)	70	Older patients (>55 years of age) Concomitant diffuse ASO in other vascular beds Ostial or proximal (2 cm) renal artery lesions
Fibromuscular dysplasia (FMD)	20	Younger to middle aged women Unclear etiology
Others		Extrinsic compression by tumor Retroperitoneal mass Arterial dissection Vasculitis Aneurysm

there is an initial increase in renin, which in turn causes an increase in AT II and aldosterone. As in the model described, resultant salt and water retention occurs, but the absence of a normal contralateral kidney prevents pressure natriuresis. Suppression of renin occurs due to volume expansion attributed to the increases in salt and water retention. This form of hypertension is considered volume mediated, whereas the 2K-1C model of unilateral RAS is renin mediated.

It has been demonstrated that oxygenation in the kidney is preserved even with a 50% reduction in blood flow to the renal arteries. However, as blood flow worsens beyond this point it leads to renal cortical hypoxia, which causes inflammation and fibrosis. As the inflammation and fibrosis progresses there is irreversible damage to the kidney even with restoration of blood flow with revascularization.

A. What Is Significant Stenosis?

Stenosis that causes hemodynamic changes with a reduction in renal perfusion pressure is called critical stenosis. In humans, hemodynamically significant stenosis is defined by more than 70% angiographic stenosis or 50–70% angiographic stenosis associated with a resting mean pressure gradient more than 10 mm Hg, systolic hyperemic pressure gradient more than 20 mm Hg or renal fractional flow reserve less than 0.8. Lesions that are not hemodynamically significant should only be considered for revascularization in rare occasions.

▶ Clinical Findings

The two major goals of the evaluation of the hypertensive patient are to recognize clinical clues for secondary forms of hypertension and to identify evidence of TOD from the hypertension. The clinical clues suggestive of RVHT are listed in Table 41–3.

A. Symptoms and Signs

RVHT should be suspected in patients presenting with severe, sudden-onset hypertension prior to 30 years of age or after 55 years of age. For reasons that are not well understood, RVHT is relatively less common in African-Americans in whom severe hypertension is most frequently essential. Because FMD occurs most frequently in younger to middle aged females, those presenting with hypertension before 30 years of age should be suspected of having RVHT. However, RVHT due to atherosclerosis is likely to present in older patients with significant hypertension in the setting of generalized atherosclerosis in other vascular beds. Malignant hypertension with neurologic symptoms and advanced fundoscopic changes with papilledema should raise the possibility of RVHT. Similarly, severe or refractory hypertension defined as hypertension requiring three or more drugs as well as severe hypertension with heart failure/flash pulmonary edema may also be one of the presenting features of RVHT. Importantly, this sudden onset of worsening azotemia after the institution of an ACE inhibitor or ARB should suggest RVHT, especially bilateral RAS or RAS with a solitary functioning kidney.

The presence of severe stage II hypertension (>160–100 mm Hg) may be a critical clue to the presence of RVHT. The presence of an abdominal bruit in the setting of increased BP is also a strong clinical clue to RAS. The bruit is systolic–diastolic in nature and is located near the epigastrium. This is seen more commonly in FMD and, in fact, correlates with surgical outcomes. However; the absence of such a bruit does not exclude RAS. The presence of stage III or IV hypertensive retinopathy on fundus examination is highly suggestive of RVHT. Evidence of diffuse atherosclerosis in the peripheral vascular, coronary, and cerebral vascular beds may be suggestive of RVHT due to ARAS in the older hypertensive population.

By definition RVHT requires an elevation of BP due to the activation of the renin–angiotensin system in the setting of renal artery occlusive disease. The diagnosis of RVHT can be made only if BP improves after a correction of RAS, thereby making RVHT a retrospective diagnosis. The primary goal in screening for RVHT is to identify a subset of patients who may have a reversible hemodynamic cause of their hypertension and/or renal dysfunction. Table 41–5 summarizes the specificity and sensitivity of these diagnostic modalities.

Table 41–5. Specificity and sensitivity.

Test	Sensitivity (%)	Specificity (%)
Plasma renin activity (PRA)	50–80	84
Functional studies		
Captopril PRA	74	89
Captopril scintigraphy/ renography	85–90	93–98
Anatomic studies		
Duplex ultrasound scanning	90	90–95
Spiral (helical) computed tomography scanning	98	94
Magnetic resonance	90–100	76–94
Angiography		

Modified with permission from Nally JV et al: Advances in non-invasive screening for renovascular disease. Cleve Clin J Med 1994;61:328.

B. Laboratory Findings

1. Electrolytes—Hypokalemia may be a surrogate marker of hemodynamically significant renal artery occlusive disease secondary to stimulation of the renin–angiotensin system with secondary hyperaldosteronism. The hyperaldosteronism results in urinary sodium retention and kaliuresis, which may be responsible for the development of hypokalemia.

2. Renal function—RVHT may be seen in patients with or without renal dysfunction. RVHT and possible ischemic nephropathy may be suspected in patients with unexplained azotemia occurring in the setting of generalized atherosclerosis and asymmetric kidney sizes (possibly due to the occlusive RAS). There may also be presence of mild-to-moderate proteinuria. As noted previously, azotemia following the administration of an ACE inhibitor or ARB is a strong clinical clue suggestive of hemodynamically significant renal artery disease.

C. Imaging Studies

1. Renal scintigraphy/renography and captopril scintigraphy/renography—These are very rarely used due to modern imaging techniques.

2. Magnetic resonance angiography—A noninvasive method of defining the renal artery vasculature includes magnetic resonance angiography (MRA), use of gadolinium MRA has been shown to significantly improve the images of the distal arteries and accessory renal arteries. Although gadolinium-enhanced MRA has previously been suggested to be an alternative non-nephrotoxic method in defining the renal artery vasculature, its use should be avoided in those with renal dysfunction (creatinine clearance <30 mL/min) due to the well-described association between gadolinium and the development of nephrogenic fibrosing dermopathy (NFD) and nephrogenic systemic fibrosis (NSF). MRA may not be as useful in detecting FMD as compared to renal angiography due to the increased spatial resolution of MRA (1 mm versus 200 vm).

3. Spiral (helical) computed tomography scanning—High quality images, as well as three-dimensional images, of the renal arteries can be obtained using CT angiography. Unfortunately, as with conventional renal angiography, contrast media must be administered and is only recommended in patients with a creatinine clearance more than 60 mL/min. CT angiography is preferred when screening for FMD.

4. Duplex ultrasound scanning—A diagnosis of RAS by Doppler ultrasound is made when there is a 3.5 times greater flow velocity at the site of stenosis. In addition, the presence of a parvus tardus velocity waveform in the artery distal to the stenosis increases the sensitivity of the study.

Renal resistive indices are also provided by duplex ultrasound. Resistive indices approximate the amount of renal arterial impedance. One study showed that in patients with RAS, an increase in renal resistive index more than 80% is associated with poorer post-revascularization outcome as well as an increased risk of progressive renal dysfunction. However, follow-up studies have showed conflicting results. Another drawback to duplex ultrasound scanning is that the procedure is operator dependent due to its high technical demands.

5. Renal artery angiography—is considered the gold standard to confirm the diagnosis of hemodynamically significant RAS and should be performed when a definitive diagnosis is required or when an interventional procedure is being considered.

▶ Treatment

The goals of therapy are optimal control of hypertension, reduction of risks of cardiovascular events and preservation of renal function, which can be achieved either through medical therapy, percutaneous renal angioplasty (PTRAS) with or (PTRA) without stenting, or renovascular bypass surgery.

A. Medical Therapy

Medical therapy is the preferred first-line treatment for RAS. The medical management of RVHT is similar to that of primary hypertension, yet three important distinctions exist: (1) hypertension may be more difficult to control and often requires multiple medications from different classes, (2) vigilant attention must be given to preserving kidney function, and (3) coexistent atherosclerotic cardiac and carotid disease are more prevalent and may require specific intervention. The response to a specific drug may be variable and highly individualized. All patients with RVHT may not readily respond to antihypertensive therapy. Current medical therapy also includes statins and antiplatelet therapy in addition to antihypertensives.

B. Antihypertensive Therapy

1. Angiotensin-converting enzyme inhibitors (ACEIs) and angiotensin II receptor blockers (ARBs)—Most research related to medical therapy of RVHT has been related to the use of ACEIs and ARBs. To achieve optimal control of hypertension, these agents are often combined with other antihypertensive agents. In patients with bilateral RAS or RAS with a single functioning kidney. Use of an ACEI or ARB should be done with caution and should have close monitoring of serum electrolytes and serum creatinine. A large cohort study involving over 3000 patients with RVHT showed that ACEI use was associated with decreased death, myocardial infarction or stroke, decreased number of hospitalizations for heart failure, and decreased number of patients requiring initiation of dialysis when compared to patients that were not prescribed an ACEI. However, use of ACEI did demonstrate twice the number episodes of acute kidney injury per 100 patient years. Even with the increased risk of acute kidney injury ACEIs and ARBs are still considered by many as the primary therapy for these patients.

2. Calcium channel blockers—Calcium channel blockers (CCBs) are effective in lowering the BP in patients with RVHT. They also maintain renal blood flow through vasodilation in the afferent arteriole. The benefit of using CCBs in RVHT is they have a more favorable effect on renal function compared to an ACE inhibitor. They can be used safely in patients with bilateral RAS without concern for a significant decline in the GFR.

C. Revascularization

1. Percutaneous renal artery intervention—Selected patients with RAS may benefit from percutaneous revascularization. Renal angiography with or without renal artery stenting has become the major form of renal revascularization. Recommendations vary as to whether the RAS is due to FMD or to atherosclerosis.

2. Percutaneous renal artery intervention for fibromuscular dysplasia—PTRA is the initial choice in younger patients with FMD. Correction is indicated to control hypertension and to prevent progressive renal disease. Results for percutaneous intervention in the majority of patients with FMD have been very good and are preferred over surgical therapy in most cases.

3. Percutaneous renal artery intervention for atherosclerotic renal artery stenosis—The current options for treatment of ARAS are medical therapy or renal artery vascularization with continued medical therapy with PTRAS as the preferred method for revascularization. There have been two large randomized clinical trials comparing these two therapies.

The Angioplasty and Stenting for Renal Artery Lesion (ASTRAL) trial involved 806 patients who were randomized to medical therapy alone or in combination with PTRAS. The study population consisted of patients with a mean age of 70 years, mean RAS percentage of 75%, mean eGFR of 40 mL/min/1.73 m^2 and mean baseline systolic blood pressure (SBP) of about 150 mm Hg. The patients were followed for 5 years and results showed no statistically significant differences in all-cause mortality, kidney function and SBP control. In addition, patients who underwent PTRAS experienced 23 serious complications, including two deaths and three amputations of toes or limbs.

The Cardiovascular Outcomes with Renal Atherosclerotic Lesions (CORAL) trial involved 947 patients who were randomized to medical therapy alone or in combination with PTRAS. The study population consisted of patients with a mean age of 69 years, mean RAS of 67% (inclusion criteria: ARAS >80% or 60–80% with a systolic pressure gradient of at least 20 mm Hg), mean eGFR 57 mL/min/1.73 m^2 and mean baseline SBP of 150 mm Hg. The patients were followed for 3.6 years and the results showed no statistically significant differences in the composite end point (death from cardiovascular or renal causes, myocardial infarction, stroke, and hospitalization for congestive heart failure, progressive renal insufficiency, or the need for renal-replacement therapy) or all-cause mortality.

There has been criticism that these two trials may have underestimated the therapeutic benefits of PTRAS in certain subsets of patients. The ASTRAL trial was criticized for having potential selection bias due to providers' likely referring patients with severe disease directly for revascularization instead of the clinical trial. The ASTRAL trial also showed lower rates of ACEI and ARB use than expected and used noninvasive imaging instead of digital subtraction angiography to determine the severity of the stenosis. The CORAL trial was also criticized for likely withdrawal of patients with severe disease and inclusion of patients with mild stenosis who were less likely to benefit from PTRAS.

A recent prospective cohort study evaluating 467 patients with RAS more than 50% found that subgroups of patients presenting with flash pulmonary or rapidly declining kidney function with refractory hypertension had reduced risk for death in those patients treated with PTRAS compared to medical therapy.

4. Renal artery bypass surgery—Earlier reports had suggested a survival benefit for RAS patients who underwent renal artery bypass surgery versus medical therapy. However, these observations came from nonrandomized studies in which there was an inherent bias for healthier patients to undergo surgery. Most patients who are referred for surgery are likely to have had unsuccessful PTRAS or show extensive atherosclerosis in the aorta that will need additional repair.

D. Current Guidelines for Treatment

The American College of Cardiology (ACC)/American Heart Association (AHA) released guidelines in 2013 for the management of RAS. They currently recommend medical therapy as the first-line treatment for RAS with effective antihypertensive therapy (ACEI, ARBs, calcium channel blockers, and beta-blockers), statins and antiplatelet agents. Careful monitoring of serum creatinine and electrolytes should be done in patients with bilateral RAS or single functioning kidney when using ACEI or ARB.

Percutaneous revascularization is recommended in patients with hemodynamically significant RAS and either (1) recurrent congestive heart failure or flash pulmonary edema, (2) accelerated, resistant or malignant hypertension and intolerance to medication, (3) asymptomatic bilateral or single functioning kidney, or (4) progressive chronic kidney disease and bilateral RAS or single functioning kidney with RAS. For patients with FMD lesions, balloon angioplasty with bailout stent placement if necessary is a class I recommendation for treatment.

Surgical revascularization is recommended in (1) FMD associated with complex disease or macroaneurysms, (2) ARAS and multiple small renal arteries or early primary branching of the main renal artery, or (3) ARAS in combination with pararenal aortic reconstruction.

The European Society of Cardiology (ESC) developed guidelines in 2014 for the management of RAS. These guidelines are similar to the ACC/AHA guidelines with a few subtle differences. First, ACEI and ARB use are contraindicated for the treatment of bilateral RAS or when the lesion affects a single functioning kidney. Second, they suggest angioplasty, preferably with stenting, may be considered in the case of more than 60% symptomatic RAS secondary to atherosclerosis. Last, they suggest consideration of surgical revascularization for patients undergoing surgical repair of the aorta, patients with complex anatomy of the renal arteries or after a failed endovascular procedure.

Currently, randomized controlled trials do not show enough evidence to support PTRAS over medical therapy alone in most patients. However, observational studies have shown that certain subsets of patients such as those with flash pulmonary edema, worsening kidney function and refractory hypertension may benefit from PTRAS. Future clinical trials should focus on patients with severe disease and characteristics of potential benefit from revascularization.

KEY READINGS

Anderson JL et al: Management of patients with peripheral artery disease (compilation of 2005 and 2011 ACCF/AHA guideline recommendations): a report of the American College of Cardiology Foundation/American Heart Association Task Force on Practice Guidelines. Circulation 2013;127:1425.

Benjamin MM et al: Prevalence of and risk factors of renal artery stenosis in patients with resistant hypertension. Am J Cardiol 2014;113:687.

Cooper CJ et al: Stenting and medical therapy for atherosclerotic renal-artery stenosis. N Engl J Med 2014;370:13.

Parikh SA et al: SCAI expert consensus statement for renal artery stenting appropriate use. Catheter Cardiovasc Interv 2014;84:1163.

Ritchie J et al: High-risk clinical presentations in atherosclerotic renovascular disease: prognosis and response to renal artery revascularization. Am J Kidney Dis 2014;63:186.

Tendera M et al: ESC Guidelines on the diagnosis and treatment of peripheral artery diseases: document covering atherosclerotic disease of extracranial carotid and vertebral, mesenteric, renal, upper and lower extremity arteries: the Task Force on the Diagnosis and Treatment of Peripheral Artery Diseases of the European Society of Cardiology (ESC). Eur Heart J 2011;32:2851.

Textor SC, Lerman LO: Renal artery stenosis: medical versus interventional therapy. Curr Cardiol Rep 2013;15:409.

Wheatley K et al: Revascularization versus medical therapy for renal-artery stenosis. N Engl J Med 2009;361:1953.

ENDOCRINE HYPERTENSION

Muriel Ghosn, MD

Several endocrine organs produce hormones that participate in the control of blood pressure (BP) by the regulation of salt and water homeostasis or vascular tone. The mechanisms of hypertension vary according to the hormonal disorder and may be direct, for example, mineralocorticoid hypertension and pheochromocytoma (PCC) or indirect, as in hyperparathyroidism or acromegaly.

The adrenal gland produces mineralocorticoids predominantly aldosterone, glucocorticoids, and androgens. Aldosterone is secreted by the zona glomerulosa of the adrenal cortex and is primarily regulated by angiotensin II (AT II) and potassium and to a lesser extent ACTH. Aldosterone exerts its actions at the level of the kidney via the activation of the mineralocorticoid receptors in the distal nephron. This results in sodium retention coupled with the secretion of potassium and hydrogen ions. Despite the fact that plasma cortisol concentration is approximately 1000 fold that of aldosterone and although the mineralocorticoid receptor has a similar affinity to cortisol and aldosterone, the enzyme 11β-hydroxysteroid dehydrogenase type 2 converts the active cortisol into its inactive form, cortisone thereby preventing cortisol from exerting its mineralocorticoid activity and conferring a relative specificity of the mineralocorticoid receptor to aldosterone. The deficiency of 11β-hydroxysteroid dehydrogenase type 2 or its inhibition by certain substrates produces the syndrome of apparent mineralocorticoid excess (AME) that is clinically identical to that of aldosterone excess; with the main difference that aldosterone is suppressed, as is its major secretagogue, AT II. Thus mineralocorticoid hypertension is defined by the excessive activation of the receptor, not the identity of the steroid, and is classified as low renin, high aldosterone hypertension and low renin, low aldosterone hypertension (Table 41–6).

Table 41–6. Causes of mineralocorticoid hypertension.

Increased mineralocorticoid secretion
  Primary aldosteronism
  Aldosterone-producing adenoma (APA)
  Idiopathic hyperaldosteronism
  Glucocorticoid-remediable aldosteronism (GRA)
  Adrenocortical carcinoma

Congenital adrenal hyperplasia
  11β-Hydroxylase deficiency
  17β-Hydroxylase deficiency

Increased mineralocorticoid action
  Apparent mineralocorticoid excess (AME)
  Congenital
  Licorice ingestion
  Ectopic corticotropin production
  Activating mutation of the mineralocorticoid receptor

Increased sodium transport in renal epithelia
  Liddle syndrome
  Pseudohypoaldosteronism type II or Gordon syndrome

PRIMARY ALDOSTERONISM

▶ General Considerations

Primary aldosteronism was originally described by Conn in the 1950s. While previously thought to be a rare condition, it is now recognized as the most common cause of secondary hypertension owing to advances in the screening procedure. Prevalence rate has been reported as high as 11% in newly diagnosed hypertensive patients and can reach 20% in patients referred for the evaluation of resistant hypertension. Primary aldosteronism has also been associated with extensive cardiovascular and renal damage independent of the degree or presence of hypertension.

▶ Clinical Findings

A. Symptoms and Signs

The most common findings in primary aldosteronism are moderate-to-severe hypertension and hypokalemia. Patients with primary aldosteronism are frequently refractory to antihypertensive medications requiring several drugs to attain control. When symptoms are present, they are the result of potassium depletion and include neuromuscular symptoms (weakness, paralysis, cramps, or tetany), fatigue, and polyuria (due to hypokalemia-induced renal concentrating defect). Potassium depletion can impair insulin secretion and cause glucose intolerance or diabetes. Edema is seldom

seen in primary aldosteronism. End-stage organ damage occurs more frequently, with a higher rate of left ventricular hypertrophy, cardiovascular and cerebrovascular events in patients with primary aldosteronism when compared to matched patients with essential hypertension. Microalbuminuria is also more common and occurs in about 30% of patients with primary aldosteronism. Fortunately, these complications are, at least partially, reversible with appropriate therapy.

Primary aldosteronism has several etiologies, the most important ones being aldosterone-producing adenoma (40–70%) and idiopathic hyperaldosteronism or bilateral hyperplasia (30–60%). Other less common causes include unilateral hyperplasia, adrenocortical carcinoma, and glucocorticoid-remediable aldosteronism (GRA), probably accounting for 1–4% of patients. The differentiation between an aldosterone-producing adenoma and idiopathic hyperaldosteronism is crucial because an adenoma can be surgically treated while idiopathic hyperaldosteronism is medically managed.

While the pathogenesis of primary aldosteronism is not completely understood, there has been a recent breakthrough in the understanding of the genetic basis of this disorder providing a better insight into the familial forms of hyperaldosteronism. There are three categories of familial hyperaldosteronism and they all follow an autosomal dominant mode of inheritance; Type 1 familial hyperaldosteronism or Glucocorticoid-remediable hyperaldosteronism is largely attributed to a hybrid *CYP11B1/CYP11B2* gene while Type 3 is due to a germline mutation in *KCNJ5* gene. The causal gene for Type 2 familial hyperaldosteronism has not been definitely identified although a linkage to 7p22 has been reported in some affected families. Furthermore, about one-third of patients with aldosterone producing adenoma carry somatic mutations of *KCNJ5* regardless of family history.

B. Laboratory Findings

Hypokalemia is not always present in patients with primary aldosteronism and the combination of hypokalemia and metabolic alkalosis is seen in about 50% of patients. The presence of normokalemia should not dissuade the physician from considering the diagnosis of primary aldosteronism.

C. Diagnostic Approach

1. Initial screening—According to the 2016 American Endocrine Society Guidelines, screening for primary aldosteronism is indicated in the following cases: patients with hypertension resistant to three conventional antihypertensive drugs (including a diuretic); BP controlled on four or more antihypertensive drugs; hypertension and spontaneous or diuretic-induced hypokalemia; hypertension and adrenal incidentaloma; hypertension and sleep apnea; hypertension and a family history of early onset hypertension or cerebrovascular accident at a young age (<40 years); and all hypertensive first-degree relatives of patients with PA.

Screening should be done by the measurement of plasma aldosterone concentration (PAC) (ng/dL) and plasma renin activity (PRA) (ng/mL/hour) and the expression of the results as the ratio (ARR). Blood sampling should be ideally taken midmorning and while assuming the sitting position. Patients should be preferably off antihypertensive drugs for at least 2 weeks prior to testing, but since this is often difficult to achieve, testing can still be done while patients are on most drugs including ACE inhibitors, AT II receptor blockers, alpha-blockers, calcium channel blockers, and less desirably on thiazide diuretics. Mineralocorticoid receptor blockers (spironolactone or eplerenone) and epithelial sodium channel inhibitors should be discontinued for at least 4 weeks prior to testing. Beta-blockers also interfere with the assay since they lower renin more than aldosterone and can spuriously increase the ratio. There is a substantial variability in the literature regarding the cutoff values for PAC and ARR for the diagnosis of primary aldosteronism; by consensus, the diagnosis is considered highly likely if ARR is greater than 30 and if PAC is greater than 15 ng/dL. However it is unlikely in patients with high ARR if PAC is lower than 9 ng/dL. Notably, PRA and PAC should be measured after correction of the hypokalemia.

2. Confirmatory testing—Further confirmatory testing should be done in patients with a positive initial screening test except those who present with spontaneous hypokalemia, suppressed PRA and elevated PAC levels above 20 ng/dL since the pretest probability in those patients is considered to be high. Four testing procedures are commonly used and currently there is insufficient evidence to recommend one test over the other. Thus, the choice of confirmatory test is determined by cost, patient compliance and local expertise. The most commonly used test is the measurement of the excretion of urinary aldosterone on the third day of a 200 mEq/day sodium diet. Twenty-four hour urine aldosterone excretion above 12 μg/day is diagnostic. A second test is the measurement of serum aldosterone at the end of the infusion of 2 L of 0.9% sodium chloride over 4 hours. A value below 6 ng/dL (or 5 ng/dL depending on the measuring technique) is normal. Less commonly used is the measurement of serum aldosterone after 4 days of a high sodium diet plus the administration of fludrocortisone 0.1 mg four times a day. A value more than 6 ng/dL confirms the diagnosis. Finally, the captopril suppression test is the least used test because of a high number of equivocal or false negative results. Patients are given 25–50 mg of captopril orally. PRA remains suppressed and PAC remains elevated when measured 1–2 hours later. Care should be taken with salt loading as often these patients have severe uncontrolled hypertension and salt loading can precipitate a hypertensive crisis.

3. Imaging studies—High-resolution computed tomography (CT) scan or magnetic resonance imaging (MRI) can usually detect adrenal masses larger than 0.5–1 cm in diameter. As such, adenomas smaller than 0.5 cm might be missed. Furthermore, many of these adenomas might be non functioning and belong to the category of incidentalomas. On the other hand, patients with idiopathic hyperaldosteronism frequently have bilateral macronodules and/or micronodules that can be uneven in size and might appear to be a unilateral adenoma. Given all these imaging limitations, adrenal vein sampling (AVS) is considered to be the gold standard procedure for the differentiation between a unilateral and a bilateral source of aldosterone excess. It is based on measurements of aldosterone and cortisol from both adrenal veins and inferior vena cava, ideally performed under ACTH stimulation to avoid fluctuations in ACTH and hence aldosterone secretion. The results are expressed as an aldosterone/cortisol ratio called the lateralization index; a ratio of aldosterone/cortisol from one side versus the opposite side that is greater than 4 establishes a diagnosis of a unilateral adrenal adenoma. The catheterization of the right adrenal vein requires considerable experience. Failure to perform AVS results in inappropriate patient selection for unilateral adrenalectomy in around 25–30% of cases. Notably, patients younger than 35 years of age with spontaneous hypokalemia, marked aldosterone excess and unilateral adrenal lesions with radiologic features consistent with an adenoma on CT (>1 cm, less than 10 Hounsfield units) can proceed directly with surgery since the likelihood of a non functioning adenoma is very low in this age group.

4. Special tests—In recent years, identification of GRA has become more common. This disorder is characterized by an uneven crossover recombination between the promoter region and the first two to four exons of the *CYP11B1* gene (11β-hydroxylase) and the last five to seven exons of the *CYP11B2* gene (aldosterone synthase) resulting in gene duplication. This gene is expressed in the zona fasciculata of the adrenal gland, is regulated by adrenocorticotropic hormone (ACTH), and synthesizes aldosterone. A genetic test is available for the diagnosis. Patients with a family history of early onset hypertension or cerebrovascular events, especially those diagnosed with hypertension at a young age should be screened for this disorder.

▶ Treatment and Prognosis

Aldosterone-producing adenomas are surgically treated via laparoscopic technique if possible. Patients with idiopathic hyperaldosteronism and those with an aldosterone-producing adenoma who are not surgical candidates or who are reluctant to undergo surgery should be treated medically with a mineralocorticoid receptor antagonist. Two agents are available. Spironolactone is administered at doses of 25–400 mg/day. Patients are started with 25 mg/day and the dose is increased to response (up to 400 mg/day). Spironolactone has multiple side effects. Since it is also an androgen receptor antagonist and progesterone receptor agonist, it can result in impotence and gynecomastia in men and menstrual irregularities and breast tenderness due to progestational effects in women. Eplerenone is a new mineralocorticoid antagonist that is more selective than spironolactone for the receptor and thus has significantly fewer side effects. It is less potent and is administered at doses of 50–200 mg/day in divided doses. In patients who do not tolerate these drugs, an epithelial sodium channel antagonist, amiloride, can also be used. Unfortunately, patients who are being medically managed frequently require multiple antihypertensive drugs before they can achieve adequate BP control.

Aldosterone synthase inhibitors and nonsteroidal dihydropyridine-based mineralocorticoid receptor antagonists are new drugs that are being developed and appear promising as alternative therapeutic options in patients with primary aldosteronism.

The cornerstone treatment for GRA is low dose dexamethasone with or without a mineralocorticoid receptor antagonist or an epithelial sodium channel blocker.

Despite the potentially curable nature of the disease, only about one third of the patients with primary aldosteronism experience cure with adrenalectomy defined by BP normalization off antihypertensive medications.

Nevertheless, in the remaining majority, BP improves with requirement of fewer medications. In addition, it appears that cardiovascular and renal complications also improve after adequate therapy, be it medical or surgical. Notably, patients with less severe hypertension (including those with shorter duration of hypertension and those requiring less medications for BP control) who lack a family history of hypertension are more likely to show a BP response after unilateral adrenalectomy.

CONGENITAL ADRENAL HYPERPLASIA

Congenital adrenal hyperplasia is the result of a deficiency in one of a multitude of enzymes leading to a dysregulation in adrenal steroid hormone synthesis. Among those enzymes, 17α-hydroxylase and 11β-hydroxylase deficiencies present with syndromes of mineralocorticoid excess (Figure 41–1).

11β-HYDROXYLASE DEFICIENCY

▶ General Considerations

11β-Hydroxylase deficiency is a rare autosomal recessive disorder that accounts for 5–8% of all the cases of congenital adrenal hyperplasia (CAH) worldwide. The prevalence of this disorder is higher in Moroccan Jews. It is due to a mutation in the *CYP11B1* gene. The defect results in a decrease in the synthesis of cortisol with an increase in the secretion of precursors, including 11-deoxycortisol and deoxycorticosterone, which have mineralocorticoid activity. The shunting of precursors to the sex hormone pathway also results in an excessive production of

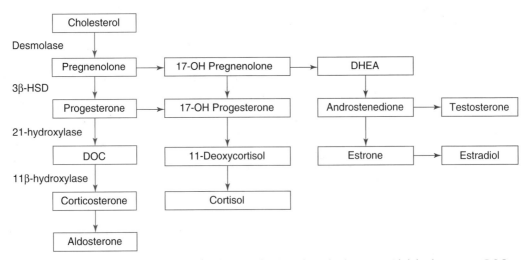

▲ **Figure 41–1.** Adrenal steroidogenesis. Abbreviations: 3β-HSD, 3 beta-hydroxysteroid dehydrogenase; DOC, deoxycorticosterone; DHEA, dehydroepiandrosterone.

17α-hydroxyprogesterone and androstenedione leading to the virilization of female children and precocious puberty of males. Patients usually present in early life with hypertension and frequently hypokalemia along with signs of androgen excess.

Clinical Findings

The disorder is more easily recognized in young girls, as they can present with virilization and early onset hypertension. Young boys usually show signs of pseudoprecocious puberty along with hypertension. The diagnosis is established by demonstrating low renin, aldosterone, and cortisol levels and high levels of deoxycorticosterone, 17α-hydroxyprogesterone and androstenedione. Genetic testing is also available.

Treatment

Treatment involves glucocorticoid supplementation with hydrocortisone ideally, to maximize growth potential in children while avoiding the development of Cushing syndrome. A mineralocorticoid receptor antagonist such as spironolactone or eplerenone can be added for better BP control. Bilateral adrenalectomy may be needed in selected cases with mineralocorticoid replacement as necessary.

17α-HYDROXYLASE DEFICIENCY

General Considerations

17α-Hydroxylase deficiency is a rare autosomal recessive disorder that accounts for less than 1% of the cases of CAH. It is due to a mutation of the *CYP17* gene resulting in the lack of formation of any 17-hydroxylated steroids including cortisol and androgens and excessive production of corticosterone and deoxycorticosterone.

Clinical Findings

Patients usually present at an early age with low renin, low aldosterone hypertension, and sexual infantilism with undervirilization in males and failure of spontaneous pubertal development in females. The diagnosis is established by the demonstration of high levels of corticosterone and deoxycorticosterone and the absence of 17β-hydroxylated steroids including 17α-hydroxyprogesterone, androstenedione, and cortisol. Genetic testing is also available.

Treatment

Treatment involves replacement with hydrocortisone and the use of mineralocorticoid receptor antagonists. Females may need estrogen replacement to promote the development of secondary sexual characteristics while males may require testosterone treatment.

APPARENT MINERALOCORTICOID EXCESS

General Considerations

Apparent mineralocorticoid excess was first described in 1977 as a potentially fatal disorder involving juvenile low-renin, low-aldosterone hypertension, hypokalemic alkalosis, low birth weight, failure to thrive, and, frequently, nephrocalcinosis. It is an autosomal recessive disorder caused by a deficiency of the enzyme 11β-hydroxysteroid dehydrogenase 2. A similar acquired syndrome has also been described in adults and is due predominantly to the ingestion of licorice. The active principle in licorice (glycyrrhizic acid) is a potent inhibitor of this enzyme. Licorice is widely used in Europe as a low-calorie sweetener in candies. Chewing tobacco in the United States is also often flavored with real licorice. Carbenoxolone and "asam boi" flavor are other compounds that also contain glycyrrhizic acid and can lead to the same syndrome. The affinity of the mineralocorticoid receptor for cortisol is similar to that for aldosterone. Furthermore cortisol normally circulates at 100–1000 times the concentrations of aldosterone. Hence the specificity of the mineralocorticoid receptor in renal transporting epithelia to aldosterone is due to the coexpression of the enzyme 11β-hydroxysteroid dehydrogenase 2, which metabolizes cortisol to inactive cortisone. A deficiency of this enzyme results in the occupancy of the receptors by cortisol and enhanced mineralocorticoid effect.

In ectopic corticotropin-secreting tumors producing Cushing syndrome, cortisol is produced in massive amounts thus saturating the 11β-hydroxysteroid dehydrogenase 2 and allowing cortisol to activate the mineralocorticoid receptor.

Clinical Findings

A. Symptoms and Signs

The severity of this disorder is variable depending on whether residual enzymatic activity is present or not. In its florid and rare form, it affects infants especially the offspring of consanguineous parents. These infants usually present with low renin, low aldosterone hypertension, hypokalemia, alkalosis, low birth weight and failure to thrive. Nephrocalcinosis is a frequent finding. In its milder form, it presents at a later age with hypertension, mildly suppressed renin levels and low plasma aldosterone concentration. A thorough dietary history should be obtained in adults with new onset AME like syndrome.

Patients with Cushing syndrome due to ectopic corticotropin (ACTH) production most often present after the diagnosis of a cancer and experience profound weakness, hypertension, and hypokalemia. Ectopic ACTH production is a late event and the phenotypic manifestations of the classic Cushing syndrome are usually absent in this particular case.

B. Laboratory Findings

The diagnosis is determined by the measurement of the ratio of urinary free cortisol to urinary free cortisone. This ratio is less than 1 in normal individuals and is clearly increased in patients with AME syndrome. The ratio of the metabolites of cortisol and cortisone, tetrahydrocortisol + allotetrahydrocortisol to tetrahydrocortisone, can be also measured in these patients. The ratio is around 1 in normal individuals and is usually higher than 2 in patients with AME. Genetic testing can further elucidate the diagnosis.

▶ Treatment

Patients with congenital AME are treated with mineralocorticoid receptor antagonists (spironolactone or eplerenone). Some patients may also benefit from treatment with dexamethasone aiming to suppress endogenous production of glucocorticoids. Acquired forms are treated by withdrawal of the offending licorice or carbenoxolone. It might take weeks to months for the syndrome to resolve following the discontinuation of these agents. Ectopic corticotropin production is treated by management of the cancer, if possible.

▶ Prognosis

The prognosis in patients with congenital AME depends on the adherence to therapy, but is relative poor, with significant morbidity and mortality at a young age. Patients with licorice-induced hypertension have a good prognosis provided that licorice intake is eliminated. Patients with ectopic corticotropin production have a poor prognosis since the syndrome usually presents late in the course of the disease.

LIDDLE SYNDROME

▶ Clinical Findings

In 1963, Liddle described a family of patients that presented with severe hypertension, hypokalemia, low PRA, and low plasma aldosterone concentrations. He demonstrated that adrenal steroids were not involved in the pathogenesis of this disorder. Affected patients responded to epithelial sodium channel blockers but not to mineralocorticoid receptor antagonists. It was not until later that a genetic defect affecting the epithelial sodium channel (ENAC) was discovered. This disorder has an autosomal dominant mode of inheritance and is due to a mutation in either the *SCNN1B* gene (coding for the β subunit of the ENAC) or *SCNN1G* gene (coding for the γ subunit of the ENAC). Both these mutations lead to an increase in the activity as well as

the surface expression of the ENAC. Affected patients usually present early in life although cases have been reported in middle aged or older adults. Patients have an increased mortality because of stroke and heart failure and end stage renal disease as a result of nephrosclerosis has been reported. Renal transplantation improves the syndrome. Notably, genetic testing is commercially available to confirm the diagnosis.

▶ Treatment

Patients are treated with salt restriction and sodium channel antagonists, primarily amiloride, at doses between 5 and 15 mg twice a day.

PSEUDOHYPOALDOSTERONISM TYPE II OR GORDON SYNDROME

▶ Clinical Findings

Pseudohypoaldosteronism type 2 is a familial autosomal dominant disorder characterized by low renin, low aldosterone hypertension, hyperkalemia, hyperchloremic metabolic acidosis, normal renal function and hypercalciuria. Affected patients have a short stature, mild mental retardation, muscle weakness, and occasionally periodic paralysis with severe hyperkalemia. This disorder is due to an increase in the activity of the sodium and chloride cotransporter in the distal convoluted tubule leading to excessive sodium retention and thus hypertension. The various families with the syndrome show linkages to chromosomes 1, 17, and 12. The ones linked to chromosome 12 have been associated with an intronic defect in the gene for WNK1 while the ones linked to chromosome 17 involve mutations in the WNK4. Both WNKs lead to the phosphorylation of SPAK and OSR1, which in turn enhance the activity, as well as the insertion of the sodium chloride cotransporter into the apical membrane of the distal convoluted tubule. Recently, two new genes have been also implicated in this syndrome, CUL3 and KLHL3. The proteins encoded by these genes contribute to the degradation of the WNKs especially WNK4 and as a result WNK levels are increased when these genes are mutated. The gene defect in syndromes associated with chromosome 1 remains unknown. Hyperkalemia is attributed to impaired distal tubular potassium secretion in the face of the loss of lumen electronegativity as a result of enhanced sodium and chloride reabsorption. It has been also recently shown that WNKs can directly affect and hence reduce ROMK expression in the collecting duct.

▶ Treatment

Patients respond to low-salt diet and the administration of thiazide diuretics.

KEY READINGS

Ardhanari et al: Mineralocorticoid and apparent mineralocorticoid syndromes of secondary hypertension. Adv Chronic Kidney Dis 2015;22:185.

Funder JW et al: The management of primary aldosteronism: case detection, diagnosis, and treatment of patients with primary aldosteronism: an endocrine society clinical practice guideline. J Clin Endocrinol Metab 2016;101:1889.

Garovic VD et al: Monogenic forms of low-renin hypertension. Nat Clin Pract Nephrol 2006;2:624.

Jain et al: Genetic disorders of potassium homeostasis. Semin Nephrol 2013;33:300.

Melcescu E et al: 11Beta-Hydroxylase deficiency and other syndromes of mineralocorticoid excess as a rare cause of endocrine hypertension. Horm Metab Res 2012;44:867.

Mulatero P et al: Long-term cardio- and cerebrovascular events in patients with primary aldosteronism. J Clin Endocrinol Metab 2013;98:4826.

O'Shaughnessy KM: Gordon syndrome: a continuing story. Pediatr Nephrol 2015;30:1903.

Rossi GP et al: PAPY Study Investigators. A prospective study of the prevalence of primary aldosteronism in 1,125 hypertensive patients. J Am Coll Cardiol 2006;48:2293.

Sechi LA, Colussi G, Di Fabio A, Catena C: Cardiovascular and renal damage in primary aldosteronism: outcomes after treatment. Am J Hypertens 2010;23:1253.

Stowasser M et al: Primary aldosteronism: changing definitions and new concepts of physiology and pathophysiology both inside and outside the kidney. Physiol Rev 2016;96:1327.

Wachtel H et al: Long-term blood pressure control in patients undergoing adrenalectomy for primary hyperaldosteronism. Surgery 2014;156:1394.

▼ PHEOCHROMOCYTOMA

Debbie L Cohen, MD

▶ General Considerations

Pheochromocytoma and paraganglioma (PGL) tumors are a rare cause of secondary hypertension and are tumors of the autonomic nervous system that arise from chromaffin tissue in the adrenal medulla and extra-adrenal ganglia, respectively. These tumors are derived from sympathetic nervous system tissue which secretes catecholamines and metanephrines. Some PGL tumors are derived from parasympathetic ganglia, especially those in the head and neck, and are often non-secretory. Even though these tumors are rare, if undiagnosed, these tumors are associated with high morbidity and mortality secondary to the elevated catecholamine secretion leading to hypertension, heart disease, stroke and even death. Of note PCC/PGL are the tumors most commonly associated with an inherited genetic mutation. Most tumors are benign but up to 25% can be malignant and are associated with a poor prognosis.

▶ Clinical Findings

A. Symptoms and Signs

PCC/PGL should be considered in patients of any age with new onset difficult to control hypertension, in patients who present with an adrenal incidentaloma and in patients with symptoms suggestive of PCC/PGL including the classic triad of headaches, palpitations and sweating, as well as anxiety, tremors, new onset or worsening of previously established diabetes mellitus, syncope or presyncope. Patients may be asymptomatic and clinicians should maintain a high level of clinical suspicion for PCC/PGL in order to make the diagnosis. BP elevation is the most common manifestation of a PCC with sustained elevation of BP being present in above 50% of patients and intermittent hypertension in about one third, while normal BP or postural hypotension is present in about 20% of patients. The most dramatic presentation of a PCC is an acute episode of severe hypertension, severe headache, palpitations, tachycardia, and diaphoresis. Arrhythmias are frequent, as is chest pain. Catecholamines can cause coronary vasospasm and acute myocarditis as well as catecholamine induced cardiomyopathy. Shock unresponsive to norepinephrine occurring after a hypertensive crisis can also be a presentation that can easily be missed. Cerebrovascular accidents occur due to the profound vasoconstriction of the cerebrovascular arteries or emboli from a catecholaminergic-dilated cardiomyopathy. Certain drugs such as tricyclic antidepressants, antidopaminergics (metoclopramide), naloxone, and beta-blockers (when not preceded by α-adrenergic blockade) can precipitate an acute hypertensive crisis in a patient with a PCC. Children with PCC usually have sustained hypertension with nausea, headaches, and sweating. Lactic acidosis in the absence of shock should be an indication for considering the diagnosis of a PCC.

B. Special Tests

Screening for PCC/PGL can be done by testing for plasma-free metanephrines or 24-hour urine fractionated metanephrines. Both plasma and urine tests have over 90% sensitivity for PCC/PGL. Plasma metanephrines are favored because this test is easier to collect and has a higher specificity compared to the 24 hour urine tests. Catecholamine and metanephrine measurements are susceptible to false positive elevations therefore guidelines recommend the plasma tests be performed with the patient resting for 20 minutes in the supine position although this is not usually practical in the clinical setting. Plasma catecholamines are particularly sensitive to this, and therefore, are not recommended as a first-line screening test due to increased likelihood of false positive results. The catecholamine and metanephrine levels for both plasma and urine tests also can be falsely elevated due to interfering medications as shown

Table 41–7. Medications that interfere with screening tests for pheochromocytoma and paraganglioma.

Acetaminophen
Levodopa
Selective serotonin inhibitors
Sympathomimetics
Monoamine oxidase inhibitors
Tricyclic antidepressants
Some beta-blockers (particularly non selective)
Some alpha-blockers (phenoxybenzamine)

in Table 41–7. Once elevated levels of catecholamines and/or metanephrines are confirmed, imaging studies should be done to localize the tumor. Cross sectional imaging with CT or MRI of the abdomen/pelvis is the first recommended imaging test since most tumors are located in the adrenal glands or in the abdomen or pelvis. PGL derived from the parasympathetic chain, usually in the head and neck region are often non-secretory, therefore, if a parasympathetic PGL is suspected, imaging should be performed regardless of biochemical testing results.

Differential Diagnosis

Multiple disorders can mimic symptoms of a PCC and some are associated with increased catecholamine secretion. Clonidine or alcohol withdrawal, cerebrovascular events, subarachnoid hemorrhages, migraines, and intracranial lesions may mimic a PCC. Drugs such as ephedrine, cocaine, phencyclidine, and LSD can also produce a similar episodic syndrome. Panic attacks, hypoglycemic episodes, or just severe hypertension with a hyperdynamic circulation might resemble episodes of PCC.

Complications

Undiagnosed PCC is associated with a high incidence of sudden death, cerebrovascular events, and dilated cardiomyopathy.

Treatment

Surgical resection is the treatment of choice for PCC/PGL and is now relatively safe with morbidity and mortality rates as low as 0–2% with use of preoperative alpha blockade. Laparoscopic adrenalectomy is the treatment of choice for adrenal PCC and is often curative for small adrenal PCC and is associated with improved outcomes. Open adrenalectomy is usually reserved for very large tumors greater than 8 cm, and extra-adrenal PGL. The entire adrenal gland is usually removed; however, cortical sparing surgery may be attempted in patients with bilateral adrenal PCC and in patients with a

genetic predisposition to bilateral PCC (such as MEN2 and vHL). If a sufficient part of the cortex can be spared, these patients can avoid lifelong glucocorticoid and mineralocorticoid replacement. There is a higher risk of recurrence with cortical sparing surgery. In preparation for surgery, patients should receive preoperative alpha-blockade for 10–14 days prior to surgery and should be instructed to take these medications on the morning of surgery. There are no standardized guidelines for the perioperative blockade regimen, and sparse data exists with no randomized controlled trials. Preoperative alpha-blockade is usually started as soon as the diagnosis is made, and surgery is usually scheduled within 2–3 weeks of the diagnosis. There are many different medical regimens used to control the effects of catecholamine hypersecretion, and these include the use of alpha-blockers, calcium channel blockers, and tyrosine hydroxylase inhibition. The typical drugs and dosing regimens are shown in Table 41–8. During surgery, patients will require either intraoperative intravenous phentolamine or nicardipine. During intubation, surgical excision and tumor manipulation, it is common to see an increase in BP; and once the tumor is removed, BP can drop precipitously due to the large decrease in catecholamine levels. After surgery, patients may require BP support with fluids, colloids, and sometimes alpha-adrenergic agonists for 24–48 hours and may need monitoring in an ICU setting. Postoperative hypotension is less common in patients who have received adequate preoperative alpha-blockade. BP usually returns to normal within a few days of surgery, but patients may remain hypertensive particularly if they have chronic underlying hypertension or widespread metastatic disease. All patients should have catecholamine biochemistries (preferably plasma metanephrines) checked about 4–6 weeks after surgery to ensure levels have returned to normal. If levels remain elevated, this may indicate residual or metastatic disease and will require further evaluation.

Prognosis and Genetic Testing

Undiagnosed and untreated PCC patients experience a high incidence of sudden death and cardiovascular and cerebrovascular events. A hypertensive crisis frequently occurs during routine procedures. Patients who are properly treated with α- and beta-blockers and surgery have a good prognosis, but there is a 10–15% incidence of recurrence. The course of malignant PCC is highly variable; some behave aggressively while others have a more indolent course. All patients should be referred for genetic testing due to the high rate of germline mutation detection. Up to 40% of patients with PCC/PGL will have a germline mutation in one of over 14 genes known to increase risk of this tumor type as shown in Table 41–9. Certain germline susceptibility gene mutations are associated with an in increased risk of recurrence or additional primary tumors, and, in the case of *SDHB* mutations, high rates of malignant or metastatic disease.

Table 41–8. Common medications for perioperative blockade for patients with pheochromocytoma and paraganglioma.

Drug	Drug Class	Mechanism of Action	Dosing	Common Side Effects
Phenoxybenzamine	Non-selective alpha-1 and alpha-2 blocker	Non-competitive antagonist	10 mg 2–3 × daily (maximum 60 mg per day)	Orthostasis, nasal congestion
Doxazosin	Selective alpha-1 blocker	Competitive antagonist	2–4 mg 2–3 × daily	Orthostasis, dizziness
Prazosin	Selective alpha-1 blocker	Competitive antagonist	1–2 mg twice daily	Orthostasis, dizziness
Terazosin	Selective alpha-1 blocker	Competitive antagonist	1–4 mg once daily	Orthostasis, dizziness
Nicardipine	Calcium channel blocker	Dihydropyridine long acting	30 mg twice daily	Headache, edema, vasodilatation
Amlodipine	Calcium channel blocker	Dihydropyridine long acting	5–10 mg daily	Headache, edema, palpitations
Metyrosine	Tyrosine hydroxylase inhibitor	Decreases catecholamine production	250–500 mg 4 × daily (dose escalated every 2 days)	Severe lethargy, extra-pyramidal neurological side effects and gastrointestinal upset
Metoprolol	Selective beta-1 blocker	Used to treat reflex tachycardia only after full alpha blockade achieved	25–50 mg 1–2 x daily	Fatigue, dizziness

Reproduced from Fishbein L, Orlowski R, Cohen D: Pheochromocytoma/Paraganglioma: Review of perioperative management of blood pressure and update on genetic mutations associated with pheochromocytoma. J Clin Hypertens (Greenwich) 2013;15:428.

Table 41–9. Pheochromocytoma and paraganglioma susceptibility genes.

Gene	Syndrome	Primary Pheochromocytoma or Paraganglioma Location
NF1	Neurofibromatosis type 1	Adrenal pheochromocytomas
VHL	von Hippel–Lindau	Adrenal pheochromocytomas
RET	Multiple endocrine neoplasia type 2	Adrenal pheochromocytomas
SDHA	Hereditary paraganglioma syndrome	Any location
SDHB	Hereditary paraganglioma syndrome	Extra adrenal paraganglioma (any location)
SDHC	Hereditary paraganglioma syndrome	Head and neck paragangliomas (thoracic paragangliomas)
SDHD	Hereditary paraganglioma syndrome	Head and neck paragangliomas (any location)
SDHAF2	Hereditary paraganglioma syndrome	Head and neck paragangliomas
TMEM127	Familial pheochromocytoma/paraganglioma syndrome	Adrenal pheochromocytoma (any location)
MAX	Familial pheochromocytoma/paraganglioma syndrome	Adrenal pheochromocytomas
FH	Hereditary leiomyomatosis and renal cell cancer syndrome	Any location

Adapted from Fishbein L, Orlowski R, Cohen D: Pheochromocytoma/Paraganglioma: Review of perioperative management of blood pressure and update on genetic mutations associated with pheochromocytoma. J Clin Hypertens (Greenwich) 2013;15:428.

KEY READINGS

Ayala-Ramirez M et al: Clinical risk factors for malignancy and overall survival in patients with pheochromocytomas and sympathetic paragangliomas: primary tumor size and primary tumor location as prognostic indicators. JCEM 2011;96:717.

Favier J, Amar L, Gimenez-Roqueplo AP: Paraganglioma and phaeochromocytoma: from genetics to personalized medicine. Nat Rev Endocrinol 2015;11:101.

Fishbein L, Orlowski R, Cohen D: Pheochromocytoma/ Paraganglioma: review of perioperative management of blood pressure and update on genetic mutations associated with pheochromocytoma. J Clin Hypertens (Greenwich) 2013;15:428.

Lenders JW et al: Pheochromocytoma and paraganglioma: an endocrine society clinical practice guideline. J Clin Endocrinol Metab 2014;99:1915.

Neary NM, King KS, Pacak K: Drugs and pheochromocytoma—don't be fooled by every elevated metanephrine. N Engl J Med 2011;364:2268.

COARCTATION OF THE AORTA

Raymond R. Townsend, MD

General Considerations

Aortic coarctations represent between 5% and 8% of congenital heart defects and typically occur in discrete segment of the aorta around the area of the ligamentum arteriosum, where the left subclavian artery originates. Coarctation occurs commonly in conjunction with other congenital abnormalities, and repair of coarctation in infancy is often attended by bicuspid aortic valve, intracardiac septal defects, subvalvular aortic stenosis and hypoplastic aortic arch. Coarctation is more common in males (66–75%). Differences in BP may clue the location of the coarctation—if it is proximal to the left subclavian artery, systolic BP is typically higher in the right arm than the left arm. More commonly, the coarctation is more distal, and the systolic BP in the right leg is lower than that in the right arm.

Clinical Findings

A. Symptoms and Signs

Although children with coarctation sometimes note dyspnea, fatigue, headache, abdominal angina, tinnitus, dizziness, cold feet, leg cramps, and leg fatigue (especially with vigorous exercise), most adults are asymptomatic. The traditional characteristic physical sign is a diminished or delayed left radial or right femoral pulse, in comparison to the right radial pulse. A loud systolic murmur, often with a thrill and occasionally heard in the back between the scapulae, may be accompanied by other murmurs, depending on the presence or absence of other cardiac abnormalities (eg, bicuspid aortic valve, present in 50–80% of children). "Notching" (typically of the inferior posterior aspects) of the ribs (third through eighth) is characteristic, and the number and location of notched ribs may provide information as to the location of the coarctation.

B. Special Tests

A transthoracic echocardiogram is typically recommended as the first test, since it can identify about 95% of coarctations through the first 8 cm of the descending aorta (which probably covers 99% of cases). CT and MRI are particularly useful to evaluate the aorta and intracranial vessels not visible by echocardiography. Angiography is sometimes not required if the other images are acceptable to a vascular surgeon.

Differential Diagnosis

The differential diagnosis includes Takayasu arteritis and Moyamoya disease (both of which can affect a major artery in one arm, which is more common than both legs and not an arm).

Treatment

A systolic pressure gradient across the coarctation of more than 20 mm Hg generally requires intervention. Sometimes extensive collateral vessel formation may be accompanied by a lower gradient in which case repair may still be indicated even when gradients are less than 20 mm Hg. A variety of surgical approaches have been successful, depending on the location of the coarctation. Postoperative elevation in systolic BP is a predictor of long-term adverse outcomes (including death). Balloon dilatation and endovascular stenting have been used, but few long-term results have been reported. Stenting may achieve better gradient reductions but re-interventions are similar when comparing balloon dilatation with stenting. Aortoplasty has also been successfully used after an initial surgical repair. Hypertension recurs in about 25–33% of patients with repaired coarctation in long-term follow-up; exercise-induced hypertension is even more common (25–56%). Recommendations for the treatment of hypertension include ACE-inhibitors, ARBs or beta-blockers.

Prognosis

Unrepaired coarctation has a mean survival to age 35 years, with about 75% mortality by age 46 years. Hypertension is common even after repair and is an important factor in premature CAD, left ventricular dysfunction and rupture of aortic or cerebral (berry) aneurysms. Follow-up imaging varies, but 2-year intervals with cardiac MRI as the imaging procedure are recommended by the European Society of Cardiology. The degree of BP lowering after a corrective procedure in patients who present with aortic coarctation in adulthood is controversial. Two of three studies indicated that most patients have a lower BP about 3 months after the operation than before it, but after 5 years about one third were hypertensive. Older age was generally associated with a higher risk for post-procedural hypertension.

KEY READINGS

Baumgartner H et al: ESC Guidelines for the management of grown-up congenital heart disease (new version 2010). Eur Heart J 2010;31:2915.

O'Sullivan J: Late hypertension in patients with repaired aortic coarctation. Current Hypertension Reports 2014;16:421.

Salcher M et al: Balloon dilatation and stenting for aortic coarctation: a systematic review and meta-analysis. Cir Cardiovasc Interv 2016;9.

Warnes CA et al: ACC/AHA 2008 guidelines for the management of adults with congenital heart disease: a report of the American College of Cardiology/American Heart Association Task Force on Practice Guidelines (Writing Committee to Develop Guidelines on the Management of Adults With Congenital Heart Disease). Developed in Collaboration With the American Society of Echocardiography, Heart Rhythm Society, International Society for Adult Congenital Heart Disease, Society for Cardiovascular Angiography and Interventions, and Society of Thoracic Surgeons. J Am Coll Cardiol 2008;52:e143.

▼ SLEEP APNEA

Raymond R. Townsend, MD

▶ General Considerations

Sleep apnea itself affects about one in five US adults, and is more common among African–Americans than whites. It is more frequently found in overweight and obese individuals (mean body mass index ~35 kg/m^2) with a mean age of about 60 years. Sleep apnea has been associated with the development of hypertension, but these results are confounded by close correlations of both hypertension and sleep apnea with age, gender, body mass index, alcohol intake, and smoking. Sleep apnea is particularly prevalent in patients with drug-resistant hypertension.

▶ Pathogenesis

The mechanisms responsible for the association of hypertension in patients with sleep apnea likely include increases sympathetic activity, inflammation, and the oxidative stress associated with periods of cyclic intermittent hypopnea/hypoxia.

▶ Clinical Findings

A. Symptoms and Signs

The typical patient with sleep apnea has daytime sleepiness and drowsiness (typically while driving), poor sleep quality (typically described as "restless sleep"), morning headache and sore throat, and excessive fatigue. Bed partners often report loud snoring and irregular breathing, and an astute observer may note cessation of breathing, gasping, and choking sounds during the night.

B. Special Tests

The Berlin Questionnaire is a validated screening tool for sleep apnea that has 86% sensitivity, 77% specificity, and 89% predictive value after evaluation in 744 primary care patients subsequently formally evaluated with polysomnography. Those who score highly are typically asked to undergo formal multichannel polysomnography to verify the diagnosis.

The STOP-Bang questionnaire also has a high sensitivity of 93%, when patients score 3 or more out of a possible 8 points.

▶ Treatment

Several options are offered to treat sleep apnea: weight loss (successful in a minority of cases in the long term), dental appliances, laryngeal surgery (if excessive pharyngeal tissue is sufficient to cause airway obstruction), and positive airway pressure (PAP) during sleep, usually delivered with a mask connected to a pressurized air-delivery system customized to a pressure that reduces a particular patient's apnea/hypopnea index (AHI). For patients who tolerate sleeping with the apparatus in place, reductions in BP are typically seen within 4 weeks. As with most long-term therapies, adherence to an initially successful intervention wanes over time. Improvements in BP are often small with therapies to manage sleep apnea. With PAP in particular, when patients wear the pressure system for more than 4 hours per night there appears to be a distinctly larger BP benefit.

Recently, several uncontrolled cohort studies have reported that spironolactone is useful in the treatment of hypertension in patients with sleep apnea.

▶ Prognosis

There is little long-term information on the effectiveness of PAP or other therapies directed to improving sleep apnea, on longitudinal BP lowering. Laryngeal surgery in appropriately selected patients improves short-term BP control. Long-term weight loss and PAP are recommended on the basis of short-term improvements in BP. Simply managing the AHI with PAP compared to usual care did not appear to reduce cardiovascular events compared in a recent long-term randomized intervention trial, though other benefits such as daytime vigilance remain as important considerations when managing sleep apnea patients.

KEY READINGS

Chung F, Abdullah HR, Liao P: STOP-Bang questionnaire: a practical approach to screen for obstructive sleep apnea. Chest 2016;149:631.

Martínez-García MA et al: Effect of CPAP on blood pressure in patients with obstructive sleep apnea and resistant hypertension: the HIPARCO randomized clinical trial. JAMA 2013;310:2407.

McEvoy RD et al: CPAP for prevention of cardiovascular events in obstructive sleep apnea. N Engl J Med 2016;375:919.

Mohsenin V: Obstructive sleep apnea and hypertension: a critical review. Curr Hypertens Rep 2014;16:482.

Yang L et al: Effect of spironolactone on patients with resistant hypertension and obstructive sleep apnea. Clin Exp Hypertens 2016;38:464.

■ CHAPTER REVIEW QUESTIONS

1. A 74-year-old white man with history of severe peripheral vascular disease and severe uncontrolled hypertension and has a renal Doppler study and is found to have a unilateral 80% stenosis of the right renal artery and 40% stenosis of the left renal artery. BP is uncontrolled on amlodipine 5 mg bid, losartan 50 mg bid, and metoprolol tartrate 50 mg bid. BP is 166/98 mm Hg, heart rate is 78 beats/min. Serum creatinine is 2.8 mg/dL with eGFR of 22 cc/min. What is the most appropriate next step in management of his BP?
   A. CT angiogram with IV contrast
   B. MR angiogram with gadolinium
   C. Add furosemide 40 mg bid and a statin
   D. Renal angiogram with percutaneous angioplasty and stent of the right renal artery
   E. Renal angiogram with percutaneous angioplasty and stent of the right and left renal arteries.

2. A 34-year-old white woman presents with sudden onset hypertension. No family history of hypertension. No other past medical history. She was started on amlodipine 10 mg daily and Lisinopril 20 mg daily and BP has remained elevated. BP is 152/92 mm Hg. Heart rate is 88 per minute. She has 1+ pedal edema present. Rest of examination is normal. She feels well but complains of lower extremity edema which is attributed to the amlodipine. CT angiogram is ordered and reveals beaded appearance of both renal arteries distally. What is the most appropriate next step in BP management for this patient?
   A. Add HCTZ 25 mg daily
   B. Add metoprolol succinate 50 mg daily
   C. Renal angiogram with angioplasty and stenting of both renal arteries
   D. Renal angiogram and angioplasty of both renal arteries

3. A 50-year-old African–American man has severe hypertension despite compliance with four medications including a diuretic. No symptoms of headaches, palpitations, or sweating. His BP is 178/96 mm Hg, HR 66 per minute, BMI = 26. Serum creatinine is 1.0 mg/dL, K is 3.3 mg/dL. Physical examination is unremarkable. Which of the following is the next most appropriate test in the work up of secondary hypertension for this patient?
   A. Plasma metanephrine levels
   B. Sleep study
   C. CT angiogram
   D. Plasma renin and aldosterone levels

4. The above patient has a renin level of 0.1 ng/dL and aldosterone level of 44 ng/dL. A CT scan of the abdomen reveals a 1.2 cm right adrenal mass consistent with an adrenal adenoma. What is the next most appropriate step in management of this patient?
   A. Right adrenalectomy
   B. MRI of abdomen
   C. Adrenal vein sampling
   D. Spironolactone 50 mg daily

5. A 22-year-old man develops an acute and severe elevation in BP to 220/140 mm Hg during tonsillectomy. The surgery is abandoned because of persistently high and uncontrolled BP. He has no prior history of hypertension, but does have a family history of hypertension. Which ONE of the following is the MOST appropriate diagnostic test to order next?
   A. Aldosterone/renin ratio
   B. Polysomnography
   C. CT angiography
   D. Plasma metanephrines
   E. Plasma catecholamines

6. A 48-year-old man with paroxysmal hypertension has recently been diagnosed with an 8 cm paraaortic PGL in the organ of Zuckerkandl observed on CT imaging. Plasma metanephrines are ten times above the upper limit of the reference range. He is referred for surgical management. In addition to adequate preoperative combined alpha- and beta-blockade before surgery, which ONE of the following is the next MOST appropriate step in management?
   A. 123-I-MIBG scan
   B. PET scan
   C. Genetic testing
   D. Plasma catecholamines

7. A 50-year-old obese hypertensive man is diagnosed with moderate-to-severe sleep apnea. Which of the following best describes the likely effects of weight loss and/or CPAP therapy in this patient?
   A. Neither weight loss nor CPAP are likely to reduce his BP.
   B. Weight loss alone will reduce BP if he complies, and CPAP will not result in additional BP reduction.
   C. CPAP alone will reduce BP if he complies, and weight loss will not result in additional BP reduction.
   D. Either CPAP or weight loss will likely reduce his BP to some degree, but if he complies with CPAP and achieves significant weight loss, BP pressure reduction will be much greater than that achieved by either therapy alone.

8. Which of the following statements is incorrect?
   A. Cross-sectional studies have shown strong evidence for an association between OSA and systemic HTN.
   B. Even in apparently normotensive OSA patients, CPAP significantly reduces BP, the frequency of prehypertension and masked HTN.
   C. Observational prospective studies consistently show that normotensive subjects with untreated OSA at baseline develop more hypertension compared to subjects who do not have OSA.
   D. OSA is present in the majority of patients with resistant hypertension.

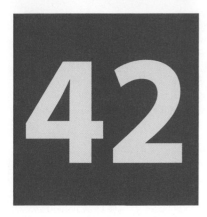

Hypertension in High-Risk Populations

David Martins, MD

Keith C. Norris, MD, PhD

Hillel Sternlicht, MD

Kisra Anis, MBBS

Anjali Acharya, MBBS

Belinda Jim, MD

▼ HYPERTENSION IN AFRICAN–AMERICANS

David Martins, MD and Keith C. Norris, MD, PhD

▶ General Considerations

At a population level increasing levels of blood pressure are associated with greater rates of adverse cardiovascular events. These events become more evident at levels greater than 120/80 mm Hg, but traditionally the term hypertension has been reserved for blood pressure levels at or above 140/90 mm Hg. Most guideline committees recommend pharmacologic treatment for blood pressure levels at or above 140/90 mm Hg in persons that have not responded to non-pharmacologic interventions or in the presence of major comorbid conditions.

The prevalence of hypertension varies with age and sex. A 2014 report of data from the National Health and Nutrition Examination Study (NHANES) estimated that 30% of adult Americans have hypertension with the prevalence increasing with age and reaching 70% in persons aged 75 years and above. At all ages and in both sexes African–Americans continue to have a higher prevalence of hypertension in the United States than all other racial/ethnic groups. In African–Americans hypertension tends to develop at an earlier age and tends to be more severe than in other racial/ethnic groups. Some patients with systemic hypertension will have a specific identifiable cause for the elevated systemic blood pressure. The estimated proportion of the cases of secondary hypertension among patients with systemic hypertension ranges from about 5% to 10% and has not been shown to exhibit racial predilection. Patients with secondary hypertension usually exhibit suggestive constellations of signs, symptoms and/or laboratory abnormalities on initial evaluation and should undergo further evaluation for specific causes of hypertension regardless of their race and/or ethnicity. Despite these differences there are no major differences in recommended target blood pressure goals or class of antihypertensive therapy for African–Americans. Although some studies demonstrated differences in level of blood pressure response to certain medications by race, there appears to be no difference in hard outcomes such as cardiovascular events and mortality. Thus a summary of key recommendations from several current reports and guidelines on the treatment of high blood pressure are shown in Table 42–1.

Hypertension is one of the major risk factors for cardiovascular disease and one of the key World Health Organization target conditions to reduce premature morbidity and mortality related to non-communicable diseases. Uncontrolled hypertension leads to specific target organ damage that contributes to overall cardiovascular morbidity and mortality. African–Americans exhibit a greater rate of target organ damage than other racial and ethnic groups. In fact, the heart disease mortality rate is 50% higher; the stroke mortality rate is 80% higher, and the incidence of hypertension-related end-stage renal disease (ESRD) is sixfold higher in African–Americans than in whites. Thus, it is apparent that hypertension along with its cardiovascular morbidity and mortality is an even greater challenge for the African–American community than it is for the rest of the nation. Many of the factors responsible for the disparities in the incidence, prevalence, detection, treatment, and control of hypertension such as education, health literacy, and access to care have been well described and can be useful in the design and development of programs and policies targeted to the diagnosis and control of hypertension within the population. Further research is needed to better understand the optimal strategies to address the sociologic issues and biologic factors that conspire to prevent the optimal control of hypertension.

▶ Pathogenesis

Blood pressure is a continuous variable determined by multiple factors and demonstrates a fairly normal distribution

Table 42–1. A summary of key recommendations for the treatment of high blood pressure (BP) from several professional organizations.

Guideline	Evidence Review Methodology	BP Target in General Adult Population	BP Target in CKD and DM
ACCF/AHA (2011)	Consensus	Age <80: ≤140/90 Age ≥80: ≤140–145/90	<130/80
NICE (2011)	Systematic review	Age <80: <140/90 Age ≥80: <150/90	<140/90
NKF-KDOQI (2012)	Consensus (Graded)	<140/90	<140/90
ESH/ESC (2013)	Consensus (Graded)	Age <80: <140/90 Age ≥80: <150/90	<140/90 (<130/80 if CKD and proteinuria)
ADA (2013)	Consensus		<140/80
ASH/ISH (2014)	Consensus	Age <80: <140/90 Age ≥80: <150/90	<140/90
CHEP (2014)	Consensus	Age <80: <140/90 Age ≥80: <150/90	<140/90 (CKD) <130/80 (DM)
JAMA "JNC 8" (2014)	Systematic review	Age <60: <140/90 Age ≥60: <150/90	<140/90

ACCF/AHA, American College of Cardiology Foundation; ADA, American Diabetes Association; ASH/ISH, American Society of Hypertension and the International Society of Hypertension; CHEP, Canadian Hypertension Education Program; CKD, chronic kidney disease; DM, diabetes mellitus; ESH/ESC, European Society of Hypertension/European Society of Cardiology; ISHIB, International Society on Hypertension in Blacks; NICE, National Institute for Health and Clinical Excellence; NKF-KDOQI, National Kidney Foundation - Kidney Disease Outcomes Quality Initiative. (Adapted from Still CH et al: Recognition and management of hypertension in older persons: focus on African Americans. *J Am Geriatr Soc* 2015;63:2130.)

within the population. Some of the factors that determine blood pressure level are genetic and these have been estimated to account for about 30–50% of the blood pressure variation in the general population. The development of primary (also called essential or idiopathic) hypertension, however, is believed to require a genetic predisposition and an environmental or psychosocial precipitation in most instances. The search for specific genes responsible for hypertension has resulted in the discovery of some rare monogenetic causes of both high and low blood pressure. While several physiologic characteristics, such as low renin levels, lower bioavailability of nitric oxide, increased salt sensitivity, and increased aldosterone levels, are more prevalent in African–Americans, specific genetic underpinnings have yet to be identified. In spite of popular expectation there is still no identified genetic basis for the excess prevalence of hypertension in the African–American community. However, several lifestyle and environmental risk factors for hypertension have been identified with important differences among racial and ethnic groups, often driven by institutionalized racism and adverse social positioning.

Excess body fat, particularly in the abdomen, is an important risk factor for hypertension. Whether expressed as overweight or obesity (or increased waist circumference

or waist to hip ratio), excess body fat is more common among African–Americans, Hispanics, and several other ethnic minorities. Dietary salt intake in the form of sodium chloride has been associated with the level of blood pressure and the rise in blood pressure with age. As a group, African–Americans have higher salt intake and have a greater sensitivity to changes in blood pressure in response to dietary salt intake, similar to that seen in older persons. In contrast low potassium intake has been associated with hypertension and there is evidence that high dietary potassium, particularly in the form of fresh fruits and vegetables, may offer protection from hypertension and perhaps reduce the need for antihypertensive drug therapy. The diets of many African–Americans are generally low in fruits and vegetables and the average dietary potassium intake among African–Americans is less than that of other major racial and ethnic groups in the United States.

Physical inactivity is a risk factor for hypertension and cardiovascular mortality. Optimum physical activity requires 20–60 minutes of rhythmic and aerobic large-muscle activity such as walking, running, and cycling 3–5 days a week for blood pressure control and cardiorespiratory fitness. Physical activity is reported to be suboptimal in over 60% of the U.S. adults, about 25% of who are totally inactive.

Physical inactivity is more common among older adults, women, a less affluent people, including both Hispanic and African–American adults.

The intake of three or more standard drinks of alcohol per day, where a standard drink is defined as 14 g of ethanol and is contained in 1.5 oz of distilled spirit, a 5-oz glass of table wine, or a 12-oz glass of beer, has been associated with serious adverse psychosocial and health consequences including hypertension. It is estimated that about 60% of Americans ages 18 years and over ingest alcohol and about 30% have five or more standard drinks on the same occasion at least once in that year. Avoidance of excess alcohol intake is prudent for all optimizing cardiovascular health for all Americans.

The high prevalence of low educational attainment and high unemployment among minority populations in the United States predisposes many minority communities, including African–American, to continued adverse political and socioeconomic conditions that contribute to environmental and psychosocial stress. In addition, increased rates of being under- or uninsured and reduced access to quality healthcare further impact cardiovascular health. Acute stress can transiently raise blood pressure, while chronic stress has been associated with sustained hypertension. The job-strain model of psychosocial conflict, designed to assess the impact of occupational stress on the health of the worker, characterizes jobs into high and low strain jobs. Workers with high decision latitudes exhibit little or no distress because they have more flexibility in deciding how best to meet their work-related demands, while those in occupations that combine high demands with low decision latitudes exhibit high stress levels and its attendant cardiovascular morbidity. African–Americans are more likely to be employed in these positions of low decision latitude. Indeed, men employed in these typically blue-collar jobs have a threefold increase in hypertension and those who remain in these jobs for 3 or more years have a reported average blood pressure that is 11/7 mm Hg higher than men in low strain jobs.

While genetic and biological differences may influence the distribution of blood pressure levels within a population, the prevailing body of evidence seems to suggest that lifestyle and socioeconomic disparities have a greater influence on the expression of hypertension and the disproportionate burden of hypertension and cardiovascular disease in African–Americans. This suggests that it is not genetics alone but the gene–environment interaction that is responsible for the higher prevalence of hypertension among African–Americans. Further evidence supporting the unique role of environment is the fact that the excess risk for hypertension in African–Americans is more strongly linked to being born and living in the United States, than with African ancestry.

Racial and/or ethnic differences in combined cardiovascular endpoints assume less significance in hypertensive-treated patients after an adjustment for differences in socioeconomic and demographic factors. The treatment and control of hypertension for optimal outcomes require an appropriate sensitivity to and an understanding of the unique sociocultural aspects of race/ethnicity to maximize effective behavioral and lifestyle recommendations, adherence to pharmacologic treatment, access to care and scheduled follow-ups. Such approaches will ultimately assist in overcoming many of the barriers to the control of hypertension and will lead to improved cardiovascular outcomes for all Americans.

▶ Treatment Strategies

A. Hypertension

Suboptimal rates of blood pressure control perpetuate severe hypertension and the disproportionate burden of cardiovascular disease (CVD) and premature death among African–Americans. While biobehavioral and socioeconomic factors are frequently cited as plausible explanations for the lack of awareness and effective treatment of high blood pressure among African–Americans, these may not fully explain the failure to achieve recommended blood pressure goals. Several large-scale multicenter studies with substantial enrollment of African–American patients have demonstrated that blood pressure can be treated to goal levels, although more aggressive therapy may be needed. African–Americans seem to have a slightly greater blood pressure response to diuretics and calcium channel blockers (CCBs) than do other ethnic groups and lesser response to angiotensin-converting enzyme inhibitors (ACEIs) and β-blockers. Nevertheless, these differences do not seem to translate into different clinical outcomes based on class of antihypertensive therapy as long as target blood pressure levels are achieved. In fact the Antihypertensive and Lipid-Lowering Treatment to Prevent Heart Attack Trial (ALLHAT) found no difference in patient outcomes by race or ethnicity in persons with hypertension randomized to treatment with diuretic, CCB or ACEIs. However, it should be noted that a fourth treatment arm with an α-blocker was discontinued early due to adverse outcomes and should not be considered for initial therapy. Thus, the search for cardiovascular risk factors and target organ damage, both of which are more prevalent among hypertensive African–Americans, and the selection of the appropriate therapeutic agent based on the coexisting comorbidities should guide the selection for blood pressure control among African–Americans. Most professional organization guidelines recommend a target blood pressure goal of less than 140/90 mm Hg with no modification by race/ethnicity.

B. Cardiovascular and Related Complications of Hypertension

Hypertension is not only a major risk factor for CVD, but often occurs in combination with one or more cardiovascular risk factors such as obesity, diabetes, and/or dyslipidemia in a constellation known as the metabolic syndrome. A race-specific role for emerging cardiovascular risk factors such as aldosterone and inflammatory mediators has yet to be determined. The clinical and laboratory search for novel cardiovascular risk factors and mediators of target-organ damage is particularly important for African–American hypertensive patients. The awareness and identification of specific end-organ damage and coexisting cardiovascular risk factors should help prioritize nonpharmacologic recommendations, the selection of compelling evidenced-based medical treatment, and the establishment of appropriate target goals. The use of statins is also recommended for patients with increased cardiovascular risk regardless of race/ethnicity. The four statin benefit groups include: (1) people with clinical atherosclerotic cardiovascular disease (ASCVD), (2) those with primary elevations of low-density lipoprotein (LDL) cholesterol more than 190 mg/dL, (3) people aged 40–75 years who have diabetes mellitus (DM) with LDL cholesterol 70–189 mg/dL and without clinical ASCVD, and (4) those without clinical ASCVD or DM with LDL cholesterol 70–189 mg/dL and estimated 10-year ASCVD risk more than 7.5%.

C. Left Ventricular Hypertrophy

Left ventricular hypertrophy is a common complication of hypertension and an independent predictor of increased mortality among hypertensive patients. It is more common among female and African–American patients with hypertension and may account for some of the ethnic and gender differences in cardiovascular mortality rates.

The treatment and control of hypertension by β-blockade and renin–angiotensin inhibition have been associated with regression of left ventricular hypertrophy. The blood pressure reduction and left ventricular mass regression associated with both of these treatments in most studies were similar in African–American and other racial and ethnic participants. A diminished response among African–Americans treated with angiotensin receptor blocker (ARB) therapy in one study may have been related to fewer African–Americans achieving target blood pressure goals, but a differential outcome based on race cannot be excluded.

D. Congestive Heart Failure

Congestive heart failure (CHF) in blacks is characterized by a higher frequency of hypertension as the etiology, a worse prognosis, and perhaps less of a response to evidenced-based CHF medical therapy in comparison to their white counterparts. There is abundant evidence that β-blockade and renin–angiotensin inhibition are beneficial for improving both mortality and hospitalization outcomes among patients with CHF, and overall these treatment strategies when adjusted for other covariates appear similar for both African–American and other racial/ethnic patients. While there are reports of higher readmission rates for African–American patients receiving these treatments, post-hospitalization mortality data suggest that when quality care is provided, the apparent racial disparities in CHF outcomes dissipate. The treatment of CHF patients should therefore encompass class-specific therapy (eg, ACEI, ARB, β-blocker) in combination with diuretics as indicated for the general population regardless of race or ethnicity. The addition of aldosterone blockade has also led to improved CHF outcomes, although there are no data on racial differences. However, it should be noted that isosorbide dinitrate and hydralazine have been shown to reduce CHF mortality by 43% compared to placebo for African–Americans. This effect is hypothesized to be related to repletion of the aforementioned low bioavailability of nitric oxide in African–Americans.

E. Stroke

African–American patients with hypertension exhibit the highest stroke rates of any racial or ethnic group. The recent decline in stroke mortality observed in other racial and ethnic groups is attenuated for African–American patients with hypertension. Blood pressure control and antiplatelet therapy remain the principal strategies for reducing stroke events among patients with hypertension. The degree of protection conferred by blood pressure control may vary for different classes of antihypertensive medications. A relative-risk reduction in stroke as high as 40% has been reported for African–Americans with diuretic therapy compared to therapy with ACEIs. Diuretics and CCBs have emerged as the preferred antihypertensive treatment for reducing stroke events for all hypertensive patients, including African–Americans. There are no reported racial and/or ethnic differences in the prevention of recurrent stroke and myocardial infarction with ticlopidine and aspirin, or apixaban in patients with nonvalvular atrial fibrillation. Aspirin is more cost effective and should therefore be the preferred agent for antiplatelet therapy. Ticlopidine should be reserved for patients with aspirin intolerance and allergy.

F. Chronic Kidney Disease

ESRD secondary to hypertension is up to six times more common in African–Americans than in the general population. The use of ACEIs in comparison to β-blockers and dihydropyridine CCBs was associated with a reduction in adverse clinical outcomes (doubling of creatinine, ESRD, or death) for African–American patients with hypertensive nephrosclerosis. Thus, the existing body of evidence suggests that optimal clinical outcomes are achieved when inhibition of the renin–angiotensin system is used as initial antihypertensive therapy with diuretics in African–Americans with hypertensive nephrosclerosis. Diabetes is the leading cause of ESRD for all racial and ethnic groups and over 90% of patients with diabetic nephropathy have hypertension. Multiple studies support the use of ACEIs or ARBs as the mainstay of therapy. The inclusion of nearly 15% African–American participants in two of the pivotal prospective randomized trial studies of the role of inhibition of the renin–angiotensin system in diabetic nephropathy, suggests that the positive outcomes extend to blacks as well as nonblacks. Thus, interruption of the renin–angiotensin system has emerged as the initial recommended therapy in combination with diuretics for treating hypertensive and diabetic nephropathy, and usually represents the minimum treatment regimen needed to achieve the more aggressive recommended treatment goal of 130/80 mm Hg for patients with chronic kidney disease (CKD) and proteinuria. Several recent randomized controlled studies support the use of either ACEIs or ARBs but not both together. Also, it should be noted the use of statins is now recommended for all patients with CKD except those on dialysis.

G. Therapeutic Lifestyle Changes

Therapeutic lifestyle changes are equally effective across racial and ethnic groups, and sometimes even more effective among African–American patients. These changes are particularly important for African–American patients with hypertension because many of the major risk factors for hypertension in these patients are behavioral and modifiable. The identification and communication of risk-attributable behaviors (such as dietary indiscretion, physical inactivity, excessive alcohol intake, and smoking), particularly within the context of the established burden of cardiovascular disease, should engage and encourage the patient to be proactive in the implementation of therapeutic lifestyle changes. Findings from the Dietary Approaches to Stop Hypertension or DASH diet have been shown to lower blood pressure with diet rich in fruits, vegetables, and low-fat dairy foods and limited sodium, sweets, sugary drinks, and red meats.

Practical suggestions for the effective implementation of therapeutic lifestyle changes are listed in Table 42–2. Many

Table 42–2. Therapeutic lifestyle changes.

Medical Target	Practical Plan to Achieve Goal
Weight loss	Lose weight gradually by making permanent changes in daily diet for the entire family. Initiate 800–1500 kcal/day diet and set a reasonable weight loss goal (1–2 lb/week for the first 3–6 months)
Dietary goals	
Low fat	Eat more broiled and steamed foods
Low sodium	Eat more grains, fresh fruits, and vegetables
High potassium	Eat fewer fats and use healthier fats, such as olive oil
Adequate calcium	Eat fewer processed foods, fast foods, and fried foods
	Read labels and pay attention to the sodium, potassium, and fat content of foods
	Do not add salt when cooking; instead use vinegar, lemon juice, or sodium substitutes such as potassium instead of standard table salt for seasoning
	Do not season foods with smoked meats, such as bacon and ham hocks
	If lactose intolerant, try lactose-free milk or yogurt, or drink calcium-fortified juices or soy milk
	No more than two beers, one glass of wine, or one shot of hard liquor per day (even less for women)
Physical fitness	Increase physical activity as part of the daily routine: eg, if currently sedentary, get off the bus six blocks from home or walk in the evening with your spouse, a friend, or a group. Gradually increase the time spent at an enjoyable physical activity to 30–45 minutes 3–5 days/week
Adapt a low stress lifestyle	Teach coping skills for specific stressors in the work and/or home environment meditation, relaxation, yoga, biofeedback, others
Additional considerations	Maintain a smoke-free environment and limit alcohol intake

Modified with permission from Douglas JG, et al: Management of high blood pressure in African Americans: consensus statement of the hypertension in African Americans working group of the International Society on Hypertension in Blacks. *Arch Intern Med* 2003;163:525.

Table 42–3. Barriers to therapeutic lifestyle changes and adherence in African–Americans.

Overweight/obese (body mass index >25/30 kg/m²)	Cultural concern that a thin body habitus is associated with poor health
High dietary intake of sodium and fat	Cultural food preparation and conditioned tasting likely were initiated or exacerbated during slavery when high salt and fat content were needed for preservation and/or palatability of suboptimal food sources (salt sensitivity is more common in African–Americans than in whites; if BP is not controlled, check 24-hour urinary sodium excretion to assess dietary adherence)
Low dietary calcium intake	Low milk and dairy intake due to high prevalence of lactose intolerance
Inactivity for women	Cultural emphasis on hair styling and relatively high cost of hair maintenance contribute to avoidance of routine exercise with increased heart rate and sweating
Low adherence to prescribed treatment plan	Assess for medication side effects (particularly impotence among males and increased cough and angioedema among African–Americans taking ACEI)
	High rate of poverty, low rates of insurance (check prescription plan) and/or ability to pay for prescribed medications (adjust therapy as needed)
	Assess biobehavioral barriers and family support structure
	Recognize distrust of the medical establishment
Missed office appointments	Transportation difficulties: Many patients may not have a car and many cities have poor mass transportation systems
	Competing priorities such as child/grandchild care and elder care (often related to extended family home structure; child care and elder care facilities are often geographically disconnected from health centers)
	Limited ability to leave work to attend healthcare appointments in many job settings

ACEI, angiotensin-converting enzyme inhibitor; BP, blood pressure.
Modified with permission from Martins D, Norris K: Hypertension treatment in African Americans: physiology is less important than sociology. *Cleve Clin J Med* 2004;71:735. Copyright © 2004 Cleveland Clinic Foundation. All rights reserved.

of the barriers to successful implementation of therapeutic lifestyle changes among African–Americans are listed in Table 42–3. The recommendations for therapeutic lifestyle changes, such as weight control, dietary salt reduction, regular physical activity, and adherence to clinic visits and pharmacotherapy, should be provided in specific detail with a patient centered approach, making it possible to break through some of these common barriers and achieve successful implementation. This may frequently necessitate the inclusion of additional healthcare professionals (eg, dietitian, pharmacist, social worker) and/or the inclusion of family members or close friends in the dialogue.

▶ Prognosis

The mainstay of hypertensive therapy for African–Americans remains diuretics and therapeutic lifestyle changes. The selection of supplemental antihypertensive agents should be tailored to the presence of coexisting risk factors, comorbid medical conditions, and/or the presence of hypertension-related target organ damage. Many of these patients will need two or more antihypertensive agents to achieve target blood pressure goals. The preference for agents that block

the renin–angiotensin system as supplemental antihypertensive agents among patients with CHF, diabetes, and kidney disease cannot be overemphasized. It is, however, pertinent to note that the use of some of these agents among African–Americans is associated with a slightly higher rate of side effects, such as cough or angioedema with ACEIs. Thus, strategies for the treatment of hypertension should be driven by the prevalence of coexisting cardiovascular risk factors and an understanding of sociocultural influences that impact access to care and adherence to evidenced-based treatment rather than minor differences in blood pressure response by racial and ethnic categories. Such approaches will ultimately reduce the disproportionate impact of hypertension and CVD within the African–American community.

KEY READINGS

Egan BM, Li J, Hutchison FN, Ferdinand KC: Hypertension in the United States, 1999 to 2012: progress toward Healthy People 2020 goals. Circulation 2014;130:1692.

Grim CE et al: Hyperaldosteronism and hypertension: ethnic differences. Hypertension 2005;45:766.

James PA et al: 2014 evidence-based guideline for the management of high blood pressure in adults: report from the panel members appointed to the Eighth Joint National Committee (JNC 8). JAMA 2014;311:507.

Julius S et al: Cardiovascular risk reduction in hypertensive black patients with left ventricular hypertrophy: the LIFE study. J Am Coll Cardiol 2004;43:1047.

Martins D, Norris K: Hypertension treatment in African Americans: physiology is less important than sociology. Cleve Clin J Med 2004;71:735.

Martins D, Norris K: Hypertension in African Americans. In: *Handbook of Black American Health: Policies and Issues Behind Disparities in Health*, 2nd ed. Livingston I (editor). The Greenwood Publishing Group, 2004.

Mozaffarian D et al: Heart disease and stroke statistics-2015 update: a report from the American Heart Association. Circulation 2015;131:e29.

Norris KC, Francis CK: Gender and ethnic differences and considerations in cardiovascular risk assessment and prevention in African Americans. In: *Practical Strategies in Preventing Heart Disease*. Wong N, Gardin JM, Black HR (editors). McGraw-Hill, 2004.

Norris KC, Brown AF: The highs and lows of blood pressure targets in the elderly and other high risk populations. J Am Geriatr Soc 2015;63:2139.

Still CH et al: Recognition and management of hypertension in older persons: focus on African Americans. J Am Geriatr Soc 2015;63:2130.

Taylor AL et al: African–American Heart Failure Trial Investigators. Combination of isosorbide dinitrate and hydralazine in blacks with heart failure. N Engl J Med 2004;351:2049. Erratum in N Engl J Med 2005;352:1276.

Wright JT Jr et al: A randomized trial of intensive versus standard blood-pressure control. N Engl J Med 2015;373:2103.

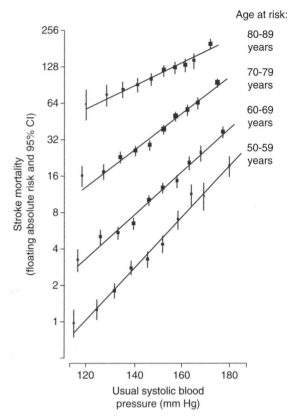

▲ **Figure 42–1.** Ten-year stroke mortality by age and systolic blood pressure. (From Lewington S et al: Age-specific relevance of usual blood pressure to vascular mortality: a meta-analysis of individual data for one million adults in 61 prospective studies. Lancet 2002;360:1903.)

▼ HYPERTENSION IN THE ELDERLY

Hillel Sternlicht, MD

▶ Introduction

Those aged 65 and older are the fasting growing age demographic in the United States. Given that age is the leading risk factor for stroke, an 80-year old with a systolic pressure of 120 mm Hg is four times more likely to suffer a stroke in the coming decade than a 50-year old with a systolic pressure of 180 mm Hg (Figure 42–1). The second leading risk factor is blood pressure with optimal control leading to marked reductions in rates of all-cause mortality, stroke, heart failure, and myocardial infarction. As such, the personal and public health implications of hypertension are incontrovertible with the elderly very much a "high risk" population.

▶ Epidemiology

Among industrialized societies, blood pressure rises linearly with age. As such, with gains in life expectancy, hypertension is nearly inevitable. According to the National Health and Nutrition Examination Survey (NHANES) for the 2011–2014 period, 65% of individuals over age 60 have blood pressures in excess of 140 mm Hg systolic or 90 mm Hg diastolic, the current (as of 2014) definition. Even if one is normotensive until the age of 60, the risk of developing hypertension over his/her remaining lifetime exceeds 85% among those who live until age 79, the current life expectancy of United States citizens. Moreover, with recent studies showing improved cardiovascular outcomes with achieved blood pressures as low as 120/80 mm Hg, the prevalence will rise further as the diagnostic threshold for hypertension falls.

While the age at one is considered "elderly" has risen along with gains in life expectancy, the phenotype of hypertension changes fundamentally with age, a process related to decreased compliance of the large vessels from atherosclerotic disease. While those less than 40 years of age suffer from combined systolic and diastolic hypertension, isolated systolic hypertension (systolic ≥140 but diastolic <90 mm Hg) is the hallmark among hypertensives above 60 years of age. This rising gradient between systolic and diastolic blood pressure, knows as the pulse pressure, is itself predictive of heightened cardiovascular event rates.

Pathogenesis

Despite a mature understanding of the epidemiology and benefits of controlling high blood pressure, the precise etiology of hypertension, including isolated systolic hypertension, remains opaque. While multifactorial, consensus exists on certain features characteristic of hypertension in the elderly, if not explaining the etiology per se. Pathologic studies of the large central vessels of such individuals show a gradual degeneration of the elastin fibers found within the arterial media leading to "cystic medial necrosis." Functionally, this results in a loss of elasticity and stiffening of the central vasculature preventing the vessels from acting as capacitance systems capable of dampening cardiac pulsation as blood moves through the arterial tree. In this milieu, the stroke volume generated by systole is rapidly propelled to peripheral vessels such that there are less blood volume in the aorta during diastole, hence the elevated systolic pressures, low diastolic pressures, and widened pulse pressure.

Among elderly individuals with hypertension, the principal risk factor for adverse clinical events is linked to systolic rather than diastolic blood pressure. Upon analysis of 25 years of longitudinal follow-up among participants in the Framingham Heart Study, Kannel found the incidence of stroke to be fourfold higher among those with systolic pressures in excess of 180 mm Hg compared to less than 140 mm Hg. In contradistinction, there was no relationship between rates of stroke and diastolic pressures ranging from less than 90 to greater than 95 mm Hg.

Benefits of Treatment and the Blood Pressures Required to Realize Them

Individual high quality studies as well as meta-analyses unequivocally demonstrate the benefit of antihypertensive therapy in reducing hard clinical endpoints among elderly hypertensives, particularly stroke, for which the principal modifiable risk factor is systolic blood pressure. A meta-analysis of 15,000 patients aged 60 or higher with isolated systolic hypertension found a 13% reduction in all-cause mortality and a 30% reduction in strokes when blood pressure was reduced by approximately 7–14/3–6 mm Hg. Moreover, despite similar relative risk reductions among all age groups with treatment of hypertension, the higher absolute rates of cardiovascular events among the elderly translate into a much lower number needed to treat to prevent one adverse outcome. For example, while 39 individuals between 60–70 years of age require treatment for 5 years to prevent one cardiovascular event, only 19 patients over the age of 70 require therapy to realize comparable benefit.

The 8th Joint National Committee (JNC-8) recommendations published in 2014 suggest a target of 150/90 mm Hg among otherwise healthy individuals over the age of 60. The 2013 European Society Hypertension Guidelines recommend systolic blood pressure goals of 140–150 mm Hg among those 70 or older. No diastolic target is mentioned. However, more recent data (see "Lifestyle and Pharmacologic Treatment Strategies") indicates improved clinical endpoints with blood pressures below these levels.

Lifestyle and Pharmacologic Treatment

The Trial of Nonpharmacologic Interventions in the Elderly (TONE) evaluated the need for ongoing antihypertensive therapy among 60–80 year olds who reduced their salt intake, weight (if obese), or both. Only individuals on drug monotherapy were included. After 7 months of lifestyle interventions, weight fell by 5% (4 kg); sodium intake fell from 3500 mg to 2300 mg. Those who achieved the aforementioned sodium or weight reduction were 60% more likely to remain off antihypertensive therapy than the control group at 30 months. Those with declines in both weight and sodium were more than 2.5 times more likely to be off antihypertensive therapy with an absolute medication resumption rate of 40% at 30 months. Given the blood pressure rises with age and the difficulty of maintaining lifestyle changes indefinitely, the long-term feasibility of these interventions remains to be seen.

Landmark studies in the field of hypertension have focused on the effects of lower blood pressure targets on improving clinical outcomes, particularly those of the cerebral and coronary systems. Prior to the publication of the Systolic Hypertension in the Elderly Program (SHEP) in 1991, no trial had directly assessed the benefits of treating isolated systolic hypertension among individuals aged 60 and above. Among 4700 individuals with a mean age of 72 and an entry blood pressure of 170/77 mm Hg, those treated primarily with a chlorthalidone based regimen achieved a final blood pressure of 143/68 mm Hg compared to 155/72 mm Hg among the placebo group (40% of whom received antihypertensives outside the study). Despite a smaller difference in blood pressure reduction between groups than anticipated, the study achieved its primary outcome by demonstrating a one third reduction in rates of stroke among those in the active treatment arm after 4.5 of follow-up. The subsequent Medical Research Council (MRC) trial compared hydrochlorothiazide/triamterene with atenolol and placebo. After 6 years, blood pressure among all treated patients was identical but only those receiving the diuretic experienced reductions in stroke (33%). The lack of benefit with β-blocker monotherapy despite comparable achieved blood pressures is addressed below. In the late 1990s, the first large trial utilizing CCBs for isolated systolic hypertension in the elderly appeared, the Systolic Hypertension in Europe (Syst-Eur).

The nearly 5000 patients had a mean age of 70 and a baseline blood pressure of 174/86 mm Hg; those randomized to the CCB nitrendipine achieved blood pressures of 151/77 compared to 161/84 mm Hg in the control arm. After 2 years of follow-up, the primary outcome of stroke was nearly 45% less likely to occur among CCB treated patients. Appearing around the same time, the Swedish Trial in Old Patients with Hypertension-2 (STOP HTN-2), assessed whether "newer" agents such as ACEIs and CCBs allowed for equal protection against cardiovascular events as "older" agents such as diuretics and β-blockers. The 6500 patients received lisinopril or enalapril, felodipine or isradipine, a β-blocker or hydrochlorothiazide. Mean age was 76. Blood pressure fell by 35/17 mm Hg from a mean initial value of 194/98 mm Hg. After over 4 years of follow-up, rates of cardiovascular outcomes were identical indicating ACEIs were equally efficacious in the treatment of isolated systolic hypertension.

With the continued gains in life expectancy achieved during the 1990s and the aforementioned trials demonstrating the unequivocal benefit of more aggressive blood pressure control among those in their 70s, investigators initiated the Hypertension in the Very Elderly Trial (HYVET) assessing the efficacy of antihypertensive therapy among those aged 80 or older. While self-evident at present, at the time some considered it unethical to undertake a study in this patient population given earlier retrospective data suggesting potential harm. With a mean age of 84 and blood pressure of 173/91 mm Hg, 3800 participants were randomized to the thiazide-like indapamide (akin to chlorthalidone) with an ACEI as needed. Upon termination at 2 years, blood pressure was 143/78 versus 158/84 mm Hg among the placebo arm. Death from any cause was decreased by 20%, stroke by 40%, and any cardiovascular event by 33%.

With a growing body of evidence demonstrating that hypertension should be treated regardless of patient age, subsequent trials turned their attention to optimal blood pressure targets. With SHEP and HYVET reporting additional benefits with blood pressures approaching 140 mm Hg systolic among those with isolated systolic hypertension, more recent trials sought to further lower blood pressure in an attempt to maximize favorable outcomes among high risk populations. For, if hypertension is defined as a blood pressure at which cardiovascular outcomes are worse compared to normotensive individuals, systolic pressures in excess of 115 mm Hg may one day be considered elevated given the risk of stroke rises linearly from this threshold upward. The initial seminal paper in the field, the effects of intensive blood pressure control in type 2 diabetes mellitus (ACCORD) randomized diabetics (mean age 62, pretreatment blood pressure 139/77 mm Hg) to more aggressive or traditional blood pressure targets with achieved systolic values of 120 and 135mm Hg systolic. Elderly patients with isolated systolic hypertension were among the study participants. After 5 years of follow-up, the study was published in 2010 showing no difference in composite cardiovascular event rates. While many found shortcomings in the study design and cohort characteristics, this "negative" trial suggested 135 mm Hg might be the lowest systolic blood pressure that resulted in cardiovascular benefit, at least among diabetics. In 2015, the Systolic Blood Pressure Intervention Trial (SPRINT) evaluated similar blood pressure targets but among non-diabetics deemed at high risk from suffering a cardiovascular event. Even among the subgroup of frail elderly, an achieved systolic pressure of 123 mm Hg resulted in a 1/3 reduction in all-cause mortality compared to those pressures of 135 mm Hg upon study completion (Figure 42–2).

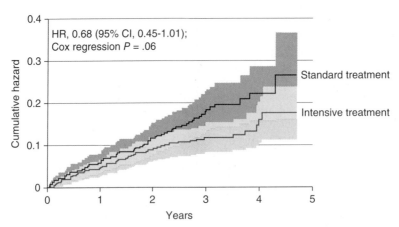

▲ **Figure 42–2.** Hazard ratio for primary cardiovascular event among frail individuals over age 75. (From Williamson JD et al: Intensive vs Standard Blood Pressure Control and Cardiovascular Disease Outcomes in Adults Aged ≥75 Years: A Randomized Clinical Trial. JAMA 2016;315:2673.)

With a strong evidence base supporting the treatment of hypertension among those in the 60–85 age range, agent selection for primary hypertension quickly comes to the fore. Apart a compelling indication for a given class of agents (ie, β-blockers for recent myocardial infarction), achieving optimal blood pressure targets supersedes considerations regarding agent selection. The following classes of agents—CCBs, angiotensin converting enzymes or angiotensin receptor blockers, and diuretics, particularly chlorthalidone and indapamide—are largely equivalent in achieving comparable clinical outcomes and recommended as initial therapy by JNC8 and the European Society of Hypertension guidelines. Their comparable efficacy was demonstrated in the influential Antihypertensive and Lipid Lowering Treatment to Prevent Heart Attack Trial (ALLHAT) which found that among the 33,000 patients who received either chlorthalidone, lisinopril, or amlodipine, all-cause mortality as well as a composite of cardiovascular events were identical after 5 years of follow-up. ALLHAT initially contained a 4th arm utilizing the α-blocker doxazosin; however, this arm was terminated prematurely given an increased rate of heart failure compared to the other medications. Nonetheless, it remains a useful antihypertensive but generally avoided as monotherapy. Beta blockers, long considered first line therapy, have fallen out of favor for those without a primary indication given their apparent inferiority to the aforementioned classes, particularly for stroke protection among the elderly.

Among those with "resistant" hypertension, defined as uncontrolled blood pressures despite triple agent therapy including an appropriately dosed diuretic, low dose spironolactone has become the preferred adjuvant therapy among those already taking a diuretic, CCB, and ACE, or ARB. Finally, the use of serum renin and aldosterone levels to guide agent selection, known as "renin profiling," may be a useful tool to guide management among those with difficult to control elevations in blood pressure. Broadly speaking, hypertension can be conceptualized as driven by one of three different pressor systems—(1) salt/volume, (2) renin–angiotensin–aldosterone system, and (3) sympathetic nervous system. While there is overlap between pathways, those with "salt sensitive" hypertension, frequently the elderly and African–Americans, achieve the largest therapeutic response with diuretics and CCBs. Such individuals are characterized by low levels of renin and aldosterone. Conversely, among the minority of patients with elevated renin and aldosterone levels, ACEIs and ARBs are the initial agents of choice. While the only randomized (but unblinded) controlled trial found improved response rates with renin profiling compared to agent selection by a hypertension specialist, retrospective analysis of larger patient cohorts have found no difference in response rates. Moreover, in an era when a majority of patients require 2-3 drugs for adequate blood pressure control, patients are treated with all three core agents regardless.

Obstacles to Implementation

While the elderly are the population most likely to benefit from antihypertensive therapy, they are, by virtue of their age, inherently more susceptible to the adverse effects of such therapies. In the SPRINT trial, those assigned to intensive therapy were 50% more likely than the usual care group to experience hypotension, acute renal failure, hyponatremia or hypokalemia. Given that clinical trials generally recruit individuals with satisfactory functional capacities, agent related complications would be more prominent among the larger aged population. Additional barriers to enhanced blood pressure control include the aggravation of pre-existing orthostasis heightening fall risk, the advisability of applying stringent blood pressure targets to the frail elderly, and the observation that attendant declines in diastolic blood pressure could compromise coronary perfusion predisposing to heightened cardiac event rates.

Using a medicare database, Tinetti retrospectively assessed the relationship between the intensity of antihypertensive therapy and serious falls. Those receiving multiple agents were at least 25% more likely to experience an injurious fall than hypertensive elderlies not on therapy. In contrast, Gangavati prospectively evaluated the relationship between orthostatic hypotension and fall risk among normotensives, controlled, and uncontrolled hypertensives (mean age 78). The author found that normotensive individuals with orthostatic hypotension did not have an increased rate of falls; among hypertensives, the more uncontrolled the blood pressure, the greater the risk of orthostatic hypotension and by extension, falls. This suggests treatment of hypertension among those with orthostatic hypotension may improve orthostasis itself.

Many have questioned whether the benefits of antihypertensive therapy, derived from clinical trials composed of individuals with higher functional statuses, are applicable to the larger elderly population. Proponents of this belief argue that frail individuals among the community are more likely to experience adverse effects—falls, hypotension—without realizing the benefits of decreased clinical event rates. Odden assessed the relationship between mortality and isolated systolic hypertension stratified by the ability to ambulate 6 meters in under 7.5 seconds, a validated protocol strongly associated with traditional measures of patient frailty. Among the 2300 participants, there was no correlation between systolic hypertension and all-cause mortality if a participants walking time exceeded the 7.5 second threshold. Consistent with this functional study's predictive value, those who were unable to complete the task under the pre-specified time limit were older, had a higher prevalence of diabetes, stroke, heart failure, and worse kidney function. In contrast, the aforementioned SPRINT trial contrasting outcomes among those with systolic pressures of 123 versus

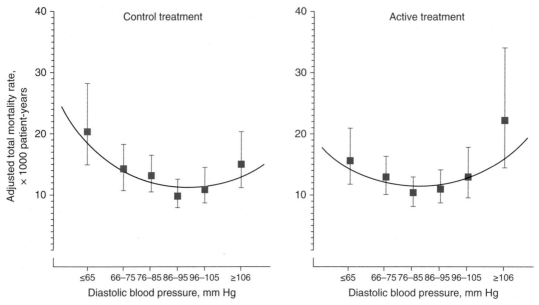

▲ Figure 42–3. Total mortality by diastolic blood pressure among untreated and treated hypertensives. (From Boutitie F et al: J-shaped relationship between blood pressure and mortality in hypertensive patients: new insights from a meta-analysis of individual-patient data. Ann Intern Med 2002;136:438.)

135 mm Hg found the benefits of such therapies preserved among frailer individuals.

Given the large pulse pressure among those with isolated systolic hypertension, achieving blood pressure targets of 120–140 mm Hg systolic often results in diastolic pressures of less than 70 mm Hg. Since tissue perfusion, particularly of the coronary arteries, occurs during diastole, studies have recorded increased numbers of cardiac events among individuals with diastolic pressures below this cut point suggesting the presence of a "J curve" such that both diastolic hyper- and hypotension enhance the rate of cardiovascular events (Figure 42–3). The larger literature offers conflicting conclusions. For example, a large meta-analysis involving 40,000 patients drawn from clinical trials evaluated the effects of antihypertensives on blood pressure found that a diastolic threshold below which adverse outcomes occurred did exist; however, this was present in both the treated and control arms suggesting that low diastolic pressures represent a higher burden of atherosclerotic disease which can explain the J curve in and of itself.

▶ Perspective

The development of several classes of potent yet well tolerated antihypertensive agents, coupled with the large and high quality trials over the last 25 years represent a major advance in the management of high blood pressure. In light of this progress, the imperative is no longer that of research and development

but rather those of patient education and treatment. While systolic blood pressure goals of 120–130 mm Hg may apply to the larger non-diabetic and otherwise high functioning elderly population, the identification of a blood pressure target and agent considerations are predicated on the assessment of each patient's particular circumstances. More frequent office visits upon initiation and modification of therapy, the use of home blood pressure measurements, and ongoing patient education to monitor for untoward effects of therapy allow patients to capture the life changing benefits of antihypertensive therapy with as few adverse effects as possible.

KEY READINGS

The ALLHAT Officers and Coordinators for the ALLHAT Collaborative Research Group: Major outcomes in high-risk hypertensive patients randomized to angiotensin-converting enzyme inhibitor or calcium channel blocker vs diuretic: The Antihypertensive and Lipid-Lowering Treatment to Prevent Heart Attack Trial (ALLHAT). JAMA 2002;288:2981.

Beckett NS et al: Treatment of hypertension in patients 80 years of age or older. N Engl J Med 2008;358:1887.

Boutitie F et al: J-shaped relationship between blood pressure and mortality in hypertensive patients: new insights from a meta-analysis of individual-patient data. Ann Intern Med 2002;136:438.

Cushman WC et al: Effects of intensive blood-pressure control in type 2 diabetes mellitus. N Engl J Med 2010;362:1575.

Egan BM et al: Plasma Renin test-guided drug treatment algorithm for correcting patients with treated but uncontrolled hypertension: a randomized controlled trial. Am J Hypertens 2009;22:792.

Franklin SS et al: Hemodynamic patterns of age-related changes in blood pressure. The Framingham Heart Study. Circulation 1997;96:308.

Franklin SS et al: Is pulse pressure useful in predicting risk for coronary heart Disease? The Framingham heart study. Circulation 1999;100:354.

Franklin SS et al: Predominance of isolated systolic hypertension among middle-aged and elderly US hypertensives: analysis based on National Health and Nutrition Examination Survey (NHANES) III. Hypertension 2001;37:869.

Gangavati A et al: Hypertension, orthostatic hypotension, and the risk of falls in a community-dwelling elderly population: the maintenance of balance, independent living, intellect, and zest in the elderly of Boston study. J Am Geriatr Soc 2011;59:383.

Hansson L et al: Randomised trial of old and new antihypertensive drugs in elderly patients: cardiovascular mortality and morbidity the Swedish Trial in Old Patients with Hypertension-2 study. Lancet 1999;354:1751.

Izzo JL: Arterial stiffness and the systolic hypertension syndrome. Curr Opin Cardiol 2004;19:341.

James PA et al: 2014 evidence-based guideline for the management of high blood pressure in adults: report from the panel members appointed to the Eighth Joint National Committee (JNC 8). JAMA 2014;311:507.

Kannel WB et al: Systolic blood pressure, arterial rigidity, and risk of stroke. The Framingham study. JAMA 1981;245:1225.

Law MR, Morris JK, Wald NJ: Use of blood pressure lowering drugs in the prevention of cardiovascular disease: meta-analysis of 147 randomised trials in the context of expectations from prospective epidemiological studies. BMJ 2009;338:b1665.

Lewington S et al: Age-specific relevance of usual blood pressure to vascular mortality: a meta-analysis of individual data for one million adults in 61 prospective studies. Lancet 2002; 360:1903.

Leotta G et al: Efficacy of antihypertensive treatment based on plasma renin activity: an open label observational study. Blood Press 2010;19:218.

Mancia G et al: 2013 ESH/ESC Guidelines for the management of arterial hypertension: the Task Force for the management of arterial hypertension of the European Society of Hypertension (ESH) and of the European Society of Cardiology (ESC). J Hypertens 2013;31:1281.

Martins D et al: Hypertension in high-risk populations. In: Current Diagnosis & Treatment: Nephrology & Hypertension, Lerma EV, Berns JS, Nissenson AR (editors). New York: McGraw Hill. 2009.

Medical Research Council trial of treatment of hypertension in older adults: principal results. MRC Working Party. BMJ 1992;304:405.

Odden MC et al: Rethinking the association of high blood pressure with mortality in elderly adults: the impact of frailty. Arch Intern Med 2012;172:1162.

Prevention of stroke by antihypertensive drug treatment in older persons with isolated systolic hypertension. Final results of the Systolic Hypertension in the Elderly Program (SHEP). SHEP Cooperative Research Group. JAMA 1991;265:3255.

Soon SS, Fryar C, Carroll M: Hypertension Prevalence and Control Among Adults: United States, 2011–2014. Hyattsville, MD: National Center for Health Statistics. 2015.

Staessen JA et al: Randomised double-blind comparison of placebo and active treatment for older patients with isolated systolic hypertension. The Systolic Hypertension in Europe (Syst-Eur) Trial Investigators. Lancet 1997;350:757.

Staessen JA et al: Risks of untreated and treated isolated systolic hypertension in the elderly: meta-analysis of outcome trials. Lancet 2000;355:865.

Tinetti ME et al: Antihypertensive medications and serious fall injuries in a nationally representative sample of older adults. JAMA Intern Med 2014;174:588.

Turnbull F et al: Effects of different regimens to lower blood pressure on major cardiovascular events in older and younger adults: meta-analysis of randomised trials. BMJ. 2008;336:1121.

Vasan RS et al: Residual lifetime risk for developing hypertension in middle-aged women and men: the Framingham Heart Study. JAMA 2002;287:1003.

Weir MR, Saunders E: Renin status does not predict the antihypertensive response to angiotensin-converting enzyme inhibition in African–Americans. Trandolapril Multicenter Study Group. J Hum Hypertens 1998;12:189.

Werner C: The Older Population: 2010. 2011 Census.gov. Accessed November 23, 2016.

Whelton PK et al: Sodium reduction and weight loss in the treatment of hypertension in older persons: a randomized controlled trial of nonpharmacologic interventions in the elderly (TONE). TONE Collaborative Research Group. JAMA 1998;279:839.

Williams B et al: Spironolactone versus placebo, bisoprolol, and doxazosin to determine the optimal treatment for drug-resistant hypertension (PATHWAY-2): a randomised, double-blind, crossover trial. Lancet 2015;386:2059.

Williamson JD et al: Intensive vs Standard Blood Pressure Control and Cardiovascular Disease Outcomes in Adults Aged ≥75 Years: A Randomized Clinical Trial. JAMA 2016;315:2673.

Wiysonge CS et al: Beta-blockers for hypertension. Cochrane Database Syst Rev 2012;11:CD002003.

Wright JT et al: A Randomized Trial of Intensive versus Standard Blood-Pressure Control. N Engl J Med 2015;373:2103.

Yusuf S et al: Blood-pressure and cholesterol lowering in persons without cardiovascular disease. N Engl J Med 2016;374:2032.

HYPERTENSIVE DISORDERS IN PREGNANCY

Kisra Anis, MBBS; Anjali Acharya, MBBS; and Belinda Jim, MD

General Considerations

Hypertensive disorders in pregnancy complicate up to 10% of all pregnancies in the United States and are responsible for 17% maternal mortality. These disorders are the dominant cause of maternal morbidity and mortality worldwide. The incidence of hypertension in pregnancy is expected to increase with the rise in obesity, metabolic syndrome, and older age of women giving birth. The diagnosis and treatment of hypertension in pregnancy also presents unique challenges due to both the physiologic changes of pregnancy and the critical balance needed for maternal and fetal well-being.

Hypertensive disorders in pregnancy are classified into four main disorders: preeclampsia-eclampsia, chronic hypertension, chronic hypertension with superimposed preeclampsia (SPE) and gestational hypertension (Table 42–4). The time of onset of hypertension along with the presence of diagnostic criteria for preeclampsia are keys to the differential diagnosis (Figure 42–4).

Table 42–4. Hypertensive disorders in pregnancy.

Hypertensive Disorder in Pregnancy	Causes	Complications	Treatment
Preeclampsia–eclampsia	Abnormal placentation leading to placental ischemia and endothelial dysfunction	• Pulmonary edema • Cerebral thrombosis or hemorrhage • PRES • Acute Kidney Injury • Hepatic dysfunction • Hepatic hematoma or rupture • Acute fatty liver of pregnancy • Thrombocytopenia • DIC • Microangiopathic hemolysis • Venous thromboembolism	Delivery of baby—taking into consideration gestational age, severity of preeclampsia and any maternal and fetal complications Treatment of hypertension *Please see Tables 42–7 and 42–8 for preferred antihypertensive medication and goal blood pressure Seizure prophylaxis with magnesium sulfate (4–6 gm IV loading dose with 1–2 gm/hour IV infusion) with clinical monitoring

Chronic hypertension	Essential hypertension
	Obesity
	OSA
	Secondary hypertension:
	  Endocrine
	  Renal artery stenosis
	  Kidney disease
	  Collagen vascular
	Disease (scleroderma and SLE)
		• Superimposed preeclampsia
		• Abruptio placenta
		• Cesarean delivery
		• Postpartum hemorrhage
		• Fetal growth restriction
		• Preterm delivery
			Treatment of hypertension
			*See Tables 42–7 and 42–8 for preferred antihypertensive medication and goal blood pressure

Chronic hypertension superimposed on preeclampsia	Essential hypertension Obesity OSA Secondary hypertension Abnormal placentation leading to placental ischemia and endothelial dysfunction *History of previous preeclampsia and MAP of 95 mm Hg or greater increases risk		

Gestational hypertension
 	
Postpartum hypertension
	Unclear but associated with development of essential hypertension later in life	• Preeclampsia
		• Postpartum hemorrhage
			Treatment of hypertension
			Avoid diuretics if lactating
			The following medications are safe to use during lactation:
			  Labetalol
			  Nifedipine
			  Enalapril
			  Captopril
			  Atenolol
			  Metoprolol

DIC, disseminated intravascular coagulopathy; MAP, mean arterial blood pressure; OSA, obstructive sleep apnea; PRES, posterior reversible leukoencephalopathy; SLE, systemic lupus erythematosus.
*Lecarpentier E, Tsatsaris V, Goffinet F, Cabrol D, Sibai B, Haddad B. Risk factors of superimposed preeclampsia in women with essential chronic hypertension treated before pregnancy. PLoS One. 2013;8(5):e62140.

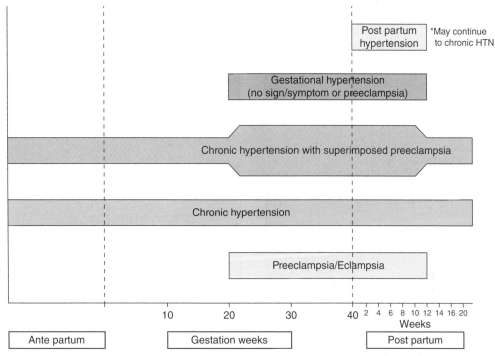

▲ **Figure 42–4.** Timeline in the differential diagnosis of hypertension in pregnancy disorders.

▶ Normal Adaptations and Blood Pressure in Pregnancy

Several hemodynamic and cardiovascular adaptations occur during normal pregnancy which impact maternal blood pressure (Figure 42–5). These include changes in the intravascular volume, cardiac output, heart rate, and systemic vascular resistance.

Many factors are involved in increasing the intravascular volume in pregnancy. Estrogen triggers increased renal renin as well as angiotensinogen production by the liver. Renin and aldosterone levels increase up to eightfold, leading to volume expansion starting at 6 weeks of gestation and peaking at 32 weeks. Other hormones contributing to volume expansion include prolactin, growth hormone, prostaglandins, deoxycorticosterone, and adrenocorticotrophic hormone. Cardiac output increases by 50% during pregnancy due to both an increase in the stroke volume and heart rate. Stroke volume rises slowly till the 26th week partly because of the increase in vascular volume. The heart rate increases by 15–20 beats by 32nd week of gestation.

Despite increase in renin and aldosterone and vascular volume, systolic blood pressure falls by 10–15 mm Hg by the second trimester. This is related to the vasodilating effects of multiple hormones and pathways, including prostacyclin,

estrogen, progesterone, renin–angiotensin–aldosterone system (RAAS), prolactin, nitric oxide, and relaxin. Estrogen and progesterone attenuate the vasoconstrictor effect of the RAAS pathway. The angiotensin-(1–7) component of the vasodilator pathway in the RAAS system is also increased in pregnancy. Relaxin, a hormone excreted by the ovary during gestation, and prostacyclin exert a direct vasodilatory effect. The overall impact is reduction in blood pressure in the second trimester and an increase back to baseline by the third trimester of pregnancy.

KEY READINGS

American College of Obstetricians and Gynecologists; Task Force on Hypertension in Pregnancy: Hypertension in Pregnancy. Report of the American College of Obstetricians and Gynecologists' Task Force on Hypertension in Pregnancy. Obstet Gynecol 2013;122:1122.

Berry C, Atta MG: Hypertensive disorders in pregnancy. World J Nephrol 2016;5:418.

Hladunewich MA et al: Course of preeclamptic glomerular injury after delivery. Am J Physiol Renal Physiol 2008;294:F614.

Moroz LA, Simpson LL, Rochelson B: Management of severe hypertension in pregnancy. Semin Perinatol 2016;40:112.

Nissaisorakarn P, Sharif S, Jim B: Hypertension in pregnancy: defining blood pressure goals and the value of biomarkers for preeclampsia. Curr Cardiol Rep 2016;18:131.

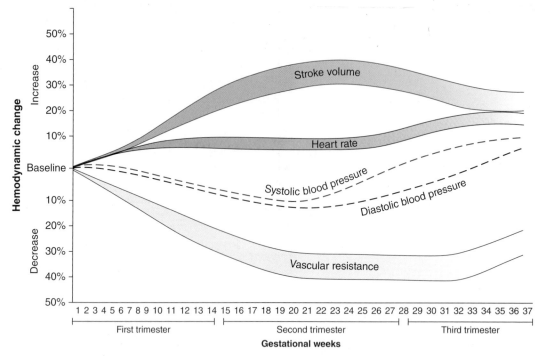

▲ **Figure 42–5.** Physiologic hemodynamic changes during normal pregnancy.

Ouzounian JG, Elkayam U: Physiologic changes during normal pregnancy and delivery. Cardiol Clin 2012;30:317.
Valdes G, Corthorn J: Challenges posed to the maternal circulation by pregnancy. Integr Blood Press Control 2011;4:45.

► Preeclampsia–Eclampsia

A. Diagnosis

Preeclampsia, a pregnancy specific condition, is defined as maternal blood pressure more than or equal to 140/90 on two occasions at least 4 hours apart after 20 weeks of gestation in a woman with a previously measured normal blood pressure with new onset proteinuria or with multisystem involvement in the absence of proteinuria. Proteinuria is defined as more than or equal to 300 mg/24 hours or urine protein to creatinine ratio of more than or equal to 0.3 in at least two random samples, or dipstick reading of 1+ (less favored). Multisystem involvement is defined by: thrombocytopenia (platelet count <100,000 /nL), renal insufficiency (serum creatinine concentrations >1.1 mg/dL or a doubling of the serum creatinine concentration), or impaired liver function (elevated blood concentrations of liver transaminases to twice the normal concentrations), pulmonary edema, or cerebral or visual symptoms. This is an updated definition of the American College of Obstetrics

and Gynecology (ACOG) and many other national societies to include consequences of other end-organs as opposed to only that of the kidney. Preeclampsia is considered severe when maternal blood pressure is more than or equal to 160/110 with end organ damage.

B. Pathogenesis

Though the pathogenesis of preeclampsia is not fully elucidated, it is believed to be a complex disease with the primary problem of defective placentation leading to overall maternal endothelial dysfunction. Traditionally, preeclampsia is thought to be a "two-stage" process, that is, abnormal placentation followed by clinical expression of the disease (Figure 42–6). In a normal pregnancy, the invasion of the muscular walls of uterine spiral arteries by the fetal-derived cytotrophoblasts leads its transformation to an endothelial phenotype, a process called "pseudovasculogenesis"; this in turn leads to the formation of low pressure, low resistance, and high capacitance dilated sac-like structures to facilitate placental blood flow. In preeclampsia, however, the trophoblastic invasion is impaired which results in insufficient spiral artery remodeling and causes placental ischemia that leads to increased production of factors such as angiotensin II, soluble fms-like tyrosine kinase 1 (sFlt-1), soluble endoglin (sEng). It is the discovery of novel angiogenic markers

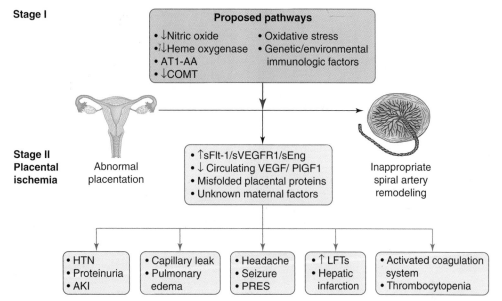

Stage I

Proposed pathways

- ↓Nitric oxide
- ↑↓Heme oxygenase
- AT1-AA
- ↓COMT

- Oxidative stress
- Genetic/environmental immunologic factors

Stage II
Placental ischemia

Abnormal placentation

- ↑sFlt-1/sVEGFR1/sEng
- ↓ Circulating VEGF/ PlGF1
- Misfolded placental proteins
- Unknown maternal factors

Inappropriate spiral artery remodeling

- HTN
- Proteinuria
- AKI

- Capillary leak
- Pulmonary edema

- Headache
- Seizure
- PRES

- ↑ LFTs
- Hepatic infarction

- Activated coagulation system
- Thrombocytopenia

▲ **Figure 42–6.** Pathogenesis of preeclampsia-two stage model. AT1-AA, autoantibody to angiotensin-1 receptor; COMT, catechol-O-methyltransferase; HTN, hypertension; LFT, liver function tests; PRES, posterior reversible encephalopathy syndrome; sVEGFR1, soluble vascular endothelial growth factor receptor 1. (Borrowed with permission from Bramham K et al: Pregnancy and kidney disease. NephSAP 2016;15:1.)

such as sFlt-1 and sEng and others that has rekindled the interest to study preeclampsia and opportunities to use them as biomarkers. We have listed the most promising biomarkers in Table 42–5.

C. Risk Factors

Risk factors for preeclampsia are many and maybe growing. Classically, preeclampsia is thought to be a disorder of first pregnancy, those with a first degree relative with preeclampsia or those with prior episodes of preeclampsia. Cardiovascular risk factors such as advanced maternal age, diabetes, chronic hypertension, CKD, obesity, multifetal gestations (especially from assisted reproductive technology) are becoming more frequent (Table 42–6). Interestingly, the incidence of pregnancy induced hypertension is decreased amongst same-paternity multigravidae as compared with new-paternity multigravidae as it is believed that exposure to paternal antigens via immune tolerance appear to offer protection against preeclampsia. Ethnicity plays a prominent role as well, since the incidence amongst women of African descent has been demonstrated to be higher in multiple studies as compared to women of European descent, Hispanics, South and East Asians, and Pacific Islanders. This finding may be the result of the higher incidence of chronic hypertension in individuals of African descent, which itself is a strong risk factor for preeclampsia.

D. Prevention and Treatment of Preeclampsia

Despite many studies on the prevention of preeclampsia, such as with calcium and antioxidants, the outcomes have been mostly disappointing. We have summarized the results in Table 42–7.

1. Low salt diet/diuretic use—Given that edema is usually seen in preeclampsia (though no longer a necessary clinical finding), the application of a low salt diet and diuretic use was studied. Neither salt restriction nor diuretic use has been found to be beneficial to prevent preeclampsia. For salt restriction, there was no difference in admissions for hypertension or obstetric outcomes, and for diuretic use there was no difference in the incidence of preeclampsia despite a decrease in edema and hypertension. In addition diuretics may have detrimental effects on the fetus by causing volume contraction.

2. Calcium supplementation—Given that there appears to be an inverse relationship between calcium intake and blood pressure, studies were undertaken to see if calcium supplementation can prevent preeclampsia. A large randomized control trial that was conducted in countries with low calcium intake showed a reduction in hypertensive disorders in patients who received two grams of elemental calcium versus placebo [OR 0.63; 95 confidence interval (CI) 0.44-0.90]. This was followed up by the Calcium for Preeclampsia

Table 42-5. Summary of biomarkers.

Name of biomarker	Use	Origin/mechanism/effects	Body fluid sampled	Type of studies	Sensitivity/specificity/predictive value	Comments
sFlt-1	Diagnosis, Prediction	Trophoblast, 200 kDa protein, binds to vascular endothelial growth factor receptor (VEGF-R), antagonistic, is antiangiogenic	Maternal serum/ plasma	Prospective, meta-analysis, nested case control	Sensitivity—26–80% Specificity—40–100%	Values varies according to time of gestation and baseline risk of population studied, may help to differentiate between preeclampsia, chronic hypertension and chronic kidney disease, less helpful in early pregnancy or low risk population
sEng	Diagnosis, Prediction	Trophoblast, 90 kDa glycoprotein, cell surface coreceptor for transforming growth factor beta, antagonistic, is antiangiogenic, prevents autophagy of syncytiotrophoblast	Maternal serum/ plasma	Prospective, meta-analysis, nested case control	Sensitivity- 18–88%, Specificity—80%	Values vary according to time of gestation and baseline risk of population studied, may help to differentiate between preeclampsia, chronic hypertension and chronic kidney disease
PlGF	Diagnosis, Prediction	Trophoblast, 60 kDa glycoprotein, binds to vascular endothelial growth factor receptor (VEGF-R), antagonistic, is proangiogenic, promotes extravillous trophoblast growth and proliferation	Maternal serum/ plasma/urine	Prospective, meta-analysis, nested case control	PlGF sensitivity 32–92.3%, Specificity—43–80%	Levels reduce naturally in third trimester, may help differentiate between preeclampsia, chronic hypertension and chronic kidney disease, its lower in smaller for gestational age fetus
sFlt-1/PlGF	Diagnosis, Prediction		Maternal serum/ plasma	Prospective, nested case control, meta-analysis	Sensitivity—78–88.5% Specificity—84–88.5% Specificity—99.4% for early onset preeclampsia, 95.4% for late onset preeclampsia	Ratio better than individual markers, elevated ratio superior to clinical diagnosis of preeclampsia in predicting adverse pregnancy outcome regardless of clinical preeclampsia a low ratio inversely correlated with prolongation of pregnancy, accuracy for screening preeclampsia moderate and high early onset preeclampsia, may assist in early diagnosis, advances in ELISA technique has improved accuracy
Podocyturia	Diagnosis, Prediction	Glomerulus, restricts protein loss in the glomerular filtration barrier	Maternal urine	Cross sectional	Sensitivity—38–100% Specificity—70–100%	Lack of standardization, as healthy pregnant women may also have podocyturia, various techniques show different results

PP-13	Diagnosis, Prediction	32 kDa, protein, binds to leucocytes and induces apoptosis T-cells	Maternal serum/plasma	Prospective, nested case control	Sensitivity—24–85% for term preeclampsia, 62–85% for preterm preeclampsia, 45–100% for early onset preeclampsia, 44–79%, Specificity—80–90%	Variable predictive value, can be used to predict small for gestational age and preterm deliveries
PAPP-A	Diagnosis	Syncytiotrophoblast, 32 kDa macroglobulin plasma protein, cleaves insulin like growth factor binding protein-4 (ILGFBP-4) to increase the availability and action of insulin like growth factor	Maternal serum/plasma	Prospective, nested case control	Sensitivity—23–24%, Specificity—80%	Variable predictive value, not so useful in late preeclampsia
Congophilia	Prediction	Placenta, marker of protein instability and misfolding	Maternal urine	Prospective	Sensitivity—85.9% Specificity—85%	Congophilia may occur in preeclampsia, chronic kidney disease and lupus nephritis
Copeptin	Prediction	Plasma, stable, inactive prosegment of arginine vasopressin contributing to reduced activity of renin-angiotensin system	Maternal serum	Prospective	AUC: 0.90, 0.90, and 0.78 for first, second, third trimester respectively	Good early biomarker in the first trimester; needs additional validation

AUC, area under the curve.

(Borrowed with permission from Nissaisorakarn P, Sharif S, Jim B: Hypertension in pregnancy: defining blood pressure goals and the value of biomarkers for preeclampsia. Curr Cardiol Rep 2016;18:131.)

Table 42–6. Risk factors for preeclampsia.

Advanced maternal age (>40 years)
Prior preeclampsia
Family history of preeclampsia
Renal disease
Chronic hypertension
Diabetes mellitus
Primiparity
Systemic lupus erythematosus
Antiphospholipid antibody syndrome
Multiple gestations
Strong family history of cardiovascular disease
Obesity (body mass index >30 kg/m²)
African ancestry

(Borrowed with permission from Bramham K, Hladunewich MA, Jim B, Maynard SE. Pregnancy and kidney disease. NephSAP 2016;15:1.)

Prevention (CPEP) trial in the United States which in 4589 nulliparous patients found no significant difference in the incidence of preeclampsia in the calcium versus placebo arms. A complementary study conducted by the World Health Organization in women with low calcium intake again demonstrated no difference in rates of preeclampsia, though there was a reduction in the severity of maternal morbidity and neonatal mortality. The recent Cochrane Review by Hofmeyr et al. found that calcium supplementation (>1 gm/day) appears to reduce the risk of severe hypertensive disorders, especially in the subgroup with low calcium intake but caution that positive results may be overestimated due to small-study effects or publication bias.

3. Antioxidants—Since part of the pathophysiology of preeclampsia is thought to be due to an imbalance between oxidant and antioxidant activity, the use of antioxidants has been studied to prevent disease. The antioxidants vitamin C and E have not shown to be beneficial in several well-conducted randomized placebo control trials. Furthermore, adverse events such as an increased number of low birth weight babies and hypertensive complications have been found in the treatment arm. Thus, supplementation with vitamins C and E is not recommended to prevent preeclampsia.

4. Antithrombotic agents—Preeclampsia is associated with a state of vasospasm, endothelial dysfunction, an activated coagulation system, as well as enhanced platelet activation with thromboxane production. Thus far, aspirin has been the most widely studied antithrombotic agent. A large meta-analysis from the Paris Collaborative Group consisting of 32,217 women from 31 randomized trials found a relative risk (RR) of developing preeclampsia to be 0.90 (95% CI 0.84-0.97), thus concluding that reduction in preeclampsia is modest. A later meta-analysis showed that aspirin significantly prevented the incidence of preeclampsia (RR 0.47, 95% CI 0.34-0.65) and intra-uterine growth restriction (IUGR) (RR 0.44, 95% CI 0.30-0.65) if administered prior to 16 weeks of gestation; these positive effects were negated if

Table 42–7. Interventions for prevention of preeclampsia.

Intervention	Evidence	Benefits	Comments
Low salt diet	Multicenter RCT (N = 361)	None	No difference in hospitalization or obstetric outcomes
Diuretic use	Meta-analysis of 9 RCTs (N = 7000)	None	Higher incidence of adverse events including nausea and vomiting May aggravate the renin-angiotensin system
Calcium supplementation	Systematic review of 13 studies (N = 15,730)	Small to moderate	Greatest benefit in women with low dietary calcium intake and women at high risk of preeclampsia
Vitamin C and E supplementation	Multicenter RCT involving 2410 women Multicenter RCT of 1877 women Multicenter RCT of 1365 women	None None None	Therapy slightly increased rate of low birth weight babies No benefit to therapy Study performed in women of low nutritional status
Aspirin	Meta-analysis of 34 RCTs involving 11,348 women	Small	Routinely recommended in high-risk women. Must be started before 16 weeks of gestation.
Heparin	Meta-analysis of 4 RCTs involving 324 women Meta-analysis of 6 RCTs involving 848 women	Moderate benefit in women with prior placental disease	Potentially useful for prevention of recurrent placenta-mediated pregnancy complications in women with a history of adverse pregnancy outcomes.

LMWH, low molecular weight heparin; RCT, randomized control trial; UFH, unfractionated heparin.
(Borrowed with permission from Bramham K, Hladunewich MA, Jim B, Maynard SE. Pregnancy and kidney disease. NephSAP 2016;15:1.)

administered after 16 weeks. Thus, it is recommended that aspirin is recommended to be given prior to 16 weeks for high-risk individuals.

Low molecular weight heparin (LMWH) has also been studied as prophylaxis for recurrent preeclampsia given the high incidence of placental thrombotic lesions. A Cochrane meta-analysis that studied antithrombotic therapy, either alone or in combination with other agents, demonstrated a reduction in the risk of preeclampsia and eclampsia in the antithrombotic group, though there was no significant difference in perinatal mortality or preterm birth. A more recent meta-analysis of more than 800 women showed a significant reduction in the composite outcome of preeclampsia, small for gestation age, placental abruption, or pregnancy loss of more than 20 weeks (RR of 0.52 with 95% CI 0.32–0.86; P = 0.01) with LMWH. The outcome of live birth rate amongst women with recurrent miscarriages however does not seem to be changed. Thus, LMWH prophylaxis should be given to women with a history of severe obstetric outcomes such as poor fetal growth, preeclampsia with IUGR, or pathologic evidence of abnormal placentation.

E. Prevention and Treatment of Eclampsia

The only agent that has been definitively proven to prevent initial seizures and recurrent seizures in preeclampsia is magnesium sulfate. When compared with standard anticonvulsants, such as phenytoin, the difference in seizure incidence was 0% versus 0.8% (P = 0.004) in favor of magnesium sulfate. An international, multicenter, randomized trial performed by The Eclampsia Collaborative Group showed that women who received magnesium sulfate had a 52% lower risk of recurrent seizures than those who received diazepam, and a 67% lower risk of recurrent convulsion compared to those who received phenytoin. Maternal mortality was also found to be lower with magnesium sulfate use. Despite known side effects of magnesium ranging from intense flushing, nausea, vomiting, muscle weakness, and respiratory depression, the benefits for the most part outweigh these risks. In patients with acute or chronic kidney injury however, close monitoring of magnesium levels is important to avoid toxicity. It is generally recommended in case of kidney injury to start with only a loading dose without a maintenance dose.

KEY READINGS

Altman D et al: Do women with pre-eclampsia, and their babies, benefit from magnesium sulphate? The Magpie Trial: a randomised placebo-controlled trial. Lancet 2002;359:1877.

American College of Obstetricians and Gynecologists: ACOG committee opinion no. 558: Integrating immunizations into practice. Obstet Gynecol 2013;121:897.

Arnadottir GA et al: Cardiovascular death in women who had hypertension in pregnancy: a case-control study. BJOG 2005;112:286.

Askie LM et al: Antiplatelet agents for prevention of pre-eclampsia: a meta-analysis of individual patient data. Lancet 2007;369:1791.

Beazley D et al: Vitamin C and E supplementation in women at high risk for preeclampsia: a double-blind, placebo-controlled trial. Am J Obstet Gynecol 2005;192:520.

Belizan JM, Villar J, Repke J: The relationship between calcium intake and pregnancy-induced hypertension: up-to-date evidence. Am J Obstet Gynecol 1988;158:898.

Belizan JM et al: Calcium supplementation to prevent hypertensive disorders of pregnancy. N Engl J Med 1991;325:1399.

Bujold E et al: Prevention of preeclampsia and intrauterine growth restriction with aspirin started in early pregnancy: a meta-analysis. Obstet Gynecol 2010;116:402.

Churchill D et al: Diuretics for preventing pre-eclampsia. Cochrane Database Syst Rev 2007;1:CD004451.

Dodd JM et al: Antithrombotic therapy for improving maternal or infant health outcomes in women considered at risk of placental dysfunction. Cochrane Database Syst Rev 2010;6:CD006780.

Gilbert JS et al: Pathophysiology of hypertension during preeclampsia: linking placental ischemia with endothelial dysfunction. Am J Physiol Heart Circ Physiol 2008;294:H541.

Hofmeyr GJ et al: Calcium supplementation during pregnancy for preventing hypertensive disorders and related problems. Cochrane Database Syst Rev 2014;6:CD001059.

Kaandorp SP et al: Aspirin plus heparin or aspirin alone in women with recurrent miscarriage. N Engl J Med 2010;362:1586.

Khalil A et al: Maternal racial origin and adverse pregnancy outcomes: a cohort study. Ultrasound Obstet Gynecol. 2013;41:278.

Knuist M et al: Low sodium diet and pregnancy-induced hypertension: a multi-centre randomised controlled trial. Br J Obstet Gynaecol 1998;105:430.

Lam C, Lim KH, Karumanchi SA: Circulating angiogenic factors in the pathogenesis and prediction of preeclampsia. Hypertension 2005;46:1077.

Levine RJ et al: Pre-eclampsia, soluble fms-like tyrosine kinase 1, and the risk of reduced thyroid function: nested case-control and population based study. BMJ 2009;339:b4336.

Levine RJ et al: Trial of calcium to prevent preeclampsia. N Engl J Med 1997;337:69.

Lucas MJ, Leveno KJ, Cunningham FG: A comparison of magnesium sulfate with phenytoin for the prevention of eclampsia. N Engl J Med 1995;333:201.

Lyall F: Priming and remodelling of human placental bed spiral arteries during pregnancy—a review. Placenta 2005;26:S31.

Myatt L, Webster RP: Vascular biology of preeclampsia. J Thromb Haemost 2009;7:375.

Murphy SR, Cockrell K: Regulation of soluble fms-like tyrosine kinase-1 production in response to placental ischemia/hypoxia: role of angiotensin II. Physiol Rep 2015;3: pii: e12310.

Poston L et al: Vitamin C and vitamin E in pregnant women at risk for pre-eclampsia (VIP trial): randomised placebo-controlled trial. Lancet 2006;367:1145.

Raijmakers MT et al: NAD(P)H oxidase associated superoxide production in human placenta from normotensive and pre-eclamptic women. Placenta 2004;25:S85.

Rasmussen K., Yaktine A: Weight Gain During Pregnancy: Reexamining the Guidelines. In: *Institute of Medicine (US) and National Research Council (US) Committee to Reexamine IOM Pregnancy Weight Guidelines.* Washington, D.C., Institute of Medicine, 2009.

Ray JG et al: Cardiovascular health after maternal placental syndromes (CHAMPS): population-based retrospective cohort study. Lancet 2005;366:1797.

Robillard PY et al: Association of pregnancy-induced hypertension with duration of sexual cohabitation before conception. Lancet 1994;344:973.

Rodger MA et al: Meta-analysis of low-molecular-weight heparin to prevent recurrent placenta-mediated pregnancy complications. Blood 2014;123:822.

Rumbold AR et al: Vitamins C and E and the risks of preeclampsia and perinatal complications. N Engl J Med 2006;354:1796.

Spinnato JA 2nd et al: Antioxidant therapy to prevent preeclampsia: a randomized controlled trial. Obstet Gynecol 2007;110:1311.

Steegers EA et al: Dietary sodium restriction during pregnancy: a historical review. Eur J Obstet Gynecol Reprod Biol 1991;40:83.

Tanaka M et al: Racial disparity in hypertensive disorders of pregnancy in New York State: a 10-year longitudinal population-based study. Am J Public Health 2007;97:163.

Vikse BE et al: Preeclampsia and the risk of end-stage renal disease. N Engl J Med 2008;359:800.

Villar J et al: World Health Organization randomized trial of calcium supplementation among low calcium intake pregnant women. Am J Obstet Gynecol 2006;194:639.

Which anticonvulsant for women with eclampsia? Evidence from the Collaborative Eclampsia Trial. Lancet 1995;345:1455.

Witlin AG, Friedman SA, Sibai BM: The effect of magnesium sulfate therapy on the duration of labor in women with mild preeclampsia at term: a randomized, double-blind, placebo-controlled trial. Am J Obstet Gynecol 1997;176:623.

Zhang S, Cardarelli K, Shim R, Ye J, Booker KL, Rust G. Racial disparities in economic and clinical outcomes of pregnancy among Medicaid recipients. Matern Child Health J 2013;17:1518.

Chronic Hypertension

Chronic or essential hypertension is defined as hypertension predating pregnancy and is seen in as many as 3% of pregnancies which has been increasing with time. It may be difficult to diagnose chronic hypertension if the pregnant woman has not sought medical care prior to pregnancy given the expected, physiologic drop in blood pressure soon after conception (see Normal Adaptations and Blood Pressure in Pregnancy). Conversely, if the woman seeks medical attention after the second trimester with elevated blood pressures, it may be difficult to differentiate that from gestational hypertension.

KEY READINGS

Chapman AB et al: Temporal relationships between hormonal and hemodynamic changes in early human pregnancy. Kidney Int 1998;54:2056.

Seely EW, Ecker J: Clinical practice. Chronic hypertension in pregnancy. N Engl J Med 2011;365:439.

Chronic Hypertension with Superimposed Preeclampsia

Superimposed preeclampsia refers to development of preeclampsia in women with underlying chronic hypertension. Maternal factors such as severity and duration of pre-pregnancy hypertension, presence of secondary hypertension, DM, obesity and history of CKD increase the risk of SPE. The incidence of SPE in women with chronic hypertension is known to be up to five times that seen in women with normotensive pregnancies. SPE is referred to as "without severe features" when there is new onset of proteinuria, or worsening of blood pressure but to less than 160 mm Hg systolic and 105 mm Hg diastolic. It is considered severe when there is sudden worsening of blood pressure to greater than 160 mm Hg systolic and 105 mm Hg diastolic, and the identification of clinical symptoms (headache, vision changes, upper abdominal pain) or development of systemic manifestations such as elevated liver enzymes, low platelets, hemolysis, the markers of HELLP syndrome, development of pulmonary congestion or development of renal insufficiency (doubling of serum creatinine or S.Cr >1.1 mg/dL). If there is preexisting proteinuria, SPE is diagnosed by a sudden increase in proteinuria or a sudden increase in blood pressure in a woman whose hypertension had previously been well controlled. The diagnosis becomes a challenge for women who present in early second trimester with undiagnosed chronic hypertension and may be mislabeled as having preeclampsia, instead of SPE, if proteinuria or new signs of end-organ dysfunction develop. It needs to be also differentiated from a rare condition called "Mirror" or "Ballantyne" syndrome which is the development of maternal edema, hypertension, and proteinuria in association with fetal hydrops where maternal symptoms may resolve without delivery if fetal hydrops resolves.

KEY READINGS

Braun T et al: Mirror syndrome: a systematic review of fetal associated conditions, maternal presentation and perinatal outcome. Fetal Diagn Ther 2010;27:191.

Hypertension in pregnancy. Report of the American College of Obstetricians and Gynecologists' Task Force on Hypertension in Pregnancy. Obstet Gynecol 2013;122:1122.

Gestational Hypertension

Gestational hypertension is the most common cause of hypertension during pregnancy and is defined by hypertension that develops after 20 weeks of gestation without proteinuria or other signs or symptoms of preeclampsia. Pregnancy may be the first instance when hypertension is diagnosed in many of these women which frequently occurs close to term. A history of preeclampsia in a previous pregnancy, multifetal gestation, and obesity increase the risk of developing gestational hypertension. When systolic blood pressure is more than or equal to 160 mm Hg and/or diastolic blood pressure is more than or equal to 110 mm Hg on two consecutive readings at least 4 hours apart, it is classified as severe gestational hypertension.

Gestational hypertension can recur in subsequent pregnancies; a meta-analysis in 2015 of 24,000 women with gestational hypertension reported that 22% developed hypertension in a subsequent pregnancy. Gestational hypertension is associated with development of hypertension later in life, and possibly associated with development of other conditions such as cardiovascular disease and CKD. Therefore, close clinical monitoring postpartum with an eye to early intervention should be the aim in women with a history of gestational hypertension.

Assessment in the postpartum period, up to 12 weeks is the definitive strategy to diagnose gestational hypertension as it should theoretically resolve within this period. If hypertension persists beyond 12 weeks postpartum, it is called chronic or preexisting hypertension. This is a critically important point in making the distinction since the natural history, management, and prognosis of these conditions are very different.

KEY READINGS

Hypertension in pregnancy. Report of the American College of Obstetricians and Gynecologists' Task Force on Hypertension in Pregnancy. Obstet Gynecol 2013;122:1122.

Magnussen EB et al: Hypertensive disorders in pregnancy and subsequently measured cardiovascular risk factors. Obstet Gynecol 2009;114:961.

van Oostwaard MF et al: Recurrence of hypertensive disorders of pregnancy: an individual patient data metaanalysis. Am J Obstet Gynecol 2015;212:624. e621–617.

▶ White Coat Hypertension

White coat hypertension (isolated office hypertension) is yet another condition to be considered. This diagnosis should be excluded by rechecking blood pressure when the patient is relaxed. Home blood pressure monitoring and ambulatory 24-hour blood pressure monitoring can help with the diagnosis.

KEY READINGS

Bellomo G et al: Prognostic value of 24-hour blood pressure in pregnancy. JAMA 1999;282:1447.

Magee LA, Ramsay G, von Dadelszen P: What is the role of out-of-office BP measurement in hypertensive pregnancy? Hypertens Pregnancy 2008;27:95.

▶ Postpartum Hypertension

Though not included in the classification of hypertensive disorders in pregnancy, postpartum hypertension is an important entity. It can occur de novo or be secondary to worsening of preexisting gestational hypertension, preeclampsia or chronic hypertension. The exact incidence of the condition is unknown as most of the women remain asymptomatic and do not have their blood pressures measured routinely in the postpartum period. Only those with symptomatic severe hypertension seek medical attention. One study reported that 0.3% of all emergency room visits in the postpartum period were due to hypertension.

Typically, blood pressure improves 24–48 hours after delivery of the fetus in preeclampsia but may rise again in 3–5 days later which results in postpartum hypertension. Delayed postpartum preeclampsia and eclampsia can also develop de novo, leading to readmission more than 2 days but less than 6 weeks after delivery. Signs and symptoms can be mild or atypical and can mimic other conditions such as cerebral vasoconstriction syndrome or even impending stroke. Risk factors for delayed postpartum preeclampsia appear to be similar to those for preeclampsia during pregnancy, but some patients may have no risk factors. Perhaps the biggest challenge to this diagnosis is the lack of awareness by both patient and providers, which untreated may lead to devastating consequences such as stroke. Thus, it is critical to educate physicians and patients of the early signs and symptoms as well as risks factors for the condition, which in addition to the above include, administration of large volumes of intravenous fluids during anesthesia, use of nonsteroidal anti-inflammatory drugs for pain, as well as ergot agents used to control uterine atony.

KEY READINGS

Al-Safi Z et al: Delayed postpartum preeclampsia and eclampsia: demographics, clinical course, and complications. Obstet Gynecol 2011;118:1102.

Clark SL et al: Emergency department use during the postpartum period: implications for current management of the puerperium. Am J Obstet Gynecol 2010;203:38. e31–36.

Sibai BM: Etiology and management of postpartum hypertension-preeclampsia. Am J Obstet Gynecol 2012;206:470.

Singhal AB, Bernstein RA: Postpartum angiopathy and other cerebral vasoconstriction syndromes. Neurocrit Care 2005;3:91.

▶ Primary Hyperaldosteronism in Pregnancy

Primary aldosteronism diagnosed in pregnancy is rare and is associated with significant adverse outcomes such as preeclampsia, abruptio placentae, HELLP, fetal growth restriction. Typically, primary aldosteronism presents as worsening signs of hypertension and hypokalemia, while surprisingly

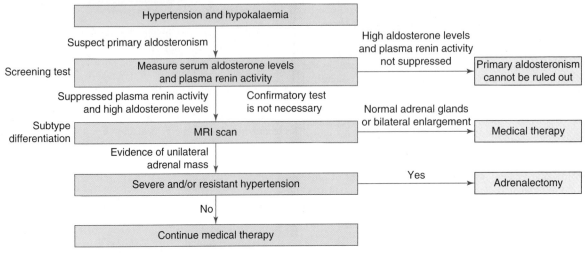

▲ Figure 42–7. The diagnosis and treatment of primary aldosteronism during pregnancy. (Borrowed with permission from Monticone S, Auchus RJ, Rainey WE: Adrenal disorders in pregnancy. Nat Rev Endocrinol 2012;8:668.)

a small number of patients may improve spontaneously before delivery. The latter phenomenon is explained by the increased levels of progesterone which acts as a mineralocorticoid receptor antagonist and masks the clinical manifestations of hyperaldosteronism. However, if these increased levels of progesterone cannot fully antagonize aldosterone, which is significantly upregulated during pregnancy, then exacerbation of symptoms occur. This clinical variability makes the diagnosis even harder during pregnancy. For diagnosis, the Endocrine Society recommends a three-step process: an initial screening test, a confirmatory test, and subtype differentiation (Figure 42–7). Once diagnosed, conservative management with potassium supplements and antihypertensive treatments are preferred, with the goal of delaying definitive surgery until after delivery (Please refer to Table 42–8 for first line blood pressure medications). Aldosterone antagonists such as spironolactone or eplerenone are not usually recommended for fear for their antiandrogenic effects on male fetuses; however, case reports of their use have not borne out these ill effects. Other potassium sparing diuretics such as amiloride and triamterene have reportedly been safe to use. Should uncontrolled hypertension and/or fetal distress ensue despite aggressive blood pressure treatment, emergent adrenalectomy may be necessary. Surgery is best performed during the second trimester where the risks for the fetus are lowest. The nine patients who underwent laparoscopic adrenalectomy between 14 and 24 weeks of gestation resulted in one case of intrauterine fetal demise at 26 weeks, two deliveries at 26 weeks due to IUGR and fetal distress, and one delivery at 34 weeks, as well as five term deliveries. Given the limited experience, is it not clear that surgery would guarantee a favorable outcome.

KEY READINGS

Al-Ali NA et al: Conn's syndrome in pregnancy successfully treated with amiloride. J Obstet Gynaecol 2007;27:730.

Ananth CV et al: Chronic hypertension and risk of placental abruption: is the association modified by ischemic placental disease? Am J Obstet Gynecol 2007;197:273. e271–277.

Aoi W et al: Primary aldosteronism aggravated during peripartum period. Jpn Heart J 1978;19:946.

Biglieri EG, Slaton PE Jr: Pregnancy and primary aldosteronism. J Clin Endocrinol Metab 1967;27:1628.

Cabassi A et al: Eplerenone use in primary aldosteronism during pregnancy. Hypertension 2012;59:e18.

Chappell LC et al: Adverse perinatal outcomes and risk factors for preeclampsia in women with chronic hypertension: a prospective study. Hypertension 2008;51:1002.

Crane MG et al: Primary aldosteronism in pregnancy. Obstet Gynecol 1964;23:200.

Funder JW et al: Case detection, diagnosis, and treatment of patients with primary aldosteronism: an endocrine society clinical practice guideline. J Clin Endocrinol Metab 2008; 93:3266.

Gordon RD, Tunny TJ: Aldosterone-producing-adenoma (A-P-A): effect of pregnancy. Clin Exp Hypertens A 1982;4:1685.

Groves TD, Corenblum B: Spironolactone therapy during human pregnancy. Am J Obstet Gynecol 1995;172:1655.

Kosaka K et al: Laparoscopic adrenalectomy on a patient with primary aldosteronism during pregnancy. Endocr J 2006;53:461.

Murakami T et al: High blood pressure lowered by pregnancy. Lancet 2000;356:1980.

Nursal TZ et al: Laparoscopic treatment of primary hyperaldosteronism in a pregnant patient. Can J Surg 2009;52:E188.

Ronconi V et al: Progesterone increase counteracts aldosterone action in a pregnant woman with primary aldosteronism. Clin Endocrinol (Oxf) 2011;74:278.

Table 42–8. Preferred medication choices in treatment of hypertension of pregnancy.

Drug (mode of administration)	Dose	Adverse Events in Pregnancy	Comments	FDA Pregnancy Category[*]
Methyldopa (PO)	500–3000 mg/day PO in 2–4 divided doses	Peripheral edema, anxiety, drowsiness, dry mouth	Large body of safety data	B
Labetalol (PO or IV)	100–1200 mg/day PO in 2–3 divided doses; 10–20 mg; repeat 20–80 mg IV every 30 min; max 300 mg/day	Fetal bradycardia	Preferred agent in CHIPS trial	C
Nifedipine (PO)	30–120 mg/day PO	Possible inhibition of labor if used in combination with magnesium sulfate,	Immediate release formulation is not recommended	C
Hydralazine (PO or IV)	50–300 mg/day PO in 2–4 divided doses; 5–10 mg IV/IM, may repeat every 20–30 min to a maximum of 45 mg; OR 0.5–1.0 mg/h for infusion	Hypotension, neonatal thrombocytopenia, lupus-like syndrome, tachycardia		C
Hydrochloro-thiazide (PO)	12.5–25 mg/day PO	Volume contraction, electrolyte abnormalities	Avoid in preeclampsia	B
Nitroprusside (IV)	0.25–0.5 mcg/kg/min to 2 mcg/kg/min, maximum duration 24–48 hours	Risk for fetal cyanide toxicity with prolonged use and higher dose	Use in shortest time and lowest dose possible	C
Nicardipine (IV)	Initial: 5 mg/hour increased by 2.5 mg/hour every 15 minutes to a maximum of 15 mg/hour	Headache, edema, tachycardia		C
Furosemide (IV)	20–40 mg IV over 1–2 minutes, may repeat every 2 hours, max dose 200 mg/d	Risk for volume depletion, electrolyte abnormalities	Use in pulmonary edema	C

[*]FDA (Federal Drug Administration) Pregnancy Category: A, adequate and well-controlled studies have failed to demonstrate a risk to the fetus in the first trimester of pregnancy (and there is no evidence of risk in later trimesters); B, Animal reproduction studies have failed to demonstrate a risk to the fetus and there are no adequate and well-controlled studies in pregnant women; C, animal reproduction studies have shown an adverse effect on the fetus and there are no adequate and well-controlled studies in humans, but potential benefits may warrant use of the drug in pregnant women despite potential risks; D, there is positive evidence of human fetal risk based on adverse reaction data from investigational or marketing experience or studies in humans, but potential benefits may warrant use of the drug in pregnant women despite potential risks.

Shigematsu K et al: Primary aldosteronism with aldosterone-producing adenoma consisting of pure zona glomerulosa-type cells in a pregnant woman. Endocr Pathol 2009;20:66.

Shiraishi K et al: Laparoscopic adrenalectomy due to primary aldosteronism during pregnancy. Hinyokika Kiyo 2014;60:381.

Sibai BM: Chronic hypertension in pregnancy. Obstet Gynecol 2002;100:369.

▶ Hypertension in Pregnancy in Renal Transplant Recipients and Donors

The success rate of pregnancy after renal allografts has improved significantly as reported by many registries. However, in a substantial number of these pregnancies, the physiologic nadir in blood pressure seen in normal pregnancy may be blunted, and hypertension is a major concern. Hypertension may either be pre-existing or develop during pregnancy, with reported rates of hypertension during pregnancy in kidney transplant recipients as high as 60–80%. In addition, the incidence of preeclampsia in renal transplant recipients is 24–38%, which is five to six times higher than the general population. Diagnosing preeclampsia in renal transplant recipients can be challenging, as an increase in blood pressure and proteinuria are common findings and changes in serum creatinine are inherently unreliable in pregnancy. Acute rejection, associated with sudden worsening of hypertension and marked increase in the proteinuria, further makes the diagnosis difficult. Hypertension may also be exacerbated by immunosuppressive drugs, such as steroids and calcineurin inhibitors. According to the American Society of Transplantation Consensus Conference, the levels of calcineurin inhibitors should be maintained at prepregnancy levels which, as per the National Transplantation Pregnancy Registry, may require higher dosages. The target blood pressure is unknown but the aim is to achieve a goal blood pressure in the normal range. Thus, antihypertensive medication should be initiated if the blood pressure is consistently higher than 140/90 mm Hg. The optimal choice of therapy in the pregnant renal transplant recipient is the same as that for the non-transplant pregnant woman. Given the high risk for preeclampsia, these women should be placed on aspirin as a preventive measure.

For many years, we had assumed that donating a kidney would not have an ill impact on future pregnancies or kidney health of the donor; this assumption was based on small observational studies. However, more recent larger studies appear to demonstrate an increased incidence of preeclampsia and/or gestational hypertension. This has been confirmed by a relatively large retrospective study of 131 kidney donors versus 788 healthy non-donors which showed an increased risk of gestational hypertension or preeclampsia (Odds Ratio 2.4, P = 0.01). The reasons behind these findings are unclear, though it may be related to older maternal age, increased incidence of hypertension, diabetes, obesity, and the use of reproductive technologies resulting in multiple gestations. Thus, it is important for the clinician to be aware of the data in counselling of woman of reproductive age for kidney donation.

KEY READINGS

Armenti VT, Radomski JS, Moritz MJ, et al. Report from the National Transplantation Pregnancy Registry (NTPR): outcomes of pregnancy after transplantation. Clin Transpl 2004:103.

Buszta C et al: Pregnancy after donor nephrectomy. Transplantation 1985;40:651.

del Mar Colon M, Hibbard JU: Obstetric considerations in the management of pregnancy in kidney transplant recipients. Advances in chronic kidney disease. 2007;14:168.

Garg AX et al: Gestational hypertension and preeclampsia in living kidney donors. N Engl J Med 2015;372:124.

Ibrahim HN et al: Pregnancy outcomes after kidney donation. Am J Transplant 2009;9:825.

Jones JW et al: Pregnancy following kidney donation. Transplant Proc 1993;25:3082.

Josephson MA, McKay DB: Considerations in the medical management of pregnancy in transplant recipients. Adv Chronic Kidney Dis 2007;14:156.

McKay DB, Josephson MA: Pregnancy in recipients of solid organs—effects on mother and child. N Engl J Med 2006;354:1281.

McKay DB et al: Reproduction and transplantation: report on the AST Consensus Conference on Reproductive Issues and Transplantation. Am J Transplant 2005;5:1592.

Podymow T, August P: Hypertension in pregnancy. Adv Chronic Kidney Dis 2007;14:178.

Reisaeter AV et al: Pregnancy and birth after kidney donation: the Norwegian experience. Am J Transplant 2009;9:820.

Rizzoni G et al: Successful pregnancies in women on renal replacement therapy: report from the EDTA Registry. Nephrol Dial Transplant 1992;7:279.

Sibanda N et al: Pregnancy after organ transplantation: a report from the UK Transplant pregnancy registry. Transplantation 2007;83:1301.

Wrenshall LE et al: Pregnancy after donor nephrectomy. Transplantation 1996;62:1934.

▶ Preconception Management and Treatment

It is important to identify and optimally manage maternal comorbidities before conception to avoid adverse outcomes including preeclampsia. Careful history should be taken to assess risk factors such as chronic hypertension, obesity, DM, connective tissue disorders and previous maternal/fetal complications. Basic laboratory studies ought to include a metabolic panel, complete blood count, HgbA1C, and urinalysis. For women with chronic hypertension, obtaining an electrocardiogram, a lipid profile, and a baseline 24-hour urine protein measurement have been recommended as well. Obese patients should aim for a body mass index (BMI) in the normal range prior to conception to improve control of blood glucose and blood pressure, since both hypertension and DM are risk factors for preeclampsia. All medications being taken need to be reviewed for teratogenic potential, with special attention to angiotensin receptor blockers, angiotensin converting enzyme inhibitors and immunosuppressive drugs. Optimization of RAAS inhibitors prior to conception in women with diabetic nephropathy has been shown to decrease proteinuria during pregnancy in small studies. RAAS inhibitors should be stopped after conception. Women with history of hypertension should be evaluated for secondary causes and end organ damage such as retinopathy, renal disease, and left ventricular hypertrophy. They must be informed about the risk of worsening hypertension, preeclampsia, and fetal complications.

▶ Postconception Treatment

Pregnant women with chronic hypertension need close follow-up since they are at risk for increased complications and up to 25% of these women can develop preeclampsia. Women with history of preeclampsia should have frequent antenatal visits to monitor for signs and symptoms of preeclampsia, follow-up blood pressure readings and have serial ultrasounds to assess fetal growth. Low dose aspirin is recommended for women who are high risk for preeclampsia. For diabetic patients, it is recommended by the American Diabetes Association that those on oral hypoglycemic should be converted to insulin for better glycemic control; HgbA1C levels above 6.5% in the second and third trimester of pregnancy are associated with a higher risk of preeclampsia. Salt restriction in women with hypertension and caloric restriction in obese women has shown no benefit in pregnancy and are not advised.

KEY READINGS

Bar J et al: Pregnancy outcome in patients with insulin dependent diabetes mellitus and diabetic nephropathy treated with ACE inhibitors before pregnancy. J Pediatr Endocrinol Metab 1999;12:659.

Barton JR, Sibai BM: Prediction and prevention of recurrent preeclampsia. Obstet Gynecol 2008;112:359.

Burke SD et al: Soluble fms-like tyrosine kinase 1 promotes angiotensin II sensitivity in preeclampsia. J Clin Invest 2016;126:2561.

Farahi N, Zolotor A: Recommendations for preconception counseling and care. Am Fam Physician 2013;88:499.

Hod M et al: Diabetic nephropathy and pregnancy: the effect of ACE inhibitors prior to pregnancy on fetomaternal outcome. Nephrol Dial Transplant 1995;10:2328.

Maresh MJ et al: Glycemic targets in the second and third trimester of pregnancy for women with type 1 diabetes. Diabetes Care 2015;38:34.

Report of the national high blood pressure education program, working group on high blood presure in Pregnancy. American Journal of Obstetrics & Gynecology. 2000;183:S1.

▶ Blood Pressure Goals in Pregnancy

In general, hypertension in pregnancy is defined as a systolic blood pressure more than or equal to 140 mm Hg or diastolic more than or equal to 90 mm Hg, with severe hypertension being systolic blood pressure more than or equal to 160 mm Hg or diastolic more than or equal to 110 mm Hg by the ACOG. The use of antihypertensive medications during pregnancy and the blood pressure goal must be carefully weighed, being cognizant of the potential pharmacologic toxicity to the fetus and effect on fetal blood flow and growth (Table 42–8). A decrease in birth weight with a drop in mean arterial pressure of 10 mm Hg has been demonstrated. There is some variation in guidelines globally as to the initiation of treatment for hypertension and the treatment goals for blood pressure during pregnancy. In general, the goal to treat chronic hypertension is to prevent maternal morbidities including cerebrovascular disease, renal failure, and long-term cardiovascular complications. The ACOG 2013 Task Force recommends initiating treatment in pregnant woman with severe hypertension (BP >160/105) with a goal blood pressure between 120–160/80–105 mm Hg. Other international societies also consider maternal comorbidities. For example, the Society of Obstetricians and Gynecologists of Canada (SOGC), the National Institute for Health and Care Excellence (NICE) from the United Kingdom, and that the European Society of Hypertension and of the European Society of Cardiology (ESC/ESH) choose their thresholds depending on presence of end-organ damage such as CKD or left ventricular hypertrophy. This is mostly due to a concern over an apparent increase in the incidence of pregnancy-related strokes in women with concurrent hypertensive disorders or heart disease. The recent landmark CHIPS trial showed that tight control of diastolic blood pressure to 85 mm Hg did not adversely affect fetal or neonatal outcomes as compared to a diastolic blood pressure of 100 mm Hg. Recommendations on blood pressure targets from six major societies are summarized in Table 42–9, but the majority agree on decreasing systolic blood pressure below 160 mm Hg and diastolic blood pressure to below 110 mm Hg.

KEY READINGS

American College of Obstetricians and Gynecologists; Task Force on Hypertension in Pregnancy: Hypertension in Pregnancy. Report of the American College of Obstetricians and Gynecologists' Task Force on Hypertension in Pregnancy. Obstet Gynecol 2013;122:1122.

Kuklina EV et al: Trends in pregnancy hospitalizations that included a stroke in the United States from 1994 to 2007: reasons for concern? Stroke 2011;42:2564.

Magee LA et al: Less-tight versus tight control of hypertension in pregnancy. N Engl J Med 2015;372:2367.

Nissaisorakarn P, Sharif S, Jim B: Hypertension in pregnancy: defining blood pressure goals and the value of biomarkers for preeclampsia. Curr Cardiol Rep 2016;18:131.

von Dadelszen P et al: Fall in mean arterial pressure and fetal growth restriction in pregnancy hypertension: a meta-analysis. Lancet 2000;355:87.

▶ Maternal and Fetal Risks

A. Maternal Risks

Despite substantial advances in our understanding of hypertensive disorders of pregnancy in the past 10 years, these conditions remain a major health concern for mothers and infants across the globe. Women with uncomplicated chronic hypertension have a higher rate of maternal complications and admissions due to uncontrolled or accelerated hypertension, especially if they have secondary hypertension, renal disease or uncontrolled hypertension pre-pregnancy. Other adverse outcomes such as cesarean deliveries and postpartum hemorrhage are also increased compared to non-hypertensive pregnancies. When women with chronic hypertension develop SPE, maternal outcomes of accelerated hypertension such as the risk of abruptio placenta and end organ damage (heart, brain and kidneys) are increased manyfold. Fatal intracerebral hemorrhage, which account for 15% of maternal deaths, may also complicate pregnancies with SPE. Women with secondary hypertension due to renal disease may experience irreversible deterioration in renal function or multi-organ system morbidity regardless of the development of SPE. If significant

Table 42–9. Blood pressure targets.

When to Start Treatment	Society	Treatment Goals	Comments
• Chronic HTN: ≥160/105 • Gestational HTN or preeclampsia: ≥160/110	ACOG	Chronic HTN: 120–160/80–105	
• Severe HTN: <160/110 • Non-severe HTN *with* co morbid conditions: 140–159/90–109 mm Hg	SOGC	Non-severe hypertension without comorbid conditions:[a] 130–155/80–105 Non-severe hypertension with comorbid conditions: <140/90 Severe HTN systolic <160 mm Hg and diastolic <110 mm Hg	Severe HTN defined as a systolic blood pressure of ≥160 mm Hg or a diastolic blood pressure of ≥110 mm Hg based on the average of at least two measurements, taken at least 15 minutes apart, using the same arm
• Uncomplicated chronic HTN/ • Gestational HTN/preeclampsia: >150/100 • With target-organ damage secondary to chronic HTN: >140/90	NICE (guidance.nice.org.uk/cg107)	Chronic hypertension: <150/80–100 Gestational hypertension and preeclampsia: <150/80–100	
• Mild to moderate HTN: ≥160/110 • Severe HTN: ≥170/110	SOMANZ	None recommended	Treatment of mild to moderate hypertension in the range 140–160/90–100 should be considered an option and will reflect local practice
• Preeclampsia: 160–170/110	ISSHP	Existing data do not permit definitive statements to be made	Maintain systolic blood pressure above 110 and diastolic blood pressure above 80
• Severe HTN in pregnancy • SBP >160 or DBP >110	ESC/ESH	None recommended	Antihypertensives may be considered in pregnant women with persistent elevation of BP ≥150/95 mm Hg, and in those with BP ≥140/90 mm Hg in the presence of gestational hypertension, asymptomatic organ damage or symptoms.

[a]Comorbid conditions: pregestational type I or II diabetes mellitus or kidney disease. Numbers indicate systolic blood pressure/diastolic blood pressure in mm Hg.
ACOG, American College of Obstetrics and Gynecology; ESC/ESH, European Society of Hypertension and of the European Society of Cardiology; HTN, hypertension; ISSHP, International Society for the Study of Hypertension in Pregnancy; NICE, The National Institute for Health and Care Excellence; SOGC, Society of Obstetricians and Gynecologists of Canada; SOMANZ, Society of Obstetric Medicine of Australia and New Zealand. (Borrowed with permission from Nissaisorakarn P, Sharif S, Jim B: Hypertension in pregnancy: defining blood pressure goals and the value of biomarkers for preeclampsia. Curr Cardiol Rep 2016;18:131.)

renal failure is present (creatinine >1.9 mg/dL, 168 μmol/L), the maternal and fetal outcomes are poor, with worsening azotemia, proteinuria, and hypertension in the mother and growth restriction in the fetus. Metabolic derangements such as increased risks of developing gestational diabetes has been reported in women with chronic hypertension, perhaps due to common predisposing factors and pathogenesis such as obesity and insulin resistance.

B. Fetal Risks

Pregnancies complicated by chronic hypertension are at risk for fetal growth restriction which is three times the rate seen in non-hypertensive women. With SPE, fetal growth restriction is even higher, as is the rate of preterm births which

may be seen in up to 35% of cases. Perinatal mortality is also higher in pregnant women with SPE.

KEY READINGS

Ankumah NE, Sibai BM: Chronic hypertension in pregnancy: diagnosis, management, and outcomes. Clin Obstet Gynecol 2017;60:206.

Jones DC, Hayslett JP: Outcome of pregnancy in women with moderate or severe renal insufficiency. N Engl J Med 1996;335:226.

Rey E, Couturier A: The prognosis of pregnancy in women with chronic hypertension. Am J Obstet Gynecol 1994;171:410.

Vanek M et al: Chronic hypertension and the risk for adverse pregnancy outcome after superimposed pre-eclampsia. Int J Gynaecol Obstet 2004;86:7.

Vigil-De Gracia P, Montufar-Rueda C, Smith A: Pregnancy and severe chronic hypertension: maternal outcome. Hypertens Pregnancy 2004;23:285.

Zetterstrom K et al: Maternal complications in women with chronic hypertension: a population-based cohort study. Acta Obstet Gynecol Scand 2005;84:419.

► Long-Term Cardiovascular Complications

There is extensive evidence to support the link between complications in pregnancy and cardiovascular disease later in life. Physiologic changes that occur during a normal pregnancy have been described as "metabolic syndrome" and "cardiac stress test"; they include insulin resistance, inflammation, hyperlipidemia, hypercoagulation and hyperdynamic circulation. These affects are heightened in women with preeclampsia, which is associated with vascular and endothelial dysfunction, and increases the risk of hypertension, ischemic heart disease, and stroke. The probability of women with history preeclampsia developing ischemic heart disease in future is related to the severity of preeclampsia and more significantly the gestation of onset. Preeclampsia before 37 weeks of gestation has been shown to increase the risk of ischemic heart disease by eightfold. The American Heart Association has included preeclampsia as a risk factor for cardiovascular disease. Multiple studies have shown an increased risk of fatal and nonfatal stroke in women who had preeclampsia with the incidence of fatal stroke being greater. Preeclampsia before 37 weeks of gestation increased the risk of stroke in general. Given the growing evidence of long-term maternal cardiovascular outcomes, the ACOG has recommends doing a screening cardiovascular profile 1 year postpartum, which includes serum electrolytes, renal function, fasting glucose, fasting lipid panel, urinalysis, and a 12-lead electrocardiography.

KEY READINGS

American College of Obstetricians and Gynecologists; Task Force on Hypertension in Pregnancy: Hypertension in Pregnancy. Report of the American College of Obstetricians and Gynecologists' Task Force on Hypertension in Pregnancy. Obstet Gynecol 2013;122:1122.

Bellamy L et al: Pre-eclampsia and risk of cardiovascular disease and cancer in later life: systematic review and meta-analysis. BMJ 2007;335:974.

Mosca L et al: Effectiveness-based guidelines for the prevention of cardiovascular disease in women—2011 update: a guideline from the American Heart Association. Circulation 2011;123:1243.

► Conclusions

As we advance our knowledge of pregnancy induced hypertension, we hope to improve our abilities to better diagnose and treat. For preeclampsia, the application of newly discovered angiogenic biomarkers would be a huge boon for this field both in terms of diagnosis and treatment. Presently, the mainstays of treatment are to remove the pregnant mother from a dangerous level of hypertension to an acceptable level for the fetus. We hope that ongoing research will soon afford us more treatment options for this growing population of at-risk women.

KEY READINGS

American College of Obstetricians and Gynecologists; Task Force on Hypertension in Pregnancy: Hypertension in Pregnancy. Report of the American College of Obstetricians and Gynecologists' Task Force on Hypertension in Pregnancy. Obstet Gynecol 2013;122:1122.

Ananth CV, Keyes KM, Wapner RJ: Pre-eclampsia rates in the United States, 1980-2010: age-period-cohort analysis. BMJ 2013;347:f6564.

Buhimschi IA et al: Protein misfolding, congophilia, oligomerization, and defective amyloid processing in preeclampsia. Sci Transl Med 2014;6:245ra292.

Bujold E et al: Prevention of preeclampsia and intrauterine growth restriction with aspirin started in early pregnancy: a meta-analysis. Obstet Gynecol 2010;116:402.

Carr DB et al: A sister's risk: family history as a predictor of preeclampsia. Am J Obstet Gynecol 2005;193:965.

Chafetz I et al: First-trimester placental protein 13 screening for preeclampsia and intrauterine growth restriction. Am J Obstet Gynecol 2007;197:35. e31–37.

Churchill D et al: Diuretics for preventing pre-eclampsia. Cochrane Database Syst Rev 2007;1:CD004451.

Clowse ME et al: A national study of the complications of lupus in pregnancy. Am J Obstet Gynecol 2008;199:127 e121–126.

Craici IM et al: Podocyturia predates proteinuria and clinical features of preeclampsia: longitudinal prospective study. Hypertension 2013;61:1289.

De Vivo A et al: Endoglin, PlGF and sFlt-1 as markers for predicting pre-eclampsia. Acta Obstet Gynecol Scand 2008;87:837.

Dodd JM et al: Antithrombotic therapy for improving maternal or infant health outcomes in women considered at risk of placental dysfunction. Cochrane Database Syst Rev 2010:CD006780.

Duckitt K, Harrington D: Risk factors for pre-eclampsia at antenatal booking: systematic review of controlled studies. BMJ 2005;330:565.

ESH/ESC Task Force for the Management of Arterial Hypertension. 2013 Practice guidelines for the management of arterial hypertension of the European Society of Hypertension (ESH) and the European Society of Cardiology (ESC): ESH/ESC Task Force for the Management of Arterial Hypertension. J Hypertens 2013;31:1925.

Eskenazi B, Fenster L, Sidney S: A multivariate analysis of risk factors for preeclampsia. JAMA 1991;266:237.

Garovic VD et al: Urinary podocyte excretion as a marker for preeclampsia. Am J Obstet Gynecol 2007;196:320. e321–327.

Hertig A et al: Maternal serum sFlt1 concentration is an early and reliable predictive marker of preeclampsia. Clin Chem 2004;50:1702.

Hofmeyr GJ et al: Calcium supplementation during pregnancy for preventing hypertensive disorders and related problems. Cochrane Database Syst Rev 2014;6:CD001059.

Jim B et al: A comparison of podocyturia, albuminuria and nephrinuria in predicting the development of preeclampsia: a prospective study. PLoS One 2014;9:e101445.

Jim B et al: Podocyturia as a diagnostic marker for preeclampsia amongst high-risk pregnant patients. J Pregnancy 2012;2012: 984630.

Khalil A, Rezende J, Akolekar R, Syngelaki A, Nicolaides KH. Maternal racial origin and adverse pregnancy outcomes: a cohort study. Ultrasound Obstet Gynecol 2013;41:278.

Khalil A et al: First trimester maternal serum placental protein 13 for the prediction of pre-eclampsia in women with a priori high risk. Prenat Diagn 2009;29:781.

Kleinrouweler CE et al: Accuracy of circulating placental growth factor, vascular endothelial growth factor, soluble fms-like tyrosine kinase 1 and soluble endoglin in the prediction of pre-eclampsia: a systematic review and meta-analysis. BJOG 2012;119:778.

Knuist M et al: Low sodium diet and pregnancy-induced hypertension: a multi-centre randomised controlled trial. Br J Obstet Gynaecol 1998;105:430.

Krotz S et al: Hypertensive disease in twin pregnancies: a review. Twin Res 2002;5:8.

Liu Y et al: Diagnostic accuracy of the soluble Fms-like tyrosine kinase-1/placental growth factor ratio for preeclampsia: a meta-analysis based on 20 studies. Arch Gynecol Obstet 2015;292:507.

Lowe SA et al: The SOMANZ Guidelines for the Management of Hypertensive Disorders of Pregnancy 2014. Aust N Z J Obstet Gynaecol 2015;55:11.

Magee LA et al: Diagnosis, evaluation, and management of the hypertensive disorders of pregnancy. Pregnancy Hypertens 2014;4:105.

McElrath TF et al: Longitudinal evaluation of predictive value for preeclampsia of circulating angiogenic factors through pregnancy. Am J Obstet Gynecol 2012; 207:407. e1–7.

Mostello D et al: Preeclampsia in the parous woman: who is at risk? Am J Obstet Gynecol 2002;187:425.

Myatt L et al: Can changes in angiogenic biomarkers between the first and second trimesters of pregnancy predict development of pre-eclampsia in a low-risk nulliparous patient population? BJOG 2013;120:1183.

Ness RB et al: Family history of hypertension, heart disease, and stroke among women who develop hypertension in pregnancy. Obstet Gynecol 2003;102:1366.

Poston L et al: Vitamin C and vitamin E in pregnant women at risk for pre-eclampsia (VIP trial): randomised placebo-controlled trial. Lancet 2006;367:1145.

Rodger MA et al: Meta-analysis of low-molecular-weight heparin to prevent recurrent placenta-mediated pregnancy complications. Blood 2014;123:822.

Romero R et al: First-trimester maternal serum PP13 in the risk assessment for preeclampsia. Am J Obstet Gynecol 2008;199:122. e121–122 e111.

Rumbold AR et al: Vitamins C and E and the risks of preeclampsia and perinatal complications. N Engl J Med 2006;354:1796.

Santillan MK et al: Vasopressin in preeclampsia: a novel very early human pregnancy biomarker and clinically relevant mouse model. Hypertension 2014;64:852.

Schneuer FJ et al: First trimester screening of maternal placental protein 13 for predicting preeclampsia and small for gestational age: in-house study and systematic review. Placenta 2012;33:735.

Spencer K et al: First-trimester maternal serum PP-13, PAPP-A and second-trimester uterine artery Doppler pulsatility index as markers of pre-eclampsia. Ultrasound Obstet Gynecol 2007;29:128.

Stepan H et al: A comparison of the diagnostic utility of the sFlt-1/PlGF ratio versus PlGF alone for the detection of preeclampsia/HELLP syndrome. Hypertens Pregnancy 2016:1.

Tanaka M et al: Racial disparity in hypertensive disorders of pregnancy in New York State: a 10-year longitudinal population-based study. Am J Public Health 2007;97:163.

Tranquilli AL et al: The classification, diagnosis and management of the hypertensive disorders of pregnancy: a revised statement from the ISSHP. Pregnancy Hypertens 2014;4:97.

Villar J et al: World Health Organisation multicentre randomised trial of supplementation with vitamins C and E among pregnant women at high risk for pre-eclampsia in populations of low nutritional status from developing countries. BJOG 2009;116:780.

Weiss JL et al: Obesity, obstetric complications and cesarean delivery rate—a population-based screening study. Am J Obstet Gynecol 2004;190:1091.

Zetterstrom K et al: Maternal complications in women with chronic hypertension: a population-based cohort study. Acta Obstet Gynecol Scand 2005;84:419.

Zhang S, Cardarelli K, Shim R, Ye J, Booker KL, Rust G. Racial disparities in economic and clinical outcomes of pregnancy among Medicaid recipients. Matern Child Health J 2013;17:1518.

■ CHAPTER REVIEW QUESTIONS

Hypertension in African–Americans

1. A 62-year-old obese African–American woman with hypertension and heart failure, on thiazide diuretic therapy and angiotensin-converting enzyme inhibitor (ACEI) presents for follow-up. CR 1.9 mg/dL, eGFR = 32 mL/min, echo-normal systolic function. Her blood pressure is noted to be elevated at 162/96 mm Hg.

   What should the treatment plan be at this point?
   A. Add a calcium channel blocker (CCB)
   B. Change thiazide diuretic to a loop diuretic
   C. Initiate dual therapy with an ACEI and angiotensin receptor blocker
   D. Add BiDil therapy (isosorbide dinitrate and hydralazine hydrochloride)

2. A 61-year-old black Puerto Rican woman, with long history of type 2 diabetes, hypertension, coronary artery disease, and hyperlipidemia presents to your office. She speaks limited English and has recently moved from Puerto Rico to join family. Current medications: Metformin, Glipizide, Losartan, Hydrochlorothiazide (HCTZ), Aspirin (ASA), Atorvastatin. Office blood pressure is 156/94. It is not clear if she is following her recommended DASH diet and prescribed medications.

   Which of the following is least likely to help address potential adherence concerns?
   A. Have her tell you about what she eats, how she prepares it and why
   B. Provide her with a quality hypertension brochure
   C. Inquire if her insurance covers her medications
   D. Inquire about her medication copayment

3. A 54-year-old black man visits his primary care provider with pain in his right knee sustained while playing basketball. He is on no medications and otherwise appears to be in good health. Blood pressure repeated twice during the examination is elevated. His body mass index (BMI) is elevated, although he is muscular and does not appear obese. He exercises regularly, is not short of breath, and appears to be fit. He has been a pack-a-day smoker since his teens and is a moderate drinker.

   ### Physical Examination
   - Height 5 ft 11 in
   - Weight 222 lb
   - BMI 31.0 kg/m^2
   - Waist circumference 40 in
   - Blood pressure (resting) 152/96 mm Hg
   - Resting heart rate 68 bpm

   Clinical Decision Point

   What should the treatment plan be at this point?
   A. Recommend lifestyle modifications
   B. Recommend lifestyle modifications, order blood work
   C. Recommend lifestyle modifications, start a thiazide diuretic
   D. Recommend lifestyle modifications, start an angiotensin-converting enzyme inhibitor (ACEI)

4. The patient in case 3 above is minimally receptive to the recommendations of lifestyle modifications. He considers himself to be slightly overweight, but not obese—and that he is active, exercises regularly, and does not have any flab. He acknowledges that he should stop or at least cut back smoking. He agrees to the blood test and the results are as follows:
   - Fasting plasma glucose (FPG) 138 mg/dL
   - HbA1C 7.5%
   - Total cholesterol (TC) 219 mg/dL
   - Low-density lipoprotein cholesterol (LDL-C) 153 mg/dL
   - High-density lipoprotein cholesterol (HDL-C) 41 mg/dL
   - Triglycerides (TG) 125 mg/dL

   What should the treatment plan be modified at this point?
   A. Initiate antihypertensive treatment with a thiazide diuretic
   B. Initiate cholesterol-lowering treatment with a statin
   C. Initiate dual therapy with an ACE inhibitor and a statin
   D. Initiate treatment of all three conditions with metformin, an ACE inhibitor, and a statin

5. The patient in cases 3 and 4 comes in for his 3-month follow-up, the patient admits to being poorly adherent with his medications, and he is only minimally following the recommended lifestyle modifications. He is intellectually aware of the risks of his conditions, but he admits that because he feels no symptoms, there is nothing to remind him that he needs to take his medications or comply with the smoking cessation, weight loss, and low-sodium diet regimen.

His laboratory values at 3 months are as follows:

- Blood pressure 147/91 mm Hg
- FPG 96 mg/dL
- A1C 6.6%
- TC 188 mg/dL
- LDL-C 103 mg/dL
- HDL-C 46 mg/dL
- TG 92 mg/dL

How should this patient's treatment be modified at this point?
A. Add a diuretic to the ACEI and reinforce adherence
B. Add a calcium channel blocker (CCB) and increase the statin dose
C. Add a β-blocker and reinforce adherence
D. Replace the ACE inhibitor with a thiazide diuretic

Hypertension in the Elderly

1. What is the etiology and distinct blood pressure profile among elderly hypertensives?
A. Combined systolic and diastolic hypertension
B. "Hyperdynamic" circulation
C. Isolated diastolic hypertension
D. Isolated systolic hypertension

2. What are some of the specific cardiovascular benefits of antihypertensive therapy; are those of advanced age more or less likely to benefit compared to the general population?
A. Decreased rates of stroke and all-cause mortality; more likely
B. Decreased rates of heart failure and dementia; less likely
C. Decreased rates of stroke and dementia: less likely
D. Decreased rates of stroke and all-cause mortality; no difference

3. What landmark papers lead to diuretics, calcium channel blockers (CCBs), and those that block the renin–angiotensin–aldosterone system (RAAS) becoming the agents of choice?
A. SHEP, Syst-Eur, CAPPP
B. PROGRESS, MRFIT, ALLHAT
C. ONTARGET, CAMELOT, MRFIT
D. STOP2, SHEP, VALUE

4. What do the most recent Joint National Committee (JNC 8) and European Society of Hypertension Guidelines (2013) advise as the goal blood pressure among the elderly?

A. ≤150/90 mm Hg, ≤140–150 mm Hg systolic (no diastolic goal proposed)
B. ≤140/90 mm Hg recommended by both
C. ≤130/80 mm Hg, ≤140 mm Hg (no diastolic goal proposed)
D. ≤140/90 mm Hg recommended by both

5. Name three obstacles that prevent widespread prescription of antihypertensives to the elderly.
A. Absence of evidence based trials in this age group, increased frailty, medication intolerance
B. Increased frailty, risk of falls, possible "J curve" effect
C. Absence of evidence based trials in this age group, possible "J curve" effect, high rates of non-adherence
D. Risk of falls, lack of comparable therapeutic benefit, increased frailty

Hypertension in Pregnancy

1. A 36-year-old woman with chronic hypertension who is 27 weeks of pregnant asks you if she should liberalize or more strictly control her blood pressure to prevent adverse pregnancy outcomes. She is currently taking nifedipine 30 mg qid for blood pressure control. Her blood pressure in the office measures 126/78 mm Hg. She has no other complaints but does exhibit 1+ bilateral ankle edema on physical examination. What is the MOST appropriate recommendation?
A. Make no changes to the current regimen
B. Implement a 2-g sodium restricted diet
C. Add hydrochlorothiazide
D. Stop nifedipine to liberalize blood pressure reading

2. A 28-year-old woman is evaluated in the immediate postpartum period after induction of labor and normal vaginal delivery for preeclampsia with severe features. Her reflexes remain brisk and she complains of a slight headache. Her medications include IV magnesium, IV labetalol. On physical examination, the BP is 152/106 mm Hg and is significant for 2+ edema of lower extremities bilaterally.

Which ONE of the following is the MOST appropriate management?
A. Discontinue IV magnesium, IV labetalol
B. Discontinue IV magnesium, but continue IV labetalol
C. Continue IV magnesium and transition to oral antihypertensive medications
D. Discontinue IV magnesium and initiate furosemide

3. A 38-year-old woman, gravida 2, para 1, is seen in follow-up for chronic hypertension at 10 weeks of gestation. She has a history of preeclampsia complicating her first pregnancy. She has been adhering to a well-balanced, Western diet. Her present medications include labetalol and a prenatal vitamin. A physical examination shows that the BMI is 34 kg/m^2. The blood pressure is 132/80 mm Hg. The abdomen is gravid, and there is no edema. She has major anxiety over developing preeclampsia again and asks for advice about how to prevent it from recurring.

Which ONE of the following is the MOST appropriate intervention to reduce her risk of preeclampsia?
A. Calcium carbonate 600 mg twice daily
B. Supplemental vitamins C and E
C. Weight loss targeting a BMI less than 30 kg/m^2
D. Aspirin 81 mg daily

4. A 35-year-old women delivered at 32 weeks for severe preeclampsia with an infant weighing 1100 grams. She is presently 6 weeks postpartum and has a blood pressure of 124/68 mm Hg, has no symptoms and an unremarkable physical examination. Though she is not on any medications, she is concerned about the impact preeclampsia on her future health.

Which ONE of the following would you advise regarding the impact of her prior episode of preeclampsia on her long-term health?
A. Reassure patient that preeclampsia is self-limited and will have no impact on her future health
B. It increases the risk of cardiovascular disease
C. It increases her risk of breast cancer
D. She has a 5% risk of developing ESRD over the next 20 years

5. A 25-year-old woman, para 1, is evaluated at 28 weeks gestation for new onset hypertension confirmed on repeat testing. She reports a new headache and blurry vision for the past 2 days. A physical examination shows a BP of 154/96 mm Hg. The remainder of the examination is normal. The complete blood count, renal function, liver chemistries, and urinalysis are normal.

Which ONE of the following is the MOST likely diagnosis?
A. Preeclampsia
B. Gestational hypertension
C. Migraine headache
D. Central venous thrombosis

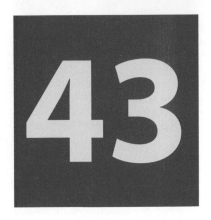

Resistant Hypertension

Julian Segura, MD, PhD

Luis M. Ruilope, MD

ESSENTIALS OF DIAGNOSIS

► Blood pressure above the recommended values (140/90 mm Hg) despite the use of greater than or equal to 3–4 antihypertensive agents, each belonging to a different class.

► Insufficient treatment prescription and lack of adherence to prescribed drugs, dietary restrictions, and lifestyle recommendations are the most frequent causes.

► Associated with obesity, sleep apnea, diabetes, chronic kidney disease, advanced age, high dietary salt intake, and black race.

Hypertension continues to be a common reason for office, urgent care center, and emergency room visits. Raised blood pressure is the leading global risk factor for cardiovascular diseases and chronic kidney disease. If not properly controlled, hypertension can lead to blindness, renal failure, heart disease, and stroke. A recent study from Rapsomaniki et al showed that the lifetime burden of hypertension remains substantial, despite modern therapy. The number of people with raised blood pressure in the world has increased by 90% during these four decades, with the majority of the increase occurring in low-income and middle-income countries, and largely driven by the growth and ageing of the population.

Common factors associated with the development of resistant hypertension include obesity, sleep apnea, diabetes, chronic kidney disease, advanced age, high dietary salt intake, and black race. Interfering substances such as nonsteroidal anti-inflammatory drugs and excessive alcohol consumption can worsen blood pressure control. However, an insufficient treatment prescription and the lack of adherence to the prescribed drug and lifestyle recommendations

(eg, the moderation of alcohol consumption, the restriction of salt intake, the reduction of body weight) seem to be the most frequent causes of uncontrolled BP. Other causes of resistance to treatment include cases of spurious hypertension, such as isolated office (white-coat) hypertension, and failure to use large cuffs on large arms. Nevertheless, a significant number of patients adequately diagnosed and treated still have uncontrolled BP. The real prevalence of resistant hypertension is difficult to determine. Published observational studies describe a prevalence that oscillates between 10% and 15%.

This review focuses on those causes of resistance to treatment that can be evaluated in the outpatient setting. These include a search for nonadherence, assessing the adequacy of the treatment regimen, and ruling out drug interactions and associated conditions. In the absence of the above factors, assessment for secondary causes of hypertension is appropriate. This careful stepwise evaluation is not only cost effective, but also capable of identifying the contributing factors in the vast majority of patients with apparently resistant hypertension.

► Definitions

Resistant hypertension is defined as high blood pressure that remains uncontrolled (>140/90 mm Hg) despite the use of effective doses of three or more different classes of antihypertensive agents, including a diuretic. The first American Heart Association Scientific Statement on resistant hypertension included patients whose blood pressure was controlled (<140/90 mm Hg) with four or more medications within the category of resistant hypertension. Refractory hypertension has been used to refer to an extreme phenotype of antihypertensive treatment failure, considering increased blood pressure levels (>140/90 mm Hg) despite the use of optimal doses of five or more different classes of antihypertensive agents, including chlorthalidone and a mineralocorticoid receptor antagonist.

Pathogenesis

Several clinical trials indicate that resistant hypertension is common, affecting 20–30% of the different study populations. Such clinical outcome studies provide good estimates of the true frequency of resistant hypertension because they employ an intensive treatment regimen mandating drug titrations if BP remained elevated, provide medications free of charge, and closely monitor adherence to the treatment regime with pill counts. In the Antihypertensive and Lipid-Lowering Treatment to Prevent Heart Attack Trial (ALLHAT) more than 33,000 subjects aged 55 years or older with a history of hypertension and one other cardiovascular risk factor were randomized to receive chlorthalidone, amlodipine, or lisinopril. The dose of the randomized medication was titrated first; non-study-related antihypertensive medications were then added as long as BP remained above 140/90 mm Hg. After a 5-year follow-up, 34% of subjects had not achieved goal BP, and overall, 27% of subjects were receiving three or more medications.

In a large cohort of treated hypertensive patients from the Spanish Ambulatory Blood Pressure Monitoring Registry including 68,045 treated patients, 8295 (12.2%) had resistant hypertension. Egan et al subdivided the NHANES data set into time periods in order to estimate trends of resistant hypertension prevalence. Resistant hypertension (BP ≥140/90 mm Hg on ≥3 medications or controlled on ≥4 medications) among all hypertensives increased from 8.5% (1999–2004) to 11.8% (2005–2008). Sim et al identified more than 470,000 persons aged elder than 17 years and diagnosed with hypertension in the Kaiser Permente Southern California health system. Results showed that 12.8% of all hypertensive individuals or 15.3% of all treated individuals met the classic definition of resistant hypertension, which includes those controlled on more than or equal to 4 medications.

Clinical Findings

A. Symptoms and Signs

Table 43–1 lists factors that have been suggested to be causes for resistance; they are often displayed as associated factors in the same patient.

1. White-coat phenomena—Some studies suggest that white-coat or isolated clinic hypertension is as least as common in patients with resistant hypertension as the general population, with a prevalence ranging from 28% to 52%. The white-coat effect is defined as an increase in BP that occurs at the time of a clinical visit and dissipates soon after. It has been known for more than 50 years that BP recorded by a physician can be as much as 30 mm Hg higher than BP taken by the patient at home, using the same technique and in the same posture. Physicians also record higher pressures

Table 43–1. Causes of resistant hypertension.

| **Inadequate treatment** |
| Noncompliance |
| Inadequate doses |
| Inappropriate combinations |
| Failure to modify lifestyle including obesity, alcohol abuse, tobacco |
| **False resistance** |
| Isolated office (white-coat) hypertension |
| Pseudohypertension |
| Improper blood pressure measurement (one measurement, failure to use large cuff on long arms) |
| **Other associated factors** |
| Volume overload due to excessive sodium intake, inadequate diuretic therapy, and/or progressive renal insufficiency |
| Sleep apnea |
| **Drug-induced resistant hypertension** |
| Nonsteroidal anti-inflammatory drugs (oral contraceptives, sympathicomimetic agents, corticosteroids, cocaine, cyclosporine, erythropoietin) |
| **Secondary hypertension** |
| Primary aldosteronism |
| Renal artery stenosis (fibromuscular dysplasia, atherosclerosis) |
| Renal parenchymal disease |
| Pheochromocytoma |

than nurses or technicians. The white-coat effect is usually defined as the difference between the clinic and daytime ambulatory pressure. The underlying mechanisms are not well understood, but may include anxiety, a hyperactive alerting response, or a conditioned response. The white-coat effect is seen to a greater or lesser degree in most if not all hypertensive patients, but is much smaller or negative in normotensive subjects or those with masked hypertension. A closely linked but discrete entity is white-coat hypertension, which refers to a subset of patients who are hypertensive according to their clinic BP but normotensive at other times. Data from the Spanish Ambulatory Blood Pressure Monitoring Registry showed that 62.5% of patients were classified as true resistant hypertensives, and the remaining 37.5% presented white-coat hypertension.

2. Secondary causes of arterial hypertension—Secondary hypertension is defined as increased systemic blood pressure due to an identifiable cause (Table 43–2). Only 5–10% of patients suffering from arterial hypertension have a secondary form, whereas the vast majority has essential hypertension. The prevalence of secondary hypertension depends mostly on age and clinical characteristics of the screened population. In patients with resistant hypertension, the prevalence of secondary forms is significantly higher than in patients with controlled BP (Table 43–2).

Table 43–2. Indicative symptoms and signs of secondary hypertension.

Secondary Cause	Prevalence[a]	Prevalence[b]	History	Screening	Clinical Findings	Laboratory Findings
Obstructive sleep apnea	>5–15%	>30%	Snoring, daytime sleepiness, morning headache, irritability	Screening questionnaire; polysomnography	↑ neck circumference; obesity; peripheral edema	Not specific
Renal parenchymal disease	1.6–8.0%	2–10%	Loss of good BP-control; diabetes; smoking; generalized atherosclerosis; previous renal failure; nocturia	Creatinine, ultrasound of the kidney	Peripheral edema; pallor, loss of muscle mass	↑ Creatinine, proteinuria; ↓ Ca^{2+}, ↑ K^+, ↑ PO_4
Renal artery stenosis	1.0–8.0%	2.5–20%	Generalized atherosclerosis; diabetes; smoking; recurrent flush pulmonary edema	Duplex, or CT, or MRI, or angiography (drive by)	Abdominal bruits; peripheral vascular disease	Secondary aldosteronism; ARR →; ↓ K^+, ↓ Na^+
Primary aldosteronism	1.4–10%	6–23%	Fatigue; constipation; polyuria, polydipsia	Aldosterone-renin ratio (ARR)	Muscle weakness	↓ K^+; ARR ↑
Thyroid disease	1–2%	1–3%	*Hyperthyroidism:* palpitations, weight loss, anxiety, heat intolerance; *Hypothyroidism:* weight gain, fatigue, obstipation	TSH	*Hyperthyroidism:* tachycardia AF; accentuated heart sounds; exophthalmus; *Hypothyroidism:* Bradycardia; muscle weakness; myxedema	*Hyperthyroidism:* TSH ↓; fT4 and/or fT3 ↑; *Hypothyroidism:* TSH ↑; fT4 ↓; cholesterol ↑
Cushing's syndrome	0.5%	<1.0%	Weight gain; impotence; fatigue; psychological changes; polidypsia and polyuria	24-h urinary cortisol; dexamethasone testing	Obesity, hirsutism, skin atrophy, Striae rubrae, muscle weakness, osteopenia	24-h urinary cortisol ↑; Glucose ↑; Cholesterol ↑; K^+ ↓
Pheochromocytoma	0.2–0.5%	<1%	Headache; palpitations; flushing; anxiety	Plasma-metanephrines; 24-h urinary catecholamine	The '5 P's': paroxysmal hypertension; pounding headache; perspiration; palpitations; pallor	Metanephrines ↑
Coarctation of the aorta	<1%	<1%	Headache; nose bleeding; leg weakness or claudication	Cardiac ultrasound	Different BP (≥20/10 mm Hg) between upper-lower extremities and/or between right-left arm; ↓ and delayed femoral pulsations; interscapular ejection murmur; rib notching on chest Rx	Not specific

AF, atrial fibrillation; ARR, aldosterone-renin ratio; BP, blood pressure; Ca^{2+}, calcium; CT, computed tomography; fT3, free triiodothyronine; fT4, free thyroxine; K^+, potassium; Na^+, sodium; PO_4, phosphate; TSH, thyroid-stimulating hormone.

[a]Prevalence in hypertensive patients.

[b]Prevalence in patients with resistant hypertension.

[c]*Kaplan's Clinical Hypertension,* 10th Edition, 2010, Lippincott Williams & Wilkins, p. 363.

3. Hyperaldosteronism—Aldosterone mediates several maladaptive changes in the nervous and cardiovascular systems that promote hypertension in addition to cardiovascular disease and chronic kidney disease. Elevated plasma aldosterone levels are reported both in hypertensive patients and animal models of hypertension, and have been correlated with increased left ventricular mass as well as established as a risk factor for developing hypertension. Primary aldosteronism, resulting from bilateral adrenal hyperplasia or an aldosterone-producing adenoma, occurs with prevalence estimated at 0.5–4.8% of the population with general hypertension, and 4.5–22% of those with resistant hypertension. Importantly, primary hyperaldosteronism leads to a greater frequency of resistant hypertension, as well as increased morbidity and mortality, compared to essential hypertension.

4. Sodium ingestion—volume overload—Excessive dietary sodium intake contributes to the development of resistant hypertension both through directly increasing blood pressure and by blunting the blood pressure-lowering effect of most classes of antihypertensive agents. With the exception of calcium channel blockers (CCBs), antihypertensive drugs show greater effectiveness when the patient follows a low sodium diet.

There is a subset of patients who are more likely to manifest increased salt sensitivity, including blacks, the elderly, and patients with underlying renal insufficiency.

Patients with resistant hypertension frequently have inappropriate volume expansion contributing to their treatment resistance such that a diuretic is essential to maximize blood pressure control. When a volume overload is suspected, 24-hour measurement of sodium urinary excretion can be insufficient to determine sodium intake. The quantification of total plasmatic volume can provide reliable information about the degree of volume overload, and can serve as a guide at the time of prescribing a diuretic.

B. Special Tests and Examinations

The auscultatory method of BP measurement with a properly calibrated and validated instrument should be used. Patients should be seated and should relax for at least 5 minutes in a chair rather than on an examination table, with feet on the floor and arm supported at heart level. Measurement of BP in the standing position is indicated periodically, especially in those at risk for postural hypotension. An appropriate sized cuff bladder (encircling at least 80% of the arm) should be used to ensure accuracy. At least two measurements should be made.

The readings should take place in a calm environment, after a rest time of 5–15 minutes, at least 30 minutes after the consumption of stimulants such as coffee or tobacco, since nicotine as much as caffeine can temporarily elevate BP readings. However, the possible alertness reaction that may take place during the consultation limits BP readings and

contributes to an increase in the prevalence of uncontrolled hypertension. The use of a correct technique with several consecutive measurements (especially by nurse personnel) offers results comparable to ambulatory measurements and provides a better evaluation of hypertensive patients. When ambulatory BP monitoring (ABPM) is used, 20–50% of patients previously diagnosed with high BP display normal BP values. Noninvasive, 24-hour ABPM has evolved over the past 25 years from a novel research tool of limited clinical use to an important and useful modality for stratifying cardiovascular risk and guiding therapeutic decisions. Early clinical uses of ABPM mostly focused on identifying patients with white-coat hypertension; however, growing evidence now points to greater prognostic significance in determining risk for hypertensive end-organ damage compared with office BP measurements. Ambulatory measurement of BP using automated devices has demonstrated the benefit in treatment resistance and borderline hypertension. On the other hand, self-measurement of BP (SMBP) at the patient's home with the correct technique and a valid and properly calibrated digital device provides very useful information on BP values of everyday life. The potential advantages of having patients take their own BP are twofold: The distortion produced by the white-coat effect is eliminated, and multiple readings can be taken over prolonged periods of time. SMBP plays an increasing role in the diagnosis of hypertension. It may be used as a first step in the evaluation of patients with suspected white-coat hypertension. There is also evidence that SMBP can improve BP control.

Pseudohypertension is another factor that can lead to a false misdiagnosis of resistant hypertension when intraarterial pressures are actually normal or below normal. It refers to the phenomenon whereby vascular stiffening results in falsely high auscultatory BP measurements. Some studies suggest that pseudohypertension may be common among the elderly, but definitive evaluation is lacking. Pseudohypertension might be suspected if some of the following occur:

1. Severe hypertension in the absence of demonstrable target-organ deterioration.

2. Symptoms of hypotension in patients with seemingly resistant hypertension.

3. Radiologic evidence of calcification of the brachial artery.

4. BP values more elevated in the brachial artery than in the legs.

5. Severe isolated systolic hypertension.

The Osler maneuver (the ability to palpate the brachial or radial artery despite ipsilateral occlusion of the artery by a BP cuff inflated to suprasystolic values) constitutes a simple screening test for pseudohypertension. Another of value when pseudohypertension is suspected is the use of ultrasonic or oscillometric measuring instruments since their readings correlate more closely with intra-arterial pressure values than those obtained by an indirect auscultatory sphygmomanometer.

▶ Complications

A. Insufficient or Inadequate Treatment

When physicians fail to prescribe lifestyle modifications, adequate antihypertensive drug doses, or appropriate drug combinations, inadequate BP control may result. Most patients with hypertension will require two or more antihypertensive medications to achieve their BP goals. The addition of a second drug from a different class should be initiated when use of a single drug in adequate doses fails to achieve the BP goal. When BP is more than 20/10 mm Hg above goal, consideration should be given to initiating therapy with two drugs, either as separate prescriptions or in fixed-dose combinations.

Likewise, the use of an inadequate drug combination, either belonging to the same pharmacologic group, or with a similar mechanism of action, or with opposing effects, can have negative consequences for obtaining adequate BP control. However, the administration of an adequate drug combination, with synergistic effects, including the administration of fixed doses, can significantly improve the observed response rates over those achieved with the use of each drug by itself. Figure 43–1 shows a model of synergistic combinations proposed in the last European

directives that can be useful in testing the adjustment of the associations. Table 43–3 gives several recommendations for optimal pharmacologic treatment.

B. Poor Patient Compliance

Poor patient compliance remains the most important reason for inadequate BP control. The lack of adherence to hypertensive treatment is one of the major determinants of the excess morbidity and mortality observed in hypertensive patients, and must be taken into account in all patients with refractory hypertension. Studies have demonstrated that in some patient groups at 1 year, fewer than 30% of patients are still taking their antihypertensive medication. There are multiple factors that influence patient compliance, including education, socioeconomic status, and drug costs. There have been numerous studies concerning the reasons for the lack of adherence to treatment and how to detect it. However, direct questioning of the patient on the correct taking of the medication continues to be the most practical measure to confirm lack of adherence to treatment. In these cases, the taking of medication under the supervision of health personnel is usually accompanied by a noticeable reduction in BP, although this measurement is not regularly made. Also, the use of electronic devices to objectively monitor following of the therapeutic treatment has contributed to an awareness of standards of behavior of patients and restores more adequate measures of control. Additionally, the role of nurse personnel in support and education programs for hypertensive patients is of great importance.

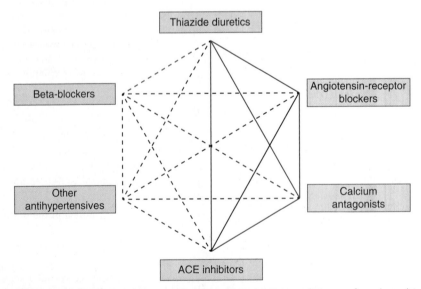

▲ **Figure 43–1.** Possible antihypertensive drug combinations. Blue continuous lines: preferred combinations; blue dashed line: useful combination (with some limitations); black dashed lines: possible but less well tested combinations; black continuous line: not recommended combination.

Table 43–3. Measures to optimize blood pressure control.

Improve compliance to treatment
Simpler regimes
One daily dose
Make the patient aware of the importance of the treatment
Build trust by empathy
Use the most efficient drugs and those best tolerated by the patient
Titrate or combine medications, when necessary
Favor the use of a fixed combination rather than multiple tablets
Use fixed drug associations that permit neutralization of the side effects of each of the drugs alone
Visits not excessively spaced apart in time

Clarify the therapeutic objective
Simple, summarized, and easy to memorize directives
Assume that blood pressure depends on the individualized risk stratification of each patient
Importance of achieving both systolic and diastolic blood pressure

Optimize the pharmacologic treatment
Use drugs in the total recommended doses
Stimulate the use of fixed associations with synergistic or additive effects
Intensive therapy is directed toward control (associate the necessary number of drugs with a synergistic or additive action, whenever they are tolerated)

The two main factors that have been shown to be most important in influencing patient compliance are the side-effect profiles of the antihypertensive agents and the convenience of the dose schedule.

1. Adverse events—The side effects that are associated with antihypertensive agents, as well as those perceived by patients to be associated with antihypertensive agents, remain by far the most important cause of poor patient compliance. It is thus crucial and almost always possible to find drugs or drug combinations that can be well tolerated by individual patients, and a concerted effort should be made to find the right drugs. It should be kept in mind that almost all side effects associated with antihypertensive agents are dose related, and utilizing smaller doses will frequently alleviate the side effects.

2. Convenience—It has been clearly demonstrated that patients who need to take antihypertensive agents twice a day take their drugs less readily than those provided with only one daily dose. Thus, wherever possible, patients should be treated with once-a-day agents. In selecting once-a-day agents, it is important to use those with a true 24-hour effect.

The risk of nonembolic strokes and of myocardial infarction peaks in the early morning and coincides with the rapid surge of BP. This occurs during arousal from sleep (typically between 6 AM and noon). Adequate BP control during this period seems to be associated with fewer cardiovascular events. Antihypertensive agents taken once daily in the morning that do not provide 24-hour efficacy may leave patients with no control at a time when they are at greatest risk of developing cardiovascular events. The duration of action of a particular antihypertensive drug can be assessed in the clinical setting by measuring BP at the trough of drug action (24–26 hours after dosing). Patients should omit taking their medication on the morning of the clinic visit so that BP is measured at trough. If BP is controlled, the agent is providing 24-hour coverage; if not, it should be replaced or two daily doses prescribed. Table 43–3 summarizes some of the keys to improving adherence to treatment.

▶ **Pharmacologic Treatment**

The best treatment for resistant hypertension is based on identification and reversal of contributing factors. Accordingly, it is mandatory to make a thorough search for noncompliance to treatment and to evaluate the adequacy of the treatment regimen, drug interactions, and associated conditions (Figure 43–2). Noninvasive 24-hour ABPM may be an important and useful modality for identifying patients with white-coat hypertension. In the absence of the above factors, assessment for secondary causes of hypertension, in particular hyperaldosteronism, is appropriate.

Addition of low-dose spironolactone (12.5–50 mg) was associated with a mean decrease in BP of 21 ± 20 mm Hg/10 ± 14 mm Hg at 6 weeks and 25 ± 20 mm Hg/12 ± 12 mm Hg at 6-month follow-up in subjects with resistant hypertension. The reduction in BP was similar to subjects with high urinary aldosterone excretion and normal or low aldosterone excretion. Also, spironolactone lowered BP equally in African–American and white subjects. More recently, the ASPIRANT trial showed that the addition of spironolactone in patients with resistant arterial hypertension using a mean of 4.5 antihypertensive drugs, led to a significant decrease of systolic BP both in the office and on ABPM after 8 weeks of treatment. Finally, the PATHWAY-2 trial shows that Spironolactone is the most effective add-on drug for the treatment of resistant hypertension. In this double-blind, placebo-controlled, crossover trial, a total of 335 patients were included. Patients rotated, in a preassigned, randomized order, through 12 weeks of once daily treatment with each of spironolactone (25–50 mg), bisoprolol (5–10 mg), doxazosin modified release (4–8 mg), and placebo, in addition to their baseline blood pressure drugs. The average reduction in home systolic blood pressure by spironolactone was superior to placebo, superior to the mean of the other two active treatments, and superior when compared with the individual treatments. These results demonstrate that an aldosterone antagonist can be effective in treating hypertension resistant to multidrug regimens that include a diuretic and an angiotensin-converting enzyme inhibitor or an angiotensin receptor blocker.

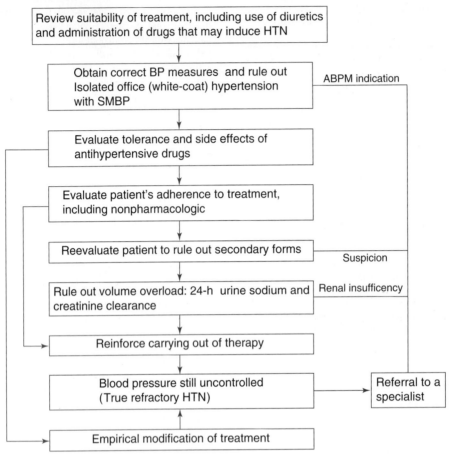

▲ **Figure 43–2.** Algorithm for the diagnostic and therapeutic management of a patient with resistant hypertension. ABPM, ambulatory blood pressure monitoring; HTN, hypertension; SMBP, self-monitoring of blood pressure.

Additional reduction in BP was also achieved in subjects without hyperaldosteronism. Benefits in such subjects may have been secondary to additional diuretic effects of the aldosterone antagonist or may reflect a broad role of aldosterone in causing resistant hypertension even in the absence of demonstrable hyperaldosteronism.

Several clinical trials document the efficacy of eplerenone, a selective aldosterone antagonist, in treating hypertension in subjects with primary hypertension. Eplerenone would likewise be effective as an additional therapy in subjects with resistant hypertension while avoiding the antiandrogenic and antiprogesteronic effects of spironolactone. Recently, in patients with resistant hypertension, add-on use of eplerenone has been effective in lowering BP, especially home and ambulatory awake BP.

Hyperkalemia or acute renal insufficiency occurs rarely, and should be monitored for, particularly in patients with chronic kidney disease and/or diabetes.

The general benefit of an aldosterone blockade in subjects with resistant hypertension suggests that aldosterone excess may be a more common cause of hypertension than previously thought. However, the aldosteronism that we are reporting as being so common is undoubtedly different from the classic syndrome of primary aldosteronism. The regulatory abnormalities, distinct from classic aldosteronism, resulting in such a high prevalence of aldosteronism are unknown. Recognition of such abnormalities may allow prevention and/or development of even more effective treatment strategies.

▶ Invasive Therapies

The presence of an enhanced sympathetic nervous system activity is frequently present in resistant hypertension and is difficult to counteract pharmacologically because of the frequent presence of side effects of the drugs acting directly on it. In 2009, the SIMPLICITY 1 study containing data from a group of 45 patients was published, which showed a reduction of BP following a catheter-mediated renal denervation (RDN). The positive effects lasted at least 24 months and the technique proved to be safe. Following this first proof-of-concept, the SIMPLICITY 2 study was started with similar inclusion criteria (systolic BP ≥160 mm Hg or 150 mm Hg for diabetic patients despite compliance with more than three antihypertensive medications). A total of 106 patients were included and randomized to denervation or to a control group. The positive effects of RDN were again observed in the absence of changes in BP in the control group during a 6-month study period. Both Symplicity HTN-1 and 2 were primarily conducted in European and Australian centers, and the positive results led to rapid acceptance of the role of RDN in the treatment of resistant HTN outside of the United States.

Symplicity HTN-3, a multicenter randomized controlled trial conducted in the United States, is the largest clinical trial examining the efficacy and safety of catheter-based RDN to date, and was the first trial to include a sham procedure as a control group. A total of 535 participants with severe resistant HTN (with a baseline mean SBP of 180 mm Hg) were randomized in a 2:1 ratio to undergo RDN or sham procedure. Although the mean SBP at 6 months was significantly lower than the baseline in both denervation and control groups (by 14.1 vs 11.7 mm Hg, respectively), the between-group difference of 2.4 mm Hg favoring denervation was not statistically significant. Similar findings were noted for the change in mean 24-hour ambulatory SBP. There were also no significant differences in safety endpoints between the two groups, with major adverse events occurring in 1.4% and 0.6% of the denervation and sham procedure group participants, respectively.

The realworld experience with RDN in patients who undergo the procedure using the Symplicity Renal Denervation System outside of clinical trials has been analyzed in the Global Symplicity Registry. Among the first 1000 consecutive patients enrolled in the registry, 1-year office SBP and 24-hour SBP reductions were similar to what was observed in the intervention arm of Symplicity HTN-3 (by 13.0 and 8.3 mm Hg, respectively). The negative results of Symplicity HTN-3 trial were a major surprise that dampened the excitement for RDN felt after the publication of Symplicity HTN-1 and 2 studies.

Data from the SPYRAL HTN-OFF MED trial, a prospective, randomized, sham-controlled trial of hypertensive patients with baseline office systolic blood pressure between 150–180 mm Hg offer new evidence. In this trial, patients are either not receiving antihypertensive medications, or drug therapy is discontinued prior to RDN study enrollment and all patients remain off medications until 3 months post randomization. A pre-specified analysis of 80 patients showed a -5.0 mm Hg difference in 24-hr ambulatory systolic blood pressure and a -7.7 mm Hg difference in office systolic blood pressure between the RDN arm compared to sham control.

Nevertheless, a number of important questions still need to be addressed in order to establish an evidence base for RDN that would permits its adoption for routine clinical use. Much of the unmet need distils down to the issue of standardization. This applies to the technology and the technique, where different systems may not work equally well in all situations. It applies to the terminology used, as well as to markers of procedural success. And perhaps most of all, standardization will be key when designing clinical trials. Treatments, populations, methods, and adherence measures need to be highly consistent to avoid inconclusive or biased results. Finally, it is urgent to delineate predictors of BP response following RDN.

Other invasive therapies as baroreflex activation therapy (BAT) via an implantable carotid sinus stimulator, BAT via carotid stenting, and creation of a percutaneous arteriovenous shunt offer exciting possibilities of future options, though at this time they continue to be investigational.

▶ Prognosis

Truly resistant hypertension, hypertension in which all known resistance causes can be excluded, could become a rarity. Nonetheless, from a practical point of view we offer a series of steps to detect, control, or diminish the conditioning factors, emphasizing the need to arrive at a correct diagnosis. For this diagnosis, the basic pillars are an adequate measuring of pressure, a guarantee of correct associations, an aceptable carrying out of the prescribed regime, and, lastly, ruling out secondary forms of hypertension. Arriving at this point, the intervention of a specialist can ensure the control of BP by means of the combined use of four or more antihypertensive agents.

KEY READINGS

Bhatt DL et al; SYMPLICITY HTN-3 Investigators: A controlled trial of renal denervation for resistant hypertension. N Engl J Med 2014;370:1393.

Böhm M et al: First report of the Global SYMPLICITY Registry on the effect of renal artery denervation in patients with uncontrolled hypertension. Hypertension 2015;65:766.

Calhoun DA et al: Resistant hypertension: diagnosis, evaluation, and treatment. A scientific statement from the American Heart Association Professional Education Committee of the Council for High Blood Pressure Research. Hypertension 2008;51:1403.

Cushman WC et al: Success and predictors of blood pressure control in diverse North American settings: the Antihypertensive and Lipid-Lowering Treatment to Prevent Attack Trial (ALLHAT). J Clin Hypertens (Greenwich) 2002;4:393.

De la Sierra A et al: Clinical features of 8295 patients with resistant hypertension classified on the basis of ambulatory blood pressure monitoring. Hypertension 2011;57:898.

Egan BM et al: Uncontrolled and apparent treatment resistant hypertension in the United States, 1988 to 2008. Circulation 2001;124:1046.

Eguchi K et al: Add-on use of eplerenone is effective for lowering home and ambulatory blood pressure in drug-resistant hypertension. J Clin Hypertens (Greenwich) 2016;18:1250.

Global Burden of Metabolic Risk Factors for Chronic Diseases Collaboration. Cardiovascular disease, chronic kidney disease, and diabetes mortality burden of cardiometabolic risk factors from 1980 to 2010: a comparative risk assessment. Lancet Diabetes Endocrinol 2014;2:634.

Grossman A et al: Drug induced hypertension: an unappreciated cause of secondary hypertension. Eur J Pharmacol 2015; 763:15.

Judd E et al: Apparent and true resistant hypertension: definition, prevalence and outcomes. J Hum Hypertens 2014;28:463.

Krum H et al: Catheter-based renal sympathetic denervation for resistant hypertension: a multicentre safety and proof-of-concept cohort study. Lancet 2009;373:1275.

Mahfoud F et al: Proceedings from the European clinical consensus conference for renal denervation: considerations on future clinical trial design. Eur Heart J 2015;36:2219.

Mancia G et al: 2013 ESH/ESC Guidelines for the management of arterial hypertension: the Task Force for the management of arterial hypertension of the European Society of Hypertension (ESH) and of the European Society of Cardiology (ESC). J Hypertens 2013;31:1281.

NCD Risk Factor Collaboration (NCD-RisC): Worldwide trends in blood pressure from 1975 to 2015: a pooled analysis of 1479 population-based measurement studies with 19.1 million participants. Lancet 2017;389:37.

O'Brien E et al: European Society of Hypertension position paper on ambulatory blood pressure monitoring. J Hypertens 2013;31:1731.

Rapsomaniki E et al: Blood pressure and incidence of twelve cardiovascular diseases: lifetime risks, healthy life-years lost and age-specific associations in 1.25 million people. Lancet 2014;383:1899.

Rimoldi SF et al: Secondary arterial hypertension: when, who, and how to screen? Eur Heart J 2014;35:1245.

Siddiqui M et al: Resistant and refractory hypertension: antihypertensive treatment resistance vs treatment failure. Can J Cardiol 2016;32:603.

Sim JJ et al: Characteristics of resistant hypertension in a large, ethnically diverse hypertension population of an integrated health system. Mayo Clin Proc 2013;88:1099.

SIMPLICITY HTN-2 Investigators. Renal sympathetic denervation in patients with treatment-resistant hypertension (the Symplicity HTN-2 Trial.): a randomised controlled trial. Lancet 2010;376:1903.

Townsend RR et al, on behalf of the SPYRAL HTN-OFF MED trial investigators: Catheter-based renal denervation in patients with uncontrolled hypertension in the absence of antihypertensive medications (SPYRAL HTN-OFF MED): a randomised, sham-controlled, proof-of-concept trial. Lancet 2017 Aug 25. DOI: 10.1016/S0140-6736(17)32281-X.

Vaclavik J et al: Addition of spironolactone in patients with resistant arterial hypertension (ASPIRANT): a randomized, double-blind, placebo-controlled trial. Hypertension 2011;57:1069.

Whaley-Connell A et al: Aldosterone: role in the cardiometabolic syndrome and resistant hypertension. Prog Cardiovasc Dis 2010;52:401.

Williams B et al: Spironolactone versus placebo, bisoprolol, and doxazosin to determine the optimal treatment for drug-resistant hypertension (PATHWAY-2): a randomised, double-blind, crossover trial. Lancet 2015;386:2059.

Yoruk A et al: Baroreceptor stimulation for resistant hypertension. Am J Hypertens 2016;29:1319.

■ CHAPTER REVIEW QUESTIONS

1. A 45-year-old woman is found to have mean office BP values around 154/96 mm Hg by her primary care doctor. She is receiving lisinopril 40 mg/day, amlodipine 10 mg/day, and hydrochlorothiazide 25 mg/day.

   Which ONE of the following is the most appropriate diagnosis at this time?
   A. Resistant hypertension
   B. Refractory hypertension
   C. Secondary hypertension
   D. Essential hypertension
   E. Normotension

2. Which ONE of the following is not considered a cause of resistant hypertension?
   A. Noncompliance
   B. Isolated office hypertension
   C. Excessive sodium intake
   D. Sleep apnea
   E. Acetaminophen

3. A 66-year-old woman is found to have mean office BP values around 158/92 mm Hg. Her home-BP measurements shows mean values of 136/82 mm Hg. She is receiving olmesartan 40 mg/day, amlodipine 10 mg/day, and chlorthalidone 25 mg/day.

   Which ONE of the following is the most appropriate approach at this time?
   A. Add bisoprolol 5 mg/day
   B. Add spironolactone 25 mg/day
   C. Perform an ambulatory BP monitoring
   D. Reevaluate secondary forms of hypertension
   E. Keep treatment and schedule a new visit in 6 months

4. A 64-year-old man diagnosed as true resistant hypertensive is found to have mena office values around 154/94 mm Hg. He is adherent to treatment and nonpharmacologic recommendations, secondary forms of hypertension have been discarded. He is receiving lisinopril 40 mg/day, hydrochlorothiazide 25 mg/day and amlodipine 10 mg/day.

Which ONE of the following is the most appropriate next step?
A. Add doxazosin
B. Add spironolactone
C. Add bisoprolol
D. Add clonidine
E. Keep treatment and schedule a new visit in 6 months

5. Which ONE of the following sentences about invasive therapies is correct?
A. Symplicity HTN-3 was a multicenter randomized controlled trial conducted in the United States, including 45 patients with resistant hypertension
B. Symplicity HTN-3 results show a clear reduction of office and ambulatory BP values in patients with resistant hypertension
C. It is urgent to delineate predictors of BP response following renal denervation
D. Global Synplicity Registry includes information about first 1000 consecutive patients and shows no reduction in BP values
E. Baroreflex activation therapy offer an adequate option for most patients presenting resistant hypertension

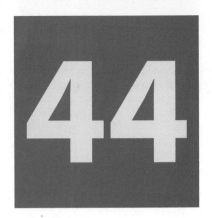

Hypertensive Emergencies and Urgencies

William J. Elliott, MD, PhD

- ▶ Emergency: Acute, ongoing target organ damage with very elevated blood pressure that should be lowered within minutes to hours.
- ▶ Urgency: Absence of acute, ongoing target organ damage with very elevated blood pressure that should be lowered over one to several hours (controversial).

▶ General Considerations

Many patients present to emergency departments or physician offices with very elevated blood pressures (BPs), but few of these constitute either hypertensive emergencies or urgencies. Hypertensive emergencies accounted for 167 of 100,000 emergency department visits across the United States in 2013, but developing nations, minority populations, economically challenged individuals, and those who are nonadherent to prescribed antihypertensive drugs have about a fourfold increased risk. The important principle to triage such patients appropriately is to identify symptoms or signs indicative of acute, ongoing target-organ damage. This usually involves examining or testing the central nervous system (including the optic fundi), cardiovascular system, kidneys, and/or uterus (see first 3 columns of Table 44–1). Patients with acute, ongoing target-organ damage are at very high risk of cardiovascular events, and generally should be treated within minutes in an intensively monitored setting with a short-acting intravenously delivered antihypertensive agent (typically sodium nitroprusside). Individuals who do not have acute, ongoing target-organ damage may be referred to a source of ongoing care for hypertension (if at low risk), or treated with orally administered antihypertensive agents (if at moderate risk), and the BP response observed.

Examples of hypertensive urgencies that would usually be treated in hospital include very elevated BPs in the perioperative period, in organ transplant recipients (especially if the transplant was recent), and in the setting of severe burns. Most other hypertensive urgencies can be diagnosed in the outpatient department; acute drug treatment in this setting has not been significantly beneficial in recent cohort studies, but is sometimes justified by local "standard of care" and traditions in a specific jurisdiction.

▶ Pathogenesis

The key pathophysiological feature to understand hypertensive emergencies is that the normal blood pressure-blood flow curve in most vascular beds is shifted to the right in patients who develop this condition. Over time, arteries in these patients adapt to the very high BPs, in order to maintain organ perfusion, a process called "autoregulation." If the BP is lowered too quickly, or to a BP that is too low to maintain autoregulation, blood flow to important organs will be compromised, and ischemia (to brain, heart, or kidneys) may result.

▶ Clinical Findings

See the first 3 columns of Table 44–1.

▶ Differential Diagnosis

Differentiation of the several neurological subtypes of hypertensive emergencies is the most difficult. This distinction is very important, since drug therapy to lower BP is often withheld in the setting of an intraparenchymal hemorrhage (although this is controversial outside the United States), whereas BP lowering is not only beneficial, but often diagnostic in hypertensive encephalopathy. The results of CT or MRI scans are often helpful.

Many other clinical syndromes include acute, ongoing target-organ damage (eg, papilledema) that could be (but is not) directly related to hypertension (eg, hematuria

Table 44–1. Common hypertensive emergencies with signs/symptoms and other findings.

Type of Emergency	Signs & Symptoms	Other Findings	Recommended Drug(s)	BP Target
Neurological emergencies				
Hypertensive encephalopathy (typically a diagnosis of exclusion)	Mental status changes, generally without focal neurological signs; Papilledema is common	No other findings to explain mental status abnormalities	Nitroprusside*	25% reduction over 2–3 hours.
Acute ischemic stroke	Focal neurological signs, headache	CT or MRI may show infarcted or ischemic area	Nitroprusside* (controversial)	BP is generally not treated unless higher than 180–220/110–120 mm Hg
Intracranial hemorrhage	Headache, focal neurological signs	CT or MRI typically shows hemorrhagic area	Nitroprusside* (controversial)	0–25% reduction over 6–12 hours (controversial)
Subarachnoid hemorrhage	Headache	Lumbar puncture shows xanthochromia and/or blood	Nimodipine	Up to 25% reduction in previously hypertensive patients, 130–160 mm Hg systolic for normotensive patients
Acute head injury/trauma	Headache, signs of external trauma	CT or MRI may show area of traumatized brain	Nitroprusside*	0–25% reduction over 2–3 hours (controversial)
Cardiovascular emergencies				
Acute myocardial infarction	Chest discomfort, dyspnea, anxiety	Electrocardiogram may show hyperacute T-wave elevation; troponin typically elevated	Nitroglycerin	Cessation of ischemia (typically only a 5–10% decrease is required)
Acute left ventricular failure/acute pulmonary edema	Dyspnea, pulmonary rales	Chest X-ray shows pulmonary vascular redistribution or worse	Nitroprusside* or nitroglycerin	Improvement in failure (typically only a 10–15% decrease is required)
Acute aortic dissection	"Tearing" chest pain, pulse deficit in legs	Widened mediastinum on chest X-ray, "intimal flap" on echocardiogram, CT, or MRI	Beta-Blocker + nitroprusside*	120 mm Hg systolic in 20 minutes (if possible; not evidence-based)
Recent vascular surgery	Tense suture lines	None	Nitroprusside*	Typically ~160/100 mm Hg
Epistaxis unresponsive to packing	Uncontrolled blood from the nose (anteriorly or posteriorly)	None	Nitroprusside*	To control bleeding (typically only a 5–10% decrease is required)
Renal emergencies				
Acute deterioration in renal function	None that are characteristic of this condition	Significant elevation of serum creatinine relative to recent level	Fenoldopam	0–25% reduction in mean arterial pressure over 1–12 hours
Hematuria (typically gross)	Red or brown urine, flank pain	4+ blood on urinalysis	Fenoldopam	To reduce bleeding rate (typically a 0–10% reduction over 1–12 hours

(Continued)

Table 44–1. Common hypertensive emergencies with signs/symptoms and other findings. (*Continued*)

Type of Emergency	Signs & Symptoms	Other Findings	Recommended Drug(s)	BP Target
Catecholamine-excess states				
Pheochromocytoma	Headache, sweating attacks, orthostatic hypotension	Elevated plasma metanephrines and urinary catecholamine metabolites; mass seen on CT or T_2 weighted images on MRI	Phentolamine	To control paroxysms and/or symptoms
Drug-related conditions (tyramine ingestion with monoamine oxidase inhibitor; withdrawal of antihypertensive drug; phencyclidine/cocaine use)	Headache, mental status change, tachycardia (often, but not always)	None characteristic of this condition	Phentolamine or withdrawn drug (if any)	Typically only one dose is necessary
Pregnancy-related conditions				
Eclampsia/ Pre-eclampsia	Seizure/headache, edema (no longer required for diagnosis)	Proteinuria (dipstick or 24-hour collection), occasionally: thrombocytopenia, elevated AST or ALT	$MgSO_4$, methyldopa, hydralazine, labetalol, nifedipine	Typically <90 mm Hg diastolic, but often lower

*Some physicians prefer an intravenous infusion of either fenoldopam or nicardipine, neither of which has potentially toxic metabolites, over nitroprusside. Acute improvements in renal function occur during therapy with fenoldopam, but not with nitroprusside. Some neurologists avoid nitroprusside because it can reduce cerebral blood flow. ALT, alanine aminotransferase; AST, aspartate aminotransferase; CT, computed tomography; MRI, magnetic resonance imaging.

from glomerulonephritis, elevation of serum creatinine in acute kidney injury exacerbating chronic kidney disease), but these generally lack the very elevated BP that is a hallmark of a hypertensive emergency.

Complications

Because of the extreme BP level and the existence of acute, ongoing target-organ damage, patients with hypertensive emergencies are at very high short-term risk for cardiovascular and renal complications if left untreated. Treatment, however, can lead to an even greater risk if carried out improperly. The most-feared complication of treatment for a hypertensive emergency is reduction of the BP too quickly or to a BP that is too low for autoregulation to be maintained. This results in reduced blood flow to important organs, and ischemia in cardiac, neurological, renal or peripheral arterial beds. This is the major reason for not using quick-acting oral hypotensive drugs (eg, nifedipine capsules), as they can precipitously lower BP, and produce major complications (myocardial infarction, stroke, acute kidney injury).

Patients with hypertensive urgencies are at much lower cardiovascular risk than patients with hypertensive emergencies. Three cohort studies have shown no significant benefit from acute treatment of BP; harm can result from aggressive treatment.

Treatment

Patients with hypertensive emergencies are most appropriately treated in a closely-monitored environment (eg, intensive care unit) with a short-acting, quickly-reversible intravenously administered drug (last 2 columns of Table 44–1). Sodium nitroprusside is the drug with the longest track record, and is very inexpensive, but carries the risk of cyanide and thiocyanate toxicity if given chronically or at high doses. After BP is maintained at the target range for several (typically 6–12) hours, oral therapy (typically with an intermediate-acting calcium antagonist) can be given, and the intravenously administered drug tapered and discontinued. Because secondary causes are more common in patients with hypertensive emergencies, appropriate screening usually begins during the hospitalization.

Prognosis

Left untreated, patients with hypertensive emergencies have a dismal prognosis (typically a 5-month mean survival); in 1928 (when the term was introduced), "malignant hypertension" reflected a prognosis as poor as patients with cancer. Since the introduction of effective antihypertensive drug therapy, the prognosis depends more on the level of renal, cardiac, and neurological function at presentation than the initial level of BP. Sufficient kidney function sometimes returns to allow discontinuation of dialysis, if it was required acutely for a hypertensive emergency, particularly if BP is well-controlled during follow-up.

KEY READINGS

Cooper CM, Fenves AZ: Hypertensive urgencies and emergencies in the hospital setting. Hosp Pract 2016:44:21.

Elliott WJ, Varon J: Evaluation and treatment of hypertensive emergencies in adults. UpToDate®, submitted 14 APR 16, posted 16 Aug 16.

Elliott WJ, Varon J: Moderate to severe hypertensive retinopathy and hypertensive encephalopathy in adults. UpToDate®, submitted 03 May 16, posted 28 Jul 16.

Elliott WJ, Varon J: Drugs used for the treatment of hypertensive emergencies. UpToDate®, submitted 03 Jun 16, posted 06 JUN 16.

Janke AT et al: Trends in the incidence of hypertensive emergencies in US emergency departments from 2006 to 2013. J Am Heart Assoc 2016:5:e004511.

Levy PD et al: Blood pressure treatment and outcomes in hypertensive patients without acute target organ damage: a retrospective cohort study. Am J Emerg Med 2015;33:1219.

Papadopoulos DP et al: Cardiovascular hypertensive emergencies. Curr Hypertens Rep 2015;17:5.

Patel KK et al: Characteristics and outcomes of patients presenting with hypertensive urgency in the office setting. JAMA Intern Med 2016;176:961.

Varon J, Elliott WJ: Management of severe asymptomatic hypertension (hypertensive urgencies) in adults. UpToDate®, submitted 12 Feb 16, posted 16 Feb 16.

■ CHAPTER REVIEW QUESTIONS

1. A 56-year-old man presents to the Emergency Department complaining of a gradually worsening headache, unresponsive to acetaminophen, over the last 2 hours. He has had hypertension for 6 years, but "ran out" of his usual medications (hydrochlorothiazide and lisinopril) 2 weeks ago. Vital signs are unremarkable except for a blood pressure of 226/128 mm Hg (right arm seated) with a regular pulse rate of 80 beats/min. Funduscopic and general physical examinations are unremarkable. Laboratory studies, including a urinalysis, are within the reference ranges. A computed tomographic scan of his head discloses no abnormalities. The most appropriate next step in the management of this patient is which of the following?

   A. Crushed captopril 25 mg dissolved in 60 mL of water, orally, now.

   B. Nifedipine 10 mg capsule, "bite and swallow" now.

   C. Oral clonidine, 0.2 mg now, and 0.1 mg each hour until the blood pressure is less than 160/100 mm Hg.

   D. Refill his chronic medications, and refer to an appropriate source of primary care.

   E. Sodium nitroprusside intravenously, starting at 0.3 μg/kg/min.

2. A 43-year-old African–American man is brought to the Emergency Department because his girlfriend says he "just faded out" over the last 4 hours. He has a 25-year history of resistant hypertension, and usually takes furosemide, lisinopril, hydralazine, and clonidine, but his girlfriend says he has not taken any for at least 2 days. His Glasgow coma scale score is 4 (no verbal response, no eye response, extension response to pain). Vital signs are unremarkable except for a blood pressure of 280/160 mm Hg (right arm supine) with a regular pulse rate of 80 beats/min. Physical examination shows bilateral papilledema and one flame-shaped hemorrhage at 3 o'clock two disc diameters from where the right nerve head should be. Laboratory studies show a serum creatinine of 4.8 mg/dL ($eGFR = 17$ mL/min/1.73 m^2), a blood urea nitrogen of 56 mg/dL; urinalysis (after placement of a Foley catheter) shows 1+ blood on dipstick and 3–5 RBCs/hpf, but no casts, white cells, or bacteria on microscopic examination. An intravenous line is placed; no acute changes are noted after administration of naloxone. The most appropriate next step in his management is which of the following?

   A. Apply a clonidine patch (0.3 mg/day) to upper thorax.

   B. Computed tomographic scan of the head.

   C. Fenoldopam mesylate intravenously, starting at 0.1 μg/kg/min.

   D. Lumbar puncture.

   E. Sodium nitroprusside intravenously, starting at 0.3 μg/kg/min.

3. A right-handed 69-year-old man with asthma is brought to the Emergency Department because he became dysarthric, dropped his spoon, and could not move his right leg while eating breakfast 30 minutes ago. He has a 10-year history of hypertension, for which he takes amlodipine, hydrochlorothiazide, and lisinopril, all of which he took 45 minutes ago. Vital signs are unremarkable except for a blood pressure of 192/114 mm Hg and a regular pulse rate of 80 beats/min. Neurological examination confirms dysarthria and right-sided weakness (3/5 upper and lower extremities). A computed tomographic scan of the head without contrast shows no blood. The most appropriate next step in his management is which of the following?
   A. Aspirin 325 mg chew and swallow, now.
   B. Nimodipine 60 mg orally now.
   C. Recombinant human tissue-plasminogen activator intravenously.
   D. Sodium nitroprusside intravenously, starting at 0.3 μg/kg/min.
   E. Subcutaneous enoxaparin 1 mg/kg q 12 hours.

4. A 65-year-old man is brought to the Emergency Department with 20 minutes of chest discomfort, described as having started between the scapulae as a "ripping" or "tearing" sensation, followed by pressure, nausea, diaphoresis and a "sense of doom." He has a 30-year history of hypertension, for which he takes chlorthalidone and lisinopril. Vital signs are unremarkable except for a blood pressure of 162/104 mm Hg (right arm supine) with a regular pulse of 88 beats/min. Physical examination shows diminished pulses at and below the femorals, bilaterally. An electrocardiogram is unremarkable. Chest X-ray shows a widened anterior mediastinum. Traditionally, the most appropriate systolic blood pressure for him (even if not properly evidence-based) is which of the following?
   A. <120 mm Hg.
   B. <130 mm Hg.
   C. <140 mm Hg.
   D. <150 mm Hg.
   E. <160 mm Hg.

5. A 34-year old man is hospitalized with a 2-week history of episodic headache, diaphoresis, and tachycardia, all of which gradually disappear over 5–10 minutes. His wife, a nurse, measured his blood pressure at 240/140 mm Hg during one "spell" last week. Last week, he was diagnosed with generalized anxiety disorder during an Emergency Department visit, and given alprazolam and atenolol. Vital signs and physical examination are unremarkable except for a right thumb subungual fibroma and two ash-leaf patches on his left flank. Six hours after admission, he spikes his regular pulse rate to 120 beats/min, his blood pressure is 260/150 mm Hg, and he is quite diaphoretic. In addition to obtaining blood and urine after the onset of symptoms, the most appropriate initial therapy for him is which of the following?
   A. Dantrolene sodium intravenously.
   B. Doxazosin orally.
   C. Esmolol intravenously.
   D. Phentolamine intravenously.
   E. Phenylephrine intravenously.

Cystic Diseases of the Kidney

Maria V. Irazabal, MD
Vicente E. Torres, MD, PhD

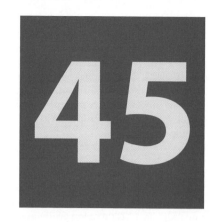

45

▶ Introduction

Renal cystic disease includes a myriad of conditions characterized by the presence of multiple hereditary or acquired renal cysts, which differ in their clinical presentation, prognosis, and management. Renal cysts are composed of smooth-walled, enclosed fluid-filled circular structures that form in the kidney by focal out pouching of renal tubules. Although the mechanism underlying cyst formation remain to be fully elucidated, defects in the primary ciliary sensing mechanisms, intracellular calcium regulation, and cellular cyclic AMP (cAMP) accumulation have been shown to contribute to cyst formation in autosomal dominant and autosomal recessive polycystic kidney diseases (ADPKD and ARPKD), which represent a significant cause of morbidity and mortality in children and young adults. Currently, there are no FDA approved treatments for ADPKD, and the existing standard of care includes risk modification, management of complications, and renal replacement therapy with dialysis or organ transplantation. Several drugs designed to slow or arrest the progression of ADPKD have shown promise in preclinical models and clinical trials, including vasopressin receptor antagonists and somatostatin analogs. The vasopressin-2 receptor antagonist Tolvaptan has been the most successful drug therapy to reduce the rate of increase in total kidney volume (TKV) and ameliorate renal functional decline in patients with ADPKD. Further elucidation of the mechanisms implicated in cyst formation and development would provide impetus for correcting the underlying abnormalities in cystic pathways.

AUTOSOMAL DOMINANT POLYCYSTIC KIDNEY DISEASE

ESSENTIALS OF DIAGNOSIS

▶ Two renal cysts unilaterally or bilaterally before age 30 years by renal ultrasound in patients with a family history of ADPKD.

▶ Two cysts in each kidney between the ages of 30 and 59 years by renal ultrasound in patients with a family history of ADPKD.

▶ Four or more cysts in each kidney after age elder than or equal to 60 years by renal ultrasound in patients with a family history of ADPKD.

▶ Genetic testing (linkage analysis and direct DNA sequencing) is available as a clinical test, and can detect *PKD1* and *PKD2* mutations in approximately 90% of confirmed cases.

▶ General Considerations

ADPKD remains one of the most frequent monogenic disorders and one of the main causes of renal insufficiency that affects 1 in 400–1000 individuals worldwide. In the United States, approximately half million people suffer from ADPKD, which accounts for an important fraction of new patients entering dialysis programs each year.

The disorder is transmitted in autosomal dominant pattern with varied expression, but nearly always with complete penetrance of mutated genes. Approximately 85% of ADPKD cases are caused by mutations in the *PKD1* gene, whereas mutations in the *PKD2* gene account for approximately 15% of the remaining mutation identified ADPKD cases. Between 7% and 10% of ADPKD cases remain genetically unresolved after genetic screening. Recent data suggest that mutations in *GANAB*, a coding gene that encodes for a glucosidase-II alpha subunit, may account for approximately 3% of the genetically unresolved ADPKD cases. However, due to the mild phenotype presentation of patients with mutations in *GANAB* it is possible that this account for a larger proportion of the missing genetic causes of ADPKD and may be underdiagnosed.

Importantly, patients with ADPKD present with a significant number of extra-renal cystic and non-cystic manifestations, including polycystic liver disease (PLD) and cysts in diverse organ systems (pancreas, arachnoid membrane, pineal gland, and seminal vesicles), intracranial saccular aneurysms, thoracic aortic aneurysms and dissections, coronary artery aneurysms, mitral and/or tricuspid valve prolapse, aortic valve insufficiency, aortic root dilation, and colonic diverticula.

Disease severity and renal dysfunction in patients with ADPKD are highly heterogeneous with significant inter-familial and intrafamilial variations. In general, mutations in the PKD1 gene are responsible for an earlier onset and more severe course of the disease. Contrarily, patients with mutations in PKD2 develop ESRD approximately 20 years later than those with mutations in the PKD1 gene. Male patients with mutations in the PKD2 gene commonly present with more extensive cystic renal dysfunction, but less liver involvement.

▶ Clinical Findings

A. Symptoms and Signs

1. Renal manifestations—In ADPKD patients, the number of cysts progresses in an exponential manner as a person ages. Enlarging cysts compress renal parenchyma and vasculature causing significant structural abnormalities that result in several manifestations of renal involvement, including pain, hematuria, hypertension, and renal dysfunction. Most of the patients present bilateral distribution of renal cysts, but in some unusual cases, cyst may develop in a unilateral or asymmetric pattern.

The Consortium of Radiologic Imaging Studies of PKD (CRISP) has shown that kidney and cyst volumes increase in most patients, and that larger kidneys are associated with a faster decline in renal function. Volumetric analyses of polycystic kidneys from CT or MR images can be used as an early means to monitor disease progression.

A. HYPERTENSION—Hypertension (HTN) is common and occurs in the majority of ADPKD patients prior to loss of renal function, with an average age of onset of HTN between 30 and 34 years.

Multiple mechanisms are responsible for the development of HTN in ADPKD, including activation of the intra-renal renin-angiotensin aldosterone system, impaired nitric oxide endothelium-mediated vasorelaxation, augmented sympathetic activity, and vascular remodeling. Importantly, hypertension in ADPKD patients is associated with the severity of kidney disease, and preceded by a reduction in the renal blood flow (RBF).

Studies have shown that early onset of HTN is associated with a poorer renal prognosis in ADPKD and increased risk for progressing toward ESRD. Additionally, early onset and/or uncontrolled HTN are significant risk factors for intracranial aneurysmal rupture and mortality from cardiac complications, including left ventricular hypertrophy and coronary artery disease.

B. PAIN—ADPKD patients commonly suffer from episodes of acute or chronic flank pains, most commonly secondary to intracystic hemorrhage, nephrolithiasis, or urinary tract infections. In some cases, massively enlarged kidneys may be the primary cause of mechanical lower back pain. Occasionally, patients with enlarged kidneys may develop chronic flank pain without an identifiable etiology. These individuals are at risk for narcotic and/or analgesic dependence and medication-related complications.

C. HEMATURIA, CYST HEMORRHAGE, AND RETROPERITONEAL HEMORRHAGE—Gross hematuria can occur in more than 40% of patients with ADPKD and may be the initial presenting symptom of the disease. Hematuria is more likely among individuals with larger kidneys, hypertension, and higher plasma creatinine concentrations, and may result from cyst hemorrhage, nephrolithiasis, infection, or renal tumors.

Cyst hemorrhage is generally self-limited and resolves within 2–7 days with conservative therapy (bedrest, hydration, and analgesics). Nephrolithiasis-induced hematuria is usually microscopic and resolves with passage or removal of the stone. First episodes or recurring hematuria in patients older than 50 years should be always investigated to rule out renal cell carcinoma. Occasionally, hemorrhagic cysts can rupture into the retroperitoneum causing severe retroperitoneal bleeding, which is associated with increased mortality rates.

D. URINARY CONCENTRATION DEFECT—Impaired urinary concentrating ability and mild polyuria are the most common and earliest manifestations of ADPKD. Renal concentrating defects correlate with the severity of cystic-induced anatomical deformities, but are independent of age and glomerular filtration rate (GFR). Changes in urinary concentration may not be clinically evident and are generally well compensated by adequate fluid intake. The mechanisms responsible for these changes remain to be elucidated, but tubular injury, defects in principal cell function, and early tubulointerstitial disease may be important contributing factors. This concentration defect in PKD is unique because it occurs despite elevated circulating levels of vasopressin, renal cAMP, and renal over expression of vasopressin V2 receptor and aquaporin 2. Some studies have suggested that elevated serum concentration of vasopressin may contribute to cystogenesis. More recently, plasma copeptin concentrations (marker of endogenous vasopressin levels) have been associated with disease severity.

E. NEPHROLITHIASIS—Nephrolithiasis occurs in approximately 20% of ADPKD patients, and should be suspected in any ADPKD patient with acute flank pain. Unlike idiopathic stone formers that present nearly always with calcium oxalate stones, more than 50% of stones observed in ADPKD patients are composed of uric acid and most of the remainders of calcium oxalate. Increased renal volume is an important contributing factor for nephrolithiasis in patients with ADPKD. In addition, low urinary volume, urinary stasis (due to distorted renal architecture), hyperuricosuria, hypercalciuria, hypocitraturia, and low urinary pH (promoting uric acid stone formation) may predispose to stone disease in these patients. Signs and symptoms of nephrolithiasis in ADPKD do not differ from those observed in non-ADPKD stone patients.

F. Urinary tract or cyst infections—Whether urinary tract infections occur more frequently in ADPKD patients is unclear, but between 30% and 50% of ADPKD patients experience some form of kidney infection during their lifetime, including cystitis, pyelonephritis, renal cyst infection, and perinephric abscesses. Importantly, the risk of complicated infections is significantly increased in ADPKD patients. Urinary tract or cyst Infections occur more frequently in women, and are primarily caused by *Escherichia coli, Klebsiella, Proteus,* and other *Enterobacteriaceae*. Patients may experience urinary frequency and urgency (cystitis), as well as fever, chills, nausea, vomiting, or flank pain (pyelonephritis, renal cyst infection, or perinephric abscesses).

G. Renal failure—ADPKD rarely progresses to ESRD in early childhood, but most commonly leads to renal failure in middle age or later in life. Patients with mutations in the *PKD1* gene have 20-year earlier onset of ESRD compared to those with mutations in *PKD2*. Once the renal clearance starts to decline, it decreases at an approximate rate of 5.0–6.4 mL/min/year. Enlarged kidneys and increased TKV are the most important risk factors for progression to ESRD. Patients with mutations located in the first half of the *PKD1* gene (5′region) are associated with a slightly earlier onset of renal failure compared to those with mutations in the second half of the gene (3′region). Other risk factors for developing kidney failure in ADPKD include male gender, episodes of proteinuria, sickle cell trait, diagnosis of ADPKD before age 30 years, first episode of gross hematuria before age 30 years, hyperlipidemia, low high-density lipoprotein (HDL), cigarette smoking, and early development of HTN (before age 35 years).

Signs and symptoms of renal dysfunction in ADPKD are noticeable when GFR is reduced to <30–40 mL/min/1.73 m², and are undistinguishable from those of non-ADPKD individuals with chronic renal failure.

2. Extrarenal manifestations

A. Polycystic liver disease—Polycystic liver disease (PLD) is the most common extrarenal manifestation of ADPKD, with cysts that become larger and more numerous as patients age. PLD is associated with both *PKD1* and *PKD2* genotypes, but also may occur as a genetically distinct disease (ADPLD), with two genes identified (*PRKCSH* in chromosome 19 and *Sec63* in chromosome 6). The occurrence of PLD in ADPKD increases with age from 0% in ADPKD children to 20% in the third decade and over 75% in the seventh decade of life. PLD tend to have an earlier onset and worse prognosis in women, particularly those with multiple pregnancies and/or on oral contraceptive or on estrogen replacement therapy. Cysts in the liver originate from small clusters of intralobular bile ductules surrounded by fibrous tissue, known as biliary microhamartomas, and from peribiliary glands.

Most PLD patients are asymptomatic and does not cause liver failure. However, some patients may present with symptoms that result from either mass effect (dyspnea, orthopnea, early satiety, gastroesophageal reflux, mechanical back pain, uterine prolapse, rib fracture, and, in severe cases, failure to thrive) or cyst-related complications, including cyst hemorrhage, rupture, or infection. Hepatic cyst hemorrhage and ruptures can present as acute abdominal pain, extrinsic bile duct compression, and liver enzyme elevation. Rarely, cysts can rupture into the peritoneum and cause acute ascites and life-threatening hemoperitoneum. In rare cases, a massively enlarged cystic liver can cause obstructions to the hepatic venous outflow tract, portal vein and/or bile duct, or the inferior vena cava, leading to portal hypertension, esophageal and/or gastric varices, ascites, and, rarely, obstructive jaundice. PLD patients with hepatic cyst infection may present with fever, chills, localized upper abdominal pain, leukocytosis, and elevation of alkaline phosphatase, frequently associated with bacteremia (Enterobacteriaceae).

B. Intracranial aneurysms and other vascular manifestations—Intracranial aneurysms (ICAs) are the most serious potential complication of ADPKD, as ICAs can rupture causing subarachnoid hemorrhage (SAH) leading to irreversible brain damage or death. The incidence of ICAs and ICA ruptures in ADPKD is increased by 5- to 10-fold compared to that in the general population. The prevalence of ICAs is 21% if someone else in the patient's family has had an ICA or SAH compared to 6% in those without such history.

ADPKD-associated ICAs may result from altered expression and/or function of the PKD gene in arterial smooth muscle cells.

Most ADPKD-associated ICAs are small (<7 mm in diameter) and approximately 90% of them are located in the anterior circulation. MR angiography (MRA) is the diagnostic imaging modality of choice. Widespread presymptomatic screening is not indicated as the risk of rupture of asymptomatic IA is comparable to that of the general population (0.05% per year for IA smaller than 10 mm). Screening is indicated in patients with previous rupture of an IA, patients with family history of IA or SAH, preparation for major surgery with potential hemodynamic instability, or high-risk occupations such as airplane pilots. If the screening MRA is negative, the recommendation is to rescreen patients with good life expectancy at 5-year intervals.

Aneurysm rupture depends on the size and location of the ICAs and whether the patient has a prior episode(s) of SAH. The yearly risk of rupture is less than 0.1% for those smaller than 7 mm in diameter, located in the anterior circulation, and in patients without a prior SAH. However, the risk is higher for ICAs larger than 7 mm in diameter, or in the posterior circulation, or in patients with a prior episode of SAH.

Most ADPKD patients with unruptured ICAs remain asymptomatic, yet focal neurologic symptoms such as cranial nerve palsy or seizure due to local compression may occur. Contrarily, ruptured ICAs present with prominent symptoms including episodes of acute onset of severe headache that often radiates to the occipital and cervical region, commonly associated with nausea and vomiting. Nuchal rigidity, photophobia, cranial nerve palsy, seizure, lethargy, and coma may be associated with the pain.

In addition of ICAs, other vascular manifestations including thoracic aortic and cervicocephalic arterial dissections, intracranial arterial dolichoectasia, coronary artery aneurysms, and central retinal vascular occlusions have also be seen (an approximately 10-fold increase) in association with ADPKD. Sign and symptoms and signs of these vascular complications are similar to those seen in non-ADPKD patients.

c. Valvular heart disease—Valvular heart abnormalities occur more frequently in ADPKD patients than in the general population, and can be detected by echocardiography in up to 25–30% of patients with ADPKD. Mild mitral valve prolapse and aortic regurgitation are the most common abnormalities seen in ADPKD patients. Less frequent valvular abnormalities include mitral insufficiency, tricuspid insufficiency, tricuspid prolapse, and aortic insufficiency often associated with aortic root dilation. Asymptomatic pericardial effusions may also occur in these patients.

The mechanisms underlying valvular heart disease in ADPKD may involve abnormalities in collagen and/or extracellular matrix. Most patients are asymptomatic, but episodic palpitations, and in rare cases, congestive heart failure may occur. Patients with audible cardiac murmurs or those with signs or symptoms of cardiac dysfunction should be always screened with echocardiography. Audible cardiac murmurs also warrants antibiotic prophylaxis against subacute bacterial endocarditis.

d. Renal cell carcinoma—It is unclear whether the overall risk of cancer is increased among patients with ADPKD. However, in ADPKD patients, RCC may present at an earlier age with frequent constitutional symptoms and a higher proportion of sarcomatoid, bilateral, multicentric, and metastatic tumors. Male and female ADPKD patients are equally likely to develop RCC. A solid mass on US, speckled calcifications on CT and contrast enhancement, and tumor thrombus and regional lymphadenopathies on CT or MRI should raise the suspicion of RCC. Because of the multiple cysts, some necrotic or cystic RCC can be difficult to detect.

B. Laboratory Findings

1. Renal pathology—Macroscopically, ADPKD is characterized by numerous spherical cysts varying in size equally distributed in cortical and medullary regions. Although enlarged kidneys generally retain their form, tubules are significantly distorted.

Substantial microscopic abnormalities are evident in patients with ADPKD and mild renal insufficiency, including interstitial fibrosis, inflammatory cell infiltration, tubular epithelial hyperplasia, flat nonpolypoid or polypoid hyperplasia, microscopic adenoma, and advanced sclerosis of preglomerular vessels.

2. Liver pathology—Macroscopically, PLD is characterized by cysts which vary in size from pinpoint to extra-large, and tend to cluster and spare segments of the remaining hepatic parenchyma.

Microscopically, cyst walls are thin and lined with a single layer of flattened or cuboidal cells of biliary origin. Biliary microhamartomas are commonly seen, associated with cysts on serial sections. Importantly, cysts derived from peribiliary glands may compress biliary ducts.

3. Urinary abnormalities—Reduction in maximal urine concentration, hypocitraturia, low urinary pH, hematuria, and mild to moderate proteinuria may be seen in patients with ADPKD.

C. Imaging Studies

Although a renal ultrasound (US) is recommended as the first diagnostic test and may reveal multiple cysts on both kidneys, it provides limited anatomic definition. In contrast, both magnetic resonance imaging (MRI) and contrast-enhanced computer tomography (CT) can accurately assess renal and cyst volume, and evaluate the preserved renal parenchyma. Additionally, CT without and with intravenous contrast possesses enough sensitivity for detecting and localizing renal stones and hemorrhages (Figure 45–1). CT and MRI can detect renal neoplasms with similar sensitivity, yet the latter is often preferred because intravenous contrast used in CT may induce nephrotoxicity.

Cysts may also be seen in the liver. Imaging studies such as abdominal CT or MRI are helpful in the diagnosis of cyst infection but have low specificity. Imaging findings associated with cyst infection include: fluid-debris levels within cysts, cyst wall thickening, intracystic gas bubbles, and heterogeneous or increased density. [18F]-fluorodeoxyglucose (FDG)

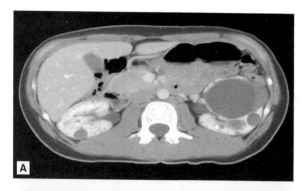

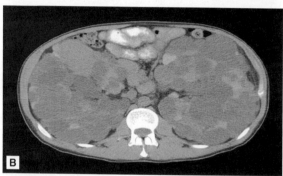

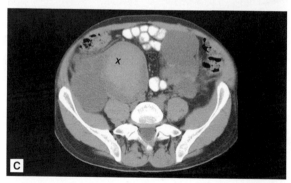

▲ **Figure 45–1.** Autosomal dominant polycystic kidney disease. **A.** Contrast-enhanced CT scan in a 26-year-old woman with early stage polycystic kidney disease. Note a dominant left renal cyst. **B.** Noncontrast CT scan in a 42-year-old male with advanced cystic disease and bilateral renal enlargement. Note innumerable renal cysts, many of which are hyperdense (hemorrhagic or with high protein content). **C.** The lower pole of the right kidney from the same patient in (B) contains a large cyst with increased and heterogeneous densities representing clots (marked by 'X') and recent hemorrhage.

positron emission tomography (PET) has become a promising agent for detection of infected cysts in the liver.

MR angiograms is considered the gold-standard methods for detecting ICAs in patients with ADPKD, with an estimated sensitivity of more than 90% for detecting aneurysms and more than or equal to 3 mm in diameters. Thin cut, noncontrast-CT is should be considered the initial test for detecting SAH, which is reflected as areas of increased density. When CT results are equivocal and clinical suspicion is high, lumbar puncture should be performed to confirm the diagnosis.

▶ **Differential Diagnosis**

In patients with atypical presentation, it should be always considered that several systemic diseases may be associated with renal cysts. Identification of extrarenal manifestations that are not typically associated with ADPKD is critical for reaching a correct diagnosis.

ADPKD must be distinguished from ARPKD and acquired cystic kidney disease (ACKD), multiple simple cysts, glomerulocystic kidney disease, tuberous sclerosis complex (TSC), and von Hippel–Lindau disease. Main distinct features that differentiate ADPKD from these conditions are outlined in Table 45–1.

▶ **Treatment**

Currently treatment options for patients with ADPKD are limited to management of renal and extra-renal complications. Patients should be advised to adopt a healthy life style. Risk factor modification, early detection and management of complications, as well as avoidance of potentially nephrotoxic agents are important steps in the management of ADPKD patients, which may limit morbidity and mortality rates.

A. Dietary Recommendations and Patient Education

Reduction in dietary sodium (<90 mEq/day), cholesterol (<200 mg/day), and protein (0.8 g/kg of ideal body weight/day) intake is recommended. Caffeine consumption should be limited, as it stimulates cAMP-mediated fluid secretion by the cyst-lining cells, promoting cyst growth. Smoking cessation is important, because it is associated with a faster decline of renal function and an increased risk of ICA rupture.

Early detection and treatment of ADPKD symptoms is associated with improved overall disease outcome. Therefore, patients should be informed about and vigilant in monitoring the occurrence of ADPKD-associated manifestations.

B. Hypertension

Antihypertensive therapy with angiotensin-converting enzyme (ACE) inhibitors or angiotensin II receptor blockers (ARBs) is recommended, as they are well tolerated and efficacious.

Table 45–1. Distinguishing features of autosomal dominant polycystic kidney disease.

Disease	Inheritance	Extrarenal Characteristics	Renal Manifestations
ADPKD	AD	Early adult onset of HTN; flank pain; gross hematuria; polycystic liver enlargement; SAH	Urine concentration defect; bilateral cystic renal enlargement; cysts arise from cortex and medullar; nephrolithiasis; renal failure with cystic disease progression
ARPKD	AR	Infantile "Potter's phenotype"; infantile HTN; portal hypertension: esophageal and gastric varices; hypersplenism	Large kidneys; bilateral fusiform collecting duct dilation; urine concentration defect; chronic renal failure
ACKD	Not inherited	Longstanding renal failure; risk of renal cancer	Normal sized or small kidneys; cysts arise from cortex; cyst wall calcification, papillary cystadenomas and renal cancer
Glomerulocystic kidney disease	AD (some)	Heterogeneous group of diseases	Cysts arise from the Bowman's capsules
Simple renal cysts	Not inherited	Associated with aging	Identified incidentally
Tuberous sclerosis complex (TSC)	AD	Prominent skin lesions; CNS: Giant cell astrocytomas and cortical tubers; cardiac rhabdomyomas; pulmonary lymphangioleiomyomatosis	Cysts; renal angiomyolipomas; renal carcinomas (rare)
von Hippel–Lindau disease (VHL)	AD	No skin lesion; retinal and CNS hemangioblastomas; pheochromocytomas; pancreatic cysts	Cysts; renal cell carcinomas (common)
Orofacial syndrome type 1	X-linked dominant	Cleft tongue and palate; broad nasal root; digital abnormalities	Cysts (may resemble ADPKD)
Medullary cystic disease	AD	Hyperuricemia	Adult onset of renal failure
Nephronophthisis	AR	Retinal degeneration (retinitis pigmentosa)	Childhood or adolescent onset of renal failure
Medullary spongy disease	Usually not familial		Papillary calcifications and renal stones; normal glomerular filtration rate

AD, autosomal dominant; ADPKD, autosomal dominant polycystic kidney disease; AR, autosomal recessive; ARPKD, autosomal recessive polycystic kidney disease; CNS, central nervous system; HTN, hypertension; SAH, subarachnoid hemorrhage.

The HALT-PKD was a clinical trial designed to evaluate whether there was a difference in the progression, or in slowing down the decline of renal function between those given dual angiotensin converting enzyme inhibitor (ACEI) and ARB therapy versus an ACEI alone, in patients with GFR more than 60 mL/min/1.73 m^2 (study A), and in patients with GFR 25–60 mL/min/1.73 m^2 (study B) respectively. In HALT-A, the study further investigated the effect of medicating to a standard (120–130/70–80 mm Hg) versus low (95–110/60–75 mm Hg) target blood pressure on renal function over time. The results from the HALT study indicated that dual blockade (Lisinopril–Telmisartan), although safe, did not show a benefit, as compared with Lisinopril alone, with regard to the change in TKV or estimated GFR. Study A showed that lowering blood pressure to levels below those recommended by current guidelines reduced the rate of increase in kidney volume by 14%, the increase in renal vascular resistance, urine albumin excretion, left ventricular mass index, and, marginally (after the first 4 months of treatment), the rate of decline in eGFR. The overall effect of low blood pressure on eGFR, however, was not statistically significant, possibly because the reduction of blood pressure to low levels was associated with an acute reduction in eGFR within the first 4 months of treatment.

C. Flank Pain

Pain management for patients with ADPKD includes non-pharmacologic therapy and physical measures. Non-opioid agents are the preferred treatment options for ADPKD patients with pain. Narcotic analgesics should be reserved for managing patients with acute and severe episodes of pain. It is important to identify treatable underlying etiologies, such as infection, renal stone, or tumors. Long-term use of potentially nephrotoxic analgesics, as well as combinations of analgesics or nonsteroidal anti-inflammatory drugs should be avoided.

Tricyclic antidepressants should be used in ADPKD patients with significant chronic pain after ruling out correctable causes. Adjunctive therapy with splanchnic nerve blockade with local anesthetics or steroids may provide prolonged pain relief. Cyst decompression should be considered when conservative measures fail, whereas cyst aspiration followed by sclerosis and surgical or laparoscopic decompression may be considered.

Alternatively, cyst aspiration followed by CT-guided alcohol sclerosis can be performed in ADPKD patients with few dominant cysts deemed to cause pain. Microscopic hematuria, localized pain, and transient fever may be minor complications of this procedure, whereas severe complications, which occur mainly after aspiration of centrally located cysts, include pneumothorax, perirenal hematoma, arteriovenous fistula, urinoma, and infections.

Patients with multiple cysts contributing to pain may be benefitted from laparoscopic or surgical cyst fenestration, which are successful in 80–90% at 1 year post-procedure and achieve sustained pain relief for 2 years or longer in 60–80% of cases. Laparoscopic or retroperitoneoscopic procedures are good alternatives with shorter and less complicated recovery that open surgical interventions.

Lastly, laparoscopic renal denervation combined with cyst fenestration, laparoscopic or retroperitoneal nephrectomy, and embolization of the renal artery may be performed in patients with end-stage renal failure.

D. Cyst Hemorrhage

Most episodes of cyst hemorrhages are self-limited and respond well to conservative therapy such as bed resting, analgesics, and adequate fluid intake. These management strategies play an important role in preventing the formation of obstructing urinary blood clots. Less frequently, bleeding episodes may be more severe favoring formation of subcapsular or retroperitoneal hematoma, which is commonly associated with decreased hemoglobin concentration and hemodynamic instability. In these patients, hospitalization is warranted, followed by CT or angiography, volume resuscitation with transfusion, and/or arterial embolization or surgery if refractory bleeding occurs.

E. Urinary Tract and Renal Parenchymal/ Cyst Infection

Symptomatic urethritis or cystitis should be immediately treated with oral antimicrobials to prevent retrograde seeding to renal parenchyma and/or cysts. Highly lipophilic antimicrobials, including trimethoprim-sulfamethoxazole, fluoroquinolones, or chloramphenicol are the preferred options to treats these patients. Blood and urine cultures should guide the selection of the correct antimicrobial agent. Parenteral therapy may be needed in acute episodes of parenchymal or cyst infection, whereas percutaneous or surgical drainage should be considered if cyst infection persists after 1–2 weeks of therapy. Recurrent fever after antibiotic treatment warrants reevaluation to rule out complications such as obstruction, perinephritic abscess, or renal stones. Antibiotic therapy may be prolonged for several months to eradicate the infection when complications are ruled out.

F. Nephrolithiasis

Management of nephrolithiasis in patients with ADPKD does not differ from management of idiopathic renal stone patients. Potassium citrate targets the three main etiologies of nephrolithiasis in ADPKD: uric acid lithiasis, hypocitraturic calcium oxalate lithiasis, and distal acidification defects. Acute stone attacks, should be treated with parenteral fluids, analgesics, and, lithotripsy or urologic procedures if indicated.

G. Renal Failure

1. Dialysis—Dialysis is generally well tolerated by patients with ADPKD, partly due to their higher production of endogenous erythropoietin and blood hemoglobin concentration. Rarely, complications may occur. For example, episodes of intradialytic hypotension may appear in ADPKD patients undergoing dialysis due to inferior vena cava compression due to medially located right renal cysts or hepatic cysts. However, this condition can be effectively managed by cyst aspiration or resection.

Peritoneal dialysis is also well tolerated in patients with ADPKD, despite the increased risk of inguinal and umbilical hernias.

2. Transplantation—Renal transplantation is the preferred treatment for patients with ADPKD that reached ESRD. Post-transplant patient and graft survival are similar between ADPKD and non-ADPKD patients. Transplantation and post-transplant immunosuppression do not affect ADPKD-related complications such as mitral valve prolapse, aortic aneurysmal rupture, and hepatic or renal cyst infection.

Cystic kidney nephrectomy is not routinely performed in ADPKD patients undergoing transplantation, because native kidneys contribute to the maintenance of postoperative hemoglobin concentration. Furthermore, in case of acute allograft failure, native kidneys may assist in fluid management. However, pretransplant nephrectomy is indicated in patients with history of cyst infection, frequent cyst hemorrhages, severe hypertension, or massive symptomatic renal enlargement.

3. Novel therapies —Advancements in understanding the pathophysiologic mechanisms responsible for the disease have provided a foundation for the development and testing of potential new therapies. Among them, vasopressin-2 receptor antagonist (Tolvaptan) has been the most successful pharmacological intervention at reducing the rate of TKV increase and renal function decline in patients with ADPKD. This drug is currently approved in Japan, Canada, the European Union, Switzerland, and South Korea for the treatment of patients with CKD stages 1–3 and rapidly progressive disease. Tolvaptan is not currently approved as a therapy for ADPKD in the United States. The somatostatin analogues Octreotide and lanreotide have shown a reduction in the average rate of TKV growth in the initial 6 or 12 months of treatment. Larger studies with somatostatin analogues are underway. mTOR inhibitors have been effective in slowing or arresting the progression of ADPKD in preclinical models, yet clinical trials in patients with ADPKD have been largely disappointing.

H. Polycystic Liver Disease

PLD is generally asymptomatic and does not require any treatment. Oral contraceptives and estrogen replacement therapy should be discontinued if the risk of cyst growth outweighs the benefit of estrogen therapy, because estrogens have the potential to contribute to cyst enlargement.

If cyst compression occurs, therapy should be directed toward reducing cyst and hepatic volume, including percutaneous cyst aspiration and sclerosis, laparoscopic fenestration, or surgical partial hepatectomy and fenestration. If cystic involvement is extensive, refractory to other treatment, and not resectable, liver transplantation should be considered.

Percutaneous aspiration should be performed to confirm the diagnosis of cyst infection, which should be treated with the combination of antibiotic therapy for at least 6 weeks and percutaneous cyst drainage. Trimethoprim-sulfamethoxazole and the fluoroquinolones have good cyst penetration and are effective against typical pathogens. Cyst-fluid culture may be used to guide the selection of the most adequate antimicrobial agent.

I. Intracranial Aneurysms

Surgical clipping or endovascular coiling are the preferred therapy for patients with ADPKD and ruptured or symptomatic ICAs. This condition is associated with high morbidity and mortality rates, so early recognition and urgent neurosurgical consultation are critical.

Treatment options for asymptomatic ICAs depend on the risk of rupture, and include observation with risk prevention and intervention such as surgical clipping or endovascular coiling.

ICAs under 7 mm in diameter located in the anterior circulation in patients without a history of aneurysmal rupture should be followed-up semiannually initially and then at less frequent intervals may be sufficient after demonstration of stability. Larger sized ICAs, and those located in the posterior circulation in patients with a prior history of SAH, should be treated. Treatment options depend on the patient's age, presence of comorbidities, local institutional experience, and expertise of care-providing physicians.

Presymptomatic ICA screening is usually not recommended for ADPKD patients without a family history of ICAs, but indicated for those with a family history of SAH, high risk occupation, prior to major elective surgeries with anticipated hemodynamic instability, and significant anxiety about ICAs.

AUTOSOMAL RECESSIVE POLYCYSTIC KIDNEY DISEASE

ESSENTIALS OF DIAGNOSIS

▸ Recessive pattern of transmission; parental consanguinity.

▸ Presentations for the neonatal period and infancy: Oligohydramnios, Potter's phenotype, pulmonary hypoplasia, and large echogenic kidneys with poor corticomedullary differentiation.

▸ Presentations for older children and adolescents: Portal fibrosis and increased hepatic echogenicity, hepatosplenomegaly, dilated intrahepatic ducts, and medullary sponge kidney (MSK) and renal cysts.

▸ General Considerations

ARPKD is a severe, recessively inherited disease caused by mutations of the *PKHD1* gene, with an estimated incidence of 1 in 20,000 live births. ARPKD affects all ethnic groups and is an important cause of perinatal morbidity and mortality. Indeed, 30% of these patients will not survive beyond infancy, and 20–45% of neonatal survivors will progress to ESRD by age 15–20 years.

Unlike ADPKD, ARPKD is presented with abnormalities confined mainly to the kidneys and biliary tract. Most patients are identified either in utero or at birth and present with a critical degree of respiratory distress due both to pulmonary hypoplasia (Potter's phenotype) from oligohydramnios and to a restricted diaphragmatic movement due to massively enlarged kidneys (Figure 45–2). A subset of patients present with late-onset ARPKD (later in childhood or adolescence) and less prominent symptoms with significant periportal fibrosis and portal hypertension, despite less severe renal involvement.

Diagnosis of ARPKD in the perinatal period is generally made by US at 20 weeks of gestation, yet some ARPKD kidneys may not show any US abnormalities until the third trimester. Therefore, normal renal US in the second or early third trimester cannot rule out the diagnosis of ARPKD. Mutation analysis is currently available.

▶ Clinical Findings

A. Symptoms and Signs

1. Neonatal and infancy—Potter's phenotype (Pulmonary hypoplasia leading to pulmonary insufficiency; specific facial characteristics including widely set eyes, a prominent inner canthus, a beaked nose, and large low-lying ears; and spine and limb contractures) is a frequent presentation in ARPKD infants. In this group of patients, morbidity and mortality are primarily due to respiratory distress and pulmonary insufficiency. Kidneys are generally enlarged and palpable, and renal function is impaired in the majority of these patients. Polyuria and renal tubular defects can be prominent, leading to dehydration, volume depletion, and metabolic acidosis, especially in patients suffering from infections or diarrhea.

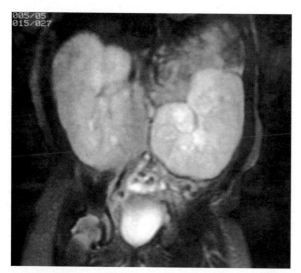

▲ **Figure 45–2.** Autosomal dominant polycystic kidney disease. Coronal T2-weighted MRI of a 1-year-old ARPKD patient. The kidneys are massively enlarged with a lobular, reniform contour.

The majority of ARPKD patients present with hypertension, which may be severe.

2. Childhood and adolescence—Biliary dysgenesis due to insufficient remodeling of the primitive intrahepatic biliary system (ductal plate), are the most common manifestations of ARPKD in childhood and adolescence, which frequently lead to congenital hepatic fibrosis and intrahepatic bile duct dilation (Caroli disease). However, hepatocytes remain unaltered. Esophageal and/or gastric varices and variceal bleeding (portal hypertension) and cytopenia (hypersplenism) may be seen.

Although renal disease may be mild, papillary collecting duct ectasia and renal cysts may be incidentally detected, and some ARPKD patients may develop chronic renal insufficiency.

3. Cholangitis—In patients with significant intrahepatic bile duct dilation, ascending cholangitis may occur at any age, which is generally presented with fever, right upper quadrant abdominal pain, leukocytosis, liver enzyme elevation, and gram-negative bacterial sepsis.

4. End-stage renal failure—ARPKD patients with ESRD commonly present with growth failure, anemia, and osteodystrophy.

B. Laboratory Findings

1. Renal pathology—Macroscopically, ARPKD kidneys from an infant or a young child are enlarged with a reniform configuration, and small cysts (1–2 mm) on the renal capsular surface.

Microscopically, kidneys are characterized by significant collecting duct ectasia, with fusiform ducts, coursing radially through the cortex, and remaining connected to the tubular system. The corticomedullary junction is not clearly demarcated.

Kidneys shrink with age, whereas both cysts and interstitial fibrosis become more prominent, which make these kidneys similar to those observed in ADPKD.

2. Hepatic pathology and functional studies—Macroscopically, the size of the liver is preserved or slightly enlarged. Biliary dilation and portal fibrosis are present, and progress with increasing age. However, liver synthetic functions (serum transaminase and albumin levels) are sustained.

C. Imaging Studies

Bilateral symmetric enlargement of the kidneys with increased echogenicity and loss of corticomedullary differentiation are common characteristic features observed in US from ARPKD patients. Tubular microcysts (2–5 mm in diameter) are also frequent. With age, kidneys shrink, but increase in echogenicity. Macrocysts (>1 cm in diameter) may be seen. These features are indistinguishable from those of observed in ADPKD kidneys. US may also assist in determining the degree of hepatobiliary involvement. In patients who progress to periportal fibrosis, the hepatic echotexture becomes coarse, associated with biliary dilation with thickened ductal walls.

The extent of hepatic and renal disease can be accurately defined by CT, yet their value is limited by the need for intravenous contrast, which may impair renal function. Under these circumstances, MRI may be helpful to evaluate kidney and cyst size, as well as the number and extent of biliary abnormalities.

▶ Differential Diagnosis

Differential diagnoses for ARPKD include childhood-onset ADPKD, glomerulocystic kidney disease, and nephronophthisis. Table 45–1 summarizes features that might help to differentiate ARPKD from other cystic renal diseases. In addition, ARPKD should be differentiated from syndromic congenital disorders such as Meckel–Gruber syndrome, Bardet–Biedl syndrome, or asphyxiating thoracic dystrophy, which present with renal abnormalities and hepatic fibrosis. Yet, these disorders can be easily differentiated because, unlike ARPKD, they are associated with other multiple congenital defects.

▶ Treatment

A multidisciplinary team of intensivists, nephrologists, gastroenterologists, specialized nurses, dietitians, social workers, and sometimes psychiatrists is recommended for the care of neonates and children with ARPKD. These specialists can also provide to support the patient's family, alleviating psychosocial stress.

A. Pulmonary Hypoplasia

Aggressive respiratory support is a critical step in the management of these patients. In ARPKD patients with severe or refractory disease, mechanical ventilation, and/or nephrectomy (to make room for ventilation) might be indicated.

B. Hypertension

Antihypertensive therapy with ACEIs and ARBs has been shown to be effective in reducing blood pressure levels in ARPKD patients. Additional therapy with α/β-blockers, calcium channel blockers, or diuretics may be indicated, depending on the clinical situation.

C. Polyuria Due to Concentration Defect

Dehydration (due to urine concentration defects) is frequent in patients with ARPKD, especially during episodes of acute febrile illness, which can be prevented by the administration of maintenance fluids.

D. End-Stage Renal Failure

Both hemotoneal and peritoneal dialysis have been successfully performed for ARPKD patients with ESRD. Renal transplant is the preferred approach, as it successfully improves survival and prevents complications such as growth retardation and osteodystrophy. ARPKD patients with massively enlarged kidneys may be benefitted from nephrectomy, whereas splenectomy may be indicated in severe cases of hypersplenism with leukocytopenia and thrombocytopenia.

E. Complications of Hepatic Fibrosis and Portal Hypertension

The degree of hepatosplenomegaly and varices should be periodically monitored by abdominal ultrasound and upper endoscopy. Bacterial cholangitis is a serious condition that should be promptly diagnosed and treated with appropriate antimicrobials. β-blockers or endoscopic variceal sclerosis or banding are useful to prevent acute variceal bleeding episodes. Additionally, portosystemic shunting may also be helpful for selected cases. Living-donor liver transplant is indicated in patients suffering from severe hepatic complications.

TUBEROUS SCLEROSIS COMPLEX

ESSENTIALS OF DIAGNOSIS

▶ Multiple cortical tubers on MRI (>2 needed for diagnosis).

▶ Radial migrating lines on head MRI (>3 needed for diagnosis).

▶ Subependymal nodules or giant cell astrocytomas (>2 needed for diagnosis).

▶ Astrocytic retinal hamartomas (>2 needed for diagnosis).

▶ Facial angiofibromas or fibrous forehead plaques (>2 needed for diagnosis).

▶ Ungual fibroma (>2 needed for diagnosis).

▶ Cardiac rhabdomyomas (fetus, infant, or child).

▶ Multiple renal cysts and angiomyolipomas or renal cell carcinoma.

▶ See Table 45–2 for diagnostic criteria.

▶ General Considerations

TSC is a multisystem disorder inherited in an autosomal dominant manner that affects 1 in 6000 individuals. TSC results from mutations in either *TSC1* (chromosomal 9) or *TSC2* (chromosomal 16) genes. De novo mutations (of which ~60% are *TSC2* mutations) account for ~60% of all

Table 45–2. Features of tuberous sclerosis complex and diagnostic criteria.

Major features

Facial angiofibromas or forehead plaques

Nontraumatic ungual or periungual fibroma

Hypomelanotic macules (more than three)

Shagreen patch (connective tissue nevus)

Multiple retinal nodular hamartomas

Cortical tuber

Subependymal nodule

Subependymal giant cell astrocytoma

Cardiac rhabdomyoma, single or multiple

Lymphangiomyomatosis

Renal angiomyolipoma

Minor features

Multiple, randomly distributed pits in dental enamel

Hamartomatous rectal polyps

Bone cysts

Cerebral white matter radial migration lines

Gingival fibromas

Nonrenal hamartomas

Retinal achromic patch

"Confetti" skin lesions

Multiple renal cysts

Diagnostic criteria[1]

Definitive tuberous sclerosis complex (TSC): Either two major features or one major feature plus two minor features probable TSC: One major plus one minor feature possible TSC: Either one major feature or two or more minor features

[1]These diagnostic criteria were adopted at the Consensus Conference on TSC held in Annapolis, Maryland, on July 10, 1998, under the auspices of the National Tuberous Sclerosis Association.

Adapted with permission from Rodriguez Gomez M (editor). *Tuberous Sclerosis Complex*, 3rd ed. Oxford University Press. 1999.

TSC cases. The *TSC2* gene is located immediately adjacent to the *PKD1* gene on chromosome 16p13.3. Therefore, deletional mutations can disrupt both the genes leading to a *TSC2-PKD1* contiguous gene syndrome, characterized by the combination of a TSC phenotype and an early-onset, and severe PKD.

TSC genes are tumor suppressor genes, and their protein products, hamartin (*TSC1*) and tuberin (*TSC2*), form a complex that deactivates small G protein (Rheb) and mammalian target of rapamycin (mTOR)-mediated cell growth and cell cycle progression. Therefore, mutations in these genes lead to abnormal cell growth and proliferation, triggering the formation of hamartomas (angiomyolipomata) in multiple organ systems, and renal neoplasms.

Many patients with TSC have angiomyolipomata, benign tumors composed of a circumscribed group of dysplastic smooth muscle cells, fat, and blood vessels, which have a poor structural organization and propensity to multiply. Furthermore, TSC mutations increase propensity to benign and malignant renal tumors.

The most frequently involved organs by angiomyolipomata in TSC are the skin, brain, retina, heart, kidney, and lung. Spinal cord lesions are rarely present, and neither the peripheral nerves nor the skeletal muscles are involved. Unlike patients with *TSC1* mutations, those with mutations in the *TSC2* gene present with a more severe clinical phenotype. Central nervous system (CNS) complications are the primary cause of death in these patients, but in the adult TSC population, the leading causes of death are renal complications, such as uremia, retroperitoneal bleeding, and metastatic renal cancers.

Clinical criteria are the quickest and the most accurate and inexpensive method to diagnose TSC. Although genetic testing is available (Athena Diagnostics, Inc.), a 20% false-negative rate limits its clinical utility. Nevertheless, the test is indicated when clinical diagnosis is unclear or when parents of an affected child are making decisions in family planning.

▶ **Clinical Findings**

A. Symptoms and Signs

TSC clinical presentation varies with age (Figure 45–3). During the perinatal period, cortical tubers and intracardiac rhabdomyomas may be detected by imaging studies (CT or MRI). Intracardiac rhabdomyomas generally reach their maximal size at birth, but regress in the postnatal years. These cardiac tumors can cause cardiac outflow tract obstruction.

Additionally, cutaneous hypomelanotic macules, facial angiofibromas (facial forehead plaques), arrhythmia due to Wolff–Parkinson–White (WPW) syndrome, and renal cysts may occur either in the perinatal or neonatal period.

Subependymal nodules may appear in early childhood, reaching their peak rate of growth at puberty, but regressing by the age of 30 years. These nodules may evolve into subependymal giant cell astrocytomas.

Seizure, regression of social-adaptive behavior, and mental retardation usually associated with seizure activity in infancy can be evident during childhood.

Retinal hamartomas may also appear during early childhood. These tumors have limited growth potential, and frequently become calcified, remaining asymptomatic.

Approximately 80% of children with TSC may present with facial angiofibromas (also known as adenoma sebaceum), shagreen patches, and ungual fibromas. Enamel pits, gingival fibromas, retinal achromic patches, confetti skin lesions, and hamartomatous rectal polyps may be also evident.

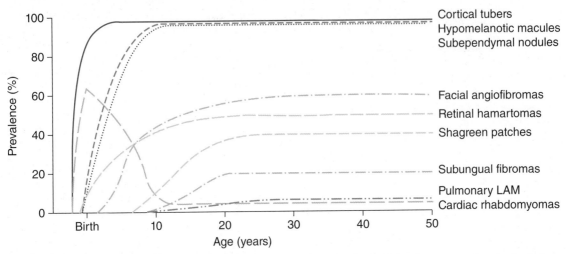

▲ **Figure 45–3.** Autosomal dominant polycystic kidney disease. Estimated age of development and age-adjusted prevalence of the main extrarenal manifestations of the tuberous sclerosis complex. LAM, lymphangioleiomyomatosis. (Reproduced with permission from Torres VE et al: Update on tuberous sclerosis complex. In: *Rare Kidney Diseases.* Schieppati A (editor). S. Karger AG, 2001.)

Pulmonary lymphangioleiomyomas (LAMs), which occur exclusively in women (up to 40%), can cause pneumothorax or chylothorax, hypoxia, and respiratory failure.

Table 45–3 summarizes the renal manifestations of TSC (angiomyolipomata, epithelioid angiomyolipomata, cysts, epithelial cell neoplasms, interstitial fibrosis associated with focal segmental glomerulosclerosis, and a variety of other lesions).

Angiomyolipomata are asymptomatic and usually accidentally diagnosed renal tumors of benign origin. These bilateral and multicentric renal tumors grow slowly and tend to be larger and more numerous in women, a predilection that might be related to the expression of estrogen and progesterone receptors on the tumor cells. Angiomyolipomata presents with hemorrhage and abdominal or flank mass and

Table 45–3. Renal manifestations of tubulosclerosis complex.

Angiomyolipomas

Cysts

Epithelioid angiomyolipomas

Renal cell carcinomas

Renal oncocytomas

Focal segmental glomerulosclerosis with interstitial fibrosis

Glomerular microhamartomas

Lymphangiomatous cysts

Rare associations (renal artery stenosis, ureteropelvic junction obstruction, nephrocalcinosis)

tenderness. Hemorrhagic episodes are sudden, painful, and life-threatening events. Hypertension, renal insufficiency, and fever of unknown origin may occur. Generally, tumors with diameters of greater than 4 cm tend present with symptoms.

Epithelioid angiomyolipomata are a variant of angiomyolipomata, characterized by non-fat-containing tumors composed of aberrant vascular smooth muscle cells bearing an epithelioid and aggressive phenotype with malignant potential. However, the natural history and clinical presentation of epithelioid angiomyolipomata have not been fully elucidated.

TSC may be also associated with epithelial neoplasms, including benign papillary adenomas and oncocytomas, as well as malignant clear cell, papillary or chromophobe carcinomas. Their clinical presentations do not differ from those of sporadic renal tumors, with the exception that TSC-associated tumors are prone to be multicentric and bilateral. Rapid growth of tumors and lack of a fat component on surveillance imaging may raise suspicion of malignancy.

Lastly, TSC is commonly associated with multiple asymptomatic renal cysts. However, in patients with contiguous TSC2-PKD1 gene syndrome, cystic renal involvement can be extensive and indistinguishable from that of ADPKD. In these patients, hemorrhage, hematuria, hypertension, and renal failure may be present.

B. Laboratory Findings

1. Renal pathology—Common renal pathologic findings in TSC include coexisting angiomyolipomata (including their epithelioid variant), cysts, and benign or malignant neoplasms.

Angiomyolipomata are characterized by proliferative mixtures of blood vessel, smooth muscle, and fatty tissues. These tumors are multicentric, wedge-shaped cortical lesions with their bases facing the surface of the kidney, and when enlarging, may penetrate into the renal parenchyma or extend to the perirenal fat becoming exophytic. Epithelioid angiomyolipomata do not contain adipose tissues, and are mostly composed of epithelioid vascular smooth muscle cells with irregular nuclei and higher mitotic activity.

Cystic renal involvement can be extensive in patients with contiguous *TSC2-PKD1* gene syndrome. Renal cancers tend to be multifocal and possess aggressive sarcomatoid features.

Other pathologic changes that can be associated with TSC include interstitial fibrosis, focal segmental glomerulosclerosis, renal vascular dysplasia, and glomerular microhamartomas.

2. Urine study—Mild to moderate proteinuria may be present.

C. Imaging Studies

Renal cysts in patients with TSC are indistinguishable from simple cysts or ADPKD cysts on US, CT, or MRI. The coexistence of angiomyolipomata distinguishes TSC from other renal cystic diseases.

The presence of fat in the tumor (increased echogenicity on US, low attenuation on CT, and high signal intensity on T1-weighted MRI) is essential to achieve the diagnosis of angiomyolipomata.

In tumors with evidence of intratumoral calcification and no identifiable fatty tissue, renal cancer should be suspected, and surgical exploration indicated.

▶ Differential Diagnosis

Differential diagnosis of TSC include ADPKD, ARPKD, ACKD, multiple simple cysts, glomerulocystic kidney disease, and von Hippel-Lindau disease. Many features may help in separating TSC from these conditions, as listed in Table 45–1.

▶ Treatment

Current therapeutic approaches for TSC renal manifestations include observation, arterial embolization, and partial or total nephrectomy.

In patients with slowly growing angiomyolipomata of less than 4 cm in diameter, semiannual or annual observational follow-up may be sufficient. In contrast, patients with larger (>4 cm) or rapidly growing angiomyolipomata, may require renal-sparing tumor resection to prevent acute hemorrhage. A decision for nephrectomy should be carefully balanced against the loss of renal function and the negative impact on the patient's long-term care. Highly

vascular lesions or those with a high risk of intraoperative bleeding may require arterial embolization (to obliterate the regional blood supply) alone or followed by renal sparing tumor resection.

Angiomyolipomata- or cyst-induced acute hemorrhage requires treatment with supportive observation, arterial embolization, and, in refractory cases, partial or total nephrectomy.

The mTOR-inhibitor rapamycin is a potential pharmacologic approach to prevent tumor formation and growth.

For TSC patients with uremia secondary to renal function from multiple renal resections, replacement of renal tissue by tumors, or severe PKD, dialysis or renal transplant is indicated. Bilateral nephrectomy is generally indicated because of the risk of bleeding and renal cancer.

VON HIPPEL–LINDAU DISEASE

ESSENTIALS OF DIAGNOSIS

- ▶ In patients with a family history of von Hippel–Lindau (VHL) disease:
  - –Cerebellar hemangioblastomas.
  - –Retinal hemangioblastomas.
  - –Renal cysts and renal cell carcinoma.
  - –Pheochromocytomas.
- ▶ In patients without a family history of this disease:
  - –Retinal hemangioblastomas (≥2).
  - –Cerebellar hemangioblastomas (≥2).
  - –Single hemangioblastomas plus a visceral tumor.
- ▶ A diagnosis can be made with one of the above findings (the number needed for diagnosis is given in parentheses).

▶ General Considerations

Von Hippel–Lindau (VHL) disease is a rare genetic disorder inherited in an autosomal dominant pattern that affects all ethnic groups worldwide, with a prevalence of approximately 1 in 35,000 individuals. VHL is caused by mutations in the *VHL* gene located on chromosome 3p25. This tumor suppressor gene encodes for pVHL, a protein that binds to a several partner proteins (Elongin B, Elongin C, Cul2, and Rbx1) and forms a stable multiprotein complex. This complex regulates the degradation of hypoxia-inducible factor (HIF), an oxygen sensor protein that induces the expression of vascular endothelial growth factor (VEGF) and erythropoietin, promoting tumor formation.

Under adequate tissue oxygenation, via ubiquitinating HIF, the pVHL complex promotes HIF degradation and thus suppresses the production of HIF-dependent protein. In VHL disease, mutant pVHL fails to degrade HIF, causing an overproduction of HIF-dependent proteins and tumorigenesis. Furthermore, the pVHL complex possesses HIF-independent tumor suppressive functions. Therefore, mutations in the *VHL* gene always lead to tumor formation.

Based on its clinical presentations, the disease may be divided into two clinical phenotypes that are correlated with the types of VHL mutations: type 1 (low risk of pheochromocytoma) and type 2 (high risk of pheochromocytoma) diseases (see Table 45–4).

Type 1 VHL disease is characterized by hemangioblastoma, renal cell carcinoma, and a low occurrence of pheochromocytoma, which is associated primarily with truncating VHL mutations. Contrarily, type 2 VHL diseases, further classified into 2A, 2B, and 2C, is almost always associated with missense mutations. Importantly, each subtype is associated with specific variants of missense mutations and presentations. VHL type 2A is characterized by a low risk of renal cell carcinoma, 2B by a high risk of renal cell carcinoma, and 2C by a sole occurrence of pheochromocytoma without significant risk of hemangioblastoma or renal cell carcinoma.

Patients with VHL disease generally develop tumors in their second to fourth decades of life. Renal cell cancer is the leading cause of death, and occurs in approximately 70% of patients during their lives.

VHL is diagnosed by its clinical presentations, yet genetic testing is available (http://www.vhl.org/dna/index.php).

▶ Clinical Findings

A. Symptoms and Signs

The most frequent earliest manifestations of VHL disease are multiple retinal and CNS hemangioblastomas. Retinal hemangioblastomas have the potential to cause local hemorrhage, retinal detachment, and blindness. Therefore, a

careful ophthalmologic examination with pupillary dilation is indicated.

The cerebellum is the primary site for CNS hemangioblastomas, followed by the spinal cord and the brain stem. These tumors do not metastasize, but their space-occupying growth at multiple locations may be associated with devastating neurologic defects.

Renal cysts, hemangiomas, benign adenomas, and renal cell carcinomas are common renal manifestations of VHL disease.

The majority of these patients develop renal cysts, which are not extensive or overtly symptomatic. However, a small fraction of them are prominent and indistinguishable from those seen in ADPKD. Cyst hemorrhage, hematuria, hypertension, and renal dysfunction may occur. Importantly, renal cysts in VHL are precursor lesions of renal cell carcinomas.

Renal hemangiomas and benign adenomas are mostly asymptomatic and are generally identified during evaluation for other clinical manifestations of VHL. However, renal clear cell type carcinomas, are commonly preceded by the growth of premalignant renal cysts, tend to be multifocal and bilateral, and have a high rate of recurrence after resection(s).

Unlike sporadic renal carcinomas, VHL-associated renal cancers have a younger age of onset (40 versus 59 years) and lack male predominance. Tumors greater than 3 cm in diameter may invade renal veins and metastasize to distant organs, such as the adrenal gland, liver, lungs, CNS, and bone.

Clinical presentation of renal cancers in VHL disease does not differ from that of sporadic ones. However, surveillance by imaging studies should be routinely performed, because of the high rate of cancer occurrence and risk of mortality.

The adrenal gland (pheochromocytomas), pancreas (cysts, adenomas, and carcinomas), inner ear (endolymphatic sac tumor), epididymis (cysts and rare hemangiomas), and spleen (angiomas) may be involved.

Pheochromocytomas in VHL disease are commonly presented as those seen in sporadic ones. Arteriography or surgery can trigger hypertensive crises in these patients, so prior to undergoing these procedures, VHL patients should be screened to rule out pheochromocytomas.

B. Laboratory Findings

1. Pathology—Macroscopically, retinal and CNS tumors depend on their composition. Microscopically, these tumors consist in vessels lined with endothelial cells, stromal cells, and pericytes.

Numerous macroscopic and microscopic tumor foci surrounded by a fibrous pseudocapsule are commonly seen in VHL kidneys, which are composed of clear cells, and sometimes focal calcifications.

Table 45–4. Classification of von Hippel–Lindau disease.

Type 1	Hemangioblastoma Renal cell carcinoma
Type 2	Pheochromocytomas (common for type 2 von Hippel–Lindau disease) Plus 2A: Hemangioblastoma Renal cell carcinoma (low occurrence) 2B: Hemangioblastoma Renal cell carcinoma (high occurrence) 2C: Pheochromocytomas (only)

2. Other laboratory abnormalities—Erythrocytosis due to the production of erythropoietin by tumor cells and elevation of 24-hour urine metanephrine may be seen in patients with pheochromocytomas (type 2 VHL disease).

C. Imaging Studies

CT and MRI are the preferred imaging studies for VHL patients with cerebellar hemangioblastomas. CT reveals round and hypodense cystic nodules, intensely enhanced by intravenous contrast administration. On MRI, the cystic part of the tumors are sharply demarcated and mural nodules can clearly be detected as high signal intensity on T2-weighted images compared to that of the surrounding gray matter. The nodules typically enhance with gadolinium administration. CT or MRI is also the preferred choice for renal cancer screening and surveillance.

▶ Differential Diagnosis

VHL disease should be distinguished from ADPKD, multiple simple cysts, and TSC (Table 45–1).

▶ Treatment

A. Central Nervous System and Retinal Hemangioblastomas

In patients with VHL disease and cerebellar hemangioblastomas, surgical resection is commonly indicated, whereas radiotherapy may be performed for symptomatic lesions that are not amenable to surgery. Post-treatment annual follow-up is necessary. Cryocoagulation or photocoagulation is the preferred treatment for retinal hemangioblastomas.

B. Renal Carcinomas

In tumors less than 3 cm in diameter, which have a low risk of metastases and are relatively slow growing, semiannual or annual follow-up with serial imaging studies, CT or MRI, is recommended. For VHL patients with larger sized renal cell cancers (>3 cm in diameter), which have a higher risk for metastasis, surgical tumor resection is indicated. When possible, renal-sparing tumor resections should be tried to preserve the patient's quality of life and prevent or delay the renal replacement therapy. All accessible renal tumors and cysts should be removed at the time of surgery. Ongoing screening after initial resection and repeated resections are generally needed, because of predictable tumor recurrence.

Alternatively, image-guided percutaneous radiofrequency ablation or cryoablation can be performed in certain cases, such as preemptive treatment of small cancers and high operative risk conditions. These procedures are minimally invasive, associated with a very low rate of complication, and can be carried out repeatedly. However, absolute contraindications of these procedures include irreversible coagulopathy and active infection (eg, sepsis).

Humanized VEGF neutralizing antibody has been shown to delay the progression of metastatic renal cancers and may be a valuable alternative for these patients.

Renal replacement therapy (dialysis or renal transplant) is indicated in patients with ESRD secondary to bilateral nephrectomy.

NEPHRONOPHTHISIS AND MEDULLARY CYSTIC DISEASE

ESSENTIALS OF DIAGNOSIS

- ▶ Small kidneys with tubular atrophy and interstitial fibrosis.
- ▶ Renal cysts located in the corticomedullary junction.
- ▶ Chronic renal failure with minimal or low-grade proteinuria.

▶ General Considerations

Nephronophthisis and medullary cystic disease constitute a rare group of inherited cystic tubulointerstitial nephritis which shares some morphological and clinical features. Nephronophthisis and medullary cystic disease have nearly identical clinical and pathologic features; however, they are considered genetically separated entities. Nephronophthisis is inherited in an autosomal recessive manner, with mutations in at least 19 different genes having been identified. Mutations in *NPHP2/INV* have been associated with development of renal failure between birth and age 3 years (infantile NPHP) and mutations in *NPHP3* and other genes, cause renal failure in the first 30 years of life (juvenile NPHP). Retinitis pigmentosa (Senior–Loken syndrome) is more frequently associated with *NPHP5/IQCB1*, *NPHP6/CEP290*, and *NPHP8/RPGRIP1L* mutations, and more rarely with mutations in other *NPHP* genes. Oculomotor apraxia (Cogan syndrome) may be observed with *NPHP1* and *NPHP4* mutations.

Contrarily, Autosomal dominant tubulointerstitial kidney disease (ADTKD), also known as medullary cystic kidney disease (MCKD), is a new term that has been proposed for a group of diseases with an autosomal dominant pattern of inheritance, characterized by small to normal size kidneys, cysts primarily located at the corticomedullary junction, associated with irregular thickening of the tubular basement membrane, tubular atrophy, and interstitial fibrosis. ADTKD is caused by mutations in at least four genes: *MUC1* (chromosome 1q22) encoding mucin-1, *UMOD* (chromosome 16p12.3) encoding uromodulin, *HNF1β* (chromosome 17q12) encoding hepatocyte nuclear factor-1β, *REN* (chromosome 1q32.1) encoding renin.

Clinical Findings

A. Symptoms and Signs

The onset of nephronophthisis and medullary cystic disease is insidious. Patients present with polyuria and polydipsia due to urinary concentration defect that precede the decline of renal function. At the early stages of renal dysfunction, renal salt wasting prevents development of hypertension. However, whit a progressive decline in renal function, hypertension, anemia, and sequelae of uremia may appear. Nephronophthisis has a childhood or adolescent onset of end-stage renal failure, whereas in medullary cystic disease real failure occurs in adulthood.

Both diseases have different extrarenal clinical manifestations, as shown in Table 45–1. Patients with nephronophthisis develop retinitis pigmentosa (1 in 10 affected individuals) while a fraction of patients with medullary cystic disease develops hyperuricemia and gouty arthritis.

B. Laboratory Findings

1. Renal pathology—Kidneys are small with cysts of variable size located mostly at the corticomedullary junction. Microscopically, tubular atrophy, irregular thickening of the tubular basement membrane, and interstitial fibrosis are diffuse. Interstitial fibrosis is commonly associated with patchy infiltrations of inflammatory cells.

2. Urinary findings—Decreased maximal urine concentration, urine salt wasting, and bland urine sediment with a mild degree or absence of proteinuria may be seen.

C. Imaging Studies

Renal US reveals normal to small-sized echogenic kidneys with a smooth contour, and small corticomedullary cysts. CT or MRI scans show small kidneys, with cysts confined to the medulla and corticomedullary junction.

Treatment

There is no specific treatment available for renal dysfunction. Yet, water and electrolyte imbalance should be corrected. Medullary cystic disease-induced hyperuricemia or gout should be treated with allopurinol. Renal transplant is preferred to chronic dialysis for patients with ESRD. There is no treatment available for visual loss secondary to retinitis pigmentosa.

MEDULLARY SPONGE DISEASE

ESSENTIALS OF DIAGNOSIS

- ▸ Precalyceal tubular ectasia with a pathognomonic "paint brush appearance" on excretory urogram.
- ▸ Usually without a positive family history and with normal renal clearance.

General Considerations

Medullary sponge disease, also known as Lenarduzzi kidney or Cacchi and Ricci disease, is a benign congenital condition generally detected incidentally during evaluation of renal colic. It may be associated with several congenital abnormalities, such as hemihypertrophy, Beckwith–Wiedemann syndrome, or Ehlers–Danlos syndrome. Although most patients maintain normal renal function, renal failure may occur due to recurrent stone-induced obstructive uropathy.

Clinical Findings

A. Symptoms and Signs

Patients with medullary sponge disease remain asymptomatic, but some may present with nephrolithiasis, recurrent urinary tract infections, and microhematuria. Calcium oxalate or calcium phosphate stones are characteristics, but the mechanisms underlying stone formation remain unclear. Tubular dilation, urinary stasis, hypercalciuria, and hypocitraturia are potential risk factors.

B. Laboratory Findings

1. Renal pathology—Macroscopically, kidneys are of normal size with papillary deformity and calcifications. Microscopically, calcified ectatic or cystic dilations of the medullary collecting ducts are present.

2. Urinary abnormalities—Microscopic hematuria, high urine pH, hypercalciuria, and hypocitraturia are common urinary abnormalities in these patients.

C. Imaging Studies

Excretory urography in patients with medullary sponge disease shows linear striated densities in one or more papillae resembling a "paint brush," which is pathognomonic of this disease.

Differential Diagnosis

Table 45–1 lists features that could separate medullary sponge disease from other renal cystic diseases.

Treatment

Nephrolithiasis is treated as the one that occurs in sporadic renal stone patients. Antimicrobial therapy for a long period of time may be required to treat the urinary tract infections.

ACQUIRED CYSTIC KIDNEY DISEASE

ESSENTIALS OF DIAGNOSIS

- ▸ Four or more cysts in each kidney by ultrasonography or CT in patients with advanced chronic renal failure or in a uremic state.
- ▸ Absence of inherited cystic renal diseases.

General Considerations

ACKD is a condition frequently seen in patients with ESRD undergoing long-term dialysis, in which a noncystic kidney develops cysts. Patients do not need to be on dialysis to have ACKD. Cystic transformations in ACKD is partly attributable to the chronic uremic milieu. The prevalence and severity of ACKD increase with the duration of end-stage renal failure, affecting 10–20% of ESRD patients at the onset of dialysis, 50% after 5 years of dialysis, and more than 90% after 10 years of dialysis.

ACKD is frequently associated with renal cancer and affecting 2–7% of patients, a more than 100-fold increase compared to the prevalence of renal cancer in the general population. The mean duration of dialysis prior to the detection of cancers is about 8 years. Renal cancer in patients with ACKD is commonly bilateral and multifocal, with a similar proportion of clear cell and papillary carcinomas. In patients with a successful renal transplant, ACKD can regress. However, preexisting renal carcinomas in native kidneys can progress and become metastatic. This may be associated with post-transplant immune suppression. ACKD and its increased risk of renal cancer can be seen on children with ESRD.

Clinical Findings

A. Symptoms and Signs

ACKD patients are generally asymptomatic, but may present with flank pain, hematuria, or perinephric hematoma due to cyst hemorrhage or renal carcinoma. In rare cases, severe retroperitoneal hemorrhage, requiring resuscitation and surgical or radiologic intervention, may occur. Paraneoplastic signs and symptoms (fever, erythrocytosis, and hypercalcemia) should raise suspicion for renal cell carcinoma.

B. Laboratory Findings

Macroscopically, ACKD kidneys are generally small with mostly cortical cysts that vary in size from pinpoint to a few centimeters. Microscopically, these cysts are lined with a single layer or multiple layers of proliferative and dysplastic renal epithelial cells. Cyst walls are often calcified, and papillary cystadenomas may be identified. Renal enlargement may occur with time.

C. Imaging Studies

Renal US or CT are commonly sufficient to define the extent of AKCD, whereas CT with intravenous contrast or MRI with gadolinium (detect enhancement) are effective to detect renal cancer.

Differential Diagnosis

Differential diagnoses of ACKD include ADPKD, ARPKD, multiple simple cysts, glomerulocystic kidney disease, TSC, and VHL disease, which can be differentiated by the features listed in Table 45–1.

Treatment

ACKD patients who develop significant complications such as retroperitoneal hemorrhage, infection, and/or renal cancer (≥3 cm in diameter) require treatment with bilateral nephrectomy.

Routine screening for renal cancer is not indicated for all patients with ACKD, because a significant proportion of them have multiple comorbidities (diabetes, hypertension, or atherosclerotic vascular diseases), which can limit their life expectancy. For those with less comorbidity, good life expectancy, and have been on dialysis for at least 3 years, screening for renal cancer is indicated.

SIMPLE RENAL CYSTS

ESSENTIALS OF DIAGNOSIS

▶ By renal US:

  –Rare in individuals less than age 30 years.

  –1.7% of individuals at age 30–49, 11.5% at age 50–70, and 22–30% at age greater than 70 years have at least one renal cyst.

▶ Conventional US underestimate the number of renal cysts compared to that of CT or MRI.

General Considerations

Unilateral or bilateral simple renal cysts are circular clear fluid-filled cysts that originate from focal dilation of renal tubules. The prevalence and the number of kidney cysts increase with age.

Clinical Findings

A. Symptoms and Signs

Simple renal cysts are nearly always asymptomatic and generally identified incidentally on abdominal imaging studies. Less frequently, flank pain, cyst hemorrhage, hematuria, or cyst infection can occur. Renin-mediated hypertension and erythropoietin-mediated erythrocytosis have been associated with the development of simple renal cysts.

B. Laboratory Findings

Simple cysts are generally located in the cortex with sizes ranging from a few millimeters to over 20 cm. Microscopically, simple cysts are lined with a single flattened layer of cyst-lining epithelia, and surrounded by normal renal parenchyma.

C. Imaging Studies

Simple cysts in renal US appear as round, smooth, and thin-walled structures with sharply defined margins, without internal echoes. CT images of simple renal cysts show round, smooth, and homogeneous cysts with densities near that of water. These images do not enhance after intravenous administration of contrast. CT images from cysts with internal echoes on US show enhancement with contrast, warrant further diagnostic evaluation with cyst aspiration and/or angiography.

▶ Differential Diagnosis

ADPKD, ARPKD, ACKD, glomerulocystic kidney disease, TSC, and VHL disease should be considered as differential diagnoses of multiple simple renal cysts, using the criteria listed in Table 45–1.

▶ Treatment

Simple renal cysts require treatment only if pain, cyst hemorrhage, or cyst infection develop (as indicated above in the ADPKD section).

KEY READINGS

Bae KT et al: Magnetic resonance imaging evaluation of hepatic cysts in early autosomal-dominant polycystic kidney disease: the Consortium for Radiologic Imaging Studies of Polycystic Kidney Disease cohort. Clin J Am Soc Nephrol 2006;1:64.

Canaud G et al: Therapeutic mTOR inhibition in autosomal dominant polycystic kidney disease: what is the appropriate serum level? Am J Transplant 2010;10:1701.

Caroli A et al: Effect of longacting somatostatin analogue on kidney and cyst growth in autosomal dominant polycystic kidney disease (ALADIN): a randomised, placebo-controlled, multicentre trial. Lancet 2013;382:1485.

Chapman AB et al: The HALT polycystic kidney disease trials: design and implementation. Clin J Am Soc Nephrol 2010;5:102.

Chapman AB et al: Renal structure in early autosomal-dominant polycystic kidney disease (ADPKD): the Consortium for Radiologic Imaging Studies of Polycystic Kidney Disease (CRISP) cohort. Kidney Int 2003;64:1035.

Chrispijn M et al: The long-term outcome of patients with polycystic liver disease treated with lanreotide. Aliment Pharmacol Ther 2012;35:266.

Hogan MC et al: Randomized clinical trial of long-acting somatostatin for autosomal dominant polycystic kidney and liver disease. J Am Soc Nephrol 2010;21:1052.

Irazabal MV et al: Imaging classification of autosomal dominant polycystic kidney disease: a simple model for selecting patients for clinical trials. J Am Soc Nephrol 2015;26:160.

Meijer E et al: Copeptin, a surrogate marker of vasopressin, is associated with disease severity in autosomal dominant polycystic kidney disease. Clin J Am Soc Nephrol 2011;6:361.

Perico N et al: Sirolimus therapy to half the progression of ADPKD. J Am Soc Nephrol 2010;21:1031.

Porath B et al: Mutations in GANAB, encoding the glucosidase IIα subunit, cause autosomal-dominant polycystic kidney and liver disease. Am J Hum Genet 2016;98:1193.

Ruggenenti P et al: Safety and efficacy of long-acting somatostatin treatment in autosomal-dominant polycystic kidney disease. Kidney Int 2005;68:206.

Serra AL et al: Sirolimus and kidney growth in autosomal dominant polycystic kidney disease. N Engl J Med 2010;363:820.

Stallone G et al: Rapamycin for treatment of type I autosomal dominant polycystic kidney disease (RAPYD-study): a randomized, controlled study. Nephrol Dial Transplant 2012;27:3560.

Torres VE et al: Renal stone disease in autosomal dominant polycystic kidney disease. Am J Kidney Dis 1993;22:513.

Torres VE et al: Tolvaptan in patients with autosomal dominant polycystic kidney disease. N Engl J Med 2012;367:2407.

van Keimpema L et al: Lanreotide reduces the volume of polycystic liver: a randomized, double-blind, placebo-controlled trial. Gastroenterology 2009;137:1661. e1661–1662.

Walz G et al: Everolimus in patients with autosomal dominant polycystic kidney disease. N Engl J Med 2010;363:830.

■ CHAPTER REVIEW QUESTIONS

1. Which ONE of the following scenarios is MOST compatible with the abdominal MRI shown in Figure 1?

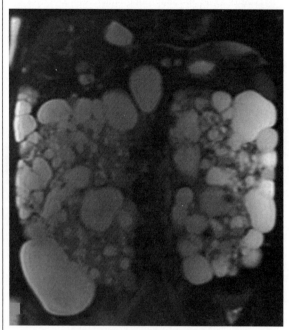

▲ **Figure 1.** Coronal T2 weighted abdominal MRI.

   A. A 17-year-old girl with a known mutation in *PKHD1* gene, a total kidney volume of approximately 5500 mL at that age.

   B. A 78-year-old woman with a hypomorphic mutation in *PKD1* gene, a total kidney volume of approximately 5500 mL at that age and eGFR of 25 mL/min/1.73 m².

   C. A 24-year-old woman with a known mutation in *PKD2* gene, a total kidney volume of approximately 5500 mL at that age, and eGFR of 25 mL/min/1.73 m².

   D. A 48-year-old woman with a known mutation in *PKD1* gene, a total kidney volume of approximately 5500 mL at that age and eGFR of 25 mL/min/1.73 m².

   E. A 48-year-old woman with a known mutation in *Sec63* gene, a total kidney volume of approximately 5500 mL at that age, and eGFR of 25 mL/min/1.73 m².

2. A 26-old-year woman consulted for sudden onset of chest pain accompanied by shortness of breath. A physical examination revealed the presence of multiple cutaneous hypomelanotic macules. A chest radiograph indicated the presence of pneumothorax and the chest CT revealed the presence of multiple thin-walled cysts of various sizes in the pulmonary parenchyma and subpleurally. An abdominal CT showed the presence of a few bilateral renal cysts and two renal masses consistent with angiomyolipomas.

Which ONE of the following is the most the most likely diagnosis?
   A. Autosomal dominant PKD
   B. Autosomal recessive PKD
   C. Tuberous sclerosis complex
   D. Multiple simple cysts
   E. Von Hippel–Lindau disease

3. A 55-old-year man with ADPKD presented with left flank pain accompanied by night sweats, anorexia and profound weight loss of 16 pounds in 7 months.

Which ONE of the following should be done next?
   A. Conservative therapy such as bed resting, analgesics, and adequate fluid intake.
   B. Refer the patient to the pain clinic for intervention such as splanchnic nerve blockade.
   C. Order an abdominal imaging study such as MRI or CT to discard the presence of renal cell carcinoma.
   D. Prescribe narcotic analgesics.
   E. Reassure the patient and refer to dietitian for dietary and lifestyle changes.

4. A 30-old-year man with a known mutation in *PKD1* and treated HTN wishes to have an estimate on the age he most likely would require a kidney transplant.

Which ONE of the following parameters would most reliably predict age at ESRD?
   A. Urine sodium excretion
   B. Total Kidney Volume as calculated by MRI or CT
   C. Age at diagnosis of HTN
   D. Urinary protein levels
   E. Serum high-density lipoprotein levels

5. A 27-year-old woman with a previous diagnosis of DM at 18 years of age consulted her OBGYN for pregnancy planning. During follow-up the patient became pregnant two times while sustaining in acceptable glycemic control but had two spontaneous miscarriages. The infertility study detected a bicornuate uterus. In addition, the patient was found to have a few bilateral renal cysts. Laboratory findings were within normal range. The patient had no family history of kidney disease or gout.

Which ONE of the following should you consider first for genetic analysis?

A. Autosomal dominant PKD; likely *PKD2* mutation
B. Autosomal recessive PKD
C. Autosomal dominant tubulointerstitial kidney disease; likely *UMOD* mutation
D. Autosomal dominant tubulointerstitial kidney disease; likely *HNF-1β* mutation
E. Autosomal dominant tubulointerstitial kidney disease; likely *REN* mutation

Familial Hematurias: Alport Syndrome and Hematuria with Thin Glomerular Basement Membranes

46

Clifford E. Kashtan, MD, FASN

▶ General Approach to Hematuria

Hematuria is a relatively common abnormality. About 0.25% of school-age children have persistent microscopic hematuria. In adults the prevalence of hematuria increases with age and is greater in women. The causes and consequently the work-up of hematuria vary with age. Glomerular disorders are responsible for most cases of pediatric hematuria, while urinary tract malignancy is an important cause of hematuria in individuals over 40 years of age.

Because most people with familial hematuria have microscopic hematuria, it is likely that these conditions are under diagnosed, and that the true prevalence of familial hematuria is higher than we might think. Familial hematuria accounts for a substantial fraction of children with isolated hematuria referred to pediatric nephrology clinics. So-called "thin basement membrane nephropathy" was diagnosed in 40–70% of patients with asymptomatic microscopic hematuria and a negative urological evaluation.

ALPORT SYNDROME

ESSENTIALS OF DIAGNOSIS

- ▶ Microscopic hematuria
- ▶ Abnormal tissue expression of collagen IV α_3, α_4, and α_5 chains, OR presence of *COL4A3, COL4A4,* or *COL4A5* mutation(s)
- ▶ Characteristic thickening and lamellation of glomerular basement membranes
- ▶ High-frequency sensorineural deafness
- ▶ Anterior lenticonus OR perimacular retinal flecks

▶ General Considerations

Alport syndrome is a disorder of the kidneys, frequently associated with sensorineural hearing loss and ocular abnormalities, that is caused by mutations in specific subspecies of collagen IV, the predominant collagenous constituent of basement membranes. These mutations result in critical defects in the structure and function of glomerular, cochlear, and ocular basement membranes.

▶ Pathogenesis

The collagen IV protein family consists of six proteins, designated $\alpha_1(IV)$-$\alpha_6(IV)$, encoded by six distinct genes, *COL4A1-COL4A6.* These genes are organized in pairs on three chromosomes: *COL4A1-COL4A2,* chromosome 13; *COL4A3-COL4A4,* chromosome 2; *COL4A5-COL4A6,* X chromosome. Within each pair the genes are oriented in a 5′-5′ fashion, separated by regulatory domains of varying length.

Collagen IV α chains associate into trimers that in turn form supermolecular networks. Three trimers have been identified in mammalian basement membranes: $\alpha_1\alpha_1\alpha_2$, $\alpha_3\alpha_4\alpha_5$ and $\alpha_5\alpha_5\alpha_6$. The $\alpha_1\alpha_1\alpha_2$ trimer is found in all basement membranes, including glomerular mesangium, but it is a relatively minor component of mature glomerular basement membranes (GBM). The predominant collagen IV species in GBM, and in the basement membrane of the Organ of Corti and certain ocular basement membranes, is the $\alpha_3\alpha_4\alpha_5$ trimer. The $\alpha_3\alpha_4\alpha_5$ trimer is also present in Bowman capsules (BC) and the basement membranes of distal (dTBM) and collecting (cTBM) tubules. The $\alpha_5\alpha_5\alpha_6$ trimer is expressed in BC, dTBM, and cTBM, but not in GBM. The $\alpha_5\alpha_5\alpha_6$ trimer is also highly expressed in epidermal basement membranes (EBM).

Alport syndrome arises from mutations in the *COL4A3*, *COL4A4*, and *COL4A5* genes. The majority of individuals with Alport syndrome (approximately 60% according to recent studies utilizing next generation sequencing) have the X-linked form of the disease (XLAS), due to mutations in *COL4A5*. Autosomal recessive Alport syndrome (ARAS) is caused by mutations in both alleles of *COL4A3* or *COL4A4*, and accounts for about 15% of people with the disease. Finally, 25% of individuals with Alport syndrome have autosomal dominant disease (ADAS), resulting from mutation in one allele of *COL4A3* or *COL4A4*. Heterozygous mutations in *COL4A3* or *COL4A4* mutations are frequently found in kindreds with apparently nonprogressive familial hematuria as well as kindreds erroneously diagnosed with familial focal segmental glomerulosclerosis.

The usual result of *COL4A5* mutations in males with XLAS is the complete disappearance of $\alpha_3\alpha_4\alpha_5$ and $\alpha_5\alpha_5\alpha_6$ trimers, and the supermolecular networks formed by these trimers, from all basement membranes. Heterozygous females with XLAS typically exhibit mosaic expression of these trimers in their basement membranes. In most patients with ARAS, $\alpha_3\alpha_4\alpha_5$ are absent from all basement membranes, but $\alpha_5\alpha_5\alpha_6$ trimers persist in BC, dTBM, cTBM, and EBM. These observations in human subjects have been confirmed in various animal models of XLAS and ARAS and have several implications that have received support from in vitro studies. First, the interactions among the six members of the type IV collagen family are specific and can only produce three trimers: $\alpha_1\alpha_1\alpha_2$, $\alpha_3\alpha_4\alpha_5$, and $\alpha_5\alpha_5\alpha_6$. Second, a mutation in a collagen IV α chain disrupts the formation and deposition of all trimers in which that chain participates. Last, since disappearance of α_3(IV), α_4(IV) and α_5(IV) chains from basement membranes is specific for Alport syndrome, immunostaining for these chains in tissues is diagnostically useful, as will be discussed below.

▶ Clinical Findings

1. Renal—Hematuria is a constant feature of Alport syndrome, occurring in 100% of affected males and about 95% of affected females. Hematuria is often detectable in infancy, and episodic gross hematuria is common during childhood.

Overt proteinuria develops in all XLAS males, often in late childhood or adolescence, and in many XLAS females. In XLAS females proteinuria is a risk factor for the development of ESRD. Onset of overt proteinuria in childhood or adolescence is typical of ARAS, with no gender difference. Overall overt proteinuria occurs later in life in individuals with ADAS.

2. Cochlear—Sensorineural hearing loss (SNHL) is detectable in 50% of males with XLAS by age 25 and 90% by age 40, while the prevalence of SNHL in females is 10% before age 40, and 20% by age 60. SNHL occurs at a relatively young age in those with ARAS, while SNHL is relatively uncommon in ADAS patients. SNHL in Alport syndrome is never congenital, always bilateral, and invariably accompanied by renal symptoms.

In XLAS males SNHL is frequently detectable by audiometry in late childhood or early adolescence, and initially affects high-frequency tones (2000–8000 Hz). Over time the hearing deficit extends into conversational speech. Recent histological studies of human Alport cochleae suggest that SNHL may be due to defective function of the basement membrane of the Organ of Corti, leading to abnormal mechanical relationships between outer hair cells and the basilar membrane, while studies of Alport mice suggest that dysfunction of the stria vascularis mediated by endothelin-1 is involved in the Alport hearing defect.

3. Ocular—Ocular defects occur in 15–30% of individuals with Alport syndrome. The pathognomonic ocular lesion of Alport syndrome is anterior lenticonus, in which the central region of the lens protrudes into the anterior chamber. Anterior lenticonus is associated with marked attenuation of the lens capsule, the basement membrane that surrounds the lens, and becomes apparent during adolescence and young adulthood. Other ocular changes associated with Alport syndrome include perimacular retinal flecks, corneal endothelial vesicles, and recurrent corneal erosions. These lesions may also arise from defective basement membranes: Bruch's membrane (perimacular flecks), Descemet's membrane (corneal endothelial vesicles) and corneal epithelial basement membrane (corneal erosions).

4. Leiomyomatosis—Coinheritance of XLAS and leiomyomatosis of the esophagus, tracheobronchial tree, and female external genitalia has been described in approximately 20 kindreds. In addition to symptoms of Alport syndrome, affected individuals may display dysphagia, postprandial vomiting, retrosternal or epigastric pain, recurrent bronchitis, dyspnea, cough and stridor, typically beginning in late childhood. Leiomyomatosis suspected by chest X-ray or barium swallow may be confirmed by computed tomography or magnetic resonance imaging.

▶ Differential Diagnosis

The cardinal symptom of Alport syndrome is persistent microscopic hematuria. In children the differential diagnosis of persistent microscopic hematuria includes Alport syndrome and related disorders, IgA nephropathy and other chronic forms of glomerulonephritis such as C3 glomerulopathy, and hypercalciuria. The clinical features of these conditions are compared in Table 46–1 and an algorithmic approach to diagnosis is presented in Figure 46–1. The differential diagnosis in adults would include these conditions as well as urologic lesions, particularly in individuals over 40 years of age.

Table 46–1. Clinical features of common causes of persistent microscopic hematuria in childhood.

	Episodic Gross Hematuria	Family History Is Frequently Positive for	Hearing Deficit	Proteinuria	Hypertension	Hypercalciuria	Low C3
Alport syndrome	Common	Hematuria ESRD hearing loss	Common[a]	Common[a]	Common[a]	Rare	Rare
Hematuria with thin glomerular basement membranes	Common	Hematuria	Rare	Rare	Rare	Rare	Rare
IgA nephropathy	Common		Rare	Rare	Rare	Rare	Rare
Hypercalciuria	Rare	Urolithiasis	Rare	Rare	Rare	Always present	Rare
C3 Glomerulopathy	Frequent		Rare	Frequent	Frequent	Rare	Common

[a]Frequency increases with age and is higher in affected males.

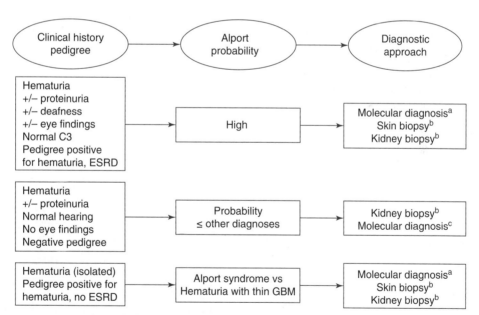

▲ **Figure 46–1.** This algorithm considers the probability of Alport syndrome as the cause of persistent glomerular hematuria, based on clinical features and pedigree.

[a]Molecular diagnosis is the initial study when suspicion of Alport syndrome is high. Next generation sequencing (NGS) of COL4A3, COL4A4, and COL4A5 is the preferred approach; sequential Sanger sequencing is an alternative method. NGS may not be feasible for some patients and families due to insurance coverage issues.

[b]Skin biopsy for diagnosis of Alport syndrome is only useful if immunostaining for the α_5 chain of collagen IV is employed. The diagnostic utility of kidney biopsy is enhanced by immunostaining for collagen IV α chains.

[c]In some centers molecular diagnosis is supplanting kidney biopsy as an early diagnostic procedure in patients with isolated glomerular hematuria.

In settings where access to molecular genetic analysis is limited by availability or insurance coverage, kidney biopsy, supplemented by clinical and pedigree data, remains the key procedure for differentiation of Alport syndrome from other glomerular causes of persistent microscopic hematuria. The presence on electron microscopy of diffuse thickening of the glomerular basement membrane (GBM) with multilamellar splitting of the lamina densa is diagnostic of Alport syndrome. However, GBM thinning due to lamina densa attenuation is typical of boys with XLAS and boys and girls with ARAS, and can be seen at any age in XLAS females and males and females with ADAS.

Immunostaining for the α_3, α_4, and α_5 chains of collagen IV is a valuable tool for confirming a diagnosis of Alport syndrome and for distinguishing the X-linked and autosomal recessive forms of the disorder. These chains are entirely absent from renal basement membranes in about 80% of males with XLAS, while 60–70% of female heterozygotes with XLAS exhibit mosaic expression of these chains. In most patients with ARAS, the $\alpha_3(IV)$ and $\alpha_4(IV)$ chains are not expressed in renal basement membranes, while the $\alpha_5(IV)$ is absent from GBM but present in Bowman's capsule and distal and collecting TBM. The heterozygous mutations in COL4A3 or COL4A4 responsible for ADAS typically cause no discernable changes in the expression of $\alpha_3\alpha_4\alpha_5$ trimers in basement membranes.

XLAS can also be diagnosed by skin biopsy, since the $\alpha_5(IV)$ chain is undetectable in epidermal basement membranes (EBM) of about 80% of XLAS males and is mosaically expressed in 60-70% of females with XLAS. In interpreting the results of type IV collagen immunostaining of skin and kidney it is important to remember that normal expression of the $\alpha_3(IV)$, $\alpha_4(IV)$, and $\alpha_5(IV)$ does not exclude a diagnosis of Alport syndrome. In XLAS males persisting expression of the $\alpha_5(IV)$ chain in skin or kidney is associated with less rapid progression to ESRD, compared to XLAS males in whom expression of $\alpha_5(IV)$ chain in skin or kidney is lacking.

Molecular genetic analysis employing next generation or whole exome sequencing is increasingly augmenting, and in some areas displacing, tissue biopsy as an early diagnostic procedure in patients with persistent glomerular hematuria, with or without a positive family history of hematuria or kidney disease. Identification of pathogenic mutation(s) in COL4A3, COL4A4, or COL4A5 provides diagnostic confirmation as well as information that can be useful in predicting prognosis and that facilitates accurate genetic counseling.

▶ Complications

Common complications of Alport syndrome include hypertension, ESRD, and SNHL. SNHL in Alport patients typically responds well to hearing aids because speech discrimination is preserved. Some patients with anterior lenticonus develop cataracts that require removal. The Alport maculopathy does not typically cause defects in visual acuity, although development of macular holes has been reported rarely. Patients with XLAS

and diffuse leiomyomatosis may need surgical treatment of esophageal and tracheobronchial smooth muscle tumors.

▶ Treatment

Studies of murine of Alport syndrome have shown that early institution of angiotensin blockade retards progression to ESRD, an observation supported by retrospective analysis of registry data. Current recommendations call for initiation of treatment in all patients with overt proteinuria, preferably prior to the onset of renal functional decline. Prospective, randomized trials of early angiotensin blockade and novel therapeutic approaches are underway or in development.

▶ Prognosis

Not surprisingly for an X-linked disorder, gender has a marked impact on the prognosis of XLAS. Fifty percent of untreated males with XLAS reach ESRD by age 25 and 90% reach ESRD by age 40. The nature of the underlying mutation in COL4A5 is an important determinant of the rate of progression to ESRD in XLAS males. While only about 12% of females with XLAS develop ESRD before age 40, the probability of ESRD increases to about 20–30% by age 60 and 40% by age 80. Risk factors for ESRD in XLAS females include a history of gross hematuria, SNHL, deafness, proteinuria and extensive GBM thickening and lamellation.

Patients with ARAS typically reach ESRD before age 40, regardless of gender. ADAS tends to advance less aggressively than XLAS or ARAS, with 50% of affected men reaching ESRD by age 50, compared to age 25 for males with XLAS.

KEY READINGS

Gross O et al: Preemptive ramipril therapy delays renal failure and reduces renal fibrosis in COL4A3-knockout mice with Alport syndrome. Kidney Int 2003;63:438.

Gross O et al: Early angiotensin-converting enzyme inhibition in Alport syndrome delays renal failure and improves life expectancy. Kidney Int 2012;81:494.

Jais JP et al: X-linked Alport syndrome: natural history in 195 families and genotype-phenotype correlations in males. J Am Soc Nephrol 2000;11:649.

Jais JP et al: X-linked Alport syndrome: natural history and genotype-phenotype correlations in girls and women belonging to 195 families: a "European Community Alport Syndrome Concerted Action" study. J Am Soc Nephrol 2003;14:2603.

Kashtan CE et al: Clinical practice recommendations for the treatment of Alport syndrome. Pediatr Nephrol 2013;28:5.

Meehan DT et al: Endothelin-1 mediated induction of extracellular matrix genes in strial marginal cells underlies strial pathology in Alport mice. Hear Res 2016;341:100.

Merchant SN et al: Temporal bone histopathology in Alport syndrome. Laryngoscope 2004;114:1609.

Savige J et al: Ocular features in Alport syndrome: pathogenesis and clinical significance. Clin J Am Soc Nephrol 2015;10:703.

Savige J et al: Alport syndrome in women and girls. Clin J Am Soc Nephrol 2016;11:1713.

Relevant Websites

A detailed review of the molecular pathogenesis and clinical features of Alport syndrome can be found on the GeneReviews website at http://www.genereviews.org/. The websites of the Alport Syndrome Foundation (www.alportsyndrome.org) and the Alport Syndrome Treatments and Outcomes Registry (www.alportregistry.org) may also be of interest.

HEMATURIA WITH THIN GLOMERULAR BASEMENT MEMBRANES

ESSENTIALS OF DIAGNOSIS

- ▶ Microscopic hematuria
- ▶ Diffuse attenuation of glomerular basement membranes
- ▶ Normal tissue expression of type IV collagen α_3, α_4, and α5 chains
- ▶ Absence of mutation in the *COL4A3, COL4A4,* and *COL4A5* genes

General Considerations

Thinning of glomerular basement membranes (GBM) is a common finding in children and adults with isolated glomerular hematuria. Patients with isolated hematuria and GBM thinning frequently have a family history of hematuria. For many years such patients were described as having "benign familial hematuria" if the family history was negative for ESRD. This diagnosis fell into disuse as evidence accumulated that patients with isolated hematuria, thin GBM and negative family history for ESRD could nevertheless develop progressive renal disease, and was replaced by "thin basement membrane nephropathy (TBMN)." This term has its own limitations, since GBM thinning is a pathological finding that does not, in and of itself, allow accurate prediction of prognosis or inheritance in an individual patient. GBM thinning may be found in young males with X-linked Alport syndrome, females of any age with X-linked Alport syndrome, males and females with autosomal recessive Alport syndrome and males and females with heterozygous mutations in *COL4A3* and *COL4A4*. GBM thinning may also be found in patients with hematuria who have no detectable pathological alterations in *COL4A3, COL4A4,* or *COL4A5*, implying the existence of other genetic loci associated with GBM thinning, as yet unidentified. Thus, in an individual patient with hematuria and thin GBM prognosis and inheritance risk are difficult to establish without specific genetic sequencing data supplemented by family history.

Patients with hematuria and thin GBM who have a mutation in *COL4A3, COL4A4,* or *COL4A5* should be considered to have Alport syndrome, with prognosis based on genotype and family history. In the absence of a mutation in *COL4A3, COL4A4,* or *COL4A5* patients should be classified as having "hematuria with thin GBM," which accurately describes their clinical and pathological findings without assigning an inappropriately specific diagnosis.

Alport syndrome and "hematuria with thin GBM" may have similar clinical presentations and pathological manifestations, especially in childhood. Patients with Alport syndrome are much more likely to develop deafness, ocular abnormalities, proteinuria, hypertension, or renal insufficiency and have a family history that is positive for relatives with kidney failure.

Pathogenesis

GBM thinning associated with mutations in the *COL4A3, COL4A4,* and *COL4A5* genes is likely due to absence or deficiency of the collagen IV network composed of α_3(IV), α_4(IV), and α_5(IV) chains, leading to an attenuated, mechanically fragile GBM. Hematuria in these patients would arise from focal, transient ruptures in the weakened GBM. The presence of some quantity of the $\alpha_3\alpha_4\alpha_5$(IV) network in the renal basement membranes of patients with heterozygous mutations in *COL4A3, COL4A4,* and *COL4A5* may ameliorate the secondary processes that lead to renal fibrosis in males with X-linked Alport syndrome and in males and females with autosomal recessive Alport syndrome. In theory GBM thinning could result from mutations in genes encoding other GBM proteins, such as the α_1(IV) and α_2(IV)chains and laminin.

Clinical Findings

The typical patient with hematuria and thin GBM has isolated microscopic hematuria, which may be persistent or intermittent. Acute infections may be associated with transient gross hematuria.

Family history is frequently positive for hematuria but negative for renal failure, and pedigree analysis often indicates that the hematuria is transmitted as an autosomal dominant trait. However, family history for hematuria may be negative or may not distinguish between autosomal and X-linked inheritance.

The development of proteinuria in a patient with hematuria and thin GBM is a risk factor for progressive renal disease. Therefore these patients should have annual urinalyses to monitor for overt proteinuria.

Differential Diagnosis

The differential diagnosis of glomerular hematuria includes Alport syndrome, IgA nephropathy, C3 nephropathy and other chronic forms of glomerulonephritis, hypercalciuria and, in adults, urologic abnormalities. A diagnostic approach is described in the previous section on Alport syndrome.

Complications

Hematuria with thin GBM is associated with good renal outcomes in patients who do not develop overt proteinuria.

Treatment

Many people with hematuria and thin GBM will not require any form of therapeutic intervention. Treatment, preferably with an agent that targets the renal-angiotensin axis, is indicated in those patients with proteinuria and/or hypertension.

Prognosis

Individuals with hematuria and thin GBM who do not develop overt proteinuria have an excellent prognosis. Annual monitoring of urinalysis and blood pressure is recommended to identify those who are candidates for angiotensin blockade.

KEY READINGS

Badenas C et al: Mutations in the *COL4A4* and *COL4A3* genes cause familial benign hematuria. J Am Soc Nephrol 2002;13:1248.

Buzza M et al: Segregation of hematuria in thin basement membrane disease with haplotypes at the loci for Alport syndrome. Kidney Int 2001;59:1670.

Deltas C et al: Carriers of autosomal recessive Alport syndrome with thin basement membrane nephropathy presenting as focal segmental glomerulosclerosis in later life. Nephron 2015;130:271.

Hall CL et al: Clinical value of renal biopsy in patients with asymptomatic microscopic hematuria with and without low-grade proteinuria. Clin Nephrol 2004;62:267.

van Paassen P et al: Signs and symptoms of thin basement membrane nephropathy: a prospective regional study on primary glomerular disease—The Limburg Renal Registry. Kidney Int 2004;66:909.

Voskarides K et al: COL4A3/COL4A4 mutations producing focal segmental glomerulosclerosis and renal failure in thin basement membrane nephropathy. J Am Soc Nephrol 2007;18:3004.

■ CHAPTER REVIEW QUESTIONS

1. A 3-year-old boy is referred to you for evaluation of microscopic hematuria. Evaluation shows normal blood pressure, renal function, urinary protein, and calcium excretion. Renal ultrasound is normal. Mother has a history of microscopic hematuria for many years and thinks her kidney function is normal. Father says he does not have hematuria. There is no family history of kidney failure or deafness.

   Which of the following statements about the child is true?
   A. Since there is no family history of kidney failure he does not have Alport syndrome.
   B. Since the father does not have hematuria this child does not have autosomal recessive Alport syndrome.
   C. The information provided by this pedigree is insufficient for establishing a diagnosis or inheritance pattern.
   D. None of the above statements is true.

2. Which of the following tests is most likely to establish a diagnosis and inheritance pattern in this family?
   A. Hearing evaluation of the child
   B. Kidney biopsy of the child's mother
   C. Kidney biopsy of the child
   D. Next generation sequencing of the child

3. If the child has X-linked Alport syndrome, which of the following statements is true?
   A. *COL4A5* genotype influences age at ESRD.
   B. There is no therapy that can delay progression to ESRD.
   C. The risk of ESRD is 25% by age 25 years.
   D. His mother is a carrier who is not at risk of developing chronic kidney disease or ESRD.

4. Identify the major collagenous network in mature mammalian glomerular basement membranes.
   A. $\alpha_1\alpha_1\alpha_2$ (IV)
   B. $\alpha_1\alpha_2\alpha_3$ (IV)
   C. $\alpha_3\alpha_4\alpha_5$ (IV)
   D. $\alpha_5\alpha_5\alpha_6$ (IV)

5. Ocular abnormalities associated with Alport syndrome include
   A. Anterior lenticonus
   B. Perimacular retinal flecks
   C. Corneal endothelial vesicles
   D. Recurrent corneal erosions
   E. All of the above

Fabry Disease

Robert J. Desnick, PhD, MD

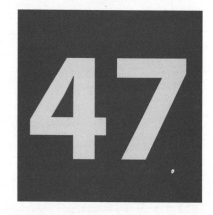

ESSENTIALS OF DIAGNOSIS

▶ Early clinical manifestations in classically affected males include angiokeratomas, acroparesthesias, hypohidrosis, and a characteristic bilateral corneal dystrophy. With advancing age, classic and later-onset males develop renal failure, cardiac disease, and strokes.

▶ The clinical diagnosis is confirmed in males by markedly deficient leukocyte α-galactosidase A (α-Gal A) activity and/or identification of a pathologic α-galactosidase gene (*GLA*) mutation.

▶ Female heterozygotes from classic and later-onset families may be asymptomatic or as severe as their affected male relatives. They are diagnosed by demonstration of the family's pathologic *GLA* mutation.

▶ General Considerations

Fabry disease is an X-linked inborn error of glycosphingolipid catabolism caused by the deficient activity of the lysosomal enzyme, α-galactosidase A (α-Gal A; Figure 47–1). This enzymatic defect results primarily in the progressive accumulation of globotriaosylceramide (Gb3 or GL-3) and related glycosphingolipids with terminal α-galactosyl moieties in the lysosomes of endothelial, epithelial, perithelial, and smooth muscle cells throughout the body.

There are two major clinical subtypes, the classic and later-onset phenotypes (Figure 47–2). Table 47–1 compares the signs and symptoms in males with the two phenotypic subtypes. In classically affected males who have little, if any, α-Gal A activity, the glycosphingolipid deposition in the vascular endothelium is responsible for the major early clinical manifestations of the disease, including angiokeratomas, acroparesthesias, and hypohidrosis

(Figure 47–3). With advancing age, the progressive vascular, cardiomyocyte, and podocyte glycosphingolipid accumulation leads to renal failure, cardiac disease, strokes, and premature demise. Based on the United States and European dialysis, and transplantation registries, most classically affected males develop renal failure between the ages of 35 and 45 years. Prior to the advent of renal transplantation and dialysis, the average age of death for classically affected males in one series was 41 years. Affected males and heterozygotes are normal intellectually. Neurologic involvement in classically affected males and symptomatic heterozygotes is primarily neuropathic pain (ie, acroparesthesias). The incidence of classical Fabry disease is estimated to be approximately 1 in 25,000–40,000 males based on recent newborn screening studies.

Males with the later-onset phenotype have residual α-Gal A activity, lack the vascular endothelial glycosphingolipid deposits, and do not have the early manifestations of classically affected males, including the acroparesthesias, angiokeratoma, hypohidrosis and corneal or lenticular lesions (see Table 47–1). Later-onset males present in the fourth to eighth decades of life with left ventricular hypertrophy (LVH) progressing to hypertrophic cardiomyopathy (HCM) and/or proteinuria and renal insufficiency leading to end-stage renal disease (ESRD). Most later-onset males have been identified by screening renal dialysis, cardiac, and stroke clinics. The incidence of the later-onset phenotype has been estimated to be approximately 1 in 4000–8000 males based on recent newborn screening studies.

Because of random X-chromosomal inactivation, heterozygous females with the classic or later-onset phenotype can have clinical symptoms of Fabry disease that range from asymptomatic to as severe as the affected males in their families. In general, heterozygous females with either phenotype are generally less severely affected and their symptoms may occur later in life than in their affected male relatives.

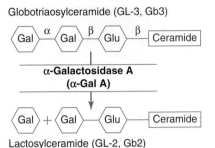

Globotriaosylceramide (GL-3, Gb3)

α-Galactosidase A (α-Gal A)

Lactosylceramide (GL-2, Gb2)

▲ **Figure 47–1.** The metabolic defect in Fabry disease. The deficient activity of α-galactosidase A (α-Gal A) results in the accumulation of globotriaosylceramide (Gb3 or GL-3) and other glycoconjugates with terminal α-galactosyl moieties.

Affected males with the classic and later-onset phenotypes can be reliably diagnosed by the demonstration of deficient α-Gal A activity in plasma and isolated leukocytes. Classically affected males typically have no α-Gal A activity (<2% of mean normal), while later-onset males have residual activity (>2% of mean normal). Identification of a pathogenic mutation in the α-galactosidase A gene (*GLA*) confirms the diagnosis and indicates the phenotypic subtype.

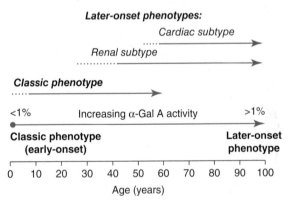

▲ **Figure 47–2.** The phenotypic spectrum of Fabry disease in affected males. There are two major phenotypic subtypes, the early-onset "classic" phenotype, which typically manifests in childhood, and the "later-onset" phenotype that presents with renal and/or cardiac disease in adulthood. There are two subtypes of the later-onset phenotype, as patients may present with primarily cardiac or renal disease, see Table 47–1 for signs and symptoms of males with the two phenotypes.

Table 47–1. Fabry disease: major manifestations in affect males with the classical and later-onset phenotypes.

Signs and Symptoms	Classical Phenotype	Later-Onset Phenotype	
		Renal Subtype	Cardiac Subtype
Age at onset	4–8 y	>25 y	>40 y
Age of death, untreated	40–45 y	>60 y	>60 y
Angiokeratoma	+++	–	–
Acroparesthesias	+++	–	–
Hypohidrosis/anhidrosis	+++	–	–
Corneal/lenticular opacity	+++	–	–
Heart:			
Arrhythmias	+++	+	+++
Valvular defects	+++	+	+++
LVH	+++	–/+	+++
HCM	+++	–/+	+++
Brain:			
Normal intelligence	+	+	+
TIAs	+	+	+
Strokes	+	+	+
Kidney:			
Isosthenuria	+++	+++	–/+
Proteinuria, >1 g/day	+++	+++	–/+
Renal insufficiency	+++	+++	–/++
Age at dialysis/transplant, untreated	35–45 y	>40 y	?
Residual α-Gal A activity	0–2%	>2%	>2%

HCM, hypertrophic cardiomyopathy; LVH, left ventricular hypertrophy; TIA, transient ischemic attack; +, present; –, absent.

Heterozygous females have markedly variable α-Gal A activities because of random X-chromosomal inactivation and, therefore, measurement of plasma and/or leukocyte α-Gal A activity may be misleading. For example, some obligate heterozygotes (daughters of affected males) may have α-Gal A activities ranging from normal to very low levels that are similar to those of affected males. Many heterozygotes (~90%) from families with the Classic phenotype have the characteristic corneal dystrophy observable by slitlamp microscopy. Accurate diagnosis of heterozygous females with either phenotype requires demonstration of the specific family mutation in the *GLA* gene. Such testing is recommended for all at-risk females.

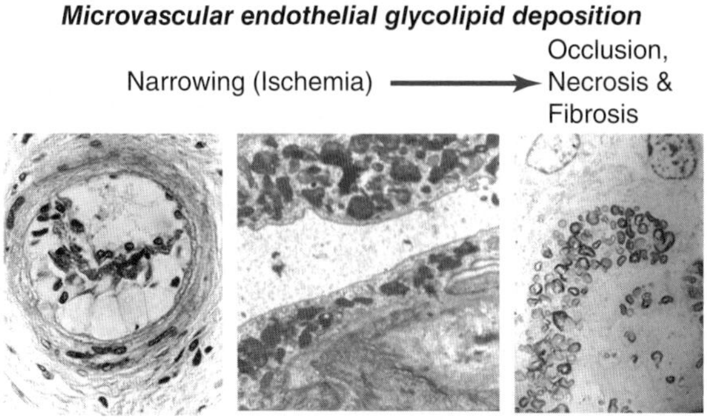

Microvascular endothelial glycolipid deposition

Narrowing (Ischemia) ⟶ Occlusion, Necrosis & Fibrosis

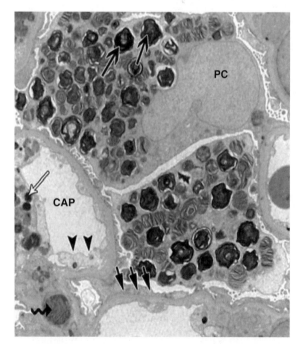

▲ **Figure 47–3.** Photomicrograph and electron micrographs showing the microvascular endothelial glycosphingolipid deposition. Left: Note the ballooned endothelial cells that narrow the lumen and are responsible for the vascular ischemia. Center: An electron micrograph showing the vessel lumen and lysosomes engorged with the glycosphingolipid substrates in the microvascular endothelial cells. Right: An occluded capillary filled with undergraded substrate. (Courtesy of Dr. R. J. Desnick.)

KEY READINGS

Desnick RJ et al: α-Galactosidase A deficiency: Fabry disease. In *The Metabolic and Molecular Bases of Inherited Disease*, 8th ed. Scriver CR et al (eds). McGraw-Hill, 2001, 3733. Available at: http://ommbid.mhmedical.com/content.aspx?bookid=971&sectionid=62644837&jumpsectionID=62644922.

Desnick RJ et al: Fabry disease, an under-recognized multisystemic disorder: expert recommendations for diagnosis, management, and enzyme replacement therapy. Ann Intern Med 2003;138:338.

Echevarria L et al: X-chromosome inactivation in female patients with Fabry disease. Clin Genet 2016;89:44.

Spada M et al: High incidence of later-onset Fabry disease revealed by newborn screening. Am J Hum Genet 2006;79:31.

▶ Pathogenesis

The pathogenesis of Fabry disease is directly related to the progressive accumulation of Gb3 and related glycosphingolipids (eg, globotriaosylsphingosine or lyso-Gb3), in tissue lysosomes and body fluids. Gb3 synthesis and its lysosomal accumulation occurs in most cell types (especially in the life-long cardiomyocytes and podocytes), Gb3 is synthesized in the liver and secreted into the plasma associated with low-density lipoprotein (LDL) particles. Early glycosphingolipid deposition in classically affected males occurs in the vascular endothelium and is greatest in the podocytes (Figures 47–3 and 47–4). In later-onset males, the vascular endothelium is usually spared, but the other renal cell types are involved, particularly the podocytes. Gb3 is taken up by vascular endothelial and smooth muscle cells by the LDL receptor-mediated pathway. In classically affected

males who have essentially no α-Gal A activity, the Gb3 accumulates in the vascular endothelium leading to the early manifestations (eg, angiokeratomas, acroparesthesias, etc.). In both classic and later-onset patients, the progressive accumulation in the cardiomyocytes and renal podocytes results in the development of left ventricular hypertrophy (LVH), hypertrophic cardiomyopathy, and progressive renal insufficiency resulting in ESRD.

In the kidney, the earliest lesions are due to the accumulation of glycosphingolipids in endothelial and epithelial cells of the glomerulus and of Bowman space and in the epithelium of the loops of Henle and of distal tubules (see Figure 47–4). In later stages, and to a lesser extent, proximal tubules, interstitial histiocytes, and fibrocytes accumulate the glycosphingolipid. Lipid-laden distal tubular epithelial cells and glomerular podocytes, desquamate and may be detected in the urinary sediment. These cells have been shown to account for about 75% of the urinary cells shed by classically affected males and heterozygotes.

▲ **Figure 47–4.** An electron micrograph of a glomerulus from an 11-year-old male with the classic phenotype. Note the glycosphingolipid deposition in the vascular endothelial cells (CAP) and the marked accumulation in the podocytes (PC). The patient had a normal glomerular filtration rate and a urine protein/creatinine ratio of approximately 40 mg/g at biopsy. (From Najafian B et al: Pediatr Nephrol 2013;28:679–687, with permission.)

Concurrently, renal blood vessels are involved progressively, and often extensively, in classically affected males and heterozygotes. An early finding is arterial fibrinoid deposits, which may result from the necrosis of severely involved muscular cells. Other histologic changes in the kidney are the sequelae of nonspecific ESRD with evidence of severe arteriolar sclerosis, glomerular atrophy and fibrosis, pseudotubular proliferation of residual glomerular epithelium, tubular atrophy, and diffuse interstitial fibrosis. Kidney size increases during the third decade of life, followed by a decrease in the fourth and fifth decades.

While classically affected males accumulate lysosomal Gb3 in endothelial, interstitial, and mesangial cells, as well as podocytes, males with the later-onset phenotype primarily have extensive deposition in podocytes and rare deposition in tubular epithelial cells, and essentially no deposition in mesangial, interstitial, and vascular endothelial and smooth muscle cells.

KEY READINGS

Meehan SM et al: Fabry disease: renal involvement limited to podocyte pathology and proteinuria in a septuagenarian cardiac variant. Pathologic and therapeutic implications. Am J Kidney Dis 2004;43:164.

Najafian B et al: AJKD atlas of renal pathology: Fabry nephropathy. Am J Kidney Dis 2015;66:e35.

Smid BE et al: Plasma globotriaosylsphingosine in relation to phenotypes of Fabry disease. J Med Genet 2015;52:262.

▶ Clinical Findings

A. Symptoms and Signs

In classically affected males, manifestations typically begin in childhood with episodes of pain and discomfort in the hands and feet (acroparesthesias) (see Table 47–1). The painful episodes may be brought on by exercise, fever, fatigue, stress, or change in weather conditions. In addition, affected males develop a dark red maculopapular skin rash, called angiokeratoma, seen most densely from the umbilicus to the knees, a decreased ability to perspire (hypohidrosis), and characteristic corneal and lenticular changes observed on slitlamp microscopy that do not affect vision. Affected males may have gastrointestinal problems, including postprandial ischemic pain and cramping, diarrhea, vomiting, and nausea. Patients also experience heat or cold, and exercise intolerance. Mild proteinuria, isosthenuria, and urinary sediment abnormalities are early evidence of renal involvement.

The disease progresses slowly and symptoms of kidney, heart, and/or neurologic involvement often do not occur until the ages of 25–45 years. In fact, many patients are first diagnosed when the accumulated storage material begins to affect kidney or heart function. Renal dysfunction leading to uremia with or without hypertension and progressing to ESRD in males is a common outcome. Cardiovascular dysfunction may include cardiac hypertrophy, valvular abnormalities, and arrhythmias while cerebrovascular complications include risk of early stroke, hemiplegia, hemianesthesia, and transient ischemic attacks. Presumably most strokes result from cardiac arrhythmias and in older patients "Holter" or "loop" monitors may reveal episodic arrhythmias. Particularly in smokers, there may be pulmonary complications like airflow obstruction and dyspnea.

Classically affected males die from complications of renal disease, cardiac involvement, and/or cerebrovascular disease. Registry studies have revealed that approximately 15% of females with Fabry disease develop renal failure. Some or all of the symptoms in classically affected males may occur in heterozygous female relatives, but typically at a later age, and to a lesser extent, than in their affected male relatives.

In males with the later-onset phenotype, manifestations typically occur in the fourth to eight decades of life with renal or cardiac manifestations (see Table 47–1). Early renal involvement presents with podocyte effacement and proteinuria. Early cardiac involvement may present with sinus bradycardia and other arrhythmias, leading to LVH and subsequently to HCM. As noted earlier, strokes may result from arrhythmias. Thus, the later-onset manifestations are similar to those that occur in males with the classic phenotype, but typically they occur at older ages in later-onset males. Of interest, some later-onset males with certain mutations will have primarily renal or cardiac disease (eg, mutations encoding p.R363H or p.N215S, respectively).

Heterozygotes from later-onset families may be asymptomatic or manifest cardiac, renal, or cerebrovascular manifestations as severe as their afflicted male relatives. Although there have been no systematic studies of the manifestations in later-onset heterozygotes, it appears that cardiac involvement is the most common manifestation.

KEY READINGS

Desnick RJ et al: α-Galactosidase A deficiency: Fabry disease. In *The Metabolic and Molecular Bases of Inherited Disease*, 8th ed. Scriver CR et al (eds). McGraw-Hill, 2001, 3733. Available at: http://ommbid.mhmedical.com/content.aspx?bookid=971&sectionid=62644837&jumpsectionID=62644922.

Hsu TR et al: Later onset Fabry disease, cardiac damage progress in silence: experience with a highly prevalent mutation. J Am Coll Cardiol 2016;68:2554.

Namdar M: Electrocardiographic changes and arrhythmia in Fabry disease. Front Cardiovasc Med 2016;3:7.

Thadhani R et al: Patients with Fabry disease on dialysis in the United States. Kidney Int 2002;61:249.

B. Laboratory Findings

1. Biochemical testing

A. MALES—The most efficient and reliable method for the diagnosis of affected males is the determination of α-Gal A activity in plasma and/or isolated leukocytes. The test is a fluorometric assay and uses the substrate 4-methylumbelliferyl-α-D-galactopyranoside. Affected males with the classic phenotype will have essentially no α-Gal A activity (<2% of mean normal), while those with later-onset phenotype have some residual activity (>2% of mean normal).

B. HETEROZYGOUS FEMALES—Measurement of plasma and/or leukocyte α-Gal A activity does not distinguish heterozygotes since they can have low to normal activities due to random X-chromosomal inactivation. Heterozygous females who have very low α-Gal A activity (<20% of mean normal) should be followed closely, as many of these females develop HCM and/or ESRD. α-Gal A mutation analysis is required for the definitive diagnosis of heterozygous females.

2. Molecular genetic testing—Mutation analysis by DNA sequencing of the *GLA* gene is the most definitive way to confirm the diagnosis in males and is required for females suspected of being heterozygotes. A mutation in the *GLA* gene has been identified in all affected males with markedly decreased α-Gal A activity. To date, almost 900 *GLA* mutations have been described; most mutations identified have been private, occurring in only a few families. There are no common mutations except IVS4+919G>A, which occurs in approximately 1 in 1000 Taiwanese and may be as common in southern parts of China.

3. Special tests—Males suspected of having Fabry disease and women suspected of being heterozygotes should have a slitlamp examination by an experienced ophthalmologist to detect the characteristic corneal and lenticular changes. The corneal opacities are found in classically affected males and most heterozygous females (~90%) from Classic families, and are typically absent in later-onset males and heterozygotes.

KEY READINGS

Desnick RJ et al: Fabry disease, an under-recognized multisystemic disorder: expert recommendations for diagnosis, management, and enzyme replacement therapy. Ann Intern Med 2003;138:338.

Nowak A et al: Plasma LysoGb3: a useful biomarker for the diagnosis and treatment of Fabry disease heterozygotes. Mol Genet Metab 2017;120:57.

Shabbeer J et al: Fabry disease: 45 novel mutations in the α-galactosidase A gene causing the classical phenotype. Mol Genet Metab 2002;76:23.

Spada M et al: High incidence of later-onset Fabry disease revealed by newborn screening. Am J Hum Genet 2006;79:31.

► Differential Diagnosis

The neuropathic pain that primarily occurs in the extremities (acroparesthesias) are similar to those of other disorders, including rheumatoid arthritis, juvenile arthritis, rheumatic fever, erythromelalgia, lupus, "growing pains," petechiae, Raynaud syndrome, fibromyalgia, and multiple sclerosis.

Differential diagnosis of the cutaneous lesions must exclude typical angiomas and the angiokeratoma of Fordyce, angiokeratoma of Mibelli, and angiokeratoma circumscriptum, none of which have the typical histologic or ultrastructural pathology of the Fabry lesion. The angiokeratoma of Fordyce is similar in appearance to that of Fabry disease, but is limited to the scrotum, and usually appears after the age of 30. The angiokeratoma of Mibelli includes warty lesions on the extensor surfaces of extremities in young adults and is associated with chilblains. Angiokeratoma circumscriptum or naeviformus can occur anywhere on the body, is clinically and histologically similar to that of Fordyce, and is not associated with chilblains.

Angiokeratoma, reportedly similar to or indistinguishable from the clinical appearance and distribution of the cutaneous lesions in Fabry disease, has been described in patients with other lysosomal storage diseases, including fucosidosis, sialidosis (α-neuraminidase deficiency with or without β-galactosidase deficiency), adult-type β-galactosidase deficiency, aspartylglucosaminuria, adult-onset α-galactosidase B deficiency, and β-mannosidase deficiency.

► Treatment

The first level of treatment for Fabry patients is preventive. The episodes of neuropathic pain generally have precipitating causes such as stress, exposure to the sun or heat, changes in temperature, physical exertion, or fever and illness. Patients should make every effort to avoid these precipitating factors, if possible. Patients with frequent severe pain may benefit from medications such as diphenylhydantoin (Dilantin), carbamazepine (Tegretol), or gabapentin (Neurontin). These medications must be taken every day to prevent the onset of pain, and to reduce the frequency and severity of painful attacks. Other preventive measures include avoidance of smoking, and in those patients with mitral valve prolapse, taking prophylactic antibiotics when undergoing dental procedures or surgery. Regular visits to a physician who will monitor general health and, in particular, urinary albuminuria and protein is a vital part of preventive therapy. For kidney health, a low-sodium, low-protein diet and presymptomatic treatment with angiotensin receptor blockers (ARBs) or angiotensin-converting enzyme (ACE) inhibitors, should be considered. For those patients with severely compromised kidney function, dialysis and kidney transplantation are available. The success of kidney transplantation offers the ability to restore kidney function in Fabry patients and has improved the overall prognosis for this disease. The disease does not reoccur in the transplanted kidney.

Enzyme replacement therapy (ERT) for Fabry disease is available in many countries. There are two preparations of recombinant human α-Gal A: agalsidase alfa (Replagal) manufactured by Shire and agalsidase beta (Fabrazyme) manufactured by the Genzyme Corporation. Both drugs were approved by the European Medicines Agency. Only Fabrazyme is approved by the Food and Drug Administration for use in the United States. Extensive preclinical, Phase 1, 2, 3, and 4 clinical trials of Fabrazyme demonstrated that recombinant human α-Gal A is well tolerated and safe, and demonstrated that the patients treated with Fabrazyme (1 mg/kg every 2 weeks) maintained Gb3 clearance from the vascular endothelium in the kidney, heart, and skin, the key sites of pathology in this disease. In addition, histologic examination of other renal, cardiac, and skin cell types revealed complete or partial clearance of accumulated Gb3. Recent studies demonstrate that dose is important for the clearance of podocytes and presumably is also true for cardiomyocytes. It is recommended for optimal outcomes to initiate ERT as early as possible in classic males.

Patients on ERT also reported improved quality of life including decreased pain and gastrointestinal problems, and increased sweating, heat tolerance, and energy. A randomized double-blind placebo-controlled Phase 4 study involving 82 Fabry patients with mild to moderate renal disease (serum creatinine >1.2, but <3.0 mg/dL), demonstrated that the patients who received 1 mg/kg of agalsidase beta every 2 weeks were 61% less likely to experience a clinically significant renal, cardiovascular, or cerebrovascular event, after an adjustment for baseline proteinuria between the treated and placebo groups. The most pronounced benefit was seen when therapy was started in patients with milder renal disease, emphasizing the importance of early treatment, even in patients with advanced disease.

A consensus report of physician experts in Fabry disease recommended that all males with Fabry disease (including those with ESRD) and heterozygous females with substantial disease manifestations should be treated by ERT as early as possible. Dialysis and transplanted patients with Fabry disease suffer from the nonrenal cardiac and cerebrovascular complications of the disease and, therefore, should be treated with enzyme replacement therapy. Studies have shown that Fabrazyme can be administered during hemodialysis as the enzyme is not filtered.

KEY READINGS

Banikazemi M et al: Agalsidase-beta therapy for advanced Fabry disease: a randomized trial. Ann Intern Med 2007;146:77.

Benjamin ER et al: The validation of pharmacogenetics for the identification of Fabry patients to be treated with migalastat. Genet Med 2017;19:430.

Desnick RJ et al: Fabry disease, an under-recognized multisystemic disorder: expert recommendations for diagnosis, management, and enzyme replacement therapy. Ann Intern Med 2003;138:338.

Eng C et al: Safety and efficacy of recombinant human alpha-galactosidase A replacement in Fabry's disease. N Eng J Med 2001;345:9.

Germain DP et al: Ten-year outcome of enzyme replacement therapy with agalsidase beta in patients with Fabry disease. J Med Genet 2015;52:353.

Germain DP et al: Treatment of Fabry's disease with the pharmacologic chaperone migalastat. N Engl J Med 2016;375:545.

Kosch M et al: Enzyme replacement therapy administered during hemodialysis in patients with Fabry disease. Kidney Int 2004;66:1279.

Najafian B et al: One year of enzyme replacement therapy reduces globotriaosylceramide inclusions in podocytes in male adult patients with Fabry disease. PloS One 2016;11:e0152812.

Schiffmann R et al: Screening, diagnosis, and management of patients with Fabry disease: conclusions from a "Kidney Disease: Improving Global Outcomes" (KDIGO) Controversies conference. Kidney Int 2017;91:284.

Tondel C et al: Agalsidase benefits renal histology in young patients with Fabry disease. J Am Soc Nephrol 2013;24:137.

▶ When to Refer/When to Admit

Affected males and at-risk female heterozygotes should be referred to a Fabry physician expert. Genetic counselors can facilitate enzyme and gene testing, and can provide counseling concerning the X-linked inheritance of the disease.

■ CHAPTER REVIEW QUESTIONS

1. A 20-year-old man presents with a history of pain in his extremities. He was referenced by his family physician as his routine urinalysis revealed only isosthenuria and microalbuminuria.

   Which ONE of the following is the MOST LIKELY diagnosis?
   A. Juvenile rheumatoid arthritis
   B. Fabry disease
   C. Alport syndrome
   D. Glomerulonephritis
   E. Nephrotic syndrome

2. Fabry disease is an X-linked disorder in which male patients are affected and female heterozygotes can be asymptomatic or have manifestations as severe as their affected male relatives.

   Which ONE is the MOST accurate method to diagnose heterozygous females?
   A. α-Galactosidase A activity in leukocytes
   B. Identification of the family mutation
   C. Slit lamp microscopy to identify the characteristic corneal opacity
   D. Measurement of the urinary glycosphingolipid accumulation
   E. Kidney biopsy revealing lysosomal glycolipid inclusions

3. Screening males in your dialysis clinic for Fabry disease by a simple enzyme assay identifies two males with marked α-galactosidase A deficiency suggesting the diagnosis of Fabry disease, a rare treatable lysosomal storage disease which progresses to renal failure.

   Which ONE of the following is the MOST effective treatment for this disease?
   A. Renal transplantation, as the normal kidney will not only correct the renal disease, but will secrete the normal enzyme.
   B. Continue the dialysis, as the toxic circulating substrate (~1000 molecular weight) will be cleared.

   C. Recombinant enzyme replacement therapy.
   D. The patient has lost his kidney function, continue dialysis or consider transplantation, and screen family members to identify at-risk young males for evaluation and treatment.
   E. Renal transplantation with a donor kidney from an unaffected family member.

4. In Fabry disease, an X-linked nephropathy, heterozygous women may be asymptomatic or may be as severely affected as their male relatives. This is also true for X-linked Alport syndrome.

   Which ONE of the following is the MOST LIKELY cause of this variable expressivity in female heterozygotes for these diseases?
   A. Gene inactivation in female heterozygotes
   B. Random X-chromosomal inactivation
   C. Modifying genes
   D. Gonadal mosaicism
   E. Cross-correction of mutant cells by normal renal cell secretions

5. In X-linked Fabry disease, most males with the severe early-onset "Classic" phenotype typically develop ESRD by ages 30–45 years, whereas many males with the "later-onset" phenotype develop ESRD or severe cardiac disease in their fifth to eighth decades of life, and are often detected by screening patients in dialysis or cardiac clinics.

   Which ONE of the following is the MOST LIKELY explanation for the two major phenotypic subtypes?
   A. Modifying genes involved in glycosphingolipid metabolism
   B. Type of mutation
   C. Polymorphisms in the gene that influence expression
   D. Epigenetic changes in the gene
   E. Mosaicism of normal and enzyme deficient cells

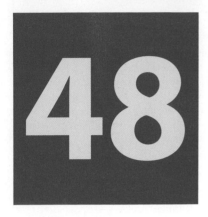

48

Sickle Cell Nephropathy

Phuong-Mai T. Pham, MD
Shaker S. Qaqish, MD
Phuong-Thu T. Pham, MD, FASN

Sickle cell disease (SCD) is an autosomal recessive hemoglobin disorder arising from the substitution of glutamate for valine at the sixth amino acid of the β-globin chain. The mutation results in poorly soluble hemoglobin S (HbS) tetramers that aggregate during cellular or tissue hypoxia, dehydration, or oxidative stress. Such aggregation can lead to red blood cell sickling deformity, premature destruction of erythrocytes, and widespread vaso-occlusive episodes, potentially leading to multiorgan damage. Various kidney complications including hematuria, renal papillary necrosis, renal tubular disorders, acute and chronic kidney injury, sickle cell glomerulopathy, and renal medullary carcinoma are reviewed in the current chapter.

HEMATURIA & RENAL PAPILLARY NECROSIS

ESSENTIALS OF DIAGNOSIS

▸ Acute painless, episodic gross hematuria or persistent microscopic hematuria.

▸ Urine microscopy typically shows isomorphic red blood cells (RBCs) but sickled erythrocytes are occasionally seen, RBC casts are absent.

▸ Ultrasound or computed tomography scan shows distinctive medullary abnormalities.

▶ General Considerations

Hematuria commonly occurs as a consequence of red blood cell sickling in the renal medulla leading to vascular obstruction and RBC extravasation into the collecting system. Hematuria may also indicate the presence of papillary necrosis, and in rare cases, renal medullary carcinoma.

▶ Pathogenesis

The low oxygen tension or relatively hypoxic, hypertonic, and acidotic environment of the inner medulla predisposes red blood cells in the vasa recta to sickle, and causes increased blood viscosity, microthrombi formation, and ischemic necrosis. Such pathologic events can cause structural changes leading to RBC extravasation into the collecting system, renal infarction, and papillary necrosis. The left kidney is affected four times more than the right due to the increased venous pressure within the longer left vein that is compressed between the aorta and the superior mesenteric artery, a "nutcracker phenomenon." The increased venous pressure leads to increased relative hypoxia in the renal medulla, hence sickling.

The renal papillary necrosis of SCD contrasts with that of the papillary necrosis observed in analgesic nephropathy, in which the vasa rectae are typically spared, and most lesions occur in peritubular capillaries.

▶ Clinical Findings

A. Symptoms and Signs

Both microscopic and macroscopic painless hematuria may be observed. Bleeding typically remits spontaneously within a few days. Hematuria is usually unilateral and originates more frequently from the left than the right due to the nutcracker phenomenon. Bilateral hematuria occurs in approximately 10% of cases. Although renal papillary necrosis typically presents with painless gross hematuria, it may be complicated by obstructive uropathy and urinary tract infections. Current data suggest that hematuria and papillary necrosis do not portend greater risk for renal failure. Acute segmental or total renal infarction may present with flank or abdominal pain, nausea, vomiting, fevers, and presumably renin-mediated hypertension.

Renal papillary necrosis (RPN) is usually discovered by radiologic investigation of patients with painless gross hematuria. However, hematuria is not invariably present in RPN. In one series, there was no difference in the incidence of RPN between symptomatic (65%) and asymptomatic (62%) patients.

Priapism in SCD patients reflects a vaso-occlusive phenomenon. The constellation of events including stasis, hypoxia, and acidosis of venous blood during a normal erection can lead to sickling of erythrocytes within the venous sinusoids of the corpus cavernosa, obstruction of the venous outflow of the corporeal bodies, and engorgement of the corpora cavernous. Patients typically present with an erect, painful, and rigid penis lasting up to 3 hours. Priapism can occur as a single acute episode or as repetitive, transient, self-limiting episodes known as stuttering priapism.

B. Laboratory Findings

A complete blood count with differential is generally consistent with chronic compensated hemolytic anemia with hemoglobin ranging between 8 and 10 g/dL. Although patients may present with a significant drop in hemoglobin, other major causes of an acute drop in hemoglobin level must be excluded. These include aplastic crisis, splenic sequestration crisis, and hyperhemolytic crisis.

C. Imaging Studies

Increased echodensity and "garland" pattern of calcification in the medullary pyramids are typical ultrasonographic findings associated with SCN. However, ultrasound is insensitive in detecting RPN in the earlier phases. Although invasive, contrast computed tomogram urography gives excellent display of anatomy and calyceal dilatation and allows early diagnosis of RPN. Papillary necrosis with sloughing can appear as "egg in a cup" or "golf ball in a club" deformity. The imaging study findings in a SCD patient presenting with hematuria is shown in Figure 48–1.

▶ Differential Diagnosis

Although continued or persistent gross hematuria in a known HbSS or HbAS patient is most likely due to renal "sickle crisis," other causes of hematuria including renal medullary carcinoma must be excluded (discussed in a later section). Urinalysis can exclude myoglobinuria associated with rhabdomyolysis. The latter can occur during strenuous exercise and dehydration or during severe sickle cell crises. Severe abdominal pain makes the diagnosis of renal sickle crisis less likely, whereas moderate discomfort often lateralizes the bleeding. Renal and bladder ultrasound can rule out bleeding from a stone or tumor and may aid in the diagnosis of RPN. Abdominal vaso-occlusive crises may be indistinguishable from acute abdominal pain from other causes or from a "surgical" abdomen. However, rebound tenderness is generally absent in sickle cell crises. Other reported causes of abdominal pain in SCD patients include hepatic or splenic sequestration, bone marrow hyperplasia, splenic hemorrhage or thrombosis, mesenteric arterial thrombosis, cholecystitis, gastroenteritis, cystitis, or pyelonephritis. Urine culture should be obtained as clinically indicated. Although rare, drug-induced hemolytic anemia and hemoglobinuria should not be overlooked. These may include sulfonamides, dapsone, rifampin, cephalosporins, and ciprofloxacin, among others.

▶ Treatment

1. Conservative measures including bed rest and oral hydration remain the cornerstone in the management gross hematuria.

2. In more severe cases, urinary alkalinization to minimize hemoglobin precipitation, loop diuretic administration to prevent microtubular obstruction, and blood transfusions to reduce HbS and sickling may be considered.

3. Refractory cases of hematuria may require high doses of oral urea to achieve blood urea nitrogen greater than 100 mg/dL for its presumed inhibitory effect on gelation of deoxygenated sickle hemoglobin or agents including vasopressin or epsilon-aminocaproic acid (EACA) to promote clotting. The latter (ie, EACA) is generally given 2–3 g daily over several days, not to exceed 12 g daily due to risk of thrombosis. It is also noteworthy that blood clot formation within the collecting system from the use of EACA may lead to tubular obstruction.

4. Angiographic embolization of the involved renal vessel or balloon tamponade for bleeding from papillary necrosis may be considered in cases of failed conservative medical therapies.

5. Unilateral nephrectomy is not recommended because bleeding can recur in the contralateral kidney.

KEY READINGS

Akingbola TS et al: Abdominal pain in adult sickle cell disease patients: a Nigerian experience. Ann Ib Postgrad Med 2011;9:100.

Kaye JD: Preliminary experience with epsilon aminocaproic acid for treatment of intractable upper tract hematuria in children with hematological disorders. J Urol 2010;184:1152.

Pham PC et al: Glomerular/vascular diseases. In: Pham PC, Pham PT (eds). *Nephrology and Hypertension Board Review*. Wolters Kluwer, Philadelphia, PA, 2017, p. 217.

Pham PC et al: Sickle cell nephropathy. Pham PC, Pham PT. Sickle cell nephropathy. In: Lerma E, Sparks M, Topf J (eds). *Neprology Secrets*, 4th ed. Mosby Elsevier (in press).

Sutariya HC et al: Renal papillary necrosis: role of radiology. J Clin Diagn Res 2016;10:TD10.

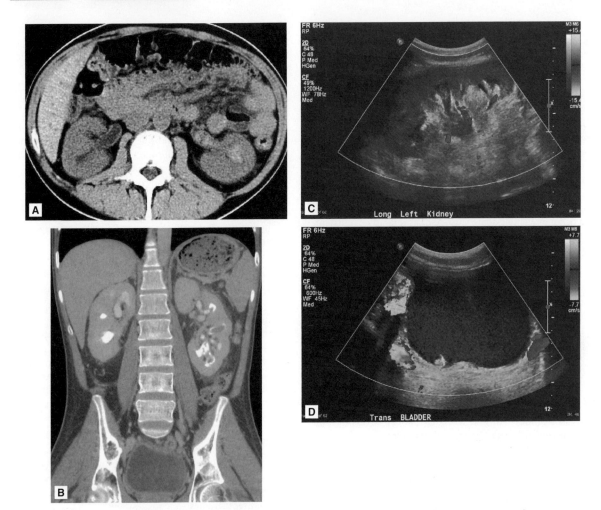

▲ **Figure 48–1.** Imaging study findings in a sickle cell disease patient presenting with hematuria. **A.** Axial non-contrast CT shows hyperdense material in left renal collecting system, consistent with blood. **B.** Coronal CTU shows hydronephrosis, filling defects in the collecting system due to blood and sloughed papillae, and calyceal "clubbing." **C.** Renal US shows dilated renal pelvis and calyces with echogenic material consistent with blood. **D.** The urinary bladder is distended with echogenic material consistent with blood, with a small clot seen dependently. (Courtesy of Dr. Matilda Jude, UCLA-Olive View Medical Center, Sylmar, California.) **(See Color Plate 26.)**

TUBULAR DYSFUNCTION

ESSENTIALS OF DIAGNOSIS

- ▶ Concentrating defect-maximum urine osmolality 400–450 mosmol/kg following water deprivation, compared with greater than 900 mosmol/kg in individuals without SCD. Urinary diluting capacity is preserved.

- ▶ Incomplete distal renal tubular acidosis (inability to lower urine pH to below 5.3 following ammonium chloride loading).

- ▶ Impaired K⁺ secretion, an aldosterone-independent process (selective aldosterone deficiency and hyporeninemic hypoaldosteronism have also been reported).

- ▶ Increased tubular secretion of uric acid and creatinine.

General Considerations

Diminished urine concentrating ability, preserved diluting capacity, and proximal tubular secretory and absorptive hyperfunctioning are characteristic of SCD. The latter is manifested by increased proximal tubular secretion of uric acid and creatinine, and increased tubular reabsorption of low molecular weight protein (β_2-microglobulins) and phosphate. Hydrogen ion and potassium secretion functions are only mildly affected.

Pathogenesis

Diminished concentrating ability: Red blood cell sickling and congestion in the vasa recta leads to ischemia and associated impairment of solute reabsorption by the ascending limb of Henle loop and the vasa recta with consequent loss of the countercurrent multiplication and exchange system of the inner medulla. The suboptimal maintenance of the high interstitial osmolality in the inner medulla reduces effective water reabsorption across the collecting tubules, hence reduced kidney concentrating ability. Vasopressin synthesis and release is normal in SCD, hence the concentrating defect is not responsive to vasopressin.

Preserved diluting capacity: Urinary dilution occurs at the water impermeable thick ascending limb of Henle loop where active sodium chloride reabsorption occurs via the Na-K-2Cl cotransporter. Since most cortical nephrons are superficial and have short loops and peritubular capillaries where vaso-occlusion is not as severe as that seen in the vaso recta in the inner medullary regions, the diluting capacity of the kidney is relatively intact.

In addition to the concentrating defect, other renal functions primarily accomplished in the renal medulla, including renal acidification and potassium secretion, are also impaired in SCD patients. Patients may develop an incomplete form of distal renal tubular acidosis via reduced H^+-ATPase activity due to hypoxemia. A blunted increase in urinary excretion of titratable acid in SCD patients compared with control subjects was demonstrated. Ammonium excretion is either normal or decreased. Hence, SCD patients are unable to lower their urine pH below 5.3 following ammonium chloride loading. This defect is not observed in patients with sickle cell trait. An intact renin–angiotensin–aldosterone axis exists, suggesting the presence of a primary defect in renal potassium secretion, presumably due to ischemic damage to the potassium secreting segment of the distal nephron. Nonetheless, selective aldosterone deficiency as well as hyporeninemic hypoaldosteronism have been described. Despite impaired potassium secretion, the serum potassium level does not increase following release of a large potassium load from sickled red blood cells. The latter suggests an increased intracellular shift of potassium, likely via β_2-adrenergic stimulation. Hence, the use of β-blockers may result in hyperkalemia.

Proximal tubular function disorders: SCD patients exhibit increased reabsorptive capacity of the proximal tubule. There is increased reabsorption of solutes such as β_2-microglobulin and phosphorus, evidenced by the frequent development of hyperphosphatemia in SCD patients. Since sodium reabsorption in the proximal tubule parallels phosphorus reabsorption, an increase in phosphorus reabsorption results in increased sodium reabsorption. Increased tubular secretion of uric acid and creatinine by the proximal tubules in SCD patients markedly increases urinary excretion of these substances. Up to 30% of the total urinary creatinine excretion results from tubular secretion in SCD patients. Hypersecretion of creatinine leads to overestimation of true glomerular filtration rate using serum creatinine-based equations.

Clinical Findings

A. Symptoms and Signs

The most common tubular abnormality in SCD is urinary concentrating defect. Affected individuals may present with nocturnal enuresis (children), nocturia, polyuria, or "hypovolemia prone" with poor oral intake. Blood transfusions of HbA-containing red blood cells can improve concentrating ability in children younger than age 15. In older adolescents and adults, medullary fibrosis and permanent destruction of collecting ducts result in irreversible concentrating defects.

B. Laboratory Findings

Diminished concentrating ability leads to hypo- or isosthenuria, where urine osmolality typically does not exceed 400–450 mosm/kg. The suboptimal acid handling in SCD patients is usually not clinically apparent under normal conditions, but can be unmasked in the setting of renal insufficiency as an incomplete form of distal RTA. Similar to the urinary acidification defect, the defect in potassium secretion is not clinically apparent under normal conditions but hyperkalemia can manifest in the presence of additional insults such as renal dysfunction, rhabdomyolysis or volume contraction during a sickle cell crisis. In essence, RTA in SCD patients resemble type IV (or aldosterone-independent) renal tubular acidosis. Other laboratory findings include hyperphosphatemia, especially in the presence of an increased phosphate load generated by hemolysis and falsely low serum creatinine. The former due to increased phosphate reabsorption and the latter due to increased creatinine secretion associated with proximal tubular hyperfunctioning (discussed above). Since sodium reabsorption in the proximal tubule parallels phosphorus reabsorption, an increase in phosphorus reabsorption results in increased sodium reabsorption. Hence, the response to diuretic therapy may be diminished in SCD patients.

Treatment

1. Patients with SCD are more prone to develop hypovolemia during painful sickle cell crisis requiring close monitoring of volume status and intravenous fluid replacement.

2. Administration of large volumes of standard sodium-containing fluids to severely anemic patients with increased sodium reabsorption may result in pulmonary edema.

3. Edema accompanying severe anemia may be difficult to manage because of diminished response to diuretics.

4. Potassium may be elevated in hemolysis, especially in the presence of renal sufficiency. Caution should be exercised when using β-blockers or angiotensin-converting enzyme (ACE) inhibitors as these drugs may aggravate hyperkalemia.

KEY READINGS

Gargiulo R et al: Sickle cell nephropathy. Disease-a-month 2014;60:494.
Pham PT et al: Renal abnormalities in sickle cell disease. Kidney Int 2000;57:1.
Scheinman JI: Sickle cell disease and the kidney. Nat Clin Pract Nephrol 2009;5:78.

ACUTE KIDNEY INJURY

Impaired kidney function occurs in 5–18% of SCD patients, and can present as acute or chronic kidney injury. In a series of 254 vaso-occlusive episodes in161 SCD patients, acute kidney injury (AKI) associated with vaso-occlusive episodes occurred in 4.3% of patients. Predisposing risk factors include volume depletion due to poor concentrating defect, sickling process, and hemolysis. Affected patients may present with acute tubular necrosis from volume depletion or sepsis, acute tubular obstruction due to accumulation of red blood cells with severe renal infarction or debris from papillary necrosis, tubular injury from ischemia-induced rhabdomyolysis, hemosiderin accumulation, or use of nonsteroidal anti-inflammatory drugs. In early SCN, increased glomerular filtration rate (GFR) and renal plasma flow (RPF) are frequently observed due to compensatory hypersecretion of vasodilator prostaglandins in response to sickling-related medullary hypoxia and ischemia. NSAID use can cause a significant decrease in GFR leading to acute or chronic kidney injury.

Although rare, AKI associated with rhabdomyolysis and disseminated intravascular coagulation can develop in patients with sickle cell trait who undergo rigorous military training.

KEY READINGS

Audard V et al: Acute kidney injury in sickle patients with painful crisis or acute chest syndrome and its relation to pulmonary hypertension. Nephrol Dial Transplant 2010;25;2524.

Wolfson JA et al: Sickle cell disease in California: a population based description of emergency department utilization. Pediatr Blood Camncer 2011;56:413.

CHRONIC KIDNEY DISEASE AND SCD-ASSOCIATED GLOMERULOPATHY

ESSENTIALS OF DIAGNOSIS

▸ The prevalence of albuminuria and proteinuria is 30% within the first 3 decades of life and increases up to 70% in older patients.

▸ Although glomerular filtration is increased in younger patients with sickle cell disease, it typically progressively declines after the age of 30.

▸ Patients with SCD generally have lower blood pressure compared with their healthy unaffected counterparts. The incidence of hypertension in SCD ranges between 2% and 6% compared with 40–45% among blacks in the United States.

▸ Glomerulopathy seen in patients with SCD: Secondary focal segmental glomerulosclerosis, membranoproliferative glomerulonephropathy, thrombotic microangiopathy, HIV nephropathy, and hepatitis-associated glomerulonephropathies.

▸ General Considerations

The incidence of chronic kidney disease (CKD) among SCD patients varies widely among different parts of the world with a reported incidence of 2.6% in Senegal, 4.3% in Brazil, 5.9% in Cuba, 11.6% in United States, and 22.5% in Saudi Arabia. The discrepancy in the incidence reported may be explained by the differences in the definition of CKD, the duration of follow-up, the age of the population studied, hospital versus clinic settings, and genetic factors or genetic modifiers, among others. The diagnosis of CKD among SCD patients generally occurs between 30 and 40 years of age, with ESRD developing in approximately 11% of patients. Progression of CKD is thought to be due in part to early glomerular hypertrophy and hyperfiltration and the eventual development of FSGS.

▸ Pathogenesis

A. Glomerular Hyperfiltration, Microalbuminuria and Proteinuria

In patients with SCD, an increase in renal blood flow and glomerular filtration frequently becomes apparent 1 year after birth. Renal blood flow and GFR decrease with age.

Glomerular changes begin as early as the first decade of life and are characterized by high renal blood flow, glomerular hyperfiltration and hypertrophy, gradual loss of permselectivity leading to micro- and macroalbuminuria, and a decrease in ultrafiltration coefficient. The decrease in ultrafiltration coefficient has been found to be associated with renal insufficiency. In addition, the ultrafiltration coefficient correlates inversely with glomerular permselectivity as assessed by the fractional clearances of albumin and IgG. In albuminuric patients with preserved GFR, the glomerular ultrafiltration coefficient is reduced compared with normoalbuminuric control subjects with SCD. Among those with depressed GFR, a severe reduction in glomerular ultrafiltration coefficient was observed, suggesting that albuminuria is a sensitive marker of early glomerular damage.

The incidence of albuminuria increases over time in patients with SCD and often precedes the elevation of creatinine. Albuminuria was correlated with age and serum creatinine concentration but not with blood pressure or hemoglobin levels, suggesting that sickle cell glomerulopathy is not solely related to hemodynamic adaptations to chronic anemia. Nonetheless, studies in children with SCD showed a significant association between the markers of hemolysis (low hemoglobin and high lactate dehydrogenase levels) and proteinuria.

Proteinuria may be associated with defects in glomerular permselectivity, tubular injury, and/or specific single nucleotide polymorphisms in the *MYH9* and *APOL1* genes.

B. Progression of CKD

Repeated cycles of sickling in the relative hypoxic inner medulla may result in ischemic injury and microinfarcts, reduced medullary blood flow, and compensatory hyperfiltration. The latter can lead to microalbuminuria, proteinuria, glomerulosclerosis, and progressive CKD, similar to that seen in other kidney diseases such as diabetic nephropathy. Furthermore, the increased filtered sodium load and tubular reabsorption of sodium associated with hyperfiltration can augment renal oxygen consumption. Such hypermetabolic states can promote tubulointerstitial injury, in part through oxidative stress. More recently, renovascular pathology related to chronic NO depletion from ongoing intravascular hemolysis has been suggested to play a role in the progression of SCN. Chronic NO synthase (NOS) inhibition caused systemic and glomerular hypertension, glomerular ischemia, glomerulosclerosis, tubulointerstitial injury, and proteinuria in experimental animal models. Studies in the general population without SCD similarly suggested that CKD-induced NO deficiency contributes to the progression of chronic kidney injury. Risk factors associated with progression of CKD to end-stage renal disease: underlying hypertension, nephrotic range proteinuria, severe anemia, vaso-occlusive crisis, acute chest syndrome, stroke, βS-gene haplotype, genetic variants of *MYH9* and *APOL1*, pulmonary hypertension, and infection

with parvovirus B19. Protective factors include coinheritance with α-thalassemia and higher fetal hemoglobin.

C. Blood Pressure

Patients with sickle cell disease generally have lower blood pressure compared with their healthy unaffected counterparts due to presumed reduced vascular reactivity, compensatory systemic vasodilatation associated with microvascular disturbances from sickling of red blood cells and thrombotic complications, elevated levels of prostaglandins and nitric oxide, and possibly renal sodium and water wasting associated with suboptimal medullary concentrating activity. Blood pressures in the "normal" range defined for the general population may thus represent hypertension in patients with sickle cell disease.

D. Glomerulopathy Seen in Patients With SCD

Secondary focal segmental glomerulosclerosis (FSGS) and its variants are major glomerular lesions observed in SCD. Both collapsing and expansive patterns of FSGS have been described. The development of FSGS is likely adaptive to the initial glomerular hyperfiltration followed by repeated episodes of ischemia and reperfusion injuries. Glomerular hypertrophy was found to be greater in HbSS patients than in idiopathic FSGS. Medullary fibrosis is prominent, suggesting that SCD-associated FSGS affects mainly the juxtamedullary nephrons supplied by the vasa recta. Membranoproliferative glomerulonephropathy and thrombotic microangiopathy may also occur, but at lower frequency than FSGS. Membranoproliferative glomerulonephritis (MPGN) with mesangial expansion and basement membrane duplication may be seen either as an isolated finding or in association with FSGS. It has been suggested that this rare form of MPGN is caused by fragmented red blood cells lodged in isolated capillary loops and phagocytosed by mesangial cells, stimulating expansion of the mesangium and new basement membrane deposition. Although MPGN was initially attributed to immune complex injury, subsequent studies demonstrated that MPGN commonly occurred without immune-complex deposits. In essence, the absence of immune complexes and electron-dense deposits differentiates SCD-associated MPGN from idiopathic MPGN. Although rare with modern screening for blood-borne pathogens, HIV nephropathy, and hepatitis-associated glomerulonephropathies may be seen.

▶ Clinical Findings

A. Symptoms and Signs

Progressive decline in GFR associated with increasing proteinuria may lead to glomerular injury and overt CKD or ESRD. The acute onset of edema and nephrotic syndrome suggest causes other than SCN such as idiopathic primary FSGS or minimal change disease. Although less common, patients with SCD may develop proteinuria due to MPGN (without immune-complex deposits), or rarely due to HIV nephropathy or hepatitis-associated glomerulonephropathies.

B. Laboratory Findings

Assessment of renal function in SCD patients based on serum creatinine (SCr) or creatinine-based equations may overestimate true GFR. Nonetheless, the progression from a seemingly "normal GFR" to an overt decrease in GFR, particularly when accompanied by proteinuria portends poor renal prognosis. Over the last decade, Cystatin C (CystC) has been extensively studied as an alternative endogenous marker of kidney function in cirrhotic patients because it is independent of muscle mass. Studies in SCD patients are currently limited. In a series of 98 subjects with homozygous SS disease (55 females: 43 males; mean age 34 ± 2.3 years), a strong association between cystatin C (Cys-C) and GFR and albuminuria was demonstrated. The Cys-C based CKD-EPI showed the greatest agreement with measured GFR using (99m)Tc-DTPA nuclear renal scan compared with other commonly used Cys-C-based or creatinine-based MDRD and CKD-EPI equations. Whether CystC-based equations may enable clinicians to more accurately assess renal function in SCD patients remain to be studied. However, it is noteworthy that CystC levels may be increased in high cell turnover states (such as hyperthyroidism, steroid use, and malignancy), advanced age, gender and ethnicity, fat mass, and diabetes, among others.

C. Imaging Studies

For clinical purposes, renal ultrasound should be adequate to estimate kidney size and to exclude the likelihood of renal medullary carcinoma. Further evaluation with computed tomography or magnetic resonance imaging studies should be performed as clinically indicated.

▶ Differential Diagnosis

The diagnosis of sickle cell nephropathy is based on clinical manifestations and is primarily a diagnosis of exclusion. Initial evaluation should include review of recent or current use of nephrotoxic medications. Common causes of proteinuria unrelated to SCN should not be overlooked. Active urine sediments suggest pathology other than SCN. Imaging studies including kidney ultrasound to rule out obstructive uropathy, bladder scanning to assess post-void retention or bladder neck obstruction, and computed tomography scan with or without contrast agent should be done as clinically

indicated. Both infectious and non-infectious serologies associated with glomerular diseases based on age, gender, and risks should be done at the discretion of the clinician. The former include HIV, hepatitis B and hepatitis C, among others. Kidney biopsy should be considered in the presence of active urinary sediment, significant proteinuria with predominant albuminuria (ie, >1 g/day), or unexplained rapid kidney function deterioration.

▶ Treatment

1. Maneuvers to reduce sickling crises are of unclear benefit, because neither the frequency of sickling crises nor the severity of anemia has consistently been shown to predict albuminuria or CKD. The theoretical benefit of nonsteroidal anti-inflammatory drugs (NSAIDs) in any patient with glomerular hyperfiltration has not consistently been shown. NSAID use in patients with SCD should be avoided due to the potential for adverse hemodynamic-related renal function deterioration, precipitation of papillary necrosis, and the development of NSAID-associated interstitial nephritis and glomerulonephropathies.

2. Although the use of angiotensin converting enzyme inhibitors and angiotensin receptor blockers are commonly used to reduce proteinuria in addition to slowing CKD progression and lowering blood pressures in nonsickle cell nephropathies, significant antiproteinuric benefits have not been proven in patients with sickle cell disease. The most updated Cochrane database review in 2015 revealed a potential for reduction in microalbuminuria and proteinuria with the use of captopril among patients with sickle cell disease compared with those without the disease. Confirmatory studies are needed.

3. The use of hydroxyurea has been suggested to reduce proteinuria and hyperfiltration.

4. All forms of renal replacement may be beneficial to patients with end-stage renal disease from sickle cell anemia. Both hemo and peritoneal dialytic therapies may be offered to patients reaching end-stage renal disease if there is no modality-specific contraindication. Both modalities may confer their own theoretical advantages. Hemodialysis can be considered in the setting of urgent or emergent need for standard and exchange blood transfusions whereas the slow rate of ultrafiltration minimizes any acute rise in hematocrit, thus a lower risk of vaso-occlusive crisis. Although survival of transplant recipients with SCD is inferior to that of matched African–American recipients without the disease, survival of sickle cell disease patients is comparable with that of matched diabetic patients. One-year graft survival exceeds 60% to 80%.

In general, patients with sickle cell disease has reduced life expectancy by 25–30 years. The median survival among patients with and without kidney failure is 29 and 51 years, respectively. Survival is substantially worse among patients with SCD receiving any form of renal replacement therapy compared with their counterpart without the disease.

KEY READINGS

Ashley-Koch AE et al: MYH9 and APOL1 are both associated with sickle cell disease nephropathy. Br J Hemaetol 2011;155:386.

Asnani M et al: Cystatin C: a useful marker of glomerulopathy in sickle cell disease? Blood Cells Mol Dis 2015;54:65.

Haymann JP et al: Glomerular hyperfiltration in adult sickle cell anemia: a frequent hemolysis associated feature. Clin J Am Soc Nephrol 2010;5:756.

Huang E et al: Improved survival among sickle cell kidney transplant recipients in the recent era. Nephrol Dial Transplant 2013;28:1039.

Nath KA, Hebbel RP: Sickle cell disease: renal manifestations and mechanisms. Nat Rev Nephrol 2015;11:161.

Pham PT et al: Chronic kidney disease and sickle cell disease. In: Kimmel PL, Rosenberg ME (eds). Chronic Renal Disease. San Diego: Elsevier, 2015, p. 513.

Sasongko TH et al: Angiotensin-converting enzyme (ACE) inhibitors for proteinuria and microalbuminuria in people with sickle cell disease. Cochrane Database Syst Rev 2015;4:CD009191.

Wang WC: Prognostic factors and the response to hydroxyurea treatment in sickle cell disease. Exp Biol Med (Maywood) 2016;241:730.

RENAL MALIGNANCY

ESSENTIALS OF DIAGNOSIS

▸ Renal medullary carcinoma occurs almost exclusively in patients with sickle cell trait (not sickle cell disease).

▸ It typically presents in young patients (20–30 years old) as an aggressive metastatic disease at the time of diagnosis.

▸ Affected individuals may present with hematuria, flank pain, abdominal mass, or weight loss.

▸ Symptomatic patients with sickle cell trait should be evaluated with an ultrasound (or other imaging studies at the discretion of the clinician).

▸ General Considerations

Chronic ischemic injuries triggering recurrent degeneration and regeneration of the epithelium of the distal collecting ducts may incite formation of renal medullary cancer, an aggressive tumor specific to patients with sickle hemoglobinopathies. Renal medullary cancer must be differentiated from a renal tubular abnormality associated with abnormal hemoglobinemia. Metastatic disease is generally present at diagnosis and portends a poor prognosis with a median survival of 3 months following diagnosis. Early diagnosis may improve morbidity and mortality.

KEY READING

Alvarez O et al: Renal medullary carcinoma and sickle cell trait: a systematic review. Pediatr Blood Cancer 2015;62:1694.

SUMMARY

Hemolysis, vasoocclusion, and ischemia reperfusion are the clinical hallmarks of sickle cell disease. The underlying mechanisms of renal injury or SCN primarily relate to hypoxia and ischemia. SCN encompasses a wide range of renal abnormalities indicating that all segments of the nephron can be affected. Functionally and clinically patient may present with hyposthenuria, isosthenuria, hematuria, hyperfiltration, proteinuria, hyperkalemia, papillary necrosis, secondary FSGS or other form of glomerulopathy, acute and chronic kidney injury, progressive decline in GRF and eventual development of ESRD. All forms of renal replacement may be beneficial to patients with end-stage renal disease from sickle cell anemia. These include hemodialysis, peritoneal dialysis and kidney transplantation. Although rare, renal medullary carcinoma should be excluded as clinically indicated, particularly in adolescents or young adults with sickle cell trait. The renal manifestations of SCD is summarized in Table 48–1. Figure 48-2 summarizes the pathogenic mechanisms of hematuria, concentrating defect, and CKD associated with FSGS in patients with SCD. The common inciting event is red blood cell sickling in the vasa recta.

Table 48–1 Renal manifestations of sickle cell disease.

Abnormalities	Comments
Hematuria	• Left 4 times more than right, 10% bilateral
Renal tubular disorders 1. Functional abnormalities in the distal nephron • Decreased concentrating ability • Incomplete form of RTA • Impaired potassium secretion (intact renin–angiotensin–aldosterone system)	• Urinary diluting capacity is preserved (see text) • RTA typically not clinically significant, but can be unmasked with reduction in GFR • Defect in potassium secretion typically not clinically apparent but hyperkalemia can manifest in the presence of additional insults (eg, renal dysfunction, rhabdomyolysis, volume contraction)
2. Supranormal proximal tubular function • Increased sodium reabsorption • Increased phosphate reabsorption • Increased β_2-microglobulin reabsorption • Increased uric acid secretion • Increased creatinine secretion	• Creatinine-based estimated glomerular filtration rate (eGFR) may be greatly overestimated
Acute and chronic kidney injury 1. Acute kidney injury 2. Chronic kidney injury and end-stage renal disease	• AKI is most commonly due to volume depletion in the setting of sickle cell crisis due to impaired concentrating ability • Glomerulopathy associated with proteinuria and CKD/ESRD – Secondary focal segmental glomerulosclerosis (most common lesion) – MPGN without immune complex deposits – Thrombotic microangiopathy (associated with history of retinitis) – HIV nephropathy and hepatitis-associated glomerulopathies (rare, likely due to blood borne viral infections from transfusions. NAT may reduce incidence further)
Renal medullary carcinoma	• Occurs exclusively in patients with sickle cell trait

CKD, chronic kidney disease; ESRD, end-stage renal disease; MPGN, membranoproliferative glomerulonephritis; NAT, nuclear acid testing.

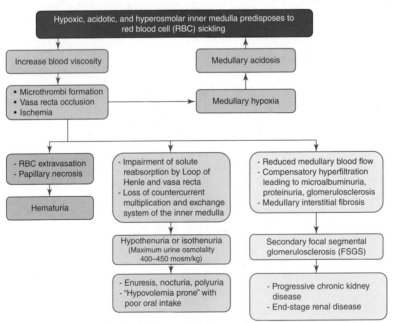

*The common inciting event is red blood cell sickling in the vasa recta.
CKD, chronic kidne disease; *SCN*, sickle cell nephropathy.

▲ **Figure 48–2** Pathogenic mechanisms of hematuria, concentrating defect and CKD associated with FSGS in patients with SCD. The common inciting event is red blood cell sickling in the vasa recta.

■ CHAPTER REVIEW QUESTIONS

1. A 21-year-old African–American man presented to the emergency room with a chief complaint of painless pinkish urine. He has no significant past medical history except for known sickle cell trait. Physical examination: afebrile, blood pressure 100/70 mm Hg, heart rate 76 beats/min, temperature 98.7°F, and respiratory rate 16 breaths/min. His examination is unremarkable. Urinalysis shows 3+ blood and >800 red blood cells per high power field. The patient was sent home on ciprofloxacin for presumed urinary tract infection. Three months later he represented to the emergency room with flank pain, recurrent gross hematuria, weight loss, chest pain, shortness of breath, and lightheadedness. Pan-body CT scan was performed to evaluate weight loss. Chest CT showed bilateral pulmonary nodules, hilar lymphadenopathy, and multiple vertebral lesions.

   Which one of the following is the most likely cause of his hematuria?
   A. Pyelonephritis
   B. Renal cell medullary carcinoma
   C. Papillary necrosis
   D. Kidney stone

2. A 19-year-old African–American man with SCD presented to your office for a preathletic physical. He described himself as healthy and physically active. He denied history of pharyngitis, tonsillitis or skin infection. He consumes 11 oz of premier protein drink with meals three times daily. His vital signs were: blood pressure 106/70 mm Hg, heart rate 76 beats/min, temperature 98.6°F, and respiratory rate 12 breaths/min. His examination was notable for pale conjunctivae and nailbeds. His lungs were clear to auscultation and percussion. He was noted to have a soft grade 1/6 systolic ejection murmur. His abdomen was soft, nondistended and nontender and he had no peripheral edema.

   Laboratory findings:
   Sodium 139 mEq/L, potassium 4.2 mEq/L, chloride 105 mEq/L, bicarbonate 24 mEq/L, blood urea nitrogen 8 mg/dL, creatinine 0.4 mg/dL, WBC count 4.2 cells/uL, hemoglobin 6.8 g/dL, hematocrit 19%, platelet count 230,000/mmol. Urinalysis: specific gravity 1.012, pH 5.5, trace blood, and trace protein. Urinary albumin to creatinine ratio is 100 ug/mg.

   The patient was advised to refrain from physical activities and return in 2 weeks for follow-up. Repeat urine studies at 2 week follow-up reveal persistent microalbuminuria.

   Which one of the following is a plausible explanation for microalbuminuria?
   A. Loss of glomerular permselectivity
   B. Protein drink
   C. Rigorous exercise
   D. Acute poststreptococcal glomerulonephritis

3. After excluding malignancy, management of gross hematuria in patients with sickle cell disease or sickle cell trait may include all of the following except:
   A. Bed rest and oral hydration
   B. Unilateral nephrectomy of the affected kidney
   C. Urinary alkalinization
   D. Blood transfusions

4. A 14-year-old African–American man with known sickle cell trait is brought to the emergency room by his mother for evaluation of transient painless reddish-colored urine. The patient reports being in good health except for a minor fall 2 days prior to his emergency room visit. He denies recent history of shortness of breath, chills, fever, joint pain, dysuria, abdominal pain, or flank pain. His vital signs are—blood pressure 110/70 mm Hg, pulse 70 beats/min, temperature 98.7°F, and respiratory rate 12 breaths/min. His physical examination is unremarkable except for a 3-cm superficial laceration on his right forearm. Urine dipstick reveals 3+ blood. Urine microscopy shows >800 red blood cells per high power field.

   Which one of the following is a plausible explanation for his hematuria?
   A. Urinary tract infection
   B. Papillary necrosis
   C. Kidney stone
   D. Rhabdomyolysis

5. Manifestations of tubular dysfunction in SCD patients include all of the following except:
   A. Diminished urine concentrating ability
   B. Diminished diluting capacity
   C. Increased proximal tubular secretion of uric acid and creatinine
   D. Increased tubular reabsorption of low molecular weight protein (β_2-microglobulins) and phosphate

Hemodialysis

Michael V. Rocco, MD, MSCE

Shahriar Moossavi, MD, PhD

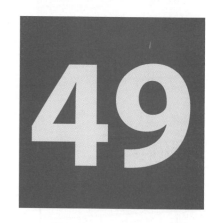

49

▶ General Considerations

The major forces responsible for solute transport across the membrane are diffusion and convection. Diffusion is influenced by the concentration gradient of the solute, the solute characteristics (eg, molecular weight and charge), and the membrane characteristics (eg, pore size and number). Removal of solutes by diffusion is enhanced by a large concentration gradient, small solute size, and a membrane with a large surface area and many large pores. The concentration gradient is maximized by using countercurrent flow of blood and dialysate.

In convection, hydrostatic or osmotic pressure forces water across the membrane. The water transport facilitates the passage of solutes across the membrane. The term ultrafiltration describes the solute and fluid removal via convection.

In hemodialysis, the predominant mechanism for solute removal is through diffusion, with a smaller amount of solute clearance occurring by convection. Thus, hemodialysis is very effective in removing solutes of small-molecular-weight, but is relatively inefficient in removing solutes of larger sizes. In addition, hemodialysis is an inefficient means of removal of protein-bound substances. Only the free portion of these solutes can diffuse across the membrane and be removed. The removal rate of protein-bound compounds thus depends on the concentration of the unbound solute, the size of the protein, and the replacement rate of the unbound solute.

In hemofiltration, the predominant mechanism for solute removal is through convection; thus, this procedure has the ability to remove solutes of larger molecular size when coupled with a dialysis membrane with a large pore size.

▶ Treatment

A. Indications for Starting Chronic Dialysis Therapy

Patients should be considered for initiation of chronic hemodialysis therapy once the estimated glomerular filtration rate

(GFR) is less than 15 mL/min. In most patients, the CKD-EPI equation can be used to estimate the GFR; the MDRD equation is also acceptable. Either a cystatin C estimated GFR or a 24-hour urine collection for creatinine and urea should be considered in those patients who have reduced muscle mass due to medical conditions such as amputations or limitation on mobility due to congestive heart failure, claudication, chronic lung disease requiring oxygen therapy, etc. There are no randomized trials that suggest an optimal time to initiate chronic dialysis therapy, so clinical judgment is important in making this decision in individual patients. The National Kidney Foundation Kidney Disease Outcome Quality Initiative (NKF-KDOQI) guidelines suggest that the decision to initiate dialysis should be based primarily on an assessment of signs and/or symptoms associated with uremia, evidence of protein-energy wasting, and the ability to safely manage metabolic abnormalities and/or volume overload with medical therapy.

1. Earlier initiation of dialysis—There are specific indications for starting chronic hemodialysis therapy at a level above a GFR of 15 mL/min. These conditions include intractable fluid overload not responsive to diuretics, hyperkalemia unresponsive to medical therapy, metabolic acidosis not fully corrected by medical therapy, malnutrition or weight loss not ascribed to other medical conditions, or decreasing functional status. It may also be desirable to start home dialysis therapies at a higher level of GFR to minimize training difficulties due to neurologic dysfunction at lower levels of GFR.

2. Later initiation of dialysis—Patients can be considered for a later initiation of dialysis if they are asymptomatic from a uremic standpoint, have adequate nutritional status, and do not have a decline in either dry weight or serum albumin levels. If renal replacement therapy is delayed, then the patient should be reassessed on a regular basis for a change in these parameters.

KEY READINGS

Inker LA et al: Estimating glomerular filtration rate from serum creatinine and cystatin C. N Engl J Med 2012;367:20.
KDOQI Clinical Practice Guideline for Hemodialysis Adequacy: 2015 update. Am J Kidney Dis 2015;66:884.
Levey AS et al: A new equation to estimate glomerular filtration rate. Ann Intern Med 2009;150:604.

B. Apparatus

The major parts of the dialysis machine are the blood pump, dialyzer, dialysate pump, safety monitors, and alarms (Figure 49–1).

1. Dialyzer— The artificial kidney or dialyzer consists of the blood compartment, the dialysate compartment, and the semipermeable membrane. The surface area of the dialyzer membrane can be increased by using either parallel plates or hollow fibers. Most dialyzers used in adults have a surface area between 1.5 and 2.4 m^2. Parallel plate dialyzers are rarely used today. Most dialysis membranes in use today are made from a variety of synthetic materials including polyamide, polyarylethersulfone, polymethylmethacrylate, polyvinylpyrrolidone, acrylonitrile-sodium methallylsulfonate (AN-69), polyacrylonitrile, polycarbonate, and polysulfone. Cellulose membranes are being used with decreasing frequency in the United States.

The contact of blood with the membrane can result in activation of the complement system, with the release of bradykinin or cytokines. The biocompatibility of the dialysis membrane depends not only on the material used but also on the degree of blood contact with the dialysate. Unsubstituted cellulose membranes activate the complement system. To decrease complement activation, the hydroxyl groups of cellulose have been replaced with acetate or a synthetic material has been added to cellulose.

2. Membrane characteristics and solute clearance— A high efficiency membrane has the ability to remove small solutes well. The removal of small solutes is a function of the membrane surface area. High-efficiency membranes have a large surface area. The efficiency of a dialyzer is measured by the clearance of urea (MW 60) and is expressed as KoA_{urea}. Larger molecular-weight solutes are removed to a greater degree by membranes with larger membrane pores. These membranes are referred to as high-flux membranes. High-flux and many high-efficiency membranes also have the ability to achieve a high ultrafiltration rate. The water permeability of a membrane is specified by its ultrafiltration coefficient (K_{uf}).

The clearance of creatinine (MW 113) by a dialyzer is usually about 20% less than the dialyzer urea clearance, despite the minimal difference in molecular weight. The removal of phosphorus (MW 31) by dialysis depends mostly on the time provided for dialysis per week, and also on the dialyzer efficiency and the predialysis phosphorus level. During dialysis, phosphorus is removed rapidly from plasma but not from the intracellular compartment. The slow equilibration between these compartments and bone is the major limiting factor of phosphorus removal.

Historically, middle molecule clearance was defined by the clearance of vitamin B_{12} (MW 1355). However, the clearance of vitamin B_{12} is low due to its high degree of protein binding. Thus, many high-flux dialyzers are now classified based on the clearance of molecules such as β_2-microglobulin (MW 11,800). With the introduction of high-flux dialyzers, the clearance of β_2-microglobulin has improved. Despite these improvements, the serum concentration of β_2-microglobulin remains markedly elevated in anuric hemodialysis patients using high-flux dialyzers. β_2-Microglobulin deposition is the cause of dialysis-associated amyloidosis.

3. Dialyzer reuse— Reuse of dialyzers is a common practice in outpatient dialysis units in the United States, but is less

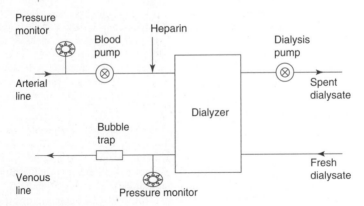

▲ **Figure 49–1.** Hemodialysis machine apparatus.

common in other countries. A method for the reuse process used in the United States has been written by the Association for the Advancement of Medical Instrumentation (AAMI). Each dialyzer should be labeled with the patient's identifying information. The total cell volume (TCV) should be measured prior to its first use. After the dialysis treatment, the membrane is rinsed with normal saline, pressure washed, and then cleansed with either bleach or a hydrogen peroxide mixture. Bleach can damage the membrane and increase protein loss with dialysis if it is used in inappropriately high concentrations. Once the membrane has been cleaned, its performance is evaluated by measuring the TCV. If the new value for TCV is >80% of the original TCV, it passes the performance test, and the membrane can be reused after disinfection and sterilization with a mixture of hydrogen peroxide, formaldehyde, or glutaraldehyde. The polysulfone membranes can also be heat sterilized. The final step of the reuse process is the removal of the germicide. Residual germicide can cause a burning sensation, itching, or other allergic reactions. The reuse of dialyzers needs an informed consent. Patients with bacteremia or hepatitis B are excluded from dialyzer reuse. HIV and hepatitis C infection are not considered contraindications to reuse. In general, membrane biocompatibility improves with dialyzer reuse. Exposure of the membrane to blood can result in the protein coating of the membrane. This protein coating may decrease complement activation. Dialyzers can be reused dozens of times without a significant loss of efficacy. A decrease in the reuse number may suggest an increased rate of clotting of the hollow fibers and can often be improved by adjusting the anticoagulation prescription.

4. Dialysis machine— The blood pump moves the blood from the arterial line through the dialyzer back to the venous line. The speed of the blood pump can be adjusted to between 200 and 600 mL/min. At any given time about 200–250 mL of blood is outside the patient. The dialysis pump sucks the dialysis fluid (dialysate) away from the dialyzer producing the transmembrane pressure. The transmembrane pressure can be adjusted to achieve the desired fluid removal. In modern dialysis machines, the transmembrane pressure is automatically adjusted by the dialysis machine based upon the amount of volume to be removed during the dialysis session and the type of ultrafiltration profiling chosen. The dialysate flow rate is usually between 500 and 800 mL/min and is usually set between 100 and 200 mL/min higher than the blood flow rate. The dialysate temperature can be adjusted. A lower temperature can cause peripheral vasoconstriction in the patient and thus improve hemodynamic stability.

The arterial and venous pressures are monitored during the dialysis treatment. The arterial pressure is measured before the blood pump to avoid excessive suction of blood and the venous pressure is measured before the blood returns to the access to avoid excessive resistance. A high

venous pressure in the access is suggestive of an impairment to flow in the venous outflow tract that could be due to stenosis in the venous outflow of the access, clotting in the venous chamber of the catheter, stenosis in native vessels through which the access drains, or kinking of the blood lines. A high negative arterial pressure is indicative of immature access, stenosis or scarring in the accessed area, suctioning against the vessel wall, or the use of long or small gauge needles or catheters.

Other safety guards included on dialysis machines are the air trap to detect air embolism, the blood leak detector to detect blood in the dialysate compartment, and the measurement of dialysate conductivity to detect a malfunction in mixing the dialysis solution. If one of these safety guards is triggered, the machine will alarm and in some cases shut down. If a blood leak is detected, the dialyzer will be replaced and the patient will be administered antibiotics to treat any possible contamination of blood with the dialysis solution.

5. Dialysis solution— The major electrolyte components of the dialysis solution are sodium, potassium, calcium, magnesium, chloride, bicarbonate, and glucose (Table 49–1). In some dialysis machines, the sodium concentration can be changed during the same treatment (sodium modeling). The concentration of potassium and calcium can be varied to some extent based on the patient's blood chemistries. Calcium and magnesium can react with the bicarbonate in an alkaline environment and precipitate as carbonate salts. These components are stored separately and the final dialysis solution is prepared during the treatment by mixing a concentrated solution of these components with treated water.

6. Water treatment— Dialysis water is obtained by processing water from the municipal water supply (Figure 49–2). The water is processed using guidelines developed by the Association for the Advancement of Medical Instrumentation (AAMI). With each dialysis treatment over 100 L

Table 49–1. Composition of dialysis solution.

Sodium 137	(135–148) mEq/L
Potassium	2.0 (0–3.0) mEq/L
Calcium	2.5 (0–3.5) mEq/L
Magnesium	0.75 mEq/L
Chloride	106 mEq/L
Bicarbonate	33 mEq/L
Acetate	4.0 mEq/L
Dextrose	100–200 mg/dL

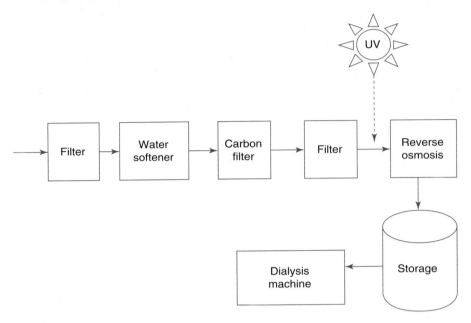

▲ **Figure 49–2.** Water treatment system.

of water is used to make the dialysis solution. Tap water is contaminated with organic and inorganic compounds, heavy metals and trace elements, bacteria, and endotoxins. In areas in which tap water is hard, a water softener can be used to facilitate calcium and magnesium removal. Organic contaminants such as chloroethylene, benzene, toluene, pesticides, herbicides, chloramine, chlorine, and other halogens are removed by a carbon filter. Chloramine is added by some municipal water agencies to help in the water cleaning process; this agent can cause hemolysis even at very low concentrations. Once the tap water is processed in these preliminary steps, the final processing for removal of contaminants occurs using either reverse osmosis (RO) or deionization. In RO, contaminants are removed by forcing water across a semipermeable membrane using high pressures. RO is very effective in removing bacteria, viruses, pyrogens, and heavy metals such as aluminum. Ultraviolet light can also damage and fragment bacteria. This bacterial debris, however, needs to be removed by the RO system. With deionization, the ionic contaminants are replaced by hydrogen or hydroxyl ions. In addition, various filters can be added to improve water quality. A 5-μm prefilter is used to remove large particles at the beginning of the water treatment system. Fine particles are removed by special filters prior to RO to protect the RO system. In addition, microfilters can be added to enhance the removal of microbial contaminants. Standard quality dialysis fluid is not free from bacteria and endotoxins. Ultrapure dialysate has a lower level of endotoxins and bacteria than AAMI standard dialysate; ultrapure dialysate is

commonly used in most Western European countries and is used in some centers in the United States.

KEY READINGS

AAMI Dialysis Standards Collection. http://www.aami.org/productspublications/ProductDetail.aspx?ItemNumber=920. Accessed December 14, 2016.

Damasiewicz MJ, Polkinghorne KR, Kerr PG: Water quality in conventional and home haemodialysis. Nat Rev Nephrol 2012;8:725.

Kasparek T, Rodriguez OE: What medical directors need to know about dialysis facility water management. Clin J Am Soc Nephrol 2015;10:1061.

C. Access

In patients with a GFR less than 30 mL/min, veins that are suitable for use for a permanent hemodialysis access should not be used for venipuncture. The placement of subclavian catheters or peripherally inserted central catheters (PICCs) should be avoided. Discussions regarding the choice of dialysis modality should begin once the patient's estimated GFR is less than 30 mL/min. Once the patient chooses hemodialysis as the preferred dialysis modality, a permanent dialysis access should be placed in a timely manner to ensure that this access is functional at the time that the patient initiates chronic hemodialysis therapy. In general, an arteriovenous (AV) fistula should be placed at least 6 months prior to the anticipated start of chronic hemodialysis treatment. This will allow adequate time for any needed intervention to promote fistula maturation, for example, angioplasty of a juxta-anastomotic stenosis or ligation of a large competing collateral vein, and still allow adequate time for AV fistula maturation. An AV graft should be placed 3–6 weeks prior to the anticipated start of hemodialysis. In addition to a history and physical examination, appropriate preoperative assessment of the patient should include an evaluation of the brachial and radial arteries and peripheral veins of the patient using Doppler ultrasound. In select cases, an evaluation of the central veins should be performed, especially if the patient has had prior internal jugular or subclavian lines.

1. Type of dialysis access

A. ARTERIOVENOUS FISTULAS—The AV fistula is the preferred type of chronic hemodialysis vascular access due to a higher primary and secondary patency rate compared to AV grafts. The preferred order of placement for an AV fistula is a wrist (radial-cephalic) primary AV fistula, any other forearm primary AV fistula, an elbow (brachial-cephalic) primary AV fistula, and a transposed brachial basilic vein fistula. This order of placement helps to maximize the number of fistulas that an individual patient can receive. The initial fistulas should be placed in the nondominant arm.

B. ARTERIOVENOUS GRAFTS—An AV graft should be placed only if an AV fistula cannot be placed due to either small veins or marked obesity of the arm that will render cannulation of an AV fistula difficult due to the depth of the access below the skin.

C. CATHETERS AND PORTS—Nontunneled central venous catheters should be used only in hospitalized patients and only temporally. A tunneled central venous catheter should be placed as soon as clinically feasible. These tunneled catheters should be placed in the internal jugular vein on the side opposite to an existing or planned AV fistula or graft in order to reduce the risk of central vein stenosis on the side of the permanent access. The position of the tip of the catheter should be verified radiologically. Catheters have a high rate of infection, and infection control measures are important to help reduce the rate of infectious complications. Catheters should be examined by trained personnel prior to each dialysis session to assess for possible infection. The catheter dressing should be changed only by dialysis staff. The catheter should not be used for any purpose other than dialysis, except in emergencies when no other blood access is available. The use of an antibiotic lock solution may decrease the rate of catheter-related blood stream infections. A lock solution consists of an antibiotic, for example, gentamicin, vancomycin, cefazolin, or ceftazidime and an anticoagulant, for example, heparin or citrate. Recent studies have shown the superiority of citrate-based lock solutions as compared to heparin-based solutions.

2. Monitoring for access dysfunction

Surveillance for access dysfunction on a regular basis may help improve access patency rates. All permanent accesses should be examined on a regular basis to detect possible stenoses. A pulsatile segment, a high-pitched bruit or an area with a decreased thrill may be suggestive of stenosis and should be evaluated by a fistulogram or other radiologic technique. There are also surveillance techniques that can be used to assess for access dysfunction. Persistent abnormalities in either the physical examination or in the surveillance techniques should result in referral of the patient for a fistulogram or other radiologic evaluation.

Several techniques can be used to assess for access dysfunction in AV fistulas and gortex grafts. Regardless of the technique used, serial observations should be used to determine changes in the functioning of the access over time. New guidelines for the monitoring of permanent accesses should be available from the National Kidney Foundation's Kidney Disease Outcomes Quality Improvement (KDOQI) in early 2018.

3. Correction of access complications

A. ARTERIOVENOUS FISTULAS—A patient should have an evaluation of an AV fistula in the presence of inadequate blood flow, hemodynamically significant venous stenosis, aneurysm formation, arm swelling, or ischemia in the access arm. A stenosis is considered to be hemodynamically significant if it is greater than 50% and is accompanied by abnormal physical findings, persistent abnormal surveillance tests, has had a previous thrombosis, or has resulted in an otherwise unexplained decrease in the measured dose of hemodialysis. Hemodynamically significant stenosis should be corrected by either surgical revision or percutaneous transluminal angioplasty. Thrombosis of an AV fistula should be performed as early as possible after the thrombus is detected in order to increase the chances of a successful declotting. Steal syndrome is often manifested by pain, but if serious and untreated can lead to loss of function and even loss of the limb. Treatment of moderate to severe ischemia is surgical and should be conducted expediently if there is loss of motor function.

B. ARTERIOVENOUS GRAFTS—A patient should have revision of an AV graft in the presence of either graft degeneration or pseudoaneurysm formation. If a graft has a 50% or greater stenosis in either the venous outflow tract or the arterial inflow tract, and the stenosis is accompanied by abnormal physical findings, decreased access flow, measured static pressure, or the presence of a past thrombosis, then the stenosis should be treated with either surgical revision or percutaneous transluminal angioplasty. Thrombosis of an AV graft should be done in an expeditious manner to increase the chances of a successful declotting. Thrombus can be treated by surgical thrombectomy, mechanical thrombolysis, or pharmacomechanical thrombolysis. An infected AV graft will need treatment with intravenous antibiotics and it will need to be resected if the infection is extensive.

C. CATHETERS— A catheter is considered to be dysfunctional if it is unable to deliver a blood flow rate of at least 300 mL/min with a prepump arterial pressure of –250 mm Hg. A dysfunctional catheter can be corrected with thrombolytics, endoluminal brush, or if the catheter is incorrectly positioned or of an inadequate length, by catheter replacement. Thrombolytics can be provided using an intraluminal lytic intradialytic lock, an intracatheter thrombolytic infusion, or an interdialytic lock.

The extent of the infection determines how an infected catheter should be treated. A catheter exit site infection, in the absence of a tunnel infection, is usually treated with topical antibiotics or oral antibiotics. All other catheter infections are treated with parenteral antibiotics. The antibiotics used should cover the suspected organisms, which are usually *Staphylococcus* or *Streptococcus*. Definitive antibiotic therapy should be chosen based on the organisms isolated by blood culture. The catheter should be removed if the patient does not have an improvement in clinical status in the first 36–48 hours after the initiation of parenteral antibiotic therapy or if the patient is clinically unstable. Catheter salvage can be attempted if the patient is clinically stable. Under these circumstances, the patient should be treated with parenteral antibiotics for 2–3 weeks.

KEY READINGS

Allon M. Novel paradigms for dialysis vascular access: Introduction. Clin J Am Soc Nephrol 2013;8:2183.

Beathard GA: How is arteriovenous fistula longevity best prolonged?: The role of optimal fistula placement. Semin Dial 2015;28:20.

Woo K, Lok CE: New insights into dialysis vascular access: What is the optimal vascular access type and timing of access creation in CKD and dialysis datients? Clin J Am Soc Nephrol 2016;11:1487.

D. Assessing the Adequacy of Hemodialysis

Providing a dose of dialysis above a certain minimal level can reduce patient mortality and morbidity. The delivered dose of dialysis should be measured monthly by obtaining a predialysis and postdialysis blood sample for blood urea nitrogen (BUN). It is critical that the post-BUN sample be obtained using a standardized method since recirculation can significantly alter the value of the postdialysis BUN. Both the stop flow or slow flow techniques are acceptable methods for obtaining the postdialysis BUN sample. These samples are then used to calculate the dose of dialysis, expressed as Kt/V, where K is the dialyzer clearance for urea, t is the number of minutes of the treatment, and V is the

volume of distribution of urea in the body, approximately equal to total body water.

1. Minimum dose of hemodialysis— Results from multiple clinical trials and observational studies suggest that the minimum dose for three times per week hemodialysis is a Kt/V of at least 1.2. To achieve this delivered dose of dialysis, the prescribed Kt/V should be at least 1.3. For patients receiving hemodialysis on a schedule other than three times per week, the minimum standardized dose of dialysis should be an sKt/V of at least 2.0. This level of sKt/V is equivalent to a single pool Kt/V of 1.2 for patients receiving hemodialysis three times per week.

2. Preservation of residual renal function— Residual kidney function is an important predictor of outcomes in hemodialysis patients. Therefore, efforts should be taken to preserve residual kidney function in chronic hemodialysis patients, including the avoidance of nephrotoxins, such as contrast dye, nonsteroidal anti-inflammatory drugs (NSAIDs), and aminoglycosides, and the use of an angiotensin-converting enzyme (ACE) inhibitor or angiotensin receptor blockers (when not contraindicated).

KEY READINGS

Daugirdas JT et al: Standard Kt/Vurea: a method of calculation that includes effects of fluid removal and residual kidney clearance. Kidney Int 2010;77:637.

Daugirdas JT et al: Improved equation for estimating single-pool Kt/V at higher dialysis frequencies. Nephrol Dial Transplant 2013;28:2156.

Mathew AT et al: Preservation of residual kidney function in hemodialysis patients: reviving an old concept. Kidney Int 2016;90:262.

E. Volume Removal in Hemodialysis

Volume removal is an important aspect of the hemodialysis prescription. Chronic volume overload leads to hypertension and left ventricular hypertrophy, which in turn contributes to increased cardiovascular mortality. Conversely, hypotension from excess fluid removal can lead to repeated bouts of regional wall motion abnormalities of the heart, which is also associated with an increase in cardiovascular events. Thus, it is imperative that the patient's dry weight, the weight that is targeted at the end of the dialysis treatment, is appropriately set.

Ideally, a patient's dry weight should be the weight at which the patient is euvolemic on a minimal number and dose of blood pressure medications. An iterative process whereby the dry weight is slowly decreased, followed by tapering of antihypertensive medications, followed by more gentle decrease of the dry weight can be used to achieve this goal. Bioimpedance has been used, typically in the research setting to determine a patient's dry weight; multifrequency measures tend to be more accurate than single frequency bioimpedance.

Sodium modeling is the conscious variation of dialysate sodium levels during a dialysis session. Typically, sodium modelling starts with a higher sodium level that is decreased during the dialysis session. Sodium modeling is no longer used as it resulted in sodium loading and an increase in interdialytic weight gains. Ultrafiltration modeling is the conscious variation of fluid removal during the dialysis session. Using this method, more fluid is typically removed early in the dialysis session, with lesser amounts removed later in the session. Most hemodialysis machines will allow for a choice of several ultrafiltration models. It is unclear if this method is beneficial in achieving the patient's dry weight while also preventing hypotensive episodes.

The patient also needs to be mindful of salt and fluid intake as, at least from epidemiologic studies, a higher inter-dialytic weight gain is associated with an increased mortality rate.

KEY READINGS

Assimon M et al: Ultrafiltration rate and mortality in maintenance hemodialysis patients. Am J Kidney Dis 2016;68:911.
Heckig M: Predialysis serum sodium level, dialysate sodium, and mortality in maintenance hemodialysis patients: the dialysis outcomes and practice patterns study (DOPPS) Am J Kidney Dis 2012;59:238.

F. Alternative Hemodialysis Therapies

Alternative schedules for hemodialysis were first developed in the 1960s. Many of the hemodialysis treatments of that era were performed at home, including nocturnal hemodialysis. These home treatments became less popular after Medicare began to cover the costs of performing hemodialysis treatments in an outpatient setting in 1973. In the past 10 years, there has been a renewed interest in both performing hemodialysis at home and performing hemodialysis more than three times per week on a routine basis.

1. In-center hemodialysis six times per week— Most studies of patients receiving dialysis six times per week (either in-center or at home) have involved small numbers of patients; the largest is the Frequent Hemodialysis Network (FHN) trials sponsored by the National Institutes of Health. In this trial, participants randomized to more frequent in-center dialysis had significant benefit in the co-primary outcome of death or increase in left ventricular mass and death and decrease in physical health composite score as well as improved control of hypertension and hyperphosphatemia.

Randomized trials of more frequent dialysis have shown that short daily dialysis using conventional dialysis machines is associated with a decrease in left ventricular mass, improvement in the physical component of quality of life, and improved control of both hyperphosphatemia and hypertension. Long-term follow-up of this cohort of patients also demonstrated improved mortality, despite patients not continuing long term on more frequent therapy.

2. Home hemodialysis— Home hemodialysis currently accounts for less than 1% of all hemodialysis treatments in the United States. It is more common in other countries such as New Zealand. Home dialysis can be performed during the day or evening 3–6 days per week or overnight for three to six nights per week. Patients receiving home hemodialysis three times per week in the United States have a lower mortality rate and fewer hospitalizations compared to patients receiving in-center hemodialysis; however, it is unclear if these results are due to selection bias, the modality itself, or some combination of the two.

Nocturnal home hemodialysis six times per week is performed in small numbers of patients throughout the developed world. Several small randomized trials of more frequent overnight home hemodialysis have shown that this modality can provide benefits in decreasing left ventricular mass and improved control of hypertension and hyperphosphatemia. Normalization of phosphorus levels was often achieved without the need for phosphorus binders. One small long-term follow-up study did not show an improvement in mortality compared to standard home hemodialysis.

3. Wearable artificial kidney— Several investigators have developed prototypes for a portable kidney that can be worn by the patient and provide for hemodialysis for short periods of time. Newer membranes, some using nanotechnology, are being developed to help minimize the risk of blood clotting. There has been very limited testing of these devices in humans thus far.

KEY READINGS

Chertow GM et al: Long-term effects of frequent in-center hemodialysis. J Am Soc Nephrol 2016;27:1830.
The FHN Trial Group. In-center hemodialysis six times per week versus three times per week. N Engl J Med 2010;363:2287.
Rocco MV et al: The effects of frequent nocturnal home hemodialysis: the frequent hemodialysis network nocturnal trial. Kidney Int 2011;80:1080.
Rocco MV et al: Long-term effects of frequent nocturnal hemodialysis on mortality: The Frequent Hemodialysis Network (FHN) Nocturnal Trial. Am J Kidney Dis 2015;66:459.

G. Hemodiafiltration

With hemodialysis, solutes are removed almost entirely by diffusive transport. The rate of diffusion decreases significantly as the molecular weight of the solute increases and is also limited due to protein binding and charged particles. Thus, hemodialysis is efficient for the removal of only a small number of the numerous uremic compounds that accumulate in end-stage renal disease.

In contrast, with hemodiafiltration, solutes are removed by convective transport, which is not dependent on the molecular weight of the solute. Thus, a larger range of uremic toxins can be remomoved with hemodialfiltration and, at least, theoretically, this removal should result in better patient outcomes. Hemodiafiltration is achieved by adding a replaement or substitution fluid to the dialysis circuit. This sterile and nonpyogenic dialysate fluid, also known as "ultrapure dialysate" can be added into the blood stream upsteam of the dialyzer, downstream from the dialyzer or both upstream and downstream.

Randomized trials of hemodiafiltration have shown conflicting results in regard to patient outcomes. Hemodiafiltration is not currently available in the United States.

KEY READINGS

Grootman MP: CONTRAST investigators. Effect of online hemodiafiltration on all-cause mortality ad cardiovascular outcomes. J Am Soc Nephrol 2012;23:1087.

Maduell F: ESHOL study group. High efficiency post-dilution online hemodiafiltratio reduces all cause mortality in hemodialysis patients. J Am Soc Nephrol 2013;24:487.

Ok E: Turkish online haemodiafiltration study. Mortality and cardiovascular events in online haemodiafiltraton compared with high-flux dialysis. Nephrol Dial Trasnsplant 2013;28:192.

▶ Complications

A. Hypotension

Hypotension is the most common complication of dialysis. It occurs in up to 30% of hemodialysis treatments. The differential diagnosis is broad. It is often related to an imbalance between fluid removal with dialysis treatment and fluid replacement by the extravascular compartment. During dialysis, fluid is rapidly removed from the intravascular space. The maintenance of blood pressure despite fluid removal is due to a fluid shift from the extravascular space back into the vascular system. A large weight gain between dialysis treatments is a major risk factor for hypotension. This factor is especially important in patients with diabetic neuropathy, low cardiac ejection fraction, and diastolic dysfunction. A low dialysate sodium concentration, elevated dialysate temperature, excessive fluid removal, or intake of antihypertensive medications prior to treatment can also cause hypotension during dialysis. Patients are advised to limit their food intake prior to or during the dialysis treatment to avoid splanchnic vasodilation and hypotension. If dialysis access is provided by a catheter, bacteremia and early sepsis syndrome need to be considered and empiric antibiotic coverage initiated. Arrhythmias, pericardiac tamponade, sepsis, hemolysis, dialyzer reactions, bleeding, and air embolus are other possible causes of hypotension. Hypotension can

result in cardiac ischemia and loss of access secondary to access thrombosis.

If a patient becomes hypotensive during hemodialysis, the ultrafiltration is stopped and the blood flow is decreased. If the patient remains hypotensive, normal saline and occasionally albumin can be infused. To prevent hypotension, intradialytic weight gain has to be limited by minimizing the fluid intake and avoiding salt intake. If the patient is anemic this needs to be corrected. Starting the dialysis with a higher sodium concentration and gradually decreasing the sodium concentration during dialysis (sodium modeling) have been reported to improve hemodynamic stability. However, sodium modeling has been linked to increased intradialytic weight gain and thirst. Increasing the dialysate calcium also improves hemodynamic stability. Lowering the dialysate temperature is also beneficial if it is acceptable to the patient. Recently, midodrine has been used to improve peripheral vasoconstriction in patients who are either not responsive to the above measures or who have autonomic dysfunction. Midodrine is a selective α_1-agonist that is given 1 hour before the initiation of dialysis. The dose can be repeated 1 hour into dialysis. Its use is contraindicated in patients with heart disease, urinary retention, and thyrotoxicosis.

B. Muscle Cramps

Muscle cramps are believed to be related to shifts in fluids and electrolytes. It is an early sign of ultrafiltration down to the patient's dry weight. Quinine is often used off-label for the treatment of leg cramps. Vitamin E intake might also be beneficial for this condition. Infusion of a hypertonic glucose solution (50 mL of 50% dextrose) can provide acute relief.

C. Nausea and Vomiting

Nausea and vomiting are common symptoms, especially during the first hour of dialysis. It is usually associated with hypotension and responds to the treatment of hypotension. It can also be an early symptom of the disequilibrium syndrome, dialyzer reaction, cardiac or intestinal ischemia, or hypercalcemia. The differential diagnosis is broad and includes reflux disease, gastroparesis, peptic ulcer disease, and gastroenteritis. The treatment is symptomatic.

D. Arrhythmias and Sudden Cardiac Death

Cardiovascular disease due to either sudden cardiac death or arrhythmias account for approximately 25% of all deaths in hemodialysis patients. The risk of sudden cardiac death is higher during the longer 3 day interdialytic interval, compared to the 2 day dialytic interval, suggesting that electrolyte and/or volume disturbances may be at least partially responsible for this entity. Many comorbid medical conditions that are prevalent in chronic hemodialysis patients are associated with an increased risk of arrhythmias, including ischemic heart disease, left atrial enlargement, left ventricular hypertrophy, and valvular abnormalities. Patients that present with acute arrhythmias should be immediately taken off of dialysis and treated for the arrhythmia per standard protocols, with dosing adjusted for end-stage renal disease.

Chronic atrial fibrillation is usually initially treated medically, either with rate control and/or rhythm control. Rate control can be achieved with one of several agents, including beta blockers, nondihydropyridine calcium channel blockers, amiodarone or digoxin, the latter two with renally adjusted doses. Anticoagulation for hemodialysis patients with atrial fibrillation remains a controversial subject with no randomized trials available for guidance. Ventricular arrhythmias should be treated the same as that in the general population.

E. Pericarditis

Uremic pericarditis is an uncommon cause of pericarditis that is usually seen either just prior to or just after the initiation of chronic dialysis therapy. These symptoms usually resolve with continuation of regular dialysis sessions. Dialysis-related pericarditis can occur at any time after the initiation of dialytic therapy and is presumed to be secondary to receiving an inadequate dose of dialysis. There are likely other etiologies, however, as the symptoms of pericarditis do not always improve with intensification of dialysis. Symptoms of pericarditis include pleuritic chest pain that is exacerbated by the recumbent position and improved by sitting up. Other symptoms of pericarditis are nonspecific and include dyspnea and cough, which may reflect the presence of a pericardial effusion, as well as fever and/or chills. Physical signs of pericarditis may include a pericardial friction rub and hypotension with volume removal on hemodialysis, a sign that may be secondary to the presence of pericardial disease. Electrocardiograms are often nondiagnostic. Echocardiography can help to identify pericardial effusions, although those patients with adhesive noneffusive pericarditis may not manifest pericardial effusions.

Pericardial effusions that are less than 100 mL in volume are considered to be hemodynamically insignificant and may be present in a minority of dialysis patients. Larger effusions require regular monitoring to ensure that they do not result in hemodynamic compromise. Initial medical management includes intensification of dialysis by increasing the number of dialysis sessions to 5 to 7 times per week. Electrolytes and volume status need to be monitoring closely to prevent volume depletion, metabolic acidosis and decreased blood levels of electrolytes. Dialysis is performed without anticoagulation to minimize the risk of hemorrhagic pericarditis. Surgical drainage of pericardial effusions should occur once the volume of the effusions is in excess of 250 mL, as hemodynamic instability can occur suddenly once pericardial volume exceeds this level. Note that glucocorticoids and nonsteroidal anti-inflammatory medications are generally ineffective in treating dialysis-related pericarditis.

F. Restless Leg Syndrome

This syndrome is of unknown etiology, although in the general population it has been associated with iron deficiency. Patients with restless leg syndrome describe an unpleasant sensation, typically in the calf muscles, but also in other muscles of the leg, that is relieved by moving the affected leg. This syndrome can result in poor quality sleep as well as delayed onset of sleep. Treatments that may be effective include massage, stretching, exercise of the affected limb, and tub baths with either hot or cold water. Medications that may be effective include benzodiazepines in renally adjusted doses as well as dopamine agonists or precursors.

G. Dialysis Disequilibrium

This entity is believed to be caused by an acute increase in brain water content. This entity is usually seen in patients with severe uremia who undergo vigorous removal of uremic toxins. In its most severe form, nausea, vomiting, and headache are followed by seizures, obtundation, and/or coma. Presence of these more severe symptoms necessitates immediate discontinuation of the dialysis session, which should result in resolution of symptoms within 24 hours. The risk of dialysis equilibrium is minimized by dialyzing acutely uremic patients with an initial short (about 2 hours) dialysis session with subsequent sessions lengthened in 15–30 minute increments.

H. Hemolysis

Massive hemolysis is considered a medical emergency as hemolyzed erythrocytes release potassium that can lead to life-threatening hyperkalemia. Manifestations of hemolysis include chest tightness, shortness of breath, and back pain. If hyperkalemia is present, muscle weakness, and electrocardiographic changes may progress to cardiac arrest. Signs of hemolysis include a "port-wine" appearance of blood in the venous blood line, plasma that is pink in color when centrifuged and a significant decline in the hemoglobin level. Hemolysis can be secondary to either physical damage to erythrocytes due to a narrowing or blockage of the blood passages, including the dialysis tubing, catheter or needle or to issues with the dialysis solution. Hemolysis can be due to hypotonic dialysis solutions, solutions contaminated by chemicals in the water supply that have not been removed during the preparation of dialysate. These chemicals include chloramine, fluoride, nitrates, zinc, and copper as well as formaldehyde, bleach, hydrogen peroxide. When signs or symptoms of hemolysis are noted, the dialysis session should be stopped immediately, with clamping of the blood lines and discarding the dialyzer circuit without returning blood to the patient in order to prevent infusion of high potassium blood back to the patient. Patients may need to be hospitalized to treat the resultant anemia and hyperkalemia, which can persist for several days after the hemolytic event.

I. Air Embolism

Air embolism is a medical emergency that can result in death if not recognized and treated emergently. The sources of air entry include the prepump arterial tubing segment, the arterial needle and a central venous catheter that is opened to air. Symptoms of air embolism are determined by the position of the patient at the time of the event as symptoms are dependent on where air accumulates in the body. In patients who lie flat, air accumulates in the heart, causing foam to accumulate in the right ventricle, with subsequent movement of air to the lungs. Air that crosses the pulmonary capillary bed is retuned to the left ventricle and can result in air embolism in the arteries of the heart, causing acute cardiac abnormalities and of the brain, causing acute neurologic events. Thus, patients present with shortness of breath and cough as well as cardiac symptoms such as chest pain and cardiac arrhythmias. In patients who are seated, air collects in the brain venous system, which results in loss of consciousness, seizures, and ultimately death. To treat this event, the venous blood line is clamped to prevent further entry of air into the patient. The patient is placed lying down with the left side of the chest and head tilted downward in order to move air to less damaging parts of the body. Oxygen at 100% concentration is administered by either mask or endotracheal tube. If there is significant air in the atria or ventricles, which can sometimes be manifested by a churning sound on auscultation, the aspiration of air via either cardiac catheterization or insertion of a percutaneous needle, may be needed.

J. Dialyzer Reactions

Dialyzer reactions can be either of the anaphylactic type (type A) or of the nonspecific type B. In its most severe form, a type A reaction is manifested by anaphylaxis, which is often heralded by dyspnea, a warm feeling that can be either at the site of the fistula or throughout the body, and a sense of an impending catastrophe. Milder forms of type A reactions can include watery eyes, coughing, sneezing, itching, urticaria as well as gastrointestinal symptoms which can include diarrhea and abdominal cramping. These symptoms usually occur with the first 5 minutes of the dialysis session, but can be delayed for up to 30 minutes after the start of dialysis. There are multiple etiologies of type A reactions. Reactions due to either ethylene oxide, a sterilant used in dialyzers, or to AN69 (acrylonitrile-sodium methallyl sulfonate) dialyzer membranes are less common than in the past, but other dialysis membranes have also been implicated. Other etiologies include contaminated dialysis solutions, inadequate reuse disinfection, and heparin. Treatment consists of immediately stopping the dialysis session, clamping the blood lines, and disconnecting the blood lines from the access without returning the blood in the system to the patient. Supportive treatment may require intravenous steroids, antihistamines and/or epinephrine as well as cardiorespiratory support. Prevention of further episodes necessitates identifying and avoiding the cause of the type A reaction. Some patients may need predialysis administration of antihistamines as well as using a reuse program, even prior to first use of a dialyzer.

Type B dialyzer reactions are usually less severe than type A reactions and typically are not seen until at least 20 minutes of dialysis have elapsed. Typical presenting symptoms include chest pain and/or back pain. The etiology of type B reactions are unclear. Treatment is supportive, including the use of supplemental oxygen. It is important to assess for other causes of chest pain, including myocardial ischemia. Symptoms usually resolve within 60 minutes of the institution of supportive therapy.

KEY READINGS

Foley RN: Long interdialytic interval and mortality among patients receiving hemodialysis. N Engl J Med 2011;365:1099.

Golper TA et al: Hemodialysis: core curriculum 2014. Am J Kidney Dis 2014;63:153.

Lemke HD, Heidland A, Schaefer RM: Hypersensitivity reactions during haemodialysis: role of complement fragments and ethylene oxide antibodies. Nephrol Dial Transplant 1990;5:264.

Parnes EL: Anaphylactoid reactions in hemodialysis patients treated with the AN69 dialyzer. Kidney Int 1991; 40:1148.

■ CHAPTER REVIEW QUESTIONS

1. Which of the following methods should be used to help minimize dialytic hypotension?
   A. Increase the time on dialysis
   B. Increase the ultrafiltration rate
   C. Use sodium modeling
   D. Increase the patient's dry weight
   E. Increase the dialysate blood flow rate

2. All of the following can be used to increase the dose of dialysis except for:
   A. Increase the blood flow rate
   B. Increase the dialysate flow rate
   C. Increase the time on dialysis
   D. Use a dialysis membrane with a larger surface area
   E. Increase the ultrafiltration rate

3. Complications of a type A dialyzer reaction include all of the following except:
   A. Anaphylaxis
   B. Dyspnea
   C. Hemolysis
   D. Urticaria
   E. Diarrhea

4. Indications to start chronic dialysis therapy includes all of the following except:
   A. Protein–calorie wasting
   B. Metabolic abnormalities
   C. eGFR of <15 mL/min
   D. Volume overload
   E. Decreasing functional status

5. The preferred order of placement for an AV fistula is
   A. Elbow (brachial-cephalic) primary AV fistula, wrist (radial-cephalic) primary AV fistula, any other forearm primary AV fistula, and a transposed brachial basilic vein fistula.
   B. Elbow (brachial-cephalic) primary AV fistula, any other forearm primary AV fistula, wrist (radial-cephalic) primary AV fistula, and a transposed brachial basilic vein fistula.
   C. Wrist (radial-cephalic) primary AV fistula, an elbow (brachial-cephalic) primary AV fistula, any other forearm primary AV fistula, and a transposed brachial basilic vein fistula.
   D. Wrist (radial-cephalic) primary AV fistula, any other forearm primary AV fistula, an elbow (brachial-cephalic) primary AV fistula, and a transposed brachial basilic vein fistula.
   E. Transposed brachial basilic vein fistula, elbow (brachial-cephalic) primary AV fistula, wrist (radial-cephalic) primary AV fistula, and any other forearm primary AV fistula.

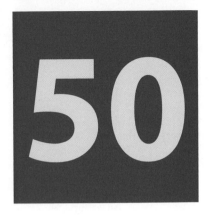

Peritoneal Dialysis

Brenda B. Hoffman, MD

▶ General Considerations

Peritoneal dialysis (PD) is an established form of renal replacement therapy that is performed primarily at home. The concept of continuous ambulatory peritoneal dialysis (CAPD) was first described by Popovich and Moncrief in 1976. During the 1980s there was rapid growth in the utilization of CAPD in the United States with the development of chronic indwelling PD catheters and the introduction of peritoneal dialysis solution in sterile, disposable plastic bags. The early 1990s witnessed an increase in the number of patients on automated peritoneal dialysis (APD) with the increased interest in dialysis adequacy and the development of simplified, automated cycler machines. Starting in the mid-1990s there was a decrease in the number of incident and prevalent PD patients, and this marked the beginning of a relatively stagnant period for PD growth in the United States. The cause of this decreased PD utilization was likely multifactorial, including lack of infrastructure and provider expertise, inadequate predialysis education, and lower reimbursement rates. More recently there has been a resurgence in PD utilization in the United States. According to the 2016 USRDS annual data report (ADR), the use of PD in 2013 was 72% higher than in 2007, with 9.5% of prevalent dialysis patients in the United States being treated with PD. This increase in PD utilization is thought to be largely due to economic incentives created by changes in reimbursement policy and the adoption of a bundled payment system. Internationally, hemodialysis (HD) still remains the most common form of treatment for end-stage renal disease (ESRD); however, the utilization of PD remains quite high in some countries such as Hong Kong (72%) and Mexico (45%), where "PD first" policies are in effect.

The selection of dialysis modality is influenced by a number of considerations such as availability and convenience, medical factors, and socioeconomic and dialysis center factors. Patients who receive predialysis education are more likely to select peritoneal dialysis. In general, the one absolute contraindication to chronic PD is an unsuitable peritoneum due to the presence of extensive adhesions, fibrosis, or malignancy. Other relative contraindications do exist (Table 50–1). PD continues to be the preferred dialysis modality for infants and young children, patients with severe hemodynamic instability on hemodialysis, and patients with difficult vascular access.

Studies investigating differences in patient mortality between PD and in-center hemodialysis have been conflicting. Variable results in these mortality studies, practically all of them retrospective and observational, have been affected by differences in patient comorbidities, inclusion of prevalent versus incident patients, and the types of analytical methods utilized.

Real differences in mortality between PD and HD can only be assessed in prospective, randomly controlled trials that have proven to be very difficult to perform. Multiple studies have found that, when compared to in-center HD, PD may provide short-term survival benefits with more comparable or decreased survival after 1 or 2 years. This initial survival advantage of PD may be related to the presence of sicker HD patients who often start dialysis urgently with a central venous catheter. Survival between the two modalities has been found to be more similar when "elective start" patients have been studied. Technique survival is shorter in PD compared to HD due to peritonitis, peritoneal membrane failure, and patient burn-out. It may be optimal to utilize a more integrative-care, "life-plan" approach to the management of ESRD patients, where incident patients initially undergo peritoneal dialysis. This affords them the independence and flexibility of a home-based modality while helping to maintain their residual renal function and preserve their veins for future vascular access. Transfer to hemodialysis can then occur later, for instance in the event of kidney transplant failure or if complications ensue with peritoneal dialysis.

Table 50–1. Contraindications to performance of peritoneal dialysis.

Absolute contraindication
Extensive abdominal adhesions or documented loss of peritoneal function

Relative contraindications
Abdominal hernias
Presence of colostomy, ileostomy, nephrostomy, or ileal conduit
Recurrent chronic backache with preexisting disc disease
Severe psychological and social problems
Severe diverticular disease of the colon
Severe neurological disease, movement disorder or severe arthritis preventing self care. (Caregivers can be trained to perform peritoneal dialysis.)
Severe chronic obstructive pulmonary disease
Malnutrition

KEY READINGS

Bargman JM: Advances in peritoneal dialysis: a review. Sem Dial 2012;25:545.

Hansson JH, Watnick S: Update on peritoneal dialysis: core curriculum 2016. Am J Kidney Dis 2016;67:151.

Hirth RA et al: The initial impact of Medicare's new prospective payment system for kidney dialysis. Am J Kidney Dis 2013;62:662.

Jain AK et al: Global trends in rates of peritoneal dialysis. J Am Soc Nephrol 2012;23:533.

Mehrotra R et al: Similar outcomes with hemodialysis and peritoneal dialysis in patients with end-stage renal disease. Arch Intern Med 2011;171:110.

Perl J et al: Hemodialysis vascular access modifies the association between dialysis modality and survival. J Am Soc Nephrol 2011;22:1113.

US Renal Data System, USRDS 2016 Annual Report: Atlas of End-Stage Renal Disease in the United States, National Institutes of Health, National Institute of Diabetes and Digestive and Kidney Diseases, Bethesda, MD, 2016.

▷ Basic Principles: Physiology of Peritoneal Transport

PD involves the transport of solutes and water across the peritoneal membrane, which separates the blood in the peritoneal capillaries and dialysis solution in the peritoneal space. The dialysis solution in the peritoneal space typically contains sodium, chloride, calcium, and lactate and is made hyperosmolar by the addition of various amounts of glucose. The peritoneal membrane as a dialyzer has a surface area that typically ranges from 1 to 2 m² in adults. It is a complex membrane comprised of the capillary endothelium and associated basement membrane, the interstitium, the mesothelium, and a stagnant fluid film that overlies the peritoneal membrane. The transport of water and solutes across this membrane best fits a model that entails the presence of three different sized pores in the peritoneal membrane. Large

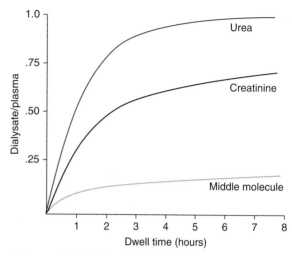

▲ **Figure 50–1.** Peritoneal dialysis diffusion curves: rate of diffusion is dependent on size.

pores that are few in number and thought to represent clefts between endothelial cells allow the transport of macromolecules such as proteins. Numerous small pores are responsible for the transport of small solutes such as urea, creatinine, cations and anions, while ultrasmall, transcellular pores or aquaporins allow the movement of electrolyte-free water.

In PD, solutes are transported by the processes of diffusion and convection. During the course of a PD dwell, smaller solutes such as creatinine, urea and potassium diffuse down a concentration gradient from the peritoneal capillary blood into the peritoneal dialysis solution. With increasing dwell time, the ratio of dialysate to serum levels approaches unity (Figure 50–1). Thus, for small solutes such as urea, the removal is maximal at the start of the dwell, when the concentration in the dialysis solution is zero, and gradually decreases during the course of the dwell. Diffusion becomes more restricted as molecular weight increases (ie, urea diffuses faster than creatinine). Glucose, lactate, and calcium will diffuse in the opposite direction, from dialysate into the blood.

Water removal or ultrafiltration, occurs as a result of an osmotic pressure gradient between the dialysis solution and the peritoneal capillary blood. The dialysis solution is made hypertonic usually by the addition of high concentrations of glucose. Ultrafiltration is maximal at the beginning of a dwell when the osmotic pressure gradient is the greatest. The osmotic pressure gradient will decrease over time due to the dilution of the glucose by ultrafiltrate and by the diffusion of glucose from the peritoneal cavity into the bloodstream (Figure 50–2). Fluid removal is maximized by using more hypertonic dialysis solutions or by doing more frequent exchanges. During ultrafiltration, solutes present in body

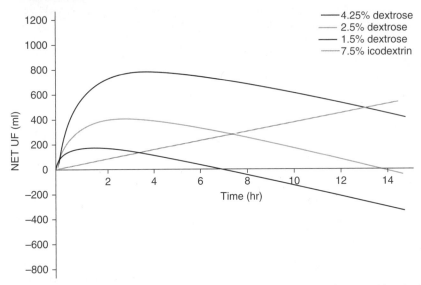

▲ **Figure 50–2.** Typical ultrafiltration (UF) profiles using 1.5%, 2.5%, 4.25% dextrose, and 7.5% icodextrin dialysate solutions.

fluids will be swept along by convection, contributing to overall solute clearance. Convective transport is relatively more important for larger rather than smaller solutes. Water and solutes are also constantly being absorbed from the peritoneal cavity into the lymphatic system, and this will counteract both solute and fluid removal.

Not all patients' peritoneal membranes transport solute at the same rate. In clinical practice, a patient's peritoneal membrane transport characteristics can be determined by measuring the creatinine equilibration curve and the glucose absorption curve during a standardized peritoneal equilibration test (PET). Conventionally, the PET involves a 2-L, 2.5% dextrose dwell with dialysate samples taken at 1, 2, and 4 hours and a plasma sample at 2 hours. Net fluid removal is also measured along with the ratio of dialysate glucose at 4 hours to dialysate glucose at time zero. Patients are classified principally into one of four transport categories: high, high-average, low-average and low (Figure 50–3).

High transporters will have the fastest equilibration of creatinine, but ultrafiltration will not be as great due to rapid absorption of glucose and dissipation of the osmotic gradient. High transporters also tend to have higher dialysate protein losses. In contrast, low transporters will have less complete equilibration of creatinine, but will have good net ultrafiltration due to the slower absorption of glucose into the bloodstream. Thus, high transporters tend to do better

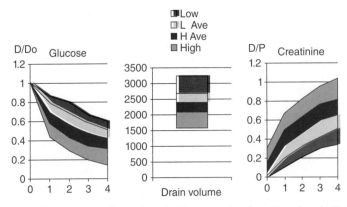

▲ **Figure 50–3.** Peritoneal equilibration test. (Reproduced with permission from Twardowski ZJ et al: Peritoneal equilibration test. Peritoneal Dial Bull 1987;7:138.)

on regimens that have frequent, short duration dwells, such as APD, whereas low transporters tend to do better on regimens with longer duration dwells, such as CAPD. Average transporters are generally able to do well on a variety of PD regimens.

KEY READINGS

Perl J, Bargman J: Peritoneal dialysis: from bench to bedside and bedside to bench. Am J Physiol Renal Physiol 2016;311:F999.
Twardowski ZJ et al: Peritoneal equilibration test. Peritoneal Dial Bull 1987;7:138.

▶ Treatment

A. Forms of Peritoneal Dialysis

Peritoneal dialysis is a form of dialysis in which dialysis solution is instilled in the peritoneal cavity, periodically drained, and exchanged with fresh solution through a single, indwelling peritoneal catheter (Figure 50–4). During each exchange there are inflow, dwell, and outflow periods. In chronic PD these exchanges are repeated according to a fixed schedule in a continuous, daily fashion such as in continuous ambulatory peritoneal dialysis (CAPD) or automated peritoneal dialysis (APD). Exchanges may also be done in a more non-continuous fashion over a fixed period of time such as in intermittent peritoneal dialysis (IPD) performed for acute kidney injury or urgent-start dialysis.

1. Continuous ambulatory peritoneal dialysis (CAPD)—In CAPD dialysis solution is constantly present in the abdomen, typically being exchanged four to five times per day, 7 days per week. The dialysis fluid is exchanged manually by the patient using the force of gravity to drain and fill the abdomen. Actual dialysis prescriptions will vary depending on the individual patient, but typical exchange volumes are usually in the range of 2–3 L with 3–4 shorter dwell periods occurring during the day and one longer dwell period overnight during sleep (Figure 50–5).

2. Automated peritoneal dialysis (APD)—In APD a cycler machine automatically exchanges fluid into and out of the abdomen for the patient. The cycler draws dialysis solution from larger bags (usually 5 L) that it warms to the desired temperature. An alarm in the cycler is set off when various monitored parameters are disrupted. APD is traditionally divided into continuous cycling peritoneal dialysis (CCPD) and nocturnal intermittent peritoneal dialysis (NIPD). A standard CCPD prescription usually has three

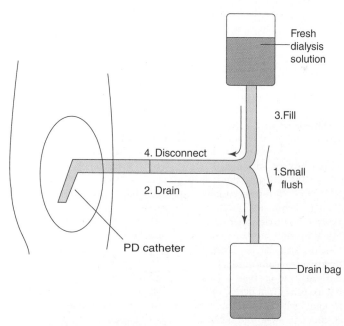

▲ **Figure 50–4.** Diagram of a continuous ambulatory peritoneal diaylsis exchange. The patient connects the peritoneal dialysis catheter to a Y-set tubing system. A small volume of fresh dialysis solution is flushed directly into the drain bag and then the abdomen is allowed to drain. This washes away any bacteria introduced into the system during the connection of the catheter. Fresh dialysis solution is then instilled and the patient disconnects the catheter from the tubing. The fluid is allowed to dwell for several hours and then the entire cycle is repeated.

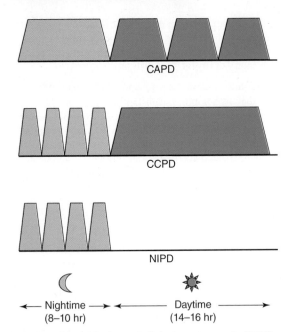

▲ **Figure 50–5.** Peritoneal dialysis regimens. In CAPD, patients perform several manual exchanges over the course of the daytime and then perform a final exchange that dwells for a longer period overnight. In CCPD, a cycler device is programmed to automatically perform several exchanges overnight, and then one last fill is delivered in the morning to dwell during the longer daytime period. In NIPD there is no last fill delivered, and the patient has a dry abdomen during the daytime period.

to four shorter nighttime dwell periods of 1.5–3.0 L. The patient usually spends between 8 and 10 hours a night on the cycler. The patient then disconnects from the cycler in the morning after a final fill is delivered and then is free to go about daily activities. In CCPD therefore the longer dwell period occurs over the daytime. In certain situations patients may also complete one or two manual exchanges during the day in order to increase solute clearance or fluid removal. In NIPD the patient drains fully at the end of the night, and the abdomen remains "dry" all day. NIPD is usually reserved for patients with significant residual renal function, as solute clearance is usually lower than in CCPD due to the absence of the long daytime dwell period. NIPD may also be employed for patients with mechanical complications such as hernias in order to avoid the increased abdominal pressure that occurs with a full abdomen during ambulation or upright posture. Tidal peritoneal dialysis (TPD) is a form of automated PD where a constant reserve volume of dialysis solution remains in the peritoneal cavity at all times while smaller tidal volumes of solution are repeatedly instilled into the abdomen by the cycler. TPD has the advantage of eliminating the non dialytic period required for filling and draining dialysis solution, but there is little evidence to suggest that TPD provides greater clearance than CCPD.

3. Intermittent peritoneal dialysis (IPD)—IPD can be performed in uremic patients who need urgent dialysis initiation immediately after catheter placement. This urgent-start PD therapy is a safe and effective alternative to starting hemodialysis with a CVC. Urgent-start PD therapy can be initiated in the hospital or the outpatient clinic and is performed for the patient by healthcare personnel, usually using an automated cycler. The initial prescription involves low-volume PD in the supine position to minimize the increase in intra-abdominal pressure and the risk for leaking. PD fill volumes are then increased incrementally over the next several weeks while the patient is being trained. The duration of treatment, number of exchanges and dwell times and the total volume of exchange fluid will depend on the individual patient. IPD can also be used in the management of acute kidney injury (AKI). In the United States, extracorporeal blood therapies are more commonly performed for patients with AKI, however the treatment of AKI using IPD and manual exchanges continues to be widespread in more low-resource areas around the world.

B. Apparatus for Peritoneal Dialysis

1. Dialysis solutions—PD solution is manufactured in clear flexible plastic bags in volumes of 1.5–5 L. Conventional PD solutions commonly have lactate as a buffer and dextrose as the osmotic agent (Table 50–2). Dialysis solutions containing 1.5%, 2.5%, and 4.25% dextrose are routinely marketed in the United States. The true anhydrous dextrose or glucose concentrations in these solutions are 1.36%, 2.27%, and 3.86%, respectively, and this is how the solutions are typically labeled outside of the United States. Glucose has been shown to be safe, effective, easily metabolized and is inexpensive. However, glucose is not an ideal osmotic agent because it is rapidly absorbed and can cause metabolic problems such as hyperglycemia, hyperinsulinemia, hyperlipidemia, and obesity. The pH of the dialysis solution must also be kept relatively low to prevent the caramelization of glucose during sterilization and production of glucose degradation products (GDPs). This unphysiologic pH, in addition to the presence of GDPs, make conventional PD solutions relatively bioincompatible and may contribute to long-term pathologic changes in the peritoneal membrane as well as impaired host defense against infection. There has been interest in developing glucose-sparing solutions that have fewer local and systemic adverse effects while improving ultrafiltration. Icodextrin is a polyglucose solution that is now widely used in the United States. Icodextrin induces ultrafiltration by an oncotic effect. It is slowly absorbed into

Table 50–2. Peritoneal dialysis solutions.

	1.5% Dextrose	2.5% Dextrose	4.25% Dextrose	7.5% Icodextrin
Dextrose, H_2O	15 g/L	25 g/L	42.5 g/L	0
Icodextrin	0	0	0	75 g/L
Sodium	132 mEq/L	132 mEq/L	132 mEq/L	132 mEq/L
Calcium	2.5–3.5 mEq/L	2.5–3.5 mEq/L	2.5–3.5 mEq/L	3.5 mEq/L
Magnesium	0.5–1.5 mEq/L	0.5–1.5 mEq/L	0.5–1.5 mEq/L	0.5 mEq/L
Chloride	95–102 mEq/L	95–102 mEq/L	95–102 mEq/L	96 mEq/L
Lactate	35–40 mEq/L	35–40 mEq/L	35–40 mEq/L	40 mEq/L
pH	5.5	5.5	5.5	5.2
Osm	347 mosm/L	413 mosm/L	486 mosm/L	282–286 mosm/L

the peritoneal bloodstream and therefore its ultrafiltration effect is more sustained than glucose (see Figure 50–2). It can be used during long dwells in patients who have high transport in order to increase ultrafiltration, and its use has also been associated with improvements in glycemic control and lipid abnormalities. Amino acids can also function as osmotic agents, and amino acid containing dialysis solutions are available. The potential benefit of these solutions is that the absorbed amino acids would replace the obligatory amino acids lost during dialysis and serve as a protein caloric source. However, long-term improvement in nutritional status has not been conclusively demonstrated with these solutions. Neutral pH solutions with low GDP content have also been developed with the goal of decreasing toxicity. These solutions employ multi-compartment bag systems where the glucose is sterilized in one compartment at lower pH in order to decrease formation of GDPs, while the buffer and electrolytes are present in another compartment at alkaline pH. Before use these solutions are mixed, resulting in neutral pH. The clinical value of these solutions remains uncertain because of inconsistent findings in trials comparing them to more conventional solutions. There is suggestion that their use may have a beneficial effect on maintaining residual renal function and may be associated with less inflow pain, however their impact on other hard outcomes such peritonitis, technique survival and patient survival are uncertain.

2. Peritoneal catheters—The peritoneal dialysis catheter must permit consistent bidirectional flow of dialysate. Most catheters are flexible silicone or polyurethane tubes with multiple ports in the intraperitoneal segment that is positioned in the pelvis. The transperitoneal portion of the catheter is implanted within the abdominal wall using one or two cuffs. With the commonly used double-cuffed catheter, the

deep cuff is secured within the rectus muscle and the superficial cuff is placed subcutaneously approximately 2 cm from the catheter exit site. Many types of catheters are available for chronic peritoneal dialysis, but the double cuff straight Tenckhoff catheter still remains one of the more commonly used catheters. The benefit of one catheter design over another has not been conclusively demonstrated, although use of straight catheters may improve outcomes and technique survival. The catheter used by a PD program primarily depends upon the experience of the clinician inserting the catheters. There are multiple insertion techniques for placing a PD catheter including percutaneous, peritoneoscopic, open surgical, and laparoscopic. Prophylactic omentopexy and adhesiolysis may be performed during laparoscopic placement. Depending on the procedure and the institution, catheters may be placed by surgeons, interventional radiologists or interventional nephrologists. PD catheters should be placed in the paramedian or lateral abdominal location with a downwardly directed tunnel to help prevent exit-site infection. The exit site should be at least 2 cm from belt lines and skin folds and should be clearly visible to the patient to permit easy exit-site care. PD catheters may also be placed with a presternal exit site. This location is often more desirable in obese patients, patients with ostomies, and children in diapers. The Moncrief–Popovich technique, where the entire extraperitoneal portion of the catheter is left embedded in a subcutaneous pocket for weeks to months and then later externalized, can be used in patients who have selected PD therapy in advance of anticipated need. Newly placed catheters are usually flushed with heparinized saline and secured with a dressing to minimize catheter movement and trauma to the exit site. To minimize the risk of fluid leak, it is preferable to wait at least 10–14 days after catheter insertion before beginning PD. However, as described above, newly placed catheters can be safely used as part of an urgent-start PD protocol.

KEY READINGS

Cho Y et al: Impact of icodextrin on clinical outcomes in peritoneal dialysis: a systematic review of randomized controlled trials. Nephrol Dial Transplant 2013;28:1899.

Cho Y et al: The impact of neutral-pH peritoneal dialysates with reduced glucose degradation products on clinical outcomes in peritoneal dialysis patients. Kidney Int 2013;84:969.

Crabtree JH: Peritoneal dialysis catheter implantation: avoiding problems and optimizing outcomes. Semin Dial 2015;28:12.

Cullis B et al: Peritoneal dialysis for acute kidney injury. Perit Dial Int 2014;34:494.

Fang JH et al: Urgent-start peritoneal dialysis and hemodialysis in ESRD patients: complications and outcomes. PLos ONE 2016;11:e0166181.

Figueiredo A et al: ISPD Guidelines/recommendations: clinical practice guidelines for peritoneal access. Perit Dial Int 2010;30:424.

Hagen SM et al: A systematic review and meta-analysis of the influence of peritoneal dialysis catheter type on complication rate and catheter survival. Kidney Int 2014;85:920.

Ivarsen P, Povlsen JV: Can peritoneal dialysis be applied for unplanned initiation of chronic dialysis? Nephrol Dial Transplant 2014;29:22016.

▶ COMPLICATIONS

A. Peritonitis and Catheter Related Infections

Peritonitis remains a leading complication of PD. It contributes to technique failure, hospitalization and patient mortality. Peritonitis is thought to occur most often by touch contamination, but may also occur in the setting of a catheter exit site or tunnel infection, by transmural migration of bacteria through the intestinal wall, or rarely by the hematogenous or transvaginal route. Patients with peritonitis usually present with cloudy peritoneal fluid and abdominal pain. When a patient presents with these complaints, the abdomen should be drained and the effluent sent for cell count with differential, Gram stain and culture. At least two of the following three conditions should be present to make the diagnosis of peritonitis: symptoms and signs of peritoneal inflammation, an effluent total white blood cell count of more than $100/mm^3$ after at least a 2-hour dwell with at least 50% polymorphonuclear neutrophil cells, and a positive culture from the dialysate. Using appropriate culture techniques an organism can be isolated from the peritoneal fluid in over 80% of cases. Infections due to gram-positive cocci (*Staphylococcus epidermidis* and *Staphylococcus aureus*) tend to be most common (60–70% episodes) compared to infections with gram-negative bacteria (15–25%) or fungi (2–3%). Infection with mycobacteria can also occur but is rare. Peritonitis with multiple organisms or anaerobes should raise the concern

of intra-abdominal pathology and lead to abdominal CT scan and surgical evaluation.

Patients who present with signs and symptoms of peritonitis should always be treated empirically with antibiotics after appropriate microbiological specimens have been obtained. Various antibiotics can be used to treat peritonitis, but empiric therapy must cover both gram-positive and gram-negative organisms (Figure 50–6). Guidelines outlining empiric antibiotic regimens are published and have changed over the years in response to concern over the development of vancomycin resistant organisms and appreciation of the importance of preservation of residual renal function. Gram-positive organisms may be covered by vancomycin or a first-generation cephalosporin, and gram-negative organisms by a third-generation cephalosporin or aminoglycoside. Numerous combinations are possible, but the choice of antibiotics should take into account the patient's infection history and the center's history of resistant organisms. Antibiotics are usually administered by the intraperitoneal route and can be given by intermittent (once daily) or continuous (in each exchange) dosing (Table 50–3). Most patients will show considerable clinical improvement within 48 hours of starting antibiotic therapy. Final antibiotic therapy should be guided by culture results and sensitivities. Treatment should be continued for a total of 2 weeks, while more severe infections due to *S aureus*, *pseudomonas*, enterococci, or multiple gram-negative organisms should be treated for 3 weeks (Figures 50–7 and 50–8). If there is no clinical improvement after 48–72 hours, then cell counts and cultures should be repeated. Refractory peritonitis is defined as failure to respond to appropriate antibiotics within 5 days and should be managed by catheter removal. Other indications for catheter removal are fungal peritonitis, relapsing peritonitis, peritonitis in the setting of severe exit-site or tunnel infection and infection due to multiple enteric organisms in the setting of a surgical abdomen. Cultures may remain negative in patients with peritonitis for various reasons, such as recent antibiotic use or technical problems obtaining proper cultures. If there is no growth by 3 days, then repeat cell count with differential should be obtained. If the patient is improving clinically, then treatment with gram-positive coverage should continue for two weeks. If the culture-negative peritonitis is not resolving at day 3, then special culture techniques should be considered for the isolation of unusual organisms such as mycobacteria, fungi, or legionella. Consultation with the microbiology laboratory would be indicated in this case. If there is no clinical improvement after 5 days of empiric antibiotic coverage, then catheter removal should be strongly considered. During peritonitis the permeability of the peritoneal membrane increases due to inflammation, and patients often will need more concentrated dialysis solution in order to maintain fluid removal. Protein losses will also increase during peritonitis. Peritonitis is also often associated with increased fibrin clot production

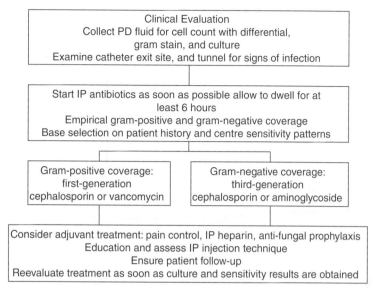

▲ **Figure 50–6.** Initial management of peritonitis. (Reproduced with permission from Li PK et al: ISPD Peritonitis Recommendations: 2016 Update on Prevention and Treatment. Perit Dial Int 2016; 36:481.)

that can occlude the dialysis catheter. Heparin can be added to each bag of dialysis solution (500–1000 units/L) in order to decrease fibrin clot production.

Catheter related infections can occur at the exit site or in the subcutaneous tunnel. An exit-site infection is defined by the presence of purulent drainage at the catheter-epidermal interface that may or may not be accompanied by erythema,

Table 50–3. Intraperitoneal antibiotic dosing for treatment of peritonitis.

	Intermittent (per exchange, once daily)	Continuous (mg/L, all exchanges)
Cefazolin	15–20 mg/kg	LD 500, MD 125
Ceftazidime/ cephalothin	1000–1500 mg	LD 500, MD 125
Ampicillin/oxacillin/ nafcillin	No data	MD 125
Vancomycin	15–30 mg/kg every 5–7 days	LD 30 mg/kg MD 1.5 mg/kg/bag
Gentamicin/netilmicin/ tobramycin	0.6 mg/kg	LD 8, MD 4
Amikacin	2.0 mg/kg	LD 25, MD 12
Aztreonam	2000 mg	LD 1000, MD 250

LD, loading dose; MD, maintenance dose.

tenderness, or crust formation. A tunnel infection may present as erythema, edema, or tenderness of the subcutaneous tunnel, but may be clinically occult. Ultrasonography may reveal a sonolucent zone around the catheter. Exit-site and tunnel infections may be caused by a variety of microorganisms, with *S aureus* and *Pseudomonas aeruginosa* being responsible for the majority. A Gram stain and culture of exit-site drainage should be performed. Empiric therapy may be initiated immediately and should always cover *S aureus*. Oral antibiotic therapy is as effective as intraperitoneal therapy. In some cases, intensified local care or a local antibiotic cream may be felt to be sufficient. A patient with an exit-site infection that progresses to peritonitis, or who presents with an exit-site infection in conjunction with peritonitis will usually require catheter removal. Patients should be taught to perform routine exit-site care in order to prevent catheter infections. Daily cleansing with antibacterial soap and water is recommended by most centers. The daily application of mupirocin or gentamicin cream to the exit site has been shown to be effective in reducing catheter infections and related peritonitis.

B. Mechanical Complications

The increased intra-abdominal pressure that occurs during PD can be associated with a variety of mechanical complications. Hernias are quite common and can be inguinal, incisional (pericatheter or other), umbilical or ventral. Risk factors for hernia formation include large dwell volumes, recent abdominal surgery, and polycystic kidney disease.

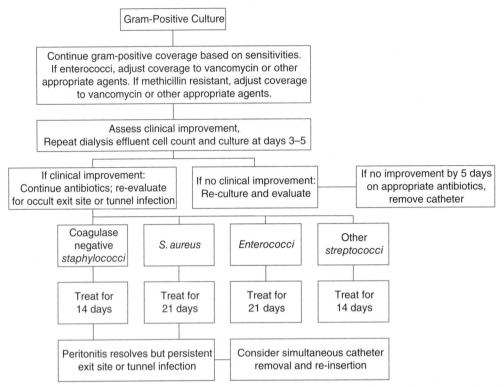

▲ **Figure 50–7.** Management of peritonitis caused by gram-positive bacteria. (Reproduced with permission from Li PK et al: ISPD Peritonitis Recommendations: 2016 Update on Prevention and Treatment. Perit Dial Int 2016; 36:481.)

Hernias usually present as painless swelling but can be associated with intestinal strangulation. The performance of a CT scan with the instillation of IP contrast can aid in the diagnosis of a hernia. Treatment usually involves surgical repair with temporary cessation of PD and conversion to hemodialysis. In some situations peritoneal dialysis can be resumed postoperatively with low volume exchanges and with the patient supine (as in NIPD) in order to maintain low intra-abdominal pressure and facilitate healing. Leaks may also occur at the catheter site or through other defects into the abdominal wall. The diagnosis of abdominal wall leaks may sometimes be difficult. Patients may present with decreased ultrafiltration and weight gain due to fluid accumulation in the tissues. Patients with leaks may also present with scrotal or labial edema which may be difficult to distinguish from fluid migration through a patent processus vaginalis. Abdominal CT with IP contrast will assist in making the proper diagnosis in this situation. Leaks can sometimes heal with conversion to NIPD or hemodialysis, but they often will require surgical repair. Hydrothorax formation due to passage of dialysate through defects in the hemidiaphragm is a rare complication of PD. Thoracentesis will yield a transudative fluid with a very high glucose concentration. Diagnosis can also be made by radionuclide scanning after technetium-labeled albumin is added to the peritoneal fluid and allowed to dwell for several hours. Definitive treatment will usually involve surgical repair of the diaphragmatic defect.

C. Encapsulating Peritoneal Sclerosis (EPS)

EPS is a rare but serious condition characterized by extensive intraperitoneal fibrosis and encasement of bowel loops. This entity should not be confused with the more benign and subclinical peritoneal fibrosis that can occur in most patients on PD. EPS is typically associated with a progressive loss of ultrafiltration and increased solute transport. Patients may present with bloody effluent, malnutrition, abdominal pain, nausea, and bowel obstruction. Diagnosis is based on clinical symptoms and the CT findings of peritoneal thickening and calcification, evidence of bowel adhesion/obstruction, and the presence of loculated fluid. Pathologic features are similar to those changes seen with long-term PD including mesothelial denudation, interstitial fibrosis, and vasculopathy. The cause of EPS is unknown but may be related to prior episodes of severe peritonitis, a reaction to foreign

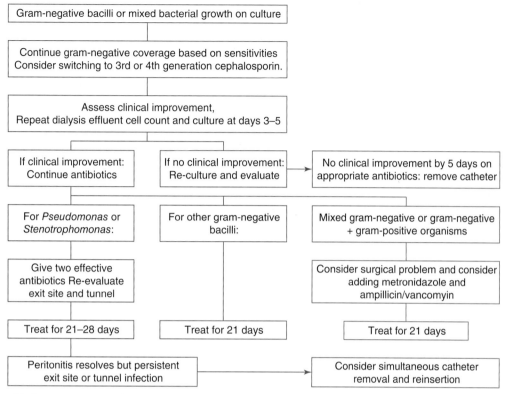

▲ Figure 50–8. Management of peritonitis caused by gram-negative bacteria. (Reproduced with permission from Li PK et al: ISPD Peritonitis Recommendations: 2016 Update on Prevention and Treatment. Perit Dial Int 2016; 36:481.)

substances such as plasticizers or disinfectants, and extended duration of peritoneal dialysis. No uniformly successful therapy for EPS exists at this time and mortality remains quite high (>50%). Described treatment strategies have included cessation of PD, bowel rest, and total parenteral nutrition. Surgery may be beneficial but can be technically difficult. Immunosuppression with corticosteroids and azathioprine and antifibrotic therapy with tamoxifen has been reported in several small series to be beneficial.

D. Ultrafiltration Failure

Fluid balance management is one of the primary functions of renal replacement therapy. Peritoneal dialysis is an excellent modality for fluid removal due to the continuous, more physiologic nature of this modality. However, there remains an unacceptably high incidence of hypertension and cardiovascular disease in the peritoneal dialysis population. Patients are trained to adjust their ultrafiltration by choosing the correct concentration of dextrose in their dialysis solution regimen depending on their dietary intake and volume status. Ultrafiltration failure can be defined as

the failure of peritoneal dialysis fluid removal to match the volume balance needs of the patient. Patients presenting with the clinical syndrome of volume overload need to be carefully evaluated prior to being labeled with ultrafiltration failure. It is important to consider the numerous factors that can alter fluid balance. Reversible causes such as dietary indiscretion, loss of residual renal function, noncompliance with dialysis, mechanical problems such as leaks or catheter malfunction, and inappropriate dialysis prescription need to initially be ruled out. Inappropriate tailoring of a PD prescription to a patient's transport type (eg, using long dwell times with low glucose concentrations in a high transporter) should not be attributed to technique failure. After these reversible causes of impaired fluid removal have been ruled out, then the next diagnostic step is to evaluate the ultrafiltration and transport functions of the peritoneal membrane in parallel (Figure 50–9). This can be accomplished by performing a modification of the standard PET using a 4.25% dextrose solution. A net ultrafiltration volume of less than 400 mL with a 4-hour dwell is considered abnormal. A net ultrafiltration volume greater than 400 mL rules out alterations in peritoneal membrane function and the

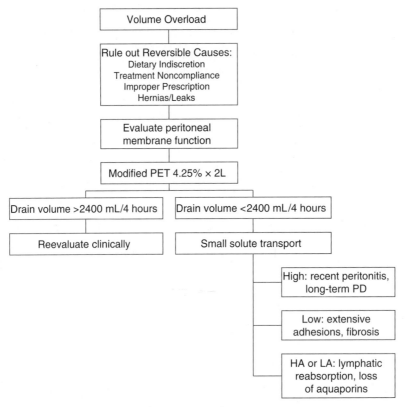

▲ **Figure 50–9.** Evaluation of volume overload in peritoneal dialysis patients.

patient should be reevaluated clinically focusing on dietary indiscretion, noncompliance, inappropriate prescription, or loss of residual renal function.

If the net ultrafiltration volume is less than 400 mL, then small solute transport characteristics should be measured. Patients with a low drain volume and high transport characteristics represent the largest group of patients with ultrafiltration failure. Patients falling into this profile include those patients with inherently high transport (approximately 10% of patients starting PD), patients with recent peritonitis, and patients who have developed high transport during long-term PD. In general it is easy to maintain solute clearance goals in these patients despite a tendency toward clinical volume overload. The combination of low ultrafiltration volume and low transport tends to be rare. This usually represents disruption of the peritoneal membrane or inadequate distribution of the peritoneal fluid such as is seen with severe adhesions or encapsulating peritoneal sclerosis. These patients will have inadequate solute clearance and fluid overload and will be difficult to maintain on PD if they have no residual renal function. Patients with low ultrafiltration volume and low average or high average transport may have

mechanical problems, high peritoneal/lymphatic absorption rates, or aquaporin deficiency.

General therapeutic strategies to prevent fluid overload include routine monitoring of desired weight, residual renal function, daily ultrafiltration volumes and PET results. Dietary counseling concerning salt and fluid intake should be ongoing. Protection of residual renal function should be a priority and high dose loop diuretics may be used in patients with residual renal function to enhance fluid removal. Hyperglycemia must be controlled in diabetic patients to allow maintenance of an osmotic gradient and adequate ultrafiltration. Preservation of peritoneal membrane function by prevention of peritonitis, the timely removal of peritoneal catheters when necessary, and the use of more biocompatible dialysis solutions should also be a priority. Specific therapeutic interventions in patients with poor ultrafiltration and high transport include converting to APD if the patient is undergoing CAPD. With CCPD the long daytime dwell may still result in fluid absorption in very high transporters in which case a manual exchange can be performed in the middle of the day. Another option is to use icodextrin in the long dwell cycle. Icodextrin is poorly absorbed and has been shown to be superior to glucose-based solutions in maintaining net ultrafiltration during long dwells. Patients with poor ultrafiltration and low solute transport will be difficult to maintain on PD if they have no residual renal function and transfer to hemodialysis is usually necessary. Therapeutic options for patients with poor ultrafiltration and low or high average transport include the use of icodextrin in long dwells and shorter dwell times for glucose based exchanges. There are no pharmacologic agents currently available to decrease lymphatic absorption.

E. Metabolic Complications

Peritoneal dialysis can be associated with a number of metabolic abnormalities. Glucose absorption will vary depending on a patients transport characteristics, but can amount to 100–150 g/day. This, in addition to the hyperinsulinemia that ensues, can lead to weight gain and possibly also increased atherosclerosis. Glucose absorption is likely responsible for the lipid abnormalities that are commonly seen in PD patients. PD patients typically have high total and LDL cholesterol, high triglycerides and low HDL cholesterol. This glucose loading may also result in hyperglycemia requiring the initiation or intensification of diabetes therapy. Protein malnutrition is common in PD patients and is partially due to protein loss across the peritoneum which can be substantial (>10 g/day) in patients with high peritoneal transport or with peritonitis. PD patients may also have a suppressed appetite due to absorption of glucose during dialysis and a feeling of abdominal fullness. A protein intake of at least 1.2 g/kg is recommended for PD patients.

KEY READINGS

Goodlad C, Brown EA: Encapsulating peritoneal sclerosis: what have we learned? Semin Nephrol 2011;31:183.
Li P et al: ISPD peritonitis recommendations: 2016 update on prevention and treatment. Perit Dial Int 2016;36:481.
Mujais S et al: Evaluation and management of ultrafiltration problems in peritoneal dialysis. Perit Dial Int 2000;20:396.

▶ Adequacy of Peritoneal Dialysis

Adequacy of dialysis should be interpreted clinically with attention to those parameters that affect quality of life such as nutritional status, anemia management, bone and mineral disorders, blood pressure control and volume status, and mental health. In addition to these clinical parameters, small solute clearances that are based on 24-hour collections of effluent and urine are still commonly used as laboratory measurements of dialysis adequacy. Urea clearance is typically reported in terms of weekly Kt/V, which is the clearance

of urea nitrogen divided by the urea distribution volume. Kt is determined by multiplying the effluent: blood urea nitrogen concentration ratio by the 24 hour total effluent volume (the sum of all dwell volumes and the daily net ultrafiltration volume). If the patient has residual renal function then the daily renal urea nitrogen clearance is added to the peritoneal clearance. This value is then divided by V, which is roughly equal to total body water (60% of weight in males, 55% weight in females) and then multiplied by 7 to give a weekly value.

The International Society of PD has published clinical practice guidelines for the adequacy of solute removal for PD. Based on the results from clinical studies, ISPD has recommended that the delivered weekly clearance should be a minimum Kt/V urea of 1.7 combining peritoneal and residual renal clearance. Renal clearance and peritoneal clearance have different effects on patient survival. In prospective observational studies, it has been residual renal function and not peritoneal small solute clearance that has been most strongly associated with patient survival. Despite this, these clearances are given equal weight and are typically added together for patient management. It is important to monitor residual renal function regularly for those patients who rely significantly on residual renal function to achieve their minimal Kt/V target.

Patients who are not doing well clinically and whose clearance is below target will need to have their dialysis dose increased. Clearance is dependent on the patient's peritoneal membrane characteristics, the length of the dwell time, and the volume of effluent drained per unit time. Four 2-L CAPD exchanges per day with 2 L of daily ultrafiltrate will represent a drain volume of 70 L/wk, which may be inadequate in the absence of renal function for many patients. As renal function is lost, patients may require larger exchange volumes (2.5 or 3 L) and may also need 5 daily exchanges to prevent uremic symptoms and maintain target clearance. Larger patients should be started on 2.5 or 3 L exchange volumes initially. To achieve increased clearance in automated PD one can increase dwell volumes and total time on the cycler, and in some cases one or two daytime dwells may need to be added. Patients should have peritoneal clearance and residual renal function monitored several times per year as part of their routine care.

KEY READINGS

Blake PG et al: Clinical practice guidelines and recommendations on PD adequacy. Perit Dial Int 2011;31:218.
Paniagua R et al: Effects of increased peritoneal clearances on mortality rates in peritoneal dialysis: ADEMEX, a prospective, randomized, controlled trial. J Am Soc Nephrol 2002;13:1307.

■ CHAPTER REVIEW QUESTIONS

1. A 60-year-old woman with ESRD on APD for 5 years develops worsening orthopnea, edema, and progressive weight gain over the last 2 months. She has been adherent to a low-sodium diet and limits her daily fluid intake to 1 L. She is anuric. Her current dialysis regimen is 4 × 2 L exchanges on the cycler over 10 hours with a last fill of 2 L. She uses all 2.5% dextrose dialysate. A recent PET test performed in the clinic shows that she has high peritoneal transport.

Which of the following changes to her PD regimen would be most appropriate?
A. Change all dialysate to 1.5% dextrose.
B. Change her regimen to CAPD.
C. Change her last fill to 7.5% icodextrin.
D. Eliminate her last fill.

2. A 50-year-old man on CAPD presents with abdominal pain and cloudy PD fluid. Examination of the catheter exit site and overlying tunnel is unremarkable. After sending appropriate fluid studies, antibiotic therapy is initiated with intraperitoneal vancomycin and gentamicin. The fluid cell count returns at 300/mm³ with 70% neutrophils and the culture grows MRSA. Gentamicin is discontinued and therapy is continued with IP vancomycin. After 5 days the patient still reports severe abdominal pain. Repeat fluid cell count is 500/mm³ and culture remains positive for MRSA.

What is the most appropriate next step in management?
A. Continue vancomycin and add back gentamicin.
B. Continue vancomycin and arrange for PD catheter removal.
C. Continue vancomycin but change to intravenous therapy.
D. Continue vancomycin and perform an abdominal CT scan.

3. A 40-year-old man with ESRD on APD for 1 year complains of worsening fatigue, poor appetite, and nausea. Despite decreased urine output and increased edema, he has lost 3 kg over the last month. His current PD regimen comprises 4 × 2 L exchanges over 10 hours on the cycler with no last fill. Three months ago in clinic his weekly total Kt/V was 1.7 = 1.2 peritoneal Kt/V and 0.5 renal Kt/V.

Which of the following is the most appropriate next step in management?
A. Transfer patient to in-center hemodialysis.
B. Switch patient to CAPD.
C. Add a daytime dwell to his APD regimen.
D. Add a loop diuretic.

4. A 35-year-old man with ESRD on CAPD presents to clinic with abdominal pain and reports of cloudy PD effluent. A sample of PD fluid is sent for cell count and culture.

Which of the following is the most appropriate next step in management?
A. Start therapy with a first generation cephalosporin.
B. Start therapy with an aminoglycoside.
C. Start therapy with vancomycin and third-generation cephalosporin.
D. Wait for results of fluid culture and sensitivities before starting antibiotics.

5. A 65-year-old woman who has been failing to thrive develops a small bowel obstruction. She has been on APD for 7 years. Her PD fluid has been blood-tinged for the last month, but fluid cultures have been repeatedly negative. An abdominal CT scan reveals dilated bowel loops with peritoneal thickening and calcification.

Which of the following is the most likely explanation for these findings?
A. Encapsulating peritoneal sclerosis
B. Adenocarcinoma with peritoneal metastases
C. Peritonitis due to mycobacteria
D. Peritonitis due to fungus

Continuous Renal Replacement Therapy

Piyush Mathur, MBBS, DNB
Ravindra L. Mehta, MD, FACP, FRCP

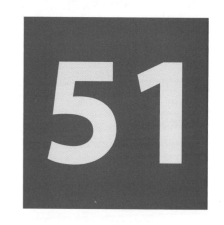

Renal replacement therapy (RRT) can be provided as hemodialysis, hemofiltration, or a combination thereof and as intermittent, or as continuous therapy. Continuous renal replacement therapy (CRRT) represents a number of technically distinct modalities characterized by slow per-minute solute clearance and ultrafiltration rates that are spread over most or all of the day to minimize wide metabolic or volume shifts. The longer duration of therapy has been associated with greater hemodynamic stability and a higher likelihood of kidney recovery compared to standard intermittent hemodialysis (IHD). CRRT encompass several methods of hemofiltration and hemodialysis and is being increasingly utilized for managing patients with AKI in the intensive care unit (ICU) setting. This chapter reviews the major terms used in the delivery of CRRT, the most prominent clinical and technical issues encountered by the healthcare teams, and promising technologies that may improve the efficacy and future applicability of the relevant modalities.

CRRT TERMINOLOGIES AND MODALITIES

Continuous renal replacement therapy is actually an umbrella term for the four different continuous modalities: slow continuous ultrafiltration (SCUF), continuous venovenous hemofiltration (CVVH), continuous venovenous hemodialysis (CVVHD), and continuous venovenous hemodiafiltration (CVVHDF). Solute removal in these techniques is achieved by either convection, diffusion, or a combination of both these methods.

Convective techniques, including ultrafiltration (UF) and hemofiltration (H), depend on solute removal by solvent drag.

Diffusion-based techniques, similar to intermittent hemodialysis (IHD), are based on the principle of a solute gradient between the blood and the dialysate.

Hemodiafiltration (HDF) processes use both diffusion and convection in the same technique. In this instance, both dialysate and a replacement solution are used, and both small and middle molecules can be removed easily.

The predominant mechanism of achieving clearance defines the modality of CRRT.

Simple diffusion: continuous venovenous hemodialysis (CVVHD)

Convection: continuous venovenous hemofiltration (CVVH)

Combination of both diffusion and convection (continuous venovenous hemodiafiltration [CVVHDF]) Table 51–1 and Figure 51–1.

CRRT PRINCIPLES

Solute removal in CRRT can be obtained by convection, diffusion, or both. Each component of the therapy can be precisely controlled, and by use of high-flux membrane filters, removal of middle and high molecules can be maximized. By removing solutes through convection, diffusion, and adsorption and replenishing depleted solutes selectively by varying the composition of the solutions used in the process, CRRT can be used to achieve solute balance to any desired level. These mechanisms can be manipulated by the type of membrane and blood and fluid flow rates to selectively influence solute clearances of molecules of different size.

▶ Diffusion

Diffusion is movement of solutes across concentration gradient through semipermeable membrane and depends on:

Concentration gradient (Cs)

Surface area of membrane (A)

Thickness of membrane (Mt)

Diffusion coefficient of the solute (D)

Temperature of solution (T)

Table 51–1. Modalities of CRRT.

	SCUF	CVVH	CVVHD	CVVHDF
Vascular access	VV	VV	VV	VV
Av. blood flow (mL/min)	100	100–200	100–200	100–200
Dialysate flow (mL/min)	0	0	10–30	10–30
Replacement fluid (L/day)	0	21.6	0	16.8
Ultrafiltrate (mL/min)	2–8	10–30	2–4	10–30
Anticoagulation	Yes/no	Yes/no	Yes/no	Yes/no
Clearance mechanism	C	C	D	C + D
Urea clearance (L/day)	1.7	16.7	21.7	30

CVVH, continuous venovenous hemofiltration; CVVHD, continuous venovenous hemodialysis; CVVHDF, continuous venovenous hemodiafiltration; SCUF, slow continuous ultrafiltration.

The gradient is affected by the dialysate infusion rate (Qd) and blood-flow rate (Qb). The dialysate runs countercurrent to the blood, so faster Qb allows for greater gradient. This is the same technique used in IHD, but Qd are much slower than Qb so there is complete saturation of the dialysate. Therefore, the Qd is the rate-limiting factor for solute removal, but it allows for enhanced clearance. The smaller the size/weight of the solute and the greater the gradient, the more efficiently solute clearance occurs.

Diffusion flux of a given solute Sd = (Cs/Mt) DTA

Convection

Convective techniques (UF and H) rely on what is known as "solvent drag," whereby dissolved molecules are dragged along with ultrafiltrated plasma water across a semipermeable membrane driven by a transmembrane pressure (TMP) gradient in response to a hydrostatic or osmotic force. The process of forcing a liquid against a membrane is called ultrafiltration; the fluid collected after it passes through a membrane is the ultrafiltrate. This can be described by the following equation:

$$Uf = Kf \times TMP$$

$$Kf = \text{coefficient of hydraulic permeability}$$

$$TMP = (Pb - Puf) - \pi$$

where Pb is hydrostatic pressure of blood, Puf is the hydrostatic pressure of the ultrafiltrate or dialysate, and π is the oncotic pressure of plasma proteins.

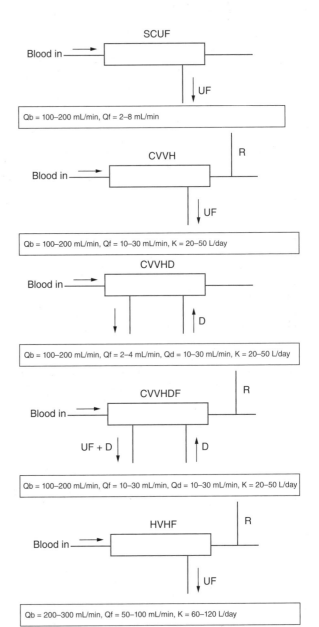

▲ **Figure 51–1.** Modalities of continuous renal replacement therapies (CRRT). Commonly available modalities in ICU. CVVH, continuous veno venous hemofiltration; CVVHD, continuous veno venous hemodialysis; CVVHDF, continuous veno venous hemodiafiltration; HVHF, high-volume hemofiltration; K, clearance; Qb, blood flow; Qd, dialysate flow; Qf, ultrafiltration rate; R, replacement; SCUF, slow continuous ultrafiltration.

The convective clearance (Cx) of a solute x will therefore depend on the following:

$$Cx = Jf \times Cs \times S$$

Jf = amount of ultrafiltration

Cs = concentration of solute in plasma water

S = sieving characteristics of membrane

Sieving coefficient (S) is the ratio of solute concentration in filtrate to solute concentration in plasma and is regulated by the reflection coefficient of the membrane (S = 1 − σ). A solute with an SC of 1 means that it can pass freely through a filter; if the SC is 0, then a solute cannot pass through the filter at all. Protein-bound solutes or those that exceed the molecular weight cutoff (generally 20,000 Da for polysulfone and polyacrylonitrile membranes) have sieving coefficients less than 1. For some molecules, adsorption across the membrane provides and additional mechanism for clearance. This is particularly relevant for poly methyl methacrylate (PMMA) membranes that can bind different cytokines.

CRRT CIRCUIT

Vascular Access

A well-functioning vascular access is a prerequisite for successful CRRT. Temporary or tunneled cuffed hemodialysis (HD) catheters are currently used as vascular access for CRRT. The Kidney Dialysis: Initiative and Global Outcomes (KDIGO) guideline recommends the use of ultrasound guidance for catheter placement because its use has been reported to reduce the failure and complication rates of central venous catheter insertion.

Blood stream infection, catheter malfunction due to thrombosis, kinking of catheter, fibrin sheath around catheter tip are some complications associated with catheters. AV fistulas and grafts are generally not recommended for CRRT due to the risk for needle displacement and high risk for injury to the access that may make it unusable in the future.

Anticoagulation

As in other extracorporeal circuits, anticoagulation is essential to prevent the activation of clotting mechanisms within the circuit and is necessary for effective delivery of CRRT. Adequate anticoagulation ensures efficacy of the filter in fluid and solute removal, overall filter longevity, and optimum patient management. Several anticoagulation methods are available and both systemic and regional anticoagulation strategies are commonly used.

A. Systemic Anticoagulation

Systemic anticoagulants have the advantage of being relatively easy to administer, especially in comparison with citrate anticoagulation. The most commonly used agents are heparins and direct thrombin inhibitors such as argatroban and hirudins.

Unfractionated Heparin

Unfractionated heparin (UFH) continues to be the most commonly used anticoagulant. It catalyses the inactivation of thrombin, factor Xa and factor IXa by antithrombin. UFH has short biologic half-life (90 minutes but can increase up to 3 hours in presence of renal insufficiency). It is mainly metabolized by the liver, with the kidney as a minor contributor to overall clearance in those patients with intact kidney function. However, neither dialysis nor hemofiltration clears heparin efficiently, and as such, the half-life of heparin is increased to roughly 40–120 minutes in patients on CRRT. UFH is usually administered as a bolus of 30 IU/kg (2000–5000 IU), followed by a continuous infusion of 5–10 IU/kg/h into arterial limb of the dialysis circuit. Careful monitoring of clotting times is necessary, with target activated clotting times (ACT) ranging from 140 to 180 seconds or activated partial thromboplastin times of 55–100 seconds. The major complication from unfractionated heparin use is hemorrhage, which occurs in roughly 25–30% of patients in whom heparin is used as the CRRT anticoagulant. Patients with minor bleeding should have their anticoagulation stopped, while patients with serious bleeding may benefit from administration of protamine. Occasionally, heparin-induced thrombocytopenia (HIT) can occur, the first sign of which may be repeated filter clotting.

Low Molecular Weight Heparin

Recently, low molecular weight heparins (LMWHs) have been shown to be safe and effective drugs for anticoagulation of CRRT circuit. These agents have higher anti-Xa/anti-IIa activity than UFH, less protein binding, more predictable pharmacokinetics, and lesser incidence of HIT. Nadroparin, dalteparin in a dose of 15–25 IU/kg as bolus followed by 5–10 IU/kg/h, and enoxaparin as 0.15 mg/kg and a maintenance infusion starting at 0.05 mg/kg/h are the agents used in various studies.

Regional Citrate

Regional citrate anticoagulation (RCA) has become increasingly popular as centers have become more familiar with its use. Its effect is based on the ability of citrate to chelate calcium (and other divalent cations), which is required at multiple levels of both the intrinsic and extrinsic coagulation cascades.

Citrate is infused into the blood at the beginning of the extracorporeal circuit which chelates ionized calcium and provides anticoagulation in the circuit. Calcium-citrate complex which is formed in the circuit is freely filtered and is lost in effluent, so calcium is infused systemically to replace the lost calcium to keep the ionized calcium within normal limits and infusion is titrated accordingly. In most protocols, the citrate infusion rate starts at a fixed fraction of blood flow and the calcium infusion starts as a fixed fraction of citrate flow. Prefilter (ie, circuit) and postfilter (ie, patient) ionized calcium levels are drawn periodically to monitor the efficacy of anticoagulation, with target levels being 0.25–0.35 and 1.1–1.3 mmol/L, respectively. The rates of the two infusions are then adjusted accordingly to meet those target ranges.

Regional citrate anticoagulation has several advantages over systemic anticoagulation. First, assuming ionized calcium levels in the patient should be normal, there is little to no bleeding risk above the patient's baseline risk. Second, citrate anticoagulation is associated with the longest filter life when compared with other anticoagulant strategies. Lastly, because citrate is metabolized by tricarboxylic acid pathway to three bicarbonate molecules in the liver, the citrate can also act as a therapeutic agent in patients with acidosis, obviating or lessening the need for anionic base replacement in the replacement fluids or dialysate. But, if the care team is not mindful that citrate is converted to bicarbonate and can represent a significant base load, severe metabolic alkalosis can occur. To decrease the risk of alkalosis, some centers have begun using high chloride dialysate.

Patients with severe liver failure and lactic acidosis may have difficulty in metabolizing citrate and may develop citrate toxicity defined as plasma total calcium/ionized calcium greater than four. Recent studies have shown that this ratio is closely related to the clinical outcome and emerged as an independent predictor of 28-day mortality. This ratio is associated with hepatic and/or multiorgan dysfunction and therefore an important therapeutic target. High ratio can be treated by attempting to increase the circuit clearance of citrate by decreasing the blood flow rate, by increasing the dialysate flow rate, and/or by decreasing the citrate infusion rate. Other complications which can occur during citrate anticoagulation are metabolic acidosis, hypernatremia

particularly with hypertonic sodium citrate and high anion gap. Figure 51–2 shows CRRT circuit with RCA.

The use of intermittent saline solution flushes in the CRRT circuit is an option when no anticoagulation is used in CRRT. Saline solution flushes every 15–30 minutes in the arterial tubing of the circuit help wash fibrin strands from the membrane. However, membrane efficacy may be compromised before the system clots and filter half-lives are generally reduced. It is thus essential to measure filter clearances on an ongoing basis through the ratio of solute concentration in effluent (Cef) to Cp. Assessment of Cef:Cp ratio can be done every 12 hours, and a ratio less than 0.8 can help predict filter clotting. The volume administered on the flushes must be included to calculate net ultrafiltration.

Other alternative methods of anticoagulation have been investigated, including regional heparin/protamine, heparinoids, thrombin antagonists (hirudin and argatroban), regional citrate, prostanoids, and nafamostat, with regional citrate anticoagulation (RCA) gaining wider acceptance with the development of simplified and safer protocols. These are summarized in Table 51–2.

▶ CRRT Solutions

All CRRT other than SCUF and CVVHD require the use of replacement fluids to compensate for the ultrafiltrate removed. A consequence of all CRRT methods is the ongoing loss of bicarbonate and electrolytes across the filter generally equivalent to the plasma concentration of these solutes times the total effluent (UF and dialysate) flow rates. Commercially prepared sterile fluids are now available as premixed dialysis and replacement solutions for

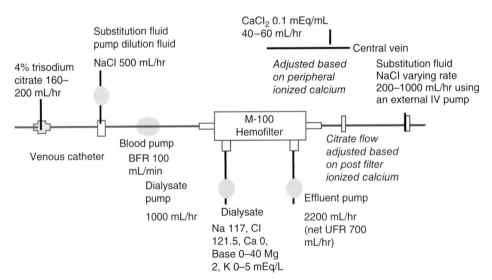

▲ **Figure 51–2.** CRRT circuit using regional citrate anticoagulation with the Gambro PRISMA machine and M-100 filter.

Table 51–2. Anticoagulation methods.

Method	Initial Dose	Maintenance Dose	Advantage	Disadvantage	Monitoring
Heparin	30 U/kg bolus	5–10 U/kg/h	Standard method; easy to use; inexpensive	Bleeding risk; thrombocytopenia	APTT 1.5–2 times of normal
LMWH Nadoparin/ Dalteparin Enoxaparin	15–25 IU/kg 0.15 mg/kg	5–10 IU/kg/h 0.05 mg/kg/h	Decreased risk of bleeding Higher anti-Xa/anti-IIa Lesser HIT	Poor reversibility with protamine Expensive Monitoring not easily available	Factor Xa levels; maintained between 0.1 and 0.41 U/mL
Regional citrate	4% trisodium citrate 150–180 mL/h	100–180 mL/h 3–7% of BFR, Ca replaced by central line	No bleeding; No thrombocytopenia Improved filter efficacy, Longevity	Complex; needs Ca monitoring; alkalosis	ACT: 200–250 maintain ionized calcium 0.96–1.2 mmol/L
Heparinoid (Danaparoid)	750–2500 U	1–2 U/kg/h	Decreased HIT	Bleeding risk Cross reactivity with heparin/ PF4 Prolonged half life in renal failure No antidote	Anti-Xa level between 0.25 and 0.35 IU/mL
Thrombin antagonist— Hirudin Argatroban	250 mcg/kg	0.005–0.01 mg/kg/h or 0.002 g/kg bolus doses 0.5–2 mcg/kg/min	Can be used in patients with HIT Can be used in patients with HIT hepatic excretion, so no dose modification in renal failure	Renal excretion-prolonged half life No antidote No antidote	Ecarin clotting test (ECT)—not easily available Target-80-100 s APTT 1–1.5 times normal
Platelet inhibiting agents prostacyclin		2–8 ng/kg/min infusion prefilter	Better circuit life	Hypotension expensive Usually needs UFH coadministration	Not required APTT when UFH used
Nafamostat		0.1 mg/kg/h	No heparin	Anaphylaxis, agranulocytosis hyperkalemia	ACT

ACT, activated clotting time; aPTT, activated partial thromboplastin time; BFR, blood flow rate; HIT, heparin induced thrombocytopenia; LMWH, low molecular weight heparin; PF4, platelet factor 4; UFH, unfractionated heparin.

CRRT which contains alkali in form of lactate or bicarbonate and electrolytes. The variable concentrations of these electrolytes allow tailoring of dialysate and replacement fluids to meet the needs of the individual patient. The choice of agent for base replacement has been a topic of some controversy, as both have significant advantages and disadvantages.

When lactate based solution is used replacement of buffer stores depends on the metabolic rate for conversion to bicarbonate. In the absence of lactic acidosis, endogenous lactate clearance does not appear to be impaired. However, the filter clearance of lactate accounts for only 2.4% of overall lactate clearance. Lactate is converted on an equimolar basis to bicarbonate in the liver and in patients with liver dysfunction, hypotension and multiorgan failure, the ability to convert lactate to bicarbonate might be impaired and could contribute to the deleterious effects of lactate accumulation. A serum lactate increase greater than 5 mmol/L during CRRT indicates lactate intolerance.

Bicarbonate, on the other hand, is physiologic and does not rely on patient's organ function for its buffering action. However, bicarbonate solutions are difficult to store because of short shelf life, and can microprecipitate with calcium if mixed in the same bag. Several studies have suggested that lactate can cause increased catabolism and worsened hemodynamics compared to bicarbonate. The KDIGO guideline suggests using bicarbonate instead of lactate as a buffer in dialysate and substitution fluid for RRT in patients with AKI, in patients with AKI and circulatory shock, and in patients with AKI and liver failure and/or lactic acidemia. In ICU patients, bicarbonate buffer in dialysate or substitution solution results in better acidosis correction, reduced lactate levels, and better hemodynamic improvement. The combination of citrate anticoagulation and bicarbonate-containing solutions has been used effectively to manage complex acid–base disorders.

The replacement fluid and/or dialysate should contain electrolytes in concentrations aiming for physiologic levels and taking into account preexisting deficits or excesses and all inputs and losses. One of the major advantages of CRRT is that the composition of replacement fluid and dialysate can be modified to achieve any specific change in plasma composition. For instance, patients with severe hypo or hypernatremia (sodium <115 or >160 mEq/L) can be managed with CRRT and the rate of correction can be adjusted by varying sodium composition in the substitution fluid and dialysate.

CRRT Membrane

The type of membrane defines the solute removal capacity and water permeability during CRRT.

Molecular weight cutoff, structure, and charge of a membrane affect the ability of a solute to convectively cross a membrane and the adsorption capacity. Inflammatory mediators (interleukin 6 [IL-6], IL-8, IL-1, and tumor necrosis factor a) can be removed by convection according to the molecular weight and degree of plasma protein binding. The ability of removing and adsorbing larger molecular-weight solutes with CVVH and CVVHDF may offer advantages in sepsis or systemic inflammatory response syndrome.

CRRT PRESCIPTION

Patient Selection and Timing

Generally, the decision to use CRRT is affected by physician beliefs as well as a number of patient and organizational characteristics. Patient characteristics may include age, gender, race, illness acuity and comorbidities. Organizational characteristics vary depending on country, type of institution, type of ICU, type of physician or insurance provider and perceived cost of therapy. Common factors responsible for the decision to delay are the risk associated with vascular access placement, anticoagulant administration, hypotension, arrhythmia, and risk for RRT dependence.

The decision to start acute RRT should be individualized and not be based solely on renal function or stage of AKI. Many small randomized control trials (RCTs), observational, cohort studies and meta-analyses have concluded that early initiation of RRT has better outcomes as compared to late initiation. However, few studies did not show any mortality benefit in early initiation of RRT. Two large RCTs (STARRT AKI and ELAIN are under way to study impact of early or accelerated initiation versus late or standard initiation of RRT.

Acute dialysis and quality initiative (ADQI) group meeting held recently on "precision CRRT" in Italy gave a consensus statement that acute RRT should be considered when metabolic and fluid demands exceed total kidney capacity (Figure 51–3). Demand for kidney function is determined by nonrenal comorbidities, the severity of the acute disease and solute and fluid burden and total kidney function is measured using a variety of different methods. Traditionally, serum creatinine and urine output are used as surrogate markers of renal function but they have their own limitations. Novel biomarkers including serum cystatin C and urine and plasma neutrophil gelatinase associated lipocalcin NGAL have emerged to predict renal damage before rise of serum creatinine and/or fall in urine output. However, these biomarkers were developed to predict AKI but not the need for RRT. Changes in kidney function and duration of kidney dysfunction can be anticipated by these markers of kidney damage.

Finally, CRRT should be initiated as renal support, instead of renal replacement, aiming to maintain normal acid base, electrolyte, and fluid status along with liberal nutritional support.

Fluid Management

Fluid management is an integral component of the care of critically ill patients to maintain hemodynamic stability and optimize organ function. The dynamic nature of critical illness often necessitates volume resuscitation and contributes to fluid overload particularly in the presence of altered renal function. Successful fluid management with CRRT depends on an accurate assessment of fluid status, an adequate comprehension of the principles of fluid management with UF, and clear treatment goals.

Fluid management in CRRT offers the opportunity to adjust plasma composition and the amount of fluid in the body. These two processes can be dissociated, thereby permitting any level of fluid balance to be coupled with a specific level of the target solute (eg, a sodium level can be kept high, normal, or low while fluid balance is kept even, negative, or positive) and maintained over time. This flexibility in therapy is achieved by manipulating the composition of the dialysate and substitution fluids and varying the amount of net ultrafiltration over a specific time.

Fluids are administered at various sites in the CRRT circuit and also intravenously. Replacement fluids are administered either prefilter (predilution), postfilter (postdilution) or intravenously. Dialysate solutions are typically administered through the dialysis port in the filter. Fluids administered before the filter (predilution) are utilized to prevent or reduce filter clotting independent of the anticoagulation used, by lowering the blood viscosity through a decrease in the hematocrit (Hct) and reducing the filtration fraction (FF). FF is expressed as follows:

$$FF = \frac{ultrafiltrate\,rate\,(UF)\,mL\,/\,min}{plasma\,flow\,rate\,(Qp)\,mL\,/\,min}$$

where Qp is the blood flow rate (Qb)(1-Hct).

An increase in UF rate and Hct or a decrease in plasma flow rate will increase FF and thus increase the risk of filter clotting. A high FF (>0.25) is typically associated with increased risk of poor filter performance and clotting due to hemoconcentration-related effects. Fluids administered prefilter decreases FF

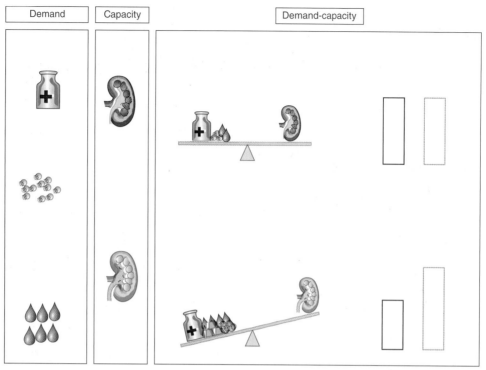

▲ **Figure 51–3.** Demand and capacity—a conceptual model. (Modified from Ostermann M et al: Patient selection and timing of continuous renal replacement therapy. Blood Purif 2016;42:224. Reprinted from Acute Dialysis Quality Initiative 17, www.adqi.org, © ADQI.)

and prevents filter clotting but at the same time solute dose is decreased because of dilution. Table 51–3 shows advantages and disadvantages of pre- and postfilter fluids.

Fluid removal in RRT is achieved through varying amounts of net ultrafiltration rate (Qnet) that can be tailored to individual need. The net ultrafiltrate is the difference between total ultrafiltrate (the plasma water removed) and total substitution (the fluid given to the patient) through the CRRT machine. CRRT machines offer the precision to balance all the fluids removed and replaced across the dialysis circuit in order to generate a net amount of fluid removal over a time. However, the CRRT machine balance does not represent the actual patient fluid balance, which includes all intakes and outputs, including the CRRT machine balance (itself determined by Qnet). Consequently, achieving patient fluid balance with CRRT requires knowledge of other intakes and outputs that need to be integrated in the prescription and delivery.

There are various techniques for achieving fluid balance with CRRT (Table 51–4 and Figure 51–4). The most common technique is to vary Qnet to meet the anticipated fluid balance needs over 8–24 hours. Net ultrafiltration can be adjusted at different intervals ranging from hourly to every

Table 51–3. Advantages and disadvantages of pre- and post-filter substitution.

Prefilter	Postfilter
Advantages –UF rate is not limited by Qb. –Enhanced elimination of urea from RBCs. –Filter life is increased as the Hct throughout the filter remains low. –Filter life is increased which may increase filter lifespan and solute clearance, even though hourly solute clearance is decreased. **Disadvantages** Solute concentrations are decreased and thus clearance is decreased.	**Advantages** –Clearance of solutes is directly related to UF rate. –A higher solute clearance rate is produced. –Delivery of specified solutes and concentrations directly to the solution. **Disadvantages** –UF rate is limited by Qb. Too much UF cannot be ordered because the end-filter Hct will be too high. –Because UF rate is limited by FF you may not reach optimal dose. –Filter life may be decreased by high end-filter Hct.

RBC, red blood cell.

Table 51–4. Two different methods for fluid balance in CRRT.

Variable	Ultrafiltration Technique	Replacement Fluid Technique
Fluid balance	Achieved by varying UF rate.	Achieved by adjusting amount of replacement fluids.
Differences	Output is varied to accommodate changes in intake and output to reach a fluid removal goal.	Output is fixed to achieve solute clearance goal and replacement fluid rates are changed to allow flexibility in reaching net fluid balance goals.
Advantages	Familiar strategy from intermittent HD. Can allow for fluid balance calculations over an extended period with calculation of a rate per unit time.	Allows for constant solute clearance. Dissociates clearance parameters from fluid balance.
Disadvantages	Solute clearance may fluctuate. Requires frequent interactions with CRRT machine to adjust UF rates to meet patient needs.	Requires hourly calculations of the amount of replacement fluid to be given with risk for fluid imbalance if rate not calculated correctly with clear appreciation of all of the inputs and outputs for the patient.

6–12 hours. Inherent to this method is that effluent volume and hence solute clearance will vary with each adjustment in net ultrafiltration. A second method of maintaining fluid balance is to keep a fixed rate of ultrafiltration that exceeds the hourly intake from all sources and to vary the amount of postdilution substitution fluid administered. This method ensures a constant effluent volume and solute clearance level. The postdilution fluid can be given outside the CRRT circuit through a peripheral intravenous line, thereby minimizing interactions with the machine. The third method is similar to the second, but fluid balance is tailored to achieve a targeted hemodynamic parameter every hour. Predefined targets are set for parameters, such as central venous pressure, mean arterial pressure (MAP), or pulmonary arterial wedge pressure, and scales are prescribed to achieve these targets.

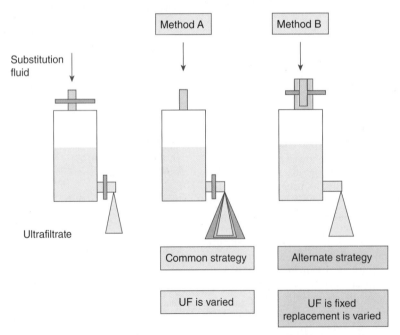

▲ **Figure 51–4.** Approaches to fluid regulation with CRRT fluid balance. (Modified from Murugan R et al: Precision fluid management in continuous renal replacement therapy. Blood Purif 2016;42:266. Reprinted from Acute Dialysis Quality Initiative 17, www.adqi.org, © ADQI.)

Acid-Base and Electrolyte Management

Derangement of acid–base and electrolyte homeostasis is a common feature of critically ill patients requiring renal replacement therapy. Ultrafiltration further disturbs blood chemistry as there is ongoing loss of bicarbonate and other electrolytes across the filter. The degree of electrolyte loss can essentially be expressed as the total ultrafiltrate/dialysate effluent rate times the plasma concentration of the individual electrolytes. For example, if the ultrafiltration rate is 2 L/h and the plasma bicarbonate concentration is 25 mEq/L, the patient will be losing 50 mEq of bicarbonate into the waste ultrafiltrate every hour. Thus, management of acid–base and electrolyte balance in CRRT requires ongoing replacement of iatrogenic bicarbonate and electrolyte losses, in addition to the correction of the patient's intrinsic metabolic abnormalities. Regulation of acid–base status is generally accomplished by adding either lactate or bicarbonate into the dialysate or replacement fluid. Control of electrolyte levels in CRRT is usually accomplished by either infusing replacement fluids containing appropriate concentrations of electrolytes and/or by diffusive exchange with the proper dialysate. The dialysate and replacement fluids differ in concentrations of potassium, magnesium, calcium, bicarbonate, and dextrose. These variable concentrations allow tailoring of dialysate and replacement fluids to meet the needs of the individual patient. For instance, a patient with serum potassium concentration of 6.8 mEq/L requiring high-dose pressors may benefit from CVVHD with a dialysate potassium concentration of 0 mEq/L and this can be modified further depending upon the patient's need and serum electrolyte concentrations.

Drug Clearance, Dosing and Intensity in Continuous Renal Replacement Therapy

A. Drug Clearance

The pharmacokinetics of drug removal in critically ill patients receiving CRRT is very complex, with multiple variables affecting clearance and both patient and CRRT technique–related factors should be considered for drug dosing in CRRT. As a result, the frequent variation on CRRT use makes generalized dosing recommendations impractical; however, some general rules apply. A fundamental concept in pharmacokinetics is drug clearance, that is, elimination of drugs from the body, analogous to the concept of creatinine clearance. Clearance can conceptually be considered to be a function of both distribution and elimination. In the simplest pharmacokinetic model,

$$Clearance = V \times K$$

V is the volume of distribution, and K is the elimination constant. V is the volume of fluid in which the dose is initially diluted, and thus, the higher the V, the lower the

initial concentration. K is the elimination constant, which is inversely proportional to the half-life, the period of time that must elapse to reach a 50% decrease in plasma concentration. When the half-life is short, K is high and plasma concentrations decline rapidly. Thus, both a high V and a high K result in relatively low plasma concentrations and a high clearance.

The larger the volume of distribution of lipid-soluble drugs, reduce the amount removed during CRRT. Drugs with limited protein binding are removed by CRRT more efficiently. Convective therapies, CVVH and CVVHDF, are expected to have higher removal of solutes with large molecular weights. The proportion of drug removal by CRRT is associated with filter pore size and is represented by the sieving coefficient of the drug. The sieving coefficient of a drug is highest during the first hours of filter use and progressively declines as protein builds up a layer on the membrane and decreases the number of unclotted fibers. Prefilter substitution fluid dilutes the blood reaching the hemodialyzer and reduces drug clearance. Increased Qb or Qd can increase drug clearance. Drug adsorption to the filter is an additional issue, especially with polyacrylonitrile filters, with the extent of adsorption being difficult to quantify. For drugs expected to be significantly removed by CRRT, extra doses are required to prevent underdosing, and when available, therapeutic drug monitoring should be used to guide drug dosing in CRRT. Table 51–5 summarizes various factors effecting drug clearances.

B. Solute Dose and Intensity

The ideal CRRT prescription for AKI should incorporate an assessment of the dose delivered. Dosing and intensity of CRRT are generally defined in terms of solute clearance and is traditionally assessed by measuring clearance of urea. Most studies considered the prescribed dose as the effluent rate represented by milliliter per kilogram per hour and reported this volume as a surrogate of solute removal. While assessing dose, various factors including water volumes, urea

Table 51–5. Factors affecting drug clearance in CRRT.

Drug and Patient Related	Dialysis Related
Bioavailability	Molecular weight of drug
Volume of distribution	Type of dialyzer
Protein binding and lipid solubility	Mode of CRRT
Drug metabolism	Flow rates
Elimination route	
Loading and maintenance dose	

generation rates, residual kidney function, and different clearance methods should be considered. Filter fouling can reduce the efficacy of solute clearance, therefore, the actual delivered dose may be substantially lower than the observed effluent rate. The prescribed dose based on the effluent rate should be incremented by 20–25%, anticipating temporary disconnections that decrease treatment time and loss of filter efficacy during the course of CRRT. Table 51–6 shows methods to assess dose.

Because effluent rate only provides an inaccurate estimate of delivered dose, in 2012 Claure-Del Granado et al actually recommend measuring and expressing delivered dose as urea clearance (K_D or K_{urea}), derived from dialysate-side kinetics. It is the ratio of mass removal rate to blood concentration and is calculated using the formula: K delivered = (FUN × EV)/BUN, where FUN is urea nitrogen in the effluent (mg/dL), BUN in urea nitrogen in the plasma (mg/dL), and EV is effluent volume (mL/min). K_D takes into account filter function and duration and effective time of treatment.

Various recent trials have assessed relationship between intensity of CRRT and outcomes of AKI. The Acute Renal Failure Trial Network (ATN) and Randomized Evaluation of Normal versus Augmented Level (RENAL) compared standard dose intensity versus high intensity. The ATN and RENAL studies have now established an upper limit of intensity for CRRT, but CRRT dose should be prescribed on the basis of patient body weight to the established effluent flow rate target of 20–25 mL/kg of body weight per hour. Based on randomized controlled trials, KDIGO guidelines recommend delivering an effluent dose of 20–25 mL/kg/h for patients with AKI; other references recommend a dose of 25–30 mL/kg/h. In most of these studies, greater than or equal to 85% of the prescribed dose was delivered to AKI patients. This is usually much more than what is delivered in clinical practice, therefore, when prescribing a treatment dose, clinicians should have about a 25% safety margin; prescribing a dose of 30–35 mL/kg/h may then deliver an adequate dose.

C. Nutritional Support

CRRT techniques allow for an unrestricted volume of nutritional support. However, it may also determine losses of nutrients that are water soluble and have low molecular weight. The estimated loss of amino acid in patients on CRRT is 10–20 g/day, depending on ultrafiltration volume. Water-soluble vitamins, micronutrients, and trace elements are also lost during CRRT and should be replaced during prolonged therapy. The KDIGO guideline recommends up to 1.7 g/kg/day of protein in patients receiving CRRT. Carbohydrates should be given at 5–7 g/kg/day, and lipids, at 1.2–1.5 g/kg/day. CRRT offers an opportunity to measure catabolic rates when steady state is achieved because effluent

Table 51–6. Methods to assess dose in CRRT.

Dialysate side

CVVH
Prescribed dose = Qs + Qnet
Delivered dose = Qef = (Qs + Qnet) × (FUN/BUN)

CVVHD
Prescribed dose = Qd + Qnet
Delivered dose = Qef = (Qd + Qnet) × (FUN/BUN)

CVVHDF
Prescribed dose = Qs + Qd + Qnet
Delivered dose = Qef + (Qs + Qd + Qnet) × (FUN/BUN)

Correcting for predilution effect
Delivered dose = Qnet × {[Qbw/(Qbw + Qs)] + Qd × [Qbw/(Qbw + Qs)]} × S

Dialysis clearance
Kd (mL/min) = [EUN (mg/mL) × Qef]/prefilter BUN (mg/mL)

Blood side

Urea clearance
KB = Qb × (BUNi [mg/dL] – BUNf [mg/dL])/BUNi [mg/dL]

Normalized clearances

CVVH, CVVHD, and CVVHDF postfilter dilution
StdKt/V5 Qef × [10.080/(W 3 0.55)] × S

CVVH and CVVHDF prefilter dilution
StdKt/V = Qef × [Qbw/(Qbw + Qs)] × [10.080/(W30.55)] × S

Equivalent renal urea clearance
EKR = G – {[(Vt × BUNt) – (V₀ × BUN₀)]/T}/TAC_BUN
where TAC_BUN = [(preBUN + postBUN) × t] + [(post BUN + post BUN)] × 60
{(pre2BUN × 0)/[2 × (t + 60 + 0)]}

BUN, blood urea nitrogen concentration; BUNf, outflow BUN concentration; BUNi, inflow BUN concentration; preBUN, pretreatment BUN; postBUN, post-treatment BUN; pre2BUN, pretreatment BUN of the next treatment; CRRT, continuous renal replacement therapy; CVVH, continuous venovenous hemofiltration; CVVHDF, continuous venovenous hemodiafiltration; EUN, amount of urea nitrogen removed (mL/min); FUN, effluent fluid urea nitrogen; G, net urea generation rate (in mg/min); Qbw, plasma flow rate, calculated as Qb 3 (1 – hematocrit), eg, when hematocrit is 0.3 and Qb is 100 mL/min, the Qbw 5 70 mL/min; Qd, dialysate flow rate; Qef, effluent flow rate (mL/min); Qnet, net ultrafiltration rate; Qs, substitution fluid rate; Quf, ultrafiltration rate; S, sieving coefficient; StdKt/V, standard Kt/V; TACBUN, time-averaged BUN concentration (mg/mL); UF, ultrafiltration; V, urea volume of distribution; subscripts 0 and t refer to values at time 0 and t; T is the duration between 0 and t; W, body weight.

solute nitrogen concentrations represent urea nitrogen generation and the associated protein breakdown as urea nitrogen is 16% of protein content. In patients with AKI receiving CRRT, normalized protein catabolic rate is known to be 1.4–1.8 g/kg/day.

Advantages of Continuous Renal Replacement Therapy

As a general group, continuous techniques enjoy theoretical advantages over IHD.

A. Improved Hemodynamic Tolerability

Hypotension is one of the most common complications associated with intermittent hemodialysis, occurring in approximately 20–30% of all treatments. In critically ill patients, the majority of whom are already hemodynamically unstable, further iatrogenic hypotensive events may lead to further organ ischemia and injury. Several prospective and retrospective studies have demonstrated better hemodynamic stability associated with CRRT, although this has not been rigorously validated.

B. Efficiency of Solute Removal

Although the clearance rate of small solutes is slower per unit time with CRRT, the continuous nature of the therapy leads to urea clearances that are more efficient after 48 hours than with alternate day intermittent hemodialysis.

C. Control Over Fluid Management

In the ICU, nutritional requirements (ie, total parenteral nutrition) and the use of intravenous medications often necessitate the administration of large amounts of fluid. The inability to severely restrict fluid intake in ICU patients can result in excessive volume overload, which may compromise tissue perfusion and has been associated with adverse outcomes. Attempts to restrict fluid in this setting may additionally compromise adequate nutrition. The ability to adjust fluid balance as often as hourly, even in hemodynamically unstable patients, is in large part responsible for the growing popularity of CRRT among intensivists.

D. Potential for Immunomodulation

In septic patients, mortality rates appear to be correlated with the levels of various inflammatory cytokines, including tumor necrosis factor (TNF)-α, interleukin (IL)-1, IL-6, and IL-8. Most of these middle-molecular-weight molecules are water soluble and are theoretically removable by plasma water purification via hemofiltration or hemodiafiltration. At present, the immunomodulatory benefits of CRRT remain theoretical and have not been shown to affect outcome in human studies.

Disadvantages of Continuous Renal Replacement Therapy

Conversely, CRRT has certain disadvantages when compared to IHD.

A. Nursing Burden

One-to-one nursing is generally required due to the more intensive monitoring necessary to manage fluid balance and metabolic parameters. A multidisciplinary approach is an essential component of CRRT delivery and requires careful care coordination that should be optimized with standardized protocols.

B. Continuous Anticoagulation

Because the patient's blood is in the extracorporeal circuit continuously, filter and circuit clotting is a serious concern and can lead to inadequate treatment. Systemic or regional anticoagulation can be used to diminish this risk but these are fraught with their own complications.

C. Patient Mobility

CRRT is by nature intended to run throughout the day. Because of the machinery and tubing involved in the typical extracorporeal circuit, mobilizing the patient for studies, procedures, etc. is often difficult. Furthermore, disconnecting patients from CRRT deprives them of dialysis and ultrafiltration time, which decreases treatment efficacy.

D. Cost

Even without considering the increased nursing costs, CRRT is roughly two to three times as expensive as traditional IHD due mostly to increased laboratory, filter, dialysate, and other equipment costs.

CRRT COMPLICATIONS

From a procedural standpoint, CRRT is generally well tolerated by patients, especially given the dire state in which most patients treated with CRRT are in. Complications pertaining to the apparatus can arise in almost any part of the circuit, ranging from vascular access failure, circuit clotting, and loss of filter efficiency to mundane problems such as line disconnection. These issues are difficult to predict and may result in significant down-time of therapy.

The most common complications of CRRT are electrolyte imbalances, hypotension, infection, bleeding, and hypothermia. Hypotension occurs when the hourly Qnet exceeds the intradialytic refilling capacity for the patient situation. In patients with compromised refilling capacity, as in diabetic neuropathy, low cardiac ejection fraction, diastolic dysfunction, and sepsis, increased fluid removal is the major risk factor for hypotension.

Patients receiving CRRT present an increased risk for hypothermia as blood circulates in the extracorporeal circulation for a prolonged time. CRRT-induced hypothermia may mask the presence of fever, and body temperature is thus an unreliable marker of inflammation and infection. Blood warmers should be used in the circuit.

Hypophosphatemia is associated with higher doses, and if severe enough can lead to decreases in cardiac output and blood pressure, rhabdomyolysis, respiratory muscle weakness, and granulocyte dysfunction with increased infection rates. Phosphate can be added to dialysate and/or replacement fluids to prevent this.

Excessive amino acid losses also occur, which can affect nutritional status. Severe protein-energy wasting ensues, leading to loss of lean body mass, reduction of fat mass, and low urea concentrations; all of these worsen in-hospital mortality, hospital stay, and infection complication outcomes. Patients should receive increased daily protein or amino acid intake to about 1.5–2.5 g/kg/day; of note, carbohydrates should be given at 5–7 g/kg/day and lipids at 1.2–1.5 g/kg/day.

Clearance of drugs may be significantly impacted. High CRRT doses influence the pharmacokinetics and pharmacodynamics of medications. Therefore, patients may be underdosed, especially with regard to antimicrobials, vasoactive drips, sedatives and paralytics, and/or antiseizure medications.

Other complications like hypomagnesemia and other electrolyte abnormalities, platelet dysfunction, increased bleeding risk and vascular access related problems can occur during CRRT and physician must be aware of all these complications while delivering CRRT. Table 51–7 summarizes complications associated with CRRT.

Table 51–7. Complications during CRRT.

Vascular access	Bleeding
	Thrombosis
	Hemothorax
	Pneumothorax
	Hematoma
	AV fistula
	Aneurysm
	Infection
Extracorporeal	Hypothermia
	Air embolism
	Reduced filter life
	Anaphylaxis and immune activation
Electrolyte and acid base disturbances	Hypophosphatemia
	Hypomagnesemia
	Hypocalcemia
	Hypokalemia
	Hypo and hypernatremia
	Metabolic acidosis
	Metabolic alkalosis
Haematological	HIT
	Hemolysis
Nutritional losses	Loss of amino acids/proteins, vitamins, and trace minerals

NONRENAL INDICATIONS OF CRRT

Continuous renal replacement therapy (CRRT) has been extensively used as renal support for critically ill patients, but active research has also been conducted on nonrenal indications for CRRT, that is, the use of CRRT for purposes other than renal support. CRRT is often used with the concept of modulating immune response and influencing circulating levels of inflammatory mediators in sepsis, hepatic failure, acute brain injury, and acute pancreatitis.

▶ CRRT in Sepsis and Multiorgan Failure

Severe sepsis and septic shock are the primary causes of multiple organ dysfunction syndrome (MODS) and is associated with AKI in 5–50% of the patients. In these patients, in addition to providing more time to achieve fluid balance and metabolic homeostasis, CRRT has been used with the concept of modulator of the immune response. With the intention of influencing circulating levels of inflammatory mediators, several modifications of CRRT have been developed over the last years. These include high-volume hemofiltration, high-adsorption hemofiltration, use of high cutoff (HCO) membranes, and hybrid systems like coupled plasma filtration absorbance. Pilot trials in septic patients using high permeability hemofilters with increased pore size, which aids the filtration of inflammatory mediators; have demonstrated positive immunomodulation, altering neutrophil phagocytosis and mononuclear cell function ex vivo. More studies are needed to confirm these effects.

▶ CRRT in Heart Failure

Although diuretics are the mainstay of therapy for acute decompensated heart failure (ADHF), improved understandings of the pathophysiology of decreased kidney function in the context of ADHF and the limitations of conventional therapy have led clinicians to use different forms of extracorporeal therapy. Intermittent isolated ultrafiltration (IUF), SCUF, and CVVH have been used as extracorporeal therapy to treat ADHF. In isolated ultrafiltration and SCUF, the extracorporeal blood circuit is adapted for isotonic fluid removal by a pressure gradient. In CVVH, the substitution fluid allows for correction of metabolic acidosis and electrolyte disturbances. In addition, recent evidence suggests that myocardial depressant factors such as IL-8 and antimonocyte chemoattractant protein 1, which is effectively removed by hemofiltration, may have adverse effects on cardiac function.

In comparison to IUF, studies have demonstrated benefits of SCUF in the treatment of ADHF. UF versus usual care for hospitalized patients with heart failure: the relief for acutely fluid-overloaded patients with decompensated congestive heart failure (RAPID-CHF) trial offered more insight into potential benefits of SCUF over usual care. This trial showed early application of UF for patients with CHF was feasible, well tolerated, and resulted in significant weight loss and fluid removal. Safety and efficacy of SCUF was demonstrated in UNLOAD study. This study was designed to compare the safety and efficacy of venovenous UF and standard intravenous diuretic therapy for hypervolemic heart failure (HF) patients and concluded that UF safely produces greater weight and fluid loss than intravenous diuretics, reduces 90-day resource utilization for HF, and is an effective alternative therapy.

▶ CRRT in Acute Brain Injury

AKI occurs in 8–23% of patients with acute brain injury (ABI) and is an independent predictor of poor outcome in these patients. In patients with acute brain injury, RRT presents a major problem because conventional IHD may exacerbate the reduction in cerebral perfusion and increase cerebral edema. Rapid urea removal from the plasma and water shift to the intracellular compartment can worsen brain edema. To maximize full potential neurologic recovery in patients requiring renal dialytic support, it is important that treatments do not themselves cause further cerebral ischemia. The goal for ABI and increased intracranial pressure (ICP) patients is to maintain CPP greater than 60 mm Hg; this is done by ensuring MAP stays up, as CPP = MAP – ICP. With IHD, intradialytic hypotension is common, leading to decreased MAP and CPP and increased ICP by compensatory cerebral vasodilation. This may result in infarction or secondary injury. Using computed tomography to measure brain density, brain water content has been shown to be increased after IHD, whereas no changes were observed after CRRT. In addition, CRRT can also be used to maintain hypernatremia and thereby reduce brain swelling. The KDIGO AKI guideline recommends "CRRT, rather than intermittent RRT, for AKI patients with acute brain injury or other causes of increased intracranial pressure or generalized brain edema."

Various other blood purification techniques have been developed and applied clinically to patients with a wide variety of diseases. Plasma exchange is used not only for the treatment of fulminant hepatic failure but also for thrombotic thrombocytopenic purpura and toxic epidermal necrolysis. Other methods like double-filtration plasmapheresis (DFPP) and plasma adsorption have been developed and applied to the treatment of autoimmune diseases, neuromuscular diseases, and other conditions.

CRRT is now the leading form of RRT for AKI in ICUs worldwide and is widely accepted as the most appropriate therapy for vasopressor-dependent patients who require RRT for AKI in the ICU. Presently, CRRT has many applications and its use can be adapted to fit different

situations beyond the classic renal indications. In the near future, technical developments in extracorporeal devices will lead to the creation of multiple organ support therapies, so that comprehensive replacement or at least support can be provided to multiple organs simultaneously.

CRRT is now the leading form of RRT for AKI in ICUs worldwide and is widely accepted as the most appropriate therapy for vasopressor-dependent patients who require RRT for AKI in the ICU. However, practice variation in the application of CRRT remains considerable owing to the absence of clear evidence-based guidelines. Presently, CRRT has many applications and its use can be adapted to fit different situations beyond the classic renal indications.

KEY READINGS

Bagshaw SM et al: Precision continuous renal replacement therapy and solute control. Blood Purif 2016;42:238.

Cerda J et al: Role of technology for the management of AKI in critically ill patients: from adoptive technology to precision continuous renal replacement therapy. Blood Purif 2016;42:248.

Claure-Del Granado R, Bouchard J: Acid–base and electrolyte abnormalities during renal support for acute kidney injury: recognition and management. Blood Purif 2012;34:186.

Claure-Del Granado R et al: Effluent volume in continuous renal replacement therapy overestimates the delivered dose of dialysis. Clin J Am Soc Nephrol 2011;6:467.

Claure-Del Granado R et al: Anticoagulation, delivered dose and outcomes in CRRT: the program to improve care in acute renal disease (PICARD). Hemodial Int 2014;18:641.

Gattas DJ et al: A randomized controlled trial of regional citrate versus regional heparin anticoagulation for continuous renal replacement therapy in critically ill adults. Crit Care Med 2015;43:1622.

Gaudry S, Hajage D, Dreyfuss D: Initiation of renal-replacement therapy in the intensive care unit. N Engl J Med 2016;375:1901.

Jain A, Agrawal N, Kazory A: Defining the role of ultrafiltration therapy in acute heart failure: a systematic review and meta-analysis. Heart Fail Rev 2016;21:611.

Joannes-Boyau O et al: High-volume versus standard-volume haemofiltration for septic shock patients with acute kidney injury (IVOIRE study): a multicentre randomized controlled trial. Intensive Care Med 2013;39:1535.

Kashani K, Mehta RL: We restrict CRRT to only the most hemodynamically unstable patients. Semin Dial 2016;29:268.

Liu C et al: Regional citrate versus heparin anticoagulation for continuous renal replacement therapy in critically ill patients: a meta-analysis with trial sequential analysis of randomized controlled trials. Crit Care 2016;20:144.

Macedo E, Claure-Del Granado R, Mehta RL: Effluent volume and dialysis dose in CRRT: time for reappraisal. Nat Rev Nephrol 2011;8:57.

Macedo E, Mehta RL: Continuous dialysis therapies: core curriculum 2016. Am J Kidney Dis 2016;68:645.

Mehta RL: Renal-replacement therapy in the critically ill—does timing matter? N Engl J Med 2016;375:175.

Murugan R et al: Precision fluid management in continuous renal replacement therapy. Blood Purif 2016;42:266.

Ostermann M et al: Patient selection and timing of continuous renal replacement therapy. Blood Purif 2016;42:224.

Passos RD et al: Lactate clearance is associated with mortality in septic patients with acute kidney injury requiring continuous renal replacement therapy: a cohort study. Medicine (Baltimore) 2016;95:e5112.

Sharma S, Waikar SS: Phosphate balance in continuous venovenous hemofiltration. Am J Kidney Dis 2013;61:1043.

Vaara ST et al: Timing of RRT based on the presence of conventional indications. Clin J Am Soc Nephrol 2014;9:1577.

Vincent JL: Serial blood lactate levels reflect both lactate production and clearance. Crit Care Med 2015;43:e209.

Wald R, Gallagher M, Bagshaw SM: Shedding new light on an old dilemma: two trials examining the timing of renal replacement therapy initiation in acute kidney injury. Am J Kidney Dis 2017;69:14.

Wald R et al: Comparison of standard and accelerated initiation of renal replacement therapy in acute kidney injury. Kidney Int 2015;88:897.

Xu Y et al: Timing of initiation of renal replacement therapy for acute kidney injury: a systematic review and meta-analysis of randomized-controlled trials. Clin Exp Nephrol, 2016. [Epub ahead of print]

Zarbock A et al: Effect of early vs delayed initiation of renal replacement therapy on mortality in critically ill patients with acute kidney injury: the ELAIN randomized clinical trial. JAMA 2016;315:2190.

■ CHAPTER REVIEW QUESTIONS

1. Solute clearances in CRRT are dependent on which of the following?
   A. Sieving coefficient of the solute
   B. Effluent flow rates
   C. Ultrafiltration rate
   D. The percent saturation of the effluent
   E. The dialysate flow rate

2. Filtration fraction in CRRT represents which of the following?
   A. The ratio of effluent volume to blood flow rate
   B. The ratio of ultrafiltration volume to blood flow rate
   C. The ratio of plasma flow rate to ultrafiltration rate
   D. The ratio of ultrafiltration rate to effluent volume
   E. The ratio of dialysate flow to blood flow rate

3. Daily fluid balance in CRRT is best represented by which of the following?
   A. The difference in effluent volume and fluids given in the circuit
   B. The difference in effluent volume and fluids given to the patient
   C. The net balance computed by the machine
   D. The total ultrafiltration volume over 24 hours
   E. The net difference in all fluids given in and removed from the patient

4. Common complications associated with CRRT include the following except:
   A. Hypophosphatemia
   B. Cardiac arrhythmias
   C. Acidosis
   D. Low albumin
   E. Hypotension

5. Which one of these statements regarding renal replacement therapy (RRT) in AKI is true?
   A. Randomized controlled trials demonstrate that early initiation of renal replacement therapy is associated with improved patient outcomes in ICU patients.
   B. Randomized controlled trials demonstrate that delayed initiation of renal replacement therapy is associated with many ICU patients not needing dialysis.
   C. The ATN and the RENAL trials have shown that the dose of dialysis is not a determinant of patient survival.
   D. All of the above.
   E. None of the above.

Kidney Transplantation

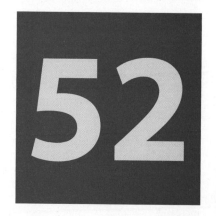

Saed Nemr, MD, FACP

William S. Asch, MD, PhD

ESSENTIALS OF DIAGNOSIS

▶ The demographic of kidney transplant candidates and recipients has increasingly shifted toward older patients with the greatest growth among recipients between 45 and 65 years of age, and especially those with a history of diabetes or hypertension. Many of these recipient candidates are frail and require a more comprehensive pretransplant evaluation to determine the appropriateness of proceeding with transplantation.

▶ Tacrolimus remains the backbone of the most commonly used immunosuppressive regimen in the United States, however, the novel intravenous costimulation blocking drug belatacept is associated with higher GFRs compared with cyclosporine. It is anticipated that allograft survival will be prolonged by belatacept as this drug is not associated with development of interstitial fibrosis and tubular atrophy in kidney transplants.

▶ The incidence and burden of malignancy development in immunosuppressed kidney transplants in increasingly a concern. It is imperative that healthcare professions caring for transplant recipients not overlook the need to continue age appropriate cancer screening.

▶ Recurrent disease remains a cause of premature allograft failure following kidney transplantation. Efforts to further characterize the putative soluble "circulating permeability factor" of FSGS have thus far been unsuccessful while C3 glomerulonephritis is associated with a high rate of recurrence and allograft loss following kidney transplantation.

▶ The decision to discontinue immunosuppression following kidney transplant failure when subsequent retransplantation is expected remains controversial. While the data indicate that survival on dialysis off immunosuppression is increased, patients who have had their immunosuppression withdrawn may be at increased risk of becoming sensitized, making identification of a subsequent compatible donor more challenging.

INTRODUCTION

Approximately 4.5 million individuals were diagnosed with chronic kidney disease (CKD) in the United States in 2014. While the majority of this group will either not progress to end stage kidney disease (ESRD), or die secondary to an etiology other than ESRD, over 100,000 individuals start on renal replacement annually. When confronted with the need for replacement therapy, affected patients have three major options to consider: hemodialysis, peritoneal dialysis, and kidney transplantation. Of course, the decision not to pursue replacement therapy is the remaining option that should always be offered and discussed with patients, particularly those who are elderly or suspected of having a low quality of life.

Kidney transplantation is a field unto itself. No single textbook, let alone single textbook chapter, can possibly cover all aspects of this complex topic. This chapter focuses on those features of kidney transplantation that a general nephrologist should be well versed and prepared to discuss with a recipient, or recipient candidate, they find under their care.

Hemodialysis and peritoneal dialysis are two options that are life-saving in ESRD patients. However, neither fully replaces the metabolic and hormonal functions of the kidney and both the length and quality of life for patients undergoing treatment was arguably rather poor. This challenged the medical profession to find a superior form of renal replacement therapy. While the concept of organ transplantation dates as far back as the Ancient Greeks, advances in surgical technique coupled with a blossoming understanding of the basic functions of the immune system led by Peter Medawar in Great Britain, led to the first successful human kidney transplant procedure by Joseph Murray at the Peter Bent Brigham Hospital in 1954.

Kidney transplantation more fully, if not nearly completely, restores kidney function to the recipient. And while superior to hemodialysis and peritoneal dialysis in maintaining both euvolemia and homeostasis, perhaps the greatest advantage of kidney transplantation is the marked improvement in the quality of life experienced by nearly all recipients. Similarly, kidney transplant recipients can expect an extension in their expected remaining lifetimes following transplantation compared to nontransplanted patients who remained on dialysis. Though, this improvement in expected lifetime is most pronounced for young recipients and steadily shrinks as the age of the recipient increases.

Kidney transplantation using a living donor remains the preferred option. Recipients of kidneys from living donors can expect longer graft survival as well as more immediate function status post transplantation (ie, with a significantly reduced rate of delayed graft function). Most importantly, recipients of kidneys from living donors can be transplanted as soon as a living donor has been approved. This is unlike recipients of deceased donor organs who frequently need to wait multiple years on the waiting list to be transplanted. While rates are variable across the United States, patients waiting for a deceased donor organ can anticipate a waiting time between 2 and 6 years depending on the region of the country in which they live. As a general rule, waiting times are longest in the United States along the coasts and are shorter in Midwest and the through the South.

KEY READINGS

Blakeslee S: Willem Kolff, inventor of kidney and heart machines, dies at 97. The New York Times. February 12, 2009.

Davis AE et al: The extent and predictors of waiting time geographic disparity in kidney transplantation in the United States. Transplantation 2014;97:1049.

Harrison JH, Merrill JP, Murray JE: Renal homotransplantation in identical twins. Surg Forum 1956;6:432.

United States Renal Data System: 2016 USRDS annual data report: epidemiology of kidney disease in the United States. Bethesda, MD: National Institutes of Health, National Institute of Diabetes and Digestive and Kidney Diseases; 2016.

IMMUNOLOGIC PRINCIPLES

T-cell activation requires three signals. The first signal, "signal 1," occurs when a peptide is displayed in the context of the major histocompatibility complex on an antigen presenting cells and is presented to a T-cell CD3 (or T-cell receptor). This receptor-ligand interaction ultimately results in NFAT (nuclear factor of activated T cells) induced nuclear activation of the T cell. This signal transduction/activation of transcription pathway includes calcineurin as a cytoplasmic intermediary. The second signal, "signal 2," or

"costimulatory signal" is not specific to any particular foreign antigen presentation to the T cell. Rather, this signal occurs when CD80 and CD86 present on the APC interact with CD28 on the T cell. Signal 3 occurs when interleukin-2, produced in either an autocrine or paracrine manner, interacts with the IL-2 receptor on the T-cell surface. Activation of the IL-2 receptor results in progression of the T cell through the cell cycle via promoting transition for G1 to the G2 phase, and thereby, leads to T-cell proliferation. The mammalian target of rapamycin (mTOR) is a cytoplasmic intermediary between the activated IL-2R and the cell cycle proteins.

KEY READING

Halloran PF: Immunosuppressive drugs for kidney transplantation. N Engl J Med 2004;351:2715.

IMMUNOSUPPRESSIVE MEDICATIONS

▶ Induction Immunosuppression

Nearly all transplant centers are using some form of induction therapy for kidney transplantation. And, the first doses are commonly given to the recipient either preoperatively or intraoperatively, prior to reperfusion of the allograft. The most commonly used agents are anti-IL2-receptor antagonists (eg, basiliximab), rabbit antithymocyte globulin (thymoglobulin), and anti-CD52 binding monoclonal antibody (alemtuzumab). Each of these agents has strengths and weakness.

Basiliximab competes with IL-2 for binding to the IL-2α receptor on the surface of T cells. As a consequence, IL-2Rα signaling is blocked and both activation and replication of the T cell is prevented. IL-2Rα is selectively expressed on T cells. Hence, basiliximab has no effect on B cells, and is therefore considered less suitable for the sensitized recipient (with an increased panel reactive antibody level) who is at an increased risk for an anamnestic antibody response. Basiliximab is given as a divided dose with the second half infused on, or around, postoperative day 4. Pharmacokinetic data indicate the complete saturation of IL-2Rα begins to decline 1–2 weeks following dosing. Additional data indicates that the beneficial effect persists for a longer period. Compared to placebo, the use of basiliximab induction significantly reduced the risk of the combined 6-month end point of allograft rejection, allograft loss, and recipient death in two studies (38–42% for basiliximab, and 55–57% for placebo). Basiliximab is extremely well tolerated with essentially no serious side effects.

Antithymocyte globulin (ATG) is a collection of antibodies raised against human T cells. The two commonly used preparations are Thymoglobulin and Atgam, from inoculated rabbits and horses, respectively. In comparison with basiliximab, ATG has a significant leukodepleting effect beyond its ability to prevent T-cell activation and replication. Indeed, this is both a benefit and common side effect of this agent. Thrombocytopenia is also commonly encountered when using ATG. The recommended dose of ATG for induction therapy varies between 4.5 and 6.0 mg/kg given over divided doses not exceeding 1.5 mg/kg. Though not used at all centers, monitoring of T-cell depletion can be achieved through the measurement of the CD3+ cell count. It is recommended that the CD3+ T-cell count remain below 20 cells/mm^3 during the early postoperative period. Note that even more significant depletion may be desired when treating a patient with ATG during an episode of rejection.

▶ Maintenance Immunosuppression

While azathioprine and prednisone were crucial to the early successes with transplantation, cyclosporine, tacrolimus, sirolimus, everolimus, and more recently Belatacept are now being used.

A. Azathioprine

Early success in kidney transplantation would not have been possible without the purine analogue azathioprine. While all cells in the body are capable of synthesizing purines for DNA synthesis *de novo*, not all cells are equally capable of scavenging purines from the outside. In particular, and fortuitous for organ transplantation, both B cells and T cells are dependent on *de novo* purine synthesis for their proliferation. Methyl-thioinosine monophosphate (MeTIMP) is the active metabolite of azathioprine that impairs purine synthesis by blocking amidophosphoribosyltransferase (the enzyme that represents the committing step in purine synthesis).

B. Calcineurin Inhibitors

Cyclosporine is a cyclic nonribosomal peptide of 11 amino acids, first identified from the fungus *Tolypocladium inflatum* in the late 1960s. Its immunosuppressive properties were first discovered in 1976. Within lymphocytes, cyclosporine binds to the cytoplasmic protein cyclophilin. This complex that forms between cyclosporine and cyclophilin inhibits the normal action of calcineurin, which is to dephosphorylated NFAT. In the absence of dephosphorylation, NFAT is unable to translocate from the cytoplasm to the nucleus where it would normally increase the transcription of the genes encoding interleukin-2 and other related cytokines. Blocking the transcription of these nuclear proteins prevents activation and proliferation of the T cell.

Tacrolimus is a macrolide lactone that was first identified from the bacterium *Streptomyces tsukubaensis*. Despite having extremely distinct biochemical structures, tacrolimus blocks T-cell activation in a manner similar to cyclosporine, thereby interfering with calcineurin signaled and NFAT-induced gene transcription within the T-cell nucleus.

Collectively known as the calcineurin inhibitors, these two drugs each significantly reduced the rate of acute cellular rejection compared with their predecessors. Following the introduction of cyclosporine, the rate of acute rejection in the first year after transplantation fell from approximately 60% to 45%, and 1-year allograft survival concomitantly improved from 65% to 90%. Following the introduction of tacrolimus, risk of acute rejection in the first year further declined to below 25% and raised 1-year graft survival above 90%.

The standard of care for the average risk kidney transplant is a triple immunosuppressive regimen that includes a calcineurin inhibitor. While some centers continue to use cyclosporine as the primary immunosuppressant in their regimen, most centers are now using tacrolimus. According to the 2012 report from the USRDS, 92% of kidney transplant recipients were on a tacrolimus based regimen. Furthermore, this report confirmed that the use of mycophenolate mofetil had nearly completely supplanted the use of azathioprine as the antimetabolite of choice. When confronted with the rare transplant recipient that has graft survival in excess of 30 years, the novice observer of transplantation may conclude that patients maintain on a two-drug regimen with azathioprine and prednisone (the regimen of that transplant era) have a superior outcome. Of course, this conclusion is false as nearly all transplant recipients of that era have since reached allograft failure. Only a select few, presumably those who are either tolerant of their allografts or simply do not require a significant degree of immunosuppression to prevent rejection, continue to have functioning allografts now.

C. Glucocorticoids

While the use of glucocorticoids (prednisone) remains the more common practice, many centers have opted to switch to either a steroid-free, or steroid sparing immunosuppressive strategy. Proponents of this approach point out potential benefits, including reduced bone osteopenia, reduced muscle sarcopenia, reduced rate of corneal cataract development, and potentially reduced rates of weight gain and post-transplant diabetes mellitus development. Critics of the steroid-free approach suggest that the rates of rejection are lower when steroids are used, and this reduced rate of rejection both justifies there use and outweighs the benefits associated with their avoidance. Some centers report using an immunosuppression strategy that is tailored to the immunologic risk of the recipient. By avoiding a one size fits all approach, the highly sensitized black male is likely to receive maintenance steroids, while a 65-year-old unsensitized female is likely to be deemed a candidate for a steroid avoidance protocol. Naturally, all kidney transplant recipients known to have a contraindication to the use of maintenance steroids (eg, psychiatric patients with a history of steroid-induced psychosis or acute decompensation in their mental health) are considered for steroid avoidance as well.

D. Belatacept

Belatacept is a first-in-class intravenous, biologic, immunosuppressant medication. Belatacept interferes with the costimulation between CD80/86 on antigen presenting cells and CD28 on the T cell (ie, signal-2 required for T-cell activation). As this drug was designed to specifically and avidly bind to CD80 and CD86, off target effects of significance are not expected. First approved by the FDA in June 2011 for use as a *de novo* immunosuppressive agent, Belatacept use is growing across transplant centers. Interestingly, more centers are currently using the drug in the context of a conversion for patients who are having side effects or for other reasons no longer tolerating a CNI or mTOR inhibitor.

A recent Cochrane Database review concluded that compared with both cyclosporine and tacrolimus, patients maintained on belatacept had similar risks of death, allograft failure, and acute rejection with less chronic interstitial fibrosis with tubular atrophy and higher eGFR. These findings were extended further with the final report from the BENEFIT trial. Compared with the cyclosporine control group, patients on belatacept were at a reduced risk for both death and allograft loss. Furthermore, eGFR was significantly higher in the belatacept patients, compared with the cyclosporine treated patients in whom eGFR declined during the seven years of follow up (eGFR of 70 for the belatacept treatment arms compared to 45 for patients treated with cyclosporine). Approximately 10% of treated patients with a CNI based regimen develop *de novo* DSA within the first transplant year, and 20% after the first 5 years. Belatacept treated patients in the BENEFIT trial had a significantly reduced rate of DSA development (1.9% and 4.6%, with the more-intensive and less-intensive arms of the study, respectively). In aggregate, the existing data indicate that belatacept-based immunosuppression has likely moved the field of kidney transplantation a significant step forward toward the goal of improving and extending long-term allograft survival.

Despite all its potential benefits, one concerning finding is the increased risk of PTLD development in patients treated with belatacept. Consistent with the concern raised during the phase II trials, PTLD occurred in five patients receiving belatacept in the BENEFIT trial, but only 1 patient in the cyclosporine control group. Furthermore, there was a predominance of central nervous system PTLD development in the belatacept treated patients. Not surprisingly, 5 of 6 patients that developed PTLD were considered to be at increased risk, primarily due to their Epstein–Barr virus (EBV) seronegative status at the time of transplant. For this reason, belatacept carries a black box warning advising against the use of the drug in EBV seronegative and seroindeterminate recipients.

▶ Immunosuppressive Drug Interactions

Physicians and allied health professions who do not possess training specialized in the care of the kidney transplant recipient routinely encounter situations in which dispensing of a new medication is indicated. While consideration of drug–drug interactions is always best practice, the relatively narrow therapeutic drug level ranges of the commonly used maintenance immunosuppressive agents makes avoidance of a drug–drug interaction particularly critical. The CNIs and mTORs are both primarily metabolized via the cytochrome P450 (CYP) found in the liver. Indeed, an abundance of commonly prescribed nonimmunosuppressive medications share these CYP enzymatic pathways for metabolic bioinactivation and elimination. In doing so, some drugs will up-regulate the activity of the CYP pathway, while others have the opposite effect. CYP up-regulating drugs bring the risk of accelerated immunosuppressive drug clearance, and therefore, a reduction in the level of immunosuppression. This, in turn, increases the risk of precipitating allograft rejection. In contradistinction, a drug that down-regulates CYP activity may lead to both an increased immunosuppressive drug level and state of immunosuppression. While the latter lowers the risk of rejection, it may render the transplant recipient at increased risk for opportunistic infections in the short term and malignancies in the long term. Perhaps more important, increased immunosuppressive drug levels bring with them the potential for drug toxicities, both within and beyond the kidney transplant (eg, acute tubular injury, reduced GFR, hyperkalemia, tremor, diarrhea, and altered cognition). Drugs are not alone in their ability to affect CYP activity. Several foods and herbal supplements share this property. A list of common drug–drug, and food/herb–drug interactions can be found in Table 52–1.

KEY READINGS

Baquero A et al: Basiliximab: a comparative study between the use of the recommended two doses versus a single dose in living donor kidney transplantation. Transplant Proc 2006;38:909.

Gaston RS: Current and evolving immunosuppressive regimens in kidney transplantation. Am J Kidney Dis 2006;47:S3.

Halloran PF: Immunosuppressive drugs for kidney transplantation. N Engl J Med 2004;351:2715.

Masson P et al: Belatacept for kidney transplant recipients. Cochrane Database Syst Rev 2014(11):CD010699.

Mourad G et al: The role of Thymoglobulin induction in kidney transplantation: an update. Clin Transplant 2012;26:E450.

United States Renal Data System: 2012 USRDS annual data report: epidemiology of kidney disease in the United States. Bethesda, MD: National Institutes of Health, National Institute of Diabetes and Digestive and Kidney Diseases; 2012.

Vincenti F et al: A phase III study of belatacept-based immunosuppression regimens versus cyclosporine in renal transplant recipients (BENEFIT study). Am J Transplant 2010;10:535.

Vincenti F et al: Belatacept and long-term outcomes in kidney transplantation. N Engl J Med 2016;374:333.

Table 52–1. Common inhibitors and inducers of the CYP-3A4 metabolic pathway.

Inhibitors of CYP-3A4	Inducers of CYP-3A4
Strong Inhibitors	*Unspecified Potency*
Clarithromycin	Rifampin
Telithromycin	Rifabutin
Indinavir	Phenytoin
Nelfinavir	Fosphenytoin
Ritonavir	Carbamazepine
Saquinavir	Topiramate
Itraconazole	Phenobarbital
Ketoconazole	Butalbital
Voriconazole	St. John's wort
Nefazodone	Efavirenz
Suboxone	Nevirapine
Chloramphenicol	Pioglitazone
Grapefruit Juice (furanocoumarins)	Troglitazone
Intermediate Inhibitors	Glucocorticoids
Aprepitant	
Erythromycin	
Fluconazole	
Verapamil	
Diltiazem	
Weak Inhibitors	
Azithromycin	
Cimetidine	
Ciprofloxacin	
Buprenorphine	
Gabapentin	
Valproic acid	

Table 52–2. Contraindications to kidney transplantation.

Coronary disease unsafe for anesthesia and (noncardiac) surgery.
Congestive heart failure at risk for decompensation.
Untreated malignancy.
Treated malignancy, but within the period of increased risk for recurrence.
Peripheral vascular disease that precludes successful allograft anastomosis.
Medication nonadherence.
Frailty (though no recognized maximum chronologic age has ever been codified).
Active illicit substance abuse that impacts activities of daily life.
Cirrhosis (though, simultaneous liver kidney transplantation may be acceptable).
Lack of a social support system.
Lack of adequate insurance coverage, or plan to cover costs of post-transplant care.
Advanced stage chronic obstructive pulmonary disease (due to both operative concerns as well as a reduced post-transplant survival).
Systemic diseases that bring a high risk the transplant will also be affected (eg, amyloidosis).
Severe systemic infections (eg, active tuberculosis).
Patients not expected to have a high probability of surviving 5 years after transplantation.
Patients for whom the risks exceed the potential benefits.

KIDNEY TRANSPLANT RECIPIENT EVALUATION

Not all patients with CKD and ESRD are appropriate candidates for kidney transplantation. The reasons for being declined placement on the waiting list vary widely for patients and between centers. Mindful of the fact that they are charged with the task of allocating a scare societal resource, kidney transplant centers may decline recipient candidates on the basis of preexisting medical conditions that either unacceptably increase their operative risk, or reduce their likelihood of a meaningful post-transplant survival (both of the allograft and the individual). Absolute and relative contraindications to kidney transplantation are noted in Table 52–2.

▶ Universal Assessment of Kidney Transplant Candidates

Surgical and anesthetic techniques have improved considerably. And while the risk of an operative death is very low for the general population, patients with advanced CKD and ESRD as a group have a higher than average risk. Furthermore, death from cardiovascular disease now exceeds the risks of major infection and is the leading cause of mortality in kidney transplant recipients. Therefore, a cardiac risk assessment needs to be a component of every recipient's pretransplant listing evaluation. Cardiac assessment is both for the purpose of determining candidate suitability, as well as for best managing patients with acceptable levels of cardiovascular disease through the postoperative experience. For example, some centers choose to accept only organs with a very low risk for delayed graft function for their recipients identified as having an increased cardiovascular risk.

Patients with diabetes and peripheral vascular disease (PVD) are at a particularly high risk for cardiovascular events post-transplantation. Furthermore, the patient with PVD will likely be referred for imaging or noninvasive studies of their lower extremities in an effort to determine if their iliac vessels are sufficiently patent and appropriate for the anastomosis of a kidney allograft. A tenuous vascular supply to the lower extremity is also of concern given the possibility that a steal syndrome could develop following transplantation. Though there is debate as to whether allograft anastomosis exacerbates limb ischemia in a meaningful way. Additional historical factors to incorporate into the candidate's cardiovascular risk assessment include obesity, hypertension (particularly if uncontrolled), hyperlipidemia, angina, congestive heart failure symptoms, prior cardiovascular events, tobacco use, and any family history significant for cardiac events. Of course, every reasonable effort should be made to address all modifiable risk factors identified.

All recipient candidates should also be up to date with all cancer screenings recommended for their age. Furthermore, candidates should also be screened for renal cell carcinoma during their evaluation given the increased risk associated with ESRD and acquired cystic disease.

Assessment of Kidney Transplant Candidates for Thrombotic Complications

Development of a vascular thrombosis is a feared complication of kidney transplantation. Frequently occurring rapidly and without warning, thrombosis of a renal vessel is a significant insult to the allograft and is generally uncorrectable unless intervened upon as quickly as possible. To reduce the risk of such an event, the detailed history obtained from the recipient candidate should include inquiring about a prior history of thrombosis. Unless clearly associated with a predisposing factor or situation, any recipient candidate identified as having a history of an unprovoked thrombotic event should be screened for states leading to hypercoagulability, or referred to a hematologist for this purpose. Moreover, it is best to determine during the evaluation phase if an anticoagulant is going to be used perioperatively and postoperatively.

Assessment of Kidney Transplant Candidates for Chronic Viral Infections

Screening for common infectious conditions in recipient candidates, such as syphilis, tuberculosis, HIV, hepatitis B, and hepatitis C is also a good practice given the concern that these conditions may be exacerbated under the influence of immunosuppression post-transplant. In the case of viral hepatitis, a thorough investigation looking for evidence of underlying liver disease is critical as some recipients are at risk for acute hepatic decompensation during the early postkidney transplant experience. Moreover, a subset of candidates will be identified for whom simultaneous liver kidney transplantation needs to be considered. Similarly, while HIV positive serostatus is no longer an absolute contraindication to kidney transplantation, suitable candidates should have an undetectable viral load and a CD4 count exceeding the threshold for opportunistic infections (ie, CD4 <200 cells/uL). In contrast to concerns for increased rates of serious infections, early trials with HIV seropositive recipients showed higher rates of acute rejection than expected, potentially a consequence of an effect HIV has on the immune system. Regardless, studies confirm that HIV infected patients have improved survival with kidney transplantation compared to matched controls that remain on dialysis.

Chronic Hepatitis C Virus Infected Recipient Candidates

Until recently, antiviral treatment for kidney recipient candidates infected with HCV was recommended prior to transplantation. However, this has changed in the era of the direct-acting antiviral (DAA) inhibitors alongside a change in demand for HCV positive organs. Presently, stable HCV seropositive patients who do not appear to be at significant risk for complications associated with a delay in HCV eradication are encouraged to wait until after transplantation to be treated. In doing so, the HCV infected recipient remains a candidate for transplantation from a similarly HCV infected donor. As candidates on the waiting list not infected with HCV are not at the present time considered safe candidates for transplantation from an HCV infected donor, the HCV infected recipient (for the moment) has a competitive advantage. Whether the high efficacy rates of the DAAs will translate into the ability to safely transplant HCV naive recipients with organs from a HCV infected donor is actively being investigated.

Each transplant center determines their minimum criteria testing and recipient candidate requirements for placement on the waiting list and for transplantation. Nonetheless, a generally agreed upon set of core tests is provided (Table 52–3).

Table 52–3. Generally accepted minimal criteria testing required for wait listing.[a]

Evidence of advanced stage kidney disease (GFR <20 mL/min)
Electrocardiogram
Chest radiograph
Tissue typing to determine recipients HLA
Tissue typing to identified anti-HLA antibodies in the candidate's serum
Social worker evaluation and clearance
Financial/insurance authorization and clearance to proceed
Ultrasound imaging of the native kidneys and bladder
Transplant nephrologist evaluation
Transplant surgeon evaluation
Registered dietician evaluation
Pharmacist specialist evaluation
Routine basic laboratory testing (CBC, BMP, LFTs, PT/PTT/INR)
ABO determination (must be independently repeated for validation)
Viral hepatitis virus screening
HIV screening
Syphilis screening
Tuberculosis screening
Colonoscopy for all candidates over age 50
PSA for all male candidates over age
Mammography for female candidates over age 40
Cervical cancer screening for female candidates between ages 21–65

[a]Each kidney transplant center is required to have criteria for the selection of both recipients and donors. But, it is at the discretion of program to determine what testing comprises its core criteria. Very frequently, cardiovascular testing and formal clearance from a cardiologist is required (ie, a candidate with longstanding diabetes, vascular disease, and an extended dialysis vintage time). But, cardiac testing beyond an ECG may not be a stipulated criterion for listing at many centers.

Assessment of Transplant Candidates with a Prior History of a Malignancy

Recipient candidates with a prior history of malignancy will need to have a period of cancer disease-free survival elapse before they can be safely transplanted. Indeed, many centers have listed these patients, but inactive status ("status 7") while they wait for this time to pass. The duration of this interval varies according to the particular type, and aggressiveness of cancer the patient experienced (Table 52–4). Clearance from the patient's treating hematologist or oncologist is highly recommended before proceeding with placement on the waiting list and transplantation. Moreover, a careful review of the chemotherapeutic agents administered during the patient's cancer treatment is important. The history of exposure to agents known to be toxic to the bone marrow is especially important as it may (and likely should) impact both the plan for which induction agent is selected and the goal level of maintenance immunosuppression following transplantation.

Transplant Education and the Psychosocial Assessment of Candidates

A significant portion of each visit a recipient candidate makes to a transplant center is spent on education. This educational process is geared toward ensuring the recipient candidate has a working understanding of the complications and expectations associated with the transplant procedure. During this portion of the visit, the recipient candidate and their family members present will be educated about the benefits derived when the donation comes from a living individual. Many centers will also offer some guidance about how to utilize the recipient's network of friends and family members, as well harness the power of social media, to aid in identifying a suitable living donor.

The candidate is interviewed by a transplant professional to assess if the candidate is appropriate for transplantation from a psychosocial perspective. In addition, a thorough evaluation into the recipient candidate's planned support system for the postoperative recovery period is also made during the visit. Finally, the team will work to determine how the recipient candidate is going to manage any out of pocket costs associated with the transplant procedure, the required immunosuppressive medications, follow-up visits, and laboratory studies.

Once the evaluation process is complete and all data and testing results have been collected, the recipient candidate is presented at the Medical Review Board (MRB), where a determination will be made to place the patient on the deceased donor waiting list. Alternatively, at the MRB meeting the decision may be to deny the candidate listing or recommend that the evaluation be expanded to include additional testing and specialist referrals to further confirm the candidate is a safe individual to transplant and immunosuppress.

Table 52–4. Treated malignancy minimum recommended waiting times before transplantation.

Selected Malignancies	Recurrence-Free Waiting Interval
Superficial bladder cancer	0
In situ cancer of the cervix	0
Nonmetastatic, nonmelanoma skin cancers	0
Prostatic cancer microscopic	0
Asymptomatic T1 renal cell carcinoma with no suspicious histological features	0
Monoclonal gammopathy of undetermined significance (MGUS)	0
Invasive bladder cancer	2
In situ breast cancer	2
Stage A and B colorectal cancer	2
Lymphoma	2
Leukemia	2
In situ melanoma	2
Kaposi's and other sarcomas	2
Prostatic cancer	2
Renal cell carcinoma (lesion <5 cm)	2
Testicular cancer	2
Thyroid cancer (and other endocrine tumors)	2
Wilm tumor	2
Uterine cancer	2
Stage II breast cancer	5
Extensive cervical cancer	5
Colorectal cancer stage C	5
Melanoma (malignant)	5
Symptomatic renal cell carcinoma	5
Renal cell carcinoma (lesion >5 cm)	5
Uncontrolled or untreated malignancies	Transplantation not recommended
Multiple myeloma	Transplantation not recommended
Advanced breast cancer (stage III)	Transplantation not recommended
Colorectal cancer (stage D)	Transplantation not recommended
Liver cancer	Kidney transplant alone not recommended

Polycystic Kidney Disease—Native Nephrectomy Consideration

In evaluating patients with PKD for renal transplantation, one challenge the physician faces is whether pretransplant native nephrectomy is indicated or not. For most patients, pretransplant nephrectomy is not routinely required. However, bilateral or unilateral nephrectomy might be indicated in situations like chronic renal parenchymal infections, recurrent symptomatic bleeding, or large kidneys extending into the lower abdominal quadrants (required to make room for the transplant). Advantages associated with preserving native kidneys include maintaining a better quality of life with keeping urine production, preserving endogenous erythropoietin production, and avoiding the need for multiple operations.

Nephrectomy should be considered for all patients with PKD that are experiencing symptoms attributable to burdensome size of their kidneys. For example, patients with early satiety, breathlessness related to impaired diaphragmatic excursion, and significant constipation secondary to crowding of the intestinal tract are valid indications for nephrectomies in patients with PKD. Absent these suggestive symptoms, a determination that there is sufficient space in the pelvis (iliac fossa) is required before proceeding. In general, if the examiner upon palpation determines that the inferior border of the PKD kidney is above the level of the anterior superior iliac spine, there is likely to be sufficient space to accommodate implantation of the allograft. In those cases where the inferior border of the PKD kidney position is not easily determined, or is definitively below the anterior iliac spine, then axial imaging (CT or MRI) should be obtained to investigate further if nephrectomy is warranted.

The timing, type of surgical approach, and whether unilateral or bilateral nephrectomy is indicated have been topics of debate in the literature. If pretransplant nephrectomy is required, it should be done at least 6 weeks before transplantation. The disadvantage of doing pretransplant nephrectomy(ies) is that the patient will require multiple operations. One other disadvantage is the risk of requiring blood transfusions in the perioperative period resulting in the development of alloantibodies that can reduce the patient's chances of finding a matching donor.

Simultaneous nephrectomy and renal transplantation procedures have also been historically associated with potential risks discouraging this approach. Reported risks include prolonged cold ischemia time, increased risk for delayed graft function, massive fluid shifts, hypotension, graft torsion, and sepsis from ruptured infected cysts. On the other hand, one of the benefits of performing simultaneous nephrectomy and renal transplantation is that it decreases total length of hospitalization and can be done using one incision.

Glassman et al compared patients with simultaneous bilateral nephrectomy and kidney transplantation to patients who underwent kidney transplantation alone and staged bilateral nephrectomy with kidney transplantation; their study showed increase intraoperative blood loss and transfusion requirements in the first group compared to the other two groups but significant decrease in length of hospitalization. The total operative time increased by about 160 minutes in the first group compared to kidney transplantation alone and about 50 minutes compared to the staged approach. Kramer et al, reported 20 cases of combined procedures with

no significant difference in graft survival at 5 years follow-up compared to historical control of patients who underwent only kidney transplant.

Unilateral simultaneous native nephrectomy has the advantage of being done using one incision that is associated with shorter length of stay and is cosmetically more satisfactory to the patients. Luca et al compared simultaneous unilateral versus kidney transplantation groups; there were no statistical difference in operative time, estimated blood loss, and creatinine at hospital discharge. However, bilateral nephrectomy groups showed greater estimated blood loss (125 vs 50 mL) and increased operative time (270 vs 180 minutes) compared to unilateral nephrectomy group.

In summary, most ADPKD patients will not require transplant nephrectomy. However, if indicated, multiple options including the staged nephrectomy and kidney transplantation approach versus simultaneous unilateral or bilateral nephrectomy can be offered.

KEY READINGS

Asch WS, Bia MJ: Oncologic issues and kidney transplantation: a review of frequency, mortality, and screening. Adv Chronic Kidney Dis 2014;21:106.

Frasca GM et al: Renal cancer in kidney transplanted patients. J Nephrol 2015;28:659.

Glassman DT et al: Bilateral nephrectomy with concomitant renal graft transplantation for autosomal dominant polycystic kidney disease. J Urol 2000;164:661.

Goldberg D, Reese PP: Open-labeled trial of zepatier for treatment of hepatitis C negative patients who receive kidney transplants from hepatitis C positive donors. In: *ClinicalTrials.gov* [internet] https://clinicaltrials.gov/show/NCT02743897 NLM Identifier: NCT02743897, 2000.

Irish A: Hypercoagulability in renal transplant recipients. Identifying patients at risk of renal allograft thrombosis and evaluating strategies for prevention. Am J Cardiovasc Drugs 2004;4:139.

Ismail HR et al: Simultaneous vs. sequential laparoscopic bilateral native nephrectomy and renal transplantation. Transplantation 2005;80:1124.

Kasiske BL et al: The evaluation of renal transplantation candidates: clinical practice guidelines. Am J Transplant 2001; 1 Suppl 2:3.

Kirkman MA et al: Native nephrectomy for autosomal dominant polycystic kidney disease: before or after kidney transplantation? BJU Int 2011;108:590.

Kramer A et al: Simultaneous bilateral native nephrectomy and living donor renal transplantation are successful for polycystic kidney disease: the University of Maryland experience. J Urol 2009;181:724.

Lucas SM et al: Staged nephrectomy versus bilateral laparoscopic nephrectomy in patients with autosomal dominant polycystic kidney disease. J Urol 2010;184:2054.

Norman SP, Kommareddi M, Kaul DR: Update on kidney transplantation in HIV-infected recipients. AIDS Rev 2012;14:195.

Northcutt A et al: Does kidney transplantation to iliac artery deteriorate ischemia in the ipsilateral lower extremity with peripheral arterial disease? Vascular 2015;23:490.

Ojo AO et al: Long-term survival in renal transplant recipients with graft function. Kidney Int 2000;57:307.

Schmitges J et al: Higher perioperative morbidity and in-hospital mortality in patients with end-stage renal disease undergoing nephrectomy for non-metastatic kidney cancer: a population-based analysis. BJU Int 2012;110:E183.

Vukas D et al: Renal transplantation—a possible factor in the development of circulatory insufficiency in the lower extremities. Acta Chir Iugosl 1989;36 Suppl 1:143.

Wagner MD, Prather JC, Barry JM: Selective, concurrent bilateral nephrectomies at renal transplantation for autosomal dominant polycystic kidney disease. J Urol 2007;177:2250; discussion 2254.

LIVING DONOR EVALUATION

It is widely recognized that recipient outcomes are superior when the transplanted kidney comes from a living donor. Furthermore, there is currently a significant shortage in deceased donor candidates and this has led to a significant increase in the time a recipient can expect to wait on the list. And with this time comes the increased attendant complications associated with an extended dialysis vintage time. For these reasons, as well as others, transplantation from a living donor is the preferred option.

▶ Universal Assessment of Living Donor Candidates

Living donor candidates are put through an extensive evaluation before they are allowed to proceed with the donation procedure. This evaluation is multifaceted and is not limited to a medical review. Rather, donor candidates are evaluated by transplant surgeons, nephrologists with specialization in transplantation, social workers, and more recently, independent living donor advocates. Each member of the donor evaluation team is charged with a different set of tasks. All must be completed before the potential candidate can be brought to a medical review board for clearance for donation.

The nephrologist takes an extensive history from the donor candidate focusing on the prior medical history. Laboratory testing accumulated as part of the donor evaluation, or preexisting and collected from the primary care physician records, is frequently evaluated by the transplant nephrologist. As one might expect, the focus of this evaluation is determining whether or not the donor candidate has a history, or findings concerning for preexisting kidney disease. Moreover, the nephrologist seeks to identify any sentinel findings, which may predict development of kidney disease in the future. Alternatively, the evaluation may reveal underlying medical conditions, which secondarily bring with them the risk of development of kidney disease in the future following the donor nephrectomy.

Candidates for living donation should expect during their evaluation to have their current kidney function measured through both blood and urinary testing. Estimated glomerular filtration rate (eGFR) will be calculated. But, in many cases a 24-hour urinary collection will be required to more accurately determine the donor's level of renal clearance. Though all centers are allowed to create their own protocols in this regard, most centers will not allow a donor candidate with an estimated glomerular filtration rate below 80 mL/min to proceed as a donor candidate. As donor nephrectomy is associated with loss of GFR (around 30%), candidates with GFRs less than 80 mL/min generate concern that they will have insufficient renal function following the nephrectomy. In particular, the goal is to avoid having the donor left with only stage III level of kidney function (ie, GFR <60 mL/min) following the nephrectomy procedure. Naturally, donors will be extensively screened for evidence of microalbuminuria and proteinuria as these are all but universally considered sentinel markers of an abnormality in renal function.

Living donor candidates are also extensively tested for evidence of diseases, which may be transmitted to the recipient at the time of transplantation. These diseases include tuberculosis, syphilis, viral hepatitis, and HIV. It is worth noting that for these infectious agents there is both risk to the recipient and potentially to the donor as well should they be allowed to proceed. For example, donor candidates determined to have viral hepatitis may develop cirrhosis, which could with some predictable rate be accompanied by development of hepatorenal syndrome. Though no studies have directly addressed this issue, we can anticipate that the development of renal disease in the future life of the donor would be more significant following donor nephrectomy on the basis of reduced renal mass. Donor candidates are carefully evaluated for the presence of hereditary kidney disease, diabetes, and hypertension.

▶ Evaluation of the Donor Candidate from a Family with PKD

ADPKD is the most common inherited form of kidney disease. ADPKD is fully penetrant. As such, nearly all individuals who inherit a mutated PKD gene will develop disease. But, the timing of disease presentation and tempo of disease progression are extremely variable, both between families with ADPKD and between affected individuals from the same family. Similarly, the age of onset of ESRD, and the spectrum of extrarenal manifestations also vary widely between affected individuals. Therefore, careful attention to exclude ADPKD, particularly disease early in its course, is essential. This is most critical when the donor candidate is a blood related family member of the recipient who is also genetically at risk for having inherited the same disease forming allele. Traditionally, screening for ADPKD included ultrasound imaging of the kidneys for donor candidates over the age of 30. Unlike the established criteria for formally making a diagnosis of PKD, most transplant centers consider the discovery of even a single cyst a relative, perhaps even absolute, contraindication to providing an at risk individual clearance to donate.

Patients under the age of 30 who have ADPKD may not yet have cysts that are sufficiently sized to be detected by ultrasound imaging. CT imaging offers an enhanced level of resolution that should be considered for these younger individuals. Genetic testing for ADPKD can also be considered when the donor and recipient are consanguineous but is most helpful when a disease causing mutation is identified in the affected recipient. Isolating and sequencing the *PKD-1* and *PKD-2* genes from the recipient and screening for pathogenic variants known to cause ADPKD accomplishes this. Presence of this same mutation in the donor candidate should prevent the donation from occurring while absence of the disease mutation provides reassurance. While the cataloged database of ADPKD causing mutations is quite extensive and continues to grow, there is still the potential of screening an affected individual in whom a disease-causing variant is never identified. This remains one of the significant limitations of the direct sequencing approach for ADPKD screening. An alternative genetic approach involves linkage analysis, whereby the segregation of chromosomal markers flanking the disease gene is determined across multiple affected and unaffected family members ideally spanning multiple generations. There are several limitations to the linkage analysis approach and for this reason direct sequencing has become the preferred approach.

▶ Screening Living Donor Candidates for Predisposition to Diabetes

All living donor candidates should be screened for predisposition to develop diabetes. How to accomplish this screening, and what screening results should be interpreted as absolute versus relative contraindications to donation are not fully agreed upon. Moreover, the same findings judged to be a contraindication for one donor candidate may not be exclusionary for another candidate coming from a lower risk ethnicity or age group. Most centers rely on obtaining a detailed history and family history for diabetes and a fasting blood glucose determination. If either is positive, testing will be expanded to include measurement of a hemoglobin A1C and an oral glucose tolerance test. Situations where these tests ought to be performed are in donor candidates with a personal history of hyperglycemia and overt diabetes (eg, gestational, steroid induced, or in the context of prior obesity) and in donor candidates with first-degree relatives who are known to have diabetes. Many centers will allow a candidate with impaired fasting glucose (IFG) to proceed, while diagnosing impaired glucose tolerance (IGT) is likely to be exclusionary for all but the lowest risk individuals. The progression from IFG and IGT to overt diabetes occurs over several years, perhaps even decades. And, a minority of diabetics develops diabetic kidney disease, with an even smaller

fraction leading to ESRD. Older donor candidates may be allowed to donate after they have been informed of the long-term risks. The concept being that such a donor's timeline for the development of significant diabetic kidney disease may exceed their estimated remaining lifetime.

▶ Donor EBV and CMV Screening

EBV and cytomegalovirus represent unique concerns in transplantation, as there is the fear that these viruses might be transmitted as passengers in the kidney from the donor to the unprotected seronegative recipient. Recipient disease resulting from EBV and CMV are discussed in detail to follow.

▶ Psychosocial and Independent Living Donor Advocate Assessment of the Donor Candidate

Similar to the recipient evaluation, the living donor candidate is also evaluated by a social worker. The goals of this encounter are to determine if the candidate has a sufficient support system in place for the donation to occur. The social worker will also confirm that there will not be any unexpected consequences to the donor from an employment perspective due to the missed hours from work, and from lost wages. A focus is often placed on ascertaining whether all close family and friends are comfortable with the donor candidate proceeding with the kidney donation. And if any close contacts or relations are not, exploring the details surrounding their objections and providing guidance to resolve uncomfortable situations.

To promote the safety and care of the living donor throughout the process of evaluation and donation, it is now a federal requirement in the United States that all living donor transplant programs have an independent living donor advocate (ILDA). The ILDA is charged with the role of being the advocate for the donor's autonomy. And given the magnitude of the decision to donate, to ensure that the donor has sufficiently understood any finding uncovered during the evaluation, educational materials provided, and the potential for both short- and long-term consequences related to kidney donation, before completing the informed consent process. Though ILDAs require specialized training and possess a unique set of skills, it is common for a social worker generally knowledgeable about transplantation to serve in this capacity.

▶ Donor Risks

Performed on carefully selected candidates, donor nephrectomy remains a safe procedure with a low risk for long-term consequences. All major surgical procedures have an associated risk of death. For donor nephrectomy, the risk of perioperative mortality is approximately 1 in 3000 (0.03%). Similar to other surgeries, common complications include development of an incisional seroma, superficial wound infection, deep wound infection, intra-abdominal bleeding, need for reoperation, pneumonia, deep venous thrombosis, etc.

Collectively, the rate of a postoperative complication (major or minor) is approximately 15% for living donor nephrectomies.

While all transplant programs fear a major operative complication, the long-term consequences of nephrectomy to the living donor remains the paramount concern and a focus of ongoing research worldwide. Prior to 2014, living donor candidates during the informed consent process were largely told that there was no known long-term risk associated with the procedure. Unfortunately, no large-scale effort to prospectively monitor donors following nephrectomy has ever been established to directly confirm this assertion. Rather, this belief was based largely, if not entirely, on the observation that patients who required a nephrectomy for treatment of disease or trauma do not appear to be at an increased risk for the development of ESRD.

Two retrospective cohort studies published a few months apart, the first from Norway and the second from the United States, subsequently reached the conclusion that there was an increased long-term risk of ESRD in living donors. Both studies reported similar data indicating that while the absolute risk of ESRD was quite low for living donors, it was significantly increased relative to well matched healthy nonkidney donors in the respective general population. More specifically, the lifetime risk of developing ESRD following donor nephrectomy is estimated at 90 per 10,000 living donors compared to 14 per 10,000 healthy nondonors (a relative risk of 6.5; based on the data from the United States). Consistent with earlier and smaller studies, this increased risk was not uniform across all demographic backgrounds. Notably, black males had the highest estimated risk (96 per 10,000 at 15 years postnephrectomy) followed by black women (58.5 per 10,000) and white men (34 per 10,000). White females had the lowest estimated risk (14.6 per 10,000) of ESRD 15 years following living donor nephrectomy.

KEY READINGS

Abecassis M et al: Consensus statement on the live organ donor. JAMA 2000;284:2919.

Hays RE et al: The independent living donor advocate: a guidance document from the American Society of Transplantation's Living Donor Community of Practice (AST LDCOP). Am J Transplant 2015;15:518.

Kasiske BL et al: The evaluation of renal transplantation candidates: clinical practice guidelines. Am J Transplant 2001; 1 Suppl 2:3.

Matas AJ et al: 2202 kidney transplant recipients with 10 years of graft function: what happens next? Am J Transplant 2008;8:2410.

Mjøen G et al: Long-term risks for kidney donors. Kidney Int 2014;86:162.

Muzaale AD et al: Risk of end-stage renal disease following live kidney donation. JAMA 2014;311:579.

Najarian JS et al: 20 years or more of follow-up of living kidney donors. Lancet 1992;340:807.

Patel N et al: Renal function and cardiovascular outcomes after living donor nephrectomy in the UK: quality and safety revisited. BJU Int 2013;112:E134.

Pei Y: Practical genetics for autosomal dominant polycystic kidney disease. Nephron Clin Pract 2011;118:c19.

Torres VE, Harris PC, Pirson Y: Autosomal dominant polycystic kidney disease. Lancet 2007;369:1287.

Vigneault CB et al: Should living kidney donor candidates with impaired fasting glucose donate? Clin J Am Soc Nephrol 2011;6:2054.

Wynn JJ, Alexander CE: Increasing organ donation and transplantation: the U.S. experience over the past decade. Transpl Int 2011;24:324.

Zhao X et al: Molecular diagnostics in autosomal dominant polycystic kidney disease: utility and limitations. Clin J Am Soc Nephrol 2008;3:146.

KIDNEY TRANSPLANT SURGERY

▶ Standard Operating Procedure

The majority of kidney transplants are implanted anteriorly into the pelvis without disturbing the native system. More specifically, the allograft is inserted into the iliac fossa (more commonly the right iliac fossa for first time recipients) via a curved inguinal Rutherford Morrison ("hockey stick") incision. The allograft renal vein is anastomosed with the recipient's external iliac vein followed by anastomosis of the allograft renal artery with the recipient's external iliac artery. At this point, the vascular clamp is removed and reperfusion of the transplant occurs. Provided that allograft function is immediate, urine production is noted from the allograft ureter, which is not yet anastomosed with the recipient's bladder. Attention is then turned to the recipient's bladder where a ureteroneocystostomy (UNC) is performed, allowing for implantation of the allograft ureter into the lateral wall of the bladder. Every effort is made to fashion the UNC such that the connection effectively forms a valve-like mechanism sufficiently tight to prevent urine refluxing, but not overly tight as to cause hydroureteronephrosis.

As the native urinary system is not disturbed during a kidney transplant, patients with residual renal function preceding transplantation will produce urine that is a composite representing the collective output from all three kidneys. While the transplant is anticipated to have the highest GFR of the three, and therefore more significantly contribute to the total urine output, this may not be the case when there is delayed allograft function. In this setting, monitoring the decline in the serum creatinine may better reflect allograft function. In addition, and especially in the case of a recipient with a history of FSGS that is believed to be at risk for immediate post-transplant disease recurrence, monitoring the urine for proteinuria development can be complicated by residual renal function making it difficult to ascertain the proteinuria source. Some transplant surgeons will consider ligating the native ureters preemptively in select cases to avoid this source of uncertainty.

Ureteral Stenting During Kidney Transplantation

Though not a universal practice, most programs insert a "double-J" internal ureteral stent at the time of kidney transplantation to hold the ureter open and maintain proper flow of urine, and allow the UNC to heal. Note that individual study data is conflicting regarding whether use of a ureter stent reduces the risks of a urine leak and other major urologic complications developing from the UNC. But, a meta-analysis concluded that universal stenting, while associated with a higher risk of post-transplant urinary tract infection, significantly reduced the risk of major ureteral complications and recommended their use become universal practice. Timing of the ureteral stent removal varies between programs, but most are removed between 4–8 weeks following transplantation. The ureteral stent is removed in the conventional manner via cystoscopy generally performed in an office based setting.

Pediatric En Bloc Kidney Transplantation

Though ever effort is made to allocate pediatric donor organs to a pediatric recipient on the waiting list, in cases were no suitable pediatric recipient can be identified, pediatric organs can be allocated to an adult recipient. A single kidney from a very young, or very small (<15 kg), pediatric donor may not provide sufficient functional renal mass to meet the metabolic needs of the adult recipient. Therefore, younger pediatric kidneys allocated to adult are frequently procured and transplanted en bloc. That is to say, rather than procuring the right and left kidneys individually, they are removed as a group along with their adjacent segment of the donor aorta and inferior vena cava. One end of these vessels is ligated, and the other ends are used to make the anastomoses with the adult recipient's external iliac artery and vein. As there will be two ureters, a decision is made to implant them either individually (ie, two UNCs) into the bladder, or to first join them together resulting in a single shared UNC. Outcomes using pediatric en bloc transplantation are excellent for carefully selected recipients and are comparable to adults receiving a kidney from a living donor.

Multiorgan Transplantation Involving Kidneys

A comprehensive discussion of the use of kidney transplants as part of a multiorgan transplant (MOT) procedure is beyond the scope of this chapter. However, as a general principle, kidneys will first be considered for allocation with other organs for the purpose of MOT before they are available for allocation to a recipient waiting for a kidney alone on the kidney transplant waiting list. As this practice for some results in a sense of inequity and unfairness, which until recently was made worse by an absence of regulatory guidelines and oversight to ensure that the use of kidneys for MOT was not being abused, it is not without critics.

Kidneys are the organ most commonly used in the setting of MOT. This practice has fallen under criticism, particularly in the context of a simultaneous liver kidney (SLK) transplant. Profession societies, nephrologists, and advocacy groups representing patients with ESRD argue that the number of kidneys allocated to patients with liver disease is excessive, and an unfair practice that bypasses those who have waited for many years on the kidney transplant wait list. On the other side of the issue are hepatologists and transplant surgeons, who argue that the patient with combined liver and kidney disease has the best chance for survival when transplanted simultaneously with a liver and a kidney. Recently, the UNOS SLK working group published their guidelines on how to regulate the practice of SLK transplantation. Prior to this set of guidelines, there was no official set of guidelines and the rates of SLK transplants varied widely across UNOS regions, donor service areas, and even between programs within the same cities.

The SLK work group did not approach this issue from the perspective of determining the number of kidneys allocated to OLT recipients. Rather, they sought to view the patient with ESLD and CKD or AKI as a unique group of individuals, different from both patients requiring an OLT or a DDKT alone. Based on their review of the literature and a critical assessment of the UNOS data collected on liver transplant recipients (both those who received an SLK and those who received a liver transplant alone) they drafted a set of guidelines to govern the practice of listing for SLK (Table 52–5).

An important feature of these new guidelines is "safety net," a provision that allows patients transplanted with a LTA who do not recover native kidney function to be listed for a DDKT. This provision requires that the listing for the DDKT occur within the year following LTA and affords the patient a higher rank in the kidney allocation system (KAS) ranking schema (Table 52–6). At present, it is not clear whether this new set of guidelines will lead to an increased

Table 52–5. Medical eligibility criteria for SLK.

CKD (must be confirmed by a nephrologist)
- GFR <60 for 90 consecutive days and
- eGFR or CrCl <30 at or after registration on kidney wait list or
- Dialysis (in setting of ESRD)

AKI (must be confirmed by a nephrologist)
- Dialysis for 6 consecutive weeks
- eGFR/CrCl <25 for 6 consecutive weeks
- Combination of above two criteria

Metabolic disease (must be confirmed by a nephrologist)
- Atypical HUS from mutations factor H or factor I
- Hyperoxaluria
- Familial nonneuropathic systemic amyloidosis
- Methylmalonic aciduria

Table 52–6. The "safety net" for liver recipients.

Sequence A KDPI ≤20%	Sequence B KDPI >20% but <35%	Sequence C KDPI >35% but <85%	Sequence D KDPI >85%
Highly sensitized	Highly sensitized	Highly sensitized	Highly sensitized
0-ABDR mismatch	0-ABDR mismatch	0-ABDR mismatch	0-ABDR mismatch
Prior living donor	Prior living donor	Prior living donor	Local SLK safety net
Local pediatrics	Local pediatrics	Local SLK safety net	Local + regional
Local top 20% EPTS	Local SLK safety net	Local candidates	National candidates
0-ABDR mismatch (all)	Local adults	Regional candidates	
Local (all)	Regional pediatrics	National candidates	
Regional pediatrics	Regional adults		
Regional (top 20%)	National pediatrics		
Regional (all)	National adults		
National pediatrics			
National (top 20%)			
National (all)			

Prioritization of the liver alone transplant recipient who subsequently qualifies for a deceased donor kidney transplant under the safety net provision of the UNOS SLK Proposal is a function of the donors KDPI (kidney donor profile index).

or decreased rate of SLK transplantation. However, it is clear that stakeholders are watching these DDKT utilization results closely and that modifications to these guidelines may be required.

Similar guidelines do not exist for MOT involving other combinations of organs. But, kidneys are also commonly allocated in the context of simultaneous pancreas–kidney (SPK) and simultaneous heart–kidney transplants. It is anticipated that guidelines similar to those for SLK transplants will be drafted for heart–kidney transplants in the near future.

KEY READINGS

Asch WS, Bia MJ: New organ allocation system for combined liver-kidney transplants and the availability of kidneys for transplant to patients with stage 4-5 CKD. Clin J Am Soc Nephrol 2017;12:848.

Formica RN et al: Simultaneous liver-kidney allocation policy: a proposal to optimize appropriate utilization of scarce resources. Am J Transplant 2016;16:758.

Sharma A et al: En bloc kidney transplantation from pediatric donors: comparable outcomes with living donor kidney transplantation. Transplantation 2011;92:564.

Wilson CH et al: Routine intraoperative stenting for renal transplant recipients. Transplantation 2005;80:877.

PUBLIC HEALTH SERVICE (PHS) INCREASED RISK DONORS

Transplant centers in the United States are required to notify recipients of donors who are at "increased risk" for the transmission of HIV, HBV, and HCV. While there is always some risk of infectious disease transmission through organ transplantation, both living and deceased donors with an appropriate history of behaviors (or those deceased donors for whom an accounting from a family member or close acquaintance is unobtainable) receive this designation. Additionally, deceased donors whose testing may be falsely negative secondary to hemodilution (either of the sample, or the potential donor secondary to significant IVF infusion or transfusion of blood products) are also categorized as PHS increased risk. At the time of writing, no less than one-third of deceased donors in the United States meet the criteria for the PHS increased risk donor designation (Figure 52–1). In the United States, every year since 2008 drug overdose death has been the leading cause of injury related death, exceeding death related to motor vehicle accidents. This is a consequence of a simultaneous reduction in motor vehicle deaths and dramatic increase in drug overdose deaths in the last decade, primarily fueled by an increased use of heroine (Figure 52–2). Many factors contributed to this heroine epidemic, including an increased potency product sold at a

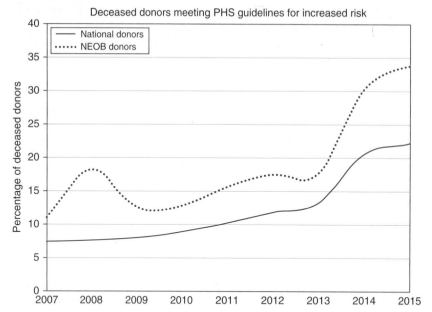

▲ **Figure 52–1.** The percentage of deceased donors in the United States meeting criteria for the PHS increased risk designation significantly increased between 2007 and 2015. In the New England Organ Bank (NEOB) Donor Service Area (within UNOS Region 1), this increase has been even more significant. Across the United States, this increase is attributed to the significantly increased use of heroin and heroin overdose deaths. (OPTN/UNOS and courtesy of the NEOB.)

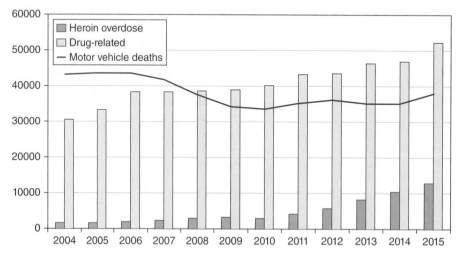

▲ **Figure 52–2.** Drug-related deaths now exceed motor vehicle deaths in the United States. Starting in 2008, drug-related deaths have exceeded the number of deaths attributable to motor vehicle accidents in the United States. Though only about a quarter of these deaths are directly linked to heroin, the rate of heroin overdose death has increased nearly 10-fold over the past decade. (DEA Strategic Intelligence Section: 2015 National Drug Threat Assessment Summary. In: Department of Justice DEA, ed. 2015.)

historically relatively reduced cost. This is often achieved as a result of mixing heroin with the synthetic opioid fentanyl. While heroine is most commonly used via the intravenous route of delivery, a significant number of abusers now use the drug via an inhalational route (sniffing, snorting, or smoking). This increased potency of the currently available heroine enables users to experiment more easily via the inhalation route, particularly users initially reluctant to make the leap to an intravenous drug of abuse. Subsequently progressing from inhalational to intravenous use is anticipated to be less of a transition. Notwithstanding the above factors, the role increased use and abuse of prescription opiates has played in the rise of heroin use in the United States cannot be overlooked.

Due to the social stigmas that carry forward from the 1980s, recipients are generally most fearful of HIV transmission. But, the risk of donor derived HIV infection is lower than for HBV and HCV. This lower risk is secondary to the lower prevalence of HIV positive individuals in the population and the very short "eclipse" or "window" period during which a potential donor who recently contracted HIV continues to test negative for disease (the latest generation assays can now consistently detect HIV positivity in as few as 5 days following infection). With the exception of transplantation to HIV seropositive recipients, which now occurs only on a selected basis under the HIV Organ Policy Equity (HOPE) Act, organs from donors who test positive for HIV are not knowingly transplanted into HIV negative recipients.

KEY READINGS

Dodd RY, Notari EPt, Stramer SL. Current prevalence and incidence of infectious disease markers and estimated window-period risk in the American Red Cross blood donor population. Transfusion 2002;42:975.

Health Resources and Services Administration (HRSA) Department of Health and Human Services. Organ procurement and transplantation: implementation of the HIV Organ Policy Equity Act. Final rule. Fed Regist 2015;80:26464.

Rudd RA et al: Increases in drug and opioid-involved overdose deaths—United States, 2010–2015. MMWR Morb Mortal Wkly Rep 2016;65:1445.

Seem DL et al: PHS guideline for reducing human immunodeficiency virus, hepatitis B virus, and hepatitis C virus transmission through organ transplantation. Public Health Rep 2013;128:247.

KIDNEY TRANSPLANT COMPLICATIONS

▶ Infections After Kidney Transplantation

It is an inescapable reality that immunosuppressed transplant recipients are at an increased risk for infection development. A major focus of the early post-transplant experience is prophylaxis against selected pathogens, and active surveillance for infection development.

In addition to their immunosuppressive medications, kidney transplant recipients are discharged on multiple agents to prevent infection. Fungal, bacterial, and viral infections can all occur early after transplant, albeit there are some characteristic times these infections are likely to occur within this window of time. Immediately following transplantation (ie, during the first month), donor-derived, operative, and nosocomial sources of infection predominate. Routine perioperative infection prophylaxis is administered at each center according to the recommendations of the hospital's epidemiology program. Furthermore, it is not uncommon for a culture collected from the deceased donor to result positively after a transplant has occurred. In these instances, there is a heightened level of concern over the possibility a donor-derived pathogen has been transmitted to the recipient. Additional prophylaxis may be warranted, and consultation with the center's infectious disease specialists is advisable when this occurs.

▶ Candidiasis

As might be expected, oropharyngeal and esophageal candidiasis is a common infection very early after kidney transplantation owing, in part, to the high doses or corticosteroids used during the period of immunosuppression induction. Candidiasis is easily diagnosed on physical examination of the oropharynx, and should always be suspected when a recipient presents with dysphagia early after transplant even in the absence of overt thrush. In cases of suspected candida esophagitis, an esophagogastroduodenoscopy should be performed to confirm the diagnosis, and evaluate for alternative causes of dysphagia such as reflux esophagitis and gastritis. Candidiasis prophylaxis is routinely provided to transplant recipients. Regimens using nystatin oral suspension or fluconazole orally are both acceptable. Though, as gastrointestinal absorption of nystatin is insignificant, it will not treat more distant sources of fungal infection. In contrast, fluconazole is well absorbed and potentially superior on this basis.

▶ *Pneumocystis jiroveci* Pneumonia (PJP)

Pneumocystis pneumonia is caused by the ubiquitous, yeast-like, fungus *Pneumocystis jiroveci*. Indeed, nearly every individual has been exposed to, and successfully combated, *P jiroveci* by the age of 4. Immunosuppression weakens host defenses against *P jiroveci*. Accordingly, while not nearly as high a concern as during earlier eras when increased doses of corticosteroids were maintained for an extended period following transplantation, PJP remains a concern for the modern transplant recipient. Though PJP can occur at any time following transplantation, the peak time for appearance is between 1 and 6 months following transplantation.

A diagnosis of PJP should be entertained for all transplant recipients presenting with symptoms of pneumonia and hypoxemia that appears disproportional to the objective findings. Furthermore, in the context of a suggestive

CXR showing a fine reticular interstitial pulmonary pattern, often occurring in a perihilar distribution, PCP should be strongly suspected. Bronchoscopy is recommended for confirmation in all cases where PJP is suspected. Trimethoprim-sulfamethoxazole is the treatment of choice for PJP, but intravenous pentamidine is equally efficacious. Other treatment regimens exist, but when studied proved inferior choices (in patients with HIV/AIDS infection).

▶ *Pneumocystis jiroveci* Pneumonia Prophylaxis

Though the questions as to whether post-transplant prophylaxis against PJP remains necessary in the modern era, it remains widely in use. The most common regimen uses trimethoprim/sulfamethoxazole (TMP/SMZ) either single strength (80 mg/400 mg) orally daily, or double strength (160 mg/800 mg) orally every other day. Even single strength dosed thrice weekly has been reported to be successful. Alternative agents, typically reserved for either the sulfa-drug allergic or hyperkalemia prone recipient, include inhalation pentamidine administered monthly, atovaquone, and dapsone. All of these agents have relative strengths and weakness, and may not be appropriate in all cases. In general, post-transplant PCP prophylaxis is offered during the first 4–6 months following transplantation, though a minority of programs continues to offer prophylaxis for the entire first year.

▶ Cytomegalovirus

Cytomegalovirus (CMV) is a ubiquitous virus found across the world. The seroprevalence of CMV is directly related to the age of the population. Approximately one-third of children below the age of 12 are seropositive due to viral infection. By early adulthood, seropositivity increases to about 50% and continues to rise by approximately 1% annually to greater than 90% above age 80. Hence, primary exposure of seronegative transplant recipients may occur at any time after kidney transplantation.

CMV can be clinically subdivided into three distinct categories: CMV viremia, CMV syndrome, and CMV tissue invasive disease. CMV viremia is a subclinical finding and is typically discovered either when "preemptive therapy" is chosen over "universal prophylaxis," and when CMV screening is done for other clinical purposes. Indeed, low grade viral reactivation in the seropositive recipient can occur in many clinical settings and is generally not felt to be significant. Preemptive therapy involves routine, protocol based, monitoring of recipients for development of CMV viremia in place of providing prophylactic therapy. Though there are benefits and shortcomings to each approach, both strategies have been shown to be safe and effective.

The CMV syndrome typically presents as a "flu-like" illness with fever, malaise, and lethargy. These symptoms are frequently associated with leucopenia or thrombocytopenia. Pharyngitis and lymphadenopathy are possible, but not seen nearly as frequently or significantly as with infectious mononucleosis from EBV. Depending on the severity of the presentation, CMV syndrome in the kidney transplant recipient can be managed on an outpatient basis.

Most concerning is the kidney transplant recipient that presents with signs or symptoms of CMV tissue invasive disease. While virtually every internal organ can become infected with CMV at the tissue level, the most commonly affected organs are in the gastrointestinal tract, particularly, the colon. Tissue invasive disease commonly occurs in the allograft independent of the organ transplanted. Indeed, CMV hepatitis occurs more commonly in liver transplant recipients, CMV pancreatitis in pancreas transplant recipients, and CMV pneumonitis in lung transplant recipients, and nephritis in kidney transplant recipients. This is believed to be a consequence of altered immune mechanisms occurring at the interface between the allograft and the host. In the kidney allograft, CMV tissue invasive disease can lead to a glomerulonephritis with intraglomerular viral inclusions frequently seen on histologic evaluation. CMV glomerulonephritis likely occurs more commonly than is generally appreciated. Patients with CMV colitis present with profuse diarrhea, the acute kidney injury that accompanies this presentation may be multifactorial and not simply a consequence of the attendant hypovolemia. Allograft biopsy is generally deferred early in the course of CMV infection as treatment for rejection (if discovered) is ill-advised in this context.

There is a well-appreciated, bidirectional relationship between CMV infection and rejection. In addition to antiviral therapy, a reduction in immunosuppression is recommended, and frequently necessary, to successfully treat a patient with significant CMV viremia or CMV tissue invasive disease. In addition to the increased risk of rejection that occurs as a consequence of this partial host immune system reconstitution, the CMV virus has been speculated to have the ability to trigger rejection. But, this ability to spawn rejection has been difficult to confirm in prospective trials. Of course, the increased level of immunosuppression that results from the treatment of active rejection raises the risk for subsequent CMV infection.

It is common to see the CMV quantitative PCR result rise when initially starting a patient on treatment for CMV viremia, syndrome, or tissue invasive disease. This rise may be the consequence of further viral replication that occurred between the time the first diagnostic sample was collected and the time treatment commenced. Increased levels of viremia secondary to therapy induced infected cell lysis and release of viral particles was suggested, but available evidence suggests the opposite is the case. More importantly, following 10–14 days of therapy without evidence of a decline in the viremia or improvement in the patient's clinical status, infection with a drug resistant strain of CMV should be suspected.

The two main treatments for CMV are ganciclovir IV (5 mg/kg twice daily) and valganciclovir orally (900 mg/kg twice daily), dose adjusted for renal insufficiency. Once suspected, testing to confirm the presence of a drug resistant strain of CMV should be undertaken and an adjustment to the therapy considered. Two mutations account for the majority of ganciclovir and valganciclovir resistance, UL97 and UL54. The former occurs in a phosphotransferase, the latter in a DNA polymerase. UL97 mutations may be overcome by increasing the dose of ganciclovir. UL54 mutations are less common, indicate resistance to high dose ganciclovir, and may result in cross-resistance to both foscarnet and cidofovir. In cases where treatment with foscarnet or cidofovir is required, development of drug induced renal injury is possible if not probable. Volume expansion with IV fluids can mitigate some of the nephrotoxic effects of these two drugs.

In life-threatening cases of CMV, reconstitution of the host immune system may be necessary. The allograft may need to be sacrificed to save the life of the host.

▶ Cytomegalovirus Prophylaxis

While primary exposure from an outside source can occur, the greater concern for kidney transplant recipients is infection from within. Indeed, reactivation of latent virus in the seropositive recipient (deemed intermediate risk), and primary infection for the seronegative recipient who received an organ from a seropositive donor (high risk), are the major sources of infection. For these reasons, the generally accepted practice is to provide CMV prophylaxis to both the intermediate and high risk kidney transplant recipients. While still at risk for primary exposure from an outside source, seronegative recipients who received an organ from a seronegative donor are at relatively low risk for CMV infection. CMV prophylaxis can be deferred for this subgroup of recipients. Non-CMV viral prophylaxis is typically provided in lieu of CMV specific prophylaxis for these recipients (Table 52–7).

▶ Polyoma BK Virus

The association between immunosuppressed states and opportunistic infections has been long appreciated. While this is true for all solid and hematologic transplants, the relationship between the BK virus and kidney transplant recipients is a unique one. Aside from bone marrow recipients, for whom this virus can be a cause of hemorrhagic cystitis, no other organ transplant other than the kidney is at risk for allograft loss due to BK. Discovered in 1971 in the urine of a kidney transplant recipient who developed a ureteral stenosis (and whose name comes from the initials of that patient), BK is a small, nonenveloped, double-stranded DNA polyoma virus. Seropositivity for BK is widespread in the population, both indicating that

Table 52–7. Postkidney transplant infection CMV prophylaxis recommendation.

CMV Donor seronegative, recipient seronegative:
Low risk for CMV infection
CMV specific antiviral prophylaxis is acceptable, but not required
Antiviral prophylaxis with acyclovir PO for three months preferred
CMV donor seronegative, recipient seropositive and
CMV donor seropositive, recipient seropositive
   Intermediate risk groups for CMV infection
   Valganciclovir prophylaxis recommended for 3 months as follows:
      CrCl >60 mL/min: 450 mg orally twice a day
      CrCl 40–59 mL/min: 450 mg orally once a day
      CrCl 25–39 mL/min: 450 mg orally every other day
      CrCl 10–24 mL/min: 450 mg orally twice a week
   Ganciclovir (renal dose adjusted) can also be used in lieu of
      valganciclovir.
CMV donor seropositive, recipient seronegative
   High-risk group for CMV infection (recipient is naive)
   Valganciclovir prophylaxis recommended for 6 months as follows:
      CrCl >60 mL/min: 450 mg orally twice a day
      CrCl 40–59 mL/min: 450 mg orally once a day
      CrCl 25–39 mL/min: 450 mg orally every other day
      CrCl 10–24 mL/min: 450 mg orally twice a week
   Ganciclovir (renal dose adjusted) can also be used in lieu of
      valganciclovir.

transmission between hosts is highly effective and highly unlikely to be a cause of significant illness in the general (nonimmunosuppressed) population. The exact mode of transmission is not definitively known, and there is reason to believe that more than one route of transmission is possible. A case for respiratory transmission is supported by the isolation of BKV from nasopharyngeal aspirate samples collected from infants. There is also evidence that BK reactivates in a significant percentage of pregnant woman, and that the virus is capable of transplacental transmission to the developing fetus. Once acquired, BKV has a significant tropism for renal tubular epithelial cells and transitional epithelial cells of the ureter and bladder. In these select tissues, it lies dormant and is presumably kept in check by the immune system.

BKV is, arguably more than rejection, the scourge of kidney transplantation. Most kidney transplant centers now report that a universal screening protocol is in place to monitor the recipients. Indeed, the American Society of Transplantation 2013 consensus guideline recommended that kidney transplant recipients be screened quarterly for 2 years, and then annually for an additional 3 years following transplantation.

PCR is the universal method for detection, but whether to screen the blood, urine, or both is center dependent. BKV titers are much greater in the urine than in the blood (presumably due to the tropism of the virus to the urinary system). Hence, urine offers the highest sensitivity. However, only a fraction of patients positive for BK viruria test positive for viremia, with an even smaller fraction discovered to have BKV associated nephropathy. For this reason, many transplant centers have adopted a screening protocol that tests the recipient's blood.

Once detected, management of BKV is suboptimal. No antiviral agent has ever been developed specifically to combat the BKV. The WHO reports that just under 70,000 kidney transplants are performed annually worldwide. Approximately 10–15% of all recipients will develop detectable viremia with a further subset advancing to manifest BK nephropathy. Hence a drug designed specifically to treat BK will likely only be of benefit to fewer than 10,000 patients annually, presumably making it not profitable for the pharmaceutical industry to pursue development of a drug solely for this disease. Nonetheless, efforts to identify an existing agent developed for another indication that has anti-BK activity continue. Hence the mainstay of BKV management involves a stepwise reduction in antirejection therapy thereby allowing for a partial immune system reconstitution. Of course, while the increased activity of the immune system associated with this reduced level of immunosuppression may be sufficient to allow for BKV clearance and return to senescence, this strategy always increases the risk of rejection in the allograft. Fortunately, rejection occurs in a minority of patients who have their immunosuppression reduced secondary to BK viremia. This may reflect the fact that most kidney transplant recipients have an idealized level of immunosuppression that is sufficient to prevent rejection, but not so sufficient as to allow for BKV replication and spread.

While a reduction in immunosuppression remains the center of BKV management, multiple existing drugs have been tested (particularly, *in vitro*) and determined to have activity against BKV. Though none has proven to have widespread efficacy in human transplant recipients. Ciprofloxacin, leflunomide, cidofovir, and IVIG have received the most attention for this disease.

Fluoroquinolones prevent and treat bacterial infections by blocking the prokaryotic DNA gyrase necessary for bacterial genome replications. Early *in vitro* studies showed that the nalidixic acid and oxolinic acid, predecessors to the modern fluoroquinolones, were able to inhibit BK virus replication. Subsequent studies confirmed that the modern fluoroquinolones were able to block SV40, a related polyoma virus found in monkeys, replication *in vitro* as well. Use of ciprofloxacin for BKV prophylaxis in kidney transplant recipients is reported to reduce the rate of early BK viremia (3 months), but to have no significant effect at one year compared to controls. Furthermore, a subsequent study looking at the use of ciprofloxacin to prevent BK viremia in a group of highly immunosuppressed kidney transplant recipients did not find the prophylactic treatment to have a beneficial effect at three months following transplantation. One recent study did report that addition of ciprofloxacin as adjuvant therapy with immunosuppression reduction had a positive impact. But, this study was not randomized and seems contradictory to the earlier studies indicating that ciprofloxacin fails as a BKV prophylactic agent.

Leflunomide is an attractive agent to trial for the treatment of BKV given that this drug is known to possess both antiviral as well as immunosuppressive properties. Indeed, leflunomide is approved for the treatment of rheumatoid arthritis. Therefore, clinicians may take comfort that they are achieving two treatment goals by exchanging the antiproliferative in use for leflunomide. Retrospective studies and case reports, which universally combine the strategies of immunosuppression reduction with the use of leflunomide, suggest a treatment benefit. However, in the absence of a randomized controlled trial the use of leflunomide is not recommended for the treatment of BKV.

Cidofovir, a nucleoside analogue, is known to inhibit BKV replication *in vitro*. Several case reports and small patient series have been reported using cidofovir for the treatment of BKV. However, none has been randomized to control for the effect of concomitant immunosuppression reduction. Furthermore, cidofovir is a highly nephrotoxic agent when used at conventional doses, prompting attempts to use cidofovir between 0.25 and 0.50 mg/kg, a significantly lowered dose compared to the standard 5 mg/kg dose used for the treatment of adenoviral infections. But, pharmacokinetic data indicate that this approach is unlikely to be effective as the resulting measured serum concentrations of cidofovir following low dose administration are in the range of 1 μg/mL, significantly less than the 36 μg/mL 50% effective concentration required to block BKV replication *in vitro*.

▶ Norovirus

While norovirus is the most common cause of viral gastroenteritis in humans, it warrants additional discussion in the setting of kidney transplantation. Diarrhea is an extremely common complaint following kidney transplantation and may have multiple potential explanations. Infection and drug-induced diarrhea (eg, from supratherapeutic levels of tacrolimus or mycophenolic acid) are both likely in this group of patients. In addition to screening for *Clostridium difficile* infection, norovirus should be part of the initial screen for all kidney transplant recipients presenting with significant diarrhea.

No specific therapy for norovirus exists. Therefore, most transplant recipients will need to have their level of immunosuppression reduced to clear this common infection. In the absence of partial immune reconstitution, this virus can establish a persistent infection leading to significant malnutrition, deconditioning, and ultimately disability.

Malignancy After Kidney Transplantation

Kidney transplant recipients are at increased risk for development of malignancy compared with the general population, and statistically these malignancies occur at an earlier age. Two separate, but related, mechanisms explain the increased risk for malignancy in transplant recipients. First, some cancers are known to occur under the influence of an oncogenic virus, which can lead to cancer development through insertion of viral oncogenes into the host cell DNA, or to up-regulate the effect of proto-oncogenes naturally occurring in the human genome. Other viruses, an example being HCV, lead to malignancy development only after years of nonspecific inflammation. Second, independent of a viral mediator, immunosuppression by itself increases the risk of developing a malignancy. As a significant protective effect of the host's immune system is to search throughout the body for cells that have undergone malignant transformation and eliminate them before they have an opportunity to significant replicate, immunosuppression interferes with this host defense.

A significant body of research exists looking at the rate of malignancy development on an individual cancer level. Most recent publications express this risk of malignancy development as a standard incidence ratio (SIR), which is a ratio of the incidence compared with aged matched controls. Nonmelanomatous skin cancer, PTLD Kaposi's sarcoma, penile, vulvar, and anogenital malignancies are among the cancers with the highest SIRs (Table 52–8).

Table 52–8. The standardized incidence ratio (SIR) of selected malignancies after kidney transplantation.

SIR >5	SIR 2–5	SIR <2
Nonmelanomatous skin	Cervical	Lung
PTLD/NHL	Thyroid	Breast
Kaposi sarcoma	Melanoma	Ovarian
Renal cell carcinoma	Esophageal	Uterine
Vulvar	Multiple myeloma	Pancreatic
Penile	Leukemia	Brain
Anogenital	Oropharyngeal	Prostate
Liver	Bladder	Testicular
Lip	Colon	

NHL, non-Hodgkin lymphoma; PTLD, post-transplant lymphoproliferative disorder; SIR, standard incidence ratio.
The SIR reflects the fold-increased risk of a malignancy in the kidney transplant recipient compared with the general population.

Nonmelanomatous Skin Cancer

Nonmelanomatous skin cancer (NMSC), and in particular squamous cell carcinoma, is the most commonly occurring malignancy in kidney transplant recipients. Estimates for the SIR range between 33 and 100. Furthermore, while the incidence of basal cell carcinoma exceeds that of squamous cell carcinoma in the general population (by a ratio of about 4:1), the reverse is true for immunosuppressed recipients. NMSC is highly preventable with appropriate attention to screening recommendations. All kidney transplant recipients should be referred to a dermatologist for a total body skin exam. During this visit, they will both be screened for skin cancer and have an assessment made regarding their unique risk for future development of skin cancer. Based on this assessment, which incorporates key factors such as the patient's prior dermatologic history and sun exposure history, the dermatologist will schedule the patient to return on a roughly annual basis. Patients deemed at a uniquely high risk for skin cancer return more frequently.

Management of NMSC when it develops does not differ from how this disease is managed in the general population. In particular, all suspicious appearing lesions should be biopsied and surgically removed to reduce the risk of metastatic disease development. For patient's receiving azathioprine as part of their immunosuppression regimen, discontinuation of this agent should be considered following development of skin cancer. Furthermore, for the rare patient who has multiple skin cancer identified and removed in a short period of time or has a skin cancer with a very aggressive course, switching from a calcineurin inhibitor to a mammalian target of rapamycin inhibitor should be considered. Though, there is neither guideline nor consensus regarding the threshold annual number of NMSC lesions that should prompt consideration of drug conversion.

All recipients on immunosuppression should be reminded and encouraged to follow best practices for the prevention of NMSC. Hats with a wide brim sufficient to cover the top of the ears, long sleeved shirts, and pants are common sense recommendations. In addition, application of a sunscreen with a sun protection factor (SPF) of 30 or higher is recommended for skin-exposed areas. Patients should all be taught of the greater importance of sunscreen reapplication compared with application of a higher SPF product, especially during extended periods in direct sunlight or swimming. Many patients will incorrectly assume that a higher SPF sunscreen provides a significantly enhanced level of protection, but this is not the case. For example, a SPF 30 product is expected to block 97% of the harmful radiation from the sun, while a SPF 50 product only extends this level of protection to 98%. While this small difference in products may prove important to some high skin cancer risk individuals, neither product is expected to remain effective much beyond 2 hours without reapplication.

Post-Transplant Lymphoproliferative Disorder

Transplantation using a kidney from an EBV seropositive donor into a EBV seronegative recipient brings with it the risk of acute infectious mononucleosis following transplantation, as well as post-transplant lymphoproliferative disorder (PTLD). This condition is more common in children for the reason that they are frequently seronegative recipients receiving an organ from an older (frequently parent) seropositive donor. It is estimated that between 80% and 85% of the adult population is seropositive for EBV. Therefore, it is difficult to avoid this phenomenon when adults donate to children. As PTLD is directly related to EBV viremia in the seronegative recipient, this condition frequently occurs during the first post-transplant year secondary to both the higher level of recipient immunosuppression as well as the fact that the recipient's immune system is naive to this infection.

PTLD can manifest across a spectrum ranging from simple lymphoproliferation to a monomorphic lymphoproliferative disorder that is essentially indistinguishable from a non-Hodgkin lymphoma. Accordingly, the World Health Organization subclassifies PTLD into three distinct pathologic categories: early lesions, polymorphic lymphoproliferation, and monomorphic proliferation. The early lesion category includes a reactive plasmacytic hyperplasia, and is the least virulent form of the disease. Monomorphic lymphoproliferation can present as either a B- or T-cell lymphoma, and is pathologically indistinguishable from a non-Hodgkin lymphoma occurring in a nonimmunosuppressed individual. The B-cell lymphomas can be further subclassified into the diffuse large B-cell lymphoma, Burkitt or Burkitt like lymphoma, and the plasma cell myeloma. The T-cell lymphomas can be subdivided into the peripheral T-cell lymphoma as well as some other rarer forms of disease. Additionally, other forms of proliferation can be seen such as Hodgkin disease like as well as plasmacytoma-like manifestations. The polymorphic form of this disease distinguishes itself from the monomorphic form by being characterized by premalignant hyperplasia.

The majority of PTLDs are of B-cell origin and are typically associated with EBV, with a minority of T-cell origin, which are commonly EBV negative. PTLDs of T-cell origin can be further distinguished by their later occurrence following transplantation. While most B-cell PTLDs occur in the first 1–2 years following transplantation, T-cell PTLDs occur at a median onset of 50–60 months following transplantation. Furthermore, the T-cell forms of PTLD as a group are more aggressive than their B-cell counterparts.

PTLD can manifest in virtually any body location and is commonly not confined to either the lymph nodes or other lymphatic areas such as the spleen. Rather, extranodal presentations of the disease are the norm. Over 80% of patients will present with extranodal and extrasplenic manifestations of PTLD.

A significantly higher incidence of disease is seen in pediatric recipients secondary to their EBV seronegativity. For this reason, most pediatric kidney transplant centers monitor their recipients for EBV viremia via protocolized screening, but this is not a universal component of routine adult post-transplant care. As the majority of seronegative adult recipients who receive a kidney from a seropositive donor who develop EBV viremia do so in the first post-transplant year, monitoring during this high-risk period should be considered. Rapid detection of EBV viremia in seronegative recipients should prompt a reduction in the intensity of immunosuppression, and consideration of antiviral therapy, rituximab, IVIG, infusion of EBV-specific cytotoxic T lymphocytes (or some combination of the above). These interventions, triggered by EBV viremia–based monitoring protocols, lead to a reduction in the incidence of PTLD in this high-risk patient population.

Management of this disease can be quite variable and is tailored to the severity of illness with which the patient presents. Treatment for the simple forms of this disease where there is only evidence of lymphoproliferation typically is limited to immunosuppression reduction. More significant presentations will require CHOP-R chemotherapy.

ALLOGRAFT COMPLICATIONS AFTER KIDNEY TRANSPLANTATION

Acute Cellular Rejection

With the rare exception of when the donor is an identical twin, rejection remains an inherent risk of kidney transplantation. Indeed, the first successful kidney transplant in 1953 was between the identical twin brothers Ronald and Richard Herrick. Immunosuppression makes transplantation possible between nonidentical individuals. But, despite significant advances and improvements in the immunosuppressant drugs available, rejection still occurs. Of course, rejection remains a significant issue for patients who are nonadherent with their prescribed regimen. Moreover, there is growing evidence that patients taking their immunosuppressants, but found to have more variable drug levels, have inferior outcomes.

Hyperacute rejection is a form of antibody-mediated rejection. It is when a recipient has preformed antibodies in their serum that come into contact with the allograft immediately upon reperfusion, or within the hours to days that follow. This form of rejection is frequently immediately obvious to the transplant surgeon, who sees a change in the allograft from a pink color to a modeled and cyanotic appearance. This change in the gross appearance of the allograft is secondary to widespread glomerular capillary thrombosis, necrosis, and intraparenchymal hemorrhage. Fortunately, with advances in pretransplant tissue typing and preimplantation cross matching, the rate of hyperacute rejection has significantly declined. Though not apparent immediately after transplantation, some patients will experience an anamnestic response. These recipients possessed the ability to produce injurious antibodies directed against the allograft through exposure to an antigen in the past. This delayed form of accelerated acute rejection occurs when transplantation reexposes the recipient's immune system to this antigen, and the response is vigorous antibody production mediated by memory B cells. Hyperacute rejection cannot be medically managed. Allografts afflicted in this manner will never function, and are at significant risk for development of a fracture with hemorrhage occurring. For this reason, kidney transplants diagnosed with hyperacute rejection should be removed as soon as possible.

After the transplant recipient progresses beyond the immediate post-transplant period, acute, but no longer hyperacute, forms of rejection become the concern. Acute rejection can be further divided into rejections that are strictly cellular in nature, and those that are associated with donor specific antibody (DSA) development. DSAs in this context are more commonly *de novo* than a result of memory B-cell activation leading to an anamnestic response. Though clinicians tend to distinguish between these two forms of acute rejection for treatment purposes, it is important to recognize that they can, and frequently do, coexist. In particular, AMR is commonly accompanied by an element of cellular rejection.

Acute cellular rejections are classified according to the Banff schema (Table 52–9). Cellular rejections classified as Banff level 1A (tubulitis and interstitial infiltrates) are most commonly treated with a pulse of high dose corticosteroids (methylprednisolone 500 mg IV daily three doses) followed by a prednisone taper. Banff 2 (vascular rejections) and 3 (a rejection with evidence of transmural arteritis or fibrinoid necrosis) lesions are more severe, and therefore treated with a combination of high-dose corticosteroids and antithymocyte immunoglobulin (ATG). The exact mechanism of ATG's beneficial effect is not fully known, but it is clear that part of the effect is secondary to significant T-cell depletion. Many Banff 1B rejections are treated with corticosteroids alone, while others that look more significant are treated with corticosteroids and ATG. Rapid recurrence of rejection following a corticosteroid pulse suggests steroid resistance. Therefore, Banff borderline, 1A, and 1B lesions first managed with a corticosteroid pulse unsuccessfully will usually be treated with a combination of corticosteroid and ATG on subsequent attempts.

▶ Acute Antibody Mediated Rejection

Acute antibody mediated rejection is diagnosed when an allograft biopsy shows findings compatible with endothelial injury, evidence of compliment activation (C4d positivity), and detection of a donor specific antibody. While under established guidelines only 2 of these 3 findings are required

Table 52–9. Banff kidney allograft rejection classification.

T-cell mediated rejection	
Borderline	Characterized by infiltration of mononuclear cells (<25% of the parenchyma) or foci of mild tubulitis (1–4 mononuclear cells/tubular cross-section)
Banff IA	Cases with significant interstitial infiltration (>25% of parenchyma affected) and foci of moderate tubulitis (>4 mononuclear cells/tubular cross section or group of 10 tubular cells)
Banff IB	Cases with significant interstitial infiltration (>25% of parenchyma affected) and foci of severe tubulitis (>10 mononuclear cells/tubular cross section or group of 10 tubular cells)
Banff 2A	Cases with mild to moderate intimal arteritis
Banff 2B	Cases with severe intimal arteritis comprising >25% of the luminal area
Banff 3	Cases with "transmural" arteritis and/or arterial fibrinoid change and necrosis of medial smooth muscle cells
Acute antibody mediated rejection	
Type (grade) I	C4d+, ATN like with minimal inflammation
Type (grade) II	C4d+, capillary margination and/or thrombosis
Type (grade) III	C4d+, transmural arteritis
Chronic antibody mediated rejection	
	Development of donor specific antibodies Deposition of C4d in the allograft Chronic graft dysfunction Graft pathology (subclinical rejection)
	Transplant glomerulopathy (with interstitial fibrosis and tubular atrophy)
	Transplant capillaropathy (with interstitial fibrosis and tubular atrophy)
	Transplant arteriopathy (with interstitial fibrosis and tubular atrophy)

to make the diagnosis, the certainly of the diagnosis is most convincing when a DSA is present. Some hypothesize that the inability to detect a DSA in all cases of suspected AMR is related to non-HLA antibodies (eg, MHC class I-related chain A [MICA] antigens, and angiotensin II type 1 receptor antibodies HLA antibodies), anti-HLA antibodies directed against antigens that are not represented in the solid phase microbead arrays, or complete absorption of the offending antibodies by the allograft.

Acute AMR is more likely to occur in patients who present with a prolonged period of immunosuppressive medication nonadherence. Treatment for AMR is less successful than those available for ACR.

Though centers will differ in their protocols for the treatment of AMR, a common strategy involves starting the treatment with a pulse of corticosteroids and ATG. Thereafter, the treatment strategy involves a combination of approaches to both remove and neutralize the injurious antibodies. Plasmapheresis can clear the antibodies already present, but will not have a durable effect if antibody production is ongoing.

Plasmapheresis sessions are paired with IVIG infusions. IVIG is pleiotropic with benefits extending well beyond simply replacing the immunoglobulin fraction removed by the plasmapheresis treatments. Potential benefits include: neutralization of complement fixing antibodies, disrupting the activity of complement cascade, blocking effector cell Fc receptor recognition of DSAs bound to the allograft, and nonspecific down regulation of T and B lymphocyte activity.

Successful treatment of acute rejection is dependent on the severity of the lesion. A recent systematic review of the literature attempted to categorize the response rates to therapy with cellular rejection subcategorized using the Banff classification system. This was only partly successful as there are no standards to define what represents a complete versus partial therapeutic response to treatment. Nonetheless, in this review the rate of functional recovery absence occurred in 4% of Borderline, 15% of Banff 1A, 25% of Banff 1B, up to 20% of Banff 2A, and 38% of Banff 2B cases of cellular rejection.

Chronic Rejection

Though death with a functioning allograft is now the primary reason for allograft loss, many recipients outlive the functional lifetime of their transplant. Indeed, this is now a leading cause for return to the kidney transplant waiting list. In 2015, patients returning to the list for repeat transplantation comprised nearly 14% of the total waiting list. The terms "chronic rejection" and "chronic allograft nephropathy" have historically been used to describe a failing transplant. Though incomplete, we increasingly have an improved understanding of the processes that underlie these descriptive findings.

The use of CNIs and mTOR inhibitors, while excellent at preventing T-cell activation and rejection, comes at a cost. CNIs act through off-target vasoconstrictive effects to promote relative ischemia within the kidney. The result is interstitial fibrosis with tubular atrophy development. This fibrosis commonly extends along the medullary rays leading to the characteristic finding of "striped" fibrosis. As no drugs are available to reverse interstitial fibrosis and tubular atrophy, these changes result in a permanent decrement in allograft function. Unlike the CNIs, mTOR inhibitors in a minority of patients (2–3%) will lead to podocyte effacement

evidenced by significant proteinuria development. If biopsied early in its course, the glomeruli will have an appearance similar to minimal change disease. Resolution of the proteinuria is expected following withdrawal of the mTOR inhibitor early after proteinuria develops, but the lesions are expected to progress to focal sclerosis if the drug is continued.

▶ Significance of Donor Specific Antibody (DSA) Development

Development of DSAs is increasingly linked to chronic allograft failure. These antibodies, through both complement dependent and complement independent mechanisms, progressively result in allograft injury and failure. Though significant advances have been made in the ability to detect DSAs, the ability to determine which DSAs (and at what titer) are injurious remains a challenge. Furthermore, while a DSA at any given titer may be injurious in one recipient it may be inconsequential to another. C1q binding to distinguish complement fixing and nonfixing antibodies, and thereby determine which DSAs are likely to be injurious has been attempted. But, further study now indicates that C1q binding activity may simply be a reflection of antibody strength, rather than an assessment of a functionally distinct DSA with clinical significance.

How to best manage a recipient who has developed a DSA remains a challenge. If the DSA is detected prior to the discovery of rejection on kidney biopsy, a biopsy should strongly be considered at this time to assess for this possibility. If acute rejection features are identified, then treatment for acute rejection should commence. If there is histologic evidence of allograft injury outside the Banff criteria for a diagnosis of acute AMR, then chronic AMR is a possible diagnosis. Indeed, there is increasing evidence to suggest that chronic AMR is a significant, and initially underappreciated, contributor to late allograft loss. How to retard the progressive allograft injury that occurs with chronic AMR remains a clinical challenge. IVIG in combination with rituximab has been attempted with some success. This is despite the fact that the culprit plasma cells producing the DSA due not display CD20, the target for rituximab, on their surface. Hence, it is inferred that rituximab may be acting in this context through depleting plasmablasts, the short lived, immature, form of the plasma cell.

Additional attempts to treat chronic AMR are being actively pursued using plasma cell depleting agent bortezomib and the alternative pathway complement activation inhibitor eculizumab. While acutely effective in reducing or eliminating DSA, the beneficial effect of bortezomib does not appear to be sufficiently sustained. And unfortunately, prolonged use of bortezomib has been associated with significant peripheral neurotoxicity.

It is generally believed that DSAs bind to HLA on the surface of allograft endothelial cells. And as a result of this binding, complement activation occurs. Eculizumab is a humanized monoclonal antibody that binds to complement factor C5 and inhibits activation of the terminal complement pathway (shared by the classical, alternative, and lectin pathways). Thus, while eculizumab is unable to deplete either DSA or DSA producing plasma cells, it may have the ability to block the injury they may cause. A pilot study from our institution has shown that eculizumab treatment may stabilize kidney function in patients with chronic AMR. But, endothelial cell associated transcripts (EndATs) predictive of antibody-mediated injury were not reduced in the eculizumab treated patients. Though underpowered, this preliminary work confirms that DSA-mediated allograft injury occurs at least partially through complement dependent mechanisms, and that terminal complement inhibition may slow the pace of this injury.

Recurrent Disease in Kidney Transplant Recipients

For those diseases, known or unknown, caused by defects intrinsic to the kidney, transplantation offers a definitive cure (eg, polycystic kidney disease, Alport syndrome). But for most other etiologies, recurrent disease is a possibility. Depending on the likelihood, recipient candidates should be counseled about this possibility as a component of their listing evaluation. For this reason, it behooves us to obtain a biopsy confirmed diagnosis as often as possible prior to transplantation. FSGS, MPGN (in particular, the C3 glomerulonephritis subtype of MPGN), IgA nephropathy, lupus nephritis, and DM nephropathy can all recur following transplantation, and will be discussed in detail (Table 52–10).

Focal Segmental Glomerulosclerosis

Recurrence of focal segmental glomerulosclerosis (FSGS) following transplantation is the most dramatic manifestation of disease recurrence. Patients with an at risk for recurrence history, namely patients with a rapid progression (under 3 years) from native kidney FSGS discovery to development of ESRD, and patients with diagnosis younger than 15 years of age, should be screened immediately following transplantation for evidence of disease recurrence. As the histological findings of FSGS will likely not be present for weeks to months following recurrence, quantitative assessment of the urine for proteinuria is the best screening approach and should be rapidly followed by an allograft biopsy with samples sent for electron microscopy. Complete foot process effacement, the earliest visible manifestation of an FSGS recurrence has been detected 24 hours following transplantation.

This immediate recurrence of FSGS following transplantation is consistent with a hereto date unidentified recipient derived, blood borne, substance, referred to as the "permeability factor." Efforts to identify this permeability factor, or complex, have been extensive spanning multiple decades. Several candidates have been proposed. Most recently suPAR, the soluble form of the urokinase type plasminogen activated receptor (uPAR) was implicated as being the causative factor in recurrent FSGS. Indeed in mice, circulating suPAR led to foot process effacement and an FSGS-like glomerulopathy. And, this proteinuric effect could be blocked *in vitro* with the addition of inactivating antibodies. Despite this preclinical data, and much excitement that the elusive circulating permeability factor had finally been identified, these findings have not been supported in humans. Though suPAR levels are high in patients with FSGS, the range of this elevation is variable between individuals leading to significant overlap with suPAR levels found in a wide variety of renal diseases. Furthermore, elevated suPAR levels have be found in a wide range of clinical conditions such as pneumonia, sepsis, and some malignancies, but none of these disease states is classically associated with proteinuria.

Table 52–10. Recurrence of selected disease after kidney transplantation.

	Recurrence Rate	Mean Time to Recurrence	Likelihood That Recurrence Will Lead to Allograft Failure (after 10 years)
Focal segmental glomerulosclerosis	20–30%	10–18 days	15–30%
IgA nephropathy	20–50%	7 years	10%
Dense deposit disease and C3 nephropathy	90%	8 months	45–55% (5 year survival)
Membranous glomerulonephritis	10–30%	10 months	10–15%
Membranoproliferative glomerulonpheritis type 1	20–50%	3–4 months	15%
Lupus nephritis	2.5%	4 years	95%
ANCA glomerulonephritis	20%	Never reported	10%

Thus, it would appear that for the present time the search for the ever-elusive circulating permeability factor continues.

Despite not having identified the biochemical culprit, multiple treatment options with varying efficacy exist. Most transplant centers will aggressively treat the transplant recipient with postoperative FSGS recurrence with plasmapheresis to remove the circulating factor. Along with routine use of antiproteinuric agents, such as the renin angiotensin system antagonists, rituximab, and injectable ACTH gel have been reported to have some role in the treatment of this disease. Success in retarding the destructive impact of FSGS recurrence is variable.

Membranoproliferative Glomerulonephritis

Membranoproliferative glomerulonephritis (MPGN) reoccurs in kidney transplant recipients. As with a diagnosis of MPGN in native kidney disease, a thorough search to identify an underlying cause for the secondary form of this disease should always be undertaken. Furthermore, it is important to make the distinction between MPGN and transplant glomerulopathy. Indeed, these two pathologic entities appear similar at the level of the light microscope. However, MPGN-1 is characterized with subendothelial electron-dense deposits on electron microscopy and TG is notable for duplication of the glomerular basement membrane with central electron-lucent zones filled with finely flocculent material but without deposits. In idiopathic MPGN, the likelihood of recurrence is predicted by the presence of polyclonal versus monoclonal immunoglobulins in the glomerular deposits. With monoclonal Igs, the rate of recurrence is 50%, while only 10% for the polyclonal form of the disease. Note that IgG3-κ is the most common Ig associated with monoclonal MPGN. Given the presence of Ig deposits in many forms of recurrent MPGN, therapies targeting suppression of antibody production have been tested. In particular, there may be a role for rituximab.

The realization that MPGN with C3 predominant staining represented a distinct subclassification of disease, newly called C3 glomerulonephritis (C3GN), is recent. Furthermore, it is clear that C3GN has at its crux dysregulation of the alternative complement pathway. Ideally, all patients with C3GN should have a thorough evaluation of their complement regulatory proteins to determine if a known mutation or deficiency is present, as this may help guide therapy following transplantation. Furthermore, measurement of the serum level of the membrane attack complex (MAC, C5b-C9) should be considered pretransplant and in patients with recurrent C3GN. Patients with C3GN and high levels of MAC appear to have greater responsiveness to eculizumab, a humanized monoclonal antibody that binds to and inhibits the cleavage of C5 to C5a and C5b by the C5 convertase. Given the high costs of eculizumab, and a lack of an understanding about when the drug can safely be discontinued, determining the willingness

of the patients insurance to cover the costs of this drug are an important component of the pretransplant evaluation and informed consent process. C3GN has an extremely high rate disease recurrence, and in the absence of an effective form of therapy the expectation should be for relatively rapid progression toward allograft failure.

Membranous Glomerulonephritis

Membranous glomerulonephritis (MGN) also can recur after kidney transplantation. Like MPGN, it is important to distinguish between the idiopathic and secondary forms of disease when considering the risk for recurrence. The discovery that antiphospholipase-A2-receptor (PLA2R) autoantibodies in the majority of patients with idiopathic MGN was a tremendous breakthrough in our understanding of this disease. Unfortunately, between 10% and 30% of patients with MGN, most of whom will be positive for anti-PLA2R autoantibodies, will experience disease recurrence after transplantation. Furthermore, anti-PLA2R positive patients are more likely to have a disease recurrence that is resistant to treatment. No published literature exists examining the efficacy of cyclophosphamide and high-dose steroid (ie, modified Ponticelli regimen) for recurrent MGN after transplantation. This is likely owing to the fact that the resulting level of immunosuppression achieved with cyclophosphamide used concomitantly with routine transplant immunosuppression would be excessive and unsafe. Furthermore, a pilot study investigating mycophenolate mofetil and prednisone compared with historically matched controls treated for one year with oral cyclophosphamide and corticosteroids concluded that the efficacy of the two regimens was similar (approximately 70% rate of remission), but that the relapse rate was higher in the MMF-treated patients. They speculated that a prolonged course of MMF might reduce the relapse rate. As kidney transplant recipients are typically on a stable immunosuppression regimen that includes MMF indefinitely, one might conclude from this study that treating transplant recipients with a MGN recurrence would derive no added benefit through the addition of cyclophosphamide.

KEY READINGS

Amore A: Antibody-mediated rejection. Curr Opin Organ Transplant 2015;20:536.

Andresdottir MB et al: Immunohistological and ultrastructural differences between recurrent type I membranoproliferative glomerulonephritis and chronic transplant glomerulopathy. Am J Kidney Dis 1998;32:582.

Bhowmik DM et al: The evolution of the Banff classification schema for diagnosing renal allograft rejection and its implications for clinicians. Indian J Nephrol 2010;20:2.

Braun MC et al: Recurrence of membranoproliferative glomerulonephritis type II in renal allografts: The North American Pediatric Renal Transplant Cooperative Study experience. J Am Soc Nephrol 2005;16:2225.

Briganti EM et al: Risk of renal allograft loss from recurrent glomerulonephritis. N Engl J Med 2002;347:103.

Contreras G et al: Recurrence of lupus nephritis after kidney transplantation. J Am Soc Nephrol 2010;21:1200.

Cravedi P, Kopp JB, Remuzzi G: Recent progress in the pathophysiology and treatment of FSGS recurrence. Am J Transplant 2013;13:266.

Einecke G et al: Antibody-mediated microcirculation injury is the major cause of late kidney transplant failure. Am J Transplant 2009;9:2520.

Hart A et al: OPTN/SRTR 2015 Annual Data Report: Kidney. Am J Transplant 2017;17 Suppl 1:21.

Kattah A et al: Anti-phospholipase A(2) receptor antibodies in recurrent membranous nephropathy. Am J Transplant 2015;15:1349.

Kulkarni S et al: Eculizumab therapy for chronic antibody-mediated injury in kidney transplant recipients: a pilot randomized controlled trial. Am J Transplant 2017;17:682.

Lamarche C et al: Efficacy of acute cellular rejection treatment according to Banff score in kidney transplant recipients: a systematic review. Transplant Direct 2016;2:e115.

Lorenz EC et al: Recurrent membranoproliferative glomerulonephritis after kidney transplantation. Kidney Int 2010;77:721.

Martin F, Chan AC: B cell immunobiology in disease: evolving concepts from the clinic. Annu Rev Immunol 2006;24:467.

Nijim S et al: Recurrent IgA nephropathy after kidney transplantation. Transplant Proc 2016;48:2689.

Pham P-TT et al: Diagnosis and therapy of graft dysfunction. In: Chronic Kidney Disease, Dialysis, and Transplantation, 3rd ed, Himmelfarb J, Sayegh MH, (editors). Philadelphia, PA: Saunders; 2010.

Ponticelli C: Recurrence of focal segmental glomerular sclerosis (FSGS) after renal transplantation. Nephrol Dial Transplant 2010;25:25.

Racusen LC et al: The Banff 97 working classification of renal allograft pathology. Kidney Int 1999;55:713.

van Gelder T: Within-patient variability in immunosuppressive drug exposure as a predictor for poor outcome after transplantation. Kidney Int 2014;85:1267.

Yell M et al: C1q binding activity of de novo donor-specific HLA antibodies in renal transplant recipients with and without antibody-mediated rejection. Transplantation 2015;99:1151.

MANAGEMENT OF THE FAILED KIDNEY TRANSPLANT

▶ Outcomes of Kidney Transplantation

Though it remains the goal of all transplant professionals to ensure that a kidney transplant functions as long as possible, the harsh reality remains that many recipients will face allograft failure. To date, advances in immunosuppression have dramatically reduced the rate of early rejection and have simultaneously improved 1-year graft survival. But, not nearly as significant advances have been made with long-term graft survival. As noted above, belatacept treated patients have improved eGFR after 7 years, suggesting that this drug may afford a significant improvement in long-term graft survival. At present, kidney transplant recipients

of deceased donor organs can expect an average allograft survival of 15 years. Some will function only a few months, while others will still be functioning 30, or more, years after transplantation. And, it is well established that kidneys from living donors have superior survival compared to those procured from deceased donors.

Management of the patient with a failing allograft is uniquely challenging. Unlike the patient with progressive CKD in their native kidneys, kidney transplant recipients recall first hand their experiences with replacement therapy. Most will report that they felt restored and rejuvenated after transplantation. The prospect of having to return to a state of health and lifestyle that they associate with lethargy, strict dietary and fluid restrictions, impediments to work and travel, and a burdensome dialysis treatment schedule, is nearly universally a cause for depression. Many patients may choose comfort measures over returning to renal replacement therapy. The transplant specialist needs to remain cognizant of these mindsets.

While many kidney transplants suddenly cease to function for reasons known (eg, rejection), and others without warning decline unexpected without an apparent inciting event, the majority will slowly decline. Similar to patients with native kidney disease, transplant recipients should always be aware of the status of their allograft, especially during periods of functional decline.

The factors that lead to the decision to start a patient with allograft failure on dialysis are indistinct from those for native kidney disease. Once allograft failure has occurred, there are decisions to be made with respect to subsequent immunosuppression management. Preservation of residual renal function, prevention of graft intolerance syndrome, and reduced sensitization to alloantigens (if repeat transplantation is anticipated) need to be considered. And, the value of achieving these goals needs to be weighed against the increased risks associated with immunosuppression while on renal replacement therapy for infection, cardiovascular events, and malignancy. With the exception of early allograft loses (eg, due to a vascular thrombosis or a hyperacute rejection) which are typically managed with a transplantectomy and immediate discontinuation off immunosuppression, whether to perform a transplantectomy is another important consideration.

▶ Sensitization Following Immunosuppression Withdrawal

The data supporting continuation of immunosuppression with the goal of preserving residual allograft renal function is limited. One study looking at patients on peritoneal dialysis showed a modest benefit to maintaining immunosuppression versus cessation (eg, life expectancy was 5.8 years vs 5.3 years, respectively). A second study analyzing USRDS registry data concluded that survival was increased for patients on PD maintained on immunosuppression for the first 2 years compared to hemodialysis. But with further increase in vintage time, this survival advantage was no longer present. Though unproven, one can speculate that preservation of residual allograft renal function mechanistically explains this observation. Further research is required to confirm that continuing immunosuppression after allograft failure reduces mortality on dialysis.

Prevention of allosensitization is a paramount concern for the patient who desires repeat transplantation. And, withdrawal of immunosuppression after allograft failure is associated with sensitization. This phenomenon appears to occur independently of whether the kidney is explanted, and does not appear linked to the recipient receiving blood transfusions. Moreover, a retrospective study of patients awaiting retransplantation compared the peak PRA level of patients who had their first kidney removed to those with a retained failed allograft. Peak PRA levels were significant higher in the allograft nephrectomy group. But, this difference resolved by the time the patients received their second allograft. Note that this difference achieved statistical significance when the median, but not the mean peak PRA (29.7% vs 22.5% for the nephrectomy and nonnephrectomy groups, respectively), was compared. Consistent with other studies, transplant nephrectomy was associated with an improved patient survival.

Possible mechanisms to explain the increase in PRA associated with nephrectomy are postulated. It has been suggested that the retained failed allograft acts as a sponge, absorbing any donor specific antibodies generated from the serum. Hence, removal of the allograft eliminates the sponge and allows the antibodies to accumulate and be detected. Other authors suggest that the process of performing the allograft nephrectomy reveals to the recipient's immune system alloantigens that were previously hidden.

Therefore, maintaining recipients with failed allografts on immunosuppression to avoid sensitization is beneficial. Whether the immunosuppression needs to be maintained indefinitely, or can be safely discontinued months to years later without development of allosensitization, remains unknown. Similarly, whether immunosuppression maintained for a long time at a reduced intensity would suffice in allosensitization suppression is also not known.

▶ Allograft Nephrectomy

Allograft nephrectomy (also referred to as transplantectomy) may neither be necessary, nor advisable, with the exception of cases of early allograft failure. The morbidity and mortality rates reported for allograft nephrectomy vary widely, likely owing to the indication and surgical technique utilized (eg, extracapsular vs intracapsular dissection).

Signs and symptoms that an allograft which experienced late failure should be consider for nephrectomy include fever or unclear origin, gross hematuria, allograft tenderness, hypoalbuminemia, erythropoietin resistance, and elevated serum markers of inflammation without an otherwise obvious source. When a patient presents with these symptoms, it is important to exclude other common causes, such as infection. Also, given that most kidney transplants are placed in the right iliac fossa in close proximity to the appendix, appropriate imaging (CT scan) should be obtained to exclude appendicitis. If the failed allograft appears swollen and enlarged on imaging, the diagnosis of graft intolerance syndrome is likely. It is a common practice to treat patient with a short course of high-dose methylprednisolone to reduce the degree of inflammation before proceeding with the nephrectomy. By doing so, hemostasis is more readily achieved during the nephrectomy.

KEY READINGS

Adeyi OA et al: Serum analysis after transplant nephrectomy reveals restricted antibody specificity patterns against structurally defined HLA class I mismatches. Transpl Immunol 2005;14:53.

Augustine JJ et al: Independent of nephrectomy, weaning immunosuppression leads to late sensitization after kidney transplant failure. Transplantation 2012;94:738.

Jassal SV et al: Continued transplant immunosuppression may prolong survival after return to peritoneal dialysis: results of a decision analysis. Am J Kidney Dis 2002;40:178.

Perl J et al: Is dialysis modality a factor in the survival of patients initiating dialysis after kidney transplant failure? Perit Dial Int 2013;33:618.

Tittelbach-Helmrich D et al: Impact of transplant nephrectomy on peak PRA levels and outcome after kidney re-transplantation. World J Transplant 2014;4:141.

■ CHAPTER REVIEW QUESTIONS

1. What clinical syndrome has gained prominent attention and is now frequency screened for during the candidate evaluation for kidney transplantation?
   A. Metabolic syndrome
   B. Frailty syndrome
   C. Antiphospholipid antibody syndrome
   D. Painful bladder syndrome (interstitial cystitis)
   E. Loin pain hematuria syndrome

2. In addition to death secondary to infection and cardiovascular disease, which of the following is the most common (and rising) cause of post-transplant morbidity and mortality in the kidney transplant recipient?
   A. BK viremia
   B. Accidental death
   C. Chronic allograft failure with patient opting not to return to renal replacement therapy
   D. Malignancy

3. All of the following have a significantly high likelihood of recurrence after transplantation EXCEPT:
   A. Lupus nephritis
   B. Focal segmental glomerulosclerosis

   C. C3 glomerulonephritis
   D. IgA nephropathy
   E. Dense deposit disease

4. Which therapeutic strategy is currently available to treat patients with chronic antibody mediated rejection?
   A. Reduction in Immunosuppression
   B. Infliximab
   C. Basiliximab
   D. Rituximab with IVIG infusion
   E. Everolimus

5. All of the following are potential consequences of complete discontinuation of immunosuppression in the patient with a failed kidney transplant EXCEPT:
   A. Acute rejection
   B. Graft intolerance syndrome
   C. Resistance to erythropoiesis-stimulating agents (ESAs)
   D. Sensitization
   E. Higher probability of premature death

Diabetic Kidney Disease

Raymond C. Harris, MD

ESSENTIALS OF DIAGNOSIS

► Can afflict as many as 30% of patients with both type 1 and type 2 diabetes

► Most common cause of end-stage renal disease (ESRD) in the western world, with >90% of patients having type 2 diabetes mellitus (DM)

► Characterized by initial period of hyperfiltration, followed by development of increasing proteinuria and progressive decline in glomerular filtration rate (GFR)

► Current therapy includes glycemic and blood pressure control and the use of renin–angiotensin–aldosterone system inhibitors

General Considerations

Diabetes mellitus has become the single leading cause of chronic kidney disease in the world, and is the most common cause of ESRD in industrialized countries. The incidence and prevalence of diabetes has increased over the past 25 years, due almost entirely to increases in type 2 diabetes. In the United States, the prevalence of diabetes has increased from 6% of the population in 1988–1994 to 9.8% in 2009–2014. This rise in the prevalence of diabetes worldwide is multifactorial and has been attributed to increasing obesity due to decreased physical activity, institution of Western diets in developing countries and the increased use of high fructose corn syrup as a sweetener. Despite the improved care of patients with diabetes, both the incidence and prevalence of ESRD secondary to diabetes continue to rise. Over 26% of individuals in the United States with diabetes have evidence of diabetic kidney disease, and more than 30% of patients undergoing either dialytic therapy or renal transplantation have ESRD as a result of diabetic nephropathy. Almost 50% of the new (incident) cases of

ESRD are attributable to diabetes. Currently, more than 200,000 patients receive ESRD care as a result of diabetic nephropathy.

In developed countries, more than 90% of patients with diabetes have type 2 rather than insulinopenic type 1 diabetes. Type 2 diabetes carries a similar risk for development of renal disease as Type 1, and over 80% of the ESRD secondary to diabetes is attributable to type 2 diabetes. The demographics of ESRD secondary to type 2 diabetes mirror the prevalence of type 2 diabetes in the US population, with a higher relative prevalence in African–Americans, Hispanic–Americans, Native Americans, and Asian–Americans and a peak incidence in the fifth to seventh decade. Recent epidemiologic studies have indicated that much of the increased mortality seen in patients with either type 1 or type 2 diabetes is associated with the prevalence of nephropathy. Diabetic patients with ESRD have a 1.5–2.5 fold increase in mortality compared to nondiabetic ESRD patients. The economic and social burden on the health care system of caring for patients with diabetic kidney disease is enormous. Given that the worldwide prevalence of obesity has increased more than fivefold in the past 20 years, an increasing incidence of diabetic nephropathy is being appreciated across the globe. These trends are especially worrisome in populations at increased risk of developing diabetes, especially Southeast Asians and Pacific Islanders.

Clinical Findings

The natural history of diabetic nephropathy is best exemplified in patients with type 1 diabetes because the onset of diabetes is more clearly definable and typically occurs at an early enough age to permit long-term follow-up. In addition, type 1 diabetes usually afflicts a younger population that do not usually initially have comorbid essential hypertension, atherosclerotic cardiovascular disease, obesity, and other conditions that are often associated with type 2 diabetes and that may independently produce chronic renal injury. However, Pima Indians, who exhibit a strong genetic predisposition for the development of type 2 diabetes by the fourth decade of life, exhibit a similar time course in progression of disease as is seen in type 1 diabetic patients. However, for the majority of patients with type 2 diabetes, the onset of nephropathy development is more variable.

Patients with both type 1 and type 2 diabetes may exhibit an increased glomerular filtration rate (GFR), so-called hyperfiltration, at the initial presentation of disease (Figure 53–1). This hyperfiltration is mediated by proportionately greater relaxation of the afferent arteriole than the efferent arteriole and results in increased glomerular blood flow and elevated glomerular capillary pressure. The GFR can be as much as 50% greater than normal, and the kidney's glomeruli and tubules hypertrophy compared with age- and weight-matched normal control subjects. Institution of intensive insulin replacement to normalize the hyperglycemia corrects the hyperfiltration in a majority of patients. However, there is a significant minority of patients (~25–40%) who have continued hyperfiltration even with

insulin therapy, and this subgroup may be at increased risk for the development of nephropathy.

The earliest clinical sign of the development of diabetic kidney disease is usually the onset of microalbuminuria. Initially, transient or intermittent microalbuminuria can be measured by radioimmunoassay, enzyme-linked immunosorbent assay, or special dipsticks, especially when induced by stress, physical exertion, concurrent illness, or poor glycemic control.

The daily urinary excretion of albumin in a health adult is normally less than 25 mg. Microalbuminuria is defined as a urinary albumin excretion of 30–300 mg/24 h in a timed collection or 30–300 µg/mg creatinine in a random urine sample. Overt nephropathy is defined as greater than 300 mg/24 h. Corresponding values for total protein excretion are less than 150 mg/24 h (control); less than 500 mg/24 h (microalbuminuria); and greater than 500 mg/24 h (overt nephropathy). Microalbuminuria may be transient and reversible during the first few years after onset of diabetes.

Approximately 30% of diabetic patients progress to a point where they develop fixed microalbuminuria of at least

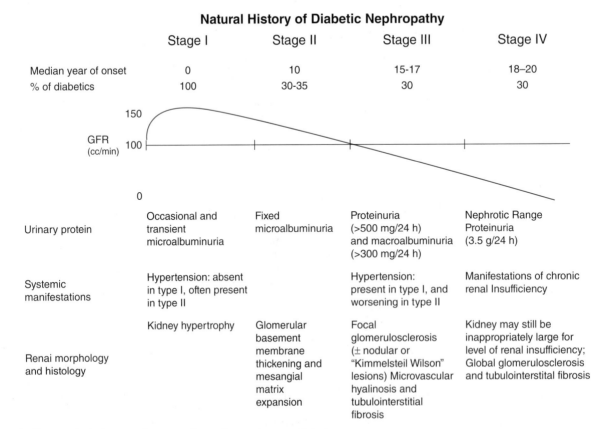

Natural History of Diabetic Nephropathy

	Stage I	Stage II	Stage III	Stage IV
Median year of onset	0	10	15-17	18–20
% of diabetics	100	30-35	30	30
Urinary protein	Occasional and transient microalbuminuria	Fixed microalbuminuria	Proteinuria (>500 mg/24 h) and macroalbuminuria (>300 mg/24 h)	Nephrotic Range Proteinuria (3.5 g/24 h)
Systemic manifestations	Hypertension: absent in type I, often present in type II		Hypertension: present in type I, and worsening in type II	Manifestations of chronic renal Insufficiency
Renai morphology and histology	Kidney hypertrophy	Glomerular basement membrane thickening and mesangial matrix expansion	Focal glomerulosclerosis (± nodular or "Kimmelsteil Wilson" lesions) Microvascular hyalinosis and tubulointerstitial fibrosis	Kidney may still be inappropriately large for level of renal insufficiency; Global glomerulosclerosis and tubulointerstital fibrosis

▲ **Figure 53–1.** Primary diagnoses for patients who start dialysis.

30 mg/24 h. In patients with type 1 diabetes, this persistent microalbuminuria occurs after a median of about 10 years of diabetes. In patients with type 1 diabetes, blood pressure may increase by 10 years after onset of disease. However, the majority (>70%) of patients with type 2 diabetes have systemic hypertension, and this percentage rises to 90% in those with documented microalbuminuria. The American Diabetes Association (ADA) recommends screening for microalbuminuria in type 1 diabetes 5 years after the initial diagnosis and then yearly. Because of the uncertainty of onset of disease in type 2 diabetes, the ADA recommends yearly screening at the time of diagnosis. Microalbuminuria is a more specific sign of diabetic nephropathy in type 1 diabetes than in type 2 diabetes because of the high incidence of hypertension, which itself may lead to microalbuminuria.

Not all patients who develop persistent microalbuminuria progress to overt nephropathy. Studies have reported that anywhere from approximately 15–40% of patients develop overt proteinuria within 5–6 years after onset of the microalbuminuria. However, not only do the majority of patients remain with microalbuminuria, but a significant percentage may revert to normoalbuminuria, especially with effective blood pressure control and the use of renin–angiotensin–aldosterone system blockade.

Patients with fixed microalbuminuria that progresses to overt nephropathy (stage III) usually do so within 5–7 years after onset of the microalbuminuria. In this stage, patients have overt proteinuria (>500 mg of total protein per 24 hours) and macroalbuminuria (>300 mg/24 h), which are detectable with a routine urinary protein dipstick. With the onset of stage III, eGFR is usually below normal levels for age and continues to decrease as the disease progresses. Blood pressure begins to rise in type 1 diabetic patients with stage III nephropathy. In type 2 diabetic patients, who frequently have preexistent hypertension, blood pressure commonly becomes more difficult to control.

Classic diabetic nephropathy, which is seen at a median time of 17 years after onset of diabetes in type 1 diabetes, is associated with overt proteinuria, a progressive decrease in glomerular filtration rate (GFR) and characteristic pathologic findings (see below). There is also frequently evidence of other microvascular disease, especially diabetic retinopathy, with 90–95% of patients with type 1 diabetic nephropathy and 60–65% in type 2 having proliferative retinopathy. The diagnosis of overt diabetic nephropathy is therefore made by three main criteria: the presence of proteinuria within an appropriate time frame, the presence of retinopathy and the absence of other causes of nephrotic syndrome or renal insufficiency. Although microalbuminuria does not always progress to overt proteinuria in these patients, it always precedes overt proteinuria in those patients who do progress. Patients who present with a natural history and clinical presentation consistent with diabetic kidney disease are not routinely biopsied at most medical centers,

and it is usually the patient who has an atypical presentation or suggestion of another kidney-related disease who will undergo renal biopsy. Since there is evidence that a number of patients with diabetic kidney disease do not have "typical" presentations, with decreases in eGFR in the face of minimal or absent proteinuria so there is an increased awareness among nephrologists that diabetes as a potential cause of kidney dysfunction should never be discounted.

Advanced diabetic nephropathy is characterized by a relentless decline in renal function and progression to ESRD. Patients typically develop heavy or nephrotic-range proteinuria (>3.5 g/24 h) and have systemic hypertension. Their urine does not contain inflammatory glomerular (red blood cell casts) or tubulointerstitial (white blood cells, white blood cell casts) lesions. The kidneys may be inappropriately large for the observed degree of renal insufficiency. However, there is increasing evidence that a subset of patients with type 2 diabetes may develop chronic kidney disease with only microalbuminuria or even normalbuminuria. At present it remains uncertain whether these patients have classic diabetic nephropathy per se or diabetes associated with other causes of renal function decline, such as hypertensive nephrosclerosis.

KEY READINGS

Afkarian M et al: Kidney disease and increased mortality risk in type 2 diabetes. J Am Soc Nephrol 2013;24:302.
Steele AM et al: Prevalence of vascular complications among patients with glucokinase mutations and prolonged, mild hyperglycemia. JAMA 2014;311:279.

PATHOLOGY

An early finding in patients with poorly controlled diabetes is enlargement of the kidneys, which represents predominantly hypertrophy of the existing structures rather than growth of new nephrons or cellular hyperplasia. Renal biopsy at the time of onset of microalbuminuria indicates glomerular and tubular basement membrane thickening and the inception of mesangial matrix expansion. Microalbuminuria is more likely in patients who also have evidence of other microvascular insults, especially proliferative retinopathy.

Renal biopsy in patients who develop overt proteinuria reveals diffuse or nodular (Kimmelstiel–Wilson) glomerulosclerosis. Although the Kimmelstiel–Wilson lesion is considered pathognomonic of advanced diabetic nephropathy, only approximately 25% of patients manifest this lesion. A nodular pattern of glomerulopathy mimicking Kimmelstiel–Wilson lesions may also be seen in light-chain nephropathy, and historic descriptions of "diabetic nephropathy without overt hyperglycemia" based solely on light microscopic analysis actually may have represented light-chain disease. Nodular glomerular lesions can also be observed in amyloidosis and membranoproliferative glomerulonephritis type 2. Diabetic nephropathy patients with Kimmelstiel–Wilson lesions have been reported to be more likely to have diabetic retinopathy and a more rapid decline in renal function. A pathologic classification of glomerular lesions in diabetic nephropathy has recently been adopted and stratifies the lesions indicated above into distinct classes. An additional pathognomonic feature of diabetic nephropathy is the finding of both afferent and efferent arteriolar hyalinosis, which can be distinguished from the isolated afferent arteriolar lesion of essential hypertension. Progressive tubulointerstitial fibrosis correlates most closely with the decline in renal function in patients with diabetic nephropathy.

KEY READING

Tervaert TW et al: Pathologic classification of diabetic nephropathy. J Am Soc Nephrol 2010;21:556.

PATHOBIOLOGY

▶ Hyperglycemia

Hyperglycemia and its metabolic sequelae are considered to be the proximate causative factor in the development of diabetic nephropathy. Hyperglycemia can induce numerous metabolic and structural abnormalities (Table 53–1) that have been implicated in the pathogenesis of diabetic nephropathy. These include generation of reactive oxygen species, activation of the polyol pathway, which can lead to de novo synthesis of diacylglycerol and increased protein kinase C activity, alterations in the hexosamine pathway, and nonenzymatic protein glycation (advanced glycosylation end products). Although experimental studies have indicated that each of these alterations can be causative in animal models of diabetic nephropathy, their role in human diabetic nephropathy remains incompletely determined.

Better glucose control does generally reduce the risk of nephropathy and other microvascular complications, especially in type 1 diabetes. Studies from Sweden and Finland, as well as epidemiologic studies in the United States have found that better glycemic control has led to a progressive

Table 53–1. Pathogenesis of diabetic nephropathy.

- Genetic predisposition
- Glomerular hemodynamic injury
- Hyperglycemia
- Nonenzymatic glycation of proteins (AGE)
- Metabolic stress-mitochondrial dysfunction
- High intrarenal angiotensin II
- Systemic hypertension

decrease in the incidence of both albuminuria and CKD in type 1 patients. Randomized interventional studies also clearly demonstrated that relatively better control of blood sugar decreased the development of nephropathy in type 1 diabetes, and observational studies with repeat renal biopsies found that the renal lesions of diabetic nephropathy could reverse after patients received a pancreas transplantation. In addition to glycemic control, better control of blood pressure and a decreased prevalence of smoking have also been attributed as contributing factors for this improved outlook for these patients.

Unlike type 1 patients, the benefit of tight glycemic control is less clear in type 2 compared to type 1 diabetes. Although patients who had glucokinase mutations, which are associated with milder hyperglycemia (average hemoglobin A_{1c} [HbA_{1c}] levels 6.9%), have less proteinuria, microalbuminuria, or nephropathy than patients with longstanding type 2 diabetes with HbA_{1c} levels averaging 7.8%, randomized multicenter trials have failed to find statistically significant improvements in either cardiovascular or all cause mortality, and current ADA recommendations for this patient population are to maintain HbA_{1c} levels less than 7% with individualization depending on the patient.

▶ Hemodynamics

Patients with type 1 and, to a lesser extent, type 2 diabetes, exhibit an increased glomerular filtration rate (GFR), which is mediated by proportionately greater relaxation of the afferent arteriole than the efferent arteriole. This hyperfiltration leads to increased glomerular blood flow and elevated glomerular capillary pressure. With poorly controlled diabetes, patients also develop glomerular hypertrophy, with an increased glomerular capillary surface area. These intraglomerular hemodynamic and structural alterations may contribute to the development or progression of diabetic renal injury. Because angiotensin-converting enzyme (ACE) inhibitors and decreased dietary protein reduce this elevated intraglomerular capillary pressure in experimental animals, the hyperfiltration hypothesis provides one rationale for the success of these interventions in slowing the progression of diabetic nephropathy.

▶ Hormones and Cytokines

Studies in experimental animals have implicated a number of cytokines, hormones, and intracellular signaling pathways in either development or progression of diabetic nephropathy, including transforming growth factor β, connective tissue growth factor, angiotensin II, vascular endothelial growth factor, endothelin, prostaglandins, and nitric oxide. Because these factors have also been implicated in progression of injury in nondiabetic kidney diseases, they are not specifically pathologic for diabetic nephropathy. However, agents that interrupt angiotensin II production and signaling have proven to be very effective in slowing the progression of diabetic nephropathy, and there is also preliminary evidence that blockade of endothelin signaling may be an additional therapeutic option. Interruption of intracellular pathways activated by these factors or by other consequences of hyperglycemia may also provide future therapeutic opportunities.

Genetics

At present, it is not possible to predict which patients will develop diabetic nephropathy. Although poor glycemic and blood pressure control clearly are contributing factors, nephropathy may or may not develop in an individual patient even after many years of hypertension and hyperglycemia. Both type 1 and type 2 diabetes cluster in families. Type 1 diabetics with siblings who have diabetic nephropathy have a greater than 70% lifetime risk of diabetic nephropathy developing in themselves. Patients with type 2 diabetes also appear to have a hereditary predisposition for or against the development of diabetic nephropathy.

However, predisposition for the development of diabetic nephropathy may represent a polygenic condition with inheritance of multiple polymorphisms with variable effect sizes. There is also increasing evidence for epigenetic modifications, likely as a result of hyperglycemia or its metabolic sequelae. In this regard, there is a possible "memory effect" in the development of diabetic kidney disease, since patients whose type 1 diabetes was poorly controlled in the past may develop nephropathy at an increased rate despite subsequent improved glycemic control.

Other Renal Complications

Patients with diabetes experience an increased rate of other kidney and genitourinary abnormalities. Type 4 (hyporeninemic, hypoaldosteronemic) metabolic acidosis with hyperkalemia is commonly encountered in patients with diabetes and mild to moderate renal insufficiency. These patients should be carefully monitored for the development of hyperkalemia in response to volume depletion or after the initiation of drugs that interfere with the renin-angiotensin system, such as ACE inhibitors, AT1 receptor blockers (ARBs), β-adrenergic blockers, both nonselective and selective cyclooxygenase-2 (COX-2) nonsteroidal antiinflammatory agents, and heparin, as well as potassium-sparing diuretics.

Patients with diabetes have an increased incidence of bacterial and fungal infections of the genitourinary tract. In addition to lower urinary tract infections, they have an increased risk for pyelonephritis and intrarenal and perinephric abscess formation.

Unilateral or bilateral renal artery stenosis is more frequent in the type 2 diabetic population than in age-matched nondiabetic individuals and should be considered if a diabetic patient has intractable hypertension or a rapidly

rising serum creatinine level immediately after initiation of therapy with an ACE inhibitor or AT1 receptor blocker. Other causes of acute deterioration in renal function include papillary necrosis with ureteral obstruction owing to sloughing of a papilla, obstructive uropathy caused by bladder dysfunction as a result of autonomic neuropathy, and contrast media–induced acute tubular necrosis. In addition, prerenal azotemia or acute tubular necrosis may develop in diabetic patients as a result of heart failure or volume depletion owing to vomiting induced by gastroparesis or diarrhea from autonomic neuropathy.

PREVENTION AND TREATMENT (See Figure 53–2)

Glycemic control significantly lessens the incidence of nephropathy in patients with type 1 diabetes for at least 20 or more years but does not completely eliminate the risk. However, tight glycemic control to reduce to a $HgBA_{1c}$ target level of 6.5% or less in patients with type 2 diabetes does not reduce the risk of nephropathy compared with standard therapy to a goal of 7–7.9%. Metformin is a mainstay for glycemic control in patients with type 2 diabetes but should be used with caution in patients with decreased eGFR because it is renally cleared. Although there is a concern for increased risk for development of lactic acidosis, a recent systemic review suggests that for patients with eGFR greater than 30 mL/min, there is minimally increased risk.

Newer agents for treatment of type 2 diabetes, DPP-4 inhibitors and SGLT2 inhibitors have also been utilized successfully in patients with mild-moderate diabetic kidney disease. Of the currently available DPP-4 inhibitors, lingagliptin is eliminated by the enterohepatic system, and no adjustment for CKD is necessary. There are recent studies suggesting that both DPP-4 inhibitors and SGLT2 inhibitors have beneficial effects to slow progression of diabetic kidney disease beyond their ability to control blood sugar, and multicenter clinical trials are in progress.

Hypertension is an important risk factor in the progression of diabetic nephropathy, and it is clear that treatment with antihypertensive agents can slow progression. However, there remains controversy about what should be the optimal blood pressure reduction to be achieved, and current recommendations are to aim for moderate blood pressure control with systolic blood pressures 130–140 mm Hg.

With decline of renal function to an eGFR less than 45 mL/min, sulfonylurea oral hypoglycemic agents become contraindicated because of the increased risk of prolonged hypoglycemia. Treatment guidelines for metformin are in flux, and there is evidence that the previous strict prohibition against the use of this agent with decreased renal function may not be indicated. Similarly, newer oral hypoglycemic agents, DPP4 inhibitors and SGLT2 inhibitors appear to be safe in patients with eGFR greater than 30 mL/min.

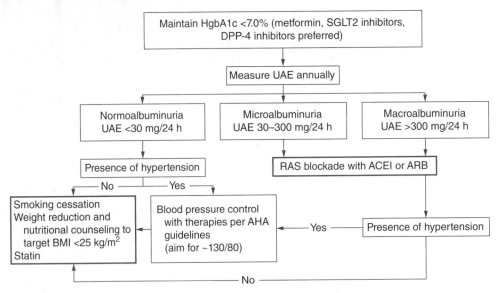

▲ **Figure 53–2.** Treatment algorithm for patients with type 2 diabetes and kidney disease.

As GFR declines, insulin requirements may decrease owing to reduced insulin degradation and clearance by the failing kidney.

Medications that interfere with the renin–angiotensin–aldosterone system, either ACE inhibitors or AT1 receptor blockers (ARBs), have additional benefits to decrease proteinuria and slow progression of nephropathy, beyond lowering systemic blood pressure. However, the combination of an ACE inhibitor and an ARB is contraindicated because of increased side effects. There is also evidence that mineralocorticoid receptor blockers (aldosterone and eplerenone) are effective in slowing progression of diabetic nephropathy. There is some evidence that addition of a mineralocorticoid receptor blocker to an ACEI or ARB provides additional benefit, although there is an increased risk for development of hyperkalemia.

Patients treated with a RAS blocker should have their serum potassium and creatinine levels monitored closely in the first week after the initiation of therapy because of the increased prevalence of type 4 renal tubular acidosis and renal artery stenosis. If blood pressure control is not achieved with these agents, diuretics and other antihypertensive agents, including cardioselective β-blockers, α-blockers, and nondihydropyridine calcium channel blockers, which do not produce arteriolar vasodilation, can be added.

Cigarette smoking has been linked to acceleration of loss of renal function in diabetic nephropathy, and patients should be encouraged to quit. Because of the increased risk of cardiovascular disease with diabetes and diabetic nephropathy, patients should be of statins for patients for hyperlipidemia.

There is an awareness of a critical need for further new therapies to combat diabetic kidney disease, and there has been investigation of a number of possible new therapies in the past few years, including endothelin A antagonists (atrasentan), NRF2 antagonists (bardoxolone), antifibrotics (sulodexide, pirfenidone) PPARγ agonists (thiazolidines), TGF-β antibodies, JAK inhibitors, vitamin D activators, protein kinase C inhibition (ruboxistaurin). Unfortunately, most of these trials failed because of futility or significant side effects of the drugs. However, the aforementioned studies with SGLT2 inhibitors and DPP-4 inhibitors hold promise that there will soon be additional therapies that can slow progression of diabetic kidney disease.

KEY READINGS

ACCORD Study Group et al: Effects of intensive blood-pressure control in type 2 diabetes mellitus. N Engl J Med 2010;362:1575.

The DCCT/EDIC Research Group Intensive diabetes therapy and glomerular filtration rate in type 1 diabetes. N Engl J Med 2011;365:2366.

Fried LF et al: Combined angiotensin inhibition for the treatment of diabetic nephropathy. N Engl J Med 2013;369:1892.

Lv J et al: Antihypertensive agents for preventing diabetic kidney disease. Cochrane Database Syst Rev 2012;12:Cd004136.

Navaneethan SD: Aldosterone antagonists for preventing the progression of chronic kidney disease: a systemic review and metaanalysis. Clin J Am Soc Nephrol 2009;4:542.

Panchapakesan U, Mather A, Pollock C: Role of GLP-1 and DPP-4 in diabetic nephropathy and cardiovascular disease. Clin Science 2013;124:17.

Vallon V, Thomson SC: Targeting renal glucose reabsorption to treat hyperglycaemia: the pleiotropic effects of SGLT2 inhibition. Diabetologia 2017;60:215.

RENAL REPLACEMENT THERAPY

The majority of patients who with end-stage diabetic nephropathy on dialysis for renal replacement therapy receive hemodialysis as compared with peritoneal dialysis. The mortality of diabetic patients who receive either type of dialysis is 1.5–2.0 times worse than in nondiabetic patients because of their associated cardiovascular, cerebrovascular, and peripheral vascular disease as well as their increased risk for infection. The 5-year survival rate is less than 20% in diabetic patients undergoing maintenance dialysis.

Patients with stage III DN or higher should be under the care of a nephrologist, and planning should be initiated for the modality of dialysis. Although dialysis is routinely initiated when the GFR declines to less than 10 mL/min, earlier initiation of dialysis is sometimes necessary in diabetic patients because their volume-dependent hypertension or hyperkalemia is not otherwise manageable or when their uremia and gastroparesis lead to malnutrition or uncontrollable recurrent emesis.

Approximately 25% of renal transplants performed in the United States are in diabetic patients. Long-term survival and quality of life are generally superior after transplantation compared with chronic dialysis. However, the other microvascular (retinopathy, neuropathy) and macrovascular complications are not improved by renal transplantation alone. Pancreas and combined kidney-pancreas transplantation can significantly improve the quality of life of patients with diabetic nephropathy by improving autonomic neuropathy, by retarding or possibly correcting retinopathy, and by avoiding the potential complications of insulin administration. However, all transplantation options remain limited by organ availability.

■ CHAPTER REVIEW QUESTIONS

1. A 64-year-old man with moderately controlled type 2 diabetes, hypertension and CKD with nephrotic range proteinuria and sCr of 2.4 is admitted to the hospital because he has suffered a cerebrovascular accident. Which is the best single answer concerning this patient?
   A. Intensive glycemic control of type 2 diabetes does not decrease incidence of nephropathy and cardiovascular mortality.
   B. Type 2 diabetic patients with CKD always have nephrotic range albuminuria.
   C. In type 2 diabetes, proteinuria correlates with increased incidence of coronary heart disease but not with stroke.
   D. In both type 1 and type 2 diabetes, hypertension usually indicates evidence of diabetic nephropathy.

2. Which is the best single answer concerning structural changes to the kidney during the course of diabetic nephropathy?
   A. Afferent and efferent arteriolar hyalinosis are nonspecific findings and are found in a variety of glomerular diseases.
   B. Greater than 90% of patients with type 2 diabetes have evidence of retinopathy at the time of diagnosis of overt nephropathy.

   C. Kimmelstiel Wilson lesions are observed in a minority of patients diagnosed with diabetic nephropathy.
   D. Thickening of the glomerular basement membrane is a late finding in diabetic nephropathy.
   E. Kidney hypertrophy always indicates that the patient will develop overt nephropathy.

3. A 47-year-old Hispanic woman is referred because of detection of dipstick positive proteinuria. She is obese and has carried the diagnosis of diabetes for the past 7 years. She also has moderately controlled hypertension and osteoarthritis. She smokes one pack of cigarettes per day but does not use other drugs or alcohol. Of note, her mother and one of her three siblings also have diabetes. Which is the best answer concerning this patient?
   A. Because she has only been diagnosed with diabetes for 7 years, her proteinuria is probably not due to diabetic nephropathy.
   B. Type 1 but not type 2 diabetic nephropathy demonstrates Mendelian inheritance.
   C. Smoking and hypertension have often been associated with increased risk for progression of diabetic nephropathy.

4. A 59-year-man patient with type 2 diabetes for greater than 12 years is referred to the nephrology clinic because of declining renal function. He is found to have a blood pressure of 146/87, an eGFR of 39 and an HBA_{1c} of 8.1. He is also found to have proteinuria of 2.1 g/24 h. What is the best single answer relating to his therapy?
   A. With progressive nephropathy, insulin requirements usually increase in diabetics.
   B. Metformin is contraindicated with renal insufficiency.
   C. There is a clear benefit for all diabetics in reducing HBA_{1c} to less than 7.5%

5. True or False: Every patient with diabetes who develops microalbuminuria invariably progresses to develop macroalbuminuria and progressive CKD.
   A. True
   B. False

Pregnancy and the Kidney

Samantha L. Gelfand, MD
Ursula C. Brewster, MD

PHYSIOLOGIC CHANGES OF PREGNANCY

General Considerations

Pregnancy is a transient physiologic state that alters kidney anatomy and physiology. It also causes changes in electrolytes, hemodynamics, water balance, and acid–base homeostasis that must be accounted for when evaluating a pregnant woman.

ANATOMIC CHANGES

In a normal pregnancy, the kidneys increase in size by approximately 1 cm from dilation of the collecting system. Hormonal and urodynamic factors result in this physiologic hydronephrosis of pregnancy as early as 6 weeks' gestation. Dilation of the renal calyces, renal pelvis, and ureters increases the capacity for urine volume in the kidney, which can hold up to 300 cc of urine in pregnancy.

While physiologic hydronephrosis of pregnancy is thought to increase the risk of ascending infection, most of the time it does not. The hydronephrosis is predominantly right-sided with normal function of that dilated kidney. However, pathologic hydronephrosis is also possible and again more common on the right; there are two anatomic reasons for this. First, the right ureter crosses the pelvic brim on top of the ovarian vein, which can exert a pressure that obstructs the ureter. On the left side, the ureter and ovarian vein run in parallel. Second, the rectosigmoid colon descends on the left side of the abdomen, which pushes the uterus slightly to the right (uterine dextrorotation), increasing its proclivity to directly obstruct the right ureter.

HEMODYNAMIC CHANGES

Pregnancy affects systemic and intrarenal hemodynamics. There is a dramatic rise in cardiac output and a fall in systemic vascular resistance and mean arterial pressure.

An increase in blood volume leads to an increase in cardiac output (by up to 50% above baseline) and an increase in maternal heart rate. Because of the increased preload needed, cardiac output may be affected by postural changes or compression of the inferior vena cava by a gravid uterus.

At the end of the first trimester, there is a fall in systemic blood pressure, driven by a fall in systemic vascular resistance. Blood pressure decreases on average 10 mm Hg below baseline during the second trimester. By the third trimester, blood pressure returns to baseline.

Hormonal factors are responsible for these changes in vascular resistance. Specifically, diminished vascular resistance in pregnancy results from relative resistance to angiotensin II and norepinephrine, as well as increased production of vasodilatory nitric oxide and prostacyclin. With the fall in systemic blood pressure, the renin–angiotensin system (RAAS) is dramatically upregulated in pregnancy; in the first trimester, plasma renin levels can be up to four times above baseline levels. Renin continues to rise until around 20 weeks. The increased renin stimulates an increase in aldosterone levels that in turn leads to salt and water retention, resulting in the increase in blood volume.

Within the kidney, the hemodynamic changes described above lead to an increase in glomerular filtration rate (GFR) and renal plasma flow (RPF). GFR begins to rise early in pregnancy and is approximately 50% above normal by the end of the first trimester. With this rise in GFR comes an increase in creatinine clearance, and so serum creatinine concentrations normally fall to below pre-pregnancy levels. A normal serum creatinine in pregnancy is less than 0.8 mg/dL. The increased filtration also leads to a slight increase in urinary excretion of protein, glucose, uric acid, amino acids, and calcium. Because of this, abnormal proteinuria is described as greater than 300 mg/day in the setting of pregnancy. Serum uric acid levels should be lower than usual in pregnancy, and a level above 4.6 mg/dL suggests impaired GFR.

WATER BALANCE

Pregnancy is associated with a fall in serum sodium concentration of approximately 5 mEq/L and serum osmolality by 5–10 mOsm/kg. The serum osmostat is reset, and there is a decrease in the osmotic thresholds for arginine vasopressin (AVP) release and thirst. Total body water increases by 6–8 L, the vast majority of which is extracellular. One effect of this increased total body water is physiologic anemia of pregnancy; the blood becomes more dilute. Hematopoiesis does increase, but not enough to accommodate the increase in intravascular volume. Another effect of increased total body water is edema, which is compounded by increases in total body sodium of approximately 900–1000 mEq.

Vasopressinase, made in the placenta, is responsible for catabolism of AVP in pregnancy and may, in some instances, lead to overt diabetes insipidus. This may occur in cases where the woman had preexisting mild (often undiagnosed) central diabetes insipidus and cannot increase production of AVP to match its enhanced destruction, or in cases of molar or twin pregnancies where production of vasopressinase is higher. These women present later in pregnancy with high urine output, but often keep their water balance intact by enhanced water drinking. When they are admitted in labor, or made NPO for any procedure, serum sodium may rise rapidly and cause symptoms in the mother or developing fetus.

ELECTROLYTES AND ACID/BASE

Serum potassium levels remain normal during pregnancy. Total serum calcium levels fall, but the serum-ionized calcium concentration remains normal. Increased production of calcitriol by the placenta leads to increased gastrointestinal absorption of calcium and resultant hypercalciuria, which may play a role in kidney stone formation. The rise in serum calcitriol results in suppression of parathyroid hormone levels.

The hormonal milieu of pregnancy leads to a mild respiratory alkalosis and a compensatory metabolic acidosis. Progesterone affects the respiratory centers in the brain, resulting in an increase in tidal volume and, subsequently, an increase in minute ventilation. It is unclear if this is a direct effect of progesterone on the respiratory center or if progesterone confers an enhanced sensitivity to pCO_2, or both. The increased minute ventilation leads to an increase in alveolar oxygen, which is needed to meet the increased metabolic oxygen demand of the placenta and fetus. There is also an expected drop in arterial carbon dioxide levels, with a fall in $Paco_2$ from a nonpregnant level of 40 mm Hg to approximately 30 mm Hg in healthy pregnant women. This respiratory alkalosis is met by a compensatory metabolic acidosis (plasma bicarbonate levels fall by 4 mEq/L) as the kidney excretes bicarbonate, to return the serum pH to near normal (7.4–7.45).

KEY READING

Cheung KL, Lafayette RA: Renal physiology of pregnancy. Adv Chronic Kidney Dis 2013;20:209.

▼ CKD AND PREGNANCY

EFFECT OF CKD ON PREGNANCY

1. Fertility

Women with advanced CKD and ESRD have lower fertility rates. Many women on dialysis have irregular menstrual cycles due to oligomenorrhea or amenorrhea, which results from impaired cyclic gonadotropin release in the hypothalamus. Additionally, prolactin levels are elevated in both men and women on dialysis due to an increased production and reduced renal clearance of the hormone, which also contributes to a reduction in fertility.

Pregnancy in patients on dialysis is rare; when conception does occur, it is often shortly after initiation of renal replacement therapy when the woman may still have significant residual renal function. Pregnancy is more common, and the outcome more successful, in women who have undergone kidney transplantation, as their hormonal axis is restored.

2. Fetal Outcomes

Pregnancy outcomes are very good for women with mild CKD (creatinine <1.4 mg/dL) and normal blood pressure. However, for women with more advanced CKD, pregnancy can result in maternal and fetal complications.

Fetal outcomes in pregnant women with advanced CKD and ESRD have improved in recent years. Currently, approximately 40% of pregnancies in women on dialysis result in a live birth. This represents a substantial improvement, as prior to 1994 the reported rate was 27%. However, most of these infants will be born premature (mean gestation age is 32 weeks), at low birth weight (usually <2000 g), and with extensive neonatal care needs. Long-term medical and developmental problems are also common. Despite improved infant survival, the rate of perinatal death is much higher than in the general population. The overall infant survival rate is similar between women treated with hemodialysis and women treated with peritoneal dialysis.

3. Polyhydramnios

Around gestational week 16, fetal kidneys begin to produce urine. In mothers with high urea due to CKD, the fetal kidneys will respond with a fetal diuresis that results in abnormally increased amniotic fluid volume (polyhydramnios). Polyhydramnios is evident in almost half of all pregnancies in women with ESRD. Clinicians should also be aware that after parturition, infants of mothers with metabolic derangements from diabetes or CKD are born with maternal serum electrolytes; hyperglycemia and azotemia in the neonate leads to an osmotic diuresis that can result in fatal hypovolemia if not managed proactively.

EFFECT OF PREGNANCY ON CKD

▶ General Considerations

Pregnancy may alter the course of disease in women with CKD. Although outcomes are usually favorable in women with mild stable CKD and serum creatinine concentrations less than 1.4 mg/dL, there is evidence to suggest that women with creatinine levels greater than 1.5 mg/dL are likely to experience progression of their CKD at a more rapid rate than women who do not become pregnant. Women with active disease are also more likely to have renal complications during pregnancy than those with stable CKD. Obstetric complications also remain higher in women with higher serum creatinine concentrations.

1. Proteinuria and Hypertension

Because GFR increases in pregnancy, albeit to a lesser degree in women with CKD, proteinuria also increases during pregnancy. This makes it challenging to interpret progressive proteinuria in a woman with preexisting proteinuric CKD; an increase in their proteinuria during pregnancy may be a factor of their physiologic increased GFR, or it may represent a new diagnosis of preeclampsia. Hypertension will also be exacerbated, after a transient and early drop in blood pressure during the first trimester, and frequently requires pharmacologic intervention during the second and third trimesters. Table 54–1 lists of antihypertensive medications that are safe to use during pregnancy.

2. Diabetic Nephropathy

Diabetes mellitus (particularly type 2) is increasing in frequency among women of child-bearing age, and some of these women have underlying diabetic nephropathy when they become pregnant (defined by urine albumin excretion >300 mg/day).

Whether pregnancy impacts the progression of diabetic CKD remains controversial. There are conflicting studies; diabetic women with normal kidney function and normal albumin excretion usually do quite well and have lower risk for development or progression of CKD compared to those with diabetic CKD at the time of conception. The risk of progression and acceleration of diabetic nephropathy is highest in women with serum creatinine concentration greater than 2 mg/dL at the time of conception.

Table 54–1. Use of antihypertensive medications in pregnancy.

Use of Antihypertensive Medications in Pregnancy		
Medication	Safety Profile	Complications Associated
ACE-inhibitors Angiotensin receptor blockers	Contraindicated	Pulmonary hypoplasia, skeletal deformities, fetal oligohydramnios
Diuretics	Contraindicated	Maternal volume depletion, fetal thrombocytopenia, hemolytic anemia
Labetalol	Widely used	Limited data
Calcium channel blockers	Widely used	Potentiates hypotensive effect of IV magnesium
Alpha-methyldopa	Widely used	
Hydralazine	Widely used	

ACE, angiotensin converting enzyme.

Women with preexisting diabetic nephropathy have a higher rate preeclampsia, which transmits a higher rate of preterm delivery (prevalence up to 30%) and intrauterine growth restriction in the developing fetus. All women with diabetic nephropathy are considered "high risk" for developing preeclampsia and therefore should be started on a low-dose aspirin for prevention. Additionally, up to 20% of women with gestational diabetes will develop preeclampsia, and this risk increases with worsening diabetic control.

The goal of antihypertensive treatment in pregnant women with diabetic nephropathy should be less than 135/85 mm Hg.

3. Lupus and Antiphospholipid Antibody Syndrome

Systemic lupus erythematosus (SLE) often occurs in young women with preserved fertility, leading to overlap with pregnancy. Management of pregnancy in patients with lupus nephritis can be complicated. Fetal and maternal outcomes are best when renal function is preserved, blood pressure is normal, and the underlying lupus has been in remission for at least 6 months prior to conception. Ideally, prednisone dosing should be stable at less than 10 mg/day for 6 months as well.

Lupus nephritis, particularly class III or IV lesions, is prone to flairs during pregnancy or the postpartum period. It can be challenging to distinguish a lupus flair from another cause of renal impairment, including preeclampsia; renal biopsy is often necessary. However, after 32 weeks' gestation, the risks of biopsy should be carefully weighed against the risks of inducing delivery, which is often thought to be the safer option.

Lupus may also be associated with multiple antibody-mediated syndromes, including antiphospholipid antibody syndrome (APS). Diagnosis of APS depends on the presence of one clinical and one laboratory manifestation of the disease. Clinical manifestations include thrombosis, a single unexplained fetal loss after 10th week of gestation, or more than three consecutive spontaneous abortions before the 10th week of gestation. Laboratory manifestations include anticardiolipin antibodies, anti-B2 glycoprotein antibodies, or the lupus anticoagulant. Anticoagulation (low-dose aspirin and heparin) is recommended, but warfarin is contraindicated in women of child-bearing age because of associated fetal malformations. The most common pregnancy complications in women with APS include fetal loss, preeclampsia (up to 50%), premature delivery, and intrauterine growth restriction.

KEY READINGS

Bili E et al: Pregnancy management and outcomes in women with CKD. Hippokratia 2013;17:163.

Kattah AG, Garovic VD: Pregnancy and lupus nephritis. Sem in Neph 2015;35:487.

Smyth A et al: Clin J Am Soc Nephrol 2010;5:2060.

MANAGEMENT OF WOMEN ON DIALYSIS DURING PREGNANCY

1. Preconception Counseling

Women of childbearing age who are on dialysis should be offered preconception counseling if they desire a pregnancy and birth control if they do not. All pregnancies in women with ESRD are high risk. Women who wish to become pregnant should fully understand the implications for their dialysis schedule, dialysis access, and medication options. For example, most women with CKD take angiotensin converting enzyme inhibitors (ACEI) or angiotensin receptor blockers (ARBs). These drugs must be discontinued before conception because they are associated with oligohydramnios, fetal renal dysfunction, fetal growth restriction, skeletal abnormalities, and fetal pulmonary hypoplasia. Although exposure to these medications in the first trimester was once thought to be safe, more recent data has shown that exposure at any fetal development stage is deleterious. Administration of these medications early in pregnancy does not necessarily warrant termination, but detailed serial ultrasounds by maternal-fetal medicine specialists are indicated to assess the developing fetus as the abnormalities are not universal.

2. Detection of Pregnancy

ESSENTIALS OF DIAGNOSIS

▸ β-hCG measurement is unreliable in women with CKD.

▸ Pregnancy in women with CKD must be confirmed by ultrasound.

Detection of a pregnancy is challenging in women on dialysis for multiple reasons. First, irregular menses are very common in women with ESRD, many of whom do not mention them to providers or seek prompt evaluation for pregnancy. Pregnancy in this population is therefore diagnosed late, at an average gestational age of 16 weeks. Additionally, evaluation for pregnancy is complicated. Anuria often precludes urine pregnancy testing and β-hCG is cleared by the kidney and therefore chronically elevated in most women with significant kidney impairment. Since most urine and blood pregnancy tests are β-hCG assays, false-positives are common. While the trend of serial β-hCG may be informative (they double every 48 hours in a normal pregnancy with normal kidney function), confirmation of pregnancy in patients with ESRD must be done by ultrasound. Transvaginal ultrasound can confirm intrauterine pregnancy as early as 5 weeks, when the gestational sac measures 5 mm.

3. Dialysis Modality

Dialysis modality need not be changed when a woman becomes pregnant. Outcomes are similar between hemodialysis and peritoneal dialysis. For women on peritoneal dialysis, as the pregnancy progresses, exchanges may need to be lower in volume and higher in number to achieve adequate Kt/V. Since ultrafiltration is mediated by dialysate glucose concentration in peritoneal dialysis, one relative contraindication to ongoing peritoneal dialysis during pregnancy is gestational diabetes. In that situation, the risks and benefits of continuing peritoneal dialysis or converting to hemodialysis should be discussed on a case-by-case basis. Heparin may be safely used during hemodialysis as it does not cross the placenta and is not teratogenic.

4. Dialysis Prescription

Significant adjustments of dialysis dose are required in the setting of pregnancy (Table 54–2). More intensive dialysis leads to better outcomes, including reduced risk of preterm delivery, improved infant survival, and fewer maternal complications. Women who conceive before dialysis is initiated, or who have more residual renal function while on

Table 54–2. Dialysis goals during pregnancy.

Dialysis sessions per week	5–7
Dialysis hours per week	At least 20
Predialysis BUN	<50 mg/dL
Diastolic blood pressure	80–90 mm Hg
Hemoglobin	10–11 g/dL
Ferritin	200–300 µg/mL

dialysis, have better outcomes, suggesting that the uremic toxins are important to clear. A minimum of 20 hours of hemodialysis per week is recommended; the increase in number of dialysis sessions allows for less ultrafiltration at each treatment, which reduces the risk of intradialytic hypotension. Additionally, maintaining a low interdialytic blood urea nitrogen (BUN) reduces the risk of polyhydramnios, which results from intact fetal kidney filtration of azotemic maternal blood.

The increase in dialysis dose can be accomplished by more frequent daytime dialysis sessions or by nocturnal treatments. Dialysis baths need to be adjusted for the increase in dose. Potassium baths often need to be 3–4K with the increase in frequency. Bicarbonate baths may need to be decreased from the unit standard as normal pregnancy is associated with a respiratory alkalosis ($PaCO_2$ 30–35 mm Hg) which requires a compensatory metabolic acidosis for maintenance of normal blood pH. Calcium balance should be positive and levels should be monitored throughout a pregnancy, as there is an increased demand from fetal skeletal development.

Dry weight adjustments can be challenging. Most women gain 2–3 lb in the first trimester and 1 lb/wk thereafter. However, great variability exists, and the expanding plasma volume makes this difficult to assess. Monitoring closely is essential to avoid volume overload or intravascular volume depletion and hemodynamic compromise.

5. Anemia

Anemia is multifactorial in pregnant women with ESRD. Their preexistent anemia from deficient renal erythropoietin production is compounded by two factors that cause anemia during all pregnancies, namely increased total body water (which dilutes the blood) and relative iron deficiency (from the iron demands of fetal hematopoiesis).

Anemia management must be proactive. Hemoglobin levels should be kept above 8 g/dL as lower levels pose a risk to the developing fetus. Recombinant erythropoietin is safe to continue during pregnancy, and dose requirements may

increase by 50–100%. There are no reports of teratogenicity. To address iron deficiency, it is common to give low-dose infusions of intravenous iron, as oral supplementation is usually insufficient in this population.

6. Nutritional Intake

Nutritional needs on dialysis increase during pregnancy. With the increase in dialysis dosage, potassium and phosphate intake may need to be increased. Patients should also be counseled to increase protein intake, and to continue water-soluble vitamin supplements to account for losses on dialysis.

KEY READINGS

Fahy BG, Gouzd VA, Atallah JN: Pregnancy tests with end-stage renal disease. Journal of Clinical Anesthesia 2009;20:609.
Manisco G et al: Pregnancy in end-stage renal disease: how to achieve a healthy delivery. Clin Kidney J 2015;8:293.
Reddy DD, Holley JL: Management of the pregnant chronic dialysis patient. Adv Chronic Kidney Dis 2007;14:146.

PREGNANCY AFTER KIDNEY TRANSPLANTATION

General Considerations

Fertility is often restored following kidney transplantation. Fetal and maternal outcomes relate to graft function; in transplant patients with serum creatinine less than 1.5 mg/dL, the success rate of delivering a healthy infant, once past the first trimester, is over 90%.

When a woman with a kidney transplant carries a pregnancy, the allograft undergoes many of the same physiologic changes as native kidneys: GFR increases commensurate to increase in cardiac output, and low-grade proteinuria is common. There does not appear to be an increased risk of rejection during pregnancy, but immunosuppressant medications may need to be altered proactively if a pregnancy is planned. Normal vaginal delivery is possible as the pelvic kidney should not obstruct the birth canal. Obstetricians may want to review the transplant operative note, or do an ultrasound to confirm placement of the kidney and ureter, especially if caesarean section is planned for any reason.

Women with solid organ transplants are typically advised not to breastfeed as there is insufficient information about drug transmission in breast milk. The long-term effects of these medications on a developing infant are unknown.

1. Hypertension and Preeclampsia

If the patient with a kidney transplant has chronic hypertension, it should be managed proactively in pregnancy, as the risks of accelerated hypertension and preeclampsia are very high. Even if the patient has no preexisting hypertension, it is common for hypertension to develop as the pregnancy progresses.

Preeclampsia is much more common in pregnant women with kidney transplants. In fact, their preeclampsia risk up to four times higher than the general pregnant population. Interestingly, calcineurin inhibitors increase the serum uric acid level, which confounds its utility as an indicator of preeclampsia.

2. Effect of Pregnancy on Allograft Function

It is safest to delay pregnancy for a minimum of 1 year after transplantation. This decreases the risk of complications from immunosuppression and graft rejection. Fetal and maternal outcomes appear to be best in women with a serum creatinine concentration less than 1.5 mg/dL who have well-controlled blood pressure. Although there is conflicting data on the long-term effect of pregnancy on graft function, current consensus is that pregnancy is safe in women with the above parameters.

3. Infection Risk

Pregnancy in a transplant patient can be complicated by infection. Urinary tract infections (UTIs) are common in the setting of pregnancy, as is asymptomatic bacteriuria; although the latter does not constitute a significant clinical threat in nonpregnant women, in pregnancy it is associated with a much higher rate of progression to UTI and is therefore treated. Because of this, pregnant women with kidney transplants should be screened for bacteriuria with monthly urine cultures.

Opportunistic viral infections may also pose a risk to the developing fetus. Reactivation of cytomegalovirus (CMV) can have devastating fetal consequences, including microcephaly, mental retardation, and perinatal death. Treatment of CMV is reserved for severe maternal infections, however, as data does not yet support treatment of fetal infection. Another common viral infection in the transplant patient is herpes simplex virus (HSV), which most often infects the fetus during passage through the vaginal canal at birth. Mothers with evidence of HSV reactivation near the time of birth should be treated with acyclovir. Intrauterine HSV infection is rare; when it does occur, it is usually during the mother's primary infection rather than reactivation, and it often results in fetal demise. Last, chronic viral hepatitides are readily transmitted from mother to fetus. Approximately 80% of neonates born to mothers with hepatitis B virus (HBV) will become chronic carriers of the virus, which puts them at risk for complications, including cirrhosis and hepatocellular carcinoma at a young age. Fetal infection can be prevented in 95% of cases if hepatitis B immunoglobulin and vaccination are offered immediately after birth to the fetus. Hepatitis C virus has a lower rate of vertical transmission, but no studied preventive therapies exist at this time.

Opportunistic parasitic infections are much less common than viral infections. The most common parasitic infection is maternal toxoplasmosis, which results in neonatal transmission in up to 65% of cases. Immunosuppression in women with transplants increases the risk of parasitemia, which leads to intrauterine fetal infection via the placenta. Fetal sequelae may include central nervous system defects such as microcephaly, ventricular dilatation, calcifications, blindness, and epilepsy. Toxoplasmosis in a pregnant mother should be treated with spiramycin, pyrimethamine-sulfonamide, or a combination of the two medicines.

4. Immunosuppression

All common immunosuppressive medications have the potential for fetal side effects, but many are low risk and well tolerated. Immunosuppression cannot be suspended during a pregnancy.

Azathioprine and calcineurin inhibitors are the mainstay of therapy in pregnant transplant patients (Table 54–3). Azathioprine is technically FDA category D drug in pregnancy, but it has been used successfully over many years. In large meta-analyses on its use in inflammatory bowel disease during pregnancy, azathioprine had no significant harmful effects on fetal development or health; it was associated with preterm delivery but not low birth weight. Calcineurin inhibitors have been shown to cross the placenta and last 1–2 days in fetal circulation; for this reason, neonates much be monitored for hyperkalemia and renal dysfunction. Additionally, it is essential to monitor calcineurin inhibitor levels closely as the volume of distribution and hepatic metabolism of these drugs change during pregnancy. There is no preference given to cyclosporine or tacrolimus, as both appear to be well tolerated.

Prednisone in dosages under 15 mg/day is likely quite safe for the developing fetus; after birth, infants should be monitored for adrenal insufficiency. Prednisone dosages over 20 mg/day have been associated with an increased risk for gestational diabetes and opportunistic infections. Mycophenolate mofetil is known to be teratogenic; the FDA has issued a black box warning against use of the drug during pregnancy. It should be avoided in pregnancy, and stopped in advance of a planned pregnancy. Experience with the mTOR (mammalian target or rapamycin) inhibitors sirolimus and everolimus in pregnancy is limited, and not enough data exists at this time to use them in pregnant women. Newer immunosuppressive agents, such as polyclonal or monoclonal antibodies, are being used with increased

Table 54–3. Immunosuppressant medicines in pregnancy.

Immunosuppressive Agent	Associations in Pregnancy	Pregnancy Risk Factor Category[a]	Clinical Use
Prednisone	- Gestational diabetes - Neonatal adrenal insufficiency	C/D	Common
Azathioprine	- Preterm birth	D	Common
Calcineurin inhibitors	- Premature birth - Low birth weight - Neonatal AKI - Neonatal hyperkalemia	C	Common
Mycophenolate mofetil	- Pregnancy loss - Congenital defects	D	Contraindicated
Rapamycin	Limited data exists	C	Uncommon

[a]Category A, controlled human studies show no risk; category B, no evidence of risk in studies; category C, risk cannot be ruled out; category D, positive evidence of risk; category X, contraindicated in pregnancy.

frequency in transplantation, but their safety profile in pregnancy is unknown at this time.

KEY READINGS

Akbari M et al: Systematic review and meta-analysis on the effects of thiopurines on birth outcomes from female and male patients with inflammatory bowel disease. Inflammatory Bowel Dis 2013;19:15.

Coscia LA et al: Report from the National Transplantation Pregnancy Registry (NTPR): outcomes of pregnancy after transplantation. Clin Tranpl 2010;65.

Del Mar Colon M, Hibbard JU: Obstetric considerations in the management of pregnancy in kidney transplant recipients. Adv Chronic Kidney Dis 2007;14:168.

Josephson MA, McKay DB: Women and transplantation: fertility, sexuality, pregnancy, contraception. Adv Chronic Kidney Dis 2013;20:433.

◤ AKI IN PREGNANCY

▷ General Considerations

Pregnancy-related acute kidney injury (PR-AKI) is rare in the developed world where women have access to care. It is unfortunately more common in parts of the world where there may be limited access to prenatal care and illegal abortions are more common. Defining AKI can also be more complicated in pregnancy. The RIFLE and AKIN criteria used in defining AKI in the nonobstetric patient have limited utility in pregnancy. Because GFR normally increases in pregnancy, a "baseline" serum creatinine is a moving target, and often considerably lower than in the nonpregnant state. As serum creatinine concentrations are not routinely checked in pregnancy, a level of 0.8 mg/dL, which may be normal in the nonpregnant state, may actually represent a significant impairment in kidney function in the setting of pregnancy.

Although certain causes of AKI are more common in pregnancy, any of the usual causes are possible. Risk factors for AKI are listed in Table 54–4. However, the differential in pregnancy can often be narrowed substantially according to the gestational age of the fetus, which we divide by first half (<20 weeks) and latter half (>20 weeks). In the first half of the pregnancy, AKI is often related to hyperemesis gravidarum, a septic abortion, or urinary tract infection. In the latter half, the risks of hypertension-related kidney disease, preeclampsia, and the thrombotic microangiopathies are more common (Figure 54–1). It is also possible to divide the differential diagnosis in the traditional pre-renal, intrarenal, postrenal categories that are more common in pregnancy.

Table 54–4. Risk factors for AKI in pregnancy.

Underlying chronic kidney disease
Preexistent proteinuria
Hypertension
Diabetes
Lupus nephritis
History of preeclampsia or gestational hypertension
History of thrombotic microangiopathy

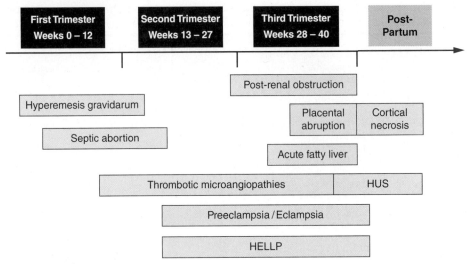

▲ **Figure 54–1.** Common causes of AKI by trimester. HUS, hemolytic uremic syndrome.

Workup of AKI in pregnancy should be targeted to the differential diagnosis. A complete history, physical examination, and a set of general chemistries, liver function tests, complete blood count, urinalysis, and urine microscopy examination can help direct the practitioner. If relevant to the differential diagnosis, further workup with a renal ultrasound, autoimmune serologic markers, blood smear, and cultures should follow.

AKI IN THE FIRST HALF OF PREGNANCY (0–20 WEEKS' GESTATION)

AKI in the early part of pregnancy is most often pre- or intrarenal in nature. Diagnosis is based on history, laboratory data, and urine sediment findings. For each of the most common causes of AKI early in pregnancy, we will discuss the presenting signs and symptoms, diagnostic approach, and management strategies.

1. Prerenal AKI

Early in pregnancy, certain causes of AKI predominate. Chief among them is hypovolemia from hyperemesis gravidarum. This clinical condition is defined as nausea and vomiting in pregnancy that is significant enough to cause volume depletion and weight loss. If volume depletion is severe enough, or if there is an additional mechanism of renal injury such use of nonsteroidal anti-inflammatory drugs, AKI from acute tubular necrosis (ATN) may result. The diagnosis of prerenal AKI in pregnancy is made the same way as in nonpregnant patients. History and physical examination findings are essential components. In the

absence of ATN, women with prerenal AKI in pregnancy will have a low urine sodium and low urine fractional excretion of sodium (FeNa) as intact tubules attempt to replenish intravascular volume. An increased BUN-to-creatinine ratio may also be seen. Treatment consists of symptomatic relief of vomiting and, if severe, repletion with intravenous fluids.

2. Acute Tubular Necrosis

▸ ATN is diagnosed by clinical suspicion.
▸ Urine microscopy may show renal tubular epithelial cells and muddy brown casts.
▸ Urine sodium tends to be above 20 mEq/L.

ATN as a cause of AKI may occur early in pregnancy as a result of a septic abortion or other infection. In the developing world, or in areas of the world where therapeutic abortion is not legal, septic abortion is more common. Usually these women will present with sepsis marked by fever, elevation in white blood cell count, and hypotension. Microscopy will reveal a urine sediment with renal tubular epithelial cells and muddy brown casts. Urine sodium will often be high (>20 mEq/L) as a result of tubular injury and subsequent inability to maximally reabsorb filtered sodium. Treatment is supportive, including hemodynamic support in the form of volume repletion, pressors, antibiotics, and electrolyte management. Renal replacement therapy may be required in some cases, but should be temporary.

3. Urinary Tract Infections

ESSENTIALS OF DIAGNOSIS

- ▸ Asymptomatic bacteriuria should be treated in pregnancy to prevent complications.
- ▸ After treatment for a urinary tract infection in pregnancy, women should be screened with monthly urine cultures.
- ▸ Pyelonephritis usually requires hospitalization and intravenous antibiotics.

Table 54–5. Commonly used antibiotics for UTIs in pregnancy.

Asymptomatic Bacteriuria and Cystitis	Pyelonephritis
Amoxicillin	Aztreonam
Amoxicillin-clavulanate	Ampicillin + gentamycin
Cephalexin	Cefepime
Nitrofurantoin	Ceftriaxone
Trimethoprim-sulfamethoxazole	Ertapenem
	Meropenem
	Piperacillin-tazobactam

Cystitis and pyelonephritis are more common in pregnancy than in the general population and may occur at any time. Progesterone-mediated smooth muscle relaxation in the ureters may contribute to the ascent of bacteria from the bladder into the kidney itself. An increase in urinary stasis in the dilated renal collecting system, as well as pressure on the bladder from the enlarging uterus, also predisposes women to ascending infections; there is a 40% increased risk of pyelonephritis in pregnant women with asymptomatic bacteriuria compared to nonpregnant women. Pyelonephritis is associated with preterm birth, low birth weight, and perinatal mortality; it therefore needs to be managed aggressively and prevented if possible.

The mainstay of prevention is screening for and treatment of asymptomatic bacteriuria. Asymptomatic bacteriuria occurs in approximately 5% of pregnant women and is most common in the first trimester. Without any suppressive antibiotic therapy, up to 40% of those women with asymptomatic bacteriuria will develop either symptomatic cystitis or pyelonephritis as the pregnancy progresses. It is for this reason that all pregnant women should be screened early in pregnancy with a urine culture. If negative, women do not need repeat screening, but those at higher risk of infection may need rescreening. A screen is positive when there are greater than 10^5 colony forming units/mL (cfu/ mL) on a clean-catch voided specimen. Guidelines suggest a repeat confirmatory test, but in practice, this is often not done. Asymptomatic bacteriuria should be treated in all pregnant women (Table 54–5). Most commonly the pathogen involved is *Escherichia coli*, but other enteric gram negative rods such as *Klebsiella* or *Enterobacter* are common, as is group B streptococcus. Antibiotic duration is 3–7 days, with a follow-up urine culture to ensure clearance at the end of the antibiotic course.

Lower urinary tract infections (cystitis) and upper urinary tract infections (pyelonephritis) may result in ATN. Acute cystitis often presents with classic symptoms of dysuria, urinary urgency and frequency, and fever. Empiric treatment should be started while the urine culture is pending. In the setting of cystitis symptoms, a positive result is a urine culture with greater than 10^3 cfu/mL of bacterial growth. Treatment is normally 3–7 days with a follow-up culture a week after treatment is completed. Screening with repeat urine cultures monthly for the duration of pregnancy may be warranted.

Pyelonephritis in pregnancy often presents the same way it does in the nonpregnant woman with fever, flank pain, vomiting, and costovertebral angle tenderness. Women often appear very ill; they are at risk for septic shock and acute respiratory distress syndrome (ARDS). Urine studies will show pyuria, but imaging studies are not routinely necessary because of radiation exposure to the developing fetus. An exception to this is when signs, symptoms, or the bacterial pathogen in the urine (such as proteus) are suggestive of obstructing stone as the etiology of the pyelonephritis; in that case, imaging with ultrasound is indicated to determine need for urologic intervention, although direct cystoscopy and ureteroscopy may be preferred. The infection may not be cleared unless the infected stone is removed.

Women with pyelonephritis in pregnancy should be admitted to the hospital and managed with intravenous antibiotics. Once afebrile for 48 hours, the women may be transitioned to oral antibiotics and treated for 10–14 days. Low-dose suppressive therapy should be offered to women for the duration of the pregnancy to prevent recurrence. Typically, nitrofurantoin or cephalexin is used.

AKI IN THE SECOND HALF OF PREGNANCY (20–40 WEEKS' GESTATION)

AKI that occurs in the second half of pregnancy is often more complicated to diagnose and treat. Preeclampsia and the thrombotic microangiopathies classically occur late in pregnancy. Renal cortical necrosis, often following an obstetric emergency, and postrenal obstruction are also possible. Acute fatty liver of pregnancy and hemolytic uremic syndrome can often look similar and must be distinguished by careful history and evaluation. For each of these causes of AKI later in pregnancy, we will discuss the presenting signs and symptoms, diagnostic approach, and management strategies.

1. Thrombotic Microangiopathies (TMAs)

ESSENTIALS OF DIAGNOSIS

▶ TMAs are defined by hemolytic anemia with schisto-cytes on peripheral blood smear.

▶ In addition to anemia, most TMAs have thrombocyto-penia and AKI.

▶ General Considerations

AKI in association with thrombotic microangiopathy usually occurs late in pregnancy. Many different diseases manifest as thrombotic microangiopathies, which is defined by thrombosis and RBC shearing in the microvasculature; these include preeclampsia/eclampsia, the hemolysis elevated liver enzymes low platelets (HELLP) syndrome, thrombotic thrombocytopenia purpura (TTP), and hemolytic uremic syndrome (HUS). There is significant overlap between many of these syndromes; most of them will appear with AKI, low platelet count, and evidence of microangiopathic hemolytic anemia (MAHA). All of them will have schistocytes on the peripheral blood smear, which reflect the common mechanism of injury in the capillary beds. Many TMAs may be acquired in the setting of pregnancy, but it is important to evaluate for genetic causes in select patients as it will impact outcomes in future pregnancies.

▶ Clinical Findings

All the thrombotic microangiopathies typically present similarly with AKI, thrombocytopenia, proteinuria, hypertension, and edema late in pregnancy. In TTP, the full clinical pentad (microangiopathic hemolytic anemia, AKI, thrombocytopenia, fever, and neurologic symptoms) is present in only a small proportion of patients. Mechanistically, we now understand that this disease results from congenital deficiency or acquired inhibitor of ADAMTS13, an enzyme which cleaves Von Willebrand factor multimers. However, pregnancy itself causes a physiologic reduction in the ADAMTS13 enzyme as well as a physiologic increase in Von Willebrand factor, which is thought to decrease the risk of bleeding at delivery. The diagnosis is confirmed by

measuring the ADAMTS13 level; an activity level less than 10% of normal is diagnostic for TTP. A mixing study can distinguish the acquired from congenital type of TTP, which will have important implications for future pregnancies.

In HUS, the most distinct aspect of the syndrome is the timing of presentation, which occurs during the postpartum period in 80% of cases. Like the other thrombotic microangiopathies, the clinical syndrome of HUS consists of renal impairment, thrombocytopenia, and microangiopathic hemolytic anemia. Although in nonpregnant patients HUS tends to follow an infectious insult, such enterocolitis from a toxigenic strains of *E Coli*, in pregnancy the trigger is unknown. There is ongoing research on the role of compliment cascade dysregulation in the pathogenesis of HUS; improved understanding of the cause of this syndrome may lead to improved therapeutics in the near future.

▶ Treatment

Treatment for the TMAs is based on the underlying etiology, so accurate diagnosis is important. Supportive therapy is essential, with dialysis sometimes required. TTP is managed with steroids and exchange plasmapheresis; in some cases, rituximab is added. Exchange plasmapheresis consists of removing the patient's plasma and replacing it with donor fresh frozen plasma and cryoprecipitate; this effectively replaces the deficient enzyme. Treatment for atypical HUS consists of supportive care and, more recently, C5-targeted therapy with eculizumab. Management of preeclampsia and HELLP syndrome consist of hypertension management, supportive care, and delivery.

▶ Prognosis

Before targeted disease specific therapy was developed for the TMAs in pregnancy, mortality was quite high. Timely diagnosis and aggressive management are critical. Currently, prognosis is quite good, although many women will be left with CKD, and more rarely ESRD.

2. Preeclampsia and Eclampsia

ESSENTIALS OF DIAGNOSIS

▶ Preeclampsia = hypertension + edema + proteinuria after 20th week of gestation

▶ Eclampsia = Preeclampsia + seizure

▶ General Considerations

Preeclampsia is defined as the new onset of hypertension and greater than 300 mg/day of proteinuria that begins after 20 weeks of gestation (Table 54–6). Preeclampsia may be

Table 54–6. ACOG diagnostic criteria for preeclampsia.

Blood pressure	Systolic > or = 140 or diastolic > or = 90 • On two occasions at least 4 hours apart • After 20 weeks' gestation • In a woman with previously normal blood pressure
AND	
Proteinuria	Any of the following: • 300 mg/24 hours urine collection[a] • Protein/creatinine ratio > or = 0.3 • Dipstick reading of 1+ proteinuria
OR any of the following:	
Thrombocytopenia	Platelets <100,000/μL
Renal insufficiency	Creatinine >1.1 or doubling of baseline
Impaired liver function	Transaminases >2 × upper limit of normal
Pulmonary edema	
Cerebral or visual symptoms	

[a]Or same amount extrapolated from a timed collection.

subdivided into early-onset preeclampsia (diagnosed before 34 weeks) and late-onset preeclampsia (diagnosed after 34 weeks) (Table 54–7). It can be accompanied by serious maternal morbidity and mortality if left untreated. HELLP syndrome may represent a severe form of preeclampsia, although this remains controversial as some women presenting with HELLP are not hypertensive. Thankfully, most cases of preeclampsia are mild and resolve with delivery, but those that are more serious require intervention.

Risk factors for preeclampsia include preexisting hypertension, chronic kidney disease, proteinuria, advanced maternal age (older than 35 years), preexisting diabetes, multiple gestations, or vascular or rheumatologic disease

Table 54–7. Early and late preeclampsia.

Early Preeclampsia (onset before 34 weeks)	Late Preeclampsia (onset after 34 weeks)
Uncommon (0.3%)	More common (2.7%)
Extensive vascular lesions of the placenta	Fewer gross placental lesions
Strong association with black race	Strong association with maternal metabolic syndrome

Table 54–8. Risk factors for preeclampsia.

Personal or family history of preeclampsia
Advanced maternal age (>35 years)
Hypertension
Proteinuria
Diabetic nephropathy
Gestational diabetes
Lupus with antiphospholipid antibody syndrome
CKD from any cause
Nulliparity
Multiple-gestation pregnancy

(Table 54–8). Although all of those risk factors are characteristics of the mother, there may also be paternal genetic factors that contribute to defective placentation and the evolution of preeclampsia. A family history of preeclampsia raises risk by two- to fivefold.

Eclampsia is recognized by the new onset of grand mal seizures in a woman with preeclampsia. It is rare, but develops more commonly in nulliparous women of low socioeconomic status. Although the cause of eclamptic seizures is not fully understood, they are usually self-limited and resolve with delivery of the fetus.

Pathogenesis

Abnormal placentation, placental ischemia, and endothelial dysfunction are critical elements in the pathogenesis of preeclampsia and HELLP. Early in gestation, abnormal trophoblasts invade the maternal endothelium and spiral arteries. These trophoblasts preclude the formation of the low resistance, highly capacitance uteroplacental circulation that is essential for a healthy placenta. Resultant placental underperfusion and hypoxia may lead to release of certain circulating anti-angiogenic factors (including soluble fms-like tyrosine kinase and soluble endoglin, among others) that lead to diffuse endothelial dysfunction. This endothelial injury manifests with multiorgan involvement, hemolysis, hypertension, and proteinuria.

Prevention

Over the years, many different agents have been tried as preventive strategies against preeclampsia. For now, the only proven preventive therapy in high-risk patients is a low-dose daily aspirin. Those characterized as high risk, include women with a history of preeclampsia, multiple-gestation pregnancy, diabetes (type 1 or 2), chronic kidney disease, hypertension, and preexisting autoimmune disease. Low-risk women should not be treated preventively.

Clinical Findings

Symptoms of preeclampsia normally develop late in the pregnancy, but may begin as early as 20 weeks. Hypertension usually develops gradually, and initially it is asymptomatic. Because most women drop their blood pressure during the first and second trimester, early preeclamptic increases in blood pressure may go unnoticed. A rise in baseline blood pressure, even to a level that remains within the normal range, may be a sign of preeclampsia. The diagnosis is confirmed by the finding of an increased blood pressure on two occasions at least 6 hours apart, but no more than 7 days apart. Edema, which often occurs in normal pregnancy, may be more abrupt or severe in preeclampsia and occurs even with a fall in intravascular volume. Neurologic signs and symptoms include headache, blurred vision, scotoma, and cortical blindness (which is very rare and represents severe preeclampsia) (Table 54–9). All signs and symptoms of preeclampsia generally resolve within 2–6 weeks of delivery.

Laboratory Findings

Proteinuria detected by urinary dipstick is often the first laboratory finding to suggest preeclampsia. One must be sure that the positive dipstick is not a false positive in the setting of a high specific gravity. Although the 24-hour urine collection remains the gold standard for proteinuria measurement, many nephrologists have shifted to the random or "spot" urine protein-to-creatinine ratio. Twenty-four hour urine collections results are plagued by incomplete collections, particularly in the setting of pregnancy, where frequent urination and habitus make the collection a challenge for women. Therefore, the spot ratio has become more routine and rapid results can allow plans to be made quickly. Urine microscopy is often benign.

Blood tests are also often abnormal in preeclampsia. Thrombocytopenia, hyperuricemia, hypocalcemia and microangiopathic hemolytic anemia are common. The latter is accompanied by an elevation in lactate dehydrogenase and a blood smear with schistocytes. Hemolysis in the setting of elevated liver enzymes suggests that preeclampsia is evolving into HELLP syndrome.

Most women with preeclampsia have normal renal function. However, if glomerular permeability is altered by vascular changes, or if preeclampsia becomes severe with features of a microangiopathic hemolytic anemia, then AKI may develop.

Much active research is being published on the utility of screening with uterine artery Doppler ultrasonography or measurement of serum or urine placental-related peptides such as soluble fms-like tyrosine kinase 1 (sFlt-1) placental growth factor (PlGF). For example, the PROGNOSIS study in 2016 reported that the ratio of sFlt-1 to PlGF is a reliable way to rule out preeclampsia in women in whom it is suspected clinically; in that study, sFlt-1: PlGF <38 had a negative predictive value of 99% for the development of preeclampsia in the subsequent week after testing. Although some of the data looks promising, these tests remain currently experimental.

Renal biopsy should not be needed to make the diagnosis of preeclampsia. If performed, it should show endothelial cell swelling with loss of fenestrations and occlusion of the capillary lumen. There is no significant podocyte effacement and there should be no deposits.

Treatment

Treatment of mild preeclampsia includes close maternal and fetal monitoring with a goal of keeping the serum blood pressure approximately 140–150/90–105 mm Hg. Medications commonly used for hypertension in pregnancy are listed in Table 54–1. Strict bed rest may predispose to lower extremity thrombosis, but it does appear that rest in the left lateral decubitus position may help lower blood pressure. Close monitoring of fetal growth and evaluation for oligohydramnios should be undertaken at the time of diagnosis and followed closely by obstetrics (Figure 54–2). Severe preeclampsia must be treated by urgent delivery, and intravenous magnesium sulfate should be given to prevent eclampsia. If delivery is early, corticosteroids should be given to enhance lung maturation in the developing fetus. Eclamptic seizures are true obstetric emergencies that pose significant risk of death or neurologic sequelae if not managed quickly. Magnesium sulfate is the drug of choice for eclamptic seizures, although phenytoin may also have a role.

Prognosis

Mild preeclampsia occurring near term is associated with a very good outcome in both mother and child. Hypertension is usually controllable with oral medications, and

Table 54–9. Features of severe preeclampsia (any of the following).

Systolic blood pressure > or = 160 mm Hg
Diastolic blood pressure > or = 110
Thrombocytopenia (platelets < 100,000/μL)
Transaminase elevation to twice the upper limit of normal
Severe right upper quadrant pain not accounted for by alternative diagnosis
Progressive renal insufficiency
Pulmonary edema
Cerebral or visual disturbances

delivery is curative. More severe preeclampsia is associated with higher morbidity as well as higher rates of recurrence. Preeclampsia is primarily a disease of nulliparous women, but women with a history of severe preeclampsia early in pregnancy are at higher risk of the disease recurring in a future pregnancy. Preeclampsia is also considered a risk factor for the development of hypertension, chronic kidney disease, and cardiovascular disease later in the mother's life. Although the prognosis for mothers with HELLP is generally very good, there is a significant (20%) risk of preeclampsia in a future pregnancy. Eclampsia is very serious with most women suffering long-term complications from the disease, particularly those who develop the disease earlier in pregnancy.

KEY READINGS

Chaiworapongsa T et al: Pre-eclampsia part 1: current understanding of its pathophysiology. Nat Rev Nephrol 2014;10:466.

Fakhouri F, Vercel C, Frémeaux-Bacchi V: Obstetric nephrology: AKI and thrombotic microangiopathies in pregnancy. Clin J Am Soc Nephrol 2012;7:2100.

Karumanchi SA, Granger JP: Preeclampsia and pregnancy related hypertensive disorders. Hypertension 2016;67:238.

Zeisler H et al: Predictive value of the sFlt-1:PlGF ratio in women with suspected preeclampsia. N Engl J Med 2016;374:13.

3. Acute Fatty Liver of Pregnancy

General Considerations

Acute fatty liver of pregnancy (AFLP) is a disorder unique to pregnancy that is characterized by fatty infiltration of hepatocytes. It is thankfully quite rare, but more common in pregnancies with multiple gestations or in women who are underweight. It often presents late in pregnancy, sometimes even in the post-partum period. Although the precise cause is uncertain, AFLP is associated with impaired mitochondrial fatty acid metabolism; deficiency in long-chain 3-hydroxyacyl CoA dehydrogenase (LCHAD) remains an area of active investigation. Because of this, both mother and newborn of those affected should undergo molecular testing for at least the most common mutation.

Clinical Findings

Women with AFLP often present with nausea, vomiting, abdominal pain, and acute hepatitis marked by elevated transaminases and bilirubin. Differentiating AFLP from HELLP may be challenging as they present with similar features. AFLP, however, is distinctive in that it can cause acute liver failure, which manifests as coagulopathy, hypoglycemia, and encephalopathy. Disseminated intravascular coagulation (DIC) is also possible. AKI is common.

Imaging by duplex ultrasonography may be undertaken to rule out hepatic infarction, venous thrombosis, or hepatoma, but is not always required.

Liver biopsy is diagnostic when it shows microvesicular fatty infiltration of hepatocytes. Fatty infiltration is most prominent in the central parts of the lobule leading to an appearance of central pallor. Liver biopsy is not always needed for the diagnosis, and should be reserved for select cases.

Treatment

It can be very difficult to separate AFLP from HELLP and often one treats for both conditions. Urgent delivery is necessary, regardless of gestational age. Maternal support with blood products (if indicated for coagulopathy), glucose infusion, and blood pressure control are essential.

Prognosis

Although in the past this condition was universally fatal, most affected women who are treated with prompt delivery and supportive care now recover fully with no long-term liver or renal impairment. AFLP may recur in future pregnancies, so women with this history should be monitored closely by maternal-fetal medicine experts. Infants who inherited an LCHAD mutation, when stressed, may develop fatal nonketotic hypoglycemia and therefore should be followed by a pediatric genetics or metabolism specialist.

4. Cortical Necrosis

General Considerations

Renal cortical necrosis is a rare but serious cause of pregnancy-related AKI. It usually presents after an obstetric emergency, such as placental abruption with massive hemorrhage or amniotic fluid embolism. Hypotension and ischemia to the kidney are frequently accompanied by DIC.

Clinical Findings

Women with cortical necrosis will normally present with acute onset of flank pain and AKI. They often have hematuria and oliguria as well. Kidney ultrasound is diagnostic by the findings of hypoechoic or hypodense areas of the renal cortex.

Treatment

Supportive therapy is all that is available at this time.

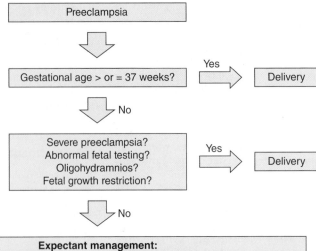

▲ **Figure 54–2.** Management of preeclampsia.

Prognosis

Many women with renal cortical necrosis will require dialysis with only some recovering some kidney function over time. Most are left with advanced CKD.

5. Postrenal Obstruction in Pregnancy

Pathogenesis

Renal obstruction may be noticed on a routine ultrasound during pregnancy. It may or may not be associated with AKI. Although true obstruction from a developing fetus and placenta compressing the outflow track is possible, it is very rare. Polyhydramnios has also been noted to cause obstructive AKI, although also rare. Clinicians should be mindful that progesterone-mediated dilation of the collecting system and ureters is common and normal in pregnancy. It is most commonly right-sided and women will have normal kidney function bilaterally. This "physiologic hydronephrosis" may result from hormonal effects on ureteral tone, or be related to the angle of the ureter as it crosses the pelvic brim on the right. Maintaining the pregnant woman in the lateral recumbent position may improve the situation. Physiologic hydronephrosis needs no direct intervention and should resolve within 3 months of delivery.

Nephrolithiasis is common in the latter half of pregnancy and may obstruct the ureter. Although calcium oxalate stones are the most common type of stone in nonpregnant individuals, calcium phosphate stones are the most common in women who are pregnant. Risk factor for stone formation includes urinary stasis in the dilated collecting system, changes in urinary pH, and increased urinary calcium excretion during pregnancy. Although AKI may result from severe unilateral obstruction due to nephrolithiasis, it is more common in the patient with a solitary functioning kidney or bilateral obstruction.

Clinical Findings

Women with the normal physiologic hydronephrosis of pregnancy will be asymptomatic. In cases where polyhydramnios causes postrenal obstruction, the most common time of detection is during routine ultrasound. Nephrolithiasis should present with renal colic and hematuria as it does in nonpregnant patients.

Treatment

Pathologic kidney obstruction should be managed quickly in pregnancy to avoid progressive AKI. The normal physiologic dilation of pregnancy needs no therapy, but obstruction from polyhydramnios would need to be treated with draining of the excessive amniotic fluid.

Kidney stones pose a challenge as imaging modalities are limited. Ultrasound is preferred. Although the sensitivity and specificity of ultrasound are inferior to those of CT scan, the radiation exposure of a CT scan should be avoided if possible. Most stones will pass on their own with conventional therapies, but consultation with urology for an obstructing stone is needed in some cases, particularly if there is clinical concern for infection.

Prognosis

Once obstruction is relieved, the prognosis for the maternal AKI is good and should be managed as in the nonpregnant patient.

KEY READINGS

Fakhouri F, Vercel C, Fremeaux-Bacchi V: Obstetric nephrology: AKI and thrombotic microangiopathies in pregnancy. C J Am Soc Nephrol 2012;7:2100.
Nwoko R, Plecas D, Garovic VD: Acute kidney injury in the pregnant patient. Clin Nephrol 2012;78:478.

■ CHAPTER REVIEW QUESTIONS

1. The upper limit of normal for serum creatinine is lower in pregnancy than in age-matched nonpregnant women because
   A. Progesterone interferes with the creatinine assay.
   B. Pregnant women have lower rates of muscle breakdown.
   C. Increased GFR leads to increased creatinine clearance.
   D. Creatinine is cleared by both maternal and fetal kidneys.

2. Which of the following is TRUE regarding pregnancy in a woman with a renal transplant?
   A. Azathioprine and cyclosporine are mainstays of immunosuppression.
   B. Women with pelvic grafts should always have cesarean sections.
   C. Reactivation of viral infections may affect fetal health.
   D. Prednisone is a teratogen.
   E. A and C.
   F. B and C.

3. Atypical HUS in pregnancy is a thrombotic microangiopathy that most often

A. Occurs in women with lupus and antiphospholipid antibody syndrome
B. Occurs after delivery of the fetus
C. Presents with acute liver failure
D. Results in seizures and permanent neurologic sequelae

4. Which of the following is TRUE about preeclampsia?
   A. Pathogenesis is related to dysfunctional placental vascularity and blood flow.
   B. It never affects nulliparous women.
   C. By definition, it does not occur in women with prepregnancy hypertension.
   D. Proteinuria in preeclampsia cannot be diagnosed by spot protein:creatinine ratio.

5. Polyhydramnios in a pregnant woman with ESRD is caused by
   A. Increased maternal total body water
   B. Decreased placental oncotic pressure
   C. Fetal nephrotic syndrome
   D. Fetal diuresis due to high maternal BUN

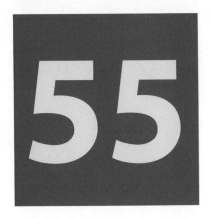

55

Aging and the Kidney

Seki A. Balogun, MBBS

Faruk H. Turgut, MD

Emaad Abdel-Rahman, MD, PhD

Aging is an inevitable biological process that affects many organ systems, of which the kidney is one of the most significantly affected. The process of aging is associated with renal changes, both physiologic and anatomical that differentiates the aged kidney from a younger one. These changes increase suspectibility to kidney injury and may lead to decline in kidney function. Apart from age associated changes in the kidney, older adults are more likely to have associated chronic medical conditions such as hypertension, diabetes mellitus (DM), issues with polypharmacy and exposure to other nephrotoxins. These conditions may further predispose older adults to chronic kidney disease (CKD) and in some cases ultimately lead to end-stage kidney disease (ESKD).

With an aging population that continues to grow, the prevalence of kidney disease tends to be higher in older adults. As a result of this, physicians increasingly have to manage older adults with acute kidney injury (AKI), various stages of CKD, as well as other renal pathologies. It is therefore imperative for clinicians, especially nephrologists, to acquire adequate knowledge about the unique characteristics of an aged kidney and its associated clinical implications in older adults.

In this chapter, we explore the structural and physiological changes that occur in the aging kidney, the common causes and treatment of kidney diseases in older adults, and unique challenges in managing older adults with kidney disease. For the purpose of this review, "older adults" will be used to describe persons age 65 years and older.

ANATOMICAL AND PHYSIOLOGICAL CHANGES IN THE AGING KIDNEY

With normal aging, structural and functional changes occur in the kidneys. These changes are different from those that are disease-mediated. The decline in kidney function noted with normal aging is associated with preserved proximal tubular function and normal serum erythropoietin, hemoglobin levels, serum urea, urinalysis as well as normal metabolic indices such as phosphorus, calcium, parathyroid hormone. This is further supported by the fact that only a small proportion of older adults with decline in kidney function progress to ESKD.

The major histological features of renal aging are arterial intimal fibrosis as well as glomerulosclerosis, tubular atrophy and interstitial fibrosis. Structural and functional changes in normal aging are summarized in Table 55–1. These structural changes in older adult kidneys result in decrease in the total kidney volume with aging especially after age 50 years. In addition, there are several radiological changes that are more evident in the aging kidney such as kidney cysts, focal scars, increased cortical surface roughness and medullary volume, and decreased parenchymal thickness.

UNIQUE CHARACTERISTICS OF RENAL DISEASES IN OLDER ADULTS

Changes in the kidney function with normal aging often overlap with pathologic processes, making the diagnosis of kidney diseases in older adults challenging. In addition, symptoms of kidney diseases can be confused with those of normal aging such as easy fatigability, sleep disturbance and cognitive changes. Furthermore laboratory tests such as serum creatinine level may remain within normal limits despite the decline in glomerular filtration rate (GFR), due to reduced muscle mass with aging. All of these factors may contribute to misdiagnosis of renal diseases in older adults.

Although older adults are prone to the same kidney diseases as younger patients, the etiology, disease course and management of kidney diseases may differ based on the age of the patient.

Table 55–1. Changes in kidney with normal aging.

Affected Parts of Kidney	Structural Changes	Functional Changes
Glomeruli	- Globally sclerosed glomeruli - Glomerular ischemia - Decrease number of functional glomeruli - Compensatory hypertrophy in remaining functional glomeruli - Thickening of glomerular basement membrane - Mesangial expansion	-Decreased GFR -Diminished renal reserve
Tubulo-interstitium	Tubule atrophies occur with fibrosis accumulating in the surrounding interstitium	- Altered tubular handling of creatinine - Reduction in sodium reabsorption and potassium secretion - Inability to maximally concentrate and dilute the urine
Vasculature	- Arteriosclerosis of the small arteries - Arterial intima becomes less smooth and displays endothelial dysfunction - Subendothelial deposition of hyaline and collagen fibers - Intimal thickening and obliteration of afferent and efferent arterioles - Vascular stiffening and atrophy of the vascular media Thickening of large vessels walls	- Decrease Renal Blood Flow - Vascular dysautonomia

ACUTE KIDNEY INJURY

General Considerations

Acute kidney injury (AKI) is more common in older patients than in younger patients. There are several risk factors that predispose older adults to AKI (Table 55–2).

Pathogenesis

In older adults, the etiology of AKI is often multifactorial and sometimes iatrogenic. While pre renal AKI may be due to hypoperfusion with volume deficiency, numerous intrarenal causes of AKI can affect older adults. The most frequent mechanisms for intrarenal AKI in these patients are prolonged hypoperfusion and sepsis leading to acute tubular necrosis (ATN). The administration of nephrotoxic agents may also cause ATN or acute interstitial nephritis (AIN). Other intrarenal causes include acute glomerulonephritis, which could be severe, requiring intensive therapy. AKI due to obstructive nephropathy is also common in older adults,

Table 55–2. Risk factors for AKI in the older adults.

Structural and functional changes with aging
Multiple comorbidities (CKD, hypertension, CHF, DM)
Polypharmacy (ACEI, ARB, NSAID)
Multiple invasive procedures (vascular and cardiac surgeries, nephrotoxic contrast dyes with procedures)

especially men with enlarged prostate from benign prostatic hypertrophy and prostate cancer.

Clinical Findings

AKI is generally detected by an increase in the serum creatinine and/or a decrease in urine output. History and physical examination is critical to narrow the differential diagnosis. The laboratory evaluation of older patients with AKI is not different from other patients. Microscopic urine examination is also a useful diagnostic tool where the presence of muddy brown casts can be diagnostic of ATN and the presence of dysmorphic red blood cells and/or red blood cell casts indicative of glomerular pathology.

Management

Management of AKI in older adults is similar to that in younger patients. It requires careful monitoring of fluid and electrolyte balance, and preventive strategies such as avoiding nephrotoxins, radiocontrast agents, and volume depletion. Urethral catheterization and/or ultrasonography should be performed to exclude possible obstructive etiologies in the initial assessment. Though volume status assessment can be challenging in this population, volume status should be carefully evaluated to guide further management. Renal function usually improves to normal levels with rehydration in older adults with prerenal AKI, provided there is no permanent kidney damage. In patients with persistent severe AKI, standard dialytic techniques including slow continuous methods should be considered. The decision on whether or not to proceed with dialysis in very elderly patients with severe AKI can be difficult. These patients frequently have multiple comorbidities that are associated with a poor prognosis. Frank discussion with patients and their families about prognosis is often warranted.

Prognosis

The prognosis of AKI in older adults depends on its severity and on the underlying disease. Multiple studies have demonstrated worse outcomes in older adults with AKI. Nonrecovery of renal function after an AKI episode in these patients is common due to their multiple risk factors stated above. Even if the kidney function recovers after an episode of AKI, these patients will need to be monitored closely as they may develop CKD.

GLOMERULAR DISEASES

General Considerations

While normal aging may be associated with decline of GFR, the presence of proteinuria and active urinary sediment should hint to the presence of renal glomerular disease rather than age-related reduction in GFR. Glomerular diseases in older adults may present with different clinical symptoms (Table 55-3), and the etiology could be either primary or secondary to various diseases (Table 55-4). Most patients present with one of two patterns, nephrotic or nephritic syndrome. The underlying etiology of nephrotic syndrome includes membranous nephropathy (MN), minimal change disease (MCD), and amyloidosis.

1. Membranous Nephropathy

Idiopathic MN is the most commonly encountered glomerular pathology in older adults. Eighty percent of MN are idiopathic and twenty percent are secondary to other causes such as solid organ tumors. Therefore, older patients should undergo a thorough examination to exclude secondary causes. While most patients with MN present with typical features of the nephrotic syndrome (>85%), few patients present with asymptomatic proteinuria, often without hematuria. Older patients with MN are more likely to

Table 55-3. The main presenting features of glomerular disease.

Asymptomatic hematuria and/or proteinuria
Nephritic syndrome
Nephrotic syndrome
Rapidly progressive glomerulonephritis
Chronic glomerular disease

Table 55-4. The common glomerular disease in older adults.

Primary Glomerular Disease	Secondary Glomerular Disease
Membranous nephropathy	Diabetic glomerulosclerosis
Minimal change disease	Systemic amyloidosis
Focal and segmental glomerulosclerosis	Systemic necrotizing and crescentic glomerulonephritis
Focal proliferative glomerulonephritis	Malignancy-related glomerulopathy
Crescentic glomerulonephritis	Lupus nephritis
Membranoproliferative glomerulonephritis	

have hypertension and hematuria compared to younger patients, they also demonstrate renal impairment at the time of kidney biopsy more frequently than younger patients.

2. Minimal Change Disease

MCD in older patients typically presents as nephrotic syndrome and the etiology of 15–20% of older individuals with nephrotic syndrome is MCD. Similar to patients with MN, older patients with MCD have microscopic hematuria, hypertension, and renal impairment more frequent at the time of presentation than in younger patients. Most common causes of MCD in older adults are medications such as nonsteriodal anti-inflammatory drugs and hematologic malignanices.

3. Proliferative Glomerulonephritis

Crescentic glomerulonephritis can be associated with circulating antiglomerular antibodies (AGBM), glomerular immune complex localization as seen in severe IgA nephropathy or lupus nephritis, or with pauci-immune disease without immune deposits as seen in antineutrophil cytoplasmic antibody (ANCA)-associated vasculitis. IgA nephropathy and lupus nephritis are uncommon in older adults. Diagnosis of lupus in older adults with or without nephritis is often delayed. Pauci-immune crescentic glomerulonephritis is a more common form of glomerular disease in older persons, and its incidence increases steadily with age.

4. Diagnosis of Glomerular Diseases

A stepwise approach to the diagnosis of the underlying condition of glomerular diseases in older adults is needed. In addition to standard laboratory testing in patients with evidence of glomerular disease, serologic testing consisting of antinuclear antibodies (ANA), ANCA, anti-GBM antibody, viral hepatitis markers and measurement of serum complement levels to detect hypocomplementemia may be included.

The systemic (extrarenal) features, the characteristics of the urine sediment and the degree of proteinuria usually help to narrow the differential diagnosis. Renal biopsy is often required for definitive diagnosis and does not carry a higher risk in older adults compared to younger patients. However, age-mediated changes in the kidney may render the interpretation of histologic findings more difficult.

5. Management of Glomerular Diseases

Treatment approaches and outcomes of glomerular diseases are similar in older and younger individuals. Conservative management (salt restriction; loop-acting diuretics; antihypertensive agents, mainly renin angiotensin aldosterone blockers) is indicated in the following situations: when proteinuria is modest (<4 g/day), the symptoms of nephrotic syndrome are tolerable, or in the absence of progression of kidney disease. If there is hypercholesterolemia, concomitant therapy with a statin may be indicated.

The treatment of lupus nephritis as well as cresentic glomerulonephritis are similar across all age groups. Treatment with a standard immunosuppressive regimen may be used in older adults with caution and appropriate dosing adjustment. Both immunosuppressants and plasmapheresis may be associated with higher risk of opportunistic infections and complications, particularly in those of very advanced age.

RENOVASCULAR DISEASE

Renovascular diseases are encountered usually in patients with atherosclerotic disease and include two entities: renal artery stenosis (RAS) or microvascular (atheroembolic) disease affecting intrarenal arteries.

1. Renal Artery Stenosis

General Considerations

RAS is often asymptomatic; however, it can be an important, potentially treatable cause of secondary hypertension. The progressive narrowing of the renal arteries and/or progressive intrinsic renal disease may cause ischemic nephropathy.

Clinical Findings

RAS should be suspected in patients who develop AKI after a mild hypotensive episode or with the use of angiotensin blockers, flash pulmonary edema, resistant hypertension, or in cases of renal impairment of unknown etiology.

Diagnosis

Several imaging studies can be used to diagnose renovascular disease; duplex doppler ultrasonography, computed tomographic angiography and magnetic resonance angiography. However, the gold standard for diagnosing RAS is renal arteriography, which can be beneficial in older patients with close follow up of kidney function. The test of choice should be based on the presence or absence of renal insufficiency, local availability and clinical expertise with each technique.

Management

Once a diagnosis of renovascular disease is made, medical therapy and risk factor reduction should be considered. Revascularization should be considered in patients with significant stenosis (usually more than 70% luminal occlusion) of both renal arteries or of one renal artery in a patient with a solitary functioning kidney.

2. Atheroembolic Disease

General Considerations

This entity may occur as a consequence of atrial fibrillation, subacute bacterial endocarditis, extensive surgery, and angiography. Cholesterol embolization after intravascular procedures or surgery may lead to acute decline in kidney function. Though microvascular disease of the kidney has not been extensively studied, it may eventually lead to ischemic nephropathy.

Clinical Findings

Patient may be asymptomatic or present with severe flank pain, hematuria, pyrexia, renal failure, and hypertension. They may also develop signs of cholesterol emobilization, including livido reticularis, change in mental status, bowel ischemia as well as peripheral eosinophilia.

Diagnosis

Small emboli may be difficult to diagnose while major emboli are defined by pyelography, renal scan, and aortography. Presence of cholesterol embolism is confirmed by renal biopsy (intravascular cholesterol crystals) and skin or muscle biopsy.

SYSTEMIC DISEASES & KIDNEYS IN THE OLDER ADULTS

Older patients frequently have comorbid conditions such as hypertension and DM that may contribute to the development of renal disease. While the incidence of primary renal diseases may decline with aging, the incidence of secondary renal diseases increases.

1. Diabetic Nephropathy (DN)

General Considerations

DM is common in older adults, as more than half of all diabetic individuals in the United States are over 60 years of age. Diabetic nephropathy (DN) is classically defined by the presence of progressive albuminuria with characteristic structural and functional changes in the kidney. DM type 2 (DMT2) is more common in older adults, with DN being a frequent finding at the time of diagnosis. DN continues to be the most common cause of ESRD in older patients.

Pathogenesis

The exact pathogenesis of DN is complex and not completely understood. Among the pathogenic factors are hyperglycemia, increased systemic and glomerular pressure, increased activity of the renin–angiotensin–aldosterone system (RAAS), and stimulation of several cytokines/growth factors by metabolic and hemodynamic factors. DN is most likely to occur in patients who have poor glycemic control and/or associated hypertension.

Management

Several therapeutic interventions targeting these mechanisms have been developed and implemented with varying degrees of success. Lifestyle modifications, optimal glycemic control, introduction of ACEIs or ARBs (as monotherapy) as first-line agents to control blood pressure (BP) optimally, and interventions for traditional cardiovascular risk factors are advised. Relatively healthy older adults with no major comorbidities may benefit from more intensive glucose control (target HBA_{1c} <7%), while more lenient targets may be more appropriate for older adults with major comorbidities, established diabetic end-organ damage or limited life expectancy. The doses of oral hypoglycemic agents and insulin may need to be decreased as the renal function declines, and more so in those of advanced age, to avoid hypoglycemia and other side effects. Several randomized controlled trials indicate that multiple antihypertensive agents, often more than three, are commonly required to achieve optimal BP control in older patients with DN. Nonpharmacologic approaches (dietary modifications, weight loss, and increased physical activity) are effective in reducing BP in nondiabetic individuals and may have similar benefits for diabetic patients. However, pharmacologic approaches remain the mainstay for controlling BP in patients with DM. Special attention should be paid in older patients with close monitoring of serum creatinine and potassium when using renin angiotensin blockers.

Prognosis

DMT2 is the leading cause of advanced CKD with mortality mostly secondary to cardiovascular disease. Approximately 40% of patients with DMT2 at the age of 45 are hypertensive; the proportion increases to 60% by the age of 75. Both systolic and diastolic hypertension markedly accelerate the progression of DN. Normotensive patients with advanced DN show slower progression compared with hypertensive patients of all ages.

2. Hypertension

General Considerations

Hypertension is very common in older adults, with prevalence as high as 60–80%. Isolated systolic hypertension is the most presentation in this age group. Older patients are more likely to be aware of their hypertension and more likely to be treated. They are, however, less likely to achieve BP control when compared with younger patients.

Management

Treatment of hypertension is crucial as untreated or poorly controlled hypertension is associated with permanent morbidity and mortality. Treating hypertension can both reduce the rate of cardiovascular complications as well as slow the progression of CKD. Many aspects of hypertension diagnosis and treatment are similar in younger and older patients; however, there are relevant issues that require attention while treating older adults. As in younger patients, the initial recommendation for older patients to achieve BP control is lifestyle modifications (eg, dietary salt restriction, weight loss in obese patients). In the absence of an indication for a specific BP medication, low-dose thiazide-type diuretic, ACEIs/ARBs, or long-acting calcium channel blocker may be started as initial monotherapy.

Currently, there is no clear consensus regarding the optimal target of BP in older adults. A recent review by Aronow on clinical practice recommendations by the American, European and Canadian associations suggest acceptable BP of less than 140/90 for patients aged 60–79 years and allowing systolic BP to be as high as 140–145 in patients 80 years and older. Intensive treatment particularly in isolated systolic hypertension may lower diastolic BP to suboptimal level that may cause coronary ischemia. Furthermore, older patients may have orthostatic hypotension, which may be aggravated by intensive antihypertensive therapy.

3. Multiple Myeloma

General Considerations

Multiple myeloma (MM) with associated renal disease is more frequent in older adults compared to younger patients. Renal disease most often occurs due to primary amyloidosis (AL type), tubular toxic effects of light chain, cast formation, and/or plasma cell infiltration. Presence of hypercalcemia, volume depletion, hyperuricemia, and nephrotoxic drugs may contribute to the development of AKI in patients in MM.

Management

Management of MM may involve use of bortezomib-based chemotherapy with renal support. Hypercalcemia and hyperuricemia secondary to chemotherapy can be prevented by adequate hydration and use of allopurinol.

Prognosis

The prognosis of MM depends on a variety of paraproteins, the stage of myeloma, and the type of chemotherapy. Patients with AKI due to dense cast formation and significant tubular damage are less likely to show improvement in kidney function. Patients with significant renal dysfunction at presentation tend to have worse outcomes.

OBSTRUCTIVE NEPHROPATHY

General Considerations

Urinary tract obstruction should always be considered in older patients with unexplained worsening renal function.

Clinical Findings

Urinary tract obstruction may be acute or chronic, partial or complete, and unilateral or bilateral. The obstruction can occur at any level of the urinary tract. In older males, the most common cause of lower urinary tract obstruction is benign prostatic hypertrophy or prostatic carcinoma. In older females, the most common cause of postrenal failure is ureteral obstruction caused by pelvic malignancy. Urethral stricture, often secondary to trauma, may also cause infravesical obstruction in those of advanced age. Patients with slowly developing obstruction typically have normal urinalysis.

Prognosis

Urinary tract obstruction may cause AKI or CKD and predispose to urinary tract infection or urosepsis.

URINARY TRACT INFECTIONS AND UROSEPSIS

General Considerations

Urinary tract infection (UTI) is very common in older adults. Older, frail, and less mobile patients are more susceptible to UTI. Predisposing factors include structural and functional abnormalities of the urinary tract, comorbid conditions such as DM, invasive instrumentation/operations, and bacterial virulence.

Clinical Findings

Common lower UTI syptoms include urgency, frequency, dysuria, and suprapubic tenderness. In addition to these symptoms, patients with upper UTI may present with impaired kidney function, fever, and costovertebral angle tenderness.

Diagnosis

The diagnosis of UTI is similar across age groups, including the presence of urinary symptoms and a positive urine culture.

Management

Trimethoprim/sulfamethoxazole, ciprofloxacin, or amoxicillin can be commenced empirically as first-line treatment for uncomplicated UTI until urine culture are available. On the other hand, acute pyelonephritis is often treated with intravenous antibiotics such as ampicillin and an aminoglycoside or a third-generation cephalosporin or a quinolone. However, over utilization of antibiotics may lead to development of multidrug resistant organisms. Therefore, a proper antibiotic selection should be based on urine culture and sensitivity results. Patients should also be evaluated for reversible causes such as obstruction, nephrolithiasis, cysts, neoplasia. Indwelling urethral catheters also play a significant role in the development of UTIs in older adults, therefore, prompt removal of the catheter is recommended when possible.

CHRONIC KIDNEY DISEASE

General Considerations

Chronic kidney disease (CKD) is of substantial concern in the older population. The prevalence and cumulative effects of risk factors for CKD such as hypertension and DM over many years increase with aging. As a result, the prevalence of ESKD requiring renal replacement therapy (RRT) has increased.

Prevalence of CKD in the adult population has gradually increased over the last three decades to peak rate of between 11% and 12% in the early 2000s, with the more recent report in 2016 showing an estimated rate of 13.6%.

Pathogenesis

The cause of CKD is often not readily apparent in many older patients. A combination of age-related structural and functional renal changes may lead to progressive reduction in GFR. Similarly, the increased prevalence of vascular diseases with advancing age contributes to the increased prevalence of CKD. Renal vascular disease may be the predominant etiology for CKD in this population as well as the presence of comorbid diseases as DM, hypertension and obesity. Longer duration and poor control of any of these comorbid diseases impose greater risk for CKD.

Another factor contributing to CKD in older adults is the frequent use of polypharmacy which may predispose to drug-induced acute or chronic tubulointerstitial nephropathy.

Clinical Findings

Older patients with CKD usually present with nonspecific symptoms, that may be confused with symptoms of the normal aging process or other comorbid conditions. This may contribute to delayed referral to the nephrologist.

The clasification of CKD based on GFR levels, is the same regardless of age. Various creatinine- and cystatin-based estimated GFR (eGFR) formulas are used to estimate kidney function; however, these formulas do not accurately estimate GFR in older adults.

Management

When managing CKD in older patients, age-related physiologic and pathophysiologic changes as well as comorbidities should be considered. Focus should be on control of hypertension, DM and proteinuria. Appropriate dietary modification may slow the progression of CKD. Salt intake should be limited with regular clinical monitoring of volume overload . Strict dietary protein restriction is often unnecessary. To avoid severe metabolic acidosis, serum bicarbonate levels should be checked regularly. Severe constipation, which is frequent in older adults, may exacerbate hyperkalemia. Starting erythropoiesis stimulating agents for anemia management in the predialysis phase (CKD stages 3–4) may improve the quality of life. Dialysis is often a valuable treatment option for ESKD, though other approaches may also be considered in that age group.

Older patients with CKD may present with two different types of metabolic bone diseases; osteoporosis with bone loss due to aging and CKD-mineral and bone disorder (CKD-MBD) due to metabolic and endocrine alterations. Mangement of CKD-MBD is similar across age groups and may include low dietary phosphorus and the use of phosphorus binders. For treatment of secondary hyperparathyroidism, vitamin D or its analogue as well as calcimemitics may be used.

Prognosis

Most older patients with CKD are less likely to progress to ESKD compared to younger age, because of slower progression in some cases and high mortality risk before developing ESKD. Regardless of the underlying cause of the CKD, proteinuria, and poorly controlled hypertension are strongly associated with more rapid progression of kidney disease. Finally, the presence of CKD increases the risk of other adverse age-related outcomes.

OPTIONS FOR RENAL REPLACEMENT THERAPY IN ELDERLY

General Considerations

Renal replacement therapy is a lifesaving treatment for patients with ESKD. An increasing proportion of individuals currently maintained on RRT include older patients. Treatment options for RRT are hemodialysis (HD), peritoneal dialysis (PD), renal transplantation, or conservative management. Nevertheless, older patients may have difficulties with dialysis vascular access and often are not candidates for renal transplantation.

1. Dialysis: Modalities/Access/Outcomes

Several factors are unique for older patients initiating dialysis compared to younger patients; they typically initiate dialysis at higher eGFR levels and lower body mass index.They also tend to have more associated comorbid conditions with higher hospital admissions and mortality rates.

The use of either HD or PD modalities in older patients is asociated with several advantages and disadvantages. Both modalities have similar mortality and hospitalization rates among older patients. Proper dialysis modality education may help guide these patients and their family members in choosing the appropriate treatment.

Hemodialysis

In-center HD is the most frequently used RRT in older patients. Although HD is a life-sustaining therapy, it may also create, increase, or prolong suffering in selected subgroups of older patients. Older patients undergoing dialysis have a much lower life expectancy in comparison with persons of the same age without ESKD. A recent systemic review by Balogun et al found similar or higher overall health-related and mental component summary quality of life (QOL) scores in older ESKD patients compared to age-matched controls or younger patients. However, the physical component summary QOL scores tended to be lower in older patients. Those with multiple comorbidities also tend to have increased risk of complications on HD which in turn can adversely affect survival.

In general, central venous catheters and polytetrafluoroethylene grafts are only recommended when arteriovenous fistula creation has been unsuccessful. A central venous catheter may be used for vascular access in emergency situations. However, a significant number of older patients continue to be dialyzed through a double-lumen catheter in many HD centers. Catheters have complications, including their dysfunction, central venous stenosis, and infections.

Peritoneal Dialysis

PD may be an alternative option for older patients who are unable to undergo HD. Yet, PD is infrequently used in these patients for multiple reasons. These reasons may include poor functional status, sensory deficits such as visual impairment, poor dexterity, and lack of social support. Still PD may be associated with good outcomes in select older patients such as nondiabetics, those with few comorbidities, and high functional capabilities. Complications of PD are similar between younger and older patients. Although the risk of peritonitis is also similar among both age groups, it is more lethal in older patients. PD may contribute to persistent malnutrition through loss of protein and free amino acids through the PD solutions.

2. Kidney Transplantation

Historically, kidney transplantation has not been considered a valid option in older patients with ESKD, due to the scarce availabilty of organs. This trend has changed. Recently, with the growing number of older patients with ESKD, kidney transplantation has increased in that age group and has been shown to demonstrate improved life expectancy and quality of life. Nevertheless, it is important to carefully evaluate older patients who are being considered for kidney transplantation using screening tools that may help identify suitable candidates for transplantation. Induction and maintenance therapy for older patients receiving kidney transplantation are similar to the therapy for younger patients.

In older adults, the long-term mortality after transplantation is higher than younger kidney recipients. The predominant causes of death among older transplant recipients are infections and cardiovascular disease. Infections usually occur in the first 6 months after the kidney transplant.

3. Conservative Management

Conservative management is a viable option for many older adults with ESKD. This can be an obvious option in certain subgroups of older adults such as the oldest old (>90 years), those with significant cogntive impairments, poor functional health and estimated life expectancy of less than 6 months. However, in certain subgroups of older patients, this decision can be difficult. Too often, many patients with ESKD view the conservative option as not having any treatment at all and fear that it would lead to a rapid demise. Contrary to this common view, several studies have shown that there is no significant survival advantage with dialysis compared to conservative management, particularly in those over 75 years and with multiple comorbidities such as DM and cardiac disease. In addition, life satisfaction and quality of life were stable in this subgroup of patients who chose conservative management. Conservative approach may include

management of volume overload, acid–base and electrolyte imbalance, treatment of anemia and CKD-MBD.

It is therefore critically important that patients with ESKD receive adequate and accurate information on the different treatment options for RRT. Specifically, it is crucial to counsel patients on what to realistically expect with the different RRT options so they can make an informed decision. The decision-making process is usually a shared one between the patient, family members and the health team, typically the primary care physician, nephrologist and nurse educator. In studies, older adults with ESKD often felt that their health team was paternalisitc and that they had little choice in the decision-making process for RRT. With the health team often guiding and assisting patients as they consider the different options, care must be taken to impart the information as objectively as possible so patients do not feel pressured to choose a particular option because they believe that is what they are expected to choose. It is also important to ensure that patients are not making these decisions based on their family members' preferences. Conservative treatment of ESKD needs to be comprehensive and utilize a strong multidisciplinary approach with a focus on medical management of symptoms, managing expectations of patients and family members, maintaining continuity of care and trust in the health team, and effective collaboration between the different disciplines in the health team. This approach greatly fosters patients' well-being and also faciliates successful conservative management of older adults with CKD, particularly in those greater than 75 years and multiple comorbidities.

UNIQUE CHALLENGES IN ELDERLY WITH KIDNEY DISEASE

Medication Management

Older patients with kidney disease are exceptionally susceptible to adverse effects from medications due to pharmacokinetic changes from aging, in additon to those due to kidney disease itself. Age-associated pharmacokinetic changes affect mostly the tissue distribution phase as a result of decreased lean muscle mass with relative increase in the fat content, the metabolism phase with age-related decrease in liver mass and the renal excretion phase with age-related decline in glomerular filtration. All of which result in reduced clearance of many medications leading to prolonged duration of drug action and/or potentiation of their effects. This often necessitates drug-dosing adjustments. Renal function of older adults is best estimated through the use of serum creatinine–based equations to calculate the eGFR, such as the Cockroft–Gault and Modification of Diet in Renal Disease (MDRD) equations as serum creatinine alone can be inaccurate due to age-related loss of muscle mass, and often overestimates kidney function in the older patients. Cystatin C–based equations have also been found to be accurate in estimating renal function, though this has not been well studied in the very old and are used to lesser degree in clinical practice. The eGFR is now automatically reported with serum creatinine levels in laboratory reports. This facilitates the use of eGFR by clinicians in determining the appropriate dose of medications in the treatment of geriatric-aged patients.

Potentially inappropriate medications for older adults such as those listed in the Beers criteria, can be especially dangerous for them and pose a high risk of adverse drug effects. These include anticholinergic agents (antihistamines, muscle relaxants), benzodiazepines, oral hypoglycemic agents, particularly those that are long acting and nonsteriodal anti-inflammatory agents, which are also nephrotoxic. In addition, older adults tend to have a higher chronic disease burden with common conditions such as DM, hypertension, osteoarthritis and are therefore prescribed multiple medications to treat these conditions. Polypharmacy also increases the risk of adverse drug effects in these adults, making their clinical management even more challenging.

Medication management of older adults with kidney disease therefore requires careful consideration of all of the potential risk factors for adverse drug effects, appropriate estimation of kidney function and renally adjusted dosing of medications when appropriate.

CLINICAL IMPLICATIONS OF KIDNEY DISEASE IN OLDER ADULTS

Certain medical conditions such as depression, frailty are common in older adults with kidney disease, particularly those with ESKD on RRT. These, in turn can lead to poor clinical outcomes and adversely affect survival. Other clinical concerns include osteoporosis, falls, sleep disturbance, cognitive impairment, and sexual dysfunction. Conditions such as osteoporosis, falls, and fractures are especially common in older adults with CKD due to the bone disease from aging and CKD-MBD, and can negatively impact quality of life. Even though older adults with CKD tend to cope better pychosocially compared to younger patients, depression is quite prevalent in older adults and predisposes to poor clinical outcomes. Prompt recognition, diagnosis, and management of these conditons in older adults with kidney disease is crucial. It is also important to closely monitor for potential adverse effects from medications used to treat some of these conditions such as antidepressants, bisphosphonates, since older adults with kidney disease are more susceptible to medication side effects. Incorporating physical therapy into the management of these patients is vital to maintain mobility, muscle strength and reducing fall risk especially in older adults with CKD on RRT as physical functioning declines significantly in this group of patients and adversely affects quality of life.

▶ Social Implications

Older adults with kidney disease tend to adjust quite well psychosocially, even those with ESKD on RRT. This can, however, impact their day to day life, particularly in older adults who live in retirement communities where RRT could interfere or limit their participation in structured daily activities. The need for strong support systems for these patients cannot be overstated.

▶ Ethical Implications

Older adults with ESKD on RRT can present an ethical dilemma in the medical community. Starting RRT in older adults raises the question of appropriateness of life-sustaining measures such as dialysis and renal transplant in those with advanced age, in light of limited health resources. Physicians and family members are faced with the difficult decision of withholding or withdrawing these life-sustaining measures particularly at the end of life. This decision often requires a multidisciplinary team, support for the patient and family, and honest discussions about prognosis and goals of medical care.

KEY READINGS

Aalten J et al: The influence of obesity on short- and long-term graft and patient survival after renal transplantation. Transpl Int 2006;19:901.

Aasen EM, Kvangarsnes M, Heggen K: Perceptions of patient participation amongst elderly patients with end-stage renal disease in a dialysis unit. Scand J Caring Sci 2012;26:61.

Abdel-Rahman EM et al: Management of diabetic nephropathy in the elderly: special considerations. J Nephrol Ther 2012;2:124.

Abdel-Rahman EM, Okusa MD: Effects of aging on renal function and regenerative capacity. Nephron Clin Pract 2014;127:15.

Abraham PA, Keane WF: Glomerular and interstitial disease induced by nonsteroidal anti-inflammatory drugs. Am J Nephrol 1984;4:1.

Al bshabshe AA et al: Pulmonary renal syndrome associated with Wegener's granulomatosis: a case report and review of literature. [Review]. Clin Exp Nephrol 2010;14:80.

American Geriatrics Society 2015: Updated beers criteria for potentially inappropriate medication use in older adults. J Am Geriatr Soc 2015;63:2227.

Aronow WS: Blood pressure goals and targets in the elderly. Curr Treat Options Cardio Med 2015;17:394.

Balogun RA et al: Association of depression and antidepressant use with mortality in a large cohort of patients with nondialysis-dependent CKD. Clin J Am Soc Nephrol 2012;7:1793.

Balogun SA et al: Quality of life, perceptions, and health satisfaction of older adults with end stage renal disease: a systematic review. J Am Geriatr Soc 2017;65:777.

Beckett NS et al: Treatment of hypertension in patients 80 years of age or older. N Engl J Med 2008;358:1887.

Buysen JG et al: Acute interstitial nephritis: a clinical and morphological study in 27 patients. Nephrol Dial Transplant 1990;5:94.

Clive DM, Stroff JS: Renal syndromes associated with nonsteroidal anti-inflammatory drugs. N Engl J Med 1984;310:563.

Da Silva-Gane M et al: Quality of life and survival in patients with advanced kidney failure managed conservatively or by dialysis. Clin J Am Soc Nephrol 2012;7:2002.

Dusseux E et al: A simple clinical tool to inform the decision-making process to refer elderly incident dialysis patients for kidney transplant evaluation. Kidney Int 2015;88:121.

Falk RJ et al: Granulomatosis with polyangiitis (Wegener's): an alternative name for Wegener's granulomatosis. J Am Soc Nephrol 2011;22:587.

Falk RJ et al: Granulomatosis with polyangiitis (Wegener's): an alternative name for Wegener's granulomatosis. Arthritis Rheum 2011;63:863.

Feinfeld A et al: Nephrotic syndrome associated with use of non-steroidal anti-inflammatory drugs: case report and review of the literature. Nephron 1984;37:174.

Ghaffar U, Maharjan N, Moore PC: Predictors of CKD and rate of decline in eGFR in the elderly: a case-cohort study. Nephrol News Issues 2016;30:38.

Glassock RJ: An update on glomerular disease in the elderly. Clin Geriatr Med 2013;29:579.

Gore JL et al: Obesity and outcome following renal transplantation. Am J Transplant 2006;6:357.

Hogan SL et al: Various forms of life in antineutrophil cytoplasmic antibody-associated vasculitis. Ann Intern Med 2006;144:377.

Jabur WL, Saeed HM: ANCA-positive pauci-immune rapidly progressive glomerulonephritis and the nephrotic syndrome. Saudi J Kidney Dis Transpl 2010;21:526.

Jennette JC et al: Nomenclature of systemic vasculitides. Proposal of an international consensus conference. Arthritis Rheum 1994;37:187.

Karsch-Völk M et al: Kidney function and clinical recommendations of drug dose adjustment in geriatric patients. BMC Geriatr 2013;13:92.

Kidney Disease: Improving Global Outcomes (KDIGO) Acute Kidney Injury Work Group: KDIGO Clinical Practice Guideline for Acute Kidney Injury. Kidney Int. 2012;2:1.

Kilbride HS et al: Accuracy of the MDRD (modification of diet in renal disease) study and CKD-EPI (CKD epidemiology collaboration) equations for estimation of GFR in the elderly. Am J Kidney Dis 2013;61:57.

Kodner CM, Kudrimoti A: Diagnosis and management of acute interstitial nephritis. Am Fam Physician 2003;67:2527

McAdams-DeMarco MA et al: Trends in kidney transplant outcomes in older adults. J Am Geriatr Soc 2014;62:2235.

Meier-Kriesche HU, Kaplan B: Waiting time on dialysis as the strongest modifiable risk factor for renal transplant outcomes: a paired donor kidney analysis. Transplantation. 2002;74:1377.

Michel DM, Kelly CJ: Acute interstitial nephritis. J Am Soc Nephrol 1998;9:506.

Murphy D et al: Trends in prevalence of chronic kidney disease in the United States. Ann Intern Med 2016;165:473.

Musso CG, Oreopoulos DG: Aging and physiological changes of the kidneys including changes in glomerular filtration rate. Nephron Physiol 2011;119:1.

Perazella MA, Markowitz GS: Drug-induced acute interstitial nephritis. [Review]. Nat Rev Nephrol 2010;6:461.

Porile J, Bakris G, Garella S: Acute interstitial nephritis with glomerulopathy due to nonsteroidal anti-inflammatory agents: A review of its clinical spectrum and effects of steroid therapy. J Clin Pharmacol 1990;30:468.

Praga M, González E: Acute interstitial nephritis. Kidney Int 2010;77:956.

Rossert J: Drug-induced acute interstitial nephritis. Kidney Int 2001;60:804.

Rule AD et al: The association between age and nephrosclerosis on renal biopsy among healthy adults. Ann Intern Med 2010;152:561.

Rutgers A et al: Pauci-immune necrotizing glomerulonephritis. [Review]. Rheum Dis Clin North Am 2010;36:559.

Sawhney S et al: Long-term prognosis after acute kidney injury (AKI): what is the role of baseline kidney function and recovery? A systematic review. BMJ Open 2015;5:e006497.

Tam-Tham H et al: Primary care physicians' perceived barriers and facilitators to conservative care for older adults with chronic kidney disease: design of a mixed methods study. Can J Kidney Health Dis 2016;3:17.

Turgut F et al: Hypertension in the elderly: unique challenges and management. Clin Geriatr Med 2013;29:593.

Verberne WR et al: Comparative survival among older adults with advanced kidney disease managed conservatively versus with dialysis. Clin J Am Soc Nephrol 2016;11:633.

Wolfe RA et al: Comparison of mortality in all patients on dialysis, patients on dialysis awaiting transplantation, and recipients of a first cadaveric transplant. N Engl J Med. 1999;341:1725.

■ CHAPTER REVIEW QUESTIONS

1. A 76-year-old Caucasian man presents with 2 months history of fatigue, nonproductive cough, hemoptysis with epistaxis, sinusitis, and nasal congestion for 5 days. Baseline serum creatinine was 1.2 mg/dL. He was evaluated by his primary care provider for symptoms of anorexia and weight loss of 5 kg (11 lb). Basic labs were collected at that time and his creatinine was found to be 3.8 mg/dL with BUN of 70 mg/dL and hemoglobin of 7.5. Chest radiograph reveals bilateral 1–2 cm nodular infiltrates' in the upper lung field. Urinalysis showed pH of 5.5, specific gravity 1.015, +1 protein. Under the microscope, urine fields showed 0 WBCs, 10–20 RBCs/hpf with some of them dysmorphic, rare RBC casts. Kidney ultrasound was unremarkable.

On examination: BP 153/74, pulse 64, respiratory rate 24, oxygen saturation was 98% on room air, temperature 37°C. The patient is a thin, chronically ill-appearing gentleman in no apparent distress. Pertinent positives on physical examination include enlarged anterior cervical nodes with large bilateral submandibular lymphadenopathy. Crackles are heard over left anterior chest.

Which of the following tests will help establish a diagnosis?
A. Serum complements and antidouble stranded DNA antibody
B. Serum angiotensin-converting enzyme
C. Antineutrophil cytoplasmic antibodies
D. Serum immune globulin A
E. Antiglomerular basement membrane antibody

2. A 74-year-old African–American man with past medical history of hypertension and osteoarthritis presents to the hospital with right arm abscess due to *staphylocoocus aureus* and is treated with antibiotic therapy. He is also on BP medication (he does not remember the name) and takes multivitamins. He improves and is discharged home. He is seen by his physician the next day with a fever—temperature 38.6°C.

His examination shows BP 118/68, pulse 78/min. Lung, heart, abdominal examinations were unremarkable. No rashes were seen and no lower extremity edema.

His laboratory data shows serum creatinine of 3.2 (a week earlier was 1.3 mg/dL). UA shows pH 6.5, specific gravity of 1.020, +1 blood, trace protein, leuko esterase and nitrite were negative. Urinalysis showed many WBCs. No RBCs. Urine sediment examination showed clumps of WBCs and few WBCs casts, and 1–5 RBCs/HPF that were homogenous.

What is the most likely cause of his acute kidney injury?
A. Acute tubular necrosis
B. Urinary tract infection
C. Acute interstitial nephritis
D. Membranoproliferative glomerulonephritis
E. Hypertensive nephrosclerosis

3. A 90-year-old woman with mild cognitive impairment, essential hypertension, diabetes mellitus type 2, degenerative joint disease of her knees and hips, and chronic kidney disease stage 5 (calculated GFR-10) was referred by her primary physician for further management of her kidney disease and discussion about options for renal replacement therapy. She ambulates with a walker and is independent of most of her activities of daily living though she lives in an assisted living facility. On physical examination, she is alert and oriented to time, place, and person. Her pulmonary and cardiac exams are stable and have no signs of fluid overload.

Regarding renal replacement options for this patient, which of the following statement is true?
A. She is not a candidate for hemodialysis as it would decrease her life expectancy and quality of life.
B. She would be a potentially good candidate for peritoneal dialysis because of her functional status.
C. Conservative management is not a viable option as it could lead to a rapid demise.
D. Conservative management could be a viable option for her as her quality of life and health satisfaction would likely be maintained.

4. The patient is a 69-year-old woman with past medical history of CKD 5. She has been diagnosed with hypertension more than 50 years, dyslipidemia, and diabetes mellitus for more than 15 years with no retinopathy or neuropathy. Seen in the renal clinic with complaints of occasional nausea and decreased appetite. Patient denies vomiting, fever, chills, chest pains, abdominal pains or any urinary symptoms. Her current is GFR 13 mL/min/1.73 m^2 and she is still making good amount of urine and is on no dialysis. Her BMI is 46. Her blood type is group A negative (waiting time for deceased kidney transplantation at her facility 4–5 years).

On examination, patient is well developed, alert, and oriented to person, place, and time.

Aside from obesity and trace lower extremity edema, her examination is unremarkable.

Which option for kidney transplantation is adequate for this patient?
A. Candidate for living related kidney transplant only
B. Candidate for living or deceased kidney transplant
C. Candidate for living or deceased kidney transplant, but needs to lose weight at first
D. Not a transplant candidate based on age

5. A 72-year-old Caucasian woman with severe arthritis of knees and hips. Pain is continuous and disabling. Patient was started on NSAID on a daily basis, which improved her pain. Three months later, the patient develops lower extremity swelling. Her BP which was originally controlled is now requiring an increase in BP medication dosing for adequate control.

On examination: BP 162/98, lungs are clear to auscultation and percussion, heart, regular rate and rhythm, normal abdominal examination with +3 lower extremity edema.

Her laboratory studies show the following: sodium 138 mEq/L, potassium 5.7 mEq/L, BUN 35 mg/dL, 2.0 mg/dL (baseline 0.9 mg/dL)

Total cholesterol: 288 mg/dL
UA: protein +4, RBCs: 1–3/hpf, WBCs: 1–3/hpf.

What is the most likely cause of the worsening of the kidney function?
A. Interstitial nephritis
B. Acute tubular necrosis (ATN)
C. Urinary tract obstruction
D. Interstitial nephritis and minimal change disease
E. Focal segmental glomerulosclerosis (FSGS)

6. An 83-year-old woman with osteoporosis and cataracts but no other health problems has a stable eGFR of 64 mL/min per 1.73 m^2 with no proteinuria, and a BP of 140/88 mm Hg. She is not taking any BP medications. Which of the following BP management strategies do you think is most appropriate?
A. Start an ACE inhibitor with a goal BP 130/80 mm Hg
B. Start a thiazide with a goal BP 130/80 mm Hg
C. Encourage her to follow a low-sodium diet
D. Continue to monitor

Interventional Nephrology

Theodore F. Saad, MD
Stephen R. Ash, MD, FACP

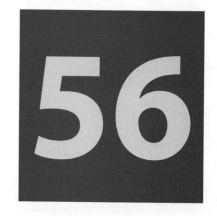

▼ ENDOVASCULAR PROCEDURES

THE ORIGINS OF INTERVENTIONAL NEPHROLOGY

The early history of dialysis was marked by advances in vascular access, conceived and developed by visionary nephrologists, including the Scribner shunt and the Brescia-Cimino arteriovenous fistula (AVF). Without a means of obtaining reliable, repeated blood access, the delivery of chronic hemodialysis would not have been possible. Few nephrologists have maintained a primary role in vascular access creation and maintenance, particularly in Europe; Konner reported a series of 748 consecutive native arteriovenous fistulae constructed by a nephrologist, with 2-year secondary patency in diabetics and nondiabetics ranging from 75% to 96%, respectively. During the 1970s and 1980s in the United States, nephrologists' interest and involvement in vascular access waned. This may have been due to progress in what were perceived as more scientifically rewarding areas of study, as opposed to the relatively mundane "plumbing" problems of vascular access. Certainly, neither technical proficiency nor a rigorous scientific approach to vascular access was emphasized at most nephrology training centers in the United States. A survey of nephrology training programs in 2008 indicated that only about 20% incorporated procedural training in vascular access.

At the same time, particularly in the United States, there was increased utilization of synthetic polytetrafluoroethylene (PTFE) grafts in favor of native arteriovenous fistulae. This shift may have been driven by device marketing, surgical reimbursement practices, limited long-term venous access catheters available for use as "bridges" to native fistulae, and increasing emphasis on short, high-efficiency hemodialysis treatments. The result was a U.S. hemodialysis patient population with a high prevalence of PTFE grafts, low utilization of arteriovenous fistulae, and not-incidentally, the highest

dialysis patient mortality of all industrialized nations. In 1999, 49% of United States' hemodialysis patients were dialyzing with AV grafts, 28% with native fistulae, and 23% with venous catheters.

During this period of a rapidly growing hemodialysis patient population, increasing PTFE graft utilization, and decreased involvement of nephrologists in the management vascular access, there was a predictable crisis in the access-related medical care of these patients. Management of access dysfunction and thrombosis was largely "reactive" and primarily utilized open surgical techniques. The role of venous stenosis contributing to arteriovenous graft thrombosis and failure was underappreciated. In the late 1980s, interventional radiologists began to recognize these problems, and became involved in the management of hemodialysis access dysfunction. In 1991, Valji et al. reported a method for declotting of arteriovenous hemodialysis grafts using pharmacomechanical thrombolysis and angioplasty. Numerous other reports and variations on this method followed, with increasing acceptance of percutaneous interventions in the management of hemodialysis access dysfunction. Largely, however, nephrologists remained on the periphery, as vascular access remained the province of the vascular surgeons, and increasingly, the interventional radiologists.

The vital role of vascular access in the comprehensive care of hemodialysis patients cannot be overemphasized. Care of the hemodialysis patient includes management of uremia, hypertension, sodium and water balance, anemia, mineral metabolism, metabolic bone disease, and nutrition. None of this can be accomplished without reliable blood access for hemodialysis. Leaving this key element of care entirely in the hands of other providers may place the patient and the nephrologist at significant disadvantage. Under ideal circumstances, when the skills and priorities of the multispecialty access team come together, patient care may be very well served. Conversely, if the appropriate surgical or interventional services cannot be delivered in a timely fashion, the patient will suffer in terms of delayed dialysis, utilization of venous hemodialysis access, unnecessary hospitalization, or other avoidable morbidity. This also will result in a significantly greater financial burden to the health care system.

In the early 1990s, this problem was recognized and confronted by Dr Gerald Beathard, a nephrologist practicing in Austin, Texas. He acquired the necessary training and skills, adapted techniques from interventional radiology, and developed a successful nephrologist-run service for percutaneous management of vascular access. He then shared this expertise, training many nephrologists from various practices and backgrounds; in fact, most interventional nephrologists practicing in the United States can trace their heritage directly back to Dr Beathard, this author included. As nephrologists incorporated these techniques to their practices, the field of "interventional nephrology" was effectively formed. Once able to master the procedures and establish suitable facilities in which to work, early interventional nephrology dealt largely with frequent percutaneous interventions directed toward day-to-day failures of PTFE grafts. This led to immediate improvements in managing episodes of care, but did little to impact the overall process of care. This realization inspired the next phase in evolution of interventional nephrology, which was to take on comprehensive vascular access management for the hemodialysis patient. These include

- Preservation of peripheral veins for native AV fistulae
- Avoidance of peripherally inserted central venous catheters and subclavian catheters
- Judicious use of internal jugular vein tunneled hemodialysis catheters
- Early referral to surgeon for construction of native AV fistula
- Education and selection of surgical colleagues willing and able to master the techniques for creation of native AV fistula
- Preoperative imaging of veins and arteries, including ultrasound vein mapping and venography
- Evaluation and treatment of poorly functioning or immature AV fistula
- Conversion from failing PTFE graft to "secondary" native AV fistula
- Maintenance of clinical database and outcome analysis
- Clinical research in techniques, medical devices, and processes of care
- Development of multidisciplinary subspecialty societies to promote education, publication, training, collaboration, and research in vascular access

Essential to provision of optimal vascular access care is the principle that for each scenario of access dysfunction, there is a "best solution." There is a tendency for vascular access solutions to follow "the path of least resistance," or worse yet, "the path of greatest reimbursement," both of which may be very different from the optimal pathway. From the perspective of the interventionist, there is the temptation to view all problems as best solved using percutaneous means. However, there are clearly situations where surgical solutions are preferable and should be employed. Conversely, there are situations where a surgical strategy alone cannot identify or correct the underlying problems. In this regard, keeping a detailed, up-to-date clinical database is essential. This allows the operator to thoroughly and efficiently assess the vascular access problem, make the most appropriate management decision based upon the history and known anatomy, and perform the optimal procedure with the lowest risk and best possibility of a successful outcome.

When a patient presents with access dysfunction, a timely solution is essential. This may represent an urgent problem such as a thrombosed arteriovenous fistula, requiring immediate intervention to salvage the access and provide dialysis. Although arguably not a true "medical emergency," restoration of fistula or graft function is of paramount importance to the care of the hemodialysis patient, with serious implications for both short-term and long-term morbidity and mortality. Other access problems may be less immediate, such as prolonged bleeding from needle puncture sites related to venous outflow stenosis; this may not prevent dialysis, but puts the patient at risk, may lead to access thrombosis, and should be dealt with before it becomes an urgent problem. Other access problems may be relatively elective in nature, such as evaluation of limb swelling associated with central venous stenosis, or a slowly enlarging pseudoaneurysm. In all cases, the goal of an interventional program should be to address each problem in an appropriate timely fashion, minimizing disruption of the patients' lifestyle and dialysis schedule. Nephrologists are in the ideal position to provide these services when equipped with the necessary tools, allowing for seamless delivery of care and management of dialysis access-related problems. Alternatively, there are many practices where excellent care and service is provided by interventional radiologists or vascular surgeons. The title of the individual responsible for the vascular access interventions is not as important as his or her knowledge, skill, availability, and willingness to work with surgeons, nephrologists, and dialysis staff as a multidisciplinary access-management team.

The Society of Vascular Surgery and Society of Interventional Radiology have long track records of addressing hemodialysis vascular access, within the context of their broad specialties. The Vascular Access Society (VAS, 1997), American Society of Diagnostic and Interventional Nephrology (ASDIN, 2000), The Vascular Access Society of the Americas (VASA, 2005) have emerged as important multidisciplinary organizations, working with similar missions to foster improved dialysis access care through education, training, and research. All three of these groups hold major annual or biannual scientific meetings, and have collaborated to support *The Journal of Vascular Access* as their official publication vehicle. VASA sponsors a biannual practicum for hands-on training of surgical techniques, interventional procedures, and ultrasound. ASDIN has developed and published standards for training, certification, and accreditation relative to diagnostic and interventional disciplines; previously there were no standards specific to the procedures of dialysis access, with tremendous variation in training, and credentialing requirements of health care facilities. With increased acceptance of these criteria in the United States and elsewhere, interventional training has become more uniform and rigorous. Interventional nephrology training programs have become established at several U.S. academic centers. As these centers develop, they will advance the standard for training, quality, and clinical research related to vascular access.

The core procedures of interventional nephrology for hemodialysis include placement and management of venous hemodialysis catheters, diagnostic imaging of arteriovenous accesses and native veins, percutaneous angioplasty, and percutaneous thrombectomy of thrombosed arteriovenous access. Other common related procedures included placement of venous stents, and ligation or embolization of native fistula accessory veins. Surgical creation of arteriovenous access by nephrologists has also become a reality in the United States in selected centers.

KEY READINGS

Asif A et al: Interventional nephrology: from episodic to coordinated vascular access care. J Nephrol 2007;20:399.

Beathard GA: Percutaneous transvenous angioplasty in the treatment of vascular access stenosis. Kidney Int 1992;42:1390.

Brescia MJ et al: Chronic hemodialysis using venipuncture and a surgically created arteriovenous fistula. N Engl J Med 1966;275:1089.

Kolesnyk I et al: Time-dependent reasons for peritoneal dialysis technique failure and mortality. Perit Dial Int 2010;30:170.

Saad TF: Training, certification, and reimbursement for nephrology procedures. Semin Nephrol 2002;22:276.

Valji K et al: Pharmacomechanical thrombolysis and angioplasty in the management of clotted hemodialysis grafts: early and late clinical results. Radiology 1991;178:243.

TUNNELED VENOUS HEMODIALYSIS CATHETERS

Venous catheters are an unavoidable necessity for many patients with acute kidney injury or advanced chronic kidney disease who require dialysis and do not have functional arteriovenous access. Insertion of tunneled hemodialysis catheters is a fundamental procedure for interventional nephrologists, building on the basic skill of temporary hemodialysis catheter placement, which is taught in nearly all nephrology training programs. Venous catheters are the least desirable means of hemodialysis access due to high risk

for infection and central venous damage leading to thrombosis, stenosis or occlusion. In a sense, every venous catheter placement represents failure: failure to prevent acute kidney injury; failure to construct a functional arteriovenous access in advance of initiating dialysis; failure to detect dysfunctional access and intervene preemptively to maintain its function or create alternative access.

The right internal jugular vein is preferred for venous catheter access, although the left can be used when necessary. The use of subclavian veins is strongly discouraged, or even contraindicated, due to the high risk of developing venous stenosis, jeopardizing future ipsilateral arteriovenous access in that limb. Less commonly, femoral, translumbar, or transhepatic catheters may be placed when other venous avenues are exhausted. A novel device is under investigation to achieve venous access in the setting of thoracic central vein occlusion. The "inside-out" technique uses the femoral vein approach to place a long vascular sheath and pass a sharp guidewire superiorly through occluded superior vena cava and right brachiocephalic vein, then out through the skin at the supraclavicular fossa. This wire is used to gain antegrade access to the right atrium and place a venous dialysis catheter or other transvenous device in the usual fashion. Preliminary results have shown high procedure success and low complication rates. This may prove to be a "game-changer" for patients who have exhausted conventional central venous access options above the diaphragm.

All long-term venous hemodialysis catheters are placed via a subcutaneous tunnel, with a cuff to securely anchor the catheter and provide a barrier to migration of bacteria. There are numerous variations of catheter design, including material, polyurethane or silicone; diameter or "French" size; cross-sectional lumen structure; tip configuration, split, stepped, or symmetrical; tunneling direction, antegrade versus retrograde; coatings, antimicrobial or antithrombotic. A detailed discussion of these variations is beyond the scope of this review. There is very little new evidence to indicate that any one catheter design is superior to another in general, although it is likely that certain properties may be advantageous based upon the anatomy of the superior vena cava and/or right atrium. No controlled study has demonstrated significant advantage or antithrombotic coating to prevent thrombosis or improve catheter function; nor has antimicrobial coating been clearly demonstrated to reduce risk for infection.

Real-time ultrasound guidance is essential for reliable, safe, and efficient venipuncture, based on higher procedure success rates and lower complications when compared with use of anatomical landmarks alone. Real-time ultrasound guidance has been promoted by multiple entities and is "standard of care" for all central venous access. Fluoroscopy is also strongly recommended for tunneled hemodialysis catheter insertions, in order to ensure passage into the intended vessel, and achieve proper catheter tip position;

this is especially important for placement left-sided insertions, and for patients who have had previous central vein catheters who are at risk for abnormal central vein anatomy. Chronic dialysis catheter performance is optimal when the catheter tips are placed into the right atrium, and Disease Outcomes Quality Initiative (DOQI) guidelines recommend this. Nevertheless, achieving the desired tip position may be challenging, even with fluoroscopy and careful attention to anatomic landmarks. A low posterior approach to the right internal jugular vein is ideal; this keeps the catheter low on the neck, with minimal patient discomfort and a good cosmetic result, while creating a smooth bend that avoids kinking. Figure 56–1A shows a poorly placed left internal jugular vein tunneled dialysis catheter, with a high vein puncture from the anterior approach, a tight bend with the catheter kinked, and its split tips extending only into the superior vena cava. This catheter did not function for dialysis. Figure 56–1B shows the catheter replaced using the right internal jugular vein puncture from a low posterior approach with a smooth bend in the neck. In Figure 56–1C, the new catheter tips are shown extending into the high right atrium, yielding excellent catheter function as required for delivery of hemodialysis.

Catheter infections require both decision making and procedural support from the interventional physician. There are three distinct types of catheter infection: exit-site, tunnel, and bloodstream. Minor exit-site infections usually respond to oral or intravenous antibiotic therapy and topical antimicrobials; removal or exchange of the catheter is not typically required. Tunnel infection, by definition extends into and above the subcutaneous cuff, and mandates immediate catheter removal; thankfully, this is relatively uncommon. Catheter-associated bacteremia is unfortunately common, and can be approached using a variety of strategies, depending upon the organism, severity of infection, and expected requirement for continued catheter access. Immediate intravenous antibiotics are essential at first suspicion for bacteremia, and must cover common gram-positive organisms including *Staphylococcus aureus*, and gram-negative organisms including pseudomonas. Typically, an initial dose of vancomycin and antipseudomonal cephalosporin are used empirically, and then tailored depending upon identified organisms. If there is not rapid resolution of acute sepsis, early catheter removal is necessary; this is especially important for patients at higher risk for complicated endovascular infection, such as those with transvenous pacemaker or defibrillator leads, prosthetic heart valves, or endografts. Once initial infection control has been achieved, leaving the catheter in place and simply treating with antibiotics is associated with poor infection outcomes and in most cases, is not appropriate. If the patient has a developing arteriovenous access or peritoneal catheter deemed suitable for use, the hemodialysis catheter may be removed and not replaced. If continued venous catheter access is unavoidable, other options for catheter management include removal and delayed replacement, exchange over a guidewire, or "locking" with antibiotic solution. The interventional physician should be knowledgeable about alternatives, risks, and benefits specific to the patient's situation, and able to guide management in concert with the dialysis nurse, nephrologist, infectious-disease specialist, and vascular surgeon.

Catheter dysfunction is another common problem, with inadequate blood flow rates leading to impaired clearance, incomplete or ineffective dialysis treatments, and consequent uremic or metabolic complications. Catheter dysfunction can occur for several reasons: improper placement or migration resulting in kink or tip malposition; intraluminal catheter thrombus; entrapment within pericatheter "fibrin-sheath"; central vein stenosis or thrombosis. Restoration of catheter function requires fluoroscopic contrast imaging of the catheter and central veins, identification and correction of underlying problems, and typically, replacement of catheter. When there is a pericatheter sheath present, this is demonstrated by retracting the catheter and gently injecting contrast, showing the residual cast of the catheter dangling in the central vein (Figure 56–2A and B). This is commonly referred to as a "fibrin-sheath," although histological studies have shown that this is composed of thrombus, collagen, smooth muscle, and endothelial cells. Typically, this is very tough, leathery material, not easily dissolved or disrupted. Various methods for removal of this sheath have been employed, including "stripping" with a snare from the femoral approach, and catheter exchange with angioplasty balloon disruption of the sheath (Figure 56–2B to E). Replacing a catheter without eliminating an existing sheath will not reliably result in long-term correction of catheter dysfunction. Nevertheless, this area has not been well-studied, and no one method has been demonstrated to be more effective than another.

KEY READINGS

d'Othée BJ, Tham JC, Sheiman RG: Restoration of patency in failing tunneled hemodialysis catheters: a comparison of catheter exchange, exchange and balloon disruption of the fibrin sheath, and femoral stripping. J Vasc Interv Radiol 2006;17:1011.

Ebner A et al: Inside-out upper body venous access. The first-in-human experiences with a novel approach using the Surfacer™ inside-out access catheter system. *Endovascular Today* June 2013.

Knuttinen MG et al: A review of evolving dialysis catheter technologies. Semin Intervent Radiol 2009;26:106.

Lata C et al: Catheter-related bloodstream infection in end-stage kidney disease: a Canadian narrative review. Can J Kidney Health Dis 2016;3:24.

Saad TF, Weiner H: Venous hemodialysis catheters and cardiac implantable electronic devices: avoiding a high-risk combination. Sem Dial 2017;30:187.

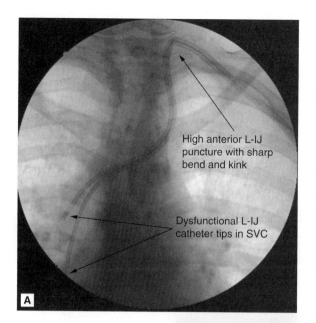

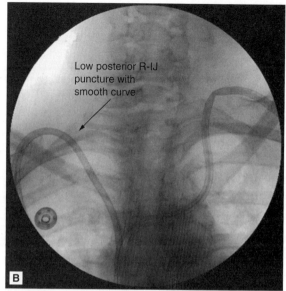

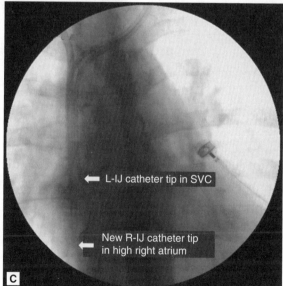

▲ **Figure 56–1. A.** Poorly placed left internal jugular vein tunneled cuffed hemodialysis catheter using a high-anterior approach. Bend is sharply kinked in the neck and tips are in the superior vena cava blood flow was insufficient to support hemodialysis. **B.** Same patient with new right internal jugular catheter using a low-posterior approach with a smooth bend in the neck, prior to removal of faulty catheter. **C.** Same patient showing the new right internal jugular vein catheter tips extending into the right atrium.

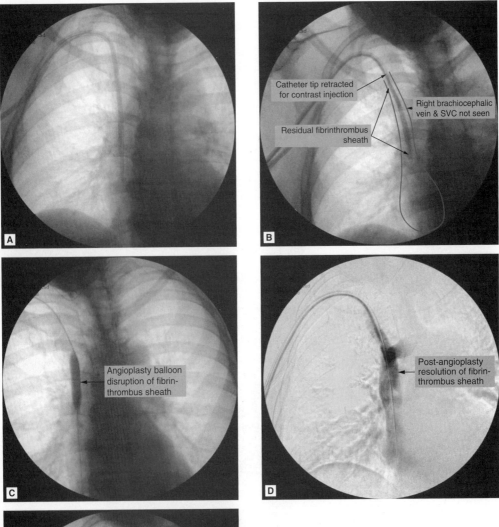

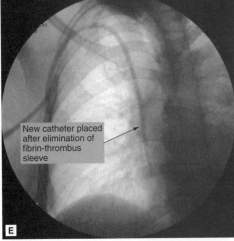

▲ **Figure 56–2.** **A.** Right internal jugular vein tunneled dialysis catheter nonfunctional for dialysis, appears properly placed, no kink, tip near high-right atrium. **B.** Catheter tip retracted to the internal jugular vein, with contrast injection demonstrating a residual fibrin-thrombus sheath, corresponding to the course of the catheter. **C.** Angioplasty balloon disruption of fibrin-thrombus sheath. **D.** Postballoon disruption, fibrin-thrombus sheath resolved, with normal superior vena cava and right atrium. **E.** Tunneled dialysis catheter replaced over wire using existing tract; functioned well for dialysis.

ARTERIOVENOUS ACCESS STENOSIS

Stenosis associated with arteriovenous grafts due to neo-intimal hyperplasia typically occurs at or near the venous anastomosis (Figure 56–3A). This may be related to turbulent blood flow, shear force on the vessel wall, or compliance mismatch between the synthetic graft and vein, ultimately triggering a variety of humoral growth factors that result in cellular proliferation and stenosis. The pathophysiology of stenosis affecting native arteriovenous fistulae is not as well studied or understood and may involve different factors, in the absence of a surgically constructed venous anastomosis or synthetic material. Vessel inflammation and cellular hypertrophy may precede construction of native AV fistulae. Trauma to the vein during surgical manipulation or from previous intravenous catheters may contribute. Stenosis may also affect any other sites in the arteriovenous access system, both native fistulae and synthetic grafts. These include the arterial anastomosis (Figure 56–4), the fistula or peripheral vein (Figure 56–5), the central veins (Figure 56–6), or the case of synthetic grafts, within the body of the graft itself. Left untreated, progressive stenosis will lead to reduction in access blood flow, ineffective hemodialysis, and ultimately access thrombosis or failure.

Numerous studies have evaluated the role of screening and preemptive intervention for stenosis associated with synthetic arteriovenous hemodialysis grafts, as a means to sustain function, prevent thrombosis, or prolong access survival. Stenosis may be detected by several methods. Physical

examination by an experienced interventional physician correctly predicts fistula stenosis in 80% of inflow, and 89% of outflow lesions. Prolonged needle site bleeding, or an excessively pulsatile quality of the access, without a prominent "thrill" may indicate outflow stenosis or poor flow and predispose to thrombosis. Thus, the utility of a good history and physical examination of the access should not be underestimated. Early studies suggested that elevated pressures measured through the venous dialysis needle during hemodialysis were predictive of PTFE graft thrombosis, and that preemptive angioplasty of these lesions was effective in reducing the rate of graft thrombosis. This may be enhanced by pressure measurement during standardized reduction of dialysis circuit flow, dynamic venous pressure screening, or by measurement of static pressures within the graft in the absence of dialysis circuit flow. Several studies have shown that periodic measurement of access flow rates is useful in detecting graft stenosis, with elective intervention leading to reduced graft thrombosis; however, other studies have failed to show a benefit of flow-screening and this question remains unsettled, at least for arteriovenous grafts. The evidence for benefit of screening and preemptive intervention based upon reduced access flow is stronger for native fistulae: One randomized-controlled study demonstrated improved fistula primary patency, reduced thrombosis, and prolonged access survival associated, based upon intervention or for access flow rate less than 750 mL/min. Although it has not been clearly demonstrated that preemptive intervention results in longer overall access survival, "active

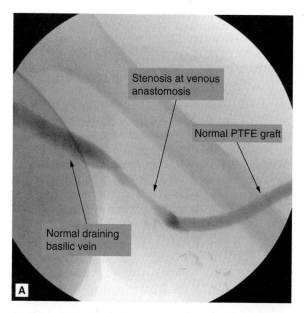
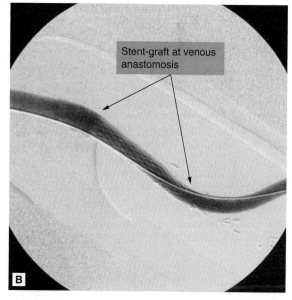

▲ **Figure 56–3. A.** Left upper-arm PTFE graft with severe stenosis at the venous anastomosis to the proximal brachial vein. **B.** Stenosis resolved after angioplasty and placement of stent-graft.

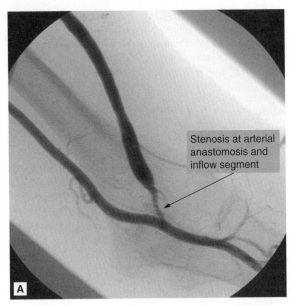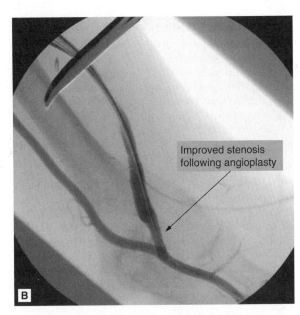

▲ **Figure 56–4.** **A.** Left upper-arm cephalic vein AV fistula with poor flow due to stenosis at the arterial anastomosis and contiguous juxta-anastomotic segment of cephalic vein. **B.** Improved stenosis following 6-mm balloon angioplasty, with improved fistula flow and performance.

surveillance" is mandated in the United States by Centers for Medicare and Medicaid Services (CMS) as a condition of coverage for dialysis.

KEY READINGS

Paulson WD, Moist L, Lok CE: Vascular access surveillance: an ongoing controversy. Kidney Int 2012;81:132.

Tessitore N et al: Can blood flow surveillance and pre-emptive repair of subclinical stenosis prolong the useful life of arteriovenous fistulae? A randomized controlled study. Nephrol Dial Transplant 2004;19:2325.

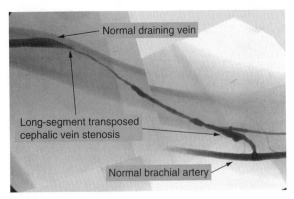

▲ **Figure 56–5.** Severe, long-segment cephalic fistula stenosis.

PERCUTANEOUS TRANSLUMINAL ANGIOPLASTY

Angioplasty of vascular stenosis is the primary tool in the management of arteriovenous hemodialysis access dysfunction. The principles and techniques of percutaneous angioplasty are well established, and must be mastered by the interventional nephrologist, radiologist, or surgeon performing the procedure. Nevertheless, there is considerable controversy over whether angioplasty alone is an "effective therapy." While it is almost always possible to successfully dilate a stenosis and achieve an immediate, anatomically improved appearance, it is not certain that this will result in a sustained resolution of stenosis, improved access performance, or prolonged access patency. Elastic recoil may occur rapidly following apparently successful angioplasty. The angioplasty procedure itself is inherently injurious to the vessel and may promote cellular proliferation leading to more rapid restenosis. Some lesions may respond more favorably to surgical correction with improved duration of patency compared with percutaneous treatment.

Some stenotic lesions in AV access are resistant to expansion using conventional angioplasty balloons, which are typically capable of delivering pressures up to 15–20 atmospheres. Nearly all of these lesions can be successfully dilated using ultrahigh-pressure angioplasty balloons, rated for pressures up to 35 atmospheres. Figure 56–7A shows a basilic vein fistula referred for evaluation of excessive dialysis needle-site bleeding. On physical examination, the fistula

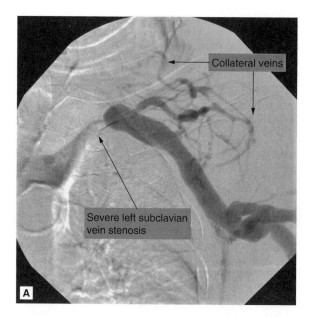

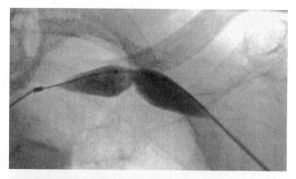

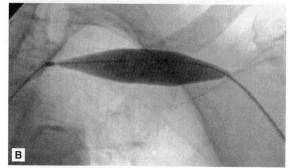

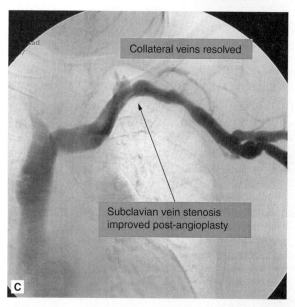

▲ **Figure 56–6. A.** Severe left subclavian stenosis with symptomatic venous hypertension, arm swelling, venous collateral engorgement. **B.** 14-mm balloon angioplasty of left subclavian vein stenosis. **C.** Resolved stenosis postangioplasty, with improved venous collateral engorgement.

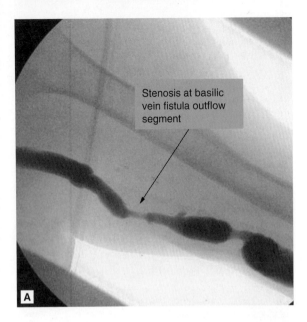

Stenosis at basilic vein fistula outflow segment

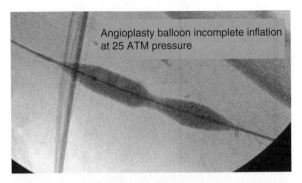

Angioplasty balloon incomplete inflation at 25 ATM pressure

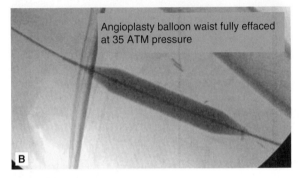

Angioplasty balloon waist fully effaced at 35 ATM pressure

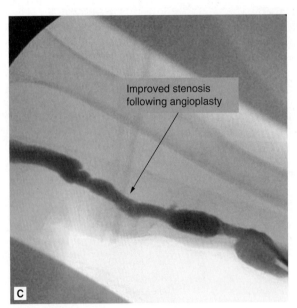

Improved stenosis following angioplasty

▲ **Figure 56–7.** **A.** Left upper-arm brachial artery to transposed basilic vein fistula with severe outflow stenosis near the surgical "swing point." **B.** Ultra high pressure 10-mm angioplasty using Conquest balloon (Bard Peripheral Vascular Inc., Tempe, AZ) waist effaced requiring 35 atmospheres. **C.** Postangioplasty image shows resolution of stenosis, associated with improved palpable thrill on examination. Note ragged appearance of vessel wall at angioplasty site.

was prominently pulsatile, with poor palpable thrill. Severe stenosis was demonstrated in the mid portion of the upper-arm basilic vein, correlating with the history and physical findings. The lesion was extremely resistant to angioplasty (Figure 56–7B), ultimately responding with sustained inflation at ultrahigh pressure, greater than 35 atmospheres. In postangioplasty there was improved angiographic appearance and flow, with restoration of a palpable thrill. Fistulogram demonstrated improved degree of stenosis, but also ragged vessel wall appearance consistent with angioplasty-induced venous injury (Figure 56–7C). This highlights the fact that angioplasty is injurious to the vessel, and may incite local factors leading to further neointimal hyperplasia, contributing to eventual restenosis.

Given the relatively poor results achieved with angioplasty alone, there has been interest in other methods to reduce the rate of restenosis and enhance clinical outcomes. One strategy was to use a "cutting-balloon," constructed with small longitudinal blades, in order to create a more controlled injury, thereby reducing vessel trauma and stimulus for cellular proliferation following angioplasty. The first large, prospective, randomized-controlled study in hemodialysis vascular access was performed to address this question. This showed no improvement in primary-patency of AV grafts using a cutting balloon versus conventional angioplasty balloon for treatment of stenosis at the venous anastomosis. However, in native AV fistulae, improved primary patency has been demonstrated using a cutting balloon for treatment of resistant stenoses.

A more attractive strategy to prevent stenosis or restenosis is to target the primary underlying pathophysiology of myointimal proliferation. Studies have shown benefit from a paclitaxel-coated angioplasty balloon on reducing restenosis following angioplasty in dialysis grafts or fistulae; based upon these data, there is approval in Europe for paclitaxel-coated balloon angioplasty in AV access stenosis. A large, multicenter, prospective-randomized trial of paclitaxel-coated balloon (Lutonix™, Bard Peripheral Vascular Inc., Tempe, AZ) versus conventional angioplasty in arteriovenous fistulae is currently underway in the United States and Canada; preliminary results show improved target lesion primary patency and reduced reintervention rate at 9 months; 1-year data are not yet available. Whether this device proves to be an important advancement in treatment of AV fistula stenosis remains to be seen, but there is an encouraging positive signal that the pathobiology of vascular restenosis may be favorably modified. More trials in this area will be needed to establish how this technology will be most effectively used for treatment of AV access dysfunction.

KEY READINGS

Portugaller RH, Kalmar PI, Deutschmann H: The eternal tale of dialysis access vessels and restenosis: are drug-eluting balloons the solution? J Vasc Access 2014;15:439.

Vesely TM: Is percutaneous transluminal angioplasty an effective intervention for arteriovenous graft stenosis? Semin Dialysis 2005;18:197.

Vesely TM, Siegel JB: Use of the peripheral cutting balloon to treat hemodialysis-related stenoses. J Vasc Interv Radiol 2005;16:1593.

VENOUS STENTS

Until recently, the role of endovascular stents in the management of stenosis associated with arteriovenous hemodialysis access has been poorly defined and controversial. This stands in sharp contradistinction to coronary and renal artery stenosis, and to some degree peripheral arterial disease, where primary stenting is standard of care. Potential sites for stent use in AV access include AV graft venous anastomosis, peripheral veins related to a native fistula or graft, or central veins.

Self-expanding "bare-metal" stents with biliary, tracheobronchial, or arterial indications have been utilized in AV access "off-label" for many years. These are primarily Nitinol (nickel-titanium alloy) stents which have advantageous radial force, flexibility, and material memory properties. Although there has been interest in bare-metal stents for treatment AV access stenosis, none has been definitively demonstrated superior to angioplasty alone, and none are FDA-approved for use in AV access. Bare-metal stents are approved for use in central veins.

Stent-grafts or "covered-stents" represent a significant advancement in stent technology, and have now been studied in multiple well-designed clinical trials of AV access stenosis. The first of these compared the Flair™ stent-graft (Bard Peripheral Vascular, Inc., Tempe, AZ) versus conventional angioplasty for treatment of stenosis at the venous anastomosis of AV grafts. This study demonstrated significantly improved 6-month target lesion primary patency and resulted in device approval in the United States. This was followed by RENOVA, a postapproval trial of the Flair™ device with 2-year follow-up; this confirmed the positive findings of the pivotal trial, and demonstrated significant sustained patency advantage of the stent-graft at 1-year and 2-year follow-up. A typical venous anastomotic lesion treated with angioplasty and Flair™ stent-graft is demonstrated in Figure 56–3.

A comparable trial, REVISE was performed using the Viabahn™ stent-graft (WL Gore, Inc, Newark, DE) for treatment of stenosis at the venous anastomosis of both thrombosed and nonthrombosed AV grafts. This also showed significant improvement in target-lesion primary patency, and reduced requirement for reintervention in the treatment group. Previous stent-graft trials had excluded thrombosed grafts, and forearm grafts requiring stent-graft to cross the elbow joint; REVISE demonstrated significantly improved patency with stent-grafts used to treat stenosis in the settings of graft thrombosis, and across the elbow. The Viabahn™ stent-graft is particularly flexible, making it suitable for the elbow where there is motion and angulation of the vein; this property also allows for use with tortuous outflow anatomy (Figure 56–8).

The Fluency™ stent-graft (Bard Peripheral Vascular, Inc., Tempe, AZ) was studied for treatment of stenosis occurring within previously placed stents at various locations in the access circuit of AV grafts or fistulae. This randomized-controlled trial, RESCUE also demonstrated improved primary patency of the target lesion and access circuit following stent-graft placement.

Prior to these large trials reporting favorable outcomes with primary stenting at the venous anastomosis, stent placement was generally considered "salvage" therapy, after failure of conventional angioplasty, due to immediate elastic

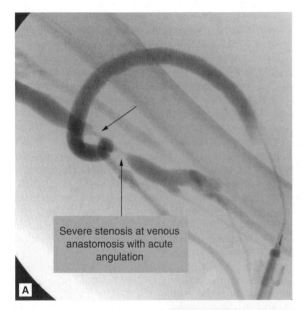

A. Severe stenosis at venous anastomosis with acute angulation

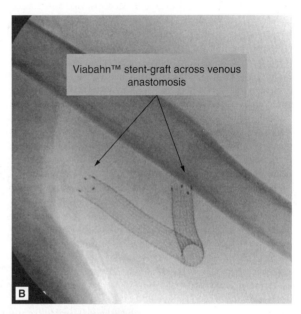

B. Viabahn™ stent-graft across venous anastomosis

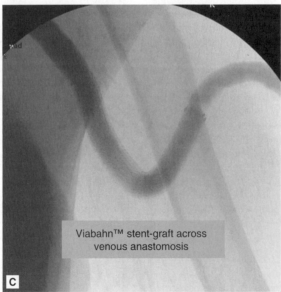

C. Viabahn™ stent-graft across venous anastomosis

▲ **Figure 56–8. A.** Left upper-arm PTFE graft with acutely angled venous anastomosis and severe stenosis extending into basilic vein. **B** and **C.** Following angioplasty and placement of Viabahn™ (WL Gore, Inc, Newark, DE) stent-graft.

recoil, rupture, or rapidly recurrent restenosis. Notwithstanding favorable primary patency results from these studies, when or whether to utilize a stent-graft for primary treatment of graft stenosis remains unsettled. Stenting will not solve other factors potentially contributing to graft failure, including arterial disease, hypotension, or hypercoagulable states. Stents should be avoided at locations where future surgical revision or secondary AV fistula construction may be a better option.

The role for stent-grafts in native AV fistulae is less well established than for AV grafts, and none are yet approved for use in native fistulae in the United States; nevertheless, there has been increasing "off-label" use of stents for treatment of fistula stenosis. Several studies have demonstrated improved patency with use of stent-grafts for treatment of cephalic arch stenosis. Figure 56–9A demonstrates severe cephalic arch stenosis, treated with angioplasty and stent-graft with excellent immediate anatomical result (Figure 56–9B). A large multicenter randomized trial is currently underway to examine the outcome of stent-grafts for treatment of stenosis in both cephalic and basilic AV fistulae; it is anticipated that this trial and others will add much-needed clarity to the role of stent-grafts in native fistulae.

Stent-grafts may be useful for treatment of graft or fistula pseudoaneurysms in uncommon situations where open surgical repair is not preferred. Figure 56–10A shows a PTFE graft with a large inflow-segment pseudoaneurysm. A stent-graft was placed, completely excluding the pseudoaneurysm (Figure 56–10B), without encroaching upon the main needle-puncture segment. While this confers an excellent immediate angiographic outcome, long-term clinical benefits of stenting pseudoaneurysms have not been demonstrated, and no stent-graft is FDA-approved for this indication. Successful use of stent-grafts in needle-puncture segments of grafts or fistulae has been reported, but remains controversial, and is generally discouraged except when no other option is deemed feasible.

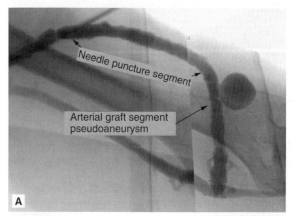

A

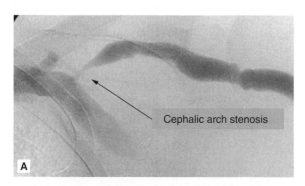

A

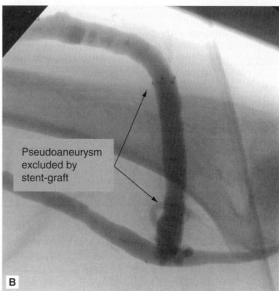

B

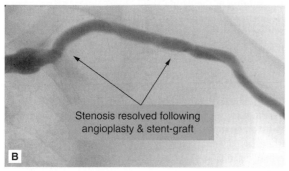

B

▲ **Figure 56–9. A.** Severe cephalic arch stenosis. **B.** Resolved cephalic arch stenosis following angioplasty and placement of stent graft.

▲ **Figure 56–10. A.** Left upper-arm graft inflow segment large pseudoaneurysm. **B.** Stent-graft placed with complete exclusion of the pseudoaneurysm.

KEY READINGS

Falk A, Maya ID, Yevzlin AS: RESCUE Investigators: a prospective, randomized study of an expanded polytetrafluoroethylene stent graft versus balloon angioplasty for in-stent restenosis in arteriovenous grafts and fistulae: two-year results of the RESCUE study. J Vasc Interv Radiol 2016;27:146576.

Haskal Z et al: Prospective, randomized, concurrently-controlled study of a stent graft vs. balloon angioplasty for treatment of arteriovenous access graft stenosis: two-year results of the RENOVA study. J Vasc Interv Radiol 2016;8:1105.

Rajan DK, Falk A: A randomized prospective study comparing outcomes of angioplasty versus Viabahn™ stent-graft placement for cephalic arch stenosis in dysfunctional hemodialysis accesses. J Vasc Interv Radiol 2015;26:1355.

Vesely T et al: Balloon angioplasty versus Viabahn stent graft for treatment of failing or thrombosed prosthetic hemodialysis grafts. J Vasc Surg 2016;64:1400.

PERCUTANEOUS THROMBECTOMY

Since the first publications of percutaneous methods for declotting AV grafts, many devices and techniques for thrombectomy of hemodialysis access have been reported. No one method has been shown to be superior others, in terms of procedure success, complications, or duration of access patency. The principal determinant of outcome is correction of underlying stenoses or other condition determined to be responsible for the thrombosis. Notable progress has been made in the management of native arteriovenous fistula thrombosis. Several studies of percutaneous native fistula thrombectomy have reported procedure success rates ranging from 76% to 94%. These reports utilized a combination of pharmacologic thrombolysis and mechanical clot extraction or maceration, with no proven difference in efficacy or safety between different methods. Secondary patency of fistulae after successful thrombectomy ranges from 50% to 86% at 24 months, comparable to results in grafts.

Thrombosed fistulae with large aneurysms present considerable challenges in management due to large thrombus burden which is difficult to clear with pharmacological thrombolysis or mechanical aspiration. These also confer higher risk for thromboembolic complications to the pulmonary or arterial circulation. In some cases, it may be necessary to abandon the fistula, or pursue an open surgical thrombectomy. A technique has been described utilizing balloon occlusion of fistula inflow and outflow, and a small incision over the fistula through which thrombus can be directly extracted. This method allows for removal of far more thrombus than other minimally invasive techniques, and may result in salvage of a fistula that would otherwise be abandoned.

It should be emphasized that to achieve long-term secondary or "assisted" patency, subsequent percutaneous interventions are commonly required after thrombectomy. Furthermore, as we attempt to create fistulae in more patients with lesser-quality veins, it is likely that the rate of native fistula dysfunction and thrombosis will be higher in these "jeopardized" fistulae than in those previously reported, using ideal arterial and venous substrate.

KEY READINGS

Joo S et al: Recanalization of thrombosed arteriovenous fistulas for hemodialysis by minimal venotomy. J Vasc Interv Radiol 2013;24:401.

Turmel-Rodrigues L et al: Treatment of failed native arteriovenous fistulae for hemodialysis by interventional radiology. Kidney Int 2000;57:1124.

FISTULA MATURATION

The term "fistula maturation" refers to a variety of biological, hemodynamic, and mechanical processes that occur from the time of fistula construction until the fistula becomes reliably usable for HD needle access. Successful maturation results in a high flow, large caliber, superficial vessel with robust wall structure suitable for repeated large-bore needle access. Criteria for assessment of maturation have been proposed by National Kidney Foundation-Kidney Disease Outcomes Quality Initiative (NKF-KDOQI) as the "rule of sixes." This stipulates that by 6 weeks after surgical creation the fistula should measure 6 mm diameter or greater, 6 mm or less deep from the skin surface, and 600 mL/min or greater blood flow. This author suggests the additional criterion for greater than 6 cm usable length. These parameters are relatively easy to quantitate, and provide a practical starting point for assessment of fistula maturity. However, there are several less easily quantified factors that may be important in achieving a mature fistula. These include patient needle tolerance; staff technical skill; quality and integrity of skin, body habitus, and anatomical accessibility of the fistula.

Numerous reports have shown poor patency of arteriovenous fistulae, with primary failure rates 15–20%, 1-year primary patency 36–63%, and secondary patency 55–66%. Only 11% of fistulae mature without requirement for further interventions. A large randomized, controlled trial of clopidogrel versus placebo for prevention of early fistula failure demonstrated reduced early thrombosis in the clopidogrel group (12.2% vs 19.5%), but no difference in fistula maturation, with failure rates of 61.8% and 59.5% in the two groups, respectively. This occurred despite additional surgical and percutaneous interventions to enhance fistula maturation.

Increased blood flow and adaptive remodeling begin immediately after successful surgical fistula construction.

Signs of maturation should be evident within 4 weeks of surgery, and it is essential that every fistula be assessed at this stage. Flow can be gauged qualitatively by the strength of palpable thrill and audible bruit. This should be low frequency and continuous through systole and diastole, but may be high-pitched and restricted to systole in the presence of stenosis. Vein diameter, depth, and usable length can be estimated and palpable stenoses and branch veins can be identified by physical examination. Duplex ultrasound may be used to complement and quantitate physical findings. When a fistula fails to develop, timely radiographic imaging is warranted to define the anatomy, and perform percutaneous interventions necessary to assist in maturation. There has been a tendency of some practitioners to wait an inordinate length of time, hoping that early fistula nonmaturation will improve over months or even years, and eventually result in a functional, mature fistula. There is no evidence to support such a protracted maturation strategy. For patients receiving hemodialysis via venous catheter, excessive delay in fistula maturation magnifies risks of catheter-related infection and central vein stenosis.

NKF-KDOQI guidelines recommend hand exercises, repeatedly squeezing a rubber ball to increase arterial blood flow and vessel size in maturing fistulae. This recommendation was based upon two very small, uncontrolled studies that demonstrated enlargement of radial artery and maximal vein diameters after a variable period of programmed hand exercises. Two randomized, controlled studies have since been published: One demonstrated measurable improvements in vein diameter, wall thickness, and blood flow rates associated with programmed tourniquet-enhanced isometric exercise; these changes correlated with improved clinical maturation. Another demonstrated no difference in flow or vein diameter, but improved clinical maturation at 1 month, particularly in distal radial-cephalic fistulae. Exercise-enhancement of fistula maturation is free and potentially beneficial, therefore remains an attractive strategy; furthermore, this activity draws the patient's attention to their fistula, encourages self-assessment for signs of maturation, and establishes an active role in the care of their "lifeline." A contrary view, however, holds that a well-constructed fistula will naturally mature based upon favorable anatomic and physiologic parameters, with or without adjunctive exercise. Conversely, if a fistula is predisposed to maturation failure due to unfavorable anatomy or biology, adjunctive exercise is unlikely to help.

There are various interventions that may assist in fistula maturation. These include balloon angioplasty of discrete stenotic lesions; balloon dilation of the intended puncture segment; ligation or coil embolization of competing accessory veins; or superficialization of deep vein. It is important to recognize that not every immature fistula can be salvaged, and in some cases, it is preferable to abandon a fistula with little hope of successful maturation. This decision must be weighed against alternative arteriovenous access options for each patient; if there is little prospect of creating a better-quality fistula, more aggressive maturation measures may be warranted. If, however the patient with a very poor quality fistula has arterial and venous anatomy well-suited to construction of a new high-quality fistula elsewhere (see Figure 56–5), the interventional physician and vascular surgeon should consider this before embarking on a serious of interventions likely to fail, or at best result in a marginal-quality, high-maintenance, low-performing fistula. Certain clinical and anatomical parameters have been found to correlate with fistula maturation; however, there is little data to help determine which established immature fistulae will respond favorably to maturation assistance maneuvers.

A meta-analysis on multiple studies of fistula nonmaturation pooled results from 12 reports comprising 745 patients treated for fistula nonmaturation. Using a variety of percutaneous and surgical methods, these demonstrated an 86% success rate in achieving a functional fistula. Primary and secondary patency rates from a subset of these papers were 51% and 76%, respectively. Several of the individual studies reviewed in this meta-analysis warrant particular attention. Beathard reported results of treating100 AVF with failure of spontaneous maturation. All had abnormalities that were clinically significant and warranted treatment, including stenosis of the venous outflow stenosis (78%), juxta-anastomotic segment (43%), arterial anastomosis (38%), or feeding artery (4%). Accessory vein ligation or embolization was performed in 46% of cases; in 12 cases the only lesion identified was an accessory vein; the results of treatment and long-term function in this subgroup were not reported separately. Successful fistula function was achieved in 92% of patients, with 68% remaining functional at 12 months. Falk reported results of treatment in 65 nonmaturing fistulae; 113 procedures were performed (1.7 per fistula), resulting in 74% functional fistulae. A high rate of subsequent interventions was also reported for matured fistulae, requiring 1.75 procedures per access-year to maintain fistula function. In a series of 119 patients with failure to mature AVF, treatments included angioplasty of the artery in 6 cases (5.1%), arterial anastomosis in 56 cases (47.1%), juxta-anastomotic segment in 35 cases (29.4%), peripheral vein in 70 cases (58.8%), and central vein in 10 cases (8.4%). Accessory veins were treated in 35 cases (29.4%). Mixed lesions were present in 85/119 cases (71.4%). Successful maturation defined by fistula use was achieved in 99/119 cases (83.2%). Numerous other papers describe similar results of various percutaneous interventions to aid in fistula maturation.

The term, "balloon maturation" has not been rigorously or uniformly defined. Miller reported results of fistula maturation utilizing a variety of interventional techniques, including "aggressive staged balloon assisted maturation" for deep and/or small caliber fistulae. This technique involves dilation of the entire fistula including the intended puncture segment. Initially 6–8-mm-diameter balloons were utilized, with sequential procedures at three week intervals, each time increasing balloon size by 2–3 mm up to a maximum of 16 mm. This technique was combined with other interventions, including ligation or coil embolization of competing vein branches. This study divided patients into two subgroups: those which met NKF-KDOQI criteria for maturity based upon size, flow, and depth were categorized as class-1 fistulae. Those not meeting NKF-KDOQI criteria based upon small size (2–5 mm diameter) or excessive depth (>6 mm) were categorized as class-2 fistulae. This study showed successful fistula maturation in 118 of 122 patients using these techniques. Class-1 patients required fewer procedures (1.6 vs 2.6) and shorter periods of time (5 vs 7 weeks) to achieve maturation when compared with class-2 patients. Primary patency for class-1 and class-2 patients, respectively, was 17% and 39% at 6 months. Secondary patency was 72% and 77% at 1 year; 53% and 61% at 2 years. These differences were not significant, and secondary patency was comparable to other reported studies. The principle importance of this paper is the description of the rather novel method of dilating veins without discrete stenosis using sequentially larger balloons ("balloon maturation") to enhance and/or accelerate their suitability for dialysis needle access.

Accessory vein obliteration by ligation or coil-embolization has been utilized in multiple series describing treatment for immature fistulae. Figure 56–11 illustrates a typical accessory vein coil-embolization procedure. In most reports, accessory vein obliteration has been combined with other percutaneous interventions to treat stenosis making it difficult to demonstrate the benefits and outcomes attributable to vein obliteration alone. There is one series reporting fistula maturation outcomes following percutaneous obliteration of accessory veins, without the presence of stenosis or use of angioplasty. In this report 17 patients underwent accessory vein obliteration using a percutaneous suture method; one to three accessory veins were ligated in each case (mean 1.7). This resulted in successful fistula maturation in 15 patients (88%) by 1.7 months (range 0.3–6 months) postintervention. Lack of a uniform, verifiable definition of clinically significant competing veins constitutes a major limitation in all reports of vein obliteration reports. This procedure has been based largely upon the operator's subjective interpretation of the physical exam, size of vessels, and angiographic appearance of flow. Distinguishing between detrimental "competing" veins, inconsequential accessory veins, and beneficial collateral veins is crucial, but not well elaborated in any trials. Collateral veins which develop in response to outflow stenosis must not be treated with vein obliteration techniques unless they are deemed to be diverting significant flow away from the fistula after definitive correction of the

outflow stenosis. No study to date has quantitated fistula flow or pressure in the primary and accessory veins before and after vein obliteration. Such quantitative measurements would be necessary to convincingly demonstrate the benefits of eliminating competing veins. Furthermore, some have argued for preservation of any/all accessory veins as potential vessels for cannulation sites or raw material for subsequent surgical revision. It is possible that premature loss of these veins may be detrimental to long-term fistula outcomes.

No discussion of fistula maturation would be complete without reference to needle access technique. Whatever the perceived quality of the fistula, response to interventions, size, and depth of the vein, or fistula blood flow, ultimately the true test of maturity is whether it can be safely, reliably, and repeatedly accessed using suitably sized dialysis needles. As with any technical skill, there is considerable variability in the experience and ability of dialysis technicians or nurses involved in fistula cannulation. Some programs and providers are experienced in the use of buttonhole needle access which may be valuable option for cannulation of selected fistulae. Substantial variability exists between programs, and even among the staff within a given facility. Thus, it is incumbent upon all programs and health care professionals to work toward improving fistula assessment and cannulation skills. It is also important to develop systems to ensure that those providers with the highest level of technical skill are utilized to cannulate the most challenging fistulae. All efforts to advance fistula maturation and usage will surely be confounded by poor cannulation technique with attendant vessel injury, infiltration, hematoma, aneurysm, or pseudoaneurysm formation. In the process, the patient will pay the price of unpleasant, painful, or prolonged dialysis sessions, frequent reinterventions, and inadequate delivery of hemodialysis. Under such adverse circumstances the patient may not appreciate the potential long-term advantages of a native fistula in the face of their personal negative experiences. For some, this may result in "fistula-phobia," refusal to accept further surgical or interventional procedures, and ultimately long-term catheter dependence.

There are special considerations applicable to angiographic evaluation and intervention for immature fistulae in patients with advanced stage chronic kidney disease who are not yet receiving hemodialysis treatment. Surgical fistula construction is recommended at least 6 months prior to the anticipated need for hemodialysis to allow sufficient time for maturation. For all the reasons discussed, these fistulae may fail to mature. Concerns about exposure to iodinated contrast media and risks for acute kidney injury may discourage some interventional physicians from performing necessary imaging studies. Carbon dioxide can be used in such cases and can provide sufficient image quality to guide intervention. However, carbon dioxide is an inherently

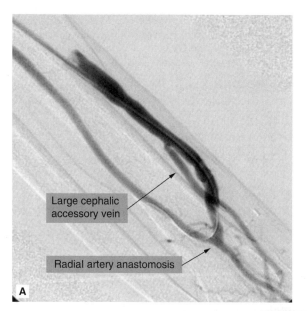

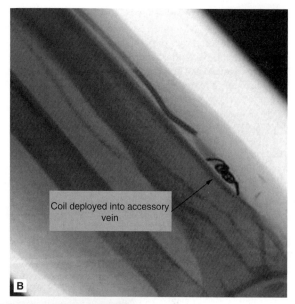

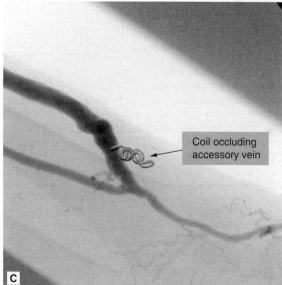

▲ **Figure 56–11. A.** Left forearm radial artery to cephalic vein fistula with a single large accessory vein diverting flow from the cephalic vein. **B.** Deployment of embolization coil into the accessory vein. **C.** Elimination of accessory vein flow following successful coil embolization.

limited imaging modality which provides less effective contrast and incomplete anatomical information compared to imaging with iodinated contrast media. Furthermore, carbon dioxide imaging of the upper-extremity arterial system is imaging is not advisable, due to risk for retrograde passage of carbon dioxide gas into the central arterial circulation.

The use of low-dose iodinated contrast (10–20 mL) for venographic imaging in 25 patients with stage IV or stage V chronic kidney disease has been reported, with no cases of acute kidney injury. Another study reported on 65 studies of immature fistula using low dose iodinated contrast (mean 7.8 mL) in 34 patients with stage IV chronic kidney disease. Mild acute kidney injury was observed in only 4.6% of studies, all spontaneously recovering to baseline without requirement for acute dialysis or other adverse clinical sequelae. Immature fistulae in chronic kidney disease patients should be studied and intervened upon as necessary to achieve functional maturation prior to the need for hemodialysis therapy.

KEY READINGS

Biuckians A, Scott EC, Meier GH, Panneton JM, Glickman MH: The natural history of autologous fistulas as first-time dialysis access in the KDOQI era. J Vasc Surg 2008;47:415.

Dember LM et al: Effect of clopidogrel on early failure of arteriovenous fistulas for hemodialysis. JAMA 2008;299:2164.

Miller GA et al: Aggressive approach to salvage non-maturing arteriovenous fistulae: a retrospective study with follow-up. J Vasc Access 2009;10:183.

Saad TF: Management of the immature autogenous arteriovenous fistula. Vascular 2010;18:316.

Voormolen EH et al: Nonmaturation of arm arteriovenous fistulas for hemodialysis access: a systematic review of risk factors and results of early treatment. J Vasc Surg 2009;49:325.

FISTULA CREATION

The creation of arteriovenous access is a surgical procedure, largely performed by vascular, transplant, or other suitably qualified general surgeons. Access creation has not been part of "mainstream" interventional nephrology in the United States, although some nephrologists in Europe have maintained this role. One U.S. nephrology group has demonstrated successful arteriovenous fistula creation by nephrologists, with maturation rate of 84%, comparable or superior to those reported in other series. It remains unclear whether other nephrologists will be willing or able to replicate this experience in their practices, overcoming substantial training, credentialing, logistical, and territorial obstacles.

Two devices are currently undergoing clinical investigation for percutaneous, nonsurgical creation of arteriovenous fistulae, each utilizing parallel catheters in adjacent peripheral artery and vein, and focally applied energy to form a direct channel between the vessels. One system utilizes magnets to approximate the adjacent catheters in the proximal ulnar artery and adjacent vein, then use a brief pulse of radiofrequency energy to create the arteriovenous fistula. Adjunctive coil embolization of the deep brachial vein was performed to encourage outflow to the superficial veins. This procedure was technically successful in 32 of 33 patients (97%). Of 27 patients available for follow-up, 24 were undergoing successful dialysis via the percutaneously-created fistula at 6 months. Two patients had patient access but did not initiate dialysis during the study; one failed due to thrombosis. Cumulative patency at 6 months was 96%.

Mean time to fistula maturation was 58 days. Comparable early results have been reported with a similar system using thermal energy.

KEY READINGS

Abdel-Aal AK, Gaddikeri S, Saddekni S: Technique of peritoneal catheter placement under fluroscopic guidance. Radiol Res Pract 2011;2011:141707.

Ash SR: Chronic peritoneal dialysis catheters: challenges and design solutions. Int J Artif Organs 2006;29:85.

Ash SR: Chronic peritoneal dialysis catheters: overview of design, placement, and removal procedures. Semin Dial 2003;16:323.

Ash SR: Chronic peritoneal dialysis catheters: procedures for placement, maintenance, and removal. Semin Nephrol 2002;22:221.

Crabtree JH et al: Peritoneal Dialysis University for Surgeons: a peritoneal access training program. Perit Dial Int 2016;36:177.

Crabtree JH: Peritoneal dialysis catheter implantation: avoiding problems and optimizing outcomes. Semin Dial 2015;28:12.

Mishler R, Yang Z, Mishler E: Arteriovenous fistula creation by nephrologist access surgeons worldwide. Adv Chronic Kidney Dis 2015;22:425.

Rajan DK et al: Percutaneous creation of an arteriovenous fistula for hemodialysis access. J Vasc Interv Radiol 2015;26:484.

Zaman F et al: Fluoroscopy-assisted placement of peritoneal dialysis catheters by nephrologists. Semin Dial 2005;18:247.

CONCLUSION

Interventional nephrology is an exciting and evolving discipline. The ability to deliver timely, efficient, high-quality, cost-effective service is central to the comprehensive care of these patients, as well as the operations of dialysis units and nephrology practices. Our role as nephrologists also allows us multiple opportunities for improvement in vascular access, including early vein preservation, creation of arteriovenous access in advance of the need for dialysis, minimization of venous catheter use, monitoring and screening for access dysfunction, and planning for creation of secondary native fistulae in anticipation of impending access failure. One of the challenges for the interventional nephrology community has been clinical research in vascular access; to this end, it is encouraging to see nephrologists involved in the design, execution, and publication of recent major interventional device trials. Working closely with surgeons, radiologists, nurses, and dialysis technicians, our challenges are to continue improving the quality of access care and outcomes for dialysis patients, lower access-related morbidity and mortality, reduce venous catheter usage, reduce hospitalizations, and reduce costs to the health care system. Dialysis access-related costs represent up to 25% of the total cost of hemodialysis care; these issues take on paramount importance in this new era of alternative payment models, where practices and dialysis providers share financial risks and incentives for the cost and quality of care.

▶ General Considerations

In addition to being a continuous daily home therapy, peritoneal dialysis (PD) offers a number of advantages for end-stage renal disease (ESRD) patients. Nevertheless, PD remains an underutilized form of renal replacement therapy. Recent data demonstrate that over 50% of ESRD patients in the United States would choose PD as the modality for renal replacement therapy if they are given the option. However, only about 12% of ESRD patients actually begin dialysis on this form of therapy. Recent attention has focused on the value of peritoneal dialysis as a convenient home therapy that is usually highly effective as long as there is some residual renal function (usually for several years after initiation of PD therapy). Slowly, the prevalence of PD therapy in the United States is increasing. A significant hindrance to its growth is the need for timely and effective placement of the chronic PD catheter. To this end, interventional nephrologists have taken the initiative in performing PD access-related procedures, including catheter insertion, catheter removal, and repositioning of a migrated catheter. The safety and success of PD access-related procedures by nephrologists have been well documented.

This chapter provides a review of PD catheter types, catheter placement procedures, and management of some catheter-related complications. It emphasizes the importance, feasibility, and advantages of PD access procedures performed with imaging techniques, as done by interventional nephrologists and radiologists.

▶ Chronic Peritoneal Catheters

A. Types

Chronic PD catheters are the most successful transcutaneous access devices in medical therapy. They have a functional lifespan measured in years, while by comparison chronic central venous catheters for dialysis often have functional problems or infectious complications within months. Chronic PD catheters constructed of soft silicone rubber material, though one prior catheter was constructed from polyurethane. The intraperitoneal portion contains 0.5–1 mm diameter side holes. One prior catheter had linear grooves or slots on its limbs rather than side holes. All chronic PD catheters have one or two extraperitoneal Dacron cuffs that promote a local inflammatory response. This produces a fibrous plug that fixes the catheter in position, preventing fluid leaks and bacterial migration around the catheter. In spite of their long term and overall success, chronic PD catheters are still imperfect. Peritoneal access failure is a source of frustration for all continuous ambulatory peritoneal dialysis (CAPD) programs, and it is the reason for about 25% of patient technique failures which

cause drop out from peritoneal dialysis therapy in the first 3 months of treatment. Increasing the success of a CAPD program requires optimal use of peritoneal catheters. Currently, the method of catheter placement has more effect on outcome than catheter design choice.

As shown in Figure 56–12, at first there appears to be a bewildering variety of chronic PDs. However, each portion of the catheter has only a few basic design options.

There are five designs of the intraperitoneal portion:

1. Straight Tenckhoff, with an 8-cm portion containing 0.5–1-mm side holes.

2. Curled Tenckhoff, with a coiled 16-cm portion containing side holes.

3. Straight Tenckhoff, with perpendicular discs (originally Toronto-Western™, now Oreopoulos-Zellerman™).

4. T-fluted catheter (Advantage™, no longer available) a T-shaped catheter with grooved limbs positioned against the parietal peritoneum.

5. Di Paolo self-locating catheter, identical to the straight Tenckhoff but with a weighted tip made of titanium (available in Europe, but not in the United States).

There are four basic shapes of the subcutaneous portion between the muscle wall and the skin exit site:

1. Straight or gently curved

2. A 150° bend or arc (Swan Neck™ or Arc™)

3. A 90° bend, with another 90° bend at the peritoneal surface (Cruz "Pail Handle" catheter, no longer available)

4. An extended catheter, with a titanium connector in the subcutaneous space connecting the internal portion to a long subcutaneous portion with Swan Neck at the outer end (Presternal™ or Exxtended™)

There are three positions and designs for Dacron™ cuffs:

1. A single cuff around the catheter, usually placed in the rectus muscle but sometimes on the outer surface of the rectus

2. Dual cuffs around the catheter, one in the rectus muscle and the other in the subcutaneous tissue

3. A disc-ball deep cuff with the parietal peritoneum sewn between the Dacron disc and the intraperitoneal silicone ball (Toronto-Western™ and Missouri™ catheters)

There are three internal diameters, each having an outer diameter of approximately 5 mm (Figure 56–13).

1. 2.6 mm, the standard Tenckhoff catheter size

2. 3.1 mm, the Cruz™ catheter

3. 3.5 mm, the Flex-Neck™ catheter

There are two materials of construction:

1. Silicone rubber (all currently available catheters)

2. Polyurethane (Cruz catheter, no longer available)

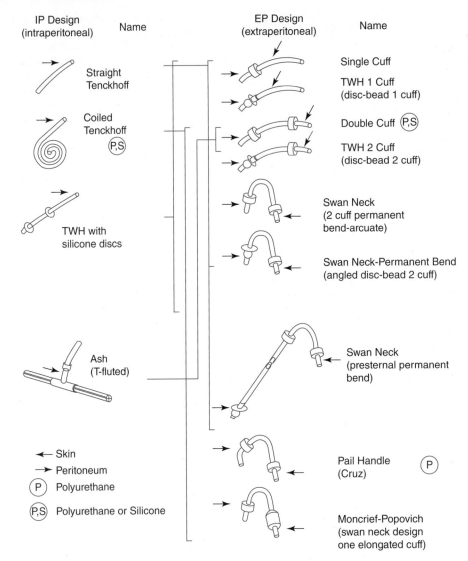

▲ **Figure 56–12.** Currently available peritoneal catheters; combinations of intraperitoneal and extraperitoneal designs.

The various intraperitoneal designs are all created to diminish outflow obstruction. The shape of the curled Tenckhoff catheter and the discs of the Toronto-Western catheter hold visceral peritoneal surfaces away from the side holes of the catheter. The grooves of the Advantage catheter distributed flow over the surface of the limbs that contact the parietal peritoneum, providing a much larger surface area for drainage than the side holes provide. An irritated omentum attaches firmly to the side holes of a catheter but only weakly to the grooves on a catheter (as demonstrated by the Blake surgical drain, with grooves on the intraperitoneal catheter surface). An older PD catheter design called

column disc (Lifecath™, no longer marketed) had a circular disc placed on the parietal peritoneal surface, with ports for fluid flow through the circumference. This catheter provided much higher outflow rates than standard Tenckhoff catheters. This catheter had to be placed and removed surgically.

The subcutaneous catheter shapes all allow creation of an exit site with a lateral or downward direction, which minimizes the risk of exit infection. An upward-directed exit site collects debris and fluid, increasing the risk of exit-site infection.

The optimal location for the standard deep cuff is within the rectus muscle. The subcutaneous cuff provides

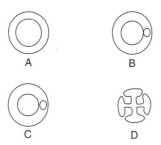

▲ **Figure 56–13.** Comparison of cross-sectional dimensions of the intraperitoneal portion of several peritoneal catheters. **A.** Flex-Neck Tenckhoff catheter (silicone). **B.** Cruz Tenckhoff catheter (polyurethane). **C.** Standard Tenckhoff catheter (silicone). **D.** One intraperitoneal limb of the T-fluted catheter (Advantage, silicone).

additional protection from bacterial contamination of the subcutaneous tunnel. The disc-ball deep cuff provides security of position of the catheter, since with the peritoneum sewn between the Dacron disc and intraperitoneal ball the catheter is fixed in position and cannot migrate outward. Similarly, the T shape of the Advantage catheter placed the intraperitoneal limbs against the parietal peritoneum, preventing outward migration of the catheter.

The larger internal diameter of the Flex-Neck catheters provides lower hydraulic resistance and more rapid dialysate flow during the early phase of outflow. In the latter part of outflow, the resistance to fluid flow is determined mostly by the spaces formed by peritoneal surfaces as they approach

the catheter, rather than the inside of the catheter. The Advantage catheter provided much larger entry ports for drainage of peritoneal fluid than the Tenckhoff catheter. This created a lower velocity of fluid entering the ports, in an attempt to diminish the tendency to draw omental tissue toward the catheter during outflow. Limited clinical studies demonstrated faster drainage of the peritoneum in the early and late phases of outflow and a decrease in residual peritoneal volume at the end of outflow. This catheter was more complicated to place than a Tenckhoff catheter, and more expensive, and so it is no longer marketed.

The material from which peritoneal catheters are constructed has not affected the incidence of complications. There was no decrease in the incidence of peritonitis or omental attachment leading to outflow failure with polyurethane catheters. They did have a weaker bond to the Dacron cuff, and loosening of this bond created pericatheter leaks and outward migration of the catheters.

B. Proper Location of Components

There is general agreement on the proper location of the components of chronic PD catheters (Figure 56–14):

1. The intraperitoneal portion should be between the parietal and visceral peritoneum and directed toward the pelvis to the right or left of the bladder.

2. The deep cuff should be within the medial or lateral border of the rectus sheath.

3. The subcutaneous cuff should be approximately 2 cm from the skin exit site.

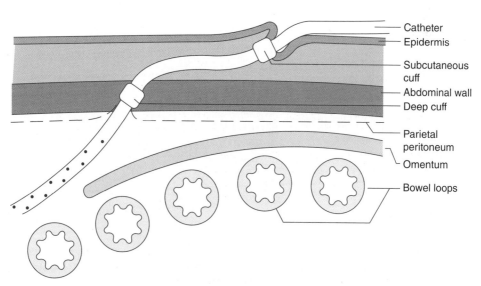

▲ **Figure 56–14.** Proper relationship of peritoneal cuffs to the abdominal musculature, parietal and visceral peritoneum, and skin exit site for the straight Tenckhoff catheter.

The parietal peritoneum is a large mostly flat surface that allows fluid to communicate with all parts of the peritoneum. Tenckhoff recommended that the intraperitoneal portion of PD catheters should be directed to lie in contact with the parietal peritoneum, to provide the best drainage of the abdomen. It should not lie between bowel loops or beneath sheets of omentum.

Placing the deep cuff within the abdominal musculature promotes firm tissue ingrowth and therefore avoids pericatheter hernias, leaks, catheter extrusion, and exit-site erosion. At the parietal peritoneal surface, the squamous epithelium reflects along the surface of the catheter to reach the deep cuff. If the deep cuff is outside the muscle wall, the peritoneal extension creates a potential hernia. At the skin surface, the stratified squamous epithelium follows the surface of the catheter until it reaches the superficial cuff. According to Tenckhoff, the subcutaneous cuff should be placed 2 cm from the exit site. If the exit-site tunnel is longer than 2 cm, the squamous epithelium progresses only partway down the tunnel and granulation tissue is left, leading to an exit site with continued "weeping" of serous fluid. T risk of exit-site infection is therefore increased.

Some peritoneal catheters have components that provide greater fixation of the deep cuff within the musculature.

When the Missouri and Toronto-Western catheters are placed, the parietal peritoneum is closed between the ball (inside the peritoneum) and disc (outside the peritoneum). With these catheters, as with the previous Advantage and column-disc catheters, outward migration of the catheter is impossible.

When placing peritoneal catheters it is best to choose a deep cuff location that is free of major blood vessels (Figure 56–15).

C. Methods of Implantation

PD catheter insertion can be accomplished by any one of five techniques: dissective (surgical), laparoscopic, blind (modified Seldinger), fluoroscopic, and peritoneoscopic. The dissective technique utilized by surgeons places the catheter by minilaparotomy, usually under general anesthesia. Laparoscopic placement is also performed by surgeons and involves entering the peritoneum with a port, infusing gas (usually CO_2), visualizing the anterior peritoneal space with a 5- or 10-mm-diameter scope, and placing the catheter through a 5- or 10-mm cannula. In the blind or modified Seldinger technique a needle is inserted into the abdomen, a guide wire is placed, a tract is dilated, and the catheter

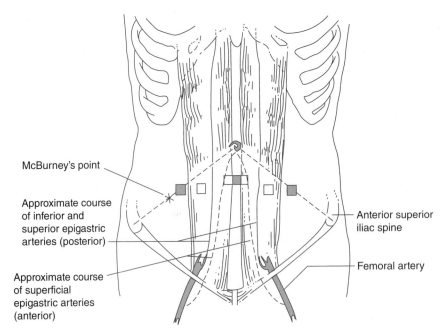

McBurney's point

Approximate course of inferior and superior epigastric arteries (posterior)

Approximate course of superficial epigastric arteries (anterior)

Anterior superior iliac spine

Femoral artery

▲ **Figure 56–15.** Major blood vessels and landmarks of the anterior abdominal wall. Open squares represent the preferred and safest points for the location of the deep cuff of a chronic peritoneal catheter within the medial or lateral border of the rectus muscle. Solid squares indicate the external landmarks used during blind insertion of a needle or cannula at the start of peritoneoscopic or blind catheter placement: One-half of the distance between the anterior superior iliac spine for the lateral border of the rectus and 2 cm below the umbilicus for the medial border of the rectus.

is inserted through a split sheath that is advanced over the wire, all without visualization of the peritoneal cavity. Fluoroscopic placement uses the same equipment, but adds use of injected dye to confirm position of the needle, guidewire, and catheter. Peritoneoscopic insertion uses a small (2.2-mm-diameter) optical peritoneoscope (Y-TEC Scope) for direct inspection of the peritoneal cavity after infusion of air, and identification of a suitable site for the intraperitoneal portion of the catheter.

There are advantages and disadvantages of each technique of catheter placement, and the overall success of the catheters is as dependent upon the skill and experience of the physician performing the procedure as the method of placement. Each procedure has unique advantages and problems.

Dissective techniques securely place the deep cuff within the abdominal musculature. The techniques can be performed without any specialized equipment except for a stylet to straighten the catheter. The incision in the abdominal musculature requires surrounding tissues to heal the wound while fibrous tissue is growing into the deep cuff. Pericatheter leaks are frequent if the catheter is used immediately after placement. Extensive dissection (incising/splitting the rectus sheath/muscle as well as incising the parietal peritoneum) in the surgical technique may lead to loose attachment of the catheter to the abdominal wall, thereby increasing the incidence of pericatheter leaks, subsequent tunnel infection and peritonitis, and catheter loss. Proper attention to technique can minimize these complications. However in general the catheter must have a "break in" period of 2–3 weeks in which PD exchanges are avoided, making early or urgent implementation of PD impossible. The dissective approach provides no visualization of adhesions and free spaces within the peritoneum. The catheter tip is advanced by "feel" and may be advanced to press against loops of bowel, or near adhesions, leading to early outflow failure of the catheter. Surgical placement is usually done under general anesthesia. General anesthesia and intubation increases risks considerably for unstable patients who are rated class IV or V. Some types of catheters require surgical placement, such as the disc-and-ball Missouri or Toronto-Western catheters.

Laparoscopic techniques allow the best visualization of the anterior peritoneal space. The course of the catheter can be carefully chosen and using instruments placed through cannulas, the catheter can be positioned to lie against the parietal peritoneum. Using other instruments, the omentum can be moved to the upper abdomen and fixed in place with sutures (omentopexy) and adhesions can be removed. Also, the tunnel of the catheter through the rectus muscle can be made at a very low angle, which helps to keep the internal part of the catheter directed toward the pelvis. These advanced techniques diminish the risk of outflow failure and improve the longevity of PD catheters. The multiple entry points each create some trauma to the peritoneum and the muscular defects must be repaired to prevent leaks. As with

dissective placement, healing of the wounds occurs at the same time as fibrous ingrowth to the Dacron cuff. Laparoscopic placement involves use of rather complex and expensive equipment, including video cameras, and it is always done under general anesthesia.

Blind placement procedures are convenient, can be performed anywhere in a hospital, and have the advantage of being low in cost. The needle, guidewire, dilators, and sheath are often packed in a kit with the peritoneal catheter. Bowel perforation is an occasional complication, usually not recognized until the catheter has been completely placed and is flushed. No visualization of the peritoneal space is provided to avoid impingement of the catheter tip on adhesions or visceral surfaces. The deep cuff is usually left just outside of the abdominal musculature, not within the rectus sheath.

Fluoroscopic placement allows injection of dye to confirm that the tip of a needle is within the peritoneal space. The dye quickly moves from the needle-point into spaces between bowel and omentum. Other pictures emerge if the needle tip is in the preperitoneal space, omentum, or bowel lumen. Fluoroscopy is used to follow the course of the guidewire when it is inserted, and the catheter as it is inserted through the peel-away sheath. Fluoroscopic techniques are very familiar to interventional radiologists and nephrologists, and the images augment the "feel" of the various steps to ensure that components are in their proper locations.

Peritoneoscopic placement allows the best visualization of the peritoneal space, of any of the above techniques except laparoscopy. In peritoneoscopy, a 2.2-mm ID cannula with internal trocar and outside spiral plastic guide is inserted through the abdominal musculature into the peritoneal space. The trocar is removed and the peritoneoscope inserted to visualize surfaces moving with inspiration. The scope is removed and 1 L of air is injected, the patient placed in Trendelenburg, and the visceral and parietal peritoneum inspected. The scope is advanced along the parietal peritoneal surface to location that is free of adhesions, and the spiral guide is left in this position. The guide directs the catheter to the chosen location, and also expands to allow the deep cuff to enter the musculature. This technique ensures placement of the catheter next to the parietal peritoneal surface, and avoids placing the catheter under bowel loops, under omentum, or against adhesions. The Y-TEC procedure can be performed in any room in the hospital. Specialized equipment must be purchased, however, and the physician must have some training in peritoneoscopic techniques. A video camera is very helpful in performing the procedure although not required. Peritoneoscopic placement varies from laparoscopic techniques by using a much smaller scope and puncture size, only one peritoneal puncture site, a device to advance the cuff into the musculature, air in the peritoneum rather than CO_2, and using local anesthetic (with mild sedation if needed) rather than general anesthesia. Peritoneoscopic insertion of a PD catheter by a nephrologist can be safely performed in a procedure room, an interventional laboratory, or an intensive care unit using standard precautions for infection control.

The preference of one technique over another for PD catheter placement must take into account the incidence of complications (such as pericatheter leakage, outflow failure, exit-site and tunnel infection), the length of catheter functional survival, the costs, ease, and timeliness of insertion, the speed at which peritoneal dialysis can be implemented, and the risks of placement (including risks of anesthesia). To this end, peritoneoscopic placement of PD catheters by nephrologists has been rigorously compared to the surgical technique. Both randomized and nonrandomized studies have documented superiority of the peritoneoscopic techniques over surgical placement, in terms of a lower incidence of catheter complications (infection, outflow failure, pericatheter leak), though catheter survival has not been proven longer with any of the techniques. The avoidance of various complications by peritoneoscopic and fluoroscopic placement may relate to the decreased tissue dissection required with this technique.

Placement by fluoroscopic techniques has the same general advantages as peritoneoscopic placement, including less trauma to tissues surrounding the catheter and placement of the internal portion of catheter against the parietal peritoneum. The deep cuff may also be placed into the muscle layer without much dissection, as long as the operator obtains good visualization of the external rectus sheath and is experienced with the techniques using a split-sheath. Outcomes of catheters placed by fluoroscopy also compare favorably to surgical techniques. Few long-term complications are seen in prospective studies. In peritoneoscopic and fluoroscopic placement, the cuff is placed securely in the muscle layer, without dissection of tissues around it and the internal portion is positioned next to the parietal peritoneum. The postoperative course is brief and the catheter can be used immediately for some schedule of PD (such as with overnight exchanges with the patient at rest, dry during the day). Thus, "early start" and "urgent" peritoneal dialysis are possible using these techniques, usually with nighttime or bedside automated machines, and the patient supine. A 2- to 3-week postoperative period for complete wound healing is recommended before implementing CAPD.

In summary, with optimal training in PD catheter insertion, a nephrologist or radiologist can perform PD catheter placement safely and successfully. The American Society of Diagnostic and Interventional Nephrology (ASDIN) has established accreditation guidelines for training centers and certification guidelines for individual physicians to obtain the necessary skills in PD catheter placement. Although two nephrologists would be ideal, a PD access placement program can be successfully initiated by a single trained nephrologist. When peritoneal catheter insertion is performed by nephrologists, a variety of advantages can occur

Table 56–1. Potential procedural advantages of peritoneal dialysis catheter insertion by an interventional nephrologist.

Interventional Nephrologist	Surgeon
Timely initiation of therapy	Unnecessary delays often present
Operating room not required	Operating room time and scheduling required
Anesthesia services not required	Anesthesia services required
Local anesthesia used	General anesthesia used (usually)
Less dissection	More dissection
Rectus sheath/muscle and peritoneum intact	Rectus sheath and peritoneum incised
Direct intraperitoneal visualization	No intraperitoneal visualization
Decreased incidence of complications	Higher incidence of complications
Longer catheter survival	Shorter catheter survival
Complete understanding of the renal disease	Minimal understanding of renal disease
Cost-effective	Higher cost
Continuity of care	Lack of continuity of care
May help to counteract peritoneal dialysis underutilization	No evidence to counteract peritoneal dialysis underutilization
Effective communication	Increased number of middle men and decreased communication

Data from Asif A et al: Semin Dial 2003;16:266. Ash SR: Semin Nephrol 2002;22:221. Ash SR: Nephrol News Issues 1993;7:33. Ash SR: Adv Perit Dial 1998;14:75. Ash SR et al: Perit Dial Bull 1983;3:8. Ash SR: Semin Dial 1992;5:199. Gadallah MF et al: Adv Perit Dial 2001;17:122. Gadallah MF et al: Am J Kidney Dis 2000;35:301.

for the patient, some related to the procedure and some related to the timeliness and continuity of care (Table 56–1). When interventional radiologists participate as a team member in care of ESRD patients, many of the same patient benefits accrue in placement of PD catheters. However, the success of the procedure is the most important patient benefit. The placement of PD catheters should be performed by the physician with the best outcomes, using whatever technique is most successful in their hands.

EFFECTS OF DESIGN ON CATHETER SUCCESS

Randomized, prospectively controlled studies have surprisingly shown little effect of catheter design on the success of peritoneal catheters. If properly placed, dual-cuff Tenckhoff catheters have a lower incidence of exit-site infection and longer lifespan than single-cuff catheters, although properly placed single-cuff catheters can work as well. Curled Tenckhoff catheters are thought to have a lower incidence of outflow failure than straight catheters but randomized studies have failed to prove a difference in frequency of this complication. Swan neck (arcuate) catheters would be expected to have a lower incidence of exit-site infection than those with straight subcutaneous segments, since the exit site is always directed downward with the Swan neck design. However, this advantage has not been proven.

A few advantages for specific PD catheters have been proven. Catheters with the best fixation of the deep cuff (such as the Missouri, Advantage, and column-disc catheters) have a very low incidence of exit-site infection. Catheters with a larger internal diameter and thinner walls, such as the Flex-Neck (see Figure 56–13) are more pliable and create less tension between deep and superficial cuffs during normal patient activities. A problem with Flex-Neck catheters is that they are prone to crimping in the subcutaneous tunnel if they are angled too sharply. If physicians follow a template to create the subcutaneous tunnel with a gentle downward curve, crimps in the subcutaneous tract are eliminated. Choosing a "swan neck" catheter shape for the subcutaneous tract minimizes the chance of kinking, for any type of catheter. Due to their pliability, Flex-Neck catheters may be somewhat more prone to migrate if omentum attaches to them, but this has not been proven. Repositioning these catheters is with the same techniques used for standard Tenckhoff catheters. Most interventionalists agree that it is easier to reposition a straight Tenckhoff catheter than a coiled Tenckhoff catheter.

All PD catheters can serve as a nidus for infection, requiring removal in cases of persistent peritonitis. None of the new designs or materials has diminished the risk of catheter infection, although extended catheters may have a higher risk of persisting peritonitis, possibly due to the length of silicone tubing or the additional titanium connector. Possibly peritoneal catheters could be constructed with long-term antibacterial surfaces, but this will probably come after such surfaces are clinically applied to central venous catheters for dialysis. Similarly if materials are found to prevent fibrous sheathing in central venous catheters for dialysis, the same materials may prevent omental attachment to peritoneal catheters. Of course, for both of these catheter types the new materials would have to be present on the inside and outside of the entire catheter, not just on the outer surface in the subcutaneous space.

BURYING THE PERITONEAL DIALYSIS CATHETER

Traditional surgical implantation of Tenckhoff catheters involves immediate exteriorization of the external segment through the skin, so that the catheter can be used for supportive PD or for intermittent infusions during the "break-in" period. To prevent blockage and to confirm function, the catheter is flushed weekly with saline or dialysate; each exchange carries the same risk of peritonitis as in CAPD therapy. The catheter must also be bandaged and the skin exit site must be kept clean in the weeks after placement to avoid bacterial contamination of the exit site. The patient must therefore be trained in some techniques of catheter care. It has always been difficult to decide when to place a PD catheter in a patient with chronic renal insufficiency. If the catheter is placed too early, the patient may spend weeks to months caring for a catheter that is not used for dialysis. If the catheter is placed after the patient becomes uremic, and early or emergent PD is implemented, there is risk of a pericatheter leak if the patient ambulates when the peritoneum is full of fluid. If PD is delayed for a 2- to 3-week "break-in" period, the uremia must be treated by hemodialysis during this period.

A placement technique has been devised in which the entire peritoneal catheter can be "buried" or "embedded" under the skin some weeks to months before it needs to be used. The catheter burying technique was first described for placement of a modified Tenckhoff catheter with a 2.5-cm-long superficial cuff (the Moncrief™ catheter), but the technique was quickly adopted for standard dual-cuff Tenckhoff catheters. In the original technique the external portion of the catheter was brought through a 2- to 3-cm skin exit site (much larger than the usual 0.5 cm incision). The catheter was then tied off with silk suture and coiled and placed into a "pouch" created under the skin. The skin exit site was then closed. Weeks to months later, the original skin exit site was opened and the free end of the catheter was brought through the skin incision and the sides of the incision were closed around the catheter. Alternatively the outer tip was brought through a newly created exit site.

The goal of burying the PD catheter was to allow ingrowth of tissue into the cuffs of the catheter without the chance of bacterial colonization and to allow a transcutaneous exit site to be created after the tissue had fully grown into the deep and subcutaneous cuffs. Burying the catheter effectively eliminated early pericatheter leaks and decreased the incidence of peritonitis. The incidence of exit-site infections was not decreased in patients with catheters that are buried and exteriorized, which may be explained by the increase in trauma near the exit site that occurred during burying and exteriorizing the catheter. An alternative method for burying the external portion of a PD catheter can be done using a small exit site incision. The catheter is placed and tunneled as usual, but the exit site is made approximately 1 cm long (rather than the usual 0.5 cm). The tip of the catheter is then blocked with a plug and brought through the exit site to lie in a linear tunnel that is created through the subcutaneous tissue. This type of tunnel can be created by making a secondary exit site and using a long tunneling tool with a removable titanium tip (Embedding® Tool). Alternatively it can be created using a split-sheath or spiral guide similar to that used in placing PD catheters. These techniques do not require a secondary exit site. The catheter plug can be fashioned from the tip of a plastic tunneling tool or any other sterile plastic instrument. In planning for hemodialysis of patients with ESRD, it is common practice to place fistulas or grafts several months before the need for initiation of dialysis, so that they can "mature" before use. PD catheters also "mature" after placement, with fibrous tissue ingrowth into the cuffs and the development of a fibrous tunnel. The fully ingrown catheter is more resistant to infection of the cuffs and the surface of the catheter. The technique of burying PD catheters after placement allows this maturation to occur before use of the catheter, much as with fistulas and grafts. It also allows the time of catheter insertion to be separated from the time of catheter use and avoids the patient having to learn how to care for the catheter site or observe the catheter site for potential complications until peritoneal dialysis is begun. At the time of initiation of dialysis, the patient and physician can focus attention on the proper performance of the technique and patient response rather than on the function of the catheter. The patient can be trained in full-volume CAPD techniques rather than in "break-in" or cycler techniques used for immediately exteriorized catheters.

A curious aspect of the burying technique is that it seems contrary to "the rules" of catheter break-in. In immediately exteriorized catheters, it is necessary to infuse and drain the dialysate or saline (with or without heparin) at least weekly to prevent outflow failure or obstruction of the catheter. However, with the completely buried catheter, there is no infusion of any fluid for periods of up to 1 year or more. This may be made possible because in the exteriorized catheter, stress and strain on the catheter and its compliance allow some fluid to enter and exit the side holes during patient movement. The buried catheter has less motion and with a secure blockage of the tip there is very little fluid inflow/outflow through the holes during normal activity. Furthermore, the infusion of saline or dialysate during break-in techniques adds a bioincompatible fluid to the abdomen at a time before the catheter is "biolized" or protein/lipid coated. The buried catheter becomes biolized in the absence of dialysate or saline in the peritoneum. Buried catheters can develop early outflow failure, but the incidence of this complication does not seem greater than for catheters placed and used in the usual manner.

CATHETER REMOVAL

In general, the physician who places a device is responsible for removing it when complications require removal or when it is no longer needed. Removal of a standard Tenckhoff PD catheter can be safely performed by nephrologists without significant discomfort under local anesthesia,

although an anxious or needle-averse patient may require conscious sedation. The procedure should be done only with a sterile technique, good lighting, antiseptic skin preparation (including the catheter near the skin), and draping typical of a procedure done in a surgical suite or outpatient surgery room. The drape to cover the primary incision, deliberately excluding the exit site, since the exit site and catheter, even when treated with antiseptic, cannot be considered clean. Here too, an operating room is not needed as the procedure can be performed in a procedure room using standard precautions for infection control.

Removal of Missouri or Oreopoulos-Zellerman type catheters is a little more complicated, since the Dacron disc rests next to the peritoneum and develops fibrous adhesions to the peritoneum and the posterior rectus sheath. The ball of the catheter is intraperitoneal. These catheters require more dissection during removal and general anesthesia may be required for their removal. These catheters are generally placed by surgeons and should be removed by the surgeons who placed them. If there is doubt regarding the type of catheter implanted, a careful ultrasound with a "vascular" probe or an X-ray can usually distinguish the various types of deep cuff.

COMPLICATIONS OF CATHETER INSERTION

Placement of a PD catheter can usually be performed safely by physicians skilled in the procedure, using any of the above techniques. However, as with any abdominal procedure, there are risks of immediate complications, including visceral perforation, bleeding, kinking of the catheter, failure of outflow, infection, pinhole leaks in the catheter, drug reaction, and postoperative pain. Other catheter complications occur weeks to days after insertion, and only indirectly relate to the method of placement. These include catheter migration, outflow failure, pericatheter leaks, pericatheter hernias, catheter breakage, infection, etc.

Bowel perforation is the most feared complication of insertion of a PD catheter and can occur with any of the above techniques (including the dissective and laparoscopic techniques). The incidence of bowel perforation is less than 1% in most studies, but over 1% in some studies using blind placement techniques. The risk is increased in patients with numerous intraperitoneal adhesions. Physicians performing this procedure should be well versed in diagnosing this complication promptly and managing the patient effectively.

Bowel perforation almost always occurs at the start of placement of a PD catheter, with the first entry to the peritoneum. By insertion of a needle or trocar, or by dissection, the physician is attempting to create a space where none existed previously (unless ascites is present). If bowel perforation occurs with a needle or small trocar (2.2 mm or less in diameter), and is immediately recognized, the procedure can be terminated and the bowel will usually heal on its own without surgical repair. It is necessary to place the patient on antibiotics and admission to the hospital is advised. Early recognition of bowel perforation is possible with fluoroscopic images (made with a few cc of dye injection) or with visual images seen through the peritoneoscope (before any fluid is infused through the cannula) or by malodorous gas with any technique. If the perforation occurs at entry of the parietal peritoneum by dissection and is recognized immediately, the bowel can be repaired at that time. However, if the bowel perforation is not recognized until after the catheter has been placed and large volumes of fluid infused (100 cc or more), then there will often be widespread peritonitis. Laparotomy, surgical repair of the bowel and drains are then required, as well as systemic antibiotics. Even with fluoroscopy or peritoneoscopy, the images can be misleading if there has been a "through-and-through" penetration of the bowel. In this case the fluoroscopic and peritoneoscopic images will demonstrate that the tip of the needle or cannula is within the peritoneum, but will not show that the proximal part of the needle or cannula passes through a bowel. A history of previous abdominal surgery can result in significant intraperitoneal adhesions and has been identified as a relative contraindication to placement of PD catheters. However, 10–20% of ESRD patients have intraperitoneal adhesions and have no history of surgery. In all patients, a careful examination of the abdominal wall by ultrasound (with a "vascular" probe) will demonstrate areas that are free of heavy or fixed adhesions. Free motion of the visceral peritoneum against the parietal peritoneum will be seen when the patient takes in a deep breath. Also, a thin double line will be seen along the parietal peritoneal surface. In patients with known adhesions or previous surgery, the best method of placing the PD catheter is by peritoneoscopy or laparoscopy. These techniques can determine the extent of adhesions, and direct the internal portion of the PD catheter toward the parietal peritoneum that is most free of adhesions.

CONCLUSIONS

PD access-related procedures can be safely and successfully performed by nephrologists with excellent catheter outcome data. There are a variety of advantages, including the timely initiation of therapy, when the catheter insertion is performed by a nephrologist. However, nephrologists must obtain optimal training and develop the necessary skills to perform these procedures. ASDIN is actively engaged in promoting the performance of PD access-related procedures by nephrologists and developing training centers at academic medical centers. At every dialysis center, selected nephrologists should consider expanding their role to perform PD access-related procedures in order to provide timely delivery of this important aspect of ESRD care.

■ CHAPTER REVIEW QUESTIONS

Endovascular Procedures

1. Real-time ultrasound guidance for central venous catheter placement is
   A. Not superior to landmark-based vein puncture
   B. Not recommended due to extra equipment and time required to perform
   C. Is recommended as "standard of care" for all central venous access procedures
   D. Is only recommended when placing tunneled, long-term venous catheters
   E. Is only recommended for jugular vein catheterization

2. Stent grafts for treatment of stenosis at AV graft venous anastomosis
   A. Have demonstrated advantage versus "bare-metal" stents
   B. Improve lesion primary patency versus angioplasty alone
   C. Increase graft secondary or cumulative patency
   D. Should only be placed as a "last resort" in the setting of failed angioplasty
   E. Should never be placed for forearm graft outflow across the elbow

3. Coil embolization of fistula branch vein should be performed
   A. For all branch veins arising from a native fistula
   B. For collateral outflow veins in the presence of venous stenosis
   C. When competing veins divert sufficient flow from the fistula to delay maturation or impair delivery of dialysis
   D. To reduce fistula flow in setting of high-output cardiac failure
   E. Never

4. Venous catheter dysfunction may be associated with
   A. Improper catheter tip position
   B. Kinking of catheter
   C. Thrombosis of catheter tip
   D. Fibrin sheath entrapment of catheter
   E. All the above

5. Which of the following may favorably alter the biology of venous hyperplasia and stenosis?
   A. Balloon angioplasty
   B. Stent grafts
   C. Paclitaxel-coated balloon angioplasty
   D. Cutting balloon angioplasty
   E. Oral antiplatelet agents

Peritoneal Dialysis Catheter Procedures

1. Peritoneal access failure accounts for what percent of patient dropout from peritoneal dialysis therapy?
   A. 5%
   B. 25%
   C. 50%
   D. 75%

2. What is the design difference between a straight and coiled Tenckhoff catheter?
   A. Coiled has larger side holes.
   B. Coiled has a 150° bend in the subcutaneous tissue.
   C. Coiled has a spiral-shaped tip within the peritoneum.
   D. There is no difference.

3. Which of the following is not a method to place PD catheters?
   A. Dissection
   B. Laparoscopy
   C. Microsurgical
   D. Blind (Seldinger)
   E. Fluoroscopy
   F. Peritoneoscopy

4. In the fluoroscopic method of PD catheter placement, how is the position of the needle tip confirmed to be intraperitoneal?
   A. Feel
   B. Fluid aspiration
   C. Rising fluid level in needle
   D. Injection of small amount of radiopaque dye
   E. Injection of small amount of air

5. Which of the PD catheter techniques are most valuable in a patient with suspected intraperitoneal adhesions?
   A. Dissection
   B. Laparoscopy
   C. Blind
   D. Fluoroscopy
   E. Peritoneoscopy
   F. B and E

Poisonings and Intoxications

James F. Winchester, MD, FRCP (Glas)

Elliot Charen, MD

Nikolas B. Harbord, MD

To underscore the importance of poisoning in modern times recent statistics reveal that the annual deaths from poisoning (47,055 in 2014) now exceed those from traffic accidents in the United States (Figure 57–1). Opioid deaths in the United States, 18,893 in 2014, (Figure 57–2) and Europe (Table 57–1) have become so serious that the antidote naloxone in the form of nasal sprays are carried by police, emergency medical services, firemen, friends, and acquaintances for emergency treatment in the event of an overdose. On the other hand, in patients obtaining advice from their local poison control center mortality is low. The latest report of the American Association of Poison Control Centers (AAPCC) for 2014 reports experience with 2,165,142 human exposures. In 2014, the majority of cases (68.1%) were managed at home, 28.3% required treatment in a health care setting and 1408 patients died; 44,713 patients were treated with single dose activated charcoal; 11,275 were treated by alkalinization; 2481 received hemodialysis; 43 received hemoperfusion; 42 received extracorporeal oxygenation, 33 "other" extracorporeal treatment and 16 had an organ transplant.

MULTIPLE-DOSE ACTIVATED CHARCOAL

One method of removing ingested toxins from the body is administration of single or multiple doses of activated charcoal per os. Charcoal given acutely decreases absorption of toxins from the gastrointestinal tract but has also been recommended in repeated doses, to capture toxic substances from the enterohepatic recirculation. However, although there is some experimental evidence that this mode of therapy can decrease the half-life of many xenobiotics, there are only a few toxic substances for which multidose charcoal administration has been shown to be effective. According to the American Academy of Clinical Toxicology, these include carbamazepine, dapsone, phenobarbital, quinine, and theophylline. One recent study in volunteers suggests that repeated doses of superactivated charcoal may

have some detoxification benefit up to 3 hours after acetaminophen ingestion. However, two other volunteer studies conclude that multiple-dose activated charcoal may not be effective more than 1 hour after acetaminophen overdose. Multiple-dose activated charcoal has also been reported to reduce death and serious arrhythmias in yellow oleander poisoning (Table 57–1).

KEY READINGS

American Academy of Clinical Toxicology: Position statement and practice guidelines on the use of multi-dose activated charcoal in the treatment of acute poisoning. Clin Toxicol 1999;37:731.

Bekka R et al: Treatment of methanol and isopropanol poisoning with intravenous fomepizole. J Toxicol Clin Toxicol 2001;39:59.

Centers for Disease Control and Prevention (CDC): Accidents or unintentional injuries. http://www.cdc.gov/nchs/fastats/accidental-injury.htm.

Cheng J-T et al: Clearance of ethylene glycol by kidneys and hemodialysis. J Toxicol Clin Toxicol 1987;25:95.

Christopherson AB et al: Activated charcoal alone or after gastric lavage: a simulated large paracetamol intoxication. Br J Clin Pharmacol 2002;52:312.

de Silva HA et al: Multiple-dose activated charcoal for treatment of yellow oleander poisoning: a single-blind, randomised, placebo-controlled trial. Lancet 2003;361:1935.

Green R et al: How long after drug ingestion is activated charcoal still effective? J Toxicol Clin Toxicol 2001;39:601.

Juurlink DN et al: Extracorporeal treatment for salicylate poisoning: systematic review and recommendations from the EXTRIP workgroup. Ann Emerg Med 2015;66:165.

Klemm A et al: Comparison of aluminum removal between hemodialysis with polycarbonate low flux membrane and hemofiltration with polysulfone high flux membrane in end-stage renal failure patients. Clin Nephrol 1997;47:133.

Mann J, Branton LJ, Larkins RG. Hyperosmolality complicating recovery from lithium toxicity. Br Med J 1978;1:1522.

Mégarbane B, Borron SW, Baud FJ: Current recommendations for treatment of severe toxic alcohol poisonings. Intensive Care Med 2005;31:189.

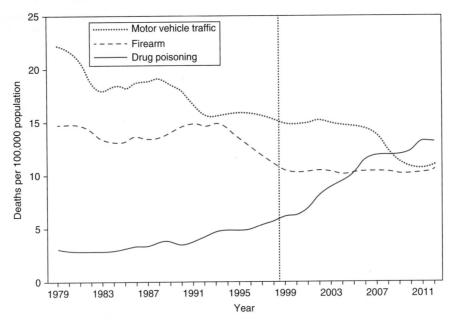

▲ **Figure 57–1.** Opioid deaths in the United States 1979–2011.

Mowry JB et al: 2014 annual report of the American Association of Poison Control Centers' National Poison Data System (NPDS): 32nd annual report. Clin Toxicol 2015;53: 962.

Sato RL et al: Efficacy of superactivated charcoal administered late (3 hours) after acetaminophen overdose. Am J Emerg Med 2003;21:189.

Simard M et al: Lithium carbonate intoxication. A case report and review of the literature. Arch Intern Med 1989;149:36.

Vodovar D et al: Lithium poisoning in the intensive care unit: predictive factors of severity and indications for extracorporeal toxin removal to improve outcome. Clin Toxicol (Phila) 2016;54:615.

Von Hartitzsch B et al: Permanent neurological sequelae despite haemodialysis for lithium intoxication. Br Med J 1972;4:757.

Zakharov S et al: Use of out-of-hospital ethanol administration to improve outcome in mass methanol outbreaks. Ann Emerg Med 2016;68:52.

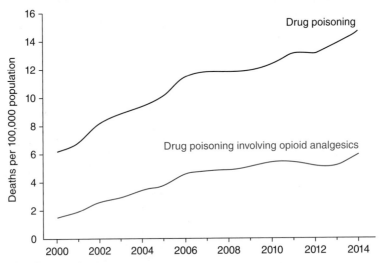

▲ **Figure 57–2.** Drug poisoning and opioid analgesic poisoning death rates in the United States 2000–2014.

Table 57–1. Substances for which multi-dose activated charcoal is indicated.

Carbamazepine
Dapsone
Phenobarbital
Quinine
Theophylline
Acetaminophen (up to 1 hour after ingestion)
Yellow oleander

Table 57–2. Dissociation constants (Pk$_a$) for various drugs.

Acids		Bases	
Drug	**pK$_a$**	**Drug**	**pK$_a$**
Acetylsalicylic acid	3.49	Amphetamine	9.9
Amobarbital	7.7	Phencyclidine	8.5
Barbital	7.91		

FORCED DIURESIS AND URINARY ALKALINIZATION

Many substances are eliminated by the kidneys if they are filtered and not reabsorbed or if they are actively secreted by the tubules into the urine. Filtration occurs freely for smaller molecules (<5000 Da) that are not highly bound to plasma proteins such as albumin. Phenobarbital is such a substance. In order for such substances to be excreted effectively, they must remain largely in the tubular fluid as they traverse the nephron.

If a substance is cleared by filtration and kidney function is good, it is important to maintain that level of function in order to continue elimination of that substance. It is therefore crucial to support the patient's extracellular fluid volume by giving appropriate intravenous saline; that is, to maintain a good diuresis. However, the concept of overhydrating a patient to "force" a diuresis has not been shown to be of benefit in poisoning and risks overloading the left ventricle. Repletion and maintenance of extracellular volume are always indicated, especially in salicylate poisoning, where there is usually a respiratory water loss of about 2 L in the adult. The patient should be monitored for signs of volume overload or depletion.

The kidneys' natural ability to clear the blood of many substances is also enhanced by their secretion of substances into the urine. The tubules take up many xenobiotics that circulate in plasma, even if they are bound to proteins, and move them into the lumen to be excreted. There are separate transport pathways for anions (such as penicillin) and cations (such as gentamicin).

Renal excretion of a particular xenobiotic can be increased if there is a form of the substance that is less readily reabsorbed back into the blood from the tubular lumen. Many drugs and toxins are weak acids or bases which diffuse back into tubular cells in their neutral form but are poorly absorbed as anions or cations. For this reason, if one can maintain the pH of the urine such that the nonreabsorbable ionized form is favored, there will be greater net excretion of that substance (Table 57–2). In general, anionic substances (such as salicylate) are best excreted at a higher urine pH (above 7), while cationic drugs (such as phencyclidine) are

best excreted at low urine pH (<5.5). This phenomenon is called "diffusion trapping." It is seen in the case of urinary ammonium, which is the main route of renal hydrogen ion excretion. Ammonia freely diffuses from the tubular lumen into the cells and the blood. However, in the relatively acid urine pH, most of the ammonia takes up hydrogen ions, and the resultant ammonium ion is trapped in the tubular lumen, to be readily excreted.

However, the clearance of many drugs and chemicals is not substantially increased by this maneuver. Not all ionizable substances have their excretion enhanced by manipulation of urine pH. This is usually because their volume of distribution (Vd) is high (Table 57–3). Substances that remain exclusively (or nearly so) in total body water will have a lower Vd than those with high affinity for lipid or protein and which appear to dissolve in a much greater quantity of water than their plasma levels indicate (digoxin is a good example). Adjusting urine pH is only effective if the Vd is low and if an altered urine pH has actually been shown to be effective in enhancing removal of the toxin.

In the case of xenobiotics which are weak bases, such as phencyclidine, no advantage has been shown in acidifying the urine to enhance the drug's excretion. Acidifying the blood in an attempt to accomplish this only leads to metabolic acidosis, which can worsen the patient's condition. On the other hand, renal excretion of a number of weak acids is markedly enhanced by urinary alkalinization (Table 57–4).

Table 57–3. Volume of distribution (L/G) and protein binding (%) of some selected drugs in a 70-kg person.

Drug	Volume of Distribution		Protein Binding (%)
	L/kg	**Liters^a**	
Acetylsalicylic acid	0.1–0.2	7–14	50–90
Amitriptyline	15	1050	95
Digoxin	6.8	476	2
Phenobarbital	0.7	49	51

Table 57–4. Substances for which urinary alkalinization improves excretion.

Salicylate
Mecoprop
2,4-D (2,4-dichlorophenoxyacetic acid)
Methotrexate
Phenobarbital (but not as effective as multi-dose activated charcoal)
Chlorpropamide (usually responds to supportive treatment)
Diflunisal (not of clinical usefulness)

Of these, the most important is salicylate, whose excretion can be quadrupled if urinary pH is 7.5 or above. It is unclear, however, why this is so, since the pK_a for salicylic acid is 3.0. At a urine pH of 6.0, 99.9% of the salicylate should already be ionized and therefore not reabsorbed. Other mechanisms besides diffusion trapping may explain the enhanced salicylate excretion at higher urine pH.

In the past, the Done nomogram has been used to estimate the toxicokinetics of salicylate in moderate to severe overdoses. Some clinicians use this nomogram to calculate the endogenous clearance of salicylate. Unfortunately, the Done calculations were established in children and assume first-order kinetic clearance of salicylate from the body, in which the excretion of a drug is proportional to the concentration of that drug in body fluids. In fact, in severe salicylate poisoning, several elimination pathways for the drug become saturated, and the clearance becomes zero-order, that is, there is a constant rate of drug removal per time, independent of concentration.

The renal excretion of two herbicides, 2,4-D (2,4-dichlorophenoxyacetic acid) and mecoprop, is also increased at higher urine pH. Alkalinizing the urine may also help eliminate overdoses of methotrexate. The excretion of phenobarbital and chlorpropamide is also augmented by urinary alkalinization, but this is rarely useful since the former is better eliminated by multi-dose activated charcoal, and the latter usually responds to supportive care with glucose infusion (Table 57–2).

KEY READINGS

Flomenbaum NE: Salicylates. In: *Goldfrank's Toxicologic Emergencies*, 7th ed. Goldfrank LR et al (eds). New York, McGraw-Hill; 2002, pp. 507–518.

Goldfarb DS, Matalon D: Principles and techniques applied to enhance elimination. In: *Goldfrank's Toxicologic Emergencies*, 10th ed. Flomenbaum NE et al (eds). New York, McGraw-Hill; 2015.

Proudfoot AT, Krenzelok EP, Vale JA: Position paper on urine alkalinization. J Toxicol Clin Toxicol 2004;42:1.

Proudfoot AT et al: Does urine alkalinization increase salicylate elimination? If so, why? Toxicol Rev 2003;22:129.

DIALYSIS TECHNIQUES USED IN POISONING

Many substances can be removed by hemodialysis and hemoperfusion.

PRINCIPLES OF DIALYSIS IN RELATIONSHIP TO DRUG REMOVAL

These principles have been discussed elsewhere in this textbook. Factors governing drug removal are: solute (or drug) size; its lipid-water partition coefficient (or lipid solubility); the degree to which it is protein bound; its volume of distribution; and the presence of a concentration gradient promoting constant removal of the drug or chemical moiety. The physical factors governing drug removal by the dialyzer are blood flow rate through the dialyzer, dialysate flow rate, dialyzer surface area, and the characteristics of the specific membrane.

For drugs (usually about 300 Da) that are diffusible across semipermeable membranes solute removal rates (clearance) increase with increasing blood flow rate. For solutes greater than 300 Da, the rate of diffusion across the membrane is less, concentration gradients across the membrane remain high, and increasing flow rates have a lesser effect on drug clearance rates. For larger drugs, the removal rate can be increased by increasing the surface area, or by choosing a high permeability membrane. The latter is the preferred method.

KEY READING

Maher JF: Principles of dialysis and dialysis of drugs. Am J Med 62:475,1977.

▶ **Clearance**

Clearance of drugs and chemicals follows the same principle as that used to calculate solute clearance by the kidney. Clearance is given by the following formula:

$$\text{Clearance} = Q_b \frac{A-V}{A}$$

where A is arterial or inlet concentration, V is venous or outlet concentration, of drug going through the dialyzer, and Q_b is blood flow rate through the dialyzer. The ratio $A-V/A$ is the drug extraction ratio (ER) across the dialyzer.

▶ **Hemodialysis**

The procedure for hemodialysis in poisoning is identical to that used in end-stage renal disease patients with one or two exceptions. Although there is a lack of randomized controlled trials (RCTs) in the treatment of poisoning, the EXTRIP workgroup has published their consensus view on the use dialysis for certain drugs using a specific methodology. The reader is referred to the EXTRIP workgroup website for the most up to date information.

In a drug intoxicated hypotensive patient who requires pressor agents to maintain an adequate blood pressure, if pressors are administered through the dialysis blood lines, they should be placed distal to the drug removing device since they are readily removed through the hemodialysis membrane or sorbent. Pressor requirements may need to be increased during the procedure even if pressors are administered in a completely separate line for the same reason.

If dialysate regeneration systems using a sorbent system (the REDY system) are used in the treatment of poisoned patients, there is the theoretical risk of sorbent saturation, and drug removal rates may decrease over time. Over the last 10 years high-efficiency dialyzers composed of synthetic membranes capable of removing drugs at higher clearances than those of early cellulosic membrane hemodialyzers, have been used in drug poisoning, with clearances approaching that of hemoperfusion devices. More recently high cutoff membrane dialysis has been associated with enhanced phenytoin removal accomplished in part by protein bound phenytoin adhering to the membrane surface. This was not the case for high cutoff membrane dialysis for tricyclic drug poisoning, being defeated by the very large volume of distribution that tricyclic drugs possess. Although several reports of the benefits of dialysis in dabigatran (an oral thrombin inhibitor anticoagulant) overdose exist, the recent approval of a monoclonal antibody against the drug has become available and approved by the Federal Food and Drug Administration.

KEY READINGS

Chen BC et al: Hemodialysis for the treatment of pulmonary hemorrhage from dabigatran overdose. Am J Kidney Dis 2013;62:591.
EXtracorporeal TReatments In Poisoning (EXTRIP) Workgroup. http://www.extrip-workgroup.org/.
Lavergne V et al: The EXTRIP (EXtracorporeal TReatments In Poisoning) workgroup: guideline methodology. Clin Toxicol (Phila) 2012;50:403.
Palmer BF: Effectiveness of hemodialysis in the extracorporeal therapy of phenobarbital overdose. Am J Kidney Dis 2000;36:640.
Pollack CV Jr: Evidence supporting idarucizumab for the reversal of dabigatran. Am J Med 2016;129:S73.
Schmidt JJ et al: Treatment of amitriptyline intoxications by extended high cut-off dialysis. Clin Kidney J 2015;8:796.
Singh T et al: Extracorporeal therapy for dabigatran removal in the treatment of acute bleeding: a single center experience. Clin J Am Soc Nephrol 2013;8:1533.

SORBENT HEMOPERFUSION

Hemoperfusion was quite popular for the treatment of poisoning in the 1970s and 1980s. Currently in the United States, activated charcoal hemoperfusion devices, but not resin hemoperfusion devices, are available for clinical use, although their availability is lacking in many medical centers.

Certain resins have been shown to be most effective for removal of lipid-soluble drugs, with drug clearance rates

Table 57–5. Available hemoperfusion devices.

Manufacturer	Device	Sorbent Type
Gambro	Adsorba	Charcoal
Braun	Haemoresin	XAD-4 resin

from blood often exceeding those achieved by charcoal hemoperfusion; these are available in Europe. Larger molecules exceeding the pore structure of even high efficiency synthetic membranes are becoming available or such use as endotoxin and cytokine removal. A partial list of the available hemoperfusion devices is given in Table 57–5. Hemoperfusion relies on the physical process of adsorption. For many drugs clearance was better than with hemodialysis. The hemoperfusion circuit for treatment of drug intoxication can but need not be combined with dialysis in certain situations (particularly when there is a serious acidosis shown to be corrected by bicarbonate dialysate). The manufacturer's "Instructions For Use" should be followed since some devices come "dry" and others need to be flushed with saline, and heparinization protocols differ. The most efficient drug removal is achieved with blood flow rates of approximately 300 mL/min. Even in the hypotensive patient lower blood flow rates achieve significant drug removal.

Removal of lipid-soluble drugs, such as glutethimide and methaqualone, was far more efficient with XAD-4 resin hemoperfusion than with activated charcoal. Modern dialyzers with high permeability may be of greater efficiency than those used in the 1970s and 1980s, and a reappraisal of dialysis versus charcoal hemoperfusion in poisoning may be called for (see Figure 57–3, showing chelated aluminum extraction ratios from treatment with a high flux dialyzer compared with charcoal hemoperfusion; as well as question 3 in Chapter Review Questions section). However, the spectrum of drugs taken in overdose situations in the 21st century is quite different from that used in the late 20th century, and studies to reexamine drugs which are obsolete may never be done.

Table 57–8 lists some drugs that have been reported to be removed by various types of hemoperfusion; again, it cannot be overstated that many of these reports are anecdotal, but critical review of drug removal rates indicates that those drugs not enclosed in parentheses are most efficiently removed.

KEY READINGS

Gelfand MC et al: Charcoal hemoperfusion in severe drug overdosage. Trans Am Soc Artif Intern Organs 1977;23:599.
Hampel G et al: Experience with fixed-bed charcoal haemoperfusion in the treatment of severe drug intoxication. Arch Toxicol 1980;45:133.

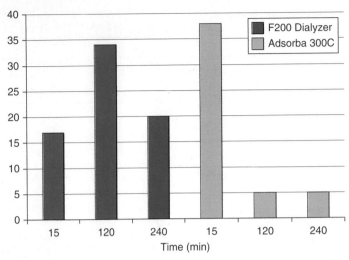

▲ **Figure 57–3.** Extraction ratios for total Al-deferoxamine complex removal: comparison of high flux dialysis and a charcoal hemoperfusion device.

Shalkham AS et al: The availability and use of charcoal hemoperfusion in the treatment of poisoned patients. Am J Kidney Dis 2006;48:239.

Verpooten GA, De Broe ME: Combined hemoperfusion hemodialysis in severe poisoning: kinetics of drug extraction. Resuscitation 1984;11:275.

Winchester JF, Harbord NB, Charen E: Sorbents, hemoperfusion devices. In: Magee CC, Tucker JK, Singh, AK (eds). *Core Concepts in Dialysis and Continuous Therapies.* Boston, MA: Springer; 2016, pp. 269–276.

COMPLICATIONS OF HEMOPERFUSION

The principal side effect of hemoperfusion with charcoal or resin preparations is platelet depletion of about 30% or greater, which may or may not give rise to clinical bleeding problems. Reductions in serum calcium and serum glucose and transient falls in white blood cell counts, usually mild may be seen. A mild reduction of 1 to 2°F in body temperature is expected, due to no rewarming in the extracorporeal circuit, and frequent body temperatures should be taken in deeply comatose patients. The falls in platelet concentration usually return to normal within 24–48 hours following a single hemoperfusion.

CRITERIA FOR HEMODIALYSIS IN POISONING

The prime consideration in the decision to employ extracorporeal techniques to remove poisons is based on the clinical features of poisoning particularly if the patient's condition deteriorates progressively despite intensive supportive therapy.

Suggested clinical criteria are outlined in Table 57–6. These criteria should be used along with the plasma concentrations of common drugs (Table 57–7), above which hemodialysis or hemoperfusion should be considered. Table 57–8 lists the reported dialyzable drugs; many of these reports are single case reports, since it has been difficult to undertake controlled studies. For further information see Matzke et al. (2011).

KEY READING

Matzke GR et al: Drug dosing consideration in patients with acute and chronic kidney disease–a clinical update from Kidney Disease: Improving Global Outcomes (KDIGO). Kidney Int 2011;80:1122.

Table 57–6. Clinical considerations for hemodialysis or hemoperfusion in poisoning.

1. Progressive deterioration despite intensive care
2. Severe intoxication with hypoventilation, hypothermia, and hypotension
3. Predisposition to complications of coma (eg, chronic obstructive pulmonary disease)
4. Impaired normal drug excretory function due to hepatic, cardiac, or renal insufficiency
5. Poisoning with agents with metabolic and/or delayed effects, eg, methanol, ethylene glycol
6. Intoxication with a drug or poison, which can be extracted at a rate exceeding endogenous elimination

Table 57–7. Plasma concentrations of common poisons above which hemodialysis (HP) or hemoperfusion (HP) should be considered.

Drug	Serum (µg/mL)	Concentration (mmol/L)	Method of Choice
Salicylates	800	5000	HD
Theophylline	400	2200	HP>HD
Paraquat	0.1	0.5	HP>HD
Methanol	50		HD

Suggested concentrations only: in mixed intoxications clinical condition may not reflect drug concentrations.

Table 57–8. Drugs and chemicals removed with hemodialysis and hemoperfusion.

Antimicrobials/Anticancer	Ampicillin	(Vancomycin)	(Secobarbital)
Cefaclor	Azlocillin	Capreomycin	
Cefadroxil	Carbenicillin	PAS	**Nonbarbiturate Hypnotics,**
Cefamandole	Clavulinic Acid	Pyrazinamide	**Sedatives, Tranquilizers,**
Cefazolin	(Cloxacillin)	(Rifampin)	**Anticonvulsants, Muscle**
Cefixime	(Dicloxacillin)	(Cycloserine)	**Relaxants**
Cefmenoxime	(Floxacillin)	Ethambutol	Carbamazepine
Cefmetazole	Mecillinam	5-Fluorocytosine	Atenolol
(Cefonicid)	(Mezlocillin)	Acyclovir	Baclofen
(Cefoperazone)	(Methicillin)	(Amantadine)	Betaxolol
Ceforanide	(Nafcillin)	Didanosine	(Bretylium)
(Cefotaxime)	Penicillin	Foscarnet	Clonidine
Cefotetan	Piperacillin	Ganciclovir	(Calcium channel lockers)
Cefotiam	Temocillin	(Ribavirin)	Captopril
Cefoxitin	Ticarcillin	Vidarabine	(Diazoxide)
Cefpirome	(Clindamycin)	Zidovudine	Carbromal
Cefroxadine	(Erythromycin)	(Pentamidine)	Chloral Hydrate
Cefsulodin	(Azithromycin)	(Praziquantel)	(Chlordiazepoxide)
Ceftazidime	(Clarithromycin)	(Fluconazole)	(Diazepam)
(Ceftriaxone)	Metronidazole	(Itraconazole)	(Diphenylhydantoin)
Cefuroxime	Nitrofurantoin	(Ketoconazole)	(Diphenhydramine)
Cefacetrile	Ornidazole	(Miconazole)	Ethiamate
Cephalexin	Sulfisoxazole	(Chloroquine)	Ethchlorvynol
Cephalothin	Sulfonamides	(Quinine)	Ethosuximide
(Cephapirin)	Tetracycline	(Azathioprine)	Gallamine
Cephradine	(Doxycycline)	Bredinin	Glutethimide
Moxalactam	(Minocycline)	Busulfan	(Heroin)
Amikacin	Tinidazole	Cyclophosphamide	Meprobamate
Dibekacin	Trimethoprim	5-Fluorouracil	(Methaqualone)
Fosfomycin	Aztreonam	(Methotrexate)	Methsuximide
Gentamicin	Cilastatin		Methyprylon
Kanamycin	Imipenem	**Barbiturates**	Paraldehyde
Neomycin	(Chloramphenicol)	Amobarbital	Primidone
Netilmicin	(Amphotericin)	Aprobarbital	Valproic acid
Sisomicin	Ciprofloxacin	Barbital	
Streptomycin	(Enoxacin)	Butabarbital	**Cardiovascular Agents**
Tobramycin	Fleroxacin	Cyclobarbital	Acebutolol
Bacitracin	(Norfloxacin)	Pentobarbital	(Amiodarone)
Colistin	Ofloxacin	Phenobarbital	Amrinone
Amoxicillin	Isoniazid	Quinalbital	(Digoxin)

(Continued)

Table 57–8. Drugs and chemicals removed with hemodialysis and hemoperfusion. (*Continued*)

Enalapril	Acetaminophen	**Plants, Animals,**	Folic acid
Fosinopril	Acetophenetidin	**Herbicides, Insecticides**	Mannitol
Lisinopril	Acetylsalicylic acid	Alkyl phosphate	Iodine
Quinapril	Colchicine	Amanitin	(Iron)*
Ramipril	Methylsalicylate	Demeton sulfoxide	(Lead)*
(Encainide)	(D-Propoxyphene)	Dimethoate	Lithium
(Flecainide)	Salicylic acid	Diquat	(Magnesium)
(Lidocaine)		Glufosinate	(Mercury)*
Metoprolol	**Antidepressants**	Methylmercury Complex	Potassium
Methyldopa	(Amitriptyline)	Oleander toxin	(Potassium dichromate)*
(Ouabain)	Amphetamines	(Organophosphates)	Phosphate
N-Acetylprocainamide	(Imipramine)	Paraquat	Sodium
Nadolol	Isocarboxazid	Snake bite	Strontium(Thallium)*
(Pindolol)	Mao Inhibitors	Sodium chlorate	(Tin)
Practolol	Moclobemide	Star fruit toxin	(Zinc)
Procainamide	(Pargylline)	Potassium chlorate	Methylprednisolone
Propranolol	(Phenelzine)		4-Methylpyrazole
(Quinidine)	Tranylcypromine	**Miscellaneous**	Sodium citrate
(Timolol)	(Tricyclics)	Acipimox	Theophylline
Sotalol		Allopurinol	Thiocyanate
Tocainide	**Solvents, Gases**	Aminophylline	Ranitidine
	Acetone	Aniline	
Alcohols	Camphor	Borates	**Metals, Inorganics**
Ethanol	Carbon monoxide	Boric acid	(Aluminum)*
2-Butoxyethanol	(Carbon tetrachloride)	(Chlorpropamide)	Arsenic*
Ethylene glycol	(Eucalyptus oil)	Chromic acid	Barium
Isopropanol	Thiols	(Cimetidine)	Bromide
Methanol	Toluene	Dabigatran	(Copper)*
Analgesics, Antirheumatics	Trichloroethylene	Dinitro-o-cresol	Formate

(Not well removed), * with chelating agent.

HEMOPERFUSION AND HEMODIALYSIS WITH CHELATING AGENTS

In dialysis patients, aluminum and iron intoxication can be treated with deferoxamine in conjunction with dialysis (continuous ambulatory peritoneal dialysis or hemodialysis) or hemoperfusion, for removal of the deferoxamine-aluminum or deferoxamine-iron complex. Clinical improvement in the osteomalacia component of renal osteodystrophy is seen after aluminum is removed. Encephalopathy, iron overload or anemia also improve.

Heavy metals and their salts are not removed efficiently by dialysis or hemoperfusion alone. During hemodialysis, metal removal may be enhanced with chelating agents, such as N-acetylcysteine or cysteine. On the other hand, removal of mercury and thallium, by hemoperfusion appears modest at best.

KEY READINGS

Chang TM, Barre P: Effect of desferrioxamine on removal of aluminum and iron by coated charcoal haemoperfusion and haemodialysis. Lancet 1983;2:1051.

Winchester JF: Management of iron overload. Semin Nephrol 1986;4:22.

IMMUNOPHARMACOLOGY IN POISONING

Digoxin antibodies, specifically the Fab fragments, neutralize digoxin and reduces any toxicity. Recrudescence of digoxin poisoning has been reported 24–48 hours after administration of Fab antibodies in renal failure patients. In a kinetic analysis of elderly and renally impaired patients with digoxin and digitoxin poisoning, it was suggested that the dose of Fab antibodies should be the same as for young patients or those with normal renal function. In digoxin poisoning the elimination halftime of digoxin in anephric patients can be substantially reduced with the addition of resin hemoperfusion, although such devices are no longer available. EXTRIP does not recommend dialysis in digoxin poisoning.

Specific antibody to dabigatran is also available to reverse the factor Xa inhibition.

KEY READINGS

Hoy WE et al: XAD-4 resin hemoperfusion for digitoxic patients with renal failure. Kidney Int 1983;23:79.

Renard C et al: Pharmacokinetics of digoxin-specific Fab: effects of decreased renal function and age. Br J Clin Pharmacol 1997;44:135.

Ujhelyi MR et al: Disposition of digoxin immune Fab in patients with kidney failure. Clin Pharmacol Ther 1993;54:388.

■ CHAPTER REVIEW QUESTIONS

1. A 32-year-old Czech man at a party in Prague had several drinks from a bottle labeled "Zubrovinka." Two of his drinking companions complained that they had headache and changes in their vision and recalled a recent newspaper article about patients in another town getting ill after drinking vodka with a label similar to theirs. He decided to go to the emergency department, where he was evaluated. His only symptom at the time was nausea without vomiting. He denied chest pain, dyspnea, headache, diaphoresis, and visual disturbances. Blood pressure was 146/86, temperature 98.7, pulse 106 and regular, and respirations 14. Examination of the head, eyes (including fundi), neck, lungs, heart, chest, abdomen, nervous system, and extremities was entirely normal. The emergency physician called a central agency and was told to start the patient on oral ethanol immediately.

Laboratory data included serum Na 138 mEq/L, K 4.8 mEq/L, Cl 99 mEq/L, CO_2 23 mEq/L, BUN 11 mg/dL, creatinine 0.8 mg/dL, glucose 96 mg/dL. Urinalysis was normal; measured serum osmolality was 390 mOsm/kg and his venous blood gas (VBG) had a pH of 7.34, pCO_2 27 mm Hg, pO_2 of 114 mm Hg, HCO_3 of 12.4 mmol/L.

The patient was begun promptly on oral fomepizole with a loading dose of 15 mg/kg and 10 mg/kg every 12 hours and sodium bicarbonate 5% in dextrose IV 500 mL every 12 hours. The following day the VBG showed the following: pH 7.2, pCO_2 30, pO_2 90, HCO_3 15. His only complaint was of "fuzzy" vision (ophthalmic exam showed no changes from the day before).

Which ONE of the following statements is correct?

A. The bicarbonate dosage should be increased.
B. He should receive hemodialysis.
C. He should receive hemodialysis AND an increase in fomepizole dosage.

2. A previously healthy 28-year-old man was hospitalized 3 hours after drinking 280 mL of antifreeze containing 95% ethylene glycol. He was tremulous and agitated but not obviously intoxicated. Blood pressure was 137/88 mm Hg, temperature 98.8°F, pulse 88 beats/min, respirations 24 breaths/min. Head, eyes, neck, lungs, heart, abdomen, neurological system, and extremities were all normal.

Laboratory data showed serum osmolality 362 mOsm/kg, Na 146, K 4.5, Cl 110, CO_2 11. BUN was 10 mg/dL and creatinine 1.1 mg/dL. Arterial pH was 7.17, pCO_2 26, pO_2 105. Urine had no protein, glucose, or cells, but contained numerous envelope- and needle-shaped crystals. The patient was loaded with saline and ethanol and subsequently hemodialyzed. At no time did the patient develop any decrease in renal function. Timed collections of blood and urine for ethylene glycol were performed before and after hemodialysis. Endogenous renal clearance of ethylene glycol was 27.5 mL/min, while hemodialysis clearance of ethylene glycol was 136.6 mL/min. By 30 hours after ingestion the patient's ethylene glycol level was zero. The patient was discharged after 72 hours with no target organ damage from the ingestion.

Was it essential to dialyze this patient?
A. Yes
B. No

3. A 75-year-old woman was admitted from another hospital 8 days following irrigation of the bladder with a 1% alum solution (aluminum potassium sulfate) for intractable hemorrhagic cystitis. Her mental status had been impaired from post-irrigation day 3, and a serum Al drawn on day 3 was reported 5 days later to be 423 μg/L. Six hours after a 500-mg infusion of deferoxamine she was dialyzed for 4 hours using a 2-M^2 high flux dialyzer for 4 hours. Because of reports that charcoal hemoperfusion was superior to hemodialysis in the past, she was treated on day 2 with a 4-hour hemoperfusion 6 hours after the same dose of deferoxamine.

Total (chelated and nonchelated) Al extraction by the devices was calculated. Although starting at a lower extraction ratio than hemoperfusion (~20% vs 38%) hemodialysis had an average extraction ratio of 24% versus an average of 16%, because of saturation of the hemoperfusion device (extraction only 5% at 2 and 4 hours). In addition the patient had no changes in platelets during hemodialysis, but profound thrombocytopenia after hemoperfusion. The patient was subsequently treated with chelation and hemodialysis alone.

Which of these methods increase dialysis efficiency for removal of any solute including removal of poisons?
A. Increase blood flow rate through device.
B. Increase dialysate flow rate through device.
C. Increase surface area of device.
D. All of the above.

4. A 22-year-old college student was found wandering in the residence hall. She was examined at student health where she was found to be irritable, confused, tachypneic, and mildly hypotensive. Her roommate called student health to report that the patient had just broken up with her boyfriend, and that the roommate had found some pills lying on the bathroom floor and an empty aspirin container. This prompted transfer to a tertiary care center, where she was found to be acidemic (pH 7.24), hypokalemic and to have a salicylate concentration of 75 mg/dL. Shortly after admission she was noticed to be somnolent. This prompted admission to the medical intensive care unit, where hemodialysis was performed via a femoral vein catheter. Within 2 hours her acidosis had improved (pH 7.34), the salicylate concentration was 35 mg/dL and by 4 hours her pH was 7.4 and the salicylate concentration was 20 mg/dL. Dialysis was discontinued.

What prompted the clinicians to initiate dialysis?
A. The pH
B. The salicylate level
C. Somnolence

5. A 62-year-old woman with bipolar disorder has been taking lithium carbonate 300 mg three times daily for several years, with effective control of symptoms at a plasma level of lithium around 0.8–1.0 mEq/L. In the summer during a routine visit to her orthopedist for knee pain she is found to have hypertension (160/95 mm Hg). Following the most recent guidelines for the treatment of hypertension the orthopedist starts her on hydrochlorothiazide 25 mg/day (HCTZ). Over the next 2 months her husband notices a gradual change in her previously mild tremor to a more coarse tremor with occasional "twitches." On the day of presentation he cannot rouse her from sleep and he calls 911.

At the emergency room she is noticed to be somnolent but arousable to pain stimuli. GCS (Glasgow Coma Scale) was 9. Her vital signs show respirations of 18, pulse 70, temperature 98.4, and blood pressure 100/70 mm Hg. There are no abnormal finding in heart, lungs, chest, and extremities except she is noticed to have myoclonic movements in the upper extremities. Chemistries are Na 135, K 3.2, Cl 100, BUN 60, Cr 1.8, HCO_3 30, Hb 12 g/L, WBC 12,000, Li 3.5 mEq/L. She is started on IV normal saline at 100 mL/h. A second lithium level 2 hours and 4 hours after receiving saline is relatively unchanged (3.3 and 3.1 mEq/L, respectively) but the plasma Na is now 145 mEq/L and Cr has risen to 2.3 mg/dL. She undergoes an 8 hour dialysis. Which of the following are correct?
A. She should not have been given HCTZ.
B. This is chronic Li toxicity.
C. She should have been given half normal saline.
D. All of the above.

Palliative Care Nephrology

Holly M. Koncicki, MD, MS

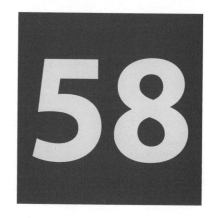

Palliative care is an approach to patient care in which there is a focus on improving the quality of life of patients and families living with complex or life limiting illnesses by ensuring that treatment is consistent with patient goals and values, as well as prompt identification and aggressive treatment of symptoms. It is often inappropriately interchanged with hospice or end of life care, though this is only a small portion of palliative care. Unlike hospice care, which is offered in the last 6 months of life, palliative care can be incorporated early, at any stage of a serious or life limiting illness and can be offered concurrently with curative or disease specific therapies (Figure 58–1). Though use has been well established in cancer and congestive heart disease, recognition of the needs in patients with chronic kidney disease (CKD) has led to a growing interest in this field of palliative care nephrology. CKD is a life-limiting condition that will necessitate the need for patients, family members, and care providers to engage in discussions regarding treatment decisions. As the number of patients with CKD increases, and as incident dialysis patients are ageing, the demand for palliative care will soon overwhelm the current availability of specialty trained physicians. There are several important palliative care skills that specialty providers should be sufficient in, in order to streamline care. These skills include the ability to engage in shared decision making including prognostication of patients with CKD and discussions regarding modality selection including conservative therapy, symptom identification and basic management, and laying the foundation for advanced care planning. Integration of nephrology and palliative care exists in certain areas of the world in which conservative care, or supportive care clinics are well established for caring for patients with CKD, some of who may opt for nondialysis, or conservative treatment of their advanced kidney disease. Referral to, or consultation with palliative care physicians is appropriate if the aforementioned needs are unable to be met by the nephrology provider, for the complicated patient or family dynamic, or for assistance with discussions and transitions for end of life care including hospice.

SHARED DECISION MAKING

The Renal Physicians Association (RPA) highlights shared decision making as the preferred approach to patient centered care when discussing treatment options for advanced renal disease. It is a meeting between the patient or surrogate decision makers, who are knowledgeable of the patient's overall goals and preferences and the nephrology provider who is able to impart medical knowledge, discuss risks and benefits, and make recommendations regarding treatments which match what the patient desires. A framework has been proposed in which four factors are evaluated: medical indications, patient preferences, quality of life and contextual features (Table 58–1). In terms of medical indications, discussion of prognosis with available treatment options, as well as preparing the patient and family for possible disease trajectories is essential. In order to elicit patient preferences, quality of life and contextual features communication tools can be utilized. Though outside the scope of this chapter, reviews and teaching programs are available to help improve communication styles of providers.

KEY READINGS

Koncicki HM, Schell JO: Communication skills and decision making for elderly patients with advanced kidney disease: a guide for nephrologists. Am J Kidney Dis 2016;67:688.

Renal Physicians Association: *Shared Decision Making in the Appropriate Initiation and Withdrawal from Dialysis*, 2nd ed. Washington, DC: Renal Physicians Association; 2010.

Schell JO, Cohen RA: A communication framework for dialysis decision-making for frail elderly patients. Clin J Am Soc Nephrol 2014;9:2014.

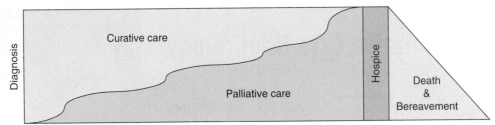

▲ **Figure 58–1.** Updated palliative care model: palliative care can be incorporated early, at any stage of a serious or life-limiting illness and can be offered concurrently with curative or disease specific therapies. Hospice is a subset of palliative care that is focused upon patients who have a prognosis of 6 months or less. (Adapted from Lynn J, Adamson DM: *Living Well at the End of Life: Adapting Health Care to Serious Chronic Illness in Old Age.* Santa Monica, CA: RAND Health, 2003. http://www.rand.org/pubs/white_papers/WP137.html.)

PROGNOSTICATION

There are benefits and limitations to prognostic tools that need to be appreciated. While these tools serve as a way to estimate prespecified outcomes in a group of patients with similar characteristics; they cannot predict who specifically will have such an outcome. The utility of these tools in caring for patients with chronic or end-stage kidney disease is to be able to identify who is at high risk for poor outcomes—whether it be mortality, hospitalizations, etc, and to use that identification as a starting point to engage in frank conversations regarding possible disease trajectories ahead, and factors that are important to the patient in terms of their overall care.

Table 58–1. A shared decision making framework.

Medical indications	• Review available therapies • Review risks and benefits of therapies • Estimate prognosis
Patient preferences	• Explore hopes and expectations of treatment • Identify worries about the future • Determine any limitations in quality or life or health status in which patient may consider forgoing a life-sustaining therapy
Quality of life	• Check in with patient at scheduled times, or have the patient reflect on current satisfaction with quality of life • Discuss what components of the patient's quality of life is most important for them to maintain
Contextual features	• Determine nonclinical factors which may play a role in decision making (eg, financial, religious or spiritual, cultural, family)
Develop a treatment plan	• Have patient and family reflect on preferences, values and quality of life and discuss what treatment best matches needs

Several prognostic tools have been developed. These tools range from the presence of clinical syndromes, to simple questions, to more involved calculations of risk.

The presence of certain clinical characteristics or syndromes can be used to guide a clinician's ability to identify those at risk of poor outcomes on dialysis, or to guide conversations with patients already on dialysis to thinking about next steps and preferences. Specifically, the presence of geriatric syndromes including the presence of falls, cognitive impairment and frailty, have all been associated with increased mortality in dialysis patients. Frailty is defined has having three of the following clinical features: unintentional weight loss, sarcopenia, weakness, poor endurance or self-reported exhaustion, slowness or low activity. This syndrome is estimated to be twice as prevalent in CKD patients over the age of 65 as compared to the general population. CKD patients with frailty are initiated on dialysis earlier, than nonfrail counterparts; however these patients have a 2.25 increased risk of death at 1 year.

An approach to prognostication, which can be done at the bedside, is "the surprise question." The "surprise question" is when a provider asks him or herself, "would I be surprised if this patient died in the next year?" A study validating the use of this screening question for prognostication in dialysis patients was completed. Of 147 patients evaluated, providers reported that they would "not" be surprised if 34 of the patient died in the next year. Patients in this group were older, had more comorbidities and lower functional status. Though overall mortality rates in the group were low, 15% at 12 months, those patients in the "no" group were 3.5 times more likely to die as compared to patients in which the provider would be surprised. Recently the surprise question was also validated in patients with stage 4 and 5 CKD, in which patients in the "no" group were approximately five times more likely to die at 1 year. This signifies an easy screening tool that can serve as a trigger to either involve the palliative care team early in a patient's course or to begin discussions about overall goals of treatment.

Table 58–2. Modified Charlson comorbidity index.

Score	Comorbid Condition
1	Coronary artery disease
	Congestive heart failure
	Peripheral vascular disease
	Cerebrovascular disease
	Dementia
	Chronic pulmonary disease
	Connective tissue disorder
	Mild liver disease
	Diabetes
2	Hemiplegia
	Moderate or severe renal disease
	Diabetes with end organ damage
	Any tumor, leukemia, or lymphoma
3	Moderate or severe liver disease
6	Metastatic solid tumor
	AIDS
+1	Age: for every 10 years over 40 years old

Low <3; moderate 4–5; high 6–7; very high 8.

Source: Adapted from Beddhu S et al: Am J Med 2000;108:609.

The prognostic value of comorbid conditions and functional status has been validated in several other studies. Patients can be risk stratified through use of the Charlson Comorbidity Score (Table 58–2). This score incorporates age, giving the patient 1 point for every 10 years over the age of 40, as well as various weights for 16 different comorbid conditions. Increases in the comorbidity score was associated with increased risk of hospital admissions, hospital days, inpatient costs, and 1 year mortality in a group of dialysis patients. An additional study evaluated elderly dialysis patients, specifically those over the age of 75 and predictors of 6 month mortality. Many of the same comorbid conditions were identified as in the Charlson Comorbidity Score, though this scoring system identified only eight conditions that were independently predictive, and additionally identified total dependency for transfers, a surrogate of poor functional status, as the most predictive of 6 month mortality.

A subanalysis of the aforementioned study identified other variables that are independent predictors of mortality at 3 months following initiation of dialysis. Of patients over the age of 75 who were initiated on dialysis, prognostic indicators included male gender, older age, presence of diabetes, heart failure, peripheral vascular disease, ischemic heart disease, cerebral vascular accident, dysrhythmia, chronic respiratory disease, cancer, cirrhosis, severe behavioral disorders, needing assistance with transfer, hypoalbuminemia, and low body mass index. This tool provides an opportunity

to predict those at high risk of mortality shortly after the initiation of dialysis. The authors suggest that for patients identified as high risk referral to a multidisciplinary team to provide comprehensive supportive care should be completed. For those at intermediate or low risk, evaluation by geriatrics for identification of geriatric syndromes may aide in optimizing care and outcomes.

An integrative tool incorporating age, three comorbid conditions (dementia, peripheral vascular disease, and hypoalbuminemia) and the surprise question has been developed into an online calculator (http://touchcalc.com/calculators/sq) that can be used to estimate 6, 12, and 18 months survival (Figure 58–2).

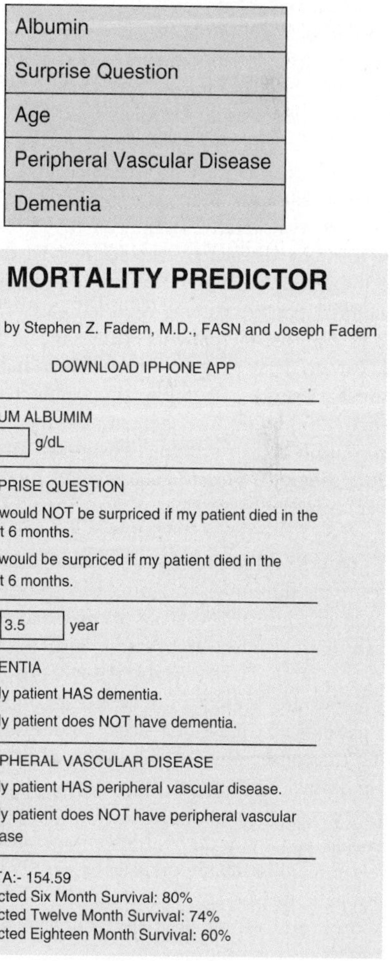

Albumin
Surprise Question
Age
Peripheral Vascular Disease
Dementia

HD MORTALITY PREDICTOR

Programmed by Stephen Z. Fadem, M.D., FASN and Joseph Fadem

DOWNLOAD IPHONE APP

SERUM ALBUMIM
3.5   g/dL

SURPRISE QUESTION

⦿ I would NOT be surpriced if my patient died in the Next 6 months.

○ I would be surpriced if my patient died in the Next 6 months.

Age 3.5   year

DEMENTIA

○ My patient HAS dementia.

⦿ My patient does NOT have dementia.

PERIPHERAL VASCULAR DISEASE

○ My patient HAS peripheral vascular disease.

⦿ My patient does NOT have peripheral vascular disease

XBETA:- 154.59
Predicted Six Month Survival: 80%
Predicted Twelve Month Survival: 74%
Predicted Eighteen Month Survival: 60%

▲ **Figure 58–2.** HD mortality predictor. (From Cohen LM et al: Predicting six-month mortality for patients who are on maintenance hemodialysis. Clin J Am Soc Nephrol 2010;5:72.)

KEY READINGS

Bao Y et al: Frailty, dialysis initiation, and mortality in end-stage renal disease. Arch Intern Med 2012;23:1071.

Beddhu S et al: A simple comorbidity scale predicts clinical outcomes and costs in dialysis patients. Am J Med 2000;108:609.

Cohen LM et al: Predicting six-month mortality for patients who are on maintenance hemodialysis. Clin J Am Soc Nephrol 2010;5:72.

Couchoud C et al: A clinical score to predict 6-month prognosis in elderly patients starting dialysis for end-stage renal disease. Nephrol Dial Transplant 2009;24:1553.

Moss AH et al: Utility of the "surprise" question to identify dialysis patients with high mortality. Clin J Am Soc Neprol 2008;3:1379.

CONSERVATIVE MANAGEMENT AS AN ALTERNATIVE TO DIALYSIS

While engaging patients in shared decision making regarding treatment options for advanced renal disease, all appropriate therapies should be discussed. For some patients, namely those who are suboptimal dialysis candidates or those patients who wish to minimize invasive procedures; an appropriate and alternative option to dialysis is comprehensive conservative management. This has recently been formally defined by the Kidney Disease: Improving Global Outcomes (KDIGO) workgroup on Supportive Care as planned holistic patient centered care, which does not include dialysis, for patients with stage 5 CKD including CKD care to delay progression of disease and minimize risk of adverse events or complications, shared decision making, active symptom management, advanced care planning, social, family and psychological support, and cultural and spiritual domains of care. The median survival of patients who are conservatively managed range from 6.3 to 23.4 months from when the estimated glomerular filtration rate (eGFR) is less than 15 mL/min/1.73 m^2. Many studies have sought to compare outcomes in terms of survival and quality of life metrics comparing dialysis to conservative management, though these studies are sought with imperfections that occur as a randomized control trial will not exist and potential bias is often present in the selection of these modalities, with patients who are older, sicker, and less functional often opting for conservative management. However, to the best of our knowledge several overarching themes are present in the results of these studies including that while dialysis will often convey a survival advantage, in certain patient populations, this advantage is less clear. This is specifically true in patients who are older than 75 with high comorbidity scores, and recent data suggesting in patients over 80 regardless of comorbidities.

A retrospective study recently showed a survival advantage with dialysis as compared to conservative therapy with patients in the dialysis group living 1.5–6.9 years as compared to 0.7–3 years. However, in certain groups this survival advantage was not seen, specifically in patients 80 years and older. In patients over the age of 70 with high comorbidity scores, a smaller survival advantage was noted. Other studies support this finding of either loss of survival advantage or a statistically insignificant survival advantage (5 months) when patients over the age of 75 years with either high comorbidity scores or cardiovascular disease were compared.

Studies looking at quality of life metrics comparing conservative to dialysis therapies are more limited. In likely that what daily life is like is vastly different between the two modalities and that this should be expressed to patients and caregivers. Dialysis, though it may be associated with longer survival involves added time interacting with the health care system, whereas conservative patients has this time limited. One study which highlighted these factors compared patients who chose dialysis versus conservative management. Though a survival advantage of over 20 months existed between the groups, it was found that of the time survived 47.5% of days were spent either in the hospital, receiving dialysis, or traveling to, from or recovering from the treatment as compared to 4.3% of days survived in the conservative care group. This suggests that though overall time survived may be less in conservative management as compared to dialysis, how that time is experienced may be very different.

KEY READINGS

Brown MA et al: CKD in elderly patients managed without dialysis: survival, symptoms, and quality of life. Clin J Am Soc Nephrol 2015;10:260.

Carson RC et al: Is maximum conservative management an equivalent treatment option to dialysis for elderly patients with significant comorbid disease? Clin J Am Soc Nephrol 2009;4:1611.

Chanda SM et al: Survival of elderly patients with stage 5 CKD: comparison of conservative management and renal replacement therapy. Nephrol Dial Transplant 2011;26:1608.

Murtagh FE et al: Dialysis or not? A comparative survival study of patients over 75 years with chronic kidney disease stage 5. Nephrol Dial Transplant 2007;22:1955.

Verberne WR et al: Comparative survival among older adults with advanced kidney disease managed conservatively versus with dialysis. Clin J Am Soc Nephrol 2016;11:633.

ADVANCE CARE PLANNING

During discussions about modality selection, and conservative management patients should also engage in discussing their values, beliefs, and care preferences which can lead to a larger conversation regarding advance care planning (ACP). This is an area in which the nephrology provider can participate to the extent which he or she feels comfortable, but can also utilize support staff including social work, and primary care physicians. Identification of a health care proxy, or a surrogate decision maker is important during modality selection to ensure that in the event the patient is cognitively impaired or unable to make decisions, there is a voice to express the patient's wishes. Discussions of larger goals including any situations in which the patient may not want to continue with a life sustaining therapy, such as dialysis should also occur. This can help to paint a picture of what the patient truly values in life, and assist in more difficult conversations about any other limitations in care, such as cardiopulmonary resuscitation (CPR). Overall, outcomes following CPR are poor with only 21.9% of end-stage renal disease (ESRD) patients surviving to discharge, and of those, a median survival post discharge of only 5 months. These discussions should begin early in the patient's course and evolve including checking in on the patient's overall health and life satisfaction with current treatment regimens, and any changes in care preferences at predefined intervals or following clinical events such as hospitalizations or at times of a new diagnosis.

END OF LIFE CARE

Advance care planning is important to ensure that the treatments patients receive up through the end of life are consistent with their preferences. Patients with ESRD on dialysis often spend the end of their life interacting with the health care system, receiving aggressive and invasive treatments. For example, of Medicare patients over the age of 65 in the last 30 days of life, ESRD patients had more hospitalizations, spent more time in an intensive care unit, and underwent more invasive procedures including feeding tube placement, being on a respirator, and resuscitation than patients with cancer or heart failure. Over 80% of ESRD patients are hospitalized during the last 90 days of life with almost 30% of these patients having 3 or more admissions in that time frame. Identification of patients who are having a clinical decline should serve as a trigger for physicians to prepare both the patient and family for the disease trajectory that may lie ahead and appropriately refer to hospice. Hospice is underutilized in the ESRD population, estimated to be used in only 25% of patient deaths. Literature surrounding management of patients at the end of life is relatively limited, but suggests that high symptom burden and rapidly changing symptoms are present which supports collaboration with palliative medicine and hospice to optimize care.

Patients with CKD stage 5 who are managed conservatively experience a higher symptom burden in the last month of life as compared to patients with advanced cancer. On average, these conservatively cared for patients report between 16 and 20 symptoms, including both physical and psychological symptoms.

Additionally, rates of dialysis discontinuation are highest among patients over the age of 85, with 34% stopping dialysis prior to death. Time of death from dialysis discontinuation will vary but has been estimated to be on average between 4 and 7 days for peritoneal and hemodialysis patients, respectively. Following dialysis discontinuation, common symptoms encountered include pain, dyspnea, and agitation. These patients can have dynamic and rapidly worsening symptoms on the days following dialysis withdrawal and work with palliative care physicians or inpatient hospice can be beneficial. Collaboration with palliative care during dialysis discontinuation should aim to fulfill four goals: to reduce the patient's suffering, both physical and psychological, to optimize patient's sense of control, to decrease burden on the family, and to optimize the patient's ability to spend meaningful time with family at the location they desire.

KEY READINGS

Cohen LM, Germain MJ, Poppel DM: Practical considerations in dialysis withdrawal: "to have that option is a blessing." JAMA 2003;289;2113.

Murtagh FE et al: Symptoms in the month before death for stage 5 chronic kidney disease patients managed without dialysis. J Pain Symptom Manage 2010;40:342.

O'Connor NR et al: Survival after dialysis discontinuation and hospice enrollment for ESRD. Clin J Am Soc Nephrol 2013;8:2117.

Wong SP, Kreuter W, O'Hare AM: Treatment intensity at the end of life in older adults receiving long-term dialysis. Arch Intern Med 2012;172:661.

Wong SP et al: Trends in in-hospital cardiopulmonary resuscitation and survival in adults receiving maintenance dialysis. JAMA Intern Med 2015;17:1028.

SYMPTOMS

Aside from symptoms at the end of life, the prevalence and severity of chronic symptoms in patients with advanced CKD is higher than that of the general population and similar to those with other serious medical conditions. Of patients with CKD and ESRD on dialysis, the number of overall symptoms reported range from 9 to 10.5, which is similar to that reported by ambulatory and inpatient cancer patients, 9.7–11.5, respectively. The most commonly encountered symptoms are sleep disorders (60%), anorexia (56%), pain (58%), nausea (46%), pruritus (40.6%), and depression (21–29%). Despite this well described prevalence, symptoms are still under-recognized, severity underestimated, and treatment inadequate. Following will be a brief summary of recommendations for treatment of depression, pain, and pruritus.

KEY READINGS

Abdel-Kader K, Unruh ML, Weisbord SD: Symptom burden, depression, and quality of life in chronic and end-stage kidney disease. Clin J Am Soc Nephrol 2009;4:1057.

Claxton RN et al: Undertreatment of symptoms in patients on maintenance hemodialysis. J Pain Symptom Manage 2010;39:211.

Davison SN: Pain in hemodialysis patients: prevalence, cause, severity, and management. Am J Kidney Dis 2003;42:1239.

Weisbord SD et al: Symptom burden, quality of life, advance care planing and the potential value of palliative care in severely ill haemodialysis patients. Nephrol Dial Transplant 2003;18:1345.

Weisbord SD et al: Renal provider recognition of symptoms in patients on maintenance hemodialysis. Clin J Am Soc Nephrol 2007;2:960.

DEPRESSION

Despite a high prevalence of depressive disorders in CKD and ESRD patients and association with adverse health outcomes, including increased mortality, depression remains under recognized and inadequately treated. It is estimated that approximately 30% of patients with CKD or ESRD meet criteria for a depression syndrome, much higher than the general population which is estimated to be 10%. Despite this prevalence, treatment with antidepressant medications has been estimated to occur in only 20% of those diagnosed with depression.

Several barriers to effective treatment exist in this population. First, diagnosis may be difficult. Though several screening tools have been validated in the CKD and ESRD population, the diagnosis of depression can be confusing as somatic symptoms that this patient population may experience, including fatigue, anorexia, loss of energy, and cognitive changes can also been seen in depression. There are specific concerns in this population, including knowledge gaps in terms of safety and efficacy of antidepressants in advanced renal disease, due to a paucity of well-designed trials. These concerns include drug–drug interactions, decreased clearance, and increased bleeding risks. From a patient perspective, some may be hesitant to add an additional medication to an already large pill burden.

Depression has been associated with several poor health outcomes in both CKD and ESRD patients. The association of depression with increased mortality has been shown in both the chronic hemodialysis and CKD population. In addition, association with increased number of hospitalizations, length of stay and cardiac events has also been shown. Lower medication adherence, dialysis noncompliance, including missed and shortened treatments and nonadherence to dietary and fluid restrictions have also been shown. The presence of depressive symptoms correlates with decreased quality of life, including decreased quality of social interaction, higher perception of burden, decreased quality of life scores on both physical and mental components of quality of life (QOL) scales. Treatment of depression has the potential to improve the aforementioned outcomes, though evidence regarding these outcomes is scarce.

Renal insufficiency may alter the pharmacokinetics of antidepressants including altered absorption through slowed gastric emptying, differences in protein binding, decreased drug excretion, and removal of medications with dialysis. Altered pharmacokinetics including prolonged half life of the parent drug or active metabolite, or reduced clearance has been shown for several classes of antidepressants, including serotonin norepinephrine reuptake inhibitors (SNRI), norepinephrine reuptake inhibitors (NRI), monoamine oxidase inhibitors (MAOI), tricyclic antidepressants (TCA), and bupropion in patients with CKD stages 3–5. Furthermore, there are specific effects of these medications that can be concerning for use in patients with advanced kidney disease. For example, TCA are associated with prolonged QTc, increased cardiac arrhythmias, and hypotension which are concerning given high rate of cardiovascular disease in this population. MAOIs have drug–drug interactions, and SNRIs have toxic metabolites that accumulate in renal insufficiency.

Based upon these considerations, an SSRI is considered to be first line in renal failure as it is hepatically metabolized into inactive metabolites which are then excreted by the kidney. The European Renal Best Practice (ERBP) recommends that treatment for Major Depression is with a selective serotonin re-uptake inhibitor as first line treatment for 8–12 weeks, after which time efficacy should be reevaluated. Sertraline is preferred as compared to other SSRIs, as medications such as citalopram, fluoxetine, and paroxetine have pharmacologic properties that require dosing adjustments in patients with renal insufficiency.

Studies evaluating use of alternative therapies for treatment of depression have also shown benefit in this population, including cognitive behavioral therapy (CBT), exercise training programs, and alterations in dialysis prescriptions. A recent crossover randomized control study by Cukor et al. evaluated use of CBT chair side during hemodialysis treatments in 65 patients over a 3-month period. CBT had improvement in depression scores, improved quality of life using the Kidney Disease Quality of Life Short Form, as well as improved compliance measured by interdialytic weight gain.

KEY READINGS

Cukor D et al: Psychosocial intervention improves depression, quality of life, and fluid adherence in hemodialysis. J Am Soc Neprhol 2014;24:196.

Hedayati SS, Yalamanchili V, Finkelstein FO: A practical approach to the treatment of depression in patients with chronic kidney disease and end-stage renal disease. Kidney Int 2012;81:247.

Nagler EV et al: Antidepressants for depression in stage 3–5 chronic kdieny disease: a systemiatic review of pharmacokinetics, efficacy and safety with recommendations by European Renal Best Practice (ERBP). Nephrol Dial Transplant 2012;27:3736.

Ossareh S et al: Prevalence of depression in maintenance hemodialysis patients and its correlation with adherence to medications. Iran J Kidney Dis 2014;8:467.

Palmer SC et al: Association between depression and death in people with CKD: a meta-analysis of cohort studies. Am J Kidney Dis 2013;62:493.

PAIN

Pain is one of the most commonly encountered symptoms, estimated to affect over 58% of CKD patients, of which 49% rate it moderate to severe in intensity. Patients can suffer from nociceptive pain, most commonly musculoskeletal, neuropathic pain, or sometimes a combination of both. In dialysis patients, uncontrolled pain is associated with worse health related quality of life, including higher rates of depression, pruritus, increased perception of burden of disease, decreased perception of social support, an increased number of shortened or missed treatments, and increased hospital visits. Treatment of pain in the CKD and ESRD population follows the World Health Organization analgesic ladder, which has been validated for use in these populations. This is a three-step ladder starting with step 1, the management of mild pain, in which use of nonopioid analgesic is preferred. In this population, acetaminophen is preferred. For pain not sufficiently controlled by acetaminophen or for pain that is moderate in intensity, opioids can be used. Preferred opioids include hydromorphone, oxycodone, and short-acting tramadol. Specific dosing recommendations exist for these medications. Overall due to impaired clearance and prolonged half life, these medications are started at lower doses and with longer dosing intervals than the general population. For pain still not controlled, or for severe pain use of higher dose hydromorphone, oxycodone or transdermal fentanyl, and methadone are preferred. Transdermal fentanyl should only be used in patients on a stable dose of short-acting opioids who need a transition to a longer acting agent. Methadone should only be prescribed by someone specifically trained in dosing and administration. Medications that are renally cleared and are at risk of accumulation should be avoided in patients with renal impairment. Several have been described to cause adverse effects in patients with decreased kidney function and are listed in Table 58–3.

For neuropathic pain, treatment follows that of the general population with special considerations of medication side effects and pharmacologic properties in patients with renal impairment. Preferred medications include gabapentin and pregabalin as these have shown potential additional benefits in treating other symptoms including sleep, pruritus,

and restless leg syndrome. Due to renal clearance of these medications, dose adjustments are recommended. As the drugs are cleared through dialysis, dosing should occur after dialysis. In elderly, frail patients or those who are conservatively managed, cautious guidelines exist regarding dosing. For example, in these patients, it is recommended to start gabapentin 100 mg every other night or pregabalin 25 mg every other night.

KEY READINGS

Barakzoy AS, Moss AH: Efficacy of the world health organization analgesic ladder to treat pain in end-stage renal disease. J Am Soc Nephrol 2006;17:3198.

Davison SN: Chronic pain in end stage renal disease. Adv Chronic Kidney Dis 2005;12:326.

Innis J: Pain assessment and management for a dialysis patient with diabetic peripheral neuropathy. CAANT J 2006;16:12.

Koncicki HM, Unruh M, Schell JO: Pain managemetn in CKD: a guide for nephrology providers. Am J Kidney Dis 2017;69:451.

Weisbord SD et al: Comparison of symptom management strategies for pain, erectile dysfunction, and depression in patietns receiving chronic hemodialysis: a cluster randomized effectiveness trial. Clin J Am Soc Nephrol 2013;8:90.

PRURITUS

Uremic pruritus is reported in over 40% of dialysis patients. Though presentation varies, it is typically described as itching that occurs bilaterally, on a daily basis in patients with CKD. Varying patient and clinical factors have been associated with increased prevalence. Some associated factors are modifiable, including low dialysis adequacy, use of low flux dialyzers, and elevated calcium and phosphors levels. Presence and severity of pruritus has been associated with decreased health-related quality of life, specifically in regards to mood, social relations, and sleep. Other studies have shown an association of pruritus with increased mortality.

Approaches to treatment have been described. For patients with CKD or ESRD on dialysis, modifying factors is this first step. This includes improving adequacy of dialysis, controlling calcium and phosphorus levels, and use of topical emollients to treat dry skin. Other nonpharmacologic treatments include use of phototherapy with UV-B light and alternative therapies, including acupuncture. Systemic therapies can also be used. Gabapentin or pregabalin is considered first line, with a potential additional benefit on other symptoms, including pain and restless leg syndrome. Several small studies have shown benefit in reducing pruritus severity with use of gabapentin in doses ranging from 100 to 400 mg post dialysis. A benefit of pregabalin over use of antihistamines, specifically doxepin, has also recently been shown.

Table 58–3. Medications to avoid in renal impairment.

Morphine
Codeine
Hydrocodone
Tapentadol
Meperidine
Tramadol extended release

KEY READINGS

Combs SA, Teixeira JP, Germain MJ: Pruritus in kidney disease. Semin Nephrol 2015;35:389.

Mathur VS et al: A longitudinal study of uremic pruritus in hemodialysis patients. Clin J Am Soc Nephrol 2010;5:1410.

Narita I, Alchi B, Omari K, et al: Etiology and prognostic significance of severe uremic pruritus in chronic hemodialysis patients. Kidney Int 2006;69:1626.

Nofal E et al: Gabapentin: a promising therapy for uremic pruritus in hemodialysis patients: a randomized-controlled trial and review of literature. J Dermatog Treat 2016;27:515.

Pisoni RL et al: Pruritus in haemodialysis patients: international results from the dialysis outcomes and practice patterns study (DOPPS). Nephrol Dial Transplant 2006;21:3495.

CONCLUSIONS

Patients with advanced renal disease represent a vulnerable population living with a chronic and life limiting illness. Collaborating care with palliative care colleagues can be helpful in caring for these patients throughout the course of their illness. As the age of patients approaching dialysis is increasing, unique considerations in this population should be taken into account and collaboration with palliative care services can be helpful. Through engaging in shared decision making and advance care planning providers can ensure that the treatment the patient receives is congruent with their overall values. Identifying patients who are having a clinical decline can lead to prompt referral to hospice for aggressive management of symptoms.

■ CHAPTER REVIEW QUESTIONS

1. While rounding the dialysis unit, you stop to speak with a long time dialysis patient who has been hospitalized three times in the last 3 months. He is an 80-year-old man with poor functional status, heart disease with stents, diabetes with peripheral vascular disease, and lower extremity amputations. His most recent admission for a nonhealing wound on his lower extremity was complicated by a prolonged stay due to the necessity for multiple debridement surgeries. Since discharge he now resides in a nursing home. He expresses that he is tired of being hospitalized and that he does not think dialysis is consistent with what he values in his life. He asks you if he stops dialysis how long could he survive. You respond:
   A. "You seem depressed. Let me arrange an appointment for psychiatry to see you."
   B. "No one can predict how long you can live."
   C. "Have you spoken to anyone about your wishes to stop dialysis?"
   D. "There is uncertainty regarding how long someone can survive, but usually it is about 7 days."

2. You are rounding on a 30-year-old woman with lupus nephritis who progressed to ESRD and now on dialysis. The dialysis nurses have alerted you that she seems sad recently, often tearful during treatments. During screening you determine that you think she is depressed. She agrees and asks you if you can start any medications to help her. First-line treatment for depression in patients with renal disease should be
   A. Cognitive behavioral therapy
   B. Selective serotonin reuptake inhibitors

   C. Serotonin norepinephrine reuptake inhibitors
   D. Monoamine oxidase inhibitors
   E. Tricyclic antidepressants

3. At the dialysis unit, a long-time patient has been complaining of pruritus. You note that he has excoriations on his legs bilaterally. He has had good clearances and calcium and phosphorous levels have been controlled. He has been trying to use an emollient, without effect. You offer to prescribe him a medication to see if it helps. What medication do you prescribe?
   A. Diphenhydramine
   B. Doxepin
   C. Gabapentin
   D. Oxycodone
   E. Cetirizine

4. At the dialysis unit you are rounding with a fellow and ask her to make sure that the patients who are at high risk for mortality have a health care proxy. She asks what is the most straightforward way to identify patients who are at high risk. You respond:
   A. Calculate their Charlson Comorbidity Score and determine if they in the "high risk group."
   B. Determine who has been hospitalized in the last 30 days.
   C. Calculate estimated 3 month mortality using 15 clinical variables.
   D. Use the "surprise question."

5. While rounding at your dialysis unit, your patient explains to you that he is having back pain that is preventing him from carrying out some of his daily activities. The back pain was from an old injury he sustained while working in construction. He has tried acetaminophen and physical therapy, per your recommendations, and while they help somewhat the pain is still moderate. He asks if there is anything stronger you can recommend. You suggest

A. Oxycodone
B. Tramadol extended release
B. Fentanyl patch
D. Morphine
E. Naproxen

Clinical Pharmacology and the Kidney

Thomas D. Nolin, PharmD, PhD

INTRODUCTION

Patients with chronic kidney disease (CKD) typically are prescribed an extraordinarily high number of medications compared to individuals without kidney disease. This is due to the presence of numerous comorbidities, including cardiovascular, hematologic, endocrine, psychiatric, and mineral and bone disorders. Notably, patients with end-stage renal disease exhibit the highest medication burden, taking an average of 12 medications (prescribed and over-the-counter) with a median pill burden of 19 per day. All CKD patients are at high risk for developing medication-related problems, including adverse drug effects and drug interactions, leading to suboptimal therapeutic outcomes, and vigilance is required to optimize drug use. Many drugs are predominantly eliminated by the kidney and can accumulate in CKD patients, and even those that are predominantly nonrenally cleared (ie, undergo hepatic metabolism) may require dose adjustment to maximize therapeutic outcomes and to minimize adverse events. As a general rule, if 30% or more of a drug is eliminated unchanged by the kidney, then it will likely require dosage regimen adjustment in CKD patients, especially those with advanced kidney disease (stages 3–5 CKD). A firm knowledge of general principles of pharmacokinetics, and especially of the effects of kidney disease on drug disposition, together with a basic understanding of processes to identify and resolve medication-related problems will facilitate improved drug selection, dosing and safety in all patients with impaired kidney function. This chapter presents clinically relevant pharmacokinetic and pharmacodynamic alterations commonly observed in patients with CKD, provides pragmatic approaches for proactively adjusting drug dosage regimens in these patients, and briefly discusses important medication safety considerations.

PHARMACOKINETIC CONSIDERATIONS

The quantitative description of individual parameters that determine drug disposition in the body, including absorption from an extravascular site of administration, distribution to various tissues, and elimination from the body, is termed pharmacokinetics. Decreased kidney function associated with kidney disease results in a reduction in the elimination of renally cleared drugs, which intuitively necessitates a corresponding modification to the dosing regimen to avoid accumulation and potential toxicity. Although renal drug dosage adjustment guidelines are commonly used for this, alterations in drug absorption, distribution, and elimination probably contribute to unpredictable and suboptimal responses.

▶ Absorption

The extent of drug absorption from an extravascular site of administration is known as bioavailability. It is presented quantitatively as the percentage of the administered dose that reaches the systemic circulation. Bioavailability may be impacted by several factors, including the route and rate of administration, and pathophysiologic changes at the site of administration. Although little quantitative information is available related to the effect of kidney disease on drug absorption, CKD patients often exhibit pathophysiological changes in the gastrointestinal (GI) tract that can influence bioavailability. For instance, delayed gastric emptying related to gastroparesis may be present in diabetic patients. GI motility may be decreased and can affect the time required to reach the maximal plasma concentration. However, this typically does not affect the maximal plasma concentrations (C_{max}) achieved and the overall extent of absorption. Conversely, increased gastric pH and concurrent medication administration can affect bioavailability of many drugs. The presence of high concentrations of urea in saliva may result in conversion of urea to ammonia by gastric urease and increased gastric pH, which in turn may alter the dissolution or ionization of a drug, leading to changes in absorption. Antacids, H_2-receptor antagonists, and proton-pump–inhibitors also may influence bioavailability by altering gastric pH. Antacids and vitamin supplements can substantially decrease the bioavailability of some drugs (eg, fluoroquinolones) by forming insoluble salts or chelates. Edema of the gastrointestinal wall has been implicated in altered bioavailability in CKD patients, particularly in patients with concomitant hepatic cirrhosis or congestive heart failure, that is, the bioavailability of furosemide may decrease from 50% to 10%. Lastly, a decrease in intestinal and hepatic first-pass metabolism may significantly influence oral drug absorption and bioavailability.

▶ Distribution

The extent to which a drug distributes throughout the body corresponds to its volume of distribution (V_D), which quantitatively describes the amount of drug in the body (A) relative to the measured concentration in plasma (C_p). The V_D is most commonly described as follows:

$$V_D = A/C_p$$

V_D does not reflect an actual anatomic space. It is a virtual space reflecting the apparent volume of plasma into which an administered dose must be distributed in order to achieve the observed concentration. V_D is useful to assess the extent of drug distribution to extravascular tissues in general, but does not provide information related to the specific tissues into which the drug has distributed. V_D is affected by several physiologic variables, including plasma protein binding, tissue binding, and total-body water, and each of these is altered in patients with kidney disease.

Plasma protein binding directly affects drug distribution. Only nonprotein bound or free drug, which represents the pharmacologically active moiety, is able to cross cellular membranes and distribute to the extravascular space. Acidic drugs bind mainly to albumin, while basic drugs bind primarily to alpha-1 acid glycoprotein (AAG). Protein binding of numerous acidic drugs, including penicillins, cephalosporins, aminoglycosides, furosemide, and phenytoin, is decreased in kidney disease likely due to hypoalbuminemia. This leads to altered relationships between unbound and total (bound + unbound) drug concentrations, and careful interpretation of the latter is necessary. For example, the unbound or free fraction of phenytoin can double from the normal of 10% to as high as 20% in the setting of advanced kidney disease, leading to increased hepatic clearance of unbound drug and a corresponding decrease in

total concentrations. Recognition of this is important, since total drug concentrations that are lower than the usual target range of 10–20 mcg/mL are necessary to achieve the target therapeutic range of unbound phenytoin, which remains constant at 1–2 mcg/mL. Qualitative changes in the albumin-binding site, and competition for albumin binding sites by other drugs, metabolites, and endogenous substances such as organic acids are also purported mechanisms of altered protein binding of acidic drugs. In general, binding of basic drugs to AAG is not altered in patients with kidney disease, despite AAG being an acute-phase reactant that is often elevated in CKD. Although changes in plasma protein binding may result in altered V_D, often these changes will be clinically insignificant because an increase in the fraction of nonprotein bound drug may result in a corresponding increase in both V_D and total clearance, resulting in no net change in systemic exposure of the drug. Clinicians are encouraged to measure and monitor unbound plasma drug concentrations, especially for drugs with a narrow therapeutic range, when possible to avoid confusion regarding interpretation of total concentrations in the setting of kidney disease.

Altered tissue binding also influences a drug's V_D in patients with kidney disease. This phenomenon is limited to few drugs however, such as pindolol, ethambutol, and classically digoxin. For instance, the V_D of digoxin is decreased by up to 50% in patients with stage 5 CKD. The reasons are unclear, but frequently cited mechanisms include competitive inhibition or displacement of digoxin from its receptor by uremic toxins or digoxin-like substances. If the digoxin loading dose is not adjusted accordingly, then the smaller V_D leads to increased serum concentrations.

In addition to alterations in binding to protein and tissues, changes in the proportion of total-body water can have a large effect on V_D. As kidney disease progresses and fluid retention leads to increased extracellular fluid volume, the V_D of hydrophilic drugs often increases, resulting in decreased serum concentrations with any given dose. Hydrophilic drugs with relatively low V_D (ie, <0.7 L/kg), such as aminoglycosides and cephalosporins are most commonly impacted by this.

▶ Nonrenal Clearance—Drug Metabolism and Transport

Nonrenal clearance (CL_{NR}) of drugs encompasses all routes of drug elimination, excluding renal excretion of unchanged drug. Historically, CL_{NR} has been assessed indirectly based on knowledge of the relationship between total systemic clearance (CL), which reflects the sum of all individual and simultaneously occurring organ clearances, and renal clearance (CL_R), as follows:

$$CL = CL_R + CL_{NR}$$

CL_{NR} is comprised primarily of clearance mediated by hepatic and extrahepatic drug metabolizing enzymes and transport proteins. In particular, several prominent oxidative (eg, cytochrome P450 [CYP]) and conjugative (eg, uridine diphosphate-glucuronosyltransferase [UGT]) enzymes and transporters, including P-glycoprotein, organic anion-transporting polypeptides (OATPs), and multidrug resistance-associated proteins in the gastrointestinal tract and hepatobiliary system are known to constitute the primary pathways of CL_{NR}. Alterations in the function of individual metabolizing enzymes and transporters and the complex interplay between them can affect the systemic exposure of nonrenally cleared drugs. In fact, the clearance of many commonly used drugs that are known substrates of these pathways (Table 59–1) is decreased in CKD patients, clearly implicating decreased CL_{NR}.

The principal site of CL_{NR} in vivo is the liver. Hepatic drug clearance is the net result of enzymatic metabolism and transport by proteins responsible for cellular uptake and efflux. Once drugs and metabolites enter the portal circulation, they may undergo active uptake across the sinusoidal membrane of the hepatocyte, followed by metabolism, then efflux across the canalicular membrane into the bile for excretion. Functional changes in any of the pathways involved can alter hepatic clearance and corresponding systemic drug exposure. That said, human CYPs appear to be minimally affected by kidney disease. Decreased hepatic CYP3A activity has been implicated in decreased clearance observed in patients with CKD. However, recent data derived from clinical studies with midazolam, a specific CYP3A probe drug, and from comprehensive reviews of pharmacokinetic data from numerous CYP3A substrates consistently demonstrate little to no effect of kidney disease on CYP3A. It is likely that alterations in transporters lead to changes in the pharmacokinetics of CYP3A substrates due to overlapping substrate specificity. Decreased activities of CYPs 2B6, 2C8, and 2D6 have also been reported in CKD patients.

The function of several other metabolic pathways may also be affected by kidney disease. For example, altered clearance of the reductase substrates naltrexone and idarubicin suggest that reduction of drugs may be altered in CKD. The clearance of morphine, which is primarily conjugated by UGT2B7 and UGT1A3, is significantly lower in CKD patients versus healthy subjects. Similarly, the antiretroviral agent zidovudine is metabolized by UGTs and is cleared more slowly in CKD than in patients with normal kidney function. N-acetyltransferase (NAT) activity may also be decreased in kidney disease, evidenced by lower clearance of the NAT substrates isoniazid and procainamide.

As mentioned above, it has become evident that the function of drug transporters is altered in kidney disease, which has confounded the interpretation of altered clearance of joint CYP3A-transporter substrates. Uptake of drugs across the sinusoidal membrane of hepatocytes regulates their access to intracellular hepatic enzymes as well as canalicular transport into the bile. Decreased clearance of the OATP substrates fexofenadine and erythromycin suggest that inhibition of hepatic uptake transporters is the likely mechanism of decreased CL_{NR} observed for several drugs that are substrates of hepatic OATPs.

In summary, overlapping substrate specificity, interplay between nonrenal clearance pathways, and the involvement of multiple organs in CL_{NR} makes identification of individual pathways that are affected by CKD challenging. It is difficult to predict with certainty which drugs will be impacted, even for structurally similar drugs within the same pharmacologic or therapeutic class. Nevertheless, it may be prudent to adjust doses of nonrenally cleared drugs, especially those with a narrow therapeutic window, in patients with advanced kidney disease in order to avoid excessive systemic exposure and to minimize the likelihood of toxicity.

▶ Renal Excretion

The most predictable and easily quantifiable determinant of renal drug clearance is kidney function. Several factors contribute to the decreased renal excretory capacity observed as kidney disease progresses, including reduction in kidney mass, the number of functioning nephrons, renal blood flow, glomerular filtration rate (GFR), and the rate of tubular secretion. CL_R of a drug is the net result of filtration or unbound drug, tubular secretion, and reabsorption, as follows:

$$CL_R = [(GFR \times f_u) + CL_{sec}] (1 - f_{reab})$$

where f_u is the fraction of the drug unbound to plasma proteins, CL_{sec} is secretory clearance, and f_{reab} is the fraction reabsorbed. Obviously, any decrease in GFR results in a corresponding decrease in CL_R, and the magnitude of the corresponding change in total systemic clearance of a drug is generally proportional to the fraction of the dose excreted unchanged (f_e) by the kidney. In other words, as the f_e increases, any decrease in renal clearance will elicit a larger reduction in systemic clearance and increase in systemic exposure.

The function of renal transporters is an important determinant of secretory clearance and net renal drug clearance. Major renal transporters involved in drug secretion include the organic anionic transporters (OAT), organic cationic transporters (OCT), P-glycoprotein, breast cancer resistance protein, and multidrug resistance associated protein transporters. Diuretics, β-lactam antibiotics, nonsteroidal anti-inflammatory drugs, and conjugated drug metabolites are secreted by OATs. Similarly, OCTs contribute to the secretion of cimetidine, famotidine, and quinidine, while P-glycoprotein is involved in the secretion of cationic

Table 59–1. Major pathways of nonrenal drug clearance and selected substrates.

CL_NR Pathway	Selected Substrates
Oxidative Enzymes	
CYP	
1A2	Caffeine, imipramine, theophylline
2A6	Coumarin
2B6	Nicotine, bupropion
2C8	Retinoids, paclitaxel, repaglinide
2C9	Celecoxib, diclofenac, flurbiprofen, indomethacin, ibuprofen, losartan, phenytoin, tolbutamide, *S*-warfarin
2C19	Diazepam, *S*-mephenytoin, omeprazole
2D6	Codeine, debrisoquine, desipramine, dextromethorphan, fluoxetine, paroxetine, duloxetine, nortriptyline, haloperidol, metoprolol, propranolol
2E1	Ethanol, acetaminophen, chlorzoxazone, nitrosamines
3A4/5	Alprazolam, midazolam, cyclosporine, tacrolimus, nifedipine, felodipine, diltiazem, verapamil, fluconazole, ketoconazole, itraconazole, erythromycin, lovastatin, simvastatin, terfenadine
Reductase Enzymes	
11β-HSD	Bupropion, daunorubicin, prednisone, warfarin
CBR	Bupropion, daunorubicin, haloperidol, warfarin
AKR	Bupropion, daunorubicin, haloperidol, ketoprofen, nabumetone, naloxone, naltrexone, warfarin
Conjugative Enzymes	
UGT	Acetaminophen, morphine, lorazepam, oxazepam, naproxen, ketoprofen, irinotecan, bilirubin
NAT	Dapsone, hydralazine, isoniazid, procainamide
Transporters	
OATP	
1A2	Bile salts, statins, fexofenadine, methotrexate, digoxin, levofloxacin
1B1	Bile salts, statins, fexofenadine repaglinide, valsartan, olmesartan, irinotecan, bosentan
1B3	Bile salts, statins, fexofenadine, telmisartan, valsartan, olmesartan, digoxin
2B1	Statins, fexofenadine, glyburide
P-gp	Digoxin, fexofenadine, loperamide, irinotecan, doxorubicin, vinblastine, paclitaxel, erythromycin
MRP	
2	Methotrexate, etoposide, mitoxantrone, valsartan, olmesartan
3	Methotrexate, fexofenadine

11β-HSD, 11β-hydroxysteroid dehydrogenase; AKR, aldo-keto reductase; CBR, carbonyl reductase; CYP, cytochrome P450 isozyme; MRP, multidrug resistance-associated protein; NAT, *N*-acetyltransferase; OATP, organic anion-transporting polypeptide; P-gp, P-glycoprotein; UGT, uridine 5'-diphosphate glucuronosyltransferase.

Source: Adapted from Nolin TD, Unruh ML: Clinical relevance of impaired nonrenal drug clearance in ESRD. Semin Dial 2010;23:482.

and hydrophobic drugs such as digoxin and *Vinca* alkaloids. Declining function of these secretory pathways as kidney disease progresses leads to decreased CL_R and necessitates renal dose adjustment to avoid toxicity.

An important consideration with respect to drug selection and dosing in patients with impaired kidney function is accumulation of drug metabolites. Metabolism of a parent drug generally leads to formation of a hydrophilic metabolite that is renally excreted. Thus, even if the parent drug itself is not excreted unchanged by the kidney, the metabolite may exhibit a high f_e and be susceptible to accumulation as kidney function declines. Metabolites of several drugs have significant pharmacologic and/or toxicologic activity, and so may elicit a clinical response. Classic examples include active metabolites of morphine and meperidine. Morphine is rapidly metabolized by hepatic UGTs into the active metabolites morphine-3-glucuronide and morphine-6-glucuronide, which cross the blood–brain barrier and appear to have more potent and longer duration of analgesic effects than morphine. Accumulation of these metabolites can lead to prolonged narcosis and respiratory depression in patients with CKD. On the other hand, the analgesic meperidine is rapidly converted to the active metabolite normeperidine, which does not exhibit analgesic effects but has central nervous system stimulatory activity. It accumulates in patients with impaired kidney function and may cause seizures. Ideally, drugs with known active metabolites should be avoided in CKD patients, assuming obviously that the metabolite is not responsible for the desirable clinical effect (ie, as with administration of prodrugs).

KEY READINGS

Nolin TD: A synopsis of clinical pharmacokinetic alterations in advanced CKD. Semin Dial 2015;28:325.

Thomson BK et al: Effect of CKD and dialysis modality on exposure to drugs cleared by nonrenal mechanisms. Am J Kidney Dis 2015;65:574.

Yeung CK et al: Effects of chronic kidney disease and uremia on hepatic drug metabolism and transport. Kidney Int 2014;85:522.

Yoshida K et al: Systematic and quantitative assessment of the effect of chronic kidney disease on CYP2D6 and CYP3A4/5. Clin Pharmacol Ther 2016;100:75.

PHARMACODYNAMIC CONSIDERATIONS

Pharmacodynamics reflects drug response, and is often described in terms of the relationship between drug concentration and its effect (Figure 59–1). While the effect of impaired kidney function on pharmacokinetics has been systematically examined for decades, pharmacodynamic assessments are rare by comparison. CKD can impact drug effects in various organs systems, leading to either an enhanced or diminished response compared to individuals

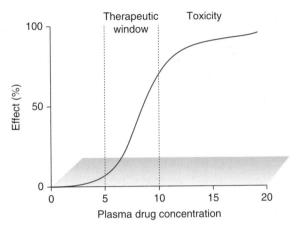

▲ **Figure 59–1.** Pharmacodynamics curve depicting a typical sigmoidal relationship observed between drug concentration and effect or response.

with normal kidney function that is not predictable based on pharmacokinetics. For example, kidney disease appears to render patients more sensitive to central nervous system effects of many drugs, including prolonged sedation with midazolam, psychomotor effects of alprazolam, and mental status changes with cimetidine. Exaggerated responses to the anticoagulant effects of enoxaparin are also reported in CKD, requiring dosage reduction to minimize the risk of bleeding.

Conversely, diminished drug effects may also be seen. Higher plasma furosemide concentrations and thus larger doses are required in CKD patients in order to ensure adequate drug reaches the site of action to elicit the desired diuretic response. The potential for altered drug responses should be carefully considered in the setting of kidney disease, particularly when prescribing drugs with questionable risk:benefit or a narrow therapeutic window.

USE OF KIDNEY FUNCTION ESTIMATES FOR RENAL DRUG DOSING

Accurate assessment of kidney function is fundamentally important in the development of drug dosing regimens. Measured GFR approaches provide accurate data, but they are impractical for routine clinical use. Estimated creatinine clearance (CL_{CR}) has been entrenched in clinical practice and commonly used as a GFR estimate for drug dosing purposes since publication of the Cockcroft–Gault equation in 1976. Moreover, the overwhelming majority of FDA approved drug labels that contain renal dosing information provide recommendations based specifically on Cockcroft–Gault derived CL_{CR}. Historically, this was based on the rationale that CL_{CR} was widely used in patient care settings as an estimate of kidney function, and was more practical than directly measuring GFR. However, estimated GFR (eGFR) is now widely reported in patient care settings, no longer rendering CL_{CR} estimates more practical (based on widespread availability alone) than other alternatives for dosage adjustment. The conundrum is that many clinicians are now arbitrarily using eGFR in place of CL_{CR} with renal dose adjustment recommendations based on the latter. Caution is warranted as the use of eGFR as a guide for drug dosage adjustment has not been systematically validated. Currently, there are limited prospective pharmacokinetic data and corresponding dosing recommendations based on eGFR. Since nearly all of the primary published literature to date has used CL_{CR} to derive the relationship between kidney function and renal and/or total body clearance of a drug (Figure 59–2), CL_{CR} remains the standard metric for drug dosing purposes. Nevertheless, widespread availability of automatically reported eGFR affords clinicians a tool that, if validated for drug dosing, could easily be incorporated into clinical practice. In the meantime, understanding the potential application and limitations of using eGFR for drug dosing is of utmost importance.

A pragmatic approach is recommended when assessing CL_{CR} and eGFR data for drug dosing purposes. Estimated GFR should not systematically replace CL_{CR} without comparing data and considering the implications. The following considerations are suggested.

- The automatically reported eGFR value provides an estimate that is normalized for body surface area (BSA) in units of mL/min/1.73 m^2. When used for drug dosing, the eGFR value should be individualized, that is, not normalized for BSA and converted to units of mL/min, particularly in patients whose BSA is considerably larger or smaller than 1.73 m^2. The individualized value may then be compared to CL_{CR} estimates expressed in equivalent units (mL/min).

- When presented with kidney function estimates that translate into different drug dosing recommendations, the regimen that optimizes the risk-benefit ratio given the patient-specific clinical scenario should be selected. Typically, more conservative kidney function estimates and corresponding doses should be used when dosing drugs with a narrow therapeutic window, particularly if therapeutic drug monitoring is not readily available. CL_{CR} estimates may be preferred when dosing narrow therapeutic window drugs, especially in high-risk subgroups, because they are more conservative and indicate the need for dose adjustment more often than eGFR. On the other hand, use of eGFR and a more aggressive dosing strategy may be acceptable for drugs with a wide therapeutic range and a broader margin of safety.

- A timed urine collection should be considered for determination of CL_{CR} when estimating equations are not expected to provide accurate measures of kidney function (ie, due to altered creatinine generation or unstable serum creatinine concentrations) and therapeutic drug monitoring is not available, particularly for narrow therapeutic window drugs with high toxicity.

- Parameters of drug response and toxicity should be carefully monitored. When possible, confirm or adjust dosing based on serum drug concentrations and prospective therapeutic drug monitoring. Adjust dosing as needed based on ongoing assessment of clinical status and risk versus benefit of current regimen.

KEY READINGS

Parsh J et al: Choice of estimated glomerular filtration rate equation impacts drug-dosing recommendations and risk stratification in patients with chronic kidney disease undergoing percutaneous coronary interventions. J Am Coll Cardiol 2015;65:2714.

Tortorici MA, Nolin TD: Kidney function assessment and its role in drug development, review and utilization. Expert Rev Clin Pharmacol 2014;7:523.

RENAL DRUG DOSING STRATEGIES IN PATIENTS WITH IMPAIRED KIDNEY FUNCTION

Several strategies may be employed to identify an appropriately adjusted dosing regimen in patients with impaired kidney function. Most FDA approved drugs that are renally cleared have been studied in patients with various levels of kidney function specifically to characterize the relationship between the drug's pharmacokinetic parameters and some measure of kidney function (usually CL_{CR}). If so, then the

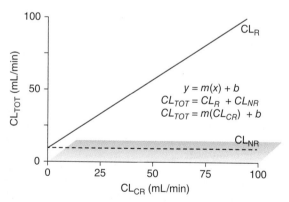

▲ **Figure 59–2.** The Dettli method of drug dosing, depicting the relationship between total systemic drug clearance (CL_{TOT}) and creatinine clearance (CL_{CR}). CL_R, renal clearance, CL_{NR}, nonrenal clearance. (Adapted from Dettli L: Individualization of drug dosage in patients with renal disease. Med Clin North Am 1974;58:977.)

manufacturer's drug label provides renal dose adjustment recommendations that generally should be followed. Often however, the recommendations are based on wide ranges of kidney function with categorical cutoffs that may not be optimal for all patients. If a more individualized dose is warranted (ie, in high-risk patient population), or if renal dosing recommendations are not provided, then tailored dosing based on pharmacokinetic principles provides the greatest likelihood achieving an optimal risk:benefit. Two basic methods have been used for this purpose, the Dettli approach and the method of Rowland and Tozer.

▶ Dettli Method

The clinical consequences of impaired kidney function on the elimination of renally cleared drugs have been appreciated for decades. Clinical studies documenting prolonged antibiotic half-lives in patients with impaired kidney function along with the relationships between drug half-lives and creatinine clearance date back to 1959. Dr Luzius Dettli published the first table of renal dose adjustment recommendations a decade later and systematically approached the issue of drug dosing in the setting of impaired kidney function. The Dettli method bases drug dosing recommendations on the linear relationship between the elimination rate constant of renally cleared drugs and a patient's creatinine clearance (see Figure 59–2), as follows:

$$k = k_{NR} + \alpha\ (CL_{CR})$$

where k is the overall elimination rate constant based on a first-order one compartment model, k_{NR} is the nonrenal elimination rate constant, and α is a constant relating the renal drug elimination rate constant to CL_{CR}. This approach assumes that the overall elimination rate constant (or CL) declines linearly with CL_{CR}, and that the nonrenal elimination rate constant (or CL_{NR}) remains constant as kidney function declines. While the first assumption generally holds true for drugs that are predominantly renally cleared, the second assumption is flawed, as the functional expression of numerous drug metabolizing enzymes and drug transporters is reduced in patients with kidney disease. Nevertheless, the Dettli method has facilitated the use of a priori estimates of CL and corresponding dosing requirements to individualize therapy based on kidney function, and is the foundation upon which dosing nomograms for renally cleared drugs are established to this day. For example, this approach was used to establish the linear relationship between the elimination rate constant of vancomycin (k_{VANC}) and creatinine clearance, and the following equation, which is commonly used to prospectively individualize vancomycin dosing was developed:

$$k_{VANC} = 0.0044 + 0.00083(CL_{CR})$$

And this is expressed in terms of vancomycin clearance (CL_{VANC}) as follows:

$$CL_{VANC} = 3.7 + 0.69(CL_{CR})$$

▶ Rowland and Tozer Method

When renal dosing recommendations or the relationship between pharmacokinetic parameters and kidney function are not available, then the CL or elimination rate constant can be estimated using the method of Rowland and Tozer, assuming the fraction of the drug that is excreted unchanged (f_e) in individuals with normal kidney function is known. Important assumptions of the method are (a) the change in CL and elimination rate constant are proportional to CL_{CR}, (b) the drug exhibits first-order (linear) kinetics, and (c) the drug's pharmacokinetics are adequately described by a one-compartment model. If these assumptions are true, then an adjustment factor (Q) can be calculated as follows:

$$Q = 1 - [f_e\ (1 - KF)]$$

where KF is the ratio of the patient's kidney function (CL_{CR} or eGFR) to the assumed normal value of 120 mL/min. So, for a drug that is 90% excreted unchanged in a patient who has a CL_{CR} of 20 mL/min, the Q adjustment factor would be

$$Q = 1 - \{0.90\ [1 - (20/120)]\}$$
$$Q = 1 - [0.90\ (1 - 0.17)]$$
$$Q = 1 - [0.90\ (0.83)]$$
$$Q = 1 - 0.75$$
$$Q = 0.25$$

The adjustment factor may then be applied to estimate the pharmacokinetic parameter in the patient. For example, the estimated clearance of a drug in the patient with impaired kidney function (CL_{PT}) is calculated as follows:

$$CL_{PT} = CL_{NORM} \times Q$$

Alternatively, the adjustment factor may be applied to the dose and/or the interval to derive an adjusted dosing regimen. Ideally, this is based on the desired goal of pharmacotherapy. That is, whether the desired goal is the maintenance of a target peak or trough, or if there is a clearly identified pharmacodynamic target, for example, time above the minimum inhibitory concentration (MIC) for β-lactams or AUC-to-MIC ratio for fluoroquinolones. If no specific target peak or trough concentrations or pharmacodynamics endpoints have been reported, then a goal of attaining the same average steady-state concentration as that in patients with normal kidney function is usually appropriate. Typically, this can be accomplished by applying the adjustment factor to either the dose, the interval, or both, described below.

1. Adjusting the dose (D):

$$D_{PT} = D_{NORM} \times Q$$

where D_{PT} is the adjusted dose in the patient with impaired kidney function, and D_{NORM} is the normal dose. If each dose is decreased and the dosing interval remains unchanged, then the average steady-state concentration will be similar, but the peak will be lower and the trough will be higher compared to the patient with normal kidney function.

2. Adjusting the interval (τ):

$$\tau_{PT} = \tau_{NORM}/Q$$

where τ_{PT} is the adjusted interval in the patient with impaired kidney function, and τ_{NORM} is the normal interval. If the dosing interval is increased (ie, increased length of time between doses) and the size of each dose administered remains the same, then the peak and trough concentrations in the patient with impaired kidney function will be similar to those in the patient with normal kidney function. This approach is often favored because less frequent drug administration is cost effective and decreases the medication burden in the patient.

3. Adjusting both the dose and the interval. This approach is generally unnecessary and is discouraged because it can lead to suboptimal dosing. However, occasionally the dose and interval may both need to be adjusted somewhat to facilitate administration of a clinically feasible dose or a practical dosing interval.

It should be noted that Q also can be calculated when the relationship between the elimination rate constant of the drug and kidney function is already established, that is, based on the Dettli approach. In this case, Q is calculated as the ratio of the drug CL estimated in the patient (CL_{PT}) relative to drug CL in patients with normal kidney function (CL_{NORM}):

$$Q = CL_{PT}/CL_{NORM}$$

Q is then applied to either the dose and/or the interval to derive an adjusted dosing regimen in the same manner described above.

MEDICATION SAFETY CONSIDERATIONS

Patients with advanced kidney disease are prescribed an extraordinarily high number of drugs. The optimal use of medication strives to maximize efficacy and safety, and this becomes increasingly difficult in the setting of polypharmacy as the number of concurrently prescribed drugs increases. Identification of the appropriate drug and dosing regimen to optimize the risk:benefit ratio is perhaps the most critical aspect of medication safety. More than two-thirds of all prescription medications are excreted by the kidney and require dosing adjustments in patients with impaired kidney function. Without appropriate safeguards in place for this purpose, CKD patients are prone to experience medication-related problems such as adverse effects, toxicity, drug interactions, or worsening of kidney function.

Generally speaking, implementation of three processes are considered vital for the prevention and resolution of the medication-related problems and to reduce polypharmacy. Medication reconciliation involves creation of an accurate medication list that reflects all medications a patient is currently receiving along with how they are being taken. Medication review is the process of specifically evaluating the medication list for appropriateness, effectiveness, safety, and convenience in conjunction with the patient's health status. Lastly, ongoing patient-centered medication therapy management facilitates development of treatment plans focused on an individual patient's medication-related goals.

KEY READINGS

Gabardi S, Abramson S: Drug dosing in chronic kidney disease. Med Clin North Am 2005;89:649.

Hartmann B, Czock D, Keller F: Drug therapy in patients with chronic renal failure. Dtsch Arztebl Int 2010;107:647.

Matzke GR et al: Drug dosing consideration in patients with acute and chronic kidney disease-a clinical update from Kidney Disease: Improving Global Outcomes (KDIGO). Kidney Int 2011;80:1122.

Matzke GR, Frye RF: Drug administration in patients with renal insufficiency. Minimising renal and extrarenal toxicity. Drug Saf 1997;16:205.

Naud J et al: Current understanding of drug disposition in kidney disease. J Clin Pharmacol 2012;52:10S.

Nyman HA et al: Comparative evaluation of the Cockcroft-Gault Equation and the Modification of Diet in Renal Disease (MDRD) study equation for drug dosing: an opinion of the Nephrology Practice and Research Network of the American College of Clinical Pharmacy. Pharmacotherapy 2011;31:1130.

Pai AB et al: Medication reconciliation and therapy management in dialysis-dependent patients: need for a systematic approach. Clin J Am Soc Nephrol 2013;8:1988.

St Peter WL: Management of polypharmacy in dialysis patients. Semin Dial 2015;28:427.

Talbert RL: Drug dosing in renal insufficiency. J Clin Pharmacol 1994;34:99.

Verbeeck RK, Musuamba FT: Pharmacokinetics and dosage adjustment in patients with renal dysfunction. Eur J Clin Pharmacol 2009;65:757.

SUMMARY

Medications are critically important in the treatment of kidney disease, offering tremendous benefits to patients with CKD when used optimally. However, inherent risks associated with suboptimal medication use in this tenuous population must be recognized. Clinicians must take into consideration the alterations in pharmacokinetics, which often require dosing adjustments and the careful selection of medications to optimize the risk:benefit ratio.

Pharmacokinetic changes in absorption, distribution, and renal clearance are well characterized and generally predictable, while changes in CL_{NR} are not. A firm knowledge of general principles of pharmacokinetics, implications of using various kidney function estimates for drug dosing, together with a basic understanding of processes to identify and resolve medication-related problems will facilitate improved drug selection, dosing and safety in all patients with impaired kidney function.

■ CHAPTER REVIEW QUESTIONS

1. A 65-year-old African–American man with a long-standing history of uncontrolled diabetes mellitus and chronic kidney disease is admitted with volume overload, dyspnea, and hypertension (160/95). His BUN and serum creatinine are 45 mg/dL and 3.8 mg/dL, respectively, and his corresponding eGFR is 18 mL/min/1.73 m². Urine dipstick is positive for protein (+++) and serum albumin is 2.5 g/dL.

   Which ONE of the following statements is CORRECT regarding the *oral bioavailability* of drugs in this patient?
   A. Diabetes may lead to slowed gastric emptying, but generally this does not affect oral bioavailability.
   B. Hypoalbuminemia leads to reduced protein binding and thus decreased oral bioavailability.
   C. Volume overload leads to edema of the GI tract, which may result in a significant increase in oral bioavailability.
   D. Concurrent administration of antacids facilitates absorption and oral bioavailability.
   E. First pass metabolism in the GI tract has no clinically significant effects on oral bioavailability.

2. Which ONE of the following statements is CORRECT regarding possible alterations in volume of distribution (V_D) in the patient described in question 1?
   A. Hypoalbuminemia leads to decreased V_D of protein bound drugs.
   B. Uremia may lead to decreased tissue binding and decreased V_D of digoxin.
   C. Increased total body water may lead to volume overload and decreased V_D of hydrophilic drugs such as aminoglycosides.
   D. V_D of drugs with large baseline V_D (ie, >2 L/kg) are most commonly affected by acute changes in volume status.
   E. V_D does not change until renal replacement therapy is initiated.

3. Drug X is a new analgesic with limited pharmacokinetic and dosing data. The recommended dose in normal healthy individuals is 500 mg Q8 hours. You are questioned about renal drug clearance in this patient, and asked to recommend a dose for a patient with stable chronic kidney disease.

   Assuming your patient has a creatinine clearance (CL_{CR}) of 50 mL/min, and the fraction of Drug X normally excreted unchanged is 0.9, what is the most appropriate (and practical) initial dosage regimen?
   A. 250 mg Q12 hours
   B. 250 mg Q24 hours
   C. 250 mg Q48 hours
   D. 500 mg Q12 hours
   E. 500 mg Q24 hours

4. Which ONE of the following statements is CORRECT regarding renal drug clearance in the patient described in question 3?
   A. Renal drug clearance is only affected by glomerular filtration, so the Dettli method of drug dosing cannot be used for drugs which are hepatically metabolized.
   B. The Dettli method of drug dosing assumes that nonrenal clearance remains constant as kidney disease progresses, so it is the preferred method for dosing hepatically metabolized drugs in patients with ESRD.
   C. The Dettli method of drug dosing assumes that renal drug clearance declines linearly with creatinine clearance, so it is most useful for drugs undergoing primarily glomerular filtration.
   D. The Dettli method of drug dosing assumes that renal drug clearance declines linearly with creatinine clearance, so it is most useful for drugs undergoing primarily tubular secretion.
   E. Renal drug clearance should only be assessed using measured urinary clearance.

5. A 52-year-old woman presents with complaints of dysuria and urgency to urinate for the last 3 days. Her past medical history is significant for stage 3 chronic kidney disease with an eGFR of 50 mL/min/1.73 m^2 noted 6 months ago. She is allergic to sulfa. Physical examination is noncontributory. Urinalysis shows yellow, cloudy urine with 10–15 WBC/hpf, leukoesterase (+), and many gram (−) rods consistent with *Escherichia coli* UTI. Ciprofloxacin is recommended, and the pharmacy suggests dosing based on creatinine clearance.

Which ONE of the following statements is CORRECT regarding use of kidney function estimates for drug dosing?

A. Creatinine clearance estimates and eGFR are virtually identical, so they can be used interchangeably for drug dosing purposes.
B. eGFR values should be converted to units of mL/min for direct comparisons to creatinine clearance.
C. When presented with kidney function estimates that translate into different drug dosing recommendations, always use the estimate providing the most aggressive dosing regimen.
D. eGFR equations have rendered creatinine clearance and timed urine collections obsolete.
E. Most FDA-approved dosing recommendations are based on eGFR.

Appendix A: Answers to Chapter Review Questions

Chapter 1

1. **The answer is A.** The most likely cause of acute kidney injury in this patient is volume depletion causing pre-renal acute kidney injury. The fractional excretion of sodium (FENa) is a useful tool to differentiate whether a cause of acute kidney injury is due to prerenal or intrinsic causes. It is calculated as follows: (Urine sodium × plasma creatinine)/(urine creatinine × plasma sodium) × 100. A FENa below 1% suggests a prerenal cause; however, in the setting of diuretics, it may have limited value, as urine sodium may not be accurately reflected. When this situation is encountered, a fractional excretion of urea can be performed. It is calculated as (urine urea × plasma creatinine)/(urine creatinine × plasma urea) × 100. A value of less than 35%, suggest a prerenal cause. In this patient, with a FE urea of 7.5%, the most likely cause of acute kidney injury is volume depletion as he has gastrointestinal fluid losses.

   Acute interstitial nephritis (AIN) has a multifactorial cause and could be related to medications most of the time, however, based on the patient's history, volume depletion is the most common cause. Diagnosis of AIN is usually made with kidney biopsy.

   Patient did not have any symptoms or signs of obstruction such as lower abdominal discomfort, urinary retention, or history of BPH. This clinical scenario is, therefore, less likely in this patient.

2. **The answer is E.** The cause of elevated creatinine and hyperkalemia in this patient is likely secondary to trimethoprim, which is typically combined with sulfamethoxazole. It inhibits a cationic transporter in the proximal convoluted tubule, causing an artifactual elevation of creatinine. It also inhibits the epithelial sodium channel (ENaC), thereby causing hyperkalemia.

   Although, a laboratory error is a possibility, based on the patient's history; there is a plausible explanation for her elevated creatinine and hyperkalemia.

   Interstitial nephritis is included in the differential diagnosis of her current clinical presentation. However, it is prudent to rule out more common causes first.

   Urinary tract infections typically do not cause elevated creatinine per se.

3. **The answer is C.** The most likely cause of hematuria in this patient is thin basement membrane nephropathy (benign familial hematuria). It is diagnosed in less than 1% of the population and the long-term prognosis is excellent. A family history is typical and it exhibits an autosomal dominant pattern. It could present as either microscopic or macroscopic hematuria. Given the excellent prognosis, reassurance without any further interventions is required.

   A kidney biopsy is not required at this moment, unless there is evidence of proteinuria.

   Abdominal and pelvis tomography is not indicated at this time based on the patient's age and no risk factors for malignancy or any other renal or ureteral problems.

   There are no indications to perform a drug screening test on this patient.

4. **The answer is C.** The next step is to perform a split 24-hour urine collection to diagnose orthostatic proteinuria. The diagnosis is made by demonstrating a normal protein excretion in the recumbent position and increased protein excretion while standing. The test should be performed after 24 hours of not performing strenuous exercises. Orthostatic proteinuria is a benign condition and tends to resolve overtime.

   Repeating a 24-hour urine collection would not help to reveal orthostatic proteinuria.

   A urine protein-to-creatinine ratio would not be helpful in this situation; however, a split protein-to-creatinine ratio performed in the recumbent and upright position would be.

   Orthostatic proteinuria is diagnosed with a split 24-hour urine collection and does not require a kidney biopsy.

5. **The answer is B.** The presence of obesity, especially if it is severe (BMI >40 kg/m^2), has been associated with proteinuria and FSGS. It is though that intraglomerular hypertension with hyperfiltration may be the cause of FSGS, associated with obesity and the majority of patients have subclinical disease. In this case, the most likely risk factor contributing to FSGS is obesity. Weight loss and RAAS blockade appear to decrease protein excretion.

   NSAIDs have been associated with minimal change in disease in addition to acute interstitial nephritis (AIN). It is unlikely that the occasional use of NSAIDs, like in this patient, causes FSGS.

   Age is not a risk factor to develop FSGS, as it could present at any age.

HIV is a risk factor to develop HIVAN (HIV-associated nephropathy), and histologically, HIVAN is a collapsing type of FSGS. The patient was screened for HIV and he does not have risk factor to suspect HIV infection.

Chapter 2

1. **The answer is E.** Determination of clinical volume status hinges on extracting key historical information and a skillfully performed physical examination, yet an accurate assessment of ECF volume status remains a challenge in clinical medicine. Choices A and B are more characteristic of mild-moderate losses, and these patients can be treated with ORS. All patients would be expected to have poor skin turgor and a FENa less than 1%, so these do not discriminate. Patients who have a decreased level of consciousness, however, are more likely to have suffered more losses that may still be ongoing and probably will be unable to drink. Such patients should be diagnosed as having more severe and probably life-threatening hypovolemia and should receive prompt and aggressive IVF therapy.

2. **The answer is D.** Patients who are hypovolemic need to always receive isotonic solution, which excludes all choices except C and D. Recent literature has suggested that using high [Cl] solutions in large volume resuscitation may increase the probability of acute kidney injury, so giving the half NaCl/half Na-bicarbonate solution may be the better choice of isotonic saline. Importantly, the rate of volume repletion needs to be commensurate with the volume already lost and exceed the rate of ongoing losses. Therapy should be monitored by following the physical examination. For example, as volume is repleted, blood pressure should increase, tachycardia should slow, and orthostasis should improve along with skin turgor, urine output, and mentation. The latter signs give a reliable readout that the patient is responding appropriately to the administration of sodium and that ECF volume is expanding toward baseline.

3. **The answer is D.** This patient with chronic heart failure has symptoms and signs of acute decompensated heart failure (ADHF), most likely exacerbated by dietary nonadherence with sodium (over Thanksgiving) and the use of ibuprofen. Loop diuretics depend on prostaglandin production for their maximal effect so, in addition to causing renal vasoconstriction, NSAIDs decrease the efficacy of loop diuretics. Patients with ADHF and evidence of ECF volume overload should be treated with IV diuretics without delay. If there is no response within 30–60 minutes, the dose should be doubled until an effective dose is found or the maximal IV dose is reached. This dose is higher (up to 200 mg) in patients with reduced GFR compared to the 40 mg in patients with normal GFR. Patients on chronic loop diuretic therapy may require up to 2.5 times their daily oral dose to be administered intravenously. For example, this patient is taking 40 mg of furosemide daily, so it is reasonable to initiate IV diuretic therapy at 100 mg. If ineffective, this dose may be doubled to 200 mg IV bolus (over 50 minutes). Although continuous IV dosing (5–40 mg/h) can be used (associated with less side effects), a recent meta-analysis has not proven superior to bolus therapy. Importantly, a continuous infusion should only be used after a threshold bolus has been identified as effective. It should not be used in those in whom bolus therapy has failed. Bolus dosing may be needed 2–3 times daily. Aldosterone antagonism with spironolactone can help minimize K loss and may be of overall cardiovascular benefit. It also helps reduce secondary hyperaldosteronism, which promotes diuretic resistance.

   Diuretic resistance is said to occur when edema is refractory to the maximum dose of a loop diuretic. The potential causes and approach to diuretic resistance is discussed at length in the chapter text. Reasons for diuretic resistance include (1) continued high salt intake, which can be assessed by measuring the amount of sodium in a 24-hour urine collection, (2) decreased secretion of diuretic due to renal hypoperfusion in heart failure and/or kidney disease, or due to the presence of an agent that blocks or competes for tubule secretion. One of these is cimetidine, which this patient is taking, and (3) extreme Na avidity of the tubule due to activation of the SNS and RAAS. Na avidity of the proximal tubule in increased by norepinephrine and Ang II, by flow-dependent hypertrophy of the cells in the DCT, and the effects of secondary hyperaldosteronism in the collecting duct. The ACEI may help reduce Ang II levels in the PT, and combination therapy with a thiazide can be added to loop diuretic therapy, which can be bolused 2–3 times a day.

4. **The answer is C.** This patient has developed resistance to furosemide and functional hypertrophy of the DCT cells is likely playing a key role. Although metolazone and HCTZ are both DCT diuretics, their oral potency will likely not be as high as IV chlorothiazide, which will be 100% bioavailable. The aim of combination therapy is to take advantage of the synergism of the loop and thiazide drugs to overcome diuretic resistance. Spironolactone can be added to this regimen to help reduce the effect of secondary hyperaldosteronism and to mitigate hypokalemia induced by the loop/thiazide combination. Patients on this regimen must be carefully monitored to ensure continued diuresis, maintain normokalemia, and avoid ototoxicity.

5. **The answer is D.** This patient is now presenting for the first time with ascites, indicating likely progression

to cirrhosis with portal hypertension. He has not yet been tried on any diuretic therapy and does not have tense ascites, although he may have gained up to 7-kg of ascites. The combination of spironolactone with furosemide given together (rather than sequentially) at a 100:40 ratio is superior to either one alone, effective in most patients, establishes that they are diuretic responsive, and maintains normokalemia. In the patient with ascites but without peripheral edema (as in this case) the rate of net fluid removal using diuretics should not exceed 500 mL per day because mobilization of peritoneal (3rd space) fluid is much slower than that for interstitial fluid. In the presence of peripheral edema, net fluid removal can be up to 2 L/day. It is important to avoid intravenous furosemide in patients with cirrhosis as it can acutely worsen kidney function and give the impression that the patient is developing the hepatorenal syndrome. A large volume paracentesis is not necessary unless the patient has tense ascites or there is a pressing need to remove the fluid quickly. Larger volume paracenteses (>5 L) should be done with caution in patient who have ascites in the absence of peripheral edema (as in this case), and such patients should receive a postprocedure albumin infusion. Over time and as the liver disease progresses, he will likely become less responsive to diuretics, so the dose should be maximized to 400 mg spironolactone with 160 mg of furosemide before diuretic resistance is diagnosed. If no other cause for diuretic resistance can be found (eg, nonadherence with a low sodium diet or other factor discussed in the chapter text), then large volume paracenteses (with postprocedure albumin infusion when >5.5 L) or a TIPS should be used to manage the ascites.

Chapter 3

1. **The answer is E.** The patient has acute hyponatremia with symptoms that reflect life-threatening cerebral edema. Unlike chronic hyponatremia, there is no risk of injury from rapid correction, so desmopressin is not indicated. Because hyponatremia may worsen as ingested water is absorbed, and because there is a risk of herniation, emergency therapy is needed without waiting for the results of laboratory tests. Transient SIADH is common in this setting and isotonic saline is contraindicated; it may lower the serum sodium concentration due to excretion of the infused sodium in a smaller volume of hypertonic urine, leading to net water retention. Although furosemide will partially block the excretion of concentrated urine, it will not reliably increase the serum sodium sufficiently. Hypertonic saline, best administered as a bolus is the most definitive way to raise the serum sodium concentration; the 100 mL bolus can be repeated up to two times if symptoms persist.

2. **The answer is E.** The patient presents from home with severe symptomatic hyponatremia. Although the duration of the disturbance is unknown, it must be presumed to be chronic, with a risk of injury from excessive correction. Several factors are present that are thought to increase the risk of osmotic demyelination: serum sodium <105 mEq/L, hypokalemia, alcoholism, and liver disease. In patients with a high risk of osmotic demyelination syndrome the desired rate of correction is 4–6 mEq/L/day and correction by >8 mEq/L should be scrupulously avoided. The patient's serum sodium concentration has already increased by 6 mEq/L in the first 4 hours after administration of isotonic saline. Because the predicted increase in sodium from 2 L of saline is only 2 mEq/L, it is likely that the infused saline has eliminated a hypovolemic stimulus for ADH release and that a water diuresis has begun. Therefore, all efforts to raise the serum sodium concentration (conivaptan or saline infusion) should cease. Desmopressin is indicated to stop urinary water losses to prevent excessive correction. Replacement of urinary water losses, with D5W would be another option.

3. **The answer is E.** The patient is excreting dilute urine despite hypernatremia. A water deprivation test is both unnecessary and dangerous as the serum sodium is already high enough to stimulate endogenous vasopressin secretion. A diagnosis of diabetes insipidus can be made, and, given the history of bipolar disease; it is likely that the patient has nephrogenic diabetes insipidus caused by lithium. The patient requires replacement of ongoing water losses and repletion of his water deficit to correct acute hypernatremia. As the loss of 2 L of water (30 mL/kg) will raise the serum sodium concentration by approximately 10 mEq/L, the serum sodium concentration of 158 mEq/L reflects a free water deficit of nearly 4 L. Assuming that urine creatinine excretion is at least 1 g in 24 hours, the urine creatinine concentration of 20 mg/dL indicates that urine output is at least 5 L in 24 hours. As there is no hypotension, a bolus infusion of isotonic saline is unnecessary and it may accelerate urinary water losses. As there is no evidence of fluid overload, furosemide is not indicated, and it will not prevent additional free water losses. Administration of 0.45% saline at 100 mL/h will not provide enough free water to replace ongoing losses and it will provide unneeded sodium. Administration of D5W at 300 mL/h is the best choice, as it will provide 7.2 L if continued for 24 hours, enough to replace ongoing losses and partially correct the water deficit. The rate of infusion should be adjusted based on frequent serial measurements of the serum sodium concentration.

4. **The answer is D.** The first step in determining the cause of polyuria is to estimate the rate of urine solute excretion. In this patient, each liter of urine

contains 500 milliosmoles (mOsm) of solute, and, with a urine output of 4.5 L/day, urine solute excretion is 2250 mOsm/24 hours, three times the solute excretion expected on a Western diet; therefore, the cause of polyuria is a solute diuresis. Urine osmolality is higher than plasma osmolality, so the cause of polyuria is not diabetes insipidus. Each liter of urine contains 30 mmol of sodium so the rate of sodium excretion is only 135 mmol/day; therefore, a diagnosis of cerebral salt wasting is not warranted. As the blood glucose is not high enough to cause glycosuria, the excess solute is likely urea. Excess urea excretion was caused by catabolism due to steroids.

5. **The answer is A.** Discussion: The laboratory findings are consistent with a diagnosis of SIADH. Conivaptan and tolvaptan, which are vasopressin receptor antagonists, are effective in raising the serum sodium concentration in this condition. Oral urea will also be effective, as it will be eliminated in the urine, increasing electrolyte-free water excretion. The urine to plasma electrolyte ratio is greater than 1 (150 mEq/L ÷ 120 mEq/L = 1.25). A ratio greater than 1 indicates that water restriction will be relatively ineffective, unless fluid intake is drastically reduced. However, isotonic saline will be the *least* effective of the choices. The sodium infused in an isotonic saline solution can be expected to be excreted in a smaller volume of hypertonic urine; the net effect will be water retention which will lower the serum sodium concentration.

Chapter 4

1. **The answer is B.** The trimethoprim component of trimethoprim-sulfamethoxazole locks the epithelial sodium channel (ENaC) in the distal tubule and thereby has an effect similar to triamterene or amiloride. This reduces Na reabsorption and the secretion of both protons and potassium by the kidney. The other medications do not directly affect potassium handling by the kidney.

2. **The answer is D.** The rapid increase of RBC mass in response to vitamin B_{12} in patients with severe pernicious anemia markedly increases the mass of cells, which contain potassium. This shift of potassium from the ECF to the cytoplasm of red cells can generate hypokalemia.

3. **The answer is A.** This patient has most likely developed acute colonic pseudo-obstruction (Ogilvie syndrome). These patients typically lose large amounts of very K-rich fluid into the colonic fluid and in the watery diarrhea.

4. **The answer is B.** Patients with loss of HCl-rich gastric fluid via NG suction or vomiting usually develop metabolic alkalosis and hypokalemia. The metabolic alkalosis is largely the direct effect of the loss HCl from the body. However, gastric fluid does not generally have a high K concentration. The K deficit, typically of these patients, is generated by renal K losses. They develop because ECF volume contraction causes secondary hyperaldosteronism, which exists simultaneously with distal tubule delivery of NaHCO$_3$. The Na, which is delivered to the distal tubule sites, is reabsorbed in exchange for Na and K.

5. **The answer is B.** Hypertension combined with otherwise unprovoked hypokalemia and metabolic alkalosis should raise the possibility of primary hyperaldosteronism. However, this patient's aldosterone levels (and renin levels) were low. Diagnostic possibilities should include nonaldosterone mineralocorticoids (DOCA or fludrocortisone); Liddle syndrome (a genetic disorder which mimics hyperaldosteronism because the ENaC in the distal tubules are constitutively open and active); and syndromes associated with inhibition of the enzyme (11β-hydroxysteroid dehydrogenase type 2) which inactivates cortisol and prevents it from stimulating the mineralocorticoid receptor. Chronic licorice ingestion can inhibit that enzyme and generate a pseudohyperaldosteronism syndrome.

Primary hyperaldosteronism should have a high aldosterone level; Bartter syndrome causes hypotension not hypertension and the renin and aldosterone levels are elevated; periodic paralysis is short lived and does not cause hypertension.

6. **The answer is B.** Patiromer releases calcium which is partially absorbed and partially excreted in the stool.

Chapter 5

1. **The answer is C.** Clearly response D is incorrect because the arterial pH is high, not low. Taken together, the laboratory values clearly suggest a metabolic alkalosis (low [tCO$_2$], elevated arterial pH, and an increased Pco$_2$). How does one determine if the increase in the Pco$_2$ to a value of 50 mm Hg, is the expected compensatory response or, in other words, is there a concomitant respiratory acidosis (response B)? The easiest approximation of the expected Pco$_2$ can be obtained by simply adding the number 15, to the measured tCO$_2$ concentration; or, as in this case 38 + 15 = 53 (mm Hg). This approach can be used in the range of serum [tCO$_2$] values from 10 to 40 mEq/L and is reasonably accurate within a range of ±3. Also, it's important to note, that values of Pco$_2$ above 50 mm Hg in compensation for metabolic alkalosis are unusual as the hypercapnic response becomes limited by the associated hypoxia, and the age of the patient, as well as whether there is lung disease present. Therefore, response B, is not correct and by elimination, the most accurate response is response C (pure metabolic alkalosis). Now, how does

one place the obvious hypokalemia into perspective; what is the cause in this case? Examination of the urine electrolytes reveals that the urine [K⁺] of 42 mEq/L is inappropriately high (>10 mEq/L) for the prevailing hypokalemia. If desired, the TTKG can be calculated from the data available. The value for TTKG is 11, indicating therefore, that there is inappropriate secretion of K⁺ by the DCT2 and principal cells of the CCD, in this patient with severe hypokalemia. The ECF volume contraction; and relative hypotension with orthostasis, and an elevated TTKG, suggests renal loss of K, moreover, since the urine [Cl⁻] is also elevated, there is an inappropriately high level of Cl⁻ excretion. The differential diagnosis in this situation might include surreptitious diuretic abuse, Bartter or Gitelman syndrome (since the urine [Cl⁻] is high, not low, surreptitious vomiting seems highly unlikely). Therefore, to be sure, you consider additional laboratory data. A screen of the urine for diuretics was obtained and was negative. However, and most importantly a spot urine for [Ca⁺²] and [Cr], indicated significant hypocalciuria (Ca/Cr = 32 which is <44 mg/g). The additional features of hypermagnesuria, and hypomagnesemia, along with the history and concurrent hypokalemic metabolic alkalosis with hypocalciuria, indicate that the correct diagnosis is Gitelman syndrome.

2. **The answer is C.** This patient has a nongap metabolic acidosis with a measured $Paco_2$ that corresponds to the value predicated from the Winter equation (1.5 × 15 + 8 = 30). The differential for the numerous causes of nongap metabolic acidoses are covered in the text, but in general, may be simplified into two categories: nonanion gap of renal origin or nonanion gap of nonrenal origin. Therefore, the urine anion gap should be calculated. In this case, the urine anion gap is clearly positive (35 + 40 − 18 = +57); a positive value indicating a nonanion gap of renal origin. Therefore, renal tubular acidosis should be considered in this circumstance. This patient presented with a nonanion gap metabolic acidosis (AG = 10 mEq/L) associated with severe hypokalemia causing flaccid paralysis. The positive **urine anion gap** is indirect evidence of an abnormally low excretion of ammonium in the face of systemic acidosis. The urine pH was inappropriately alkaline, yet there was no evidence of hypercalciuria, nephrocalcinosis, or bone disease. With more careful questioning and a thorough review of systems, it was evident that the patient exhibited the typical features of the sicca syndrome (xerostomia and keratoconjunctivitis sicca, but without synovitis, arthritis, or rash, or evidence of another collagen vascular disease). The patient was subsequently shown to have hyperglobulinemia, and the positive anti-Ro/SS-A, and anti-La/SS-B, confirmed the diagnosis of Sjögren syndrome.

These findings, taken together, indicate that the cause of this patient's hypokalemia and nongap metabolic acidosis was a renal tubular disease. The hypokalemia and abnormally low excretion of ammonium, as estimated by the positive urine anion gap, in the absence of glycosuria, phosphaturia, or aminoaciduria (Fanconi syndrome), defines the entity, **classical distal renal tubular acidosis (dRTA)**, also known as type 1 RTA.

Classical distal renal tubular acidosis is often acquired in patients with Sjögren syndrome. Several auto-antibodies have been associated with Sjögren syndrome; and it is likely that some of these auto-antibodies prevent the normal trafficking of the H⁺-ATPase to the apical membrane of the type A intercalated cell of the collecting tubule. As a result, the H⁺-ATPase remains confined to the intracellular compartment and is inactive. Defective H⁺-ATPase function also occurs in certain inherited forms of classical distal RTA, in which there may be inherited abnormalities of the genes that encode for one of the subunits of the H⁺-ATPase. There was no family history in the present case and other family members were not affected, nor was there a family history of deafness. While proximal RTA has also been reported in patients with Sjögren syndrome, it is much less frequent and there were no features of proximal tubule dysfunction (Fanconi syndrome) in this patient. The hypokalemia associated frequently with cDRTA, is due to secondary hyperaldosteronism from volume depletion.

The long-term renal prognosis for patients with classical distal RTA due to Sjögren syndrome has not been established. Nevertheless, the metabolic acidosis and the hypokalemia respond to alkali replacement with either sodium citrate solution (Shohl solution) or sodium bicarbonate tablets (1–2, 650 mg tablets bid). The long-term goal is to correct the serum bicarbonate to the normal value of 25 mEq/L. Obviously, potassium deficits must be replaced initially, but chronic potassium replacement is often not required in distal RTA patients because sodium bicarbonate (or citrate) therapy corrects the secondary hyperaldosteronism associated with volume depletion. A consequence of the interstitial infiltrate seen in patients with Sjögren syndrome and classical distal RTA is progression of chronic kidney disease. Cytotoxic therapy plus glucocorticoids has been the mainstay of therapy in Sjögren syndrome for many years, and the B-lymphocyte infiltration in salivary gland tissue subsides and urinary acidification improves after treatment with rituximab, suggesting resolution or improvement in the interstitial nephritis.

3. **The answer is C.** This patient presented with a normal [HCO₃⁻], pH, and Pco₂, but the anion gap is 20 mEq/L, and confirms the presence of a high anion gap acidosis.

Nevertheless, by comparing the delta values (ΔAG and ΔHCO$_3^-$) or (20–10 = 10 versus 25–25 = 0), it is immediately obvious that the patient has highly disparate Δ values. When the ΔAG exceeds the ΔHCO$_3^-$ by more than 4 mEq/L, a mixed metabolic alkalosis coexists with the high anion gap acidosis. In this case, protracted vomiting was the presenting complaint. Vomiting results in the expulsion of gastric contents (eg, NaCl, HCl, and KCl), and when HCl is not transmitted to the small bowel, HCO$_3^-$ secretion cannot proceed. Thus, the HCO$_3^-$ is retained in the ECF and metabolic alkalosis is "generated." The loss of NaCl and KCl results in volume depletion and hypokalemia, as well as hypochloremia, all of which impair the ability of the kidney to excrete the excess HCO$_3^-$. Therefore, until the volume depletion and hypokalemia are corrected, the kidney will retain bicarbonate inappropriately ("maintenance phase" of metabolic alkalosis). The severe volume depletion in this patient with established CKD, also resulted in acute on chronic renal failure, as evidenced by the documented increase in BUN and Cr. Since ketones were not elevated and the lactate was normal in this case, the most likely cause of the high anion gap acidosis was assumed to be renal failure. The patient improved with fluid administration as IV 0.9% NaCl with KCl (20 mEq/L) and the BUN and Cr returned to baseline.

4. **The answer is D.** This case illustrates a patient with obvious alkalemia (arterial pH = 7.54), an elevated [HCO$_3^-$], in the electrolyte panel, and as well, severe hypokalemia and hypochloremia and a Pco$_2$ that is elevated. With this information, it should be clear that a metabolic alkalosis is present. Therefore, response C and response A are both incorrect. Predicting the respiratory compensatory response for metabolic alkalosis is imprecise when the [HCO$_3^-$] is raised to levels over 40, because, the response by the respiratory center to metabolic alkalosis (alveolar hypoventilation) is limited by the offsetting response to hypoxia as the Pco$_2$ climbs significantly. Therefore, the limitation of the hypercapnic response is usually to a value of no more than a Pco$_2$ of 55 in healthy adults. This level is subject to downward adjustment for numerous comorbidities, such as chronic lung disease, advanced age, and muscle wasting. Moreover, with hypokalemia, it is often assumed that the respiratory compensatory response is also subdued. However, using the standard formula for prediction of the Pco$_2$ in metabolic alkalosis (the Pco$_2$ increases 0.6 mm Hg for each 1.0 mEq/L increase in [HCO$_3^-$]), the expected Pco$_2$ in this case would be equal to 50 mm Hg. Therefore, a mixed respiratory disorder is not present and responses A and B are incorrect, and response D is correct. This patient has a pure metabolic alkalosis. In addition to the high values for [HCO$_3^-$] and pH in this

case, attention should also be paid to the value for the serum [Cl$^-$], of 85 mEq/L. In this example, the serum [Cl$^-$] is low while the value for serum [Na$^+$] is in the normal range. A value for [Cl$^-$] that is disproportionally low in comparison to the [Na$^+$] heralds the coexistence of a metabolic alkalosis or respiratory acidosis. Since the latter is clearly not the case, the disproportionately low [Cl$^-$] is further evidence for a metabolic alkalosis. Unfortunately, in many clinical situations little attention is paid to the serum [Cl$^-$].

5. **The answer is B.** This patient presented with obtundation and a concerning history, but with a documented high anion gap. Together, these findings suggest ingestion of a toxin. With an anion gap of 25 mEq/L, it should be observed that the ΔAG of 15 was equal to the ΔHCO$_3^-$ of 15. The fact that the Δ values were not significantly disparate indicates that a mixed high anion gap metabolic acidosis and a metabolic alkalosis (answer D), was not present. Furthermore, the respiratory compensatory response (Pco$_2$ = 23 mm Hg) is precisely what would be predicted from the Winter equation (1.5 × [HCO$_3^-$] + 8 = (1.5 × 10) + 8 = 23). Therefore, answer C is incorrect. The correct diagnosis is a simple high anion gap metabolic acidosis (answer B). Renal failure is not causative since the BUN and Cr are normal. Since neither the plasma ketones nor the L-lactate level were elevated, another cause of the high anion gap must be considered. The presence of an elevated **osmolar gap** in this case, raises the possibility of toxic alcohol ingestion. The osmolar gap of 33 (difference in measured and calculated osmolality or 325–292) in the face of a high anion gap metabolic acidosis, is diagnostic of the presence of an osmotically active metabolite in plasma; a difference of more than 10 mOsm/kg indicates a significant concentration of an unmeasured osmolyte. Examples of toxic osmolytes include toxic alcohols, such as ethylene glycol, diethylene glycol, methanol, and propylene glycol.

Several caveats apply to the interpretation of the osmolar and anion gaps in the differential diagnosis of toxic alcohol ingestions. First, unmeasured, neutral osmolytes can also accumulate in lactic acidosis and alcoholic ketoacidosis, that is, an elevated osmolar gap is not specific to anion gap acidoses associated with toxic alcohol ingestions. Second, patients can present having extensively metabolized the ingested toxin, with an insignificant osmolar gap but a large anion gap, that is, the absence of an elevated osmolar gap does not rule out toxic alcohol ingestion. Third, the converse can also be seen in patients who present earlier after ingestion of the toxin, that is, a large osmolar gap with minimal elevation of the anion gap. Ethylene glycol is commonly available as antifreeze or solvents and may be ingested accidently or in a suicide attempt, as was implied in this case. The metabolism of ethylene glycol by alcohol dehydrogenase generates acids such as glycolaldehyde, glycolic acid, and oxalic acid. The initial effects of intoxication are on the central nervous system, and in the earliest stages mimic inebriation, but may quickly progress to full-blown coma. Delay in treatment is one of the most common causes of mortality with toxic alcohol poisoning. The kidney shows evidence of acute tubular injury with widespread deposition of calcium oxalate crystals within tubular epithelial cells. Cerebral edema is common, as is crystal deposition in the brain; the latter is irreversible.

The concurrent crystalluria, as evident on the urinalysis in this case, is typical of ethylene glycol intoxication; both needle-shaped monohydrate and envelope-shaped dihydrate calcium oxalate crystals can be seen in the urine as the process evolves. Circulating oxalate can also complex with plasma calcium, reducing the ionized calcium, as seen in this case.

Although ethylene glycol intoxication should be verified eventually by measuring ethylene glycol levels, therapy **must be initiated immediately** in this life-threatening situation. While therapy can be initiated with confidence in cases of known or witnessed ingestions, such histories are rarely available. Therapy should thus be initiated in patients with severe metabolic acidosis and elevated anion and osmolar gaps, when the other causes of a high anion gap acidosis are not operative. Other diagnostic features, for example, hypocalcemia or acute renal failure with crystalluria, can provide important confirmation for urgent, empiric therapy.

Since all the osmotically active toxic alcohols, ethylene glycol, diethylene glycol, methanol, and propylene glycol are metabolized by alcohol dehydrogenase to generate toxic products, competitive inhibition of this key enzyme is common to the treatment of all four intoxications. The most potent inhibitor of alcohol dehydrogenase, and the drug of choice in this case, is fomepizole (4-methyl pyrazole). Fomepizole should be administered intravenously as a loading dose (15 mg/kg) followed by doses of 10 mg/kg every 12 hours, for four doses, and then 15 mg/kg every 12 hours thereafter until ethylene glycol levels have been reduced to less than 20 mg/dL and the patient is asymptomatic with a normal pH. Additional very important components of the treatment of toxic alcohol ingestion include fluid resuscitation, thiamine, pyridoxine, and folate administration. Initially, one or two ampules of $NaHCO_3$ should be administered. Acute hemodialysis is almost always indicated in the comatose patient with high ethylene glycol levels. Hemodialysis is used to remove both the parent compound and toxic metabolites, but also removes administered fomepizole, necessitating adjustment of dosage frequency. Gastric aspiration, induced

emesis, or the use of activated charcoal is only effective if initiated within 30–60 minutes after ingestion of the toxin. When fomepizole is not available, ethanol, which has more than 10-fold affinity for alcohol dehydrogenase compared to other alcohols, may be substituted. Ethanol must be administered i.v. to achieve a blood level of 22 mEq/L (100 mg/dL). A disadvantage of ethanol is the obtundation that follows its administration, which is additive to the CNS effects of ethylene glycol. Furthermore, if hemodialysis is utilized, the infusion rate of ethanol must be increased because it is rapidly dialyzed. In general, hemodialysis is indicated for all patients with ethylene glycol intoxication when the arterial pH is less than 7.3 or the osmolar gap exceeds 20 mOsm/kg H_2O. Isopropanol is also a toxic alcohol and is the primary component of "rubbing alcohol," windshield de-icer fluid, and some antifreezes. It is also metabolized by alcohol dehydrogenase. However, it is important to recognize that isopropanol intoxication is an exception to the treatment paradigm outlined above because, although ingestion of isopropyl alcohol also causes an increase in the osmolar gap, it **does not increase the anion gap** because isopropanol is metabolized primarily to acetone. Therefore, isopropanol ingestion is typically not life threatening as fatality is very rare. One caution in isopropyl alcohol ingestion is that it should not be over treated and the indications for and specific type of therapy understood. The hallmark of isopropanol intoxication is marked ketonemia and ketonuria without metabolic acidosis. Fomepizole is not indicated. Isotonic fluids should be administered to induce a significant increase in urine output. Nevertheless, massive propranolol ingestion may cause coma when isopropyl alcohol levels exceed 500 mg/dL (80 mmol/L). In such severe cases, the clinician should consider tracheal intubation to protect the airways. Hemodialysis may be recommended for patients who are persistently unstable hemodynamically. However, dialysis is very rarely required, even when measured serum levels are greater than 500 mg/dL, if the patient maintains a stable BP and tissue perfusion.

6. **The answer is A.** In evaluating the electrolytes available in this case, it is clear that because of the normal anion gap of 10 mEq/L, a high anion gap acidosis cannot be present, eliminating response B. However, the $[HCO_3^-]$ and pH are low, documenting the presence of a metabolic acidosis. Furthermore, the predicted P_{CO_2} is approximately to the measured value of 30 mm Hg, so that response C is not correct. Therefore, this case is an example of a nongap metabolic acidosis. The differential diagnosis for this disorder is covered in the text, but the finding of a negative urine anion gap ([15 + 10] − 45), indicating that the nongap metabolic acidosis is of nonrenal origin. With the history of diarrhea, it

appears safe to conclude that the acid base disorder is due to chronic diarrhea. Note however, that the urine pH is 6.0, an alkaline value. Is not an inappropriately alkaline urine pH in a patient with a nongap metabolic acidosis, indicative of a renal tubular disorder such as renal tubular acidosis? However, this is not always the case. With chronic loss of bicarbonate precursors from the GI tract in a patient with normal kidney function, one should expect to observe an increase in urine ammonium excretion, which is precisely why the urine anion gap is negative. As more NH_4^+ is excreted, because of its buffering properties, the urine pH will be required to increase (pK of NH_4^+ = 9.0). Therefore, be cautious when relying only on the urine pH to diagnose renal tubular acidosis.

Chapter 6

1. **The answer is B.** The most common causes of hypercalcemia are either primary hyperparathyroidism or secondary to malignancies. In general, patients with primary hyperparathyroidism have relatively minor increase in serum calcium, generally less than 12.5–13.0 mg/dL. In this patient, because of the hypoalbuminemia, his corrected calcium would be approximately 14.9 mg/dL (an increase of 0.8 mg/dL for every decrease of 1 g/dL of albumin). In addition, with primary hyperparathyroidism, there is generally hypophosphatemia and rarely is there renal insufficiency. Although vitamin D toxicity can cause marked hypercalcemia, you need to have excessive intoxication with blood levels of vitamin D of greater than 150 ng/dL, which would be very hard to achieve with this dosing regimen. It is generally seen when patients are taking excessive doses of activated vitamin D, such as calcitriol. Thiazide diuretics can cause mild hypercalcemia by increasing distal tubule calcium reabsorption. Prostate cancer generally causes osteoblastic metastasis and more commonly may cause hypocalcemia. In this patient, the hypercalcemia is most likely due to malignancy, with multiple myeloma being the best option. He has anemia, acute renal failure associated with marked hypercalcemia, complaining of bone pain, and in particular, the low anion gap of 3 are all consistent with multiple myeloma.

2. **The answer is C.** Acute kidney injury is frequently associated with increase in serum phosphate with a compensatory decrease in serum calcium. Hypomagnesemia is associated with disorders in parathyroid hormone and hypocalcemia. Both acute pancreatitis and rhabdomyolysis is associated with sequestration of calcium into necrotizing tissue. Metabolic alkalosis is associated with hypocalcemia as it causes an increase in the binding of calcium with albumin. Whereas metabolic acidosis may cause hypercalcemia by decreasing the binding of calcium from albumin as well as increasing bone resorption and thus release of calcium from bone.

3. **The answer is E.** This is an otherwise healthy young female with mild hypercalcemia, with no other laboratory abnormality. Although both a high normal parathyroid hormone concentration and a low serum phosphate are consistent with primary hyperparathyroidism, they are not diagnostic. A low vitamin D concentration could be a cause of secondary hyperparathyroidism, however, in that case the serum calcium should be low. A magnesium concentration is not helpful as hypomagnesemia is associated with hypocalcemia and not hypercalcemia. A 24-hour urine calcium would be required to confirm the diagnosis of hypercalcemia caused by hyperparathyroidism. With primary hyperparathyroidism, in addition to hypercalcemia, relatively low serum phosphate or hypophosphatemia, an elevated urine calcium should be present to confirm the diagnosis. Although, parathyroid hormone increases the reabsorption of calcium by the kidney, the filtered load of calcium is greatly increased, thus the net effect would be hypercalciuria. In contrast, familial hypocalciuric hypercalcemia, is a nonpathological condition caused by mutations in the calcium sensing receptor gene resulting in loss-of-function mutations in the calcium sensing receptor. These patients generally excrete significantly less than 100 mg (frequently as low as 50 mg) of calcium per 24 hours. In order to regulate parathyroid hormone production and secretion, a higher ionized serum calcium is required to inhibit the parathyroid gland. This is an autosomal dominant condition, which is relatively rare. Since these patients do not have any pathology, surgery should not be performed, as it may result in patients becoming hypoparathyroid.

4. **The answer is E.** This patient has moderate hypercalcemia with appropriately maximally suppressed parathyroid hormone. The differential would include malignancy, hypervitaminosis D, vitamin D intoxication, or granulomatous disease. He likely has mild renal insufficiency from hypercalcemia. There does not appear to be any evidence of underlying malignancy. Measurement of the active hormonal form of vitamin D, calcitriol, would confirm the diagnosis of hypervitaminosis D and an ACE level would differentiate whether there is a granulomatous disease or if negative, would suggest there was an underlying lymphoma. Measurement of vitamin D would not be helpful as in order for the vitamin D to cause increase in serum calcium, the calcitriol concentration would need to be elevated.

5. **The answer is D.** Thiazide diuretics increase the distal tubular reabsorption of calcium, thus may cause mild hypercalcemia. The hungry bone syndrome occurs in patients who have moderate to severe

hyperparathyroidism and then have a parathyroidectomy. During the immediate postoperative period, there is excessive bone formation with sequestration of calcium from the blood into the bone, resulting in hypocalcemia, which could be rather severe and symptomatic. The binding of calcium to albumin is fixed and though with decrease in serum albumin concentration, the total calcium will fall, the ionized calcium will stay the same. Serum calcium concentration represents less than 1% of the total body calcium with the bone comprising approximately 99%, thus changes in serum calcium have no impact on the total body calcium content.

Chapter 7

1. **The answer is D.** Given the elevated serum calcium concentration, hyperphosphatemia and a suppressed PTH the best option would be to stop the calcium-containing binder and switch to a noncalcium-containing binder. Paricalcitol would not be optimal given the suppressed PTH and hypercalcemia. Cinacalcet would also not be a good option given the suppressed PTH. Alendronate would also not be a good option given the suppressed PTH.

2. **The answer is C.** An FGF-23 level would be the next test to order. The patient has severe hypophosphatemia and urinary phosphate wasting likely as a result of oncogenic osteomalacia. Severe hypophosphatemia is seen in patients with this disorder due to removal of sodium phosphate cotransporters from the luminal membrane of the proximal tubule and a decrease in 1,25 dihydroxyvitamin D_3 concentration due to downregulation of 1α-hydroxylase and upregulation of 24-hydroxylase mediated by FGF-23. PTH generally does not cause severe hypophosphatemia because renal phosphate loses are to some degree mitigated by the actions of PTH on bone and intestine. PTH upregulates 1α-hydroxylase and increases intestinal calcium reabsorption. The same is true of PTHrP. 1,25(OH)$_2$ vitamin D_3 level would not be the best option. Bone biopsy is not the best option at this early point in the evaluation.

3. **The answer is B.** Of these options egg whites are the best choice they have the lowest phosphorus to protein ratio about 1.4 mg of phosphorus per gram of protein whereas dairy products are the highest in the range of 30 mg of phosphorus per gram of proteins. Meats are intermediate. Nut butters are high in phosphorus.

4. **The answer is E.** This patient has acute respiratory alkalosis. The most common electrolyte abnormality associated with metabolic alkalosis is hypophosphatemia, which occurs as a result of stimulation of glycolysis with a resultant shift of phosphorus into cells. In a classic study by Mostellar et al. Eleven healthy adults aged 20–40 years showed a decline in serum phosphorus concentration to less than 1.0 mg/dL in 90 minutes with voluntary hyperventilation to a Pco$_2$ of 13–20 mm Hg. This was associated with a marked reduction in urinary phosphate excretion as would be expected with intracellular shift of phosphorus.

5. **The answer is A.** This patient has Fanconi syndrome as evidenced by nongap metabolic acidosis associated with hypophosphatemia, hypokalemia and glycosuria with a normal serum glucose concentration. Of the drugs listed only tenofovir has been associated with Fanconi syndrome.

Chapter 8

1. **The answer is C.** Amiloride is used as an adjuvant treatment of hypomagnesemia. By inhibiting sodium transport via ENaC, it establishes a negative membrane potential in the distal convoluted tubule cells and therefore favors Mg^{2+} reabsorption.

2. **The answer is C.** Normal intracellular magnesium levels will inhibit K$^+$ efflux via the ROMK channel. Low intracellular magnesium levels are believed to relieve this inhibition, thereby causing ROMK-mediated potassium secretion.

3. **The answer is A.** Epidermal growth factor receptor (EGFR) activation is essential for the expression of TRPM6, the main apical Mg^{2+} transporter in the DCT. Monoclonal antibodies against EGFR such as cetuximab are associated with significant hypomagnesemia.

4. **The answer is D.** If the etiology of hypomagnesemia is not readily apparent, obtaining a 24-hour urine for magnesium or a spot urine sample to determine the fractional excretion of magnesium should distinguish whether the hypomagnesemia is due to gastrointestinal losses/malabsorption versus inappropriate urinary losses of magnesium. In the setting of magnesium depletion, conservation of magnesium by normal kidneys can decrease the usual fractional excretion of magnesium from 3% (approximately 100 mg/day) to very low levels (ie, sometimes <0.5% or 12 mg/day). Therefore, demonstrating an inappropriately high rate of renal magnesium excretion in the setting of hypomagnesemia confirms the diagnosis of renal magnesium wasting, whereas appropriate conservation would suggest a gastrointestinal etiology.

5. **The answer is D.** High levels of magnesium decrease transmission of neuromuscular messages by inhibiting acetylcholine at the neuromuscular endplate. This ultimately leads to decreased deep tendon reflexes, muscle weakness progressing to flaccid skeletal muscle paralysis, respiratory depression, and apnea. The combination of high dose magnesium infusion and development of renal dysfunction (oliguria) likely resulted in the development of severe hypermagnesemia.

Chapter 9

1. **The answer is C.** Continuous renal replacement therapy is able to provide greater net volume removal than intermittent hemodialysis with less hemodynamic instability. Despite this benefit, continuous therapy has not been demonstrated to provide a survival benefit as compared to intermittent hemodialysis.

   Large studies did not show any survival benefits between with CRRT and conventional intermittent hemodialysis.

2. **The answer is C.** Several studies in cardiac surgery patients have associated low-dose dopamine therapy with increased incidence of atrial arrhythmias, presumably mediated by β-adrenergic stimulation. Low-dose dopamine has not been found to have any of the above benefits (decreased duration of dialysis-dependence, increased diuretic-responsiveness, lower mortality) in prospective studies.

3. **The answer is E.** Trimethoprim-mediated blockade of collecting duct apical Na channels and increase in creatinine.

   Reabsorption of sodium without chloride in the collecting duct generates lumen negative potential enhancing the gradient for K secretion.

   Trimethoprim blocks creatinine secretion but has no effect on GFR; therefore, the rise in creatinine reverses with discontinuation of the drug.

4. **The answer is B.** Patients undergoing bypass grafting with CKD, off-pump bypass was associated with a decreased risk of AKI.

   There is no evidence that dopamine, furosemide, N-acetylcysteine or normal saline decrease the risk of AKI following coronary artery bypass grafting. In a randomized controlled trail of low-dose dopamine, furosemide, no benefit was observed with dopamine and furosemide infusion was associated with an increased incidence of acute kidney injury.

5. **The answer is D.** Aggressive volume replacement is the most important strategy after crush injury to prevent or attenuate the development of rhabdomyolysis and AKI.

   Fluids resuscitation should be initiated as soon as possible to replace intravascular volume deficits and maintain a high urine output.

   No benefit for dopamine, furosemide, N-acetylcysteine or norepinephrine has been shown in controlled studies in this setting.

Chapter 10

1. **The answer is A.** The patient had developed acute kidney injury (AKI) because her serum creatinine had risen by ≥50% from a stable baseline in the previous 3 months. The International Ascites Club has defined AKI in cirrhosis as either a rise in serum creatinine by 0.3 mg/dL in ≤48 hours, or if a baseline serum creatinine is not available within 48 hours, the a ≥50% increase in serum creatinine from a stable baseline reading will also be acceptable.

   An AKI diagnosis in cirrhosis does not require any abnormal urine findings or the use of a fluid challenge.

   Such a small rise in serum creatinine cannot be ignored, as we can see that the patient subsequently had further rise in her serum creatinine.

2. **The answer is E.** While it is appropriate to try to find out the etiology of her AKI by checking her urine for casts or abnormal findings, or enquire about potential nephrotoxic agents or diuretic use, or monitoring her for systemic hypotension, the first step in differentiating the various causes of her AKI would be to give her a fluid challenge, preferably in the form of albumin, as albumin does not only have oncotic properties, it also has anti-inflammatory, antioxidant, endothelial stabilizing properties, as well as scavenging functions that can reduce the extent of inflammation in cirrhosis.

   It would not be wise to perform a large volume paracentesis, as this tends to induce postparacentesis circulatory dysfunction by exaggerating the reduction in the effective arterial blood volume and worsens the renal dysfunction.

3. **The answer is B.** This patient has nonalcoholic steatohepatitis as a cause of her cirrhosis. Diabetes is a common association with nonalcoholic steatohepatitis. Therefore, it is not surprising that she has a mildly elevated random serum glucose and glycosuria. While it is good clinical practice to refer her to the diabetic clinic for education about her diabetes, these will not help to improve her serum creatinine. It is paramount to get her serum creatinine to decrease, as failure to do so will significantly worsen her prognosis.

   She should be rehydrated immediately. Saline would normally be the fluid of choice. However, in patients with cirrhosis, the salt load will greatly increase her ascites, especially when there is still some residual portal hypertension from a stenosed TIPS. Therefore, rehydration with albumin would be more appropriate, as albumin has more than just oncotic properties as outlined in the answer for Question 2.

4. **The answer is B.** According to the International Ascites Club's revised definition of AKI-HRS, this patient has had a 2-fold increase in her serum creatinine from a stable baseline serum creatinine within the past 3 months, while fulfilling all the other diagnostic criteria of hepatorenal syndrome (Table 10-3). A threshold of serum creatinine is no longer required for the diagnosis of AKI-HRS, nor is the 14-day time constraint required for the diagnosis. In order to make the diagnosis of AKI-HRS, the patient should have received a fluid challenge

and should have been shown to be nonresponsive to the fluid challenge with no reduction of her serum creatinine.

TIPS should not be used as a treatment of AKI-HRS, and opening up of the stenosed TIPS will tend to worsen the systemic vasodilatation, and exaggerate the reduction in the effective arterial blood volume with the potential of worsening the renal dysfunction.

5. **The answer is D.** This patient is clearly deteriorating. It appears that the insertion of her TIPS had worsened her liver function significantly, possibly by inducing liver ischemia when a significant volume of the splanchnic blood volume is being shunted to the systemic circulation without passing through the hepatic microcirculation. She therefore needs urgent referral for liver transplant assessment despite her normal liver enzymes. She is developing acute-on-chronic liver failure, which is usually accompanied by other organ failures, and in this scenario, the extra-hepatic organ failure is renal failure. Liver transplantation is the definitive treatment for AKI-HRS. Vasoconstrictor therapy can also be tried. However, terlipressin is not available commercially in North America. The combination of midodrine, octreotide, and albumin is inferior to terlipressin, and is only given when no other options are available. Norepinephrine infusion can be tried, but it requires admission into intensive care unit, which is not always available. Renal replacement therapy in the form of dialysis should only be considered when the patient is already on the liver transplant waiting list, and the patient has an indication for dialysis.

Chapter 11

1. **The answer is B.** The history of exertional trauma, myoglobinuria (positive dipstick for blood, negative microscopy) and acute kidney injury most likely points to rhabdomyolysis. Polymyositis is excluded based on acute presentation following exercise. IgA nephropathy and other acute glomerulonephritis are unlikely diagnoses given negative urine microscopy.
2. **The answer is A.** This patient most likely has statin induced rhabdomyolysis, given recent addition of atorvastatin to medication regimen. Discontinuation of offending medication would be most appropriate at this time. Normal saline infusion is not applicable in this situation, given mild CK elevation, and low risk for developing acute kidney injury. Similarly, sodium bicarbonate infusion is not indicated at this time. Cardiology evaluation is not indicated, given the rise in CK levels after addition of atorvastatin. Measurement of serum troponin levels is more specific for cardiac work up and can be tested if indicated.
3. **The answer is B.** This patient most likely has a glycogen storage disease, given recurrent rhabdomyolysis during high intensity exercise. Further evaluation for metabolic myopathies would be the appropriate diagnostic step. Given no symptoms during exercise free periods, hypothyroidism, diabetes, and adrenal insufficiency are less likely.
4. **The answer is B.** Though there are differing opinions on types and rates of resuscitation fluid used, initial volume repletion with normal saline has been recommended. Albumin has not been studied or recommended. Given severity of crush injuries, and cell damage with potential hyperkalemia, Lactated Ringer's is not the immediate choice for initial fluid used.
5. **The answer is B.** Aggressive fluid resuscitation with isotonic saline is the recommended initial management of rhabdomyolysis. Continuation of fluids is recommended till plasma CK levels are stable and not increasing. Intravenous fluids not only replete the intravascular volume depletion, but also serve to increase urinary flow and prevent myoglobin from forming tubular casts. Initiation of renal replacement therapies for removal of myoglobin has not been established. Sodium bicarbonate infusions theoretically improve urine alkalinization but there is no clear evidence supporting use of alkaline diuresis versus saline diuresis. Use of mannitol to increase diuresis is also not recommended due to conflicting results.

Chapter 12

1. **The answer is D.** Prophylactic hemodialysis has not been demonstrated to prevent CIN. The prophylactic value of statins is limited by size and demand of studies of statin's value in this setting. Thus date too preliminary to recommend statins as prophylaxis for CIN at present time. Although many studies of *N*-acetylcysteine on prophylaxis of CIN, some are positive and others negative. No consensus on value of *N*-acetylcysteine with some guidelines recommending use while others do not recommend this agent. There is universal agreement that volume expansion with intravenous saline is the single most important prophylactic measure for prevention of CIN.
2. **The answer is B.** There is nothing to support acute interstitial nephritis as the cause of acute kidney injury—no eosinophilia, rash, unexplained fever, sterile pyuria, or eosinophiluria. No hemodynamic data is given to support prerenal azotemia and the urine sediment does not show just hyaline casts, a finding of prerenal azotemia. Cholesterol crystal embolization is always a concern after intra-arterial contrast administration but there are no clinical findings such as embolic lesions on the toes (blue toe syndrome), livedo reticularis venous pattern of the abdominal skin, or bright refractile cholesterol lesions in the retina (Hollenhorst plaques) or laboratory

findings such as hypocomplementemia to support this diagnosis. The findings of granular casts suggesting acute tubular necrosis and the timing of acute kidney injury within 48 hours of contrast exposure are typical for CIN.

3. **The answer is D.** Neither peripheral artery disease or hypertension are considered "risk factors" for CIN. Chronic kidney disease is a significant risk factor—the more severe the chronic kidney disease, the greater the risk. Diabetes is not a risk factor by itself—however, when coupled with chronic kidney disease; it becomes a risk factor in addition to the chronic kidney disease. For example, a patient with both diabetes and chronic kidney disease (eGFR 25 mL/min) is at greater risk than a patient with chronic kidney disease (eGFR 25 mL/min) and no diabetes.

4. **The answer is C.** There does not exist enough supporting evidence to recommend theophylline as a prophylactic measure for CIN. The value of *N*-acetylcysteine is controversial and has been addressed in the answer explanation of Question 1. The issue of whether intravenous fluids are effective prophylaxis for CIN even with mild impairment of eGFR as in this patient has not been the subject of well-designed clinical studies. Also, the risk of CIN appears to be greater with intra-arterial contrast compared to intravenous contrast at any given level of eGFR. It is the authors' opinion that intravenous fluid prophylaxis is indicated for eGFR <60 mL/min for intra-arterial contrast administration and for eGFR <45 mL/min for intravenous contrast administration.

5. **The answer is D.** Allergic interstitial nephritis is not likely given the absence of rash, unexplained fever, sterile pyuria, and eosinophiluria. Acute glomerulonephritis can be excluded primarily by a urinalysis which shows no microscopic hematuria with dysmorphic red blood cells and no proteinuria. Contrast induced nephropathy is rarely oliguric and usually the urinalysis shows a pattern of acute tubular necrosis with granular casts and renal tubular epithelial cells. The finding of oliguria and distal phalanges which are mottled and dusky—so called "blue toe syndrome," along with peripheral eosinophilia is classic for atheroembolic renal disease.

Chapter 13

1. **The answer is B.** The electrolyte disturbances found in TLS are due to the massive release of intracellular contents. Intracellular potassium is as high at 120 mEq/L and phosphorus concentrations can be up to four times higher intracellularly in malignant cells than in nonmalignant cells, resulting in hyperkalemia and hyperphosphatemia during cell lysis. Hypocalcemia develops in TLS as a result of calcium-phosphorus complexes in the setting of hyperphosphatemia.

2. **The answer is B.** The patient has a high risk malignancy and upon presentation presents with laboratory tumor lysis syndrome (uric acid >8 mg/dL, phosphorus >6.5 mmol/L, calcium <7.0 mg/dL, though potassium is no >6.0 mg/dL). Due to patient's diagnosis, once chemotherapy is initiated he is at highest risk for developing clinical tumor lysis (AKI, cardiac arrhythmia, and/or neurologic events) which is why preventative measures are critical in this patient. Volume expansion is essential to support intravascular volume, renal blood flow and maintain glomerular filtration in an effort to optimize excretion of potassium, uric acid, and phosphate. Rasburicase is warranted as patient uric acid is elevated >8 mg/dL and his hyperuricemia is expected to worsen with treatment of his ALL. Allopurinol is generally used for patients with low or intermediate risk TLS, this patient has high risk TLS. Patient potassium is slightly elevated without any ECG abnormalities, close monitoring is needed but treatment with kayexalate or hemodialysis is not yet warranted.

3. **The answer is C.** The patient correctly received crystalloid IVF for volume expansion with 0.9% NS and his uric acid after one dose of rasburicase markedly improved; however, the use of bicarbonate rich fluids for maintenance fluids most likely alkalinized the urine, thereby exacerbating calcium-phosphorus precipitation and deposition, leading to nephrocalcinosis, tubulointerstitial nephritis, and end-organ damage. The IVF of choice in TLS is 0.9% NS, and urinary alkalinization is not recommended in the management. The patient's uric acid markedly improved with a single dose of rasburicase, therefore reducing the risk of urate nephropathy and with a presumed newly alkaline urine pH is unlikely to now be developing uric acid intratubular crystallization. There clinical scenario of otherwise hemodynamically stable patient does not support acute tubular necrosis as primary cause of AKI.

4. **The answer is C.** Rasburicase is a recombinant urate-oxidase enzyme that promotes the conversion of uric acid to carbon dioxide, hydrogen peroxide, and allantoin, all of which are highly soluble and readily excreted when compared to uric acid.

5. **The answer is D.** TLS depends on the type of malignancy, stage of the disease, disease bulk, and presence/absence of renal injury. Burkitt-type leukemia confers a high-risk TLS. Solid tumors and multiple are considered low risk, if presented with renal injury would be raised to intermediate risk. ALL in this example, especially when compared to Question 2, is considered intermediate risk because the LDH is within normal limits.

Chapter 14

1. **The answer is A.** The accumulation of sucrose inside the PCT cells increases the osmolarity and draws the fluid into the cells. Kidney failure occurs as a result of cell swelling, vacuolization, and tubular luminal occlusion from swollen tubular cells.

2. **The answer is D.** Volume depletion and exposure to NSAIDs may increase the risk of kidney injury. Since serum creatinine was elevated slightly, and K is in normal range it is best to stop NSAIDs and observe this patient.

3. **The answer is B.** Proton pump inhibitors have been proposed as a potential cause of drug-induced AIN. The use of proton pump inhibitors have been reported to be four to five times more likely to experience AIN compared to nonproton pump inhibitors users.

4. **The answer is C.** Switching from tenofovir disoproxil fumarate to tenofovir alafenamide was associated with a significant improvement in proteinuria, albuminuria, proximal renal tubular function, and bone mineral density. In early evidence of kidney impairment patients should be switch from tenofovir disoproxil fumarate to tenofovir alafenamide.

5. **The answer is D.** Potential explanations: although not clear, it seems vancomycin-induced ATN occurs as a result of decreased clearance of vancomycin by piperacillin-tazobactam-induced AIN, resulting in an accumulation of vancomycin.

Chapter 15

1. **The answer is D.** Diarrhea can induce intravascular volume depletion and subsequently make the kidney dependent on vasodilating prostaglandins (PGs) to maintain renal perfusion and GFR. In addition to true intravascular volume depletion, states of "effective volume depletion" like heart failure, cirrhosis, and nephrotic syndrome also make the kidney PG dependent. When a NSAID is administered in this setting, vasodilating PGs are decreased and a form of prerenal azotemia can develop. As seen in this patient, acute kidney injury resolved rapidly with indomethacin discontinuation. At times, however, severe volume depletion with hypotension along with NSAID use can cause ischemic acute tubular injury. None of the other options are correct, although NSAID use in patient with hypertension can cause worsening of BP control.

2. **The answer is E.** All of the answers noted are complications of NSAIDs. The clinical renal syndromes associated with NSAIDs include both acute and chronic kidney issues. As PGs are important for many functions in the kidney (renal perfusion, GFR, and sodium,

potassium, and water excretion), these complications can develop at a patient at risk (like the patient in this case).

3. **The answer is B.** The CKD patient in this case has prerenal azotemia from the NSAID. The urine studies that best support this diagnosis is B. Answer A is more consistent with acute tubular injury, answer C is more consistent with glomerulonephritis, answer D is more consistent with acute interstitial nephritis, and answer E is consistent with a glomerular lesion causing nephrotic syndrome.

4. **The answer is C.** Only acute interstitial nephritis is an idiosyncratic adverse reaction to NSAIDs. The other choices are dose dependent with larger doses of NSAIDs more likely to cause each one of the adverse reaction.

5. **The answer is D.** The selective cyclooxygenase (COX) inhibitors were thought to be less nephrotoxic than nonselective NSAIDs due to their more selective inhibition of COX-2 but not COX-1 in the kidney. However, it was subsequently shown that COX-2 is upregulated in the kidney to produce PGs in settings of true or effective volume depletion and to maintain normal water, sodium, and potassium balance. Numerous clinical reports described the same renal syndromes that occurred with nonselective NSAIDs. Thus, the selective COX-2 inhibitors drugs have the same nephrotoxicity as nonselective NSAIDs. The patient in this case is at high risk to develop adverse renal effects with either of these drugs and should not receive them. Another analgesic should be utilized to control her pain.

Chapter 16

1. **The answer is A.** Pyelonephritis in obstructed kidney requires drainage of collecting system. Observation (B) is not correct because patient is at risk of worsening sepsis if source of infection is not drained. Shock wave lithotripsy (C) is not indicated as there is no mention of ureterolithiasis and lithotripsy is not performed during active infection. A CT urogram (D) would not be the next step because serum creatinine is not provided and must be obtained prior to administering IV contrast. CT urogram may be considered once hydronephrosis is drained, but once drain is in place, antegrade urogram can be performed without exposing patient to intravenous contrast.

2. **The answer is B.** Patient may be experiencing postobstructive diuresis. The treatment of postobstructive diuresis should involve replacing urine output with intravenous fluids at a rate less than urine output to prevent replacement fluids from contributing to diuresis. In addition, many patients with chronic bladder outlet obstruction may be volume overloaded, and diuresis

may be appropriate response. DDAVP (C) is used to diagnose and/or treat central diabetes insipidus, which is unlikely in this patient. Observation (D) puts patient at risk for volume depletion.

3. **The answer is A.** Kidney stones <5 mm often pass spontaneously. Initial treatment of nephrolithiasis includes increased fluid intake, pain medication, and α_1-blockers. Extracorporeal shockwave lithotripsy, ureteroscopic stone extraction, and percutaneous nephrostomy are treatments reserved for patients with complicated nephrolithiasis or stones that do not pass spontaneously.

4. **The answer is C.** Hydronephrosis is normal in pregnancy. Renal ultrasound 2–3 months postpartum can be performed to document resolution of hydronephrosis. Other options are incorrect. There is no pyuria present and no indication for prophylactic antibiotic administration. There is no need for repeat renal ultrasound during pregnancy or induction of labor, as hydronephrosis in pregnancy is normal.

5. **The answer is B.** This patient most likely has congenital ureteropelvic obstruction. The finding of thin echogenic cortex makes significant renal recovery unlikely and percutaneous nephrostomy (A) is therefore not indicated. There is no reason to perform a nephrectomy (C) and radionuclide scanning (D) would not change management.

Chapter 17

1. **The answer is E.** Cetuximab, a monoclonal antibody against epithelial growth factor receptor (EGFR) is known to cause hypomagnesemia. This happens as a result of reduction in the transport of transient receptor potential melastatin (TRPM) 6/7 ion channels to the apical membrane of the distal renal tubule. Filtered magnesium (Mg) is reabsorbed mainly in the thick ascending limb of Henle and the distal tubule, where most of the EGFR is located in the kidney. Epidermal growth factor is an autocrine paracrine hormone that regulates renal Mg reabsorption by regulating the activity and transport of TRPM6. Blocking EGFR with cetuximab blunts the movement of TRPM6/7 channel, which leads to renal Mg wasting and hypomagnesemia. The main risk factors for developing hypomagnesemia are duration of treatment, age, and baseline Mg values. Hence, choice E is correct.

2. **The answer is B.** This is a case of spurious hyperkalemia and hypokalemia. For patients with very elevated WBCs, the cells can lyse in the test tube, producing hyperkalemia. Pseudohypokalemia can also occur since the cells are metabolically active and can take up potassium while in the test tube. A plasma sample should provide a more accurate read of the serum potassium. Choice B is correct.

3. **The answer is A.** Given the pathology findings demonstrating electron dense deposits, diagnosis of membranous nephropathy is correct. Choice A is the correct answer. Nephrotic syndrome after HSCT is considered to represent a kidney manifestation of GVHD. In a case series of patients with nephrotic syndrome after HSCT, the most common etiology identified was membranous nephropathy followed by minimal change disease and close to half of these patients developed the nephrotic syndrome concurrently with onset of other GVHD manifestations. A diagnosis of minimal change disease should prompt the nephrologist to rule out relapse of a primary hematologic malignancy. Unlike idiopathic membranous nephropathy, patients who develop membranous nephropathy post HSCT are rarely anti-PLA2R antibody positive. The mainstay of treatment varies on the pathology noted. Treatment options described in the literature varies and ranges from high-dose steroids, calcineurin inhibitors, (CNIs) mycophenolate mofetil, or rituximab.

4. **The answer is A.** The two most common glomerular diseases noted with paraproteinemia are MIDD and AL amyloidosis. Choice B is incorrect as AA amyloidosis is usually seen with chronic inflammatory conditions. C3 GN can be seen with paraproteinemias but is a rare finding mostly with MGUS or smoldering myeloma. Minimal change disease has not been reported with paraproteinemias. MIDD is the most likely finding given the kappa predominance and progressive renal disease overtime in the above patient. The correct answer is A.

5. **The answer is B.** Nivolumab is a PD-1 inhibitor used for treatment of melanoma. Renal injury with this form of check point inhibitor is not uncommon. Acute interstitial nephritis is the known pathologic presentation with this agent. It usually can be subtle with no urinalysis findings. Usually, the injury can happen anywhere from 3 to 12 months from start of therapy. ATN and TMA have not been reported with this agent. The correct answer is B.

Chapter 18

1. **The answer is B.** The 67-year-old male with two simple cysts in the right kidney, without albuminuria or hematuria, and an estimated GFR of 68 mL/min, does not fulfill KDIGO criteria of CKD. Although the patient has structural abnormalities detected by imaging studies (specifically two simple renal cysts), they virtually carry no risk of subsequent renal function decline. Moreover, the eGFR is >60 mL/min and there are no markers of kidney damage, such as albuminuria or hematuria.

Option A, the 28-year-old male with a persistently elevated serum creatinine of 6 mg/dL over the past

4 months, most likely has CKD because that degree of elevation of the serum creatinine most likely reflects an eGFR of <60 mL/min. Furthermore, the serum creatinine elevation has persisted for >3 months, which excludes acute kidney injury.

Option C, the 58-year-old female with a 15-year history of diabetes, albumin-to-creatinine ratio of 258 mg/g, and an estimated GFR of 54 mL/min and declining over the past year, has CKD because her eGFR is <60 mL/min and has been dropping over 1 year. Additionally, as expected by her history of diabetes, she has A2 albuminuria.

Option D, the 70-year-old male with a history of poorly controlled chronic hypertension, a slowly rising serum creatinine, and symptoms felt to be due to uremia, has CKD because of the symptoms of uremia and the slowly rising serum creatinine over the past several years.

2. **The answer is D.** The three listed factors contribute to the pathophysiology of the anemia of CKD. The most import one is decreased erythropoietin production by the failing kidneys. Accelerated hemolysis associated with uremia, nutritional deficiencies (ie, folic acid) due to reduced dietary intake, and iron losses due to easy bleeding related to platelet dysfunction, are additional contributing factors.

3. **The answer is C.** CKD screening is only cost-effective in populations that are at high risk for developing CKD, such as people with diabetes or hypertension. In the general population, CKD screening has not been shown to be cost-effective because only a few cases of CKD would be detected by screening a large population, with what this implies regarding cost and need for repeat testing among those with false-positive results. Secondary prevention should start with early detection of CKD among asymptomatic individuals. The recommended tests for CKD screening are the evaluation of proteinuria preferably with a urine albumin-to-creatinine ratio in an early morning urine sample, and a serum creatinine to estimate GFR with an accepted equation (preferably, the CKD-EPI equation). Secondary prevention will be incomplete if early detection is not followed by interventions that have been shown to slow the progression of CKD, such as glycemic and blood pressure control, as well as the use of ACE inhibitors or angiotensin-receptor antagonists (ARAs).

4. **The answer is C.** It has been shown that an adequate glycemic control slows the progression of CKD in patients with diabetes. The recommended target hemoglobin A_{1c} is approximately 7%. It can be even higher in patients with multiple comorbidities and those at high risk for developing hypoglycemia. Concomitant use of ACE inhibitors and angiotensin-receptor antagonists is not recommended because it has not associated with slower

progression of CKD compared to the effect each agent alone, and there is an increased risk of complications, such as acute kidney injury and hyperkalemia. Likewise, concomitant use of direct renin inhibitors, such as aliskiren, and ARAs, is of no benefit. KDIGO recommends lowering blood pressure to <130/80 in patients with urine albumin-to-creatinine ratio >30 mg/g.

5. **The answer is A.** Diabetes mellitus is the leading cause of end-stage renal disease in the United States, accounting for approximately 45% of cases. Systemic hypertension is the second most frequent cause. Together with diabetes explains close to two-thirds of the new cases of treated ESRD in the United States. Glomerulonephritis and polycystic kidney disease are less frequent causes of CKD.

Chapter 19

1. **The answer is D.** This patient's CKD does not explain the significant drop in hemoglobin and the reader should be cognitive of coexisting etiologies of anemia in CKD patients. Specifically in this patient the higher likelihood of a GI malignancy resulting in blood loss and iron deficient anemia in addition to the relatively mild (hemoglobin 11 g) anemia of CKD.

2. **The answer is D.** Given the results of CHOIR & CREATE the FDA has specifically recommended caution in both the initiation and anemia therapy (Hbg <10 g) and the avoidance of "targets." Management of anemia rather should focus on transfusion avoidance.

3. **The answer is C.** This is a difficult case as she has progressive anemia due to her CKD and also compounded by her chronic ulcer and is symptomatic. Although you could make a case to initiate therapy with an ESA and see if there is some improvement in her hemoglobin levels this is fraught with risk. First, the time to improvement given her symptoms is worrisome. Second, she will most likely have some degree of ESA resistance and may require higher dosing putting her at greater risk of a cardiovascular or cerebral vascular event. Finally, given these risk factors for a cardiac event, not offering treatment with dropping hemoglobin makes a transfusion the best option.

4. **The answer is D.** As mentioned, up to 50% of patients receiving ESA therapy will become iron deficient making monitoring of serum iron levels critically important. This patient presents a classic case of exactly this. Although it had been a common practice to initiate iron replacement and continue ESA treatment, this is not the best answer. Rather it is most appropriate to hold ESAs and replace iron. The reasoning for this is that there is already some degree of ESA resistant given the lower availability of iron so there is some ESA wastage, therefore you cannot justify the additional cost or higher ESA

dosage risk. C is also correct since given the patient's age, one must always be concerned of GI malignancies. As far as the method or iron replacement, given his levels, IV replacement would trump oral replacement give the immediate iron requirements.

5. **The answer is B.** Statistically the presence of anemia of CKD in stages 1 and 2 are less than 10%. This should prompt and aggressive work-up for other causes of anemia including hemoglobinopathies (sickle-cell disease, thalassemia, etc).

Chapter 20

1. **The answer is E.** Patients with impaired kidney function are more likely to die than to progress to ESRD requiring renal replacement therapy. Additionally, both decrease in GFR and increase is albuminuria >30 mg/g are associated with an increased risk of all-cause mortality and cardiovascular event.

2. **The answer is D.** The main benefit of ESAs is decreasing the transfusion need. The four major randomized-controlled trials that looked at ESA use failed to show cardiovascular or mortality benefits.

3. **The answer is C.** Statins are effective for the primary prevention of cardiovascular disease in the nondialysis CKD population and according to the KDIGO guidelines, they should be prescribed for patients above 50 years of age. It is unclear whether the benefit of aspirin for primary prevention in the nondialysis CKD population outweighs the risk of bleeding. KDIGO does not recommend the use of aspirin for that purpose. There is no specific circumstance or reason justifying referral to a specialist.

4. **The answer is A.** Kidney disease is an independent cardiovascular risk factor and the major cause of mortality in dialysis patients. The patient should be subjected to a proper cardiac evaluation. Cardiac troponins may be elevated in ESRD but still offer useful information, particularly if the levels are troponins are higher than baseline or rising. For this reason, patients suspected of having an acute coronary syndrome should be followed with serial cardiac troponin assessment, and the finding of an elevated troponin concentration should not necessarily be dismissed as a false-positive result. Aspirin loading dose can be prescribed if the initial evaluation reveals an acute coronary syndrome.

5. **The answer is C.** In patients on dialysis, the target hemoglobin currently recommended by KDIGO is 10–11.5 g/dL. Targeting normal or near-normal hemoglobin values has been associated with an increased rate of cardiovascular events in several randomized controlled trials. KDIGO recommends against the use of erythropoiesis-stimulating agents to intentionally increase the hemoglobin levels above 13 g/dL.

Chapter 21

1. **The answer is C.** If the patient continues to eat nonprocessed foods and has difficulty tolerating binders, daily or nocturnal dialysis is the best option. Lanthanum is contraindicated if she cannot chew, and calcimimetics and calcitriol are not indicated at her level of PTH.

2. **The answer is D.** Phosphorus levels can vary widely due to dietary intake and diurnal variation. There is no data that phosphate binders impact clinical outcomes at this stage of CKD, and thus interventions are indicated only to lower a biochemical value. Thus, care should be taken to ensure the level is clearly abnormal prior to implementing drug therapy. However, given her stage of CKD, she would benefit from avoiding processed foods as a mechanism to lower both dietary phosphorus and sodium intake.

3. **The answer is E.** The patient has sustained and refractory hyperparathyroidism. Her calcium is elevated and thus calcitriol and vitamin D analogs are contraindicated. The rate of nausea with the IV calcimimetics is the same with oral calcimimetics. Bisphosphonates will lower the calcium level, but would also be retained in bone. Lowering the dialysate calcium concentration will reduce ionized calcium levels during dialysis and increase PTH. After 5 years on the transplant list she would likely be receiving a kidney transplant in the near future. The risk of a new transplant with severe hyperparathyroidism is significant hypercalcemia (due to new kidney being responsive to PTH). Such hypercalcemia can put the new kidney at risk of AKI due to hypercalcemia. Thus, parathyroidectomy is the definitive treatment, and the best for the new kidney.

4. **The answer is D.** These t scores put the patient at considerable fracture risk. DXA scores in patients with this stage of kidney disease are predictive of fracture. Her kidney disease is early stage, and without proteinuria progression is likely to be slower. Her PTH is normal for this stage of kidney disease and thus calcitriol is not indicated. The patient already consumes approximately 500 mg of calcium per day and thus the addition of 1000 mg of calcium would put her in positive calcium balance. Although her 25(OH) vitamin D level is slightly low, it is unlikely this is a major cause of her bone loss, and 50,000 U/week is excessive. The patient has osteoporosis and needs treatment to prevent fracture. Given her PTH level, she does not have CKD-MBD; therefore, she is similar to patients in randomized trials of antiosteoporosis agents, and could receive any of a number of treatments, including bisphosphonates and denosumab.

5. **The answer is C.** Although the patient may not become hypercalcemic or hyperphosphatemic, both ions will have increased intestinal absorption induced by calcitriol.

Calcitriol directly inhibits PTH at the parathyroid gland. Calcitriol is also a potent stimulator of FGF23 secretion from osteoblasts/osteocytes.

Chapter 22

1. **The answer is B.** A low-protein diet (LPD) is traditionally defined as 0.6–0.8 g/kg/day of daily protein intake; it is recommended to nondialysis dependent CKD patients with stage 3b to 4 CKD or any CKD stage and substantial proteinuria. LPD may slow CKD progression rate, mitigate uremic symptoms and ensure adequate protein intake, especially if at least 50% of it is high biologic value protein. The Institute of Medicine recommends 0.8 g/kg/day as the required daily protein intake, while 0.9–1.1 g/kg/day range is generally recommended by dietitians and other practitioners. The 1.2–1.4 g/kg/day is considered high-protein diet and usually recommended to prevalent dialysis patients on standard dialysis dose and frequency and minimal to no residual kidney function. Any protein intake >1.5 g/kg/day is considered very high protein intake, and it may be required for hypercatabolic states such as patients under critical care conditions.

2. **The answer is E.** Megestrol acetate (Megace) is a steroidal progestin that has been used as an appetite stimulant in patients with cancer cachexia or AIDS and also occasionally in anorectic or malnourished dialysis patients. Dronabinol (Marinol) is a cannabinoid (similar to marijuana, which is herbal cannabis) and may be used to treat loss of appetite. Mirtazapine (Remeron, or under other brand names) is an antidepressant agent which may lead to substantial weight gain and which has been occasionally used as an appetite stimulant in dialysis patients. Dihydroxycholecalciferol (Calcitriol) is active vitamin D and is often administered for correction of secondary hyperparathyroidism, it has no known effect on improving appetite.

3. **The answer is D.** Explanation to Question 3: As reviewed under Question 1, a protein intake in the range of 1.2–1.4 g/kg/day is considered high-protein diet and usually recommended to prevalent dialysis patients on standard dialysis dose and frequency, who have minimal to no residual kidney function, given high catabolic rate of dialysis treatment that may be combined with some protein loss during dialysis therapy. A low protein diet is traditionally defined as 0.6–0.8 g/kg/day and recommended for management of nondialysis dependent CKD patients. A very high-protein intake of >1.5 g/kg/day may be required for more hypercatabolic states such as patients under critical care conditions but not stable dialysis patients.

4. **The answer is C.** Evidence suggests that peritoneal dialysis patients have on average 0.2–0.3 g/dL lower serum albumin level than their hemodialysis counterparts of the same age, gender, and comorbid states. This is believed to be due to higher loss of protein via peritoneal membrane or because peritoneal dialysis patients may have longer preservation of residual kidney function than thrice-weekly hemodialysis patients. However, despite a lower level of serum albumin and despite the consistent finding that a low-serum albumin is the strongest predictor of mortality in dialysis patients, peritoneal dialysis patients do not have inferior survival to hemodialysis patients. Other statements are correct.

5. **The answer is D.** Phosphorus in plants is often in form of phytate and is less readily absorbable (30–50%) since human gastrointestinal tract lacks the enzyme phytase to degrade and release phosphorus; whereas phosphorus in animal-based protein is more absorbable (50–70%). Inorganic phosphorus the preservatives added to the food is much more readily absorbable (up to 100%) and, hence, may play a major role in dietary phosphorus burden. There are consistent data that hyperphosphatemia especially >6 mg/dL is associated with incrementally worse survival in CKD patients.

   The only correct statement is about the association of higher protein intake with higher likelihood of hyperphosphatemia in CKD patients.

Chapter 23

1. **The answer is D.** In this case, the patient has diabetic nephropathy and has persistent microalbuminuria on RAAS blockade. The most important intervention would be to increase her RAAS inhibitor to maximally suppress her proteinuria. Her blood pressure is at goal by ACCORD standards, and increasing the metoprolol dose the same antiproteinuric effects seen with RAAS blockade. Control of blood glucose in type 2 diabetes has not been definitively linked with improved renal outcomes. Her mild metabolic acidosis does not require therapy.

2. **The answer is C.** In this case, the chronic use of nonsteroidal anti-inflammatory drugs (NSAIDs) in association with worsening control of hypertension may signal a decline in renal function. The monitoring of renal function in certain high risk patient subgroups is useful in order to enhance patient counseling. Certainly, in a patient with gout, a serum uric acid may shed light on the likelihood of a gout flare as a potential explanation for his symptoms, but given the examination of his knee which does not suggest an acute inflammatory condition; it is likely of lower yield than a serum creatinine. Urine sodium and interrogation of bone density with DEXA scanning are not indicated.

3. **The answer is C.** The DCCT trial definitively showed that tight control of blood glucose values led to decreased

incidence of developing microalbuminuria and other microvascular complications. Since the earliest changes in diabetic nephropathy—namely hyperfiltration—are challenging to detect, microalbuminuria serves as the earliest clinical detector of nephropathy in these patients. In order to detect that, current guidelines recommend that diabetic patients (both type 1 and type 2) undergo yearly monitoring for the development of albuminuria. Unfortunately, the initiation of RAAS blockade before the detection of microalbuminuria has not been definitively linked to decreased rates of developing diabetic nephropathy; though once detected it has shown to decrease the pace of CKD progression.

4. **The answer is D.** The hyperfiltration that occurs with parenchymal loss is adaptive with early disease, but as disease progresses, this can lead to maladaptive increases in the intraglomerular pressures that can become maladaptive. Given that the use of RAAS blockade can impede mediators of the neurohumoral cascade that lead to progression of disease, there is biological plausibility for its use in all advanced renal disease that is born out in many clinical trials, including those examining both proteinuric and nonproteinuric renal diseases. The avoidance of new renal injuries is important. While there may be risk of progression once a certain stage of disease is reduced due to the factors noted above, acute kidney injuries can lead to a need for renal replacement sooner than would be otherwise needed. While lacking trial level evidence, this is likely of greatest importance in people of advanced age. In this patient group, the pace of disease progression and potential need for dialysis needs to be balanced against overall longevity, with a goal of extending the life of native renal mass.

5. **The answer is D.** Diabetic patients benefit from blood pressure management. Trial level evidence in type 2 diabetes mellitus subjects has shown that a systolic blood pressure target of <140 mm Hg led to improved cardiovascular benefits, though tighter control (<120 mm Hg) led to unfavorable cardiovascular events. Multiple studies have demonstrated a benefit in diabetic patients, both type 1 and 2, from employing maximal tolerated RAAS blockade.

Chapter 24

1. **The answer is B.** This patient's clinical history, family history, and laboratory findings are very concerning for nephrotic syndrome related to focal segmental glomerulosclerosis and kidney biopsy is the only means by which this disease can be diagnosed.

Antinuclear antibody and anti-dsDNA antibody assay would help to determine serologic evidence of systemic lupus erythematosus. Lupus nephritis is more commonly associated with a nephritic syndrome. Since this patient has severe proteinuria and no evidence of hematuria, his presentation is more consistent with nephrotic syndrome. Furthermore, positivity of ANA and anti-dsDNA does not always equate to lupus nephritis a kidney biopsy would need to be performed for a diagnosis.

Antiphospholipase A_2 receptor antibody assay is a test used in diagnosis and to monitor treatment response of primary membranous nephropathy. Though this patient's presentation would be consistent with a membranous induced nephrotic syndrome, his age and being African–American makes FSGS more likely. Also, Antiphospholipase A_2 receptor antibody is only present in approximately 70% of patient with primary membranous nephropathy, thus a kidney biopsy is still gold standard for diagnosis of membranous nephropathy.

Serum protein electrophoresis (SPEP) is not warranted in this patient since he has no history or serologic abnormalities concerning for multiple myeloma or amyloidosis. Additionally, myeloma is even less likely given his age and lack of family history for malignancy.

2. **The answer is D.** Mycophenolate mofetil with corticosteroids with and without tacrolimus as well as cyclophosphamide plus corticosteroids have been shown to be effective first-line treatments for lupus nephritis. Plasmapheresis only has not been shown to be effective in lupus nephritis when used without the additional of another immunosuppression agent.

3. **The answer is A.** Treatment with an ACEI or ARB is first-line therapy in someone with proteinuria. In this individual, who has significant proteinuria and hypertension, using an ACEI or ARB would help with both these issues. Using NSAIDs or combination ACEI and ARB are not recommended in the treatment of proteinuria unless the proteinuria is excessive to the points it is causing malnutrition. In this individual, his nutrition status seems good and does not have an indication either of these. Thus, starting ACEI or ARB monotherapy is the more appropriate option.

Increasing his furosemide dose may help improve his edema and hypertension but would not help treat his proteinuria.

4. **The answer is D.** This patient has findings of uncontrolled diabetes mellitus including elevated HgbA1c, glycosuria, neuropathy, and diabetic retinopathy. Since diabetic nephropathy is the leading cause of nephrotic syndrome in the United States and given the patient's clinical and laboratory findings, particularly the diabetic retinopathy, diabetic nephropathy is the most likely cause. Systemic lupus erythematous and hepatitis C–related MPGN are unlikely in the setting of a negative ANA and hepatitis C antibody, respectively. Primary focal segmental glomerulosclerosis can present

as a nephrotic syndrome but given the patient's age, ethnicity, and stigmata of systemic diabetic disease, FSGS is less likely.

Chapter 25

1. **The answer is C.** This child is very likely to have minimal change nephrotic syndrome. He is in the peak age group of presentation, and at his age there is a 2:1 prevalence of boys to girls with MCD. The absence of hematuria makes the likelihood of an inflammatory glomerular lesion such as post infectious glomerulonephritis highly unlikely. However, a C3 and ANA are typically ordered for completeness sake, though the yield is very low. An echocardiogram is not indicated as the anasarca can be explained on the basis of his nephrotic syndrome. Although not necessary, a chest radiograph should confirm the suspicion of pleural effusions. Children presenting with nephrotic syndrome have a greater than 95% chance of having minimal change disease so a kidney biopsy is not necessary before starting empiric therapy with corticosteroids.

2. **The answer is B.** This woman fulfills the diagnostic criteria for nephrotic syndrome with nephrotic range proteinuria (urine total protein/creatinine ratio >3.5), hypoalbuminemia, hypercholesterolemia, and edema. As an adult, MCD is in the differential, but a kidney biopsy is required to diagnose her renal lesion in order to guide therapy. Membranous nephropathy and FSGS are also in the differential. The presence of microscopic hematuria (which is seen in a minority of patients with MCD) broadens your differential to include other forms of glomerulonephritis such as IgA nephropathy. Hepatitis B and C testing might be indicated if the biopsy findings show a lesion that might be associated with those chronic infections. It is always a good idea to test for TB prior to starting immunosuppressive therapy, but steroids should not be used empirically in an adult nephrotic patient without a diagnostic kidney biopsy. Diuretics should be used with caution, especially if the patient is not uncomfortable, as it can worsen the intravascular volume depletion seen in some patients.

3. **The answer is D.** This young boy has developed signs of steroid toxicity with hypertension, weight gain, slowed growth and Cushingoid features. It is time to consider alternative treatments. Since he has always responded promptly to steroids, the results of a kidney biopsy are unlikely to guide your treatment choices. Studies have shown that the response to steroids in children with nephrotic syndrome is a better prognostic indicator than glomerular histology—even if he were to have FSGS on biopsy, you would offer him the same treatment options as you would if he had MCD. If his C3 and ANA were negative at diagnosis, he is highly

unlikely to have developed lupus or hypocomplementemic glomerulonephritis. There are several second line immunosuppressive treatments available. All of their benefits and potential side effects should be explained to his family in detail and weighed against the complications of steroid therapy that he has experienced. One family might be put off by and the required weekly CBCs and the very low potential risk of gonadal toxicity presented by a 12-week course of cyclophosphamide, while another family would welcome the possibility that cyclophosphamide could induce a prolonged remission. Another family might be concerned about the frequent blood tests to follow through tacrolimus levels. If you are concerned about the ability of the family to follow up closely with clinical monitoring, you might recommend rituximab. Since childhood nephrotic syndrome is a chronic disease, it is important to participate in shared decision making with the family.

4. **The answer is D.** While the overall prognosis for a child with MCD is excellent, they are at risk for the life-threatening complications of sepsis (especially pneumococcal) and thrombosis. This child has a high fever, left shift on WBC and ascites with abdominal tenderness, concerning for peritonitis. While pneumococcus is the most common cause of peritonitis, other organisms such as *Haemophilus influenza* type B and gut organisms can also cause peritonitis so the initial empiric choice of antibiotics should cover these organisms. While acute kidney injury (AKI) is more common in adults with MCD, it is also seen in children with MCD, especially at times of crisis. Typically during relapse the patient has intravascular volume contraction that increases the risk of AKI. For the critically ill patient the team will want to preserve renal perfusion by expanding the intravascular volume. However, if a patient has AKI and the urine output is compromised, he is at risk of developing pulmonary edema during vigorous volume expansion. Checking a fractional excretion of sodium to check for AKI is helpful in guiding fluid management. Since this patient has a low serum albumin, the use of intravenous 25% albumin is beneficial in maintaining the intravascular volume and will help with diuresis. Typically, the intravenous albumin is followed by intravascular furosemide to augment the diuresis, but it should be used with caution in a patient who is hemodynamically unstable. This child also has a high hematocrit and an elevated platelet count which are risk factors for thrombosis. Expanding the intravascular volume may help reduce the risk of thrombosis. While the team is always tempted to place a central line in a critically ill child, if possible, that should be avoided in the nephrotic child as they are prone to develop clots in these lines. Because of the risk of sagittal sinus thrombosis, it is also necessary to monitor for changes in neurologic status.

5. **The answer is C.** Only about 3% of MCD children followed into adulthood develop ESRD and up to 42% will continue to relapse into adulthood. Children with frequent relapses and those who required steroid-sparing medications are the most likely to continue to have relapses as adults. In one long-term study only 8 of 42 patients followed for a median of 22 years after diagnosis had had children, with cytotoxic therapy identified as a risk factor for childlessness. However, the longer a child goes off therapy without a relapse, the more likely he is to maintain a remission.

Chapter 26

1. **The answer is C.** In this otherwise healthy individual, the finding of nephrotic range proteinuria, hypoalbuminemia, elevated serum creatinine and no evidence of infection, suggest that the etiology is kidney disease with a requirement to assess the renal tissue for diagnosis.

2. **The answer is E.** In adults with FSGS and no family history of disease, genetic testing may be considered as part of the FSGS recurrence post-transplant risk assessment. Specifically, causative genetic polymorphisms confer a lower risk for FSGS recurrence. Genetic testing has been incorporated in many research studies that support discovery of disease mechanisms, novel therapeutic targets, and phenotype/genotype associations.

3. **The answer is B.** The kidney biopsy of FSGS, subtotal podocyte foot process effacement and medical history of sickle-cell disease suggest that this patient has secondary FSGS. In this setting angiotensin-converting enzyme inhibitor or angiotensin-receptor blocking agents may reduce proteinuria and slow the decline of kidney function. Immunosuppression agents are not indicated in the setting of secondary FSGS. This patient has well preserved kidney function based on normal serum creatinine therefore a kidney biopsy is not indicated.

4. **The answer is A.** In this setting of congenital nephrotic syndrome, over 80% of infants will have a genetic mutation in a podocyte protein. This testing will provide more precise information about the cause of the disease, prognosis, and treatment.

5. **The answer is D.** The overall risk of recurrent FSGS is approximately 25%. A rapid decline in GFR from disease onset is associated with a greater likelihood of this complication. Elevated blood pressure and type of donor are not predictive factors. APOL1 genotype may impact on outcome for the donor but not on recurrence in the recipient.

Chapter 27

1. **The answer is B.** The patient has newly diagnosed MN. Although he is anti-PLA2R positive, the long history of smoking makes it imperative that lung cancer is rule out by performing a chest CT. He is hypertensive and thus should be started on angiotensin II blockade, which may also reduce proteinuria. The fact that he is severely nephrotic with a serum albumin of 11 g/L raises consideration for anticoagulation prophylaxis, unless contraindicated. We do not have information on serum anti-PLA2R levels and they are crucial in ascertaining probability for spontaneous remission and to guide introduction of immunosuppression (De Vriese, et al. *J Am Soc Nephrol.* 2017;28(2):421–430). As such, initial therapy in this case should be maximizing conservative therapy with low-sodium and low-protein diet, angiotensin II blockade and blood pressure control.

2. **The answer is B.** The patient has developed a complication of severe nephrotic syndrome, namely a DVT. As such anticoagulation should be started. In view of the severity of the disease, the patient should also be started on immunosuppression therapy (Hofstra JM, Fervenza FC, Wetzels JF. *Nat Rev Nephrol.* 2013;9(8):443–458).

3. **The answer is D.** This is a typical presentation of membranous lupus nephropathy (class V). In these cases, complement levels are normal, as opposed to class III and IV where complement levels are usually decreased. Inflammatory markers are also absent in class V lupus, while immunofluorescence typically shows a "full house" pattern. Many patients with membranous lupus have negative anti-DNA antibodies at diagnosis although they may become positive on follow up. Anti-PLA2R antibodies are typically negative (Austin HA, Illei GG. *Lupus.* 2005;14(1):65–71).

4. **The answer is D.** Current recommendations are to continue calcineurin inhibitors for at least 12 months in patients that are responding to the therapy. Early discontinuation, especially in a patient who is in partial remission since early discontinuation of therapy is likely to result in a relapse (Cattran, et al. *Kidney Int.* 2007;72(12):1429–1447). Several studies have shown that nadir of proteinuria, in patients who are responding to therapy, may not be achieved until after 18–24 months (Ruggenenti, et al. *J Am Soc Nephrol.* 2012;23(8):1416–1425; Ponticelli, et al. *J Am Soc Nephrol.* 1998;9(3):444–450). There is no role for repeating a renal biopsy at this stage. Monitoring serum anti-PLA2R levels may also help in tailoring immunosuppressive therapy in patients with a positive antibody (De Vriese, et al. *J Am Soc Nephrol.* 2017;28(2):421–430).

Chapter 28

1. **The answer is C.** The most likely diagnosis in IgA nephropathy. While the blood could be coming from the genital tract, this is unlikely. A CT contrast scan is more than is needed and it is too soon for a biopsy given normal renal function. Since she is a smoker, there

are possible bladder lesions, and also possible kidney stones, so a renal ultrasound is the best screening test with the fewest possible complications. Although not listed here as one of the choices, a cystoscopy would be reasonable given concern for transitional cell cancer in setting of smoking, as well as trial of cessation of running and birth control pills since they can cause hematuria as well.

2. **The answer is B.** Given the presence of gross hematuria and acute kidney failure in the setting of "synpharyngitic hematuria" (hematuria occurring at the same time as upper respiratory tract infection, the most likely diagnosis is IgA nephropathy, with potential for crescentic presentation. However, lupus nephritis (less likely given gender and no other systemic symptoms to suggest lupus), and other diseases that cause rapidly progressive glomerulonephritis, such as antiglomerular basement disease and renal limited vasculitis (less likely given age) are in the differential diagnosis. Although poststreptococcal glomerulonephritis is also in the differential diagnosis, it is less likely because of the short time elapsed from upper respiratory tract symptoms to gross hematuria (hence "synpharyngitic"). A kidney biopsy is indicated to determine the diagnosis and guide treatment.

Empiric corticosteroid treatment should not be pursued since some of the diseases in the differential diagnosis require cytotoxic treatment as well (eg, cyclophosphamide, mycophenolate), and such treatment may not be indicated if patient has acute kidney failure from hematuria-induced acute tubular necrosis in the setting of IgA nephropathy. Quantifying the proteinuria is indicated but has little prognostic use unless the disease becomes chronic. Antistreptolysin O (ASO) antibody level is only useful if the diagnosis of antistreptococcal glomerulonephritis is being entertained, and is more effective in ruling out the disease if it is negative. If ASO antibodies are present, may be indicative of prior infection and not current infection. At this time, serum IgA levels are neither sensitive nor specific enough for diagnosis. Serum IgA1 levels, specifically looking for galactose-deficient IgA1, may be useful for the future, but would require further study and validation.

3. **The answer is D.** All of the treatments above except for IgA1 protease and topical budesonide have been studied, some in randomized control fashion, and have not yielded consistently favorable results. In particular, tonsillectomy may be effective in the Japanese population, but has not been shown to be of benefit in European populations, which would be more applicable to this patient. Anticoagulation treatment, if beneficial, may be so only in the pediatric population. IgA1 protease treatment of mice reduces IgA deposits in the mesangial, directly targeting the disease mechanism.

4. **The answer is D.** It is most likely that this 18-year-old male with extremity rash, abdominal pain, and glomerulonephritis has Henoch–Schonlein purpura. The renal biopsy suggests that he has an IgA dominant lesion as well. Henoch–Schonlein purpura with a relapsing and remitting course usually does not require therapy. The majority of these patients usually have long spontaneous remissions, thus immunomodulating drugs including glucocorticoids, mycophenolate mofetil, or azathioprine are not indicated. The patient is hypertensive and has some proteinuria, thus it is reasonable to suggest that he be treated with an angiotensin converting enzyme inhibitor to lower blood pressure and to decrease his proteinuric state. Thus, the correct answer is D, an angiotensin converting enzyme inhibitor.

5. **The answer is E.** This patient has IgA nephropathy with advanced chronic renal disease. At a serum creatinine 3.5 mg/dL, he has likely reached the "point-of-no-return" where no specific therapy, other than control of blood pressure, will reverse the condition. Thus none of the options involving immunosuppressive therapy are correct. He should be vigorously treated with angiotensin II inhibition in an attempt to reduce his blood pressure to around 120/80 mm Hg and his protein excretion rate to less than 1.0 g/day, if possible.

6. **The answer is A.** The patient has IgA nephropathy with severe features indicative of a "poor" prognosis, including proteinuria >2.5 g/day despite combined ACE inhibitor and angiotensin II inhibitor therapy (Note: This combination of medications should only be used in patients with severe proteinuria and relatively preserved kidney function given risk for hyperkalemia and worsening kidney function.) Based on these considerations, treatment is indicated. Controlled clinical trials have suggested that a steroid regimen similar to that described in option A may be best approach. No controlled trails demonstrate benefit with cyclosporine or MMF in the circumstances described by this patient. Aggressive immunosuppression would be best limited to those patients who demonstrate progressive renal disease. Fish oil is not indicated as meta-analysis of reported trials has shown that any benefits are inconsistent.

Chapter 29

1. **The answer is C.** Abnormal activation of the alternate pathway of complement has been documented in patients with MPGN. It can be due to genetic mutations that alter the activity of complement regulatory proteins. The kallikrein system is involved in blood pressure control but is not specific for MPGN. The pituitary-adrenal axis is normal in patients with MPGN, interaction between AVP and the V2 receptor

contribute to autosomal dominant polycystic kidney disease but not MPGN. There is no evidence of a specific disturbance in the Th1 or any other lymphocyte subset in patients with MPGN.

2. **The answer is B.** This older man has no pulmonary or hepatic complaints making sarcoidosis and hepatitis unlikely. The absence of travel makes malaria an unlikely diagnosis. He has no fever or murmur which would exclude endocarditis. The presence of MPGN with nephrotic range proteinuria is most consistent with the presence of a monoclonal gammopathy.

3. **The answer is D.** Serum amyloid protein is a nonspecific acute phase reactant. ANCA associated vasculitis is not associated with hypocomplementemia. IgA nephropathy rarely presents with nephrotic syndrome and the serum IgA levels are usually normal. NGAL is a marker of tubular injury and is not a diagnostic test in patients with glomerular disease. C3 nephritic factor is often present in patients with MPGN, especially type II or dense deposit disease.

Chapter 30

1. **The answer is D.** The patient has combined renal and respiratory failure—or pulmonary renal syndrome—which has many causes. These can be segregated into six broad groups: immune mediated; directly caused by infection; fluid overload caused by acute tubular necrosis; left heart failure with pulmonary oedema and renal hypoperfusion; direct toxicity from paraquat; and rarely caused by an assortment of other conditions. Usually the critical distinction is between immune-mediated and infection-mediated disease. None of the diagnoses is excluded by the information given in the clinical vignette but the rate of rise serum creatinine together with urinary dipstick results and active urine sediment make acute tubular necrosis or tubulointerstitial disease extremely unlikely which makes answers A, C, and E wrong. Instead, they strongly suggest glomerulonephritis with a rapidly progressive clinical course of which anti-GBM disease or ANCA-associated vasculitis (AAV) with pauci-immune focal necrotizing glomerulonephritis are the most likely. Both cause severe crescentic glomerulonephritis but the rate of deterioration of renal function is more typical of AAV since the evolution of anti-GBM disease is usually more explosive. More decisively, palpable purpura indicative of leukocytoclastic vasculitis is not a feature of anti-GBM disease but occurs commonly in AAV. Accordingly answer B is wrong and answer D is correct. The facts favor a diagnosis of pauci-immune focal necrotizing glomerulonephritis caused by AAV and positive ANCA. Given the findings the ANCA is most likely to be specific

for myeloperoxidase and the clinical diagnosis to be microscopic polyangiitis.

2. **The answer is B.** Immunoassays for autoantibodies for NC1 domain of the α3 chain of type IV collagen (α3 (IV) NC1) in the GBM are the hallmark of classic anti-GBM disease. In this context, they correlate closely with linear IgG deposition along the GBM, and are easily distinguished from low levels of background staining for IgG is often visible along to GBM. This background staining is accentuated when the GBM is thickened (as for example in diabetes) or with heavy proteinuria, but it is never of the +++ intensity in the present case; accordingly answer A is wrong. The IgG deposits in early fibrillary glomerulonephritis can lie along the GBM and mimic linear staining on fluorescence but the fibrillary deposits are easily visible on electron microscopy; such deposits were absent in the present case and so answer C is wrong. In rare cases anti-GBM antibodies specific for α3 (IV) NC1 are predominantly IgG4 subclass that are barely if at all detected in standard anti-GBM immunoassays. These individuals present with classic anti-GBM disease, but often with severe pulmonary hemorrhage and relatively mild focal necrotizing glomerulonephritis (FNGN). The individual had chronic membranoproliferative glomerulonephritis with nephrotic range proteinuria rather than acute focal necrotizing glomerulonephritis and so answer D is wrong. By contrast the present case has the characteristics of atypical anti-GBM disease associated with antibodies that have affinity for the GBM but which do not bind α3 (IV) NC1. Some cases these are autoantibodies specific for a conformational epitope in intact NC1 hexamers similar to that recognized by alloantibodies in patients with Alport syndrome after renal transplantation. In most however the specificity is unknown and indeed the affinity for the GBM could be due to the biophysical properties of the IgG rather than recognition of a specific antigen.

3. **The answer is C.** Alport syndrome is caused by mutations in the α3, α4, or α5 chains of type IV collagen that together form the collagen network in the GBM. Consequently these chains are deficient or severely poorly expressed in glomeruli of an Alport kidney and appear as alloantigens in transplanted kidneys. The gene encoding α5 chain is encoded on the X chromosome and α5 mutations account for around 85% of cases. Missense mutations are usually associated with low levels of α5 whereas deletions favor complete absence and a greater chance of developing alloimmune anti-GBM disease. Accordingly answer A is false. Anti-GBM alloantibodies do not recognize the classic Goodpasture antigen (α3 [IV] NC1) but instead a conformational epitopes involving the NC1 domains all three chains. Consequently they are recognized poorly if at all by standard anti-GBM

antibody assays. Consequently a negative immunoassay does not exclude the diagnosis and Answer B is false. Alport anti-GBM disease with focal necrotizing glomerulonephritis is uncommon and occurs in no more than 5% of allografts and perhaps far fewer but transient linear IgG deposition without glomerular inflammation is more common. Accordingly answer C is correct whilst answer D is false. The diagnosis requires intense linear staining and focal necrotizing glomerulonephritis.

Chapter 31

1. **The answer is B.** The immunofluorescence figure shows bright coarsely granular glomerular capillary wall and mesangial staining for C3 and IgA ("starry-sky" pattern), supporting a diagnosis of IgA-dominant bacterial infection associated glomerulonephritis. The vast majority of cases of IgA-dominant bacterial infection associated glomerulonephritis are due staphylococcal infection (most commonly associated with *Staphylococcus aureus*).

2. **The answer is D.** Subepithelial humps are far more common in bacterial infection–associated glomerulonephritis than IgA nephropathy. Other clinical and pathologic features that favor IgA-dominant staphylococcus-associated glomerulonephritis over IgA nephropathy are initial presentation at an older age, presence of hypocomplementemia, and presence of exudative glomerulonephritis on light microscopy.

3. **The answer is E.** The figure shows a trichrome stain of renal biopsy section. The two glomeruli shown exhibit large cellular crescents which compress the underlying tufts. While crescents can be seen in any form of bacterial infection–associated glomerulonephritis, they are usually more common and affect a higher percentage of glomeruli in infectious endocarditis-associated glomerulonephritis.

4. **The answer is D.** Streptococcus-associated glomerulonephritis typically begins after the pharyngeal or skin infection has resolved (spontaneously or with effective antibiotic therapy). In contrast, bacterial infection–associated glomerulonephritis caused by other bacteria (including staphylococcus) usually develops when the infection is still present. In about a third of cases of acute poststreptococcal glomerulonephritis, immunofluorescence shows bright glomerular staining for C3 only (with negative or trivial staining for IgG, IgA, and IgM). The incidence of acute poststreptococcal glomerulonephritis has decreased dramatically in the developed countries likely due to the accessibility to early medical care and antibiotic treatment resulting from improvements in living standards. Generally, renal biopsy is needed to confirm the diagnosis of sporadic acute poststreptococcal glomerulonephritis in adults

as the differential diagnosis is wide and includes IgA nephropathy, C3 glomerulonephritis, lupus nephritis, and ANCA-associated pauci-immune crescentic glomerulonephritis. The most common causative bacterium in bacterial infection-associated glomerulonephritis in the elderly is staphylococcus (46%) followed by streptococcus (16%).

5. **The answer is A.** *Staphylococcus epidermidis* is the most frequent responsible bacterium in shunt nephritis, followed by *Propionibacterium acne*. Shunt nephritis develops in patients with infected ventriculoatrial or ventriculojugular shunts and only rarely occurs in patients with ventriculoperitoneal shunts. Patients present with hematuria (microscopic or gross), proteinuria, renal insufficiency, and hypertension. As crescentic phenotype is uncommon, a presentation with rapidly progressive glomerulonephritis is exceptional. Contrary to other types of bacterial infection–associated glomerulonephritis, light microscopy typically exhibits a membranoproliferative glomerulonephritis pattern of injury likely reflecting the chronic antigenemia and indolent disease course in these patients. On electron microscopy, there are mesangial and subendothelial electron dense deposits. Subepithelial humps are uncommon.

Chapter 32

1. **The answer is A.** This patient is presenting with features of ANCA-associated vasculitis. Serological tests show only ANCA-positivity. In such patients the kidney biopsy is typically negative or only shows trace staining for antibodies on immunofluorescence ("pauci immune"). The presence of linear glomerular basement (GBM) staining is suggestive of anti-GBM antibody disease. This entity is typically associated with positive anti-GBM antibodies. Similarly, granular staining suggests immune complex disease. The presence of multiple antibodies and complement components being positive suggests lupus nephritis which is unlikely given the negative lupus serologies and complements. The finding of immunoglobulin with only kappa or lambda light chains suggest a monoclonal gammopathy–related kidney disease. In the presence of a negative peripheral monoclonal gammopathy workup, this is unlikely.

2. **The answer is B.** In a patient with clinically suspected ANCA-vasculitis, the presence of frank hemoptysis with respiratory failure is an indication for pulse steroids and plasma exchange. These treatment should be started even if the kidney biopsy results are pending since the pretest probability of ANCA vasculitis with the above presentation is high. In patients without a classic presentation, a bronchoscopy may be performed to determine whether the patient has hemoptysis from diffuse alveolar hemorrhage or other etiologies (eg, infection).

Cardiac catheterization is not indicated in this patient who does not show evidence of active ischemia on ECG and troponin levels.

3. **The answer is C.** The patient in this case has worsening pulmonary symptoms and infiltrates in the setting of improving parameters of ANCA-vasculitis. The main concern here is pulmonary opportunistic infection with *Pneumocystis jiroveci* or other organisms. Thus escalating immunosuppression is not correct and rapid diagnosis with bronchoscopy and bronchoalveolar lavage is the next step. A lung biopsy is not indicated at this stage.

4. **The answer is C.** In this patient with kidney biopsy-proven pauci immune glomerulonephritis, the underlying diagnosis is likely ANCA-associated vasculitis. However, there a few atypical features in her clinical presentation. The presence of a positive ANA and anti-histone antibodies suggest a drug-induced vasculitis. Among the drugs implicated, propylthiouracil, TNF-blocking agents, sulfasalazine, D-penicillamine, and hydralazine are the most closely associated with this syndrome. The treatment would involve immunosuppression and withdrawal of hydralazine.

5. **The answer is B.** The patient being discussed presented with severe ANCA-associated disease involving the lungs and kidneys. She is currently in full remission on a minimal dose of steroids and monthly IV cyclophosphamide, which had been started as part of her induction regimen. This is the time to de-escalate immunosuppression and switch to a maintenance protocol. The risk of relapse in ANCA-associated vasculitis is high in the absence of maintenance therapy. Current guidelines favor azathioprine over other maintenance therapies.

Chapter 33

1. **The answer is B.** There is rather broad experience showing that proteinuric flares can arise during maintenance therapy. In cases such as this, the renal pathology may reflect attenuated expression (related to the ongoing immunosuppression) of flares arising from the same original class of proliferative disease. Quite often, proteinuric flares in such cases may represent transition to class V lupus membranous nephropathy, or a combination of mixed membranous and proliferative LN. Renal biopsy is usually needed to distinguish these pathways, to assess the degree of cumulative damage, and to redirect therapies.

2. **The answer is D.** Endorsing the patient's desire to proceed with pregnancy after 1-year-long period of sustained remission of SLE is supported by recent data on relative risks to mother and fetus. However, it is essential that the patient understand the necessity of discontinuation (and replacement with effective

substitutes if necessary) of potentially teratogenic drugs such as lisinopril and mycophenolate.

3. **The answer is C.** Lupus podocytopathy is an uncommon manifestation of LN that occurs as a subset within class I or class II LN. It is unknown whether lupus podocytopathy arises from a unique pathogenic mechanism related to SLE, or whether it represents a rare coincidence of LN and an unrelated nephropathy such as minimal change disease and/or focal segmental glomerulosclerosis. In both class I and II LN, deposits of immune complexes confined to mesangial regions and the manifestation of concurrent lupus podocytopathy is recognized by the presence of widespread effacement of podocytes without capillary loop deposits as would be typical of minimal change disease. Compared to classic class I or II LN, lupus podocytopathy is manifested clinically by rapid appearance of nephrotic-range proteinuria and often responds to corticosteroids alone.

4. **The answer is C.** A high chronicity index reflects the degrees of loss of renal reserve (compensation) capacity and the amount of irreversible cumulative damage; hence, the chronicity index is a useful predictor of long-term prognosis in LN. A high activity index is commonly used to tailor the indications for high-intensity induction therapy. Per se, the activity index is a relatively poor predicator of outcome because its components may heal by regression under the influence of effective therapy.

5. **The answer is B.** True. The natural history of SLE and LN is manifestly different among diverse populations. This makes reliable extrapolation of treatment effects among different groups very tenuous.

Chapter 34

1. **The answer is D.** Both of these have been shown in large studies to predict the development of acute renal failure and cast nephropathy. A contains new definitions for symptomatic multiple myeloma but not cast nephropathy. B and C are parts of the CRAB criteria that define symptomatic multiple myeloma but not for cast nephropathy. E contains risk factors that could increase the risk of cast nephropathy but would not precipitate cast nephropathy on their own with the other risk factors.

2. **The answer is C.** The recovery of renal function from cast nephropathy is predicted by the percent reduction of serum-free light chain and the speed at which that is accomplished. None of the other has been shown to have any prognostic value.

3. **The answer is B.** Studies have shown a minimum of VGPR is necessary for improvement of organ dysfunction in AL amyloidosis including the kidney. D and E are not response criteria in AL amyloidosis.

4. **The answer is B.** In two recent studies, symptomatic multiple myeloma was diagnosed in 20% of patients with MIDD. In older literature where smoldering multiple myeloma was included, the rate increases to 56–65%.

5. **The answer is D.** In a recent study, all patients with a positive immunofixation and an abnormal serum-free light chain ratio had a pathologic clone identified. The presence of IgG3 actually decreases the chance of identifying a pathologic clone.

CHAPTER 35

1. **The answer is D.** This patient's findings are consistent with thrombotic thrombocytopenic purpura. ADAMTS13 activity should be measured in a sample collected prior to plasma exchange, but treatment with plasma exchange should not be delayed while awaiting the results. Corticosteroids may be beneficial, but rituximab can be reserved for patients with refractory or recurrent disease. Alternative diagnoses should be considered, including autoimmune disease, infections, and cancer. Transfusion of packed red blood cells or platelets can be performed if necessary, but should not be undertaken based on lab values.

2. **The answer is E.** Treatment with eculizumab increases the risk of meningococcal infections. All patients treated with the drug should be immunized for meningococcus. Antibiotic prophylaxis should also be used if treatment is going to start before the immunization can take effect. Corticosteroids and plasma exchange are first line therapy for thrombocytopenic thrombotic purpura. Plasma exchange may be effective in some cases of atypical hemolytic uremic syndrome, but it is not necessary in patients treated with eculizumab. Atypical hemolytic uremic syndrome is a clinical diagnosis, and a renal biopsy is usually not helpful for distinguishing this disease from other causes of thrombotic microangiopathy.

3. **The answer is A.** Quinine is the most common cause of drug-induced thrombotic microangiopathy, and it causes antibody-mediated disease. Although the Food and Drug Administration has warned against using quinine containing pills to treat leg cramps, antimalarial medications still contain quinine and it is present in some supplements and in beverages. Although avoidance of quinine is the most important intervention, plasmapheresis may remove pathogenic autoantibodies. It is important to start plasma exchange as quickly as possible in patients with possible thrombotic thrombocytopenic purpura, but administration of fresh frozen plasma would violate this patient's religious beliefs. A decreased C3 level is a nonspecific finding. There is no evidence to support the use of drugs to protect the vasculature or prevent thrombosis in drug-induced thrombotic microangiopathy.

4. **The answer is D.** In general, patients with renal failure from Shiga-toxin induced hemolytic uremic syndrome do well after renal transplantation. Although calcineurin inhibitors have been linked with the development of *de novo* thrombotic microangiopathy, there is no evidence that they increase the risk of disease recurrence after transplantation. Although there may be genetic predispositions to hemolytic uremic syndrome in patients infected with Shiga-toxin producing bacteria, kidneys can be donated by relatives. Eculizumab is recommended for patients with complement-mediated hemolytic uremic syndrome to prevent disease recurrence in the peritransplant period.

5. **The answer is A.** Although thrombotic thrombocytopenic purpura is possible, this patient's laboratory tests and history are more consistent with scleroderma renal crisis. Scleroderma renal crisis is a medical emergency, and treatment with an angiotensin converting enzyme inhibitor is appropriate for this patient. ADAMTS13 activity should be measured, and testing for other causes of thrombotic microangiopathy should also be performed but empiric treatment for other diseases should not be started unless specific findings point to an alternative diagnosis.

Chapter 36

HIV-ASSOCIATED RENAL DISEASE

1. **The answer is D.** The patient in the question has heavy proteinuria without hypertension or edema. Patient has advanced kidney failure that occurred rapidly but without a nephritic presentation. The patient's clinical history suggests long standing HIV infection that has progressed to AIDS and African–American race suggests that he is may have genetic susceptibility to developing HIVAN. The most effective treatment for HIVAN is cART (choice D). While prednisone and ACE-i may also provide benefits for some patients with HIVAN, they should be considered only after starting cART. Rituximab (choice C) has no known therapeutic effect on HIVAN.

2. **The answer is A.** The patient in the question had stable renal function while on a tenofovir-containing cART regimen. The addition of cobicistat in the new regimen was associated with an increase in serum creatinine. Cobicistat impairs tubular creatinine secretion resulting in a small, stable, and reversible increase in serum creatinine. Conservative monitoring is the most desirable option.

3. **The answer is D.** The patient in the question demonstrates a Fanconi-like syndrome most likely due to tenofovir toxicity. His high total protein is due to an HIV-related polyclonal gammaglobulinemia (no

monoclonal detected) and his weakness and electrolyte deficiencies can best be explained by hypophosphatemia rather than other medications in his regimen.

4. **The answer is A.** Atazanavir use is associated with elevated risk of nephrolithiasis especially in patients with liver disease because atazanavir is cleared primarily by the liver. Needle shaped crystals suggestive of atazanavir crystalluria which is more likely than uric acid in this patient. Tenofovir does not cause nephrolithiasis and the findings of a stone on renal ultrasound, crystalluria, and hematuria in the setting of atazanavir use does not merit renal biopsy.

5. **The answer is D.** The patient is Caucasian and therefore unlikely to develop HIVAN. She lacks hematuria common in the presentation HIV-associated immune complex disease. Her HIV does increase the risk of developing diabetic kidney disease and this is the most likely diagnosis in this patient. Recent evidence suggests that HIV may promote progression of diabetic kidney disease.

HEPATITIS-ASSOCIATED GLOMERULONEPHRITIS

1. **The answer is B.** HCV-associated nephrotic syndrome is apparent as reflected by nephrotic-range proteinuria, impaired renal function in the face of high circulating HCV RNA. The principal renal manifestation of HCV infection is MPGN type I, usually in the context of cryoglobulinemia, although other causes of the nephrosis cannot be excluded in the absence of renal histology. Regardless of the form of nephritis, it is important to ascertain the presence of circulating cryoglobulins as there is therapeutic implications in which plasmapheresis may be applied to remove circulating cryoglobulins, thus preventing their deposition in glomeruli and blood vessel walls. In addition, there is also evidence of cirrhosis and portal hypertension leading to cytopenia. Therefore, although confirmation by kidney biopsy is desirable, the presence of thrombocytopenia renders this a high-risk procedure. This makes choice B the correct answer.

2. **The answer is B.** The presence of renal disease (proteinuria and kidney impairment), elevated liver enzyme, cryoglobulins type II, vasculitic skin lesions and histologic features of MPGN in a high-risk individual (intravenous drug addict) with positive anti-HCV all point to a diagnosis of cryoglobulinemic glomerulonephritis. The standard of care in the era of direct acting antiviral agents should include such effective viral eradication therapy. Recent data showed that these agents can be extended to patients with CKD. Checking HCV RNA is essential in monitoring treatment response in terms

of sustained viral remission (SVR). The KDIGO recommendation in 2012 of using pegylated interferon and ribavirin should understandably be updated to include the more effective DAA treatment. The experience with corticosteroid and anti-CD20 is more anecdotal. This makes choice B the correct answer.

3. **The answer is B.** This patient is a chronic hepatitis B carrier who recently developed proteinuria suggestive of an underlying glomerulonephritis. The causative role of hepatitis B is his renal pathology needs to be established. It is important to understand that antiviral therapy for HBV infection is expensive and often lifelong.

Chapter 37

1. **The answer is E.** Faster than usual progression in the setting of existing CKD should prompt evaluation of drug-induced tubulointerstitial nephritis, particularly in the setting of an offending medication. This patient, with CKD stage 2, had fairly stable eGFR until she started taking omeprazole. She also has white blood cells in her urine, which support a diagnosis of drug-induced tubulointerstitial nephritis. Thus, the possibility of a kidney biopsy should be considered in this patient.

   Follow-up in 1 year is not recommended in this patient who has lost 26 mL/min of eGFR in a year. Urine eosinophil is not accurate for ATIN diagnosis and is often misleading. The diabetes is fairly well controlled and change in diabetes care is not necessary. The patient has known nonproliferative diabetic retinopathy and follow-up with ophthalmology is not necessary at this time.

2. **The answer is B.** Multiple studies have demonstrated that degree of interstitial fibrosis on kidney biopsy is the best predictor of renal outcomes in patients with acute tubulointerstitial nephritis. Number of eosinophils in the interstitium, presence of extrarenal manifestations such as rash, or drug responsible for acute tubulointerstitial nephritis are not associated with long-term renal outcomes.

3. **The answer is B.** NSAID-induced tubulointerstitial nephritis is often associated with massive proteinuria and associated glomerular changes of minimal change disease or membranous nephropathy on the kidney biopsy. NSAID-induced tubulointerstitial nephritis typically does not have eosinophils on the interstitium and a biopsy is required for diagnosis.

4. **The answer is C.** Medications are responsible for over 70% of acute tubulointerstitial nephritis in the developed world. In the elderly, medications are responsible for an even greater proportion of cases since autoimmune diseases are uncommon in this age group. As the renal failure in acute tubulointerstitial

nephritis is slowly progressive, these patients often do not meet the KDIGO AKI definition (SCr rise by 50% in <7 days). The degree of interstitial fibrosis is the predictor of long-term outcomes in acute tubulointerstitial nephritis.

5. **The answer is D.** PPI-related tubulointerstitial nephritis generally does not present with allergic features of rash and eosinophilia. Multiple studies have demonstrated that healthy individuals taking PPI are at higher risk of acute tubulointerstitial nephritis and chronic kidney disease. This is usually a class effect and switching to another PPI is usually not recommended. The latent period from starting a PPI to diagnosis of acute tubulointerstitial nephritis is usually weeks to months. PPIs have also been associated with hypomagnesemia.

Chapter 38

1. **The answer is C.** The patient has laboratory findings consistent with CTIN, most likely from heavy metal exposure (lead) related to restoration of old homes. His creatinine is mildly elevated most likely indicating a long standing process with moderate fibrosis. His acidosis, glycosuria, hypophosphatemia, and proteinuria can all be explained by proximal tubular dysfunction. The disparity between the urinalysis and measured protein is most likely due to the fact that a urinalysis is only specific for albuminuria. With CTIN, patients may have more low molecular weight (nonalbumin) proteinuria that will only be picked up by direct quantification of total protein or with the sulfosalicylic acid reagent.

2. **The answer is D.** The patient will most likely have acute tubular necrosis from volume depletion in the setting of his diarrhea and emesis while concurrently taking NSAIDs and his lisinopril. The time frame is not consistent with interstitial nephritis. It is unlikely that the patient has an acute glomerular process, although evaluation of the sediment would be useful to see if there are any renal tubular epithelial cells, either isolated or in casts, granular casts, or dysmorphic red blood cells.

3. **The answer is B.** The patient most likely has calcium oxalate nephropathy. With a recent history of gastric bypass surgery, a slow rise in creatinine, and crystals in the urine consistent with the morphology of dehydrate calcium oxalate crystals, the patient most likely has a chronic tubulointerstitial injury from calcium oxalate. Although uric acid can be elevated in patients with hydrochlorothiazide, the morphology of the crystals in the sediment is more consistent with calcium oxalate. This presentation and the chronicity are not consistent with an obstructive process. Although NSAID use can predispose the patient to CTIN, oxalate nephropathy is more likely in this patient.

4. **The answer is C.** The patient is a good candidate for transplant; however, aristolochic acid nephropathy has a high prevalence of urothelial carcinomas. It is recommended that all patients undergoing transplant have a preemptive bilateral nephroureterectomy at the time of transplant consideration.

5. **The answer is A.** The patient has IgG4 related disease with kidney involvement. Given the rise in creatinine and other organ involvement, the patient should begin glucocorticoid therapy. Other regimens should be used in cases that are refractory to glucocorticoid therapy.

Chapter 39

1. **The answer is B.** There are some studies looking at exercise and kidney stones, but none of them strongly correlates in an increased risk of stones with exercise in women.

2. **The answer is B.** The stone has a low HU, so is likely to be uric acid. Medical dissolution therapy with potassium citrate is appropriate as he is nontoxic appearing and may be able to avoid surgery. A 9-mm stone is unlikely to pass even with tamsulosin.

3. **The answer is A.** This patient has both hypercalcemia and hypercalciuria. Only hyperparathyroidism would cause these two abnormalities. A distal RTA would be associated with hypocitraturia. Dent disease is primarily in men, and causes hypercalciuria but not hypercalcemia. A thiazide may cause hypercalcemia but not hypercalciuria. A loop diuretic would cause hypercalciuria but not hypercalcemia.

4. **The answer is D.** The patient likely had significant hypercalciuria due to uncontrolled hyperthyroidism from the multinodular goiter. Prolonged hypercalciuria may cause nephrocalcinosis. Although distal RTA, MSK and primary hyperparathyroidism are in the differential for nephrocalcinosis, they are unlikely as she has no history of kidney stones. Nephrocalcinosis may be associated with hereditary causes of kidney stones, but she has no stones.

5. **The answer is B.** The patient does not have hyperoxaluria so oxalate restriction is not appropriate. Low salt, high fluid intake, and high calcium intake are appropriate. High protein intake is not.

Chapter 40

1. **The answer is A.** Combinations of central α_2-agonists like clonidine and metoprolol make no pharmacologic sense for lowing BP and can lead to severe bradycardia. Moreover, the tartrate preparation of metoprolol should be given at least three if not four times a day and increasing the dose will increase side effects while not providing additive BP reduction. HCTZ is has a shorter

duration of action and is not as effective in lowering BP as chlorthalidone which is effective down to a GFR of 25 mL/min for BP reduction. Spironolactone is contraindicated due to hyperkalemia in advanced CKD. Amlodipine has been shown to have additive BP lowering effects with metoprolol as well as a thiazide-like diuretic.

2. **The answer is C.** Lifestyle is very important, such as weight gain and increased salt can easily raise BP to a higher level requiring intervention. Salt sensitivity is come with aging and more prevalent in obesity. The combination of the two conditions accentuates BP elevations periodically throughout the day. Exercise lowers BP and with significant weight loss maintains BP reduction. Many people blame stress for elevated BP, while stress can increase BP it is not responsible for the diagnosis of hypertension.

3. **The answer is C.** It is well known that people with long history of poor BP control have worse renal function than indicated by labs when BP is high. A 30% increase in serum creatinine is acceptable as long as BP is controlled and no hyperkalemia occurs. Stopping the olmesartan will deprive the patient of renoprotection as this is exactly the type of patient that will benefit from this treatment. There is NO evidence of volume depletion and so spironolactone should not be stopped. β-Blockers have not been shown to further slow progression of kidney disease independent of blood pressure reduction.

4. **The answer is D.** Increase BP variability is very common in people who get less than 6 hours of uninterrupted sleep a night consistently and is associated with increased stroke risk. Improving sleep will not only reduce heart and variability due to sympathetic over activity but will also reduce BP itself. Spironolactone may provide some help since it will reduce sympathetic tone but will not resolve the problem. Switching to a longer acting diuretic which will increase sympathetic tone if volume depletion occurs is also not the correct approach. Referring for a sleep study may be useful but this patient has no symptoms consistent with sleep apnea and clearly has poor sleep hygiene.

5. **The answer is C.** Many people do not realize how much salt is in food when eating out and even amount within 50% of what is recommended in older people can raise BP significantly until equilibrium is reached through natriuresis. While arguments certainly can raise BP during the argument in people without hypertension BP returns to normal within a short time following such events. Weight gain can certainly account for this problem but they state that clothes fit the same and no other evidence of significant weight gain. Support stocking which are very useful in cases of orthostatic hypotension can increase BP but she is not consistently wearing them. Anxiety can be a cause of BP variability and

elevated pressure but she has no significant evidence of this problem.

Chapter 41

1. **The answer is C.** This patient is a vasculopath with stage 4 chronic kidney disease and is at high risk for contrast nephropathy with IV contrast and nephrogenic systemic fibrosis form gadolinium so further imaging should be avoided if possible. There are multiple studies showing no definite benefit of percutaneous intervention as opposed to aggressive medical therapy with statin, RAAS blockade and aspirin. Only the lesion on the right would be considered significant and one would prefer not to intervene on this high risk patient. BP should improve with an addition of a diuretic.

2. **The answer is D.** This patient has radiologic features of fibromuscular dysplasia and should undergo renal angiogram and possible angioplasty of both renal arteries. There lesions usually do not require stenting as restenosis rate is very low. This is a potentially curable form of hypertension so adding additional medication is not the best long-term solution.

3. **The answer is D.** Patient has resistant hypertension and hypokalemia and most likely has primary aldosteronism and should be screened for this first. Other studies are reasonable if the renin/aldosterone levels are normal.

4. **The answer is C.** It is appropriate to refer for adrenal vein sampling before proceeding to surgery to ensure lateralization occurs on the side of the adenoma before proceeding with adrenalectomy.

5. **The answer is D.** Acute severe onset of hypertension in a young patient particularly in a stressful situation should prompt the physician to exclude an underlying pheochromocytoma. The best screening test is a plasma metanephrine level.

6. **The answer is C.** Approximately 40% of apparently spontaneous pheochromocytomas and paragangliomas are due to germline mutations and all patient should be referred for genetic testing. Plasma catecholamines would presumably be elevated but would not add anything to the diagnostic work up. MIBG and PET scanning would be appropriate if metastatic disease is suspected.

7. **The answer is D.** Studies have shown that both CPAP and weight loss reduce BP to a minor degree but the combination of both weight loss and CPAP has a more beneficial effect on reducing BP than either intervention alone.

8. **The answer is A.** There is a strong association between OSA and hypertension. OSA is present in about 40% of resistant hypertension patients. CPAP has not been effective in reducing BP in normotensive patients.

Chapter 42

HYPERTENSION IN AFRICAN–AMERICANS

1. **The answer is B.** African–Americans have a high risk of progression from chronic kidney disease (CKD) to end-stage renal disease (ESRD) and should be closely observed for such progression. The lower GFR (32 mL/min) is at the level where thiazide diuretics loss their efficacy. Adding a calcium channel blocker would lower blood pressure and may be necessary if changing thiazide diuretic to a loop diuretic does not work. Dual therapy with an ACEI and angiotensin receptor blocker has not been shown to be effective in patients with chronic kidney disease and may be harmful. BiDil or isosorbide dinitrate and hydralazine hydrochloride has been shown to be effective in improving outcomes in African–Americans with heart failure. While this patient has a history of heart failure her echo is presently normal. Bidil is worth considering but at this time the primary issue is blood pressure control which most likely necessitates changing thiazide diuretic to a loop diuretic.

2. **The answer is B.** Inquiry to discern dietary habits can be helpful especially to assess sodium intake. An understanding of her insurance coverage and related issues such as medication copayment if she does have insurance can help to better assess her ability to access prescribed medications. This is especially important for low income and minority patients who are more likely to be uninsured or underinsured.

   Providing a quality hypertension brochure is least likely to have an impact on blood pressure control

3. **The answer is B.** Initiating drug therapy at this point is an option but many clinicians would prefer to see the response to lifestyle modifications and results of a metabolic profile and lipid panel before initiating treatment. With or without drug therapy lifestyle modifications should strongly be urged, especially smoking cessation, alcohol reduction, weight loss, use of the dietary approaches to stop hypertension (DASH) diet, and sodium restriction.

   These could lower his systolic blood pressure by as much as 10–15 mm Hg.

   If drug therapy were initiated it should be remembered that African–Americans generally have a more substantial reduction in blood pressure with thiazide diuretic treatment than an ACEI. Given no overt coexisting cardiovascular disease, pending results of the metabolic profile thiazide diuretic treatment would be the recommended initial drug therapy.

4. **The answer is D.** The patient's combination of stage 1 hypertension, T2DM, and dyslipidemia suggests that the best clinical practice would be to address these three issues at the same time. Although a thiazide diuretic would be an appropriate first-line drug therapy for hypertension if his case was not complicated, the presence of T2DM suggests that a renin-angiotensin-aldosterone system (RAAS) blocker such as an ACEI is a better choice.

5. **The answer is A.** The patient's FPG and A1C levels indicate that his T2DM is well controlled with metformin despite poor adherence, and the lipid profile while not ideal is improved.

   However, his blood pressure is still elevated. For many patients with T2DM and hypertension, a second drug is often needed to attain therapeutic goals.

   In this case, the addition of a diuretic to the ACEI and reinforcing adherence to both medications and lifestyle are critical.

   The ACE inhibitor/diuretic combination works very well in most patients. The ACEI/CCB combination lowers blood pressure through two completely different mechanisms—the ACEI addresses the RAAS while the CCB reduces the contractility of vascular smooth muscle, reducing total peripheral resistance—and is a good second choice if the addition of a diuretic causes any bothersome side effects or if more potent antihypertensive lowering is needed. The ACE inhibitor/β-blocker combination is somewhat less favored, since both agents address the RAAS to some degree.

HYPERTENSION IN THE ELDERLY

1. **The answer is D.** With aging, there is a progressive loss of elasticity within the larger central vessels leading to more resistance during systole but less residual volume during diastole on account of accelerated run off of blood into the peripheral vasculature. Thus, the signature profile of hypertension in the elderly is a heightened systolic pressures accompanied by low diastolic readings.

   The resultant widening of pulse pressure (difference between systolic and diastolic blood pressure) is predictive of cardiovascular events and also renders lowering systolic pressure without causing frank diastolic hypotension challenging.

2. **The answer is A.** Effective blood pressure control results in lower rates of stroke, heart failure, all-cause mortality, end-stage renal disease, and myocardial infarction to name but a few benefits. However, the therapeutic effects of antihypertensive on dementia have yet to be conclusively demonstrated.

   While the relative benefit of treating blood pressure is identical among all age groups, age is a leading risk factor for a variety of cardiovascular events. As such, the number needed to prevent one event is often several fold lower among older patient populations.

3. **The answer is A.** The first large scale randomized trial involving diuretics dates back to the Veteran Affairs Cooperative Studies in the late 1960s. The subsequent Hypertension Detection and Follow Up Program in 1979 confirmed the cardiovascular benefit of antihypertensive therapies. Additional historical studies of import include ANBP1 (1980) and MRFIT (1982). Calcium channel blockers have shown their value not only in Syst-Eur (1997) and Syst-China (1998) but also STOP2 (1999) and ALLHAT (2002). Agents that block the RAAS system have been used for secondary prevention or for a disease specific indication since the 1990s but the original randomized trial confirming their value for primary prevention was CAPPP (1999).

PROGRESS (2001) evaluated the salutary of diuretics and angioconverting enzyme inhibitors in the secondary prevention of stroke. ONTARGET (2008) found that dual RAAS blockade failed to prevent more cardiovascular events among a high risk population with either vascular disease or diabetes. CAMELOT (2004) found that both calcium channel blockers and ACEi had a modest beneficial effect on cardiac outcomes among those with preexisting coronary artery disease and prehypertension.

4. **The answer is A.** Based on the results of the SHEP and HYVET trials where inclusion criteria and goal blood pressures were higher than those targeted among studies including younger participants, JNC 8 recommends a goal blood pressure of less than or equal to 150/90 mm Hg. However, diastolic blood pressure has never been an endpoint given that it declines with aging even without the use of antihypertensives. Consistent with trials not specifying diastolic targets, the European statement focuses on systolic pressures with nearly comparable targets. A lower limit of 140 mm Hg may have been selected given that the aforementioned trials accomplished achieved blood pressures in this range.

5. **The answer is B.** Effective treatment of hypertension in this age group presents its own set of challenges. While this population is likely to be the most adherent to medications, high fall rates, particularly upon therapy initiation, often mitigate long-term benefits of therapy. While blood pressure goals are often achieved, those with poor functional status (frail individuals) do not seem to realize similar gains in life expectancy and reductions in cardiac and cerebrovascular events. Finally, given that hypertension is exclusively limited to systolic elevations, reductions in systolic pressure also lower diastolics to levels that may paradoxically increase mortality, the so called "J curve."

HYPERTENSION IN PREGNANCY

1. **The answer is A.** The CHIPS study showed that treating women with hypertension in pregnancy to a diastolic blood pressure target of 85 mm Hg versus 100 mm Hg had no significant effect on maternal and fetal outcomes. However, the less tight control group had a higher frequency of severe maternal hypertension, and a trend toward a higher incidence of transaminases and thrombocytopenia. This woman's BP of 128/85 mm Hg is acceptable, and would not warrant intensification of her antihypertensive regimen. Dietary sodium restriction has not been shown to decrease diastolic blood pressure, hospitalizations for hypertension or adverse obstetric outcomes; therefore, option B is incorrect. Diuretics are generally not recommended as first line agents for the treatment of chronic hypertension in pregnancy because they attenuate the normal physiologic expansion of the extracellular fluid volume that accompanies normal pregnancy, thereby potentially compromising placental blood flow. A meta-analysis of nine randomized trials of diuretic use showed a decreased incidence of edema and hypertension, but not of preeclampsia. A higher frequency of nausea and vomiting were reported with diuretic use, leading to discontinuation of therapy. Lower extremity edema may be a normal, physiologic finding in pregnancy. Thus, option C, addition of hydrochlorothiazide for more stringent control of BP or management of a small amount of edema is not recommended. Stopping nifedipine would likely result in a rise in her blood pressure above the diastolic target of 85, potentially increasing her risk of adverse maternal outcomes, therefore option D is incorrect. Hence, option A is correct.

2. **The answer is C.** In the majority of women with preeclampsia, hypertension resolves over the first postpartum month. Although evidence is lacking with respect to specific targets, most women require antihypertensive therapy in the early postpartum period. Hence, option A is incorrect. The continuation of IV magnesium in the immediate postpartum period is appropriate in a young woman with ongoing neurological symptoms due to the continued risk of seizures postpartum, making A and B incorrect. Her blood pressure is no longer severe and therefore intravenous treatment could be transitioned to oral agents, therefore C is correct. Women with preeclampsia are often intravascularly depleted, therefore furosemide may cause further renal injury and is an inappropriate choice in the absence pulmonary edema, making option D incorrect.

3. **The answer is D.** Numerous trials of calcium supplementation have shown a nonsignificant difference between the incidence of preeclampsia or high blood pressure measurements for women on a Western diet. The most recent analysis from the Cochrane Review by Hofmeyr and coworkers showed that calcium supplementation (>1 gm/day) appears to reduce the risk of severe hypertensive disorders, especially in the subgroup with low calcium intake. However, these results, as the authors

stated, may be overestimated given small study effects or publication bias. Hence, it is recommended that for a woman with a well-balanced, Western diet as in the present scenario, calcium carbonate supplemetation is unlikely to be of signficant benefit; therefore, option A is not the best answer. Several well-conducted randomized placebo controlled trials of supplemental vitamins C and E demonstrated no impact on the rate of preeclampsia. Furthermore, Poston and coworkers showed an increased number of low birth weight babies in the group receiving supplemental vitamins C and E. Therefore, the antioxidant vitamins C and E are not recommended for the prevention of preeclampsia, and option B is incorrect. Weight loss during pregnancy is not recommended, even in obese individuals; option C is incorrect.

This woman is at increased risk for preeclampsia and treatment with aspirin is the most apporpriate management strategy; option D is the best answer. A meta-analysis from the Paris Collaborative Group of more than 32,000 women from 31 randomized trials found that the relative risk (RR) for developing preeclampsia was 0.90 (95% confidence interval [CI], 0.84–0.97). A later meta analysis by Bujold and colleagues showed that aspirin significantly reduced the incidence of preeclampsia and intra-uterine growth restriction (IUGR) when administered prior to 16 weeks of gestation (RR 0.47, 95% CI, 0.34–0.65) and (RR 0.44, 95% CI, 0.30–0.65), respectively. The number needed to treat is large in low-risk women. Therefore, aspirin is only recommended for the prevention of preeclampsia in high risk women such as this patient.

4. **The answer is B.** There is increasing evidence of increased adverse cardiovascular outcomes in women with a history of preeclampsia; option B is correct, and option A is incorrect. Bellamy and coworkers found an increased relative risk of ischemic heart disease and stroke at 2.16 (95% CI, 1.86–2.52) after 11.7 years, and 1.81 (95% CI, 1.45–2.27) after 10.4 years, respectively. Other studies have also shown the risk is intensified in women with preterm delivery and fetal growth restriction. Preeclampsia also increases the risk of hypertension, cerebral vascular disease, peripheral vascular disease, and end-stage renal disease. The relative risk of developing end-stage renal disease was shown to be 4.7 (95% CI, 3.6–6.1) in a Norwegian Registry database. However, the absolute incidence of ESRD was only 0.32% at a mean of 17 years after preeclampsia; option D is incorrect. Most studies have found no increased risk of cancer following preeclampsia.

5. **The answer is A.** According to the American College of Obstetrics and Gynecology, preeclampsia can be diagnosed in the absence of proteinuria if other severe features are present. This patient meets criteria for preeclampsia based on the new onset of hypertension after 20 weeks' gestation, and the presence of cerebral/visual symptoms; option A is correct. Other severe features which are diagnostic of preeclampsia in a woman with new-onset hypertension without proteinuria include thrombocytopenia, pulmonary edema, impaired liver function, or elevated serum creatinine. Gestational hypertension is present when hypertension only develops after 20 weeks of gestation in the absence of other features of preeclampsia so option B s incorrect. The visual and cerebral symptoms of preeclampsia can resemble those of migraine or central venous thrombosis; however, these entities would not be associated with new onset hypertension, making option D incorrect.

Chapter 43

1. **The answer is A.** Resistant hypertension is defined as high blood pressure that remains uncontrolled (>140/90 mm Hg) despite the use of effective doses of three or more different classes of antihypertensive agents, including a diuretic. Refractory hypertension has been used to refer to an extreme phenotype of antihypertensive treatment failure, considering increased blood pressure levels (>140/90 mm Hg) despite the use of optimal doses of five or more different classes of antihypertensive agents, including chlorthalidone and a mineralocorticoid receptor antagonist.

2. **The answer is E.** Drug-induced resistant hypertension is related with many pharmacologic classes, including non-steroidal anti-inflammatory drugs, oral contraceptives, anticancer agents, sympathicomimetic agents, corticosteroids, cocaine, cyclosporine, erythropoietin, etc. The acetaminophen effects on BP is unclear.

Noncompliance, isolated office hypertension, excessive sodium intake, sleep apnea are well-known causes of resistant hypertension.

3. **The answer is C.** The white-coat effect is seen to a greater or lesser degree in most if not all hypertensive patients. Growing evidence now points to greater prognostic significance in determining risk for hypertensive end-organ damage compared with office BP measurements. Ambulatory measurement of BP using automated devices has demonstrated the benefit in treatment resistance and borderline hypertension.

4. **The answer is B.** ASPIRANT trial showed that the addition of spironolactone in patients with resistant arterial hypertension using a mean of 4.5 antihypertensive drugs, led to a significant decrease of systolic BP both in the office and on ABPM after 8 weeks of treatment. More recently, the PATHWAY-2 trial shows that spironolactone is the most effective add-on drug for the treatment of resistant hypertension. In this double-blind, placebo-controlled, crossover trial, a total of 335 patients were included. Patients rotated,

in a preassigned, randomized order, through 12 weeks of once daily treatment with each of spironolactone (25–50 mg), bisoprolol (5–10 mg), doxazosin modified release (4–8 mg), and placebo, in addition to their baseline blood pressure drugs.

5. **The answer is C.** Simplicity HTN-3 is the largest clinical trial examining the efficacy and safety of catheter-based renal denervation to date, and was the first trial to include a sham procedure as a control group. A total of 535 participants with severe resistant HTN were randomized to undergo renal denervation or sham procedure. Although the mean SBP at 6 months was significantly lower than the baseline in both denervation and control groups (by 14.1 versus 11.7 mm Hg, respectively), the between-group difference of 2.4 mm Hg favoring denervation was not statistically significant. Similar findings were noted for the change in mean 24-hour ambulatory SBP. The real-world experience with renal denervation in patients who undergo the procedure using the Simplicity Renal Denervation System outside of clinical trials has been analyzed in the Global Simplicity Registry. Among the first 1000 consecutive patients enrolled in the registry, 1-year office SBP and 24-hour SBP reductions were similar to what was observed in the intervention arm of Simplicity HTN-3 (by 13.0 and 8.3 mm Hg, respectively). Other invasive therapies as baroreflex activation therapy offer exciting possibilities of future options, though at this time they continue to be investigational. A number of important questions still need to be addressed in order to establish an evidence base for RDN that would permits its adoption for routine clinical use. It is urgent to delineate predictors of BP response following RDN.

Chapter 44

1. **The answer is D.** The patient described has no ongoing acute target organ damage, so this **cannot** be a hypertensive emergency. Some physicians would diagnose this man with a hypertensive urgency, but several recent papers suggest that intensive or even acute drug treatment in such a situation has not improved outcomes (Patel et al, 2016; Levy et al, 2015). Others would argue that "a hypertensive urgency" is not an evidence-based diagnosis, and should be stricken from the ICD-10 codes (Heath I: Hypertensive urgency—is this a useful diagnosis [editorial]. *JAMA Intern Med.* 2016;176:988–989). The most important thing for this patient is to replenish the medications he has exhausted, and connect him with an ongoing source of primary care. Crushed tablets of, or sublingual, captopril have both been studied in this setting, despite variable oral absorption rates, variable acute effects on blood pressure (with some hypotension reported); this treatment

modality is more commonly used in Brazil than in the United States (Souza LM, et al. Oral drugs for hypertensive urgencies: systematic review and meta-analysis. *Sao Paulo Med J.* 2009;127;366–372). Nifedipine capsules have also been studied after being given sublingually or orally; sublingual absorption is minimal, whereas puncturing the capsules and delivering the medication orally can cause rapid hypotension, stroke, myocardial infarction, and death. The FDA declined to approve nifedipine capsules for acute treatment of hypertension because of this (Winker MA. The FDA's decisions regarding new indications for approved drugs: where's the evidence? *JAMA.* 1996:276:1342–1343). "Clonidine loading" was a popular treatment option in the 1980s and 1990s, and was studied prospectively by Kathleen Zeller and colleagues (Zeller KR, von Kuhnert L, Matthews C. Rapid reduction of severe asymptomatic hypertension. A prospective, controlled trial. *Arch Intern Med.* 1989;149:2186–2189), who showed no significant outcomes benefit of this regimen compared to either a single dose of oral clonidine, or a refilled prescription for the patient's chronic medications. The "clonidine loading" regimen does cause quite a lot of sedation, and usually the patient is unable to drive home after it. Sodium nitroprusside is perhaps the most versatile of the intravenous hypotensive agents commonly used for hypertensive emergencies, but can cause thiocyanate and cyanide toxicity if used at high dose or for long durations (Padilla Ramos A, Varon J. Current and newer agents for hypertensive emergencies. *Curr Hypertens Rep.* 2014;14:450).

2. **The answer is C.** Because of the very high blood pressures and bilateral papilledema, this patient likely has hypertensive encephalopathy, although this is a diagnosis of exclusion. Although one might argue that a computed tomographic scan of the head would be quite appropriate, this procedure will **delay** careful and therapeutic lowering of blood pressure. In most such cases without an identifiable focal neurological deficit, an attempt to judiciously lower blood pressure is warranted **before** the CT is done. In many such cases, the patient's mental status will improve rather quickly, after only approximately 10% reduction in mean arterial pressure, which makes the diagnosis. Lumbar puncture is **contraindicated**, because of the presence of papilledema and the risk of uncal herniation with the elevated intracranial pressure. A clonidine transdermal patch might eventually be helpful (particularly if the patient is acutely "rebounding" after sudden discontinuation of this medication), but the delivery of clonidine will be far slower than either of the two intravenously delivered options. The presence of abnormal renal function (but not the hematuria) helps make the appropriate choice between nitroprusside (somewhat less preferred,

because it often worsens kidney function acutely during treatment of hypertensive emergencies, and risks cyanide and thiocyanate toxicity) and fenoldopam mesylate (which would usually be preferred because it acutely improves renal function during treatment of hypertensive crises, and has no toxic metabolites that are renally cleared; see Shusterman NH, Elliott WJ, White WB. Fenoldopam, but not nitroprusside, improves renal function in severely hypertensive patients with impaired renal function. *Am J Med.* 1993;95:151–158).

3. **The answer is D.** According to the history, physical examination, and computed tomographic scan results, this patient appears to have an acute ischemic stroke, and would be a candidate for thrombolytic therapy, except that his blood pressure is too high (>185/110 mm Hg, according to the NINDS rtPA Stroke Study inclusion criteria, and current US stroke treatment guidelines; see: Jauch EC, et al. Guidelines for the early management of patients with acute ischemic stroke: a guideline for healthcare professionals from the American Heart Association/American Stroke Association. *Stroke.* 2013;44:870–947). If tPA were given in this setting, the patient's risk of intracranial hemorrhage would greatly increase, so efforts are traditionally focused instead to lower (and control) blood pressure so that brain-saving tPA can be administered. Although many stroke neurologists initiate this near-term therapeutic endeavor with labetalol, this agent is contraindicated in asthmatics, and does not always lower blood pressure to target in supine patients. Conversely, sodium nitroprusside is nearly uniformly effective, can be titrated rapidly to therapeutic effect, and can be discontinued without fear of rebound. The dose suggested (0.3 µg/kg/min) is a little higher than the usual preferred initial dose (of 0.1 µg/kg/min), but the primary objective is to get the blood pressure into a range that would enhance the safety of tPA (ie, <180/108 mm Hg) as quickly as possible. Nitroprusside usually takes only minutes to titrate, so downtitration is also easily and quickly accomplished. Aspirin has no useful role in acute ischemic stroke, although it significantly prevents a recurrent ischemic stroke (see Kernan WN, et al. Guidelines for the prevention of stroke in patients with stroke and transient ischemic attack. A guideline for healthcare professionals from the American Heart Association/American Stroke Association. *Stroke.* 2014;45:2160–236). Nimodipine is FDA-approved for subarachnoid hemorrhage, but was ineffective in improving outcomes after acute ischemic stroke. Enoxaparin may be useful to prevent or treat deep venous thrombosis in bedridden patients, but heparin products, in general, have shown no outcomes benefits in acute ischemic stroke, and therefore are generally not recommended for such patients.

4. **The answer is A.** The most likely diagnosis for this man is acute aortic dissection, as suggested by the description of the chest discomfort, radiation to the back, diminished pulses in the lower extremities, and widened anterior mediastinum on the chest X-ray. Because propagation of the dissection and continued ripping of the intima from the supporting structures of the aorta depends primarily on the shear stress generated by each systole, the traditional initial therapy for such patients is directed toward lowering the blood pressure to <120 mm Hg systolic, and reducing $\delta P/\delta t$, by giving a β-blocker. In today's world, clevidipine and esmolol are often begun **before** an imaging study, done to define the location and extent of the intimal tear, in order to minimize the risk of propagation. The systolic blood pressure target of <120 mm Hg (to be achieved in <20 minutes!) is based on extensive clinical experience and expert opinion, rather than randomized clinical trials (see Hiratzka LF, et al. 2010 ACCF/AHA/AATS/ACR/ASA/SCA/ SCAI/SIR/STS/SVM guidelines for the diagnosis and management of patients with thoracic aortic disease: a report of the American College of Cardiology Foundation/American Heart Association Task Force on Practice Guidelines, American Association for Thoracic Surgery, American College of Radiology, American Stroke Association, Society of Cardiovascular Anesthesiologists, Society for Cardiovascular Angiography and Interventions, Society of Interventional Radiology, Society of Thoracic Surgeons, and Society for Vascular Medicine. *Circulation.* 2010;121:e266–e369, and Tsai TT, et al. Clinical characteristics of hypotension in patients with acute aortic dissection. *Am J Cardiol.* 2005;95:48–52).

5. **The answer is D.** The most likely diagnosis for this man is pheochromocytoma, based on episodes of headache, diaphoresis and hypertension (which were present in 95% of patients with diagnosed pheochromocytoma in one large French series). The presence of the subungual fibroma and the ash-leaf patches (sometimes "shagreen patches") suggests that the patient also has tuberous sclerosis complex ("Pringle disease, de Bourneville disease"), which is one of the phakomatoses associated with pheochromocytoma. The fact that he was given atenolol for presumed generalized anxiety disorder probably explains why his blood pressure soared to even higher levels than before, since norepinephrine secreted by the tumor now has many of its β-adrenergic effects blunted, whereas its α-adrenergic vasoconstrictor effects remain unblocked. The usual and customary initial antihypertensive therapy for patients with a pheochromocytoma crisis is intravenous phentolamine, which is often transitioned to oral phenoxybenzamine before surgery is attempted. Dantrolene sodium is the most appropriate therapy for a patient having a malignant hyperthermia

APPENDIX A

mia: a review. *Orphanet J Rare Dis.* 2015;10:93 and
Litman RS, Rosenberg H. Malignant hyperthermia:
update on susceptibility testing. *JAMA.* 2005;293:
2918–2924), and is not known to have any therapeutic
efficacy for pheochromocytoma crisis. Doxazosin has
been successfully given to patients with pheochromocytoma crisis (most commonly in the Philippines), but
several cases of failure to control blood pressure and
other symptoms have been reported. Esmolol is unlikely
to be helpful here, both because the patient is already
taking atenolol, and because it will likely exacerbate the
hypertension, as it will block β-adrenergic receptors
and leave α-adrenergic receptors alone (see Aronoff SL,
et al. Norepinephrine and epinephrine secretion from
a clinically epinephrine-secreting pheochromocytoma.
Am J Med. 1980;69:321–324). Similarly, phenylephrine
will raise blood pressure due to its α-adrenergic
vasoconstrictor effects.

Chapter 45

1. **The answer is D.** The abdominal MRI shows bilateral
and diffuse distribution with marked replacement of
kidney tissue by cysts. This image is most consistent
with the typical presentation of a 48-year-old female
patient with a mutation in the *PKD1* gene (answer D).
Most commonly, adolescents with biallelic mutations
in *PKHD1* gene (answer A) present with small cysts,
and the most common liver manifestation is congenital hepatic fibrosis. Patients with *PKD1* hypomorphic
mutations (answer B) or *PKD2* mutations (answer C)
usually present with mild-moderate disease. Although
patients with *Sec63* mutations (answer E) may present
with a few renal cysts, mutations in this gene cause
autosomal dominant polycystic liver disease.

2. **The answer is C.** The presence of diffuse replacement
of the pulmonary parenchyma with thin-walled cysts
of varying sizes is highly suggestive of lymphangioleiomyomatosis (LAM). LAM is a rare, progressive, cystic
lung disease that occurs almost exclusively in females,
usually between menarche and menopause. Together
with the presence of bilateral angiomyolipomas on
the abdominal CT and accompanied by cutaneous
hypomelanotic macules is compatible with a diagnosis of Tuberous sclerosis complex (TSC) (answer C).
Autosomal dominant PKD, autosomal recessive PKD,
multiple simple cysts and von Hippel–Lindau disease
(answers A, B, D, and E) should be considered in the
differential diagnosis of TSC.

3. **The answer is C.** Pain is one of the most frequent
symptoms afflicting patients with ADPKD. The most
common causes of acute pain are renal hemorrhage,
nephrolithiasis, or urinary tract infections. RCC is a

rare cause of pain in ADPKD, and does not occur more
frequently than in the general population. However, in
ADPKD patients, RCC may present at an earlier age
with frequent constitutional symptoms and a higher
proportion of sarcomatoid, bilateral, multicentric, and
metastatic tumors. This 55-old-year patient presents
with flank pain that is accompanied by profound weight
loss and night sweats. Conservative therapy such as bed
resting, analgesics, and adequate fluid intake (answer A)
is usually the first measure in pain management. Pain
clinic interventions such as splanchnic nerve blockade
(answer B) with local anesthesia or steroids may be
helpful in the management of pain. However, exclusion
of causes that may require intervention such as RCC
should be done first (answer C). Narcotic analgesics
(answer D) should be reserved for acute episodes. Reassurance, dietary and lifestyle changes (answer E) may
aid in the long-term management of pain, but in this
context, RCC should be discarded prior to referral to a
dietitian.

4. **The answer is B.** The Consortium of Radiologic Imaging Studies of PKD (CRISP) has demonstrated that
kidney and cyst volumes increase in most patients, and
that larger kidneys are associated with a faster decline
in renal function. Volumetric analyses of polycystic
kidneys from CT or MR images, particularly when used
together with age, can be used as prognostic biomarker
in ADPKD. Although high urine sodium excretion
(answer A), development of hypertension at young age
(answer C), high urinary protein levels (answer D), and
low serum high-density lipoprotein (answer E) have
been associated with faster decline in kidney function, TKV remain the best predictor of age at ESRD
(answer B).

5. **The answer is D.** A new terminology—autosomal
dominant tubulointerstitial kidney disease (ADTKD)—
has been recently proposed for a group of diseases
caused by at least four genes: *MUC1* encoding the
mucoprotein mucin-1, *UMOD* encoding uromodulin,
HNF-1β encoding hepatocyte nuclear factor-1β, and
REN encoding renin. ADTKD-*HNF-1β* is inherited
in an autosomal dominant fashion; however, between
30% and 50% of the patients present *de novo* mutations. Patients with heterozygous mutations of *HNF-1β*
present usually with renal and extrarenal phenotypes.
The renal abnormalities include unilateral or bilateral
agenesis or hypoplasia, multicystic dysplasia, abnormal
calyces and papillae, and renal cysts. The extrarenal
abnormalities include maturity-onset diabetes of the
young type 5 (MODY5), exocrine pancreatic failure,
fluctuating liver test abnormalities, and genital tract
abnormalities. The patient in Question 5 presents
with DM, genital tract abnormalities, renal cysts and
normal uric acid levels; most likely due to a mutation

in *HNF-1β* gene (answer D). *HNF-1β* has been found to regulate the transcription of many genes including *PKHD1*, *PKD2*, and *UMOD*. However, Autosomal Recessive PKD (answer B) is a distant diagnosis in this case. Although patients with a *PKD2* mutation (answer A) may present with mild disease (few bilateral cysts) at a young age, ADPKD characterizes by progressive increase in the number of cysts and kidney size with age. ADTKD-*UMOD* (or MCKD type 2) (answer C), is frequently but not always associated with hyperuricemia and gout at an early age. ADTKD-*REN* (answer E) should be considered in patients with a history of anemia in childhood, mild hypotension, and mildly elevated serum uric acid and potassium concentrations.

Disease	Inheritance	Gene	Associated Findings	
Multiple simple cysts	Acquired	N/A	Simple cysts are rare in children but the incidence increases with age and are relatively common in the general population. Multiple bilateral simple renal cysts may be difficult to differentiate from a hereditary form. In this case, the distribution of renal cysts, presence or absence of family history, renal enlargement, and associated liver disease may aid in the diagnosis.	
Acquired cystic renal disease	Acquired	N/A	Acquired cystic renal disease is seen in patients with advanced CKD, usually on dialysis. Typically small cystic lesions are seen in small atrophic kidneys and are associated with increased risk for RCC.	
ADPKD	Dominant	*PKD1*	~85% of cases of ADPKD; more aggressive disease. Average onset of ESRD 54.3 y.o.	Bilateral macrocysts (from all parts of the nephron), liver cysts, intracranial aneurysms, cardiac valve abnormalities, abdominal wall hernias.
		PKD2	~15% of cases of ADPKD; milder disease with fewer cysts. Average onset of ERSD 74 y.o.	
ARPKD	Recessive	*PKHD1*	More frequently in newborns/young children. Bilateral microcysts (fusiform dilations of the collecting tubules); bile duct proliferation and ectasia with congenital hepatic fibrosis (CHF).	
TSC	Dominant	*TSC1, TSC2*	Renal angiomyolipomas, facial angiofibromas, nontraumatic ungual or periungual fibromas, hypomelanotic macules, shagreen patch, retinal nodular hamartomas, cortical tubers, subependymal giant cell astrocytoma, cardiac rhabdomyoma, multiple renal cysts, "confetti" skin lesions.	
VHL	Dominant	*VHL*	Hemangioblastomas of the brain, spinal cord, and retina; renal cysts and renal cell carcinoma; pheochromocytoma; and endolymphatic sac tumors.	
OFDS	X-linked Dominant	*OFD1*	Malformations of the face, oral cavity, and digits; CNS abnormalities; renal cysts, glomerulocystic kidney.	
ADTKD	Dominant	*UMOD*	Kidneys usually of small to normal size with cysts at the corticomedullary junction, irregular thickening of the tubular basement membrane, and marked tubular atrophy and interstitial fibrosis	Frequently but not always associated with hyperuricemia and gout at an early age.
		MUC-1		Hyperuricemia and gout usually at advanced stages of the disease
		HNF-1β		May present with extrarenal features including maturity-onset diabetes of the young type 5 (MODY5), exocrine pancreatic failure, hypomagnesemia, fluctuating liver test abnormalities, and genital tract abnormalities.
		REN		History of anemia in childhood, mild hypotension and mildly elevated serum potassium and uric acid concentrations.
NPHP	Recessive	*NPHP2*	ESRD 1–3 y.o., Tubulointerstitial nephritis with cortical microcysts; Senior–Løken syndrome (retinitis pigmentosa), situs inversus and ventricular septal defect, hypertension, hepatic fibrosis.	
	Recessive	*NPHP1, 3-18*	ESRD 5–25 y.o. First symptoms: Polyuria and polydipsia; Late symptoms: Related to the progressive renal insufficiency (nausea, anorexia, weakness). Small cysts in the medulla; Senior–Løken syndrome.	

(Continued)

Disease	Inheritance	Gene	Associated Findings
JBTS	Recessive	JBTS1-JBTS21	Hypo/dysplasia of the cerebellar vermis "molar tooth sign," developmental delay, retinal dystrophy, nephronophthisis, hepatic fibrosis, and polydactyly.
MKS	Recessive	MKS1, MKS3-11	Renal cystic dysplasia, central nervous system defects (typically occipital encephalocele), polydactyly and biliary dysgenesis.
BBS	Recessive	BBS1-BBS19	Obesity, polydactyly, pigmentary retinopathy, learning disabilities, various degrees of cognitive impairment, hypogonadism, renal cystic dysplasia.
MSK	Unclear		Kidneys are usually normal in size or slightly enlarged. Few to multiple bilateral renal cysts with predominantly medullary distribution. Medullary nephrocalcinosis; kidney stones; "brush" or linear striations on intravenous pyelogram.

Abbreviations: ADPKD, autosomal dominant polycystic kidney disease; ADTKD, autosomal dominant tubulointerstitial kidney disease; ARPKD, autosomal recessive polycystic kidney disease; BBS, Bardet–Biedl syndrome; *BBS1-BBS19*, Bardet–Biedl syndrome 1–19 genes; CKD, chronic kidney disease; *HNF-1β*, hepatocyte nuclear factor-1β gene; JBTS, Joubert syndrome; *JBTS1-JBTS21*, Joubert syndrome 1–21 genes; *MKS1*, Meckel syndrome 1 gene; *MKS3-11*, Meckel syndrome 3–11 genes; MSK, Meckel Syndrome; MSK, medullary sponge kidney; *MUC-1*, mucoprotein mucin-1 gene; NPHP, nephronophthisis; *NPHP1-18*, nephronophthisis 1–18 genes; *OFD1*, orofacial digital 1 gene; OFDS, oral-facial-digital syndrome; *PKD1*, polycystic kidney disease 1 gene; *PKD2*, polycystic kidney disease 2 gene; *PKHD1*, polycystic kidney and hepatic disease 1 gene; RCC, renal cell carcinoma; *REN*, renin gene; TSC, tuberous sclerosis complex; *TSC1*, tuberous sclerosis complex 1 gene; *TSC2*, tuberous sclerosis complex 2 gene; *UMOD*, uromodulin gene; *VHL*, von Hippel–Lindau tumor suppressor gene.

Chapter 46

1. **The answer is C.** First, pedigree information provided by families is not always accurate. Second, the mother may have a spontaneous rather than inherited mutation. Last, the child may have autosomal recessive Alport syndrome, in which case a family history of ESRD would typically be negative. The pedigree is consistent with any of the three genetic forms of Alport syndrome: X-linked, autosomal recessive or autosomal dominant. The information provided by this pedigree however, is insufficient for establishing a diagnosis or inheritance pattern.

   About 50% of people who are heterozygous for a mutation in the *COL4A3* or *COL4A4* gene are asymptomatic.

2. **The answer is D.** In boys with X-linked Alport syndrome and in boys and girls with autosomal recessive Alport syndrome, sensorineural deafness typically becomes detectable by audiogram after the age of 5–6 years. A 3-year-old boy with Alport syndrome is likely to have a normal audiogram.

   The kidney biopsy of the mother may show mixed thinning and lamellation of glomerular basement membranes (GBM), thinning of GBM only or no pathological changes; whereas the kidney biopsy of a 3-year-old boy with Alport syndrome is likely to show GBM thinning. Distinguishing between Alport syndrome and other causes of GBM thinning may be possible if immunostaining of the biopsy specimen for collagen IV chains is available.

Next generation sequencing of the *COL4A3*, *COL4A4*, and *COL4A5* genes is the test most likely to establish a diagnosis of Alport syndrome and identify the inheritance pattern in this family.

3. **The answer is A.** In males with X-linked Alport syndrome *COL4A5* genotype has a strong influence on age at ESRD. Early treatment with angiotensin converting enzyme inhibition or angiotensin receptor blockade has been demonstrated to delay the progression to ESRD in males and females with X-linked Alport syndrome. In males with X-linked Alport syndrome who receive no treatment, the risk of ESRD is 50% by age 25.

   Women who are heterozygous for X-linked Alport syndrome have a 20–30% risk of ESRD by age 60.

4. **The answer is C.** The major collagenous network in mature glomerular basement membranes is the α3α4α5(IV) network. The α1α1α2(IV) network is a minor component of mature glomerular basement membranes, except in the kidneys of patients with Alport syndrome. The α5α5α6(IV) network is not found in human glomerular basement membranes. There is no evidence for the existence of a α1α2α3(IV) network.

5. **The answer is E.** Each of these ocular abnormalities may be found in patients with Alport syndrome, with anterior lenticonus and perimacular retinal flecks having the greatest diagnostic specificity.

Chapter 47

1. **The answer is B.** Only answer Fabry disease accounts for the acroparesthesias (pain in the hands and feet) and

urinalysis findings, as the other diseases would have had marked proteinuria.

2. **The answer is B.** Identification of the family mutation is the best and most accurate method to diagnose Fabry disease in symptomatic and asymptomatic female heterozygotes. In female heterozygotes, the leukocyte enzyme level can be normal; and only a percentage (80–90%) of DNA-confirmed heterozygotes have the keratopathy. Urinary Gb3 levels may vary in heterozygotes from essentially normal to markedly elevated. Although the kidney biopsy would be diagnostic, it is particularly invasive.

3. **The answer is C.** With this patient already dialysis-dependent, the most appropriate and effective treatment is recombinant enzyme replacement therapy, which can protect and slow progression in the heart and other tissues. Although a renal transplant would intuitively be better than dialysis, it will only correct the renal problem. Continuing dialysis may decrease the circulating glycolipid somewhat, but would not treat the systemic accumulation. Whereas prevention for young family members is important, it does not address question about treatment for this patient.

4. **The answer is B.** Random X-chromosomal inactivation is responsible for the variable expression in heterozygotes, which can be asymptomatic to as severe as males. Gene inactivation would only make the disease more severe; while modifying genes will typically alter the manifestations only slightly. Gonadal mosaicism is the presence of a small number of mutant cells among mostly normal gonadal cells. Very rarely will a mutant egg cell be fertilized and result in a patient with the disease. There is limited cross-correction of mutant cells by normal cell secretions in Fabry disease.

5. **The answer is B.** Mutations predict enzyme activity, hence, the type of mutation is the most likely explanation for the two major phenotypic subtypes. Nonsense, frame-shift, consensus splice-site, etc. all predict the classic phenotype. Missense (amino acid substitutions) mutations can be classic, later-onset or totally benign. If there were known modifying genes, they would only alter the phenotype slightly. Polymorphisms in the introns of *GLA* gene do not cause or modify the phenotype; and no epigenetic (nongenetic) modifiers are known. Mosaicism (two different cell types, one mutant, one normal) does not alter phenotype.

Chapter 48

1. **The answer is B.** Renal medullary cancer occurs almost exclusively in patients with sickle cell trait at a relatively young age (20–30 year old) as aggressive metastatic disease at the time of diagnosis. Patient may present with hematuria, flank pain, abdominal mass, or weight loss.

2. **The answer is A.** Protein drink does not cause proteinuria and strenuous exercise-induced proteinuria usually resolves within 24–48 hours. Although acute poststreptococcal glomerulonephritis (GN) can cause mild persistent proteinuria for several months, the patient has no antecedent history of pharyngitis, tonsillitis, or skin infection. In addition his examination does not reveal any peripheral edema which is commonly seen in acute poststreptococcal GN. Glomerular changes in sickle cell disease patients begin as early as the first decade of life and are characterized by high renal blood flow, glomerular hyperfiltration and hypertrophy, gradual loss of glomerular permselectivity leading to micro- and macroalbuminuria, and a decrease in ultrafiltration coefficient.

3. **The answer is B.** Bed rest and oral hydration are the cornerstones in the management of gross hematuria in patients with SCD or sickle-cell trait. In more severe cases, urinary alkalinization, and blood transfusions may be considered to minimize hemoglobin precipitation and to reduce HbS sickling, respectively. Unilateral nephrectomy is not recommended because bleeding can recur in the contralateral kidney.

4. **The answer is B.** Both hemoglobinuria and rhabdomyolysis-induced myoglobinuria can be detected on the urine dipstick as "blood." However, urine microscopy in rhabdomyolysis only shows a few red blood cells despite strongly positive heme on a urine dipstick. The presence of >800 RBCs indicates hematuria. Papillary necrosis typically presents as self-limiting painless microscopic or macroscopic hematuria whereas urinary tract infection and kidney stone are usually associated with dysuria and flank pain, respectively.

5. **The answer is B.** Urinary dilution occurs at the water impermeable thick ascending limb of Henle loop where active sodium chloride reabsorption occurs via the Na-K-2Cl cotransporter. Since most cortical nephrons are superficial and have short loops and peritubular capillaries where vasoocclusion is not as severe as that seen in the vasa recta in the inner medullary regions, the diluting capacity of the kidney is relatively intact.

Chapter 49

1. **The answer is A.** Dialysis hypotension can be decreased by decreasing the ultrafiltration rate, which is accomplished by increasing the time on dialysis. Sodium modeling will worsen hypotension by causing larger interdialytic weight gain. Increasing the patient's dry weight is not an optimal method of minimizing hypotension as it could lead to chronic volume overload and hypertension. Increasing the dialysate flow rate should not have any significant influence on dialytic hypotension.

2. **The answer is E.** Methods that can be used to increase the dose of dialysis include increasing the blood flow rate, increasing the surface area of the dialyzer and increasing the dialysis flow rate. If these methods are ineffective, then the time on dialysis can be increased. Increasing the ultrafiltration rate will not significantly increase the dialysis dose.

3. **The answer is C.** Anaphylaxis, dyspnea, urticarial, and diarrhea can all be seen with a type A anaphylaxis reaction. Hemolysis can be secondary to either physical damage to erythrocytes due to a narrowing or blockage of the blood passages, including the dialysis tubing, catheter or needle or to issues with the dialysis solution. Hemolysis can be due to hypotonic dialysis solutions, solutions contaminated by chemicals in the water supply that have not been removed during the preparation of dialysate.

4. **The answer is C.** All of the other factors listed, if unresponsive to medical therapy, are indications to start chronic dialysis therapy. An eGFR of <15 mL/min indicates that the patient may be at risk of developing symptoms that should be treated with the initiation of dialysis therapy.

5. **The answer is D.** Fistula should be placed most distally first, then subsequent fistulas move up the arm proximally, in order to increase the number of locations that an AV fistula can be placed.

Chapter 50

1. **The answer is C.** This patient has developed worsening volume overload while on CCPD. We are told that she is compliant with sodium and fluid restriction, so we can rule out these reversible causes of volume overload. She has high peritoneal transport, and her dialysis regimen needs to be adjusted. Changing to less concentrated dialysate (ie, 1.5% dextrose) will result in decreased ultrafiltration. Changing to CAPD will also likely result in decreased daily ultrafiltration due to the increased dwell time with the manual exchanges. In the setting of high peritoneal transport and increased dwell time, the osmotic pressure gradient will dissipate and fluid will likely be reabsorbed before the next exchange. Eliminating her last fill may result in improved daily ultrafiltration because we are eliminating her longest dwell; however, this would not be the best option because she is anuric (no residual renal function) and would be at risk for under dialysis without a daytime dwell. The best answer would be to employ icodextrin during the long daytime dwell. The icodextrin will result in sustained ultrafiltration during the long dwell, despite the high peritoneal transport, due to the maintenance of an oncotic pressure gradient.

2. **The answer is B.** This patient has refractory peritonitis. There has been no clinical improvement after 5 days of appropriate antibiotic therapy. Refractory peritonitis is an indication for catheter removal in order to preserve the peritoneum for future PD and to decrease morbidity and mortality. Intravenous antibiotics are not more effective than IP antibiotics in the treatment of PD associated peritonitis. A CT scan and surgical evaluation would not necessarily be indicated for the management of this patient with peritonitis caused by a single gram positive organism, but would be appropriate if there was polymicrobial infection with gram negative organisms or anaerobes. Restarting the gentamicin would not be appropriate therapy. The peritoneal fluid is still growing MRSA, and gentamicin would not be effective therapy for this gram positive infection.

3. **The answer is C.** This patient has developed uremic symptoms in the setting of decreased residual renal function. We see that his residual renal function was previously contributing to his small solute clearance, and with this contribution his total Kt/V was just meeting the minimal recommended weekly target of 1.7. We are now told that urine output has decreased, and this is the most likely reason that he is now demonstrating signs of uremia. The addition of a diuretic may help somewhat with volume overload, but is unlikely to increase solute clearance to alleviate uremic symptoms. Solute clearance should increase with the addition of a daytime dwell, which would be relatively easy to perform by having the cycler deliver a last fill. There is no indication to switch to CAPD, which may not necessarily increase his small solute clearance if he is a rapid transporter, or to abandon PD all together and transfer the patient to HD. Adding a last fill on the cycler is a relatively simple adjustment and would be the most likely therapeutic maneuver to improve clearance and alleviate his uremic symptoms.

4. **The answer is C.** Empiric antibiotics covering both gram negative and gram positive organisms (in this case vancomycin and third-generation cephalosporin) should always be started when a patient presents with peritonitis. Treatment should never be delayed until after culture results are back. Therapy with first-generation cephalosporin alone would not be adequate coverage against gram negative bacteria, and therapy with aminoglycoside alone would not cover gram positive bacteria.

5. **The answer is A.** This vignette describes the typical clinical scenario of a patient presenting with encapsulating peritoneal sclerosis—a long-time PD patient who presents with bloody PD effluent, failure to thrive and bowel obstruction. The CT findings described above are the typical radiographic findings of EPS. Adenocarcinoma would be much less likely, and we are told that

PD cultures have been negative, making peritonitis with mycobacteria or fungus unlikely.

Chapter 51

1. **The answer is D.** Solute clearances in CRRT depend on the permeability of the membrane for the particular solute defined by its sieving coefficient (SC) (ratio of solute in the effluent versus plasma), and the transport mechanisms for the modality (convection for hemofiltration (SCUF, CVVH), diffusion for hemodialysis (CVVHD) and both convection and diffusion for hemodiafiltration (CVVHDF). Effluent volume content is determined by the modality and includes both UF and dialysate. Thus clearance = SC × effluent volume. For small solutes like urea nitrogen SC is usually 1 and consequently the clearance depends on effluent volume. However as the SC changes due to changes in filter permeability clearance will be reduced proportionally. Thus it is important to monitor the SC through the course of therapy as effluent volume alone does not reflect clearance.

2. **The answer is C.** Filtration fraction represents the proportional concentration of blood as it traverses the membrane. The ratio of ultrafiltration rate to plasma flow rate reflects the amount by which hematocrit will rise from the inlet to the outlet of the membrane. Thus FF = UFR/min/plasma flow rate/min. Plasma flow rate: The plasma flow rate = blood flow rate − hematocrit. So for a blood flow rate of 100 mL/min and a hematocrit of 30 the plams flow rate is 100 − 30 = 70 mL/in. If the ultrafiltration rate is 1000 mL/h = 16.7 mL/min the FF = 16.7/70 = 23.8. Since effluent volume includes ultrafiltration and dialysate it would overestimate FF in modalities where dialysate is used. Similarly utilizing blood flow rate in the calculation would underestimate the FF. In general it is recommended to keep the FF below 25–30% to minimize chances of filter clotting.

3. **The answer is E.** The CRRT machine balance reflects the fluids managed through the CRRT circuit and does not include any fluids eg intravenous drugs, or NG nutrition that are given outside the circuit or any outputs, eg urine, drains. Consequently patient fluid balance requires a computation of all the patient's intake and output including that through the CRRT circuit and should be computed on a flow sheet integrating these data. The frequency with which these data are captured and integrated will enable better management and control of fluid balance. The total UF volume, effluent volume and net balance shown on the machine do not account for the other fluid losses. Insensible loses are not accounted for and should be considered particularly in situations such as burns.

4. **The answer is D.** Standard membranes used for CRRT are not permeable to proteins and albumin is not removed across the filter. Although hypoalbuminemia is commonly encountered in patients on CRRT it is secondary to the underlying illness, vascular leakage and nutritional factors. It is often difficult to ascertain if hypotension and cardiac arrhythmias are secondary to the CRRT procedure or the underlying illness however should be monitored. Acidosis secondary to base loss and insufficient base replacement and hypophosphatemia are common complications that should be anticipated and corrected.

5. **The answer is D.** The single center ELAIN trial showed a mortality benefit in cardiac surgery patients initiated with RRT when they reached stage 2 AKI whereas the multicenter AKIKI trial showed that delaying initiation of RRT in patients with stage 3 AKI until they reached a life-threatening indication did not result in any difference in mortality however 50% of patients did not receive dialysis. Among those who did receive dialysis in the delayed group mortality was higher. Dialysis does as measured by effluent volume in the ATN and RENAL trials did not show any relationship to mortality, however, patient fluid balance status was associated with mortality.

Chapter 52

1. **The answer is B.** Frailty, a syndrome characterized by an elevated risk of catastrophic declines in health and function, is increasingly being screened for during recipient evaluations and follow visits while on the deceased donor waiting list. The most commonly used frailty examination is a simple to perform assessment of grip strength, walking speed, physical activity, and endurance. As the frail recipient has an elevated associated risk of mortality, transplant centers will frequently encourage "prehabilitation," followed by improvement on reassessment, before proceeding with transplantation.

2. **The answer is D.** Malignancy is now the third most common cause of death in the kidney transplant recipient. It is now well recognized that patients receiving immunosuppression are at an increased risk for malignancy development than age matched controls in the general population, and that they are more likely to die from malignancy when one occurs.

3. **The answer is A.** In contrast to focal segmental glomerulosclerosis (20–30%), C3 glomerulonephritis (90%), IgA nephropathy (20–50%), and dense deposit disease (90%) which all have a relatively high rate of recurrence following transplantation, recurrent lupus nephritis rarely occurs affecting only 2–3% of at risk recipients. However, when lupus nephritis does recur it is associated with a high likelihood that recurrence will result in allograft failure (95%).

4. **The answer is D.** Management of chronic antibody mediated rejection remains an unsolved challenge. IVIG in combination with rituximab has been attempted with some success. This is despite the fact that the culprit plasma cells producing the DSA do not display CD20, the target for rituximab, on their surface. Hence, it is inferred that rituximab may be acting in this context through depleting plasmablasts, the short lived, immature, form of the plasma cell.

5. **The answer is E.** Full immunosuppression withdrawal following kidney transplant failure is associated with an increased risk of developing an acute inflammatory state within the allograft. This immune mediated inflammatory process is indistinguishable from acute rejection at the level of the tissue. This inflammatory state can result in a constellation of findings and symptoms including fever, gross hematuria, allograft tenderness, hypoalbuminemia, resistance to ESAs, and elevated inflammatory markers—collectively referred to as graft intolerance syndrome. In contrast, one of the potential benefits to complete discontinuation of immunosuppression after allograft failure is a lower probability of premature death presumably secondary to a lower rate of infectious and oncologic complications.

Chapter 53

1. **The answer is A.** Intensive glycemic control of type II diabetes does not decrease incidence of nephropathy and cardiovascular mortality. The ACCORD trial indicated an increased risk of overall mortality with intensive glucose lowering in this population. Recent meta-analyses have indicated a decrease in cardiovascular disease outcomes, specifically nonfatal myocardial infarctions and risk of progression of nephropathy, but could not confirm that there was any decrease in nephropathy incidence or cardiovascular mortality.

2. **The answer is C.** Kimmelstiel–Wilson lesions are observed in a minority of patients diagnosed with diabetic nephropathy.

3. **The answer is C.** Hypertension is well documented to increase progression of DN. Most recent studies have indicated an association of smoking and progression, although this association has not been universally observed.

4. **The answer is B.** Metformin is contraindicated with renal insufficiency due to the potential risk for development of lactic acidosis.

5. **The answer is B.** False. Not all patients with diabetes who develop persistent microalbuminuria will progress to overt nephropathy. Studies have reported that anywhere from approximately 15–40% of patients would develop overt proteinuria within 5–6 years after onset of the microalbuminuria. However, not only do the majority of patients remain with microalbuminuria, but a significant percentage may actually revert to normoalbuminuria, especially with effective blood pressure control and the use of renin–angiotensin–aldosterone blockade.

Chapter 54

1. **The answer is C.** During pregnancy, cardiac output, total blood volume, and GFR increase significantly. The rate of creatinine production, which comes from routine muscle catabolism, remains unchanged. Steady creatinine production and increased creatinine clearance results in a lower serum creatinine level. The upper limit of normal creatinine during pregnancy is 0.8 mg/dL. Progesterone does not have an effect on the measurement of serum creatinine. Pregnant women do not have lower rates of muscle breakdown compared to nonpregnant women. Maternal serum creatinine is not cleared in any significant way by fetal kidneys.

2. **The answer is E.** Azathioprine and calcineurin inhibitors, including cyclosporine and tacrolimus, are commonly used and well-tolerated in pregnancy. Immunosuppression puts transplant patients at higher risk of infection, which has important consequences for fetal growth and development. Prednisone is not a teratogen and may be used during pregnancy, particularly at low dosages. Women with transplants may give birth vaginally or by cesarean section. Maternal fetal medicine specialists and transplant nephrologists should follow any pregnant patient who has a kidney transplant.

3. **The answer is B.** Hemolytic uremic syndrome is a thrombotic microangiopathy that occurs most commonly in the postpartum period, although it can occur in the late second or third trimester. There is no association with lupus or APS. Although HUS may cause transaminitis, it is not associated with acute liver failure, which is seen in acute fatty liver of pregnancy.

4. **The answer is A.** Preeclampsia results from endothelial dysfunction, which results in placental vasoconstriction and hypoperfusion. In recent years, preeclampsia has been found to cause increased systemic levels of antiangiogenic factors, including sFlt-1 and EGFR, and decreased systemic levels of angiogenic growth factors like PlGF and VEGF. Preeclampsia most commonly affects nulliparous women, but can recur in subsequent pregnancies. While it may be more challenging to detect preeclampsia in women who have HTN or proteinuria prior to pregnancy, those conditions are both associated with increased risk of preeclampsia. Although 24-hour urine collection is classic gold standard for proteinuria quantification, a random protein:creatinine ratio is an accurate and clinically much more timely method for proteinuria evaluation, so is widely used.

5. **The answer is D.** Fetal urine excretion is a major source of normal amniotic fluid. Polyhydramnios, or abnormally high amniotic fluid volume, is the result of fetal diuresis due to high urea content of maternal blood. Electrolytes in maternal blood are passed freely to the fetus, whose developing kidneys begin to process them during the second trimester. Although this is the most common mechanism of polyhydramnios in women with ESRD, the fetus should be evaluated for a number of other congenital problems which can result in polyhydramnios.

Chapter 55

1. **The answer is C.** Patient developed acute kidney injury that is rapidly progressive with red blood cells casts along with upper airway disease is suggestive of ANCA-associated vasculitis. Serum complement can be decreased in a variety of renal pathologies including acute interstitial nephritis, lupus nephritis, and postinfectious glomerulonephritis; there is nothing in the patient's history to support any of these entities. Increased ACE levels may be a sign of sarcoidosis as well as several other disorders. The patient's presentation, age and race are not compatible with sarcoidosis. While crescentic IgA nephropathy can present with rapidly progressive glomerulonephritis as well as hematuria, the presence of sinusitis, hemoptysis and epistaxis points towards ANCA-associated vasculitis. Antiglomerular basement membrane antibody is present with patients with Goodpasture syndrome. The disease presents with acute kidney injury and a nephritic picture like ANCA-associated vasculitis; however, it usually occurs with pulmonary symptoms in a younger age.

2. **The answer is C.** Patient received antibiotics for his abscess which caused acute interstitial nephritis (AIN). AIN from any cause may present with nonspecific signs and symptoms of acute renal dysfunction. Patients usually do not have significant proteinuria, and nephrotic syndrome occurs in <1% of patients with AIN. Though the patient did not have a rash, the history of the antibiotics and the urinalysis showing WBCs and WBCs casts are suggestive of acute interstitial nephritis. The absence of urinary symptoms and a positive nitrite or leukoesterase in the urine make the diagnosis of urinary tract infection unlikely.

Patients may present with symptoms related to the cause of the AIN. Classically, patients with drug-induced AIN were reported to have symptoms and/or signs of an allergic-type reaction, including rash, fever, and eosinophilia. However, these findings of a typical allergic response were relatively less common at presentation.

Thus, the originally described classic triad is less commonly observed than initially reported. The onset of drug-induced AIN following drug exposure typically ranges from 3 to 5 days (as occurs with a second exposure to an offending drug) to as long as several weeks to many months (as occurs following a first exposure to an offending drug).

Hypertensive nephrosclerosis can explain the chronic kidney disease but not the acute component. The absence of muddy brown casts and nephritic urine make acute tubular necrosis and membranoproliferative glomerulonephritis less likely.

3. **The answer is D.** Conservative management can be a viable option for the oldest-old (>90 years old) with multiple comorbidities. In addition, studies found that life satisfaction and quality of life were stable in this subgroup of patients who chose conservative management.

Option C is incorrect as several studies have shown that there is no significant survival advantage with dialysis compared to conservative management, particularly in those over 75 years and with multiple comorbidities such as DM and cardiac disease.

Option A is incorrect as older patients on hemodialysis typically have similar or higher overall health related and mental component summary quality of life (QOL) scores but lower physical component summary QOL life scores and life expectancy compared to younger or age-matched controls.

Option B is incorrect as peritoneal dialysis is best suited for younger patients with high functional status, few comorbidities and good social support.

4. **The answer is C.** Patients who receive a successful kidney transplant gain a survival benefit compared with remaining on dialysis across age line. Although the survival advantage of transplantation was most pronounced in younger end-stage renal disease (ESRD) patients, patients of all ages gained additional years of life with transplant compared with dialysis. Therefore, because of this mortality benefit, kidney transplantation is the treatment modality of choice for ESRD. This rule out option D. An important question for elderly patients is whether or not they have a realistic chance of obtaining a transplant.

While long waiting period for a deceased kidney transplant may be a hindrance for kidney transplant in the elderly, extended criteria donor kidney (ECD) may be an attractive option for elderly transplant candidate as it can reduce the waiting period for transplantation.

Prevalence of obesity in patients who have ESRD and register for kidney transplantation is increasing and complications and outcomes are worse in obese patients when compared with their nonobese counterparts.

5. **The answer is D.** The patient has evidence of AKI with Nephrotic syndrome, with a history of NSAID intake.

An association of NSAID with minimal change disease and acute interstitial disease is well described. Most patients with this syndrome due to NSAID do not have the triad of rash, fever and eosinophiluria. No data available linking NSAID to *de novo* FSGS. Interstitial nephritis alone and ATN do not present with nephrotic syndrome. Nothing to suggest urinary tract obstruction in the history, and is not associated with nephrotic syndrome.

6. **The answer is D.** A target of blood pressure less than 130/80 mm Hg is recommended for older hypertensive patients with CKD. In this patient who is above 80 years of age with no documented CKD, higher blood pressure is acceptable. The American College of Cardiology and the American Heart Association expert consensus document on hypertension in older adults recommends systolic blood pressure to 140–145 mm Hg if tolerated in adults aged 80 years and older.

Chapter 56

ENDOVASCULAR PROCEDURES

1. **The answer is C.** US guided venipuncture is superior to landmark puncture; simple dedicated vascular US equipment is readily available in most U.S. centers, and its use does not add significant time or expense; guided venipuncture confers the same advantages for accessing any central vein, and for any catheter, tunneled, or nontunneled.

2. **The answer is B.** Several studies have shown improved primary patency of the target lesion versus angioplasty; stent-grafts have never been compared with bare-metal stents "head-to-head"; no benefit has been demonstrated for secondary patency; studies have shown benefit as primary intervention, not just as salvage for failed angioplasty; the Viabahn stent-graft is approved for use across the elbow.

3. **The answer is C.** There is no rationale or evidence to support eliminating all vein branches; collateral veins provide necessary outflow in the setting of stenosis and should never be embolized; branch veins do contribute significantly to excessive flow in high-flow fistulae; there are some circumstances where branch vein ligation appears to be beneficial and should be performed, notwithstanding the lack of good studies in this area.

4. **The answer is E.** Each listed problem may result in catheter dysfunction.

5. **The answer is C.** Paclitaxel has been shown to reduce neo-intimal hyperplasia, active clinical trials underway to demonstrate the clinical effect of this in AV access; angioplasty alone causes vessel injury which likely accelerates cellular proliferation; stent-grafts physically block ingrowth of hyperplastic tissue, but do nothing to reduce hyperplasia; the cutting balloon has not been demonstrated to reduce hyperplasia or re-stenosis; no systemic agent has demonstrated a benefit in reducing cellular hyperplasia in AV access.

PERITONEAL DIALYSIS CATHETER PROCEDURES

1. **The answer is B.** According to Kolesnyk, Krediet et al, technique failure of peritoneal dialysis within the first 3 months is due to infections, catheter failures, psychosocial or unknown problems, underdialysis, and abdominal problems. The incident rate for all of these problems is 147 per 1000 pt-years. Catheter failure incident rate alone is 40 per 1000 pt-years, or 27% of the total of causes of technique failure.

2. **The answer is C.** The physical description of Tenckhoff catheters is somewhat complicated, since there are variations in the shape of the internal portion and the subcutaneous portion. The "curled" portion of the curled Tenckhoff is actually a spiral, with the total deflection of the tip being 540° (versus the body of the catheter). Subcutaneous sections are either "straight" or "arcuate."

3. **The answer is C.** There is no microsurgical method for placement of PD catheters, as very fine suturing and incisions are not needed. However, it might evolve someday. As it is, all of the other methods are used successfully in various centers. Some few centers around the world still use the original Tenckhoff Trocar, which includes a large metal trocar and surround metal sheath of size to pass the body of the catheter.

4. **The answer is D.** In techniques that use a trocar or a blunt needle for first entry to the peritoneum, there is the feel of a "pop" when the tip passes through the anterior and posterior rectus sheaths, and sometimes as the tip passes through the parietal peritoneum. However with a sharp needle, there is little feel as it passes through tissues. Injection of a few cc of radiopaque dye creates a "spider web" picture as the dye moves in grooves formed by bowel loops resting on the parietal peritoneum. Fluid rises in the needle placed in the peritoneum only if there is significant ascites or peritoneal dialysate present. Injecting a small amount air will not change the fluoroscopic image when the patient is supine.

5. **The answer is F.** When gas is injected into the anterior peritoneum in a supine patient, bowels and omentum tend to fall and the parietal peritoneum rises. This creates a gas-filled space in which adhesions become easily visible by laparoscopy or peritoneoscopy. Dissection, blind placement and fluoroscopy do not give visualization of adhesions. When adhesions are seen, the catheter can be directed to avoid the adhesions (with peritoneoscopy) or lysed (with laparoscopic tools). Avoiding adhesions near the catheter will diminish the risk of outflow failure.

Chapter 57

1. **The answer is C.** The toxin in question is methanol, presenting with high anion gap metabolic acidosis along with high osmolal gap. Hemodialysis was performed for 8 hours with a 1.8-m² dialyzer, since there was an inability to maintain a pH greater than 7.3 with bicarbonate and fomepizole indicating that alcohol dehydrogenase (ADH) was not completely inhibited allowing methanol metabolism to formic acid production. In addition any visual symptoms are an indication for dialysis. Fomepizole is expensive (about $1000/g, and usually 4 g is used) and many countries inhibit ADH with ethanol, oral, IV or in dialysate. Both fomepizole and ethanol are dialyzable and both require augmented dosage during dialysis. Fomepizole alone has been used in a patient who refused hemodialysis, but resulted in a prolonged hospitalization due to the fact that the renal clearance of methanol is 1 mL/min. Methanol epidemics from illegal bootlegging are common and recently occurred in the Czech Republic; oral ethanol was started immediately and prevented vision loss and deaths in those who tested positive for ethanol at hospitals in the study. The patient in this question recovered completely without vision loss.

2. **The answer is B.** This was an obvious case of ethylene glycol poisoning (history, high osmolal gap, and oxalate crystals in the urine). This case illustrates the following: prompt administration of ethanol or fomepizole, blockers of alcohol dehydrogenase (ADH), can prevent injury to the kidneys, heart, and brain; hemodialysis clearance of ethylene glycol is about five times greater than the endogenous clearance of the toxin; and because it is so much more efficient. While hemodialysis is an important means of rapidly reducing the amount of ethylene glycol and its metabolites in the body and can substantially shorten the hospital stay, ethanol administration can result in an intoxicated/uncooperative individual in the hospital. Therefore fomepizole administration is preferred alone in ethylene glycol intoxication; dialysis should be instituted if the pH is unable to be maintained above 7.3 with bicarbonate and fomepizole (see Mégarbane et al, 2005). Determination of methanol/ethylene glycol concentrations and of their metabolites are rarely measured or, are reported long after treatment is finished, except in specialized centers (see Bekka, 2001).

3. **The answer is D.** Although the correct answer to the question is all of the above there are caveats. Increasing blood flow too high (>500 mL/min) theoretically increases clearance (BFRxA-V/A) but in fact the short exposure time at the membrane surface may induce a fall in diffusion and a plateau will be reached. This of course could be increased by hydrostatic ultrafiltration which increases convection and "solvent drag." Since most drugs are around 300 Da, there is little need to increase blood flow rates higher than 200–300 mL/min, except for tightly protein bound drugs (eg, phenytoin). The caveat for increases in dialysate flow rate is that a plateau in clearance is reached at about 1.5 times the blood flow rate. The surface area of a dialyzer is critical to drug removal and an optimal drug clearance is reached about 1.8–2.0 m². The other illustrative point in this case is there is a need to reappraise older literature in light of improvements in dialysis. Chelation therapy for Al removal was particularly common in the 1990s when low flux dialyzers were the norm; with high flux membranes in use currently the deferoxamine-Al complex is removed more efficiently.

4. **The answer is C.** Blood levels of drugs should be of lower importance in triggering action. EXTRIP recommends dialysis at 90–100 mg/dL with any clinical status, but at any concentration if there is mental status changes and persistent acidosis. Central nervous system changes in the presence of acidemia reflect CNS trapping of salicylate and an urgency to correct the pH with bicarbonate dialysate; salicylate is an ideally dialyzable drug (although protein binding is high the bond is weak and the molecule traverses dialysis membranes easily).

5. **The answer is D.** Use of distal tubular diuretics (like HCTZ) was an unfortunate choice for a patient taking Li, because they induce compensatory proximal tubular reabsorption on Na and Li, whereas loop diuretics do not. There are case reports of hypernatremia with normal saline and half normal would have been appropriate. The most important reasons for dialysis: CNS symptoms, GCS less than 10, Li levels that will predictably not be below Log 0.6 in 24 hours and acute kidney injury manifested here (see Vodovar). This is chronic Li toxicity induced by diuretics and summer perspiration without increased thirst interrupting the normal fractional clearance of Li. The patient had one prolonged dialysis with a Li level 0.8 mEq/L at the end of 8-hour dialysis with slight rebound to 1.0 mEq/L. She was wide awake after dialysis but the myoclonic movements took 6 months to resolve completely.

Chapter 58

1. **The answer is D.** Explanation: When a patient asks about prognosis, it is important to always clarify exactly what the patient is asking and if the patient really wants an estimate of time. For example, asking this question may be because the patient is wondering if he would live long enough to see his granddaughter graduate from high school. If a patient expresses that they wish to know time, the correct answer is D. Though uncertainty exists, literature suggests that average life expectancy after withdrawing from hemodialysis is about 7 days, though has ranged in one study from 0 to 40 days.

2. **The answer is B.** Explanation: Altered pharmacokinetics have been described for various antidepressants in dialysis patients including for SNRI, MOAIs, and TCAs. These alterations include increased half life of either the parent drug or active metabolite and decreased clearances. This prolonged exposure places patients at increased risk of adverse effects. Conversely, SSRIs are metabolized by the liver into inactive metabolites so are believed to be more well tolerated in dialysis patients. Though CBT has shown benefit in a small study of 65 dialysis patients, it is not considered first-line therapy.

3. **The answer is C.** Several small studies have shown benefit in reducing pruritus severity with use of gabapentin in doses ranging from 100 to 400 mg post dialysis.

4. **The answer is D.** The surprise question has been validated in both patients with CKD stage 4 and 5, and dialysis patients at predicting who is at high risk of poor outcomes, specifically mortality, at 1 year.

5. **The answer is A.** Preferred opioids for pain that is not sufficiently controlled by acetaminophen or for pain that is moderate in intensity include hydromorphone, oxycodone, and short-acting tramadol. Transdermal fentanyl should only be used in patients on a stable dose of short-acting opioids who need a transition to a longer acting agent. Morphine and extended release tramadol are not recommended for use in patients with advanced renal disease.

Chapter 59

1. **The answer is A.** Delayed gastric emptying related to gastroparesis may be present in diabetic patients. GI motility may be decreased and can affect the time required to reach the maximal plasma concentration. However, this typically does not affect the maximal plasma concentrations (C_{max}) achieved and the overall extent of absorption, so bioavailability is not affected.

2. **The answer is B.** The V_D of digoxin is decreased by up to 50% in patients with stage 5 CKD. The reasons are unclear, but frequently cited mechanisms include competitive inhibition or displacement of digoxin from its receptor by uremic toxins or digoxin-like substances. If the digoxin loading dose is not adjusted accordingly, then the smaller V_D leads to increased serum concentrations.

3. **The answer is E.** The adjusted dose can be determined using the method of Rowland and Tozer using the following equation:

$$Q = 1 - [f_e (1 - KF)]$$

where KF is the ratio of the patient's kidney function (CL_{CR} or eGFR) to the assumed normal value of 120 mL/min.

Since drug X is 90% excreted unchanged in the patient has a CL_{CR} of 50 mL/min, the Q adjustment factor would be

$$Q = 1 - \{0.90\ [1 - (50/120)]\}$$
$$Q = 1 - [0.90\ (1 - 0.42)]$$
$$Q = 1 - [0.90\ (0.58)]$$
$$Q = 1 - 0.64$$
$$Q = 0.36$$

The adjustment factor may then be applied to derive an adjusted dosing regimen. Increasing the interval and less frequent administration typically is preferred unless the drug specifically requires target peak or trough concentrations. Thus, the adjusted interval can be calculated as

$$\tau_{PT} = \tau_{NORM} \div Q$$
$$\tau_{PT} = 8\ h \div 0.36$$
$$\tau_{PT} = 22\ h$$

The most practical interval then becomes Q24 hours or once daily.

4. **The answer is C.** The Dettli method bases drug dosing recommendations on the linear relationship between the elimination rate constant of renally cleared drugs and a patient's creatinine clearance. This approach assumes that the overall elimination rate constant (or CL) declines linearly with CL_{CR}, and that the nonrenal elimination rate constant (or CL_{NR}) remains constant as kidney function declines. The first assumption holds true for drugs that are predominantly renally cleared, but the second is flawed since the function of several CL_{NR} pathways decline as kidney function declines. Therefore, the Dettli method is most useful for drugs undergoing primarily glomerular filtration.

5. **The answer is B.** Automatically reported eGFR values provide an estimate that is normalized for body surface area (BSA) in units of mL/min/1.73 m². When used for drug dosing, the eGFR value should be individualized, that is, not normalized for BSA and converted to units of mL/min, particularly in patients whose BSA is considerably larger or smaller than 1.73 m². The individualized value may then be compared to CL_{CR} estimates expressed in equivalent units (mL/min).

Index

Note: Page numbers followed by *f* indicate figures; *t* indicate tables.